Dermatology for Advanced Practice Clinicians

A Comprehensive Guide to Diagnosis and Treatment

SECOND EDITION

Dermatology for Advanced Practice Clinicians

A Comprehensive Guide to Diagnosis and Treatment

SECOND EDITION

Margaret A. Bobonich, DNP, FNP-C, DCNP, FAANP

Assistant Professor
Department of Dermatology
Case Western Reserve University School of Medicine and
Frances Payne Bolton School of Nursing
University Hospitals Cleveland Medical Center
Cleveland, Ohio
Adjunct Faculty
Christine E. Lynn College of Nursing
Florida Atlantic University
Boca Raton, Florida

Mary E. Nolen, MS, ANP-BC, DCNP

Adjunct Assistant Professor
Christine E. Lynn College of Nursing
Florida Atlantic University
Boca Raton, Florida

Jeremy Honaker, PhD, MSN, FNP-C, CWOCN, DCNP

Assistant Professor
Department of Dermatology
Case Western Reserve University School of Medicine
University Hospitals Cleveland Medical Center
Cleveland, Ohio

Douglas DiRuggiero, DMSc, MHS, PA-C

Skin Cancer & Cosmetic Dermatology Center
Rome, Georgia

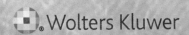. Wolters Kluwer

Philadelphia • Baltimore • New York • London
Buenos Aires • Hong Kong • Sydney • Tokyo

Acquisitions Editor: Nicole Dernoski
Development Editor: Maria M. McAvey
Senior Editorial Coordinator: Lindsay Ries
Senior Production Project Manager: Sadie Buckallew
Design Manager: Stephen Druding
Manufacturing Coordinator: Kathleen Brown
Marketing Manager: Linda Wetmore
Prepress Vendor: Aptara, Inc.

2nd edition

Library of Congress Cataloging-in-Publication Data

Names: Bobonich, Margaret A., editor. | Nolen, Mary E., editor. | Honaker, Jeremy, editor. | DiRuggiero, Douglas, editor.
Title: Dermatology for advanced practice clinicians : a comprehensive guide to diagnosis and treatment / [edited by] Margaret A. Bobonich, Mary E. Nolen, Jeremy Honaker, Douglas DiRuggiero.
Description: Second edition. | Philadelphia : Wolters Kluwer, [2021] | Includes bibliographical references and index.
Identifiers: LCCN 2021006329 | ISBN 9781975148355 (paperback)
Subjects: MESH: Skin Diseases–diagnosis | Skin Diseases–therapy
Classification: LCC RL71 | NLM WR 140 | DDC 616.5–dc23
LC record available at https://lccn.loc.gov/2021006329

shop.lww.com

Contributors

Lakshi M. Aldredge, MSN, ANP-BC

Nurse Practitioner
Portland VA Medical Center
Portland, Oregon

Margaret A. Bobonich, DNP, FNP-C, DCNP, FAANP

Assistant Professor
Department of Dermatology
Case Western Reserve University School of Medicine and
Frances Payne Bolton School of Nursing
University Hospitals Cleveland Medical Center
Cleveland, Ohio
Adjunct Faculty
Christine E. Lynn College of Nursing
Florida Atlantic University
Boca Raton, Florida

Nicole Bort, DNP, AGNP-C, DCNP

Dermatology Nurse Practitioner
Department of Dermatology
University Hospitals of Cleveland
Cleveland, Ohio

A. Matthew Brunner, MHS, PA-C

Physician Assistant
Dermatology & Skin Surgery Center P.C.
Stockbridge, Georgia

Melissa E. Cyr, PhD, ANP, FNP

Dermatology Nurse Practitioner
Dermatology & Skin Health
Peabody, Massachusetts

Melissa Davis, PA-C, MSPAS

Adjunct Faculty
Sullivan University
Louisville, Kentucky

Douglas C. DiRuggiero, DMSc, MHS, PA-C

Skin Cancer and Cosmetic Dermatology
Rome, Georgia

Elizabeth Drumm

Family Nurse Practitioner
Dermatology Nurse Practitioner
Department of Dermatology
AMITA Health Adventist Medical Center La Grange
La Grange, Illinois

Wayne Emineth, PA-C

Physician Assistant
Dermatology
Georgia Regents University/University of Georgia
AtlantaAugusta/Athens, Georgia
Physician Assistant
Dermatology
Northside Hospital
Atlanta, Georgia

Victoria Garcia-Albea, PNP, MSN, DCNP, BSN, RN

Nurse Practitioner
Department of Dermatology
Beth Israel Lahey Health
Burlington, Massachusetts

Bethany Grubb, MPH, MPAS, PA-C

Assistant Professor
Department of PA Studies
UT-Southwestern
Dallas, Texas

Gail Batissa Handwork, RN, MSN, ANP-BC, DCNP

Dermatology Nurse Practitioner
Department of Dermatology
Lahey Hospital & Medical Center
Burlington, Massachusetts

Kathleen Haycraft, DNP, FNP/PNP-BC, DCNP, FAANP

Riverside Dermatology
General Dermatology
Hannibal, Missouri

Travis M. Hayden, MPAS, PA-C

Professor of Practice, Assistant Academic Coordinator
Department of Physician Assistant Studies
Le Moyne College
Voluntary Faculty, Clinical Instructor
Physician Assistant Program
SUNY Upstate Medical University
Syracuse, New York

Jeremy Honaker, PhD, MSN, FNP-C, CWOCN, DCNP

Assistant Professor
Department of Dermatology
School of Medicine
Case Western Reserve University School of Medicine
Dermatology Nurse Practitioner
Department of Dermatology
University Hospitals of Cleveland
Cleveland, Ohio

Mark A. Hyde, PhD, PA-C
Assistant Professor
College of Health and Public Service
Utah Valley University
Orem, Utah

Victoria Lazareth, MA, MSN, NP-C, DCNP
Affiliate Professor
Department of Nursing
Simmons University
Boston, Massachusetts
Nurse Practitioner
Department of Dermatology
Southern Maine Health Care
Kennebunk, Maine

Joe R. Monroe, PA

Mary E. Nolen, MS, ANP-BC, DCNP
Adjunct Assistant Professor
Christine E. Lynn College of Nursing
Florida Atlantic University
Boca Raton, Florida

Katie B. O'Brien, MSN, ANP-BC
Nurse Practitioner
Mystic Valley Dermatology
Stoneham, Massachusetts

Theodore D. Scott, MSN, FNP-C, DCNP
Retired

Martha Sikes
Assistant Professor
Physician Assistant Program
Emory University
Atlanta, Georgia

Dorothy A. Sullivan, PhD (c), ARNP-BC
Adjunct Clinical Instructor
University of New Hampshire
Durham, New Hampshire

Susan Tofte, DNP, MS, FNP-C
Assistant Professor
Department of Dermatology
Oregon Health & Science University
Portland, Oregon

Jeffrey Viveiros, APRN, FNP-BC, DCNP

Joleen M. Volz, DMSc, MPAS, PA-C, DFAAPA
Physician Assistant
US Dermatology Partners
Waxahachie & Corsicana, Texas

Susan T. Voss, DNP, FNP-BC, DCNP, FAANP
Riverside Dermatology
Hannibal, Missouri

Mandy Wever, MSN, FNP-C, DCNP, DNC
Nurse Practitioner
Bedford, Indiana

Jennifer Winter, MSPAS, PA-C

Previous Edition Contributors

Lakshi M. Aldredge, MSN, ANP-BC

Glen Blair, RN, MSN, ANP-C, DCNP

Margaret A. Bobonich, DNP, FNP-C, DCNP, FAANP

Niki Bryn, APRN, GNP-BC, NP-C, DCNP

Susan Busch, MSN, ANP-BC

Cathleen K. Case, MS, ANP, DCNP

Janice T. Chussil, MSN, ANP-C, DCNP

Melissa E. Cyr, MSN, ANP-BC, FNP-BC

Pamela K. Fletcher, DNP, RN, FNP-BC, DCNP

Victoria Garcia-Albea, MSN, PNP, DCNP

Victoria Griffin, RN, MSN, ANP-BC, DCNP

Diane Hanna, MSN, DNP

Linda Hansen-Rodier, MS, WHNP-BC

Kathleen E. Dunbar Haycraft, DNP, FNP/PNP-BC, DCNP, FAANP

Dea J. Kent, MSN, RN, NP-C, CWOCN, DNP-C

Victoria Lazareth, MA, MSN, NP-C, DCNP

Gail Batissa Lenahan, APRN, DCNP

Mary E. Nolen, MS, ANP-BC, DCNP

Kelly Noska, RN, MSN, ANP-BC

Katie Brouillard O'Brien, MSN, ANP-BC

Theodore D. Scott, RN, MSN, FNP-C, DCNP

Diane Solderitsch, MSN, FNP

Dorothy A. Sullivan, MSN, APRN-BC, NP-C

Jane Tallent, ANP-BC

Susan J. Tofte, MS, BSN, FNP

Susan Thompson Voss, APRN, DNP, FNP-BC, DCNP

Preface

Five years ago, we created the first dermatology text specifically dedicated to advanced practice clinicians. Our goal was to fill an educational gap which existed, and still persists, between graduate school instruction and real-life clinical practice. That text, the first edition, provided an everyday reference for clinicians as they encountered simple and complex dermatologic complaints.

Content in the first edition focused on professional guidance of skin diseases that are high volume (the most common conditions), high morbidity (causing disability or high impact on the community), and high mortality (life or limb threatening). While many things have changed over the years, this focus has not. Clinicians still need evidenced-based knowledge for everyday practice. Yet, they must also recognize the urgent and emergent skin conditions that may present. As the demand for high-quality skin care continues to rise rapidly, so does the need for quality reference textbooks coupled with ongoing specialty education, training, and professional competencies. Moreover, the addition of two new editors, Jeremy Honaker, PhD, MSN, FNP-C, CWOCN, DCNP and Douglas DiRuggiero, DMSc, MHS, PA-C, has provided breadth and depth to content and structure. As dermatology clinicians, nurse practitioners (NPs) and physician assistants (PAs) work alongside each other every day, and despite differing educational paths, our clinical roles and responsibilities are similar and complimentary. As iron sharpens iron, having 12 second-edition chapters authored by NPs and PAs reflect an interprofessional collaboration that not only enriches this text but, ultimately, improves patient care. Furthermore, many new NP and PA contributors are "rising star" master clinicians. We must welcome and mentor this next generation as they bring innovative clinical acumen and new perspectives to education, publishing, and medical practice.

You will see from the table of contents that the organization of the sections and chapters in this edition has been regrouped based on visual characteristics, anatomical location of skin findings, or by symptom or patient complaints. The first two chapters are reconfigured to improve or solidify understanding of the structure and function of skin, assessment, and morphology—which creates a foundation for the rest of the text. Take some time to familiarize yourself with this information before plunging head-first into the diagnosis-based material.

Furthermore, within each chapter, content has been rearranged into a more user-friendly format. A concise, bulleted format provides a quick reference of essential information. "Differential Diagnoses" and "Clinical Pearls" boxes, new tables, and treatment algorithms have been incorporated to highlight and summarize important concepts. Lastly, due to the very visual nature of dermatology, we have enhanced and expanded our photograph collection for visual identification of skin lesions/diseases.

It is with great enthusiasm that we invite you to utilize every aspect of this textbook. Our sincerest hope is to help NPs, PAs, medical and nursing students, and physicians in primary care to develop a deeper understanding of dermatology, provide evidenced-based guidance, and optimize patient outcomes.

Margaret A. Bobonich, DNP, FNP-C, DCNP, FAANP
Mary E. Nolen, MS, ANP-BC, DCNP
Jeremy Honaker, PhD, MSN, FNP-C, CWOCN, DCNP
Douglas DiRuggiero, DMSc, MHS, PA-C

Acknowledgments

It was more than a decade ago that we began our journey as friends and colleagues to identify the gaps in dermatology education for NPs and standardize professional practice. Our ambitious undertaking to publish the first dermatology textbook for advanced practice clinicians earned us the nickname of "M&M." We are indebted to our colleagues, as our accomplishments throughout these years could not have been achieved without the hard work and support of our fellow NPs. TOGETHER, strong voices and hard work have elevated our profession. We are also thankful for our amazing dermatologist colleagues and mentors who contributed so much to our education, research, and clinical experience. There has never been a better exemplar of collaboration in interprofessional education. Our continued commitment to scholarship has not waivered. The readership of our first edition has grown tremendously over these past 5 years. We have listened to your feedback and are eternally grateful. Our belief is that dermatology education and high-quality care should not be conducted in silos, therefore we embrace the new perspectives and partnership of our PA colleagues who have joined us on this journey. Together, we can improve patient satisfaction, health care outcomes, and reduce health care costs. We remain steadfast in our efforts to not only educate novice clinicians but to prepare the next generation of educators, researchers, clinical experts, and leaders. Many of the contributors in this text are experts eager for the opportunity to teach their colleagues. We are excited to have them join us. We are grateful to be joined by Douglas DiRuggiero, PA and Jeremy Honaker, NP in editing the second edition. Their academic accomplishments are only surpassed by their passion for interprofessional education. Their skilled contributions and tireless effort have greatly enhanced our text. We also wish to extend our sincerest gratitude to all the contributors of the first edition. Their original efforts established the foundation for future work. Lastly, we appreciate all of the continued support of family, friends, and colleagues who have been the foundation for all of our achievements including this second edition. The road we have traveled has not been an easy one but our commitment to each other and our profession will not waiver. It has been an amazing experience.

—M&M

To Dr. Kevin Cooper and Dr. Neil Korman, I am deeply grateful for your mentorship. You both have always nurtured my inquisitive nature and pushed me to grow in ways I did not think possible. Thank you so much for believing in me and continuing to push me to grow academically and personally.

To Margaret and Mary, words alone cannot express my gratitude for giving me this opportunity to be an editor of such an amazing project. I could not have done this without your patience, unending support, and time spent showing me the ropes of editing. You both are amazing mentors and I am forever grateful for your imparted wisdom and continued friendship. To my wife, Jennifer, and my children, Kaiden and Kara, thank you so much for your love, support, and patience over this past year. Throughout all of my academic endeavors, you all have been so very understanding, have always encouraged me, kept me pushing forward when I was exhausted, and sacrificed so much so that I can accomplish all that I do. Most importantly, I want to thank God for the amazing mentors, wisdom, knowledge, and opportunities that he has used to shape me to be who I am. The success of this project would not have been possible without you.

—Jeremy

More than 15 years ago, I started co-teaching dermatology workshops with a PA who was my senior in both life and work experience. I took far more from him than he received from me. With patience, this PA, Joe Monroe, encouraged, corrected, molded, and informed me as a teacher and lecturer. Most importantly, he demonstrated a passion for teaching colleagues the subtleties of treating the skin—and guided my trajectory down the same path. The four physician supervisors in my 24-year career have all had a great impact on me: Gene Davidson, MD gave me an internal medicine foundation; Jason Smith, MD jettisoned me into dermatology and provided 5 years of superb training and instruction; Kavita Mariwalla, MD combined Long Island charm with powerhouse clinical acumen; and fourthly, my current 15-year employer John Chung, MD. John creates and encourages a practice environment where God is acknowledged as the giver of all knowledge and skills and as the ultimate healer. Through his tutelage and example, I have learned to practice dermatology as a ministry. Lastly, my wife and three college-aged children are my most-prized possessions. They are the everything-but-the-bagel seasoning in my life and remind me to keep laughter and adventure on the front burner. I am grateful to Mary and Margaret for asking me to join this editorial team. I hope this textbook blesses all those who utilize it and ultimately improves the lives of your patients.

—Douglas

Contents

Structure and Function of the Skin

Margaret A. Bobonich

In This Chapter

- Skin
  - Epidermis
  - Dermis
  - Subcutaneous Layer
- Adnexa
  - Eccrine Glands
  - Apocrine Glands

Dermatology is specialized care focused on conditions involving the skin, hair, nails, and mucous membranes. While healthy skin is beautiful and resilient, disease and dysfunction can cause significant morbidity and mortality. Cutaneous lesions may signal an underlying systemic process or psychological condition. This chapter will provide clinicians with essential dermatology concepts including: the structure and function of the skin, examination of the skin, and a morphology-based approach for the diagnosis of skin lesions. Mastering these fundamentals will enhance your diagnostic reasoning.

This section is an overview of the anatomy and physiology of the skin which provides a foundation for learning dermatology. It is impossible to understand the pathogenesis of skin conditions and therapeutics prescribed to treat them, if you do not understand the structure and function of the skin itself.

SKIN

The skin is the largest organ in the body as well as the most visible, allowing both patients and clinicians the opportunity to observe symptoms and changes. Although patients "wear" their disease, the structure of human skin is more complex and associated with our other body systems. Skin is comprised of the epidermis, dermis, subcutaneous tissue, adnexa or skin appendages and has regional variability in its thickness and structures (Fig. 1.1-1). Glabrous skin does not have hair follicles or sebaceous glands, is located on the palms and soles, and is generally thick. In general, thin skin over the rest of the body houses a variable number of appendages including the nails, hair, sebaceous, and sweat glands.

The skin is complex, dynamic, and provides multiple functions:

- It acts as a physical barrier against the environment.
- It provides an innate and adaptive immunity that protects the body from pathogens.
- It provides for thermoregulation.
- It is also responsible for vitamin D synthesis.
- It protects from ultraviolet radiation on non–hair-bearing skin.
- It acts as a reservoir for medication administration.
- It is a sensory organ for pain, pressure, itch, temperature, and touch.

Understanding the normal structure and function of the skin will enhance your ability to correlate clinical and histologic findings associated with skin lesions.

Epidermis

- Commonly referred to as the "dead skin" layer, the epidermis is the locus of important cellular structures including keratinocytes, Langerhans cells, Merkel cells, and melanocytes (Fig. 1.1-2).
- Nucleated *keratinocytes* differentiate as they ascend from the basal layer to the surface, filling with keratin and losing their nucleoproteins.
- *Langerhans cells* are intraepidermal macrophages responsible for phagocytosis of antigens and migration into the lymphatics and presentation to T cells.
- The immune function of the epidermis is of paramount importance.
- *Merkel cells* are believed to have a somatosensory function and responsible for light touch and possible neuroendocrine function.
- *Melanocytes* synthesize pigment which accounts for the variation in skin color among races. They are found in the dermis during fetal life and migrate to the basement membrane.

Epidermal Layers

- The layers (*strata*) of the epidermis are responsible for protecting the body from the environment as both a mechanical and chemical barrier.
- Each strata has unique characteristics and functions (Table 1.1-1).
- Flattened keratinocytes with a thickened cell membrane create the stratified layer (shingles on a roof) in the stratum corneum, which is not capable of metabolic activity.
- This cornified layer saturated in a lipid complex provides a virtually impermeable barrier and minimizes water loss. Thus, any defect or impaired function of this layer can lead to pathologic changes and diseases.

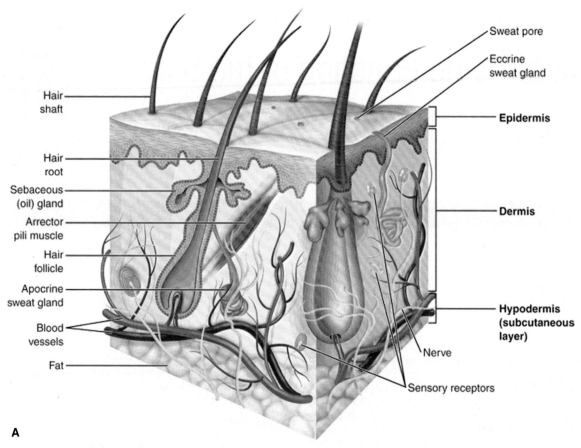

A

FIG. 1.1-1. Anatomy of skin.

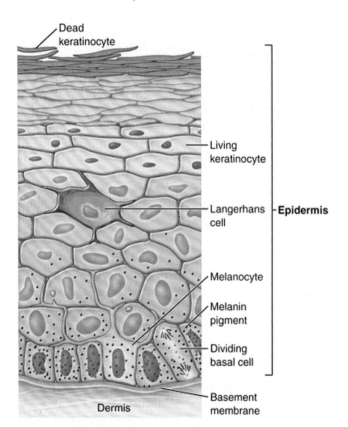

FIG. 1.1-2. Layers of epidermis.

Dermis

- The dermis is comprised of fibroblasts, histiocytes, and mast cells, and is separated from the epidermis at the *basement membrane* (dermal–epidermal junction or DEJ). It adjoins with the *papillary dermis* (upper portion) (Fig. 1.1-3).

- Fibroblasts produce collagen (90% of the dermis), elastin, and ground substances which comprise the majority of the dermis and are the supporting matrix of the skin.

- The dermis is also responsible for the continued immune response initiated in the epidermis by Langerhans cells, as well as neutrophils, lymphocytes, monocytes, and mast cells.

- Blood vessels provide essential nutrients and temperature regulation of the skin. Nerve endings provide sensory for pain, pressure, touch, itch, and temperature.

- Arrector pili muscles in the dermis contract to make hair follicles stand up, creating the "goose bumps" effect.

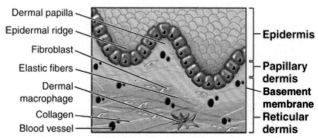

FIG. 1.1-3. The dermis.

TABLE 1.1-1	Strata of the Epidermis	
STRATUM (LAYER)	**CHARACTERISTIC**	**FUNCTION**
Corneum	Brick and mortar layer Lipid matrix and barrier Antimicrobial peptides	Mechanical protection; limits transepidermal water loss; limits penetration of pathogens (bacterial, viral, and fungal) or allergens
Lucidium	Only on soles and palms	Protection
Granulosum	Keratin and filaggrin >80% of mass of epidermis	Profilaggrin cleaved into filaggrin, and loricrin forming cornified envelop
Spinosum	Lamellar granules (containing ceramides) Langerhans cells	Found intracellularly in upper layer but migrate to corneum where most effective, responsible for lipid barrier function Defends against microbial pathogens
Basale	Cuboidal basal cells with nucleus and integrins Scattered melanocytes	Integrins responsible for adhesion to dermis Initiation of keratinocyte differentiation Migration upward to stratum corneum takes 2–4 wk

- The *reticular dermis* (lower portion) joins with the subcutaneous or fat layer of the skin.

Subcutaneous Layer

- The subcutaneous layer, also referred to as *fatty tissue* or *hypodermis*, is comprised of adipose cells and connective tissue, which varies in thickness according the body location.
- The hypodermis provides a layer of protection for the body, thermoregulation, storage for metabolic energy, and mobility of the skin.

ADNEXA

Adnexa or appendages of the skin include the hair, nails, eccrine, and apocrine glands. The structure of hair and nails along with their associated disorders are discussed later in this text (Section 11).

Eccrine Glands

- Chiefly responsible for thermoregulation of the body, the *eccrine* or *sweat glands,* are tubules that extend from the epidermis through the dermis and are triggered by thermal and emotional stimuli.
- Although they are diffusely spread over the body, most are located on the palms and soles, and can contribute to hyperhidrosis, hypohidrosis, or anhidrosis.
- Eccrine glands maintain an important electrolyte and moisture balance of the palms and soles.

Apocrine Glands

Only found in the axillae, external auditory canal, eyelids, mons pubis, anogenital surface, and areola, apocrine glands secrete a minute amount of oily substance that is odorless. The role of these glands is not clearly understood.

READINGS AND REFERENCES

Ackerman, A. B. (1975). Structure and function of the skin. Section I. Development, morphology and physiology. In S. L. Moschella, D. M. Pillsbury, & H. J. Hurley (Eds.), *Dermatology*. Saunders.

Calonje, J. E., Brennm T., Lazar, A. J., & Billings, S. D. (2020). *McKee's pathology of the skin, with clinical correlations* (5th ed.). Elsevier.

Morphology: How to Describe the Skin

Margaret A. Bobonich

Clinicians simply cannot know about every dermatosis, but they can develop assessment skills that will be the key to a timely and accurate diagnosis. Skin lesions can be described in a variety of ways and categorized by morphology, distribution, configuration, and arrangement. While experienced dermatologists may use various approaches to diagnosis, this author suggests that non-dermatology and less experienced dermatology providers establish an organized and consistent approach to diagnosis based on morphology of the primary lesions. This section is dedicated to aiding clinicians in improving their diagnostic reasoning skills through a morphology-based approach to skin eruptions. Subsequent chapters in this text will enable you to use those skills to diagnose and manage the most common skin conditions seen by primary care and dermatology providers. The remaining disease entities discussed will address atypical presentations of common diseases and those with high morbidity and mortality.

Morphology

- The characteristics or structure of a skin lesion is referred to as *morphology*. Once the clinician has identified the morphology of the *primary* or initial lesion, then one can generate a differential diagnosis.

- Often, dermatology textbooks and online resources use a morphology-based approach to categorize diseases. Therefore, clinicians who lack the ability to correctly identify the morphology of the primary lesion must resort to fanning through the color atlas of dermatologic conditions hoping that they will see a similar lesion or rash.

Primary Lesions

- The morphology of a *primary skin lesion* can provide important information about the depth of the process and the location of

the pathology, that is, the epidermis, dermis, and/or subcutaneous tissue.

- A thorough understanding of the structure and function of the skin will then allow the clinician to envision the underlying pathologic process and assist in making the clinicopathologic correlation.

- Flat lesions often represent disease located in the epidermis, while raised lesions usually involve the dermis and/or subcutis.

- All clinicians should be able to identify these basic morphologic types that provide the foundation of diagnosis for any skin condition (Fig. 1.2-1).

Secondary Lesions

- Secondary changes in the primary lesion can occur as the result of external factors, the process of healing, or complications from treatment (crusts, atrophy, purpura, scar, etc.).

- The characteristics of the *secondary skin lesions* provide further description (an adjective) about the primary lesion (noun). There are many descriptors, but there are several that are commonly used in everyday practice such as crust, ulceration, excoriation, lichenification, and fissure (Fig. 1.2-2).

Characteristics

- The *configuration* of a lesion describes the shape which can provide valuable clues. Annular plaques are characteristic of tinea and granuloma annulare (Fig. 1.2-3).

- The *arrangement* is the location of lesions relative to each other. Lesions can be solitary, satellite (set apart from the body of the eruption), or clustered.

- A red cherry angioma is typically a solitary lesion.

- The eruption of vesicles and pustules in herpes zoster are usually clustered and follow dermatomal arrangement.

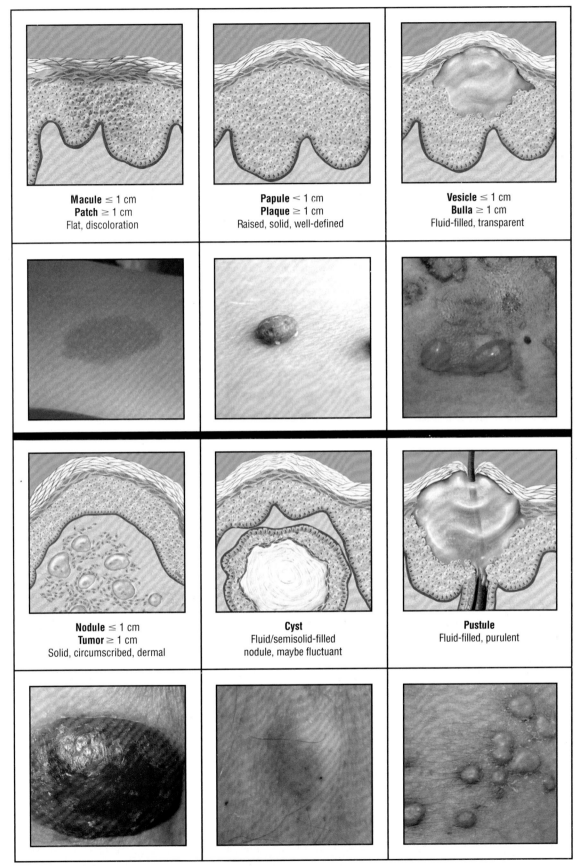

FIG. 1.2-1. Morphology of *primary* lesions. Diagram structure in the skin with corresponding clinical photos. (Photos courtesy of M. Bobonich.)

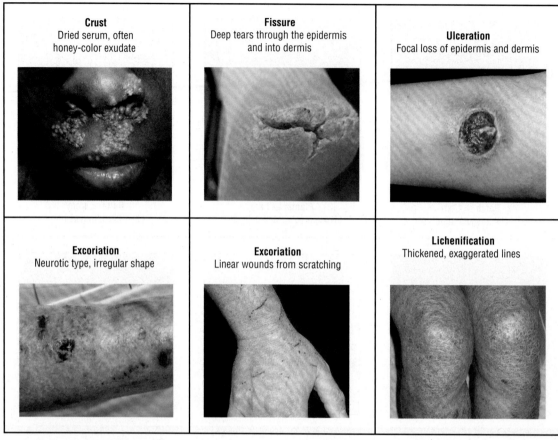

FIG. 1.2-2. Morphology of secondary lesions.

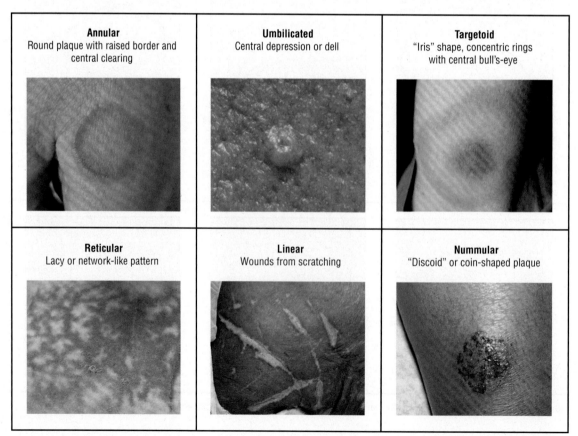

FIG. 1.2-3. Common characteristics of skin lesions.

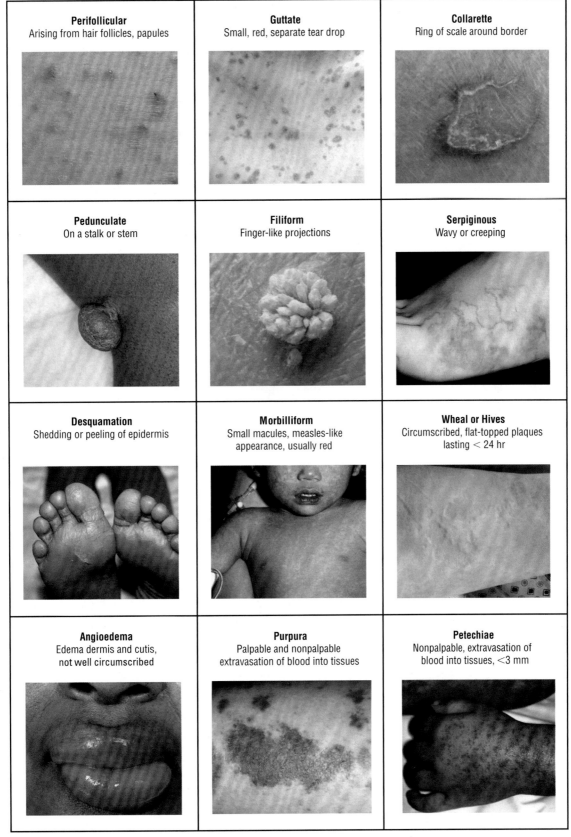

Perifollicular
Arising from hair follicles, papules

Guttate
Small, red, separate tear drop

Collarette
Ring of scale around border

Pedunculate
On a stalk or stem

Filiform
Finger-like projections

Serpiginous
Wavy or creeping

Desquamation
Shedding or peeling of epidermis

Morbilliform
Small macules, measles-like
appearance, usually red

Wheal or Hives
Circumscribed, flat-topped plaques
lasting < 24 hr

Angioedema
Edema dermis and cutis,
not well circumscribed

Purpura
Palpable and nonpalpable
extravasation of blood into tissues

Petechiae
Nonpalpable, extravasation of
blood into tissues, <3 mm

FIG. 1.2-3. (*Continued*)

Distribution

- The *distribution* of skin lesions can provide valuable diagnostic clues. Lesions may be generalized, localized, or may favor particular areas of the body such as the interdigital spaces, acral areas, or mucous membranes.
- Many cutaneous and systemic diseases have hallmark clinical presentations based on the distribution of lesions (Fig. 1.2-4).

- For example, lesions on the palms are characteristic of conditions like erythema multiforme, dyshidrotic eczema, secondary syphilis, and palmoplantar psoriasis.
- Chronic scaly and erythematous patches or plaques on the extensor aspects of the extremities would favor a diagnosis of psoriasis compared to atopic dermatitis that usually affects the flexural surfaces.

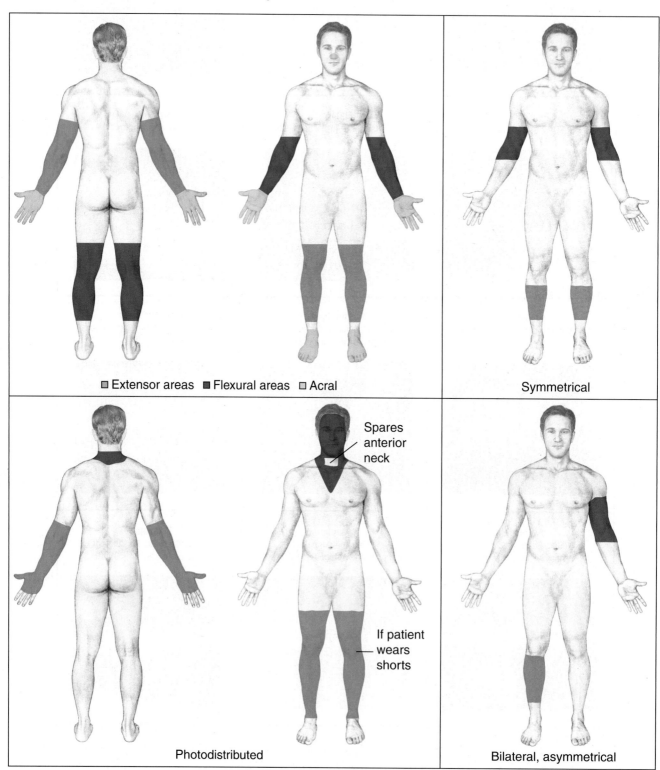

□ Extensor areas ■ Flexural areas □ Acral

Symmetrical

Spares anterior neck

If patient wears shorts

Photodistributed

Bilateral, asymmetrical

FIG. 1.2-4. Distribution of lesions.

- Care should be taken to note lesions involving the hair, nails, and mucous membrane, which can be unique for some diseases.
- Lastly, the clinician should remember that the distribution of the lesions may change as a skin eruption progresses. Drug rashes typically start on the trunk and spread to the extremities (centrifugal).
- In contrast, erythema multiforme starts on the hands and feet, and advances to the trunk (centripetal).

Color

- For most clinicians, the color of lesions is given little consideration and usually categorized as red or brown. But next time you examine a lesion, take a closer look and use tangential lighting. You will see in Section 10 of this text that colors can provide insight into the underlying pathogenesis of a lesion (Table 1.2-1).
- Red skin lesions and eruptions can be further differentiated based on whether there is scale present (Fig. 1.2-6).
- Eczematous dermatoses are characterized by red and scaling lesions that present with a disruption in the epidermis. Although papulosquamous lesions are also red and scaly, the epidermis is typically intact (Table 1.2-2). However, disease stage and secondary changes can make it difficult to appreciate the integrity of the epithelial barrier.
- Smooth red lesions are a unique morphology to a separate group of differential diagnosis (Table 1.2-3).
- Yellow and orange colors are typically the result of lipid, chemical, or protein deposition.
- Brown, black, blue colors are associated with melanin or hemosiderin.
- White lesions can be associated with a lack of pigment and a "flesh-color" lesions refer to the patient's natural skin color.

TABLE 1.2-2	Differential Diagnosis for RED and SCALY Dermatoses
ECZEMATOUS *Epithelial disruption*	**PAPULOSQUAMOUS** *No epithelial disruption*
Atopic dermatitis	<u>Papules</u>
Irritant contact dermatitis	Pityriasis rosea
Allergic contact dermatitis	Keratosis pilaris
Dyshidrotic eczema	Tinea
Nummular eczema	Lichen planus
Stasis dermatitis	Secondary syphilis
Scabies	Guttate psoriasis
Secondary lesions from scratching or friction	<u>Prominent plaques</u>
Seborrheic dermatitis	Psoriasis
Polymorphic light eruption	Tinea
Lichen planus	Lupus erythematosus
Eczematous reaction patterns	Discoid lupus erythematosus
Xerotic eczema	CTCL (mycosis fungoides)
Exfoliative erythroderma	Pityriasis rubra pilaris
	Darier disease
	Exfoliative erythroderma

Associated Signs and Symptoms

- Identifying symptoms such as pruritus, pain, and burning can be paramount in discerning a diagnosis. For example, pruritus is a classic symptom in urticaria compared to the burning sensation associated with angioedema.
- Other lesion signs and symptoms reported may include tenderness, drainage, and odor.
- Clinicians should always be alert to systemic symptoms that may have proceeded or accompanied the cutaneous lesions. This should prompt a complete review of systems and comprehensive physical examination.
- Red flag signs and symptoms such as a febrile patient with a rash, altered level of consciousness, facial edema or angioedema, purpura, oral or ocular mucosal ulcerations, bullae with mucosal involvement, chest pain or dyspnea, positive Nikolsky sign, and erythroderma (>80% body with erythema) warrant an immediate referral for further evaluation and management.

MORPHOLOGY-BASED APPROACH TO DIFFERENTIAL DIAGNOSIS

It cannot be overstated that the foundation for a diagnosis of any skin lesion or eruption begins with a thorough history and physical examination. The morphology of the primary lesion provides a critical diagnostic clue and the first step in a systematic approach for generating a differential diagnosis. After the primary morphology has been identified, then the clinician can incorporate other lesion characteristics, associated findings, and patient comorbidities to narrow the differential and arrive at the correct diagnosis.

Developing Your Diagnostic Skills

An algorithmic approach can help clinicians organize not only their assessment but improve diagnostic reasoning. Health care providers have utilized this technique to develop clinical competencies since the beginning of their health care education and training. Repeated application of tools and guidelines aids the learner's progression from novice to expert. Theorists like Benner

TABLE 1.2-1	Differential Diagnosis for Lesions with Color	
Flesh Color	**Brown**	**White**
<u>Rough surface</u>	Freckles	Pityriasis alba
Skin tags	Skin tags	Idiopathic guttate
Verruca	Lentigines	hypomelanosis
Open comedones	Nevi	Tinea versicolor
Actinic keratosis	Seborrheic keratosis	Ash leaf macule
Corns/Callus	Tinea versicolor	Milia
Epidermal nevus	Postinflammatory	Keratosis pilaris
	hyper-pigmentation	Postinflammatory
<u>Smooth</u>	Erythrasma	hypopigmentation
Molluscum	Dermatofibroma	Nevus anemicus
contagiosum	Café au lait	Morpheaform basal
Basal cell carcinoma	Mongolian spot	cell carcinoma
Verruca/HPV	Melanoma	Vitiligo
Epidermoid cysts	Pigmented basal cell	Piebaldism
Lipomas	Dysplastic nevus	Lichen sclerosus et
Keloids/hypertrophic	Congenital nevus	atrophicus
scar	Fixed-drug eruption	Morphea
Granuloma annulare	Becker nevus	Tuberous sclerosis
Neurofibromas		
Pearly penile papules		**Yellow**
Adnexal tumors		Xanthelasma
		Sebaceous hyperplasia
		Necrobiosis lipoidica
		Morphea

TABLE 1.2-3	Differential Diagnosis for RED and SMOOTH Dermatoses	
Inflammatory lesions *Monomorphic[a]* *Usually solitary* *Papules and dome shaped*	**Vascular reactions** *Polymorphic[b]* *Multiple, often confluent flat-topped*	
Macules and papules Arthropod assaults Spider and cherry angiomas Scabies Acne Keratosis pilaris Candidiasis Pyogenic granulomas Granuloma annulare Viral exanthems Early psoriasis lesions Pityriasis rosea (w/o scale) Secondary syphilis Pityriasis lichenoides Grover disease **Nodules** Furuncles/Carbuncles Epidermoid cysts Cellulitis Erythema nodosum Acne vulgaris	**Transient** Rosacea Urticaria **Purpuric/Nonblanchable** Petechiae Coagulation disorders Leukocytoclastic vasculitis Henoch–Schönlein purpura Ecchymoses Meningococcemia Rocky Mountain spotted fever Vascular ulcers	**Persistent/blanching** Kawasaki disease SSS Toxic shock syndrome Red man syndrome Angioedema Autoimmune blistering diseases Erythema multiforme Erythema nodosum Drug eruption Urticarial vasculitis

[a]Monomorphic—same size and shape.
[b]Polymorphic—varied size and shape.

(1984) and Dreyfus (1986) have provided models that assess and support the acquisition of skills and competencies for professionals.

Primary care providers aren't expected to be dermatology experts, but they should strive to achieve a competent level of knowledge and skills. The novice must rely on the "recipe" or conscious approach to their assessment because they lack experience and intuition. With time and experience, a clinician can learn about the relevance of variables (what is important or not), individualize it to the patient, develop an analytical thought process, and understand the desired outcomes/goals.

Algorithmic Approach

When faced with a patient who presents with a diffuse or intense skin eruption, the clinician might easily be overwhelmed with the diagnostic challenge. This may be coupled with the patient's perception that issues with their skin are superficial and thus should be easy to diagnose and manage. This would be the ideal situation of course, but "rashes" aren't always a clear-cut diagnosis and there may be a systemic etiology. The following algorithms and differential diagnosis groups are designed to help the clinicians develop an acceptable standard of clinical reasoning skills.

Where to Begin

There are three basic questions or characteristics of the primary lesion to begin your assessment:

1. Is the lesion **fluid-filled** or **solid?** (see Fig. 1.2-5 and Table 1.2-4)
2. If it is a solid lesion, what **color** is it?
3. If the lesion color is red, is there any **scale**? (see Fig. 1.2-6)

These are simple concepts that almost every clinician is capable of assessing. Progressing through the assessment of the

primary lesion will lead you to an associated group of potential differential diagnosis. Then, the clinician can incorporate additional characteristics and unique patient symptoms to develop a plan of care. Standardizing the approach to lesions and rashes will

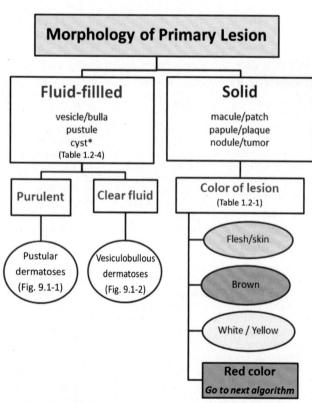

FIG. 1.2-5. Morphology-based approach to diagnosis of skin lesion.

TABLE 1.2-4	Differential Diagnosis for Fluid-Filled Dermatoses[a]		
VESICLES (≤1 cm)	**BULLAE (≥1 cm)**	**PUSTULAR**
Dyshidrotic eczema	Bullous impetigo	Acne vulgaris
Herpes simplex	Bullous tinea	Rosacea
Impetigo	Trauma/Thermal injury	Drug-induced pustular acne
Varicella/Zoster	Bullous erythema multiforme	Folliculitis–bacterial or pityrosporum
Tinea pedis	Staph scalded skin	Candidiasis
Scabies	Stevens–Johnson syndrome	Scabies
Contact dermatitis	Toxic epidermal necrolysis	Pustular psoriasis
Hand, foot, and mouth disease	Autoimmune blistering disease	Perioral dematitis
Polymorphic light eruption	Bullous drug eruption	Subcorneal pustulosis
Porphyria cutanea tarda	Lichen planus	CONSIDER infectious pathogens
Photodrug eruption	Porphyria cutanea tarda	
Grover disease	Diabetic bullae	
Autoimmune blistering disease		
Arthropod assaults		
Erythema multiforme		
Id reaction		

[a]See Chapter 9.1 for additional algorithm and differential diagnosis of pustular eruptions (Fig. 9.1-1) and vesiculobullous eruptions (Fig. 9.1-2).

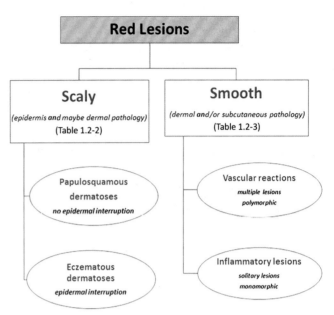

FIG. 1.2-6. Morphology-based approach to diagnosis of RED skin lesions.

enhance the clinician's ability to recognize abnormal findings, provide a precise assessment, and improve diagnostic accuracy. Keep in mind:

- The use of algorithms can be helpful and are intended as adjunctive tools accompanied by critical thinking.
- Once the category of dermatoses is identified, key characteristics such as distribution, associated symptoms, and diagnostic studies should be used narrow your final diagnosis.
- More extensive lists of differential diagnosis can be found online, in manuals, or with the aid of digital diagnostic tools.
- Ultimately, use of diagnostic tools like these algorithms requires repeated use, good clinical judgment, and individualized patient care. There are always uncommon diseases and atypical presentations that will challenge even the most experienced dermatology clinician.
- When the clinician is perplexed by the lesion or eruption, always consult with an experienced colleague or dermatology specialist to ensure diagnostic accuracy and appropriate management for optimal care.

CLINICAL PEARLS

- When there is a change in the surface of the skin, it usually indicates an epidermal process.
- Use the punch biopsy technique for inflammatory lesions.
- Vesicles can be from an immune response or infectious process.
- Pustules are most often associated with infection.
- Consider the possibility of immunosuppression in patients with chronic or recurrent skin infections or atypical presentations.
- Pathologic processes occurring deep in the dermis or subcutaneous can leave the surface of the skin smooth but result in larger plaques that are not as well circumscribed (wheals/hives compared to angioedema).
- Be aware of the *Great Mimickers* of skin disease: lupus erythematosus, tuberculosis (mycobacterium), cutaneous T-cell lymphoma, secondary syphilis, sarcoidosis, and amelanotic melanoma.
- Diffuse eruptions involving large BSA can overwhelm the clinician. ALWAYS start with the basics, the morphology of the primary lesion.

REFERENCES

Benner, P. E. (1984). *From novice to expert: Excellence and power in clinical nursing practice*. Addison-Wesley Publishing.

Dreyfus, H. L., & Dreyfus, S. E. (1986). *Mind over machine: The power of human intuition and expertise in the age of the computer*. Blackwell Publishing.

Approach to the Skin Examination

Margaret A. Bobonich

In This Chapter

- History
- Physical Examination
- Diagnostics

Primary care and nondermatology specialty clinicians see the majority of patients with initial skin complaints on a daily basis. While patients may make an appointment to see their provider for a routine physical examination or blood pressure management, they often use the opportunity to address a skin complaint. Conversely, patients may call to schedule an appointment for treatment of a "rash." This catch-all term reported by so many patients, often provides very little advance understanding regarding the nature of the eruption or complaint.

A complete and pertinent history is fundamental to any assessment of skin. Every clinician is encouraged to perform a thorough full-body skin examination despite the limitation of time and often reluctance by the patient. As you will see in later chapters, the initial chief complaint by the patient may be misleading and result in only a focused area of examination. Whenever possible, the patient should be encouraged to disrobe fully and be gowned appropriately. Practitioners are afforded very limited time to assess, diagnose, treat, and document patient care, therefore developing a systematic approach will minimize your likelihood of missing an important finding. This section details a logical sequence to history taking and skin examination and can be used as a guideline.

HISTORY

- The patient history is sometimes slighted in lieu of time available for physical examination and patient education. However, the importance of an appropriate history relative to the skin complaint should not be overlooked (Box 1.3-1).

- The history should begin with the patient's general health and proceed with a focused or complete history relative to the skin complaint and presence of systemic symptoms.

- Be aware that patients may be very cursory with details about their health history as they perceive it as inconsequential to their skin condition. For example, a female seeking treatment for acne may fail to report oral contraceptives on her medication list or past medical history of polycystic ovarian syndrome. Both can impact the clinician's ability to adequately assess, diagnose, and manage her skin condition.

- Medications are one of the most significant aspects of a history, receive the least attention, and yet has the greatest risk of impacting the patient's skin condition. Medication history should not only include prescription drugs, but over-the-counter and illicit drugs, supplements, herbals, and "borrowed" medications. Section 8.1 provides tips on taking a medication history.

- The elderly and adolescents are known for sharing drugs and may be sheepish about admitting to it.

- NSAIDs and oral contraceptives can have a significant impact on the skin, but are commonly omitted from the patient's list of medications.

- Before concluding the history of intake, it is recommended that clinicians inquire (an open-ended question) about any other specifics that the patient believes might be important about their skin condition. This invites communication and acknowledges the important role of the patient, family, and caregivers in their patient-centered care.

- Patients may express grave concerns that their symptoms are similar to the disease discussed on a television talk show or health information discovered on an internet search engine.

- Transparency in the patient's perception and expectations at the beginning of the office visit will enable the clinician to personalize care for a better patient experience.

PHYSICAL EXAMINATION

- Physical examination of the skin is a skill that is developed through repeated and systematic evaluations of your patients.

- The extent of the examination is determined by the patient's symptoms and willingness to reveal their body.

- A complete skin examination is recommended for skin cancer screenings with the patient completely disrobed and in a patient gown.

- It is also preferred for patients who come in with complaints of a skin eruption or those with systemic symptoms.

- A focused examination, however, from the waist up may be adequate for a chief complaint of acne that only requires exposure of the back and chest.

- Clinicians should encourage patients to allow maximum visualization for a thorough examination while respecting their modesty and rights to limit their physical exposure.

- A helpful guide is provided to aid in developing a systematic approach for a skin examination for either the entire body or regional areas (Box 1.3-2).

- It is not necessary to wear gloves for a skin examination, allowing the clinician to use touch to optimize their assessment.

BOX 1.3-1 Complete History for the Assessment of Skin Lesions

Demographic Data
Age, sex, race-predilection in some diseases/conditions

Allergies
Drug, environmental, and foods. Consider possible cross-reactivity.

Medications
See Section 8.1 (Drugs and Rash) if drug-related eruption is suspected

Medical and Surgical History
Personal (birth history for children) including skin cancer
Family (hereditary disease associated with genodermatoses)
Pregnancy or lactation

History of Lesion or Eruption
Onset, circumstances, and duration
Spread and/or course of skin condition
Aggravating or relieving factors
Associated symptoms—itch, pain, blisters, drainage, odor
Previous episodes, treatment, and response
Impact on sleep, eating, social activities, work, and school

Social History
Occupation and hobbies
Sunscreen use, tanning behaviors, and UVR exposure
Alcohol intake and smoking
Exposures (e.g., infectious, environmental, occupational)
Sexual behavior and orientation
Travel
Living conditions or households (important for infectious disease)
Family structure

Psychological History
Etiology or complication of disease

BOX 1.3-2 Complete Skin Examination

How to Perform a Skin Examination
- The two most important elements of a complete skin examination are exposure and lighting.
- The patient must be properly gowned so that each part of the body can be visualized. Always encourage the patient to undress completely.
- Extra lighting may be needed for examination rooms without windows.
- A dermatoscope can be very helpful in providing not just light but also magnification.
- Develop a systematic approach that you use for every examination. Begin with the patient seated in front of you; and slightly lower if possible.
- Gently glide your fingers across the skin. Your touch will comfort and may identify lesions not visible.

Scalp
- Part the hair in multiple sections to visualize the scalp and identify redness, papules, pustules, nodules, scale, and scarring.

Hair and Nails
- Observe the hair color, pattern, and texture (see Section 11.1 for details).
- Look for patterns of hair thinning or alopecia and the presence or absence of hair follicles within.
- Observe the nail unit and periungual area for presence of cuticle, discoloration or pigmentation in nail plate, or skin around the nail.
- Check for erythema or signs of infection (see Section 11.2 for details). Remember melanomas can occur beneath the nail plate.

Face
- Get an overview of face noting symmetry.
- Note the presence of scarring (acute or chronic), papules, pustules, nodules, erythema, scale, skin tags, keratoses, and dyspigmentation.

Mouth
- Look for any brown or red spots on lips.
- Dryness and scale in elderly may be related to chronic sun damage.
- Severe dryness or chapped lips may also be contact dermatitis or related to medication such as isotretinoin.
- Examine the oral cavity for lesions or erosions on palate, buccal mucosa, and tongue (see Section 11.3 for details).

Eyes
- Examine the inner and outer canthus, and orbital area for any growths.
- Note redness, scale in eyebrows, and lid margins.

Ears
- Look for scale or lesions on helix.
- Examine earlobes for keloids or cysts.
- Check the posterior sulcus and conchal bowl for scale, hyperpigmentation, scale, and scarring.

Nose
- Look and feel the bridge, sides, creases, and nasal rim.
- Note telangiectasia, ulcerations, or abnormal pigmentation.

Neck
- Note the color, texture, and distribution of discoloration, lateral aspect versus submental area (photo-distribution).

Trunk
- Visualize trunk with patient sitting, standing, and lying down, checking the umbilicus for signs of psoriasis, moles, or melanoma.
- Be sure to examine the buttocks, hips, and perianal area.
- If patient refuses genital examination, inquire about presence of lesions, rashes, and itch.

Arms and Hands
- Inspect each arm and raise to view the axilla and lateral trunk.
- Look for increased pigmentation or loss.
- The antecubital fossa may reveal presence of eczema.
- Examine the dorsal and palmar aspect of hands, fingers, and interdigital spaces.

Legs and Feet
- Examine both legs individually.
- Remove socks to check feet, toes, and interdigital spaces.
- Carefully check the plantar surface of feet for warts, corns, or pigmented lesions.

Lymphadenopathy
- Note occipital, posterior, and anterior cervical nodes in presence of scalp lesions or infections.
- In patients with a history of melanoma or SCC, careful examination of regional lymph nodes at least should be performed.

- All providers should clean their hands prior to and after examining a patient. Patients, and our society in general, have become increasingly aware of infection control and appreciate seeing the clinician cleanse their hands while in their presence.

- Universal precautions should always be observed when preforming cutaneous procedures, exposure to body fluids, or examining skin that is not intact.

- They should also be worn when infection is suspected or touching the anogenital area and then immediately discarded.

DIAGNOSTICS

- While the history and physical examination are the foundation for developing differential diagnosis, diagnostic tests may be necessary to rule out disease or support a definitive diagnosis.

- Each chapter in this text will identify the indications and recommendations for diagnostic tests relative to the disease. Section 15 provides more detail on common dermatologic procedures.

- In-office diagnostic tools that can easily be used by nondermatology clinicians include the Wood's lamp, KOH, or mineral prep.

- Diagnostic tests such as patch testing requires a skilled assessment, application, and interpretation by a dermatology specialist.

- Diagnostic aids such a dermatoscope have been increasingly utilized by dermatology clinicians especially for the evaluation of pigmented lesions. It is a noninvasive method that allows visualization of the epidermis and papillary dermis that cannot be seen by the naked eye (Fig. 1.3-1). Colors, structures, and patterns may be observed and aid in the diagnoses of cutaneous neoplasms. The skill of dermoscopy requires education, training, and time to master. Therefore, utilization of a dermatoscope, which can be quite expensive, is usually reserved for dermatology specialists.

- Biopsy is one of the most important diagnostics used in the evaluation of cutaneous lesions. Clinicians trained to perform shave and punch biopsies can send specimens for hematoxylin and eosin (H&E) stain, which provides microscopic analysis and reports on the pathologic changes in the skin.

- When indicated, immunohistology on patient tissue or sera utilizes various immunostaining techniques with light microscopy to identify antibodies. This is especially helpful in cutaneous manifestations with autoimmune diseases and is discussed in further detail in Section 9.

- Clinicians should learn to competently interpret histopathology reports to ensure that clinicopathologic correlation exists, especially in inflammatory skin conditions.

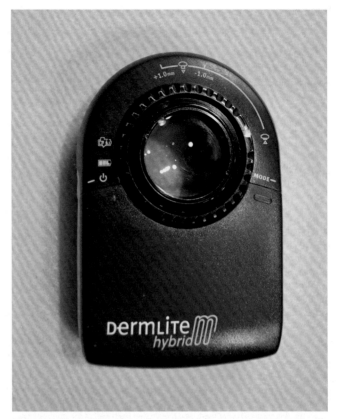

FIG. 1.3-1. The dermatoscope uses polarized and nonpolarized light to visualize pigment and vascular structures of cutaneous lesions.

- When there are questions regarding the report or interpretation, the clinician should discuss the biopsy with the pathologist. Most dermatologic specialists send tissue biopsies to a *dermatopathologist,* who is specialty trained and board certified in dermatology with a fellowship in dermatopathology. They can provide a superior histologic analysis and opinion about possible diagnoses, especially when the clinician provides pertinent history, clinical findings, and a comprehensive list of differential diagnoses.

READING

Yélamos, O., Braun, R. P., Liopyris, K., Wolner, Z. J., Kerl, K., Gerami, P., & Marghoob, A. A. (2019). Dermoscopy and dermatopathology correlates of cutaneous neoplasms. *Journal of the American Academy of Dermatology, 80*(2), 341–363. https://doi.org/10.1016/j.jaad.2018.07.073

Common Dermatologic Therapeutics

Gail Batissa Handwork and Margaret A. Bobonich

The skin is a large and complex organ that performs multiple functions allowing us to maintain a state of homogeneity. It provides a critical barrier that protects the body against chemicals, microorganisms, ultraviolet radiation (UVR), and the loss of bodily fluids. It is also a nutritive organ, supplied by a network of superficial vessels, that nourishes and repairs the skin. Another important role of the skin is for temperature regulation. Skin is regulated by dynamic vasodilation and constriction of blood vessels, along with the cooling response by the sweat glands. The hydration or moisture content in the skin is key to the percutaneous absorption and efficacy of topical preparations.

This chapter will explore the appropriate use of various topical formulations as well as both topical and systemic glucocorticosteroids in the treatment of common dermatologic conditions. Systemic corticosteroids are often used in dermatology, and we will review their optimum indications and usage. With the appropriate utilization of topical corticosteroid (TCS) therapies, oral corticosteroids can usually be avoided and therefore systemic side effects can be minimized.

SKIN HEALTH

Patients often ask about skin care recommendations. For some, their interest in learning about how to care for their skin is merely a factor of cosmesis, but many seek help because of uncomfortable and sometimes disfiguring skin conditions. Providing recommendations and accurate information about both prescription and over-the-counter skin care products aids them in making more informed decisions when faced with the myriad of options.

Cleansing and Bathing

All patients can benefit from good skin care education. Recommendations regarding bathing and hand washing may vary depending on a person's age, activity, environment, culture, and skin condition.

- To maintain hydration and proper barrier function, patients should avoid extreme water temperatures and use tepid water when cleansing.
- After bathing, patients should use care to avoid rubbing, but rather gently pat the skin dry. This will help to preserve the oils in their skin.
- Cleansing too often can contribute to worsening of certain skin conditions such as acne and eczema.

- Use of antibacterial soaps is not recommended and does not provide better efficacy than washing with plain soap and water. Actually, antibacterial soaps can have potential negative effects on both health and our environment including bacterial resistance. In 2017, the U.S. Food and Drug Administration issued a warning on topical antiseptics including triclosan which is found in many consumer products like soaps.

  "… As part of the FDA's ongoing review of topical antiseptic active ingredients used in nonprescription antiseptic drug products, the FDA has issued a final rule determining that triclosan and 23 other active ingredients are not generally recognized as safe and effective for use in certain over-the-counter (OTC) health care antiseptic products because no additional safety and effectiveness data for these ingredients were provided to the agency." (https://www.federalregister.gov/documents/2017/12/20/2017-27317/safety-and-effectiveness-of-health-care-antiseptics-topical-antimicrobial-drug-products-for)

- Abrasive materials and devices are unnecessary and can actually be harmful to the skin by contributing to irritation or allergic reactions.

Moisturizing

Throughout this text, we will discuss skin conditions that involve, in addition to other factors, a loss of the skin's barrier function. When the skin is dry, the epidermis cannot perform its protective function, allowing microbes and allergens easy access to stimulate inflammation and/or infection. Skin products marketed to treat dry skin commonly have properties of both moisturizers as well as emollients. As water quickly evaporates from the skin, it is recommended that a moisturizer or emollient be applied to the entire body within 3 minutes of bathing. Selection of these products is made on individual preferences based on texture, scent, and the area of the body being treated.

- Moisturizers technically hydrate the skin.
- Emollients soften and help the skin maintain its hydration. White petroleum, cocoa butter, and lanolin are examples of common emollients that decrease transepidermal water loss.
- Humectants such as urea, glycerin, and lactic acid work by drawing water into the stratum corneum.

Bleach Baths

Primary care providers traditionally provide bathing recommendations for care of their patients with atopic dermatitis. In a systematic review by Chopra et al. (2017), there were no significant differences between *Staphylococcus aureus* colonization in patients receiving bleach baths compared to those in regular bath water. Therefore, data do not support the routine use of bleach baths as a recommendation for all AD patients. However, the increased frequency of bathing immediately followed by emollients did result in a decrease of AD severity. PCPs should consider recommending frequent or daily bathing followed with emollients to their AD patients instead of reducing their bathing frequency. Bleach baths may be considered with concomitant mupirocin to their nares as treatment to effectively eradicate *S. aureus* in patients with community-acquired recurrent soft tissue or skin infections (Fritz et al., 2011).

Bleach Bath Recipe

- Add ¼ cup unscented household bleach to a full bathtub of warm water
- Make sure to distribute it well
- Soak in bleach bath from the neck down for 10 minutes
- Bleach bath should be limited to one or two times weekly

Lifestyle Recommendations

Healthy lifestyles help maintain a person's youthful and healthy skin appearance. Incorporating adequate sun protection, a proper diet, minimizing alcohol intake, avoiding smoking and excessive stress are key factors in maintaining skin health and protecting it from premature aging.

Irritants and Allergens

Water itself is the most common skin irritant. Hand dermatitis is often seen in occupations such as health care providers who have to wash their hands frequently or wear occlusive gloves for extended periods of time. This type of "wet work" results in repeated wet-dry cycles causing chronic inflammation of the epidermis. Symptoms of irritant contact dermatitis from water are dry, scaly, red and itching hands and fingers that crack and blister. It can be extremely painful.

Occupations where employees wash their hands frequently should be instructed that the use a gel sanitizer made with at least 60% alcohol which provides an effective, less drying alternative to soap and water. Alcohol gel sanitizers should only be used on intact skin and when hands are not visibly soiled. Frequent hand washing with soap and water is sometimes necessary, minimizing exposures and moisturizing after washing is advised. Employers often provide personal protective equipment (e.g., gloves, eyewear, and heat repellent garments) which protect the skin from the environment but conversely may trigger allergic or irritant contact dermatitis.

Patients with skin disorders should always use caution before using new topical products, as they may include ingredients that can cause allergic and/or irritant contact dermatitis. Providers should guide patients away from known allergens in products that trigger an irritant or allergic response, including products advertised as "all natural."

- Additives or inactive ingredients like sunscreen, fragrances, alcohol, preservatives, and other chemicals may be added to moisturizers, emollients, and humectants. Many of these additives can be irritating or cause an allergy and result in a skin eruption.

TABLE 1.4-1	Brand-Name Products Free of the Most Common Allergens[a]
CATEGORY	**PRODUCT**[b]
Wipes	7th Generation Free & Clear Baby Wipes
Cleansers	Aveeno Baby Cleanser Moisturizing Wash Eucerin Skin Calming Dry Skin Body Wash Free & Clear Liquid Cleanser for Sensitive Skin Vanicream Gentle Facial Cleanser VML Hypoallergenics Essence Skin-Saving Clear & Natural Soap Spring Cleaning Purifying Facial Wash for Oily Skin
Moisturizers	Aveeno Eczema Therapy Moisturizing Cream Baby Eczema Therapy Moisturizing Cream Cetaphil Oil Control Moisturizer SPF Eucerin Professional Repair for Extremely Dry Skin Lotion Vaniply Ointment for Sensitive Skin VML Hypoallergenics Red Better Daily Therapy Moisturizer
Lubricants	Fragrance- and preservative-free: Aquaphor Fragrance-, lanolin-, and preservative-free: white petrolatum or petroleum jelly

[a]Formaldehyde, fragrance (including botanicals), paraben mix/parabens, and propylene glycol.
[b]Retailers may sell old formulations of the brand. Manufacturers may change the formulation at any time and without warning or notice to consumers.

- Patient's should be made aware that labels that claim products are dermatologist recommended, hypoallergenic, natural, pure and organic, are marketing claims that are not monitored and do not guarantee that products are free from common sensitizers. If there is a suspected allergy, patients should be advised to use products with the minimal number of ingredients and avoidance of known allergens that may trigger contact dermatitis (Table 1.4-1).
- Companies are at liberty to change the inactive ingredients in their products without any label change or notifying the consumer. Thus, patients are often mystified about developing an allergic contact dermatitis because they have been using the specific brand for years or they report they aren't using anything "new."
- Referral to dermatology for patch testing may be necessary to determine if there is indeed an allergy. Please refer to Section 4.2 about contact dermatitis for more details on patch testing and known allergens in cosmetics.

TOPICAL THERAPEUTICS

Cosmetic Botanicals

Clinicians may be asked about skin care products, specifically those containing botanicals which they presume are healthier as they are "natural" ingredients. There is some evidence to suggest that botanical products may be useful, but the scientific evidence is lacking. For patients with sensitive skin, eczema, atopic dermatitis, inflammatory or pruritic conditions, products containing feverfew, colloidal oatmeal, or sunflower seed oil may provide some soothing relief. Patients with either rosacea or hyperpigmentation might benefit from products containing licorice root extract, which has both anti-inflammatory and skin lightening properties.

Botanical extracts are being used with increased frequency in the cosmetic industry, and the future of antiaging products, in particular, appears to be promising. Today many cosmetic formulations are

TABLE 1.4-2	Common Botanicals		
NAME	**ORIGIN**	**EFFECT**	**USE**
Aloe	Leaves of *Aloe vera*	Emollient, preventing infection	Eczema, wound care, ringworm, burns, insect bites
Arnica	Flowers of *Arnica montana*	Anti-inflammatory	Wound care, bruising, eczema, blisters (Avoid use on broken skin), acne, chapped lips
Calendula	Flowers of *Calendula officinalis* (pot marigold)	Antifungal, anti-inflammatory	Radiation induced burns, decubitus ulcers, bruising
Cayenne	Fruit of *Capsicum annuum*	Analgesic, warming stimulant	Neuropathic pain from shingles, massage oils, psoriasis
Chamomile	Dried flower heads and oil from *Matricaria chamomilla*	Antioxidant, antimicrobial, analgesic, anti-inflammatory	Wound care, burns
Chocolate	Seeds of *Theobroma cacao*	Antioxidant	Cocoa butter for chapped skin, burns, irritants
Dandelion	Leaves, flowers, or root of *Taraxacum officinale*	Anti-inflammatory, antioxidant, antibacterial, possible antitumor activity	Eczema, psoriasis, acne
Eucalyptus	Leaves, oil from *Eucalyptus globulus*	Antiseptic, astringent	Skin abscesses, minor wounds, bruises
Feverfew	Leaves, flowering tops of *Tanacetum parthenium*	Antioxidant, anti-inflammatory, anti-irritant, and anticancer properties. Orally, chewing leaves can cause ulceration and oral edema	Rosacea, antiaging, atopic dermatitis
Green Tea	Leaves, buds from *Camellia sinensis*	Anti-inflammatory, antioxidant	Healing wounds and photoprotection
Lavender	Flowers, essential oil from *Lavandula angustifolia*	Fragrance, antimicrobial, antianxiety	Fragrance, sleep inducer, sunburn, fungal infection, as rub form circulatory and rheumatic ailments
Lemongrass	Leaves, young stems, and oil of *Cymbopogon citratus*	Antiseptic, antibacterial, antifungal	Athlete's foot, ringworm
Licorice root extract[a]	Underground stem of *Glycyrrhiza glabra*	Antioxidant, anti-inflammatory, antiviral and antimicrobial	Skin lightening, healing for herpes blisters, canker sores, sunburn, insect bites
Patchouli	Leaf, stem of *Pogostemon cablin*	Antibacterial, antifungal	Eczema, seborrhea, acne, eczema, mosquito repellent
Resveratrol	Skin and seeds of grapes, berries, peanuts, and other foods	Antioxidant, anti-inflammatory, and antiproliferative agent	Antiaging, wrinkle reduction
Rosemary	Leaves, twigs from *Rosmarinus officinalis*	Anti-inflammatory, antioxidant, analgesic	Seborrhea, alopecia
Soy	Seeds from *Glycine max*	Antioxidant, anticarcinogenic, anti-inflammatory	Skin lightening, improve skin elasticity, moisturizer
Tea tree oil	Leaves from *Melaleuca alternifolia*	Antifungal, antimicrobial, anti-inflammatory	Acne, onychomycosis, ringworm, dandruff eczema, insect bites
Witch hazel	Leaves, bark, twigs of *Hamamelis virginiana*	Astringent, antioxidant, anti-inflammatory	Acne, contact dermatitis, bites, burns

[a]The oral form of licorice root extract can interact with angiotensin-converting enzyme inhibitors, aspirin, oral contraceptives, oral corticosteroids, diuretics, insulin, and stimulant laxatives.
Adapted from Foster, S., & Johnson, R. L. (2006). *Desk reference to nature's medicine.* National Geographic Society.

made of botanical extracts with *claims* that they improve the health, texture, and integrity of the skin, hair, and nails. Botanicals are also being used in cleansers, moisturizers, and astringents. Therefore, it is important to have some understanding of the expected benefit of these products. Table 1.4-2 includes an overview of the more popular botanical ingredients used in skin care products today but does not inclusive or an endorsement.

Strength/Frequency

A concentration of 1% indicates 1 g of drug will be contained in 100 g of the formulation. The fact that the efficacy of a topically applied drug is usually not proportionate to the concentration can be confusing to many patients. For example, a prescription of halobetasol propionate 0.05% cream prescribed for a rash may not make sense to a patient compared to the hydrocortisone 2.5% cream that they used previously was unsuccessful.

Occlusion increases the penetration and may in turn increase the potency of a topical medication. It is important for patients to know if you want them to apply a dressing after the application of their topical steroid cream. Clinicians should use caution in selecting the potency for areas of the body with natural occlusion like the intertriginous areas or underneath clothing. Of note, compounding of proprietary products with other ingredients may alter the stability of the drugs and should be done with caution if at all.

Percutaneous Absorption (PCA)

The ability of a topical medication to be effective is dependent on the transdermal delivery of the active ingredients from the stratum corneum of the epidermis to the underlying capillaries. There are many variables which can promote or impede PCA including drug concentration, frequency of administration, occlusion, surface area involved, the vehicle, age and weight of patient, location on the body, and amount of time the topical is left on the skin. PCA is increased with hydrated (moist) skin, heat or elevated temperature, and the condition of skin barrier.

PCA depends on the thickness of the skin which varies in different areas of the body. For example, the face and neck, antecubital or popliteal areas, axillae, and genital skin have a thinner epidermis and dermis where medication is quickly absorbed. Skin on the palms, soles, knees, and elbows are thicker, decreasing the rate of absorption of topical medications. There are many variables that influence PCA and should be taken into considered when prescribing the concentration, duration, frequency, and location of the therapy.

- Age—infants and children have smaller BSA to volume and therefore increase PCA
- Occlusion
- Hydration
- Inflamed, irritated, or disrupted skin barrier
- Thickness of skin

- Vascularity
- Mucosa surfaces
- Drug—potency, solubility or lipophilicity and molecular size

Vehicle

Topical agents are prepared in a variety of vehicles or bases that constitute the inactive ingredients of the medication, impacting the delivery of the drug into or through the skin (Table 1.4-3). Understanding the advantages and disadvantages of the vehicle is important for selection of the most appropriate medication for your patient.

Brand Versus Generic

Insurance companies generally incentivize patients to use generic medications in place of brand-name medications including topical preparations for cost containment. While generic products may the same active ingredients, the product's vehicle often differs. This difference may alter the drug's efficacy, and further complicate the patient's condition with contact dermatitis if the patient has an allergy to the ingredients in the product. The prices of both generic and brand name dermatologic therapeutics have increased tremendously over the past decade making it difficult for patients to afford medications prescribed by their providers. Although providers may be sensitive to this barrier to treatment and favor generic prescriptions, many of branded drugs require a time-consuming prior authorization process which may delay or prohibit patients' time to adequate treatment.

Combination Drugs

Commercially prepared TCS may be combined with drugs from a different class such as antifungal or anti-yeast agents and are not generally recommended by dermatology specialists as it may obscure the correct diagnosis. In addition, combination products may promote development of microbial resistance to topical antibiotics

TABLE 1.4-3	Vehicles for Topical Preparations	
VEHICLE	**DEFINITION**	**PREFERENCES**
Solution	Homogeneous mixture of two or more substances	Excellent for scalp/ hair-bearing areas
Lotion	Liquid preparation, thicker than solution Likely to contain oil, water, and/or alcohol	Lotions spread easily Use in large areas
Cream	Thicker than lotion Requires preservatives to extend shelf life Greater potential for allergic reactions	Use when skin is moist or exudative Can be used in any area Well tolerated
Ointment	Semisolid, mostly water-free Petrolatum-based product Spreads easily, penetrates better than creams	Choose when skin is dry or for increased penetration (thick skin) Messy in hairy areas
Gel	Aqueous, semisolid emulsion Liquefies when in contact with skin	Great for hairy areas Avoid on blistered skin, may sting
Foam	Liquid comprised of oil, solvents, and water packaged under pressure in aluminum cans	Great for scalp and thick plaques Penetrates well without mess
Spray	Liquid dispensed through an aerosol container or atomizer	Helpful for hard to reach places And scalp or hairy areas

and/or increase sensitization to ingredients. Yet TCSs have been successfully paired with a vitamin D analog, calcipotriene, in the treatment of psoriasis. Likewise, acne preparations are often combined, offering ease of use, lower costs, and assist with the compliance of younger patients.

CORTICOSTEROIDS

Corticosteroids play a significant role in the treatment of dermatologic disorders. The fact that they can be used topically, intralesionally, and systemically provides the clinician with numerous options for patient management. Corticosteroids are a synthetic derivative from the natural steroid, cortisol, which is produced by the adrenal cortex. There are two types of corticosteroids: glucocorticoids and mineralocorticoids.

Topical glucocorticoids are the most common drug prescribed in dermatology. In general, regardless of the method of administration, these drugs act as anti-inflammatory, immunosuppressive, and antiproliferative agents. When they are used topically, their vasoconstrictive properties determine their potency. TCSs are used to treat a wide range of disorders from acute allergic dermatitis to chronic immunobullous disorders. We will look more closely at these frequently used medications in the next two sections and discuss their mode of administration, indications, side effects, and recommendations for use depending on the severity of the disorder.

Topical Corticosteroids

Dermatologic conditions like atopic dermatitis, psoriasis, hand eczema, and localized vitiligo are managed in both primary care and dermatology. TCSs are indicated for the treatment of inflammatory and pruritic corticosteroid-responsive skin conditions including acute flares and rotational therapy for chronic management. They penetrate the skin and work by decreasing the inflammatory pathways that cause the skin to become red and inflamed. Within days of use, however, the production of new skin cells is suppressed, creating the risk of atrophy and striae with long-term usage. Many variables impact the efficacy of a TCS and should be considered when prescribing them.

Generic formulations of TCS vary considerably in the type and amount of inactive ingredients. Contact dermatitis may worsen if a generic product that includes an allergen is substituted for a brand-name prescription that does not contain the allergen. Vehicles can also alter the potency of the corticosteroid itself, which is why the same drug formulated in an ointment may be high potency compared to a lotion formulation that is moderate potency. Additionally, consistency or eloquence of the vehicle may be important for patient preference.

The recommendation is to use the least potent TCS that is effective; however, using a TCS that is too weak may be ineffective and decrease compliance along with patient confidence in the provider. Low-potency corticosteroid preparations can be used safely when needed on thinner skin. The risk for adverse events should be considered for any TCS but increases with potency, chronic overuse, and comorbid conditions.

Ultrapotent or high-potency TCS should be limited to a rotational schedule, with two or three daily applications for a 2-week period, followed by 1 or 2 weeks without TCS. There are some well-known exceptions for use of stronger TCS (groups I and II) used on mucosa for skin disorders such as lichen sclerosis and lichen planus.

Some clinicians advocate use of topical immunomodulators such as calcineurin inhibitors, tacrolimus 0.01% (15 years and older) and 0.03% (2 years and older) ointment b.i.d., or pimecrolimus 1% cream (2 years and older) b.i.d. which can be used for 6 weeks during this break period. Other nonsteroidal topicals that can be helpful in avoiding steroid side effects include a phosphodiesterase-4 inhibitor, crisaborole 2% (3 months and older) b.i.d. or simply use emollients. A common side effect for these topical immunomodulators is burning and irritation which can make adherence challenging. However, it usually subsides after a couple weeks of use.

Adverse Effects

- Common side effects with TCSs and their vehicles include contact dermatitis, acne-like eruptions, skin atrophy, hypopigmentation, telangiectasia, purpura, and striae, as well as ocular conditions of increased intraocular pressure, cataract formation, and glaucoma.

- When using corticosteroids under occlusion, there is also a risk for folliculitis and maceration of the skin. In addition to patient education, providers can help reduce these risks by ordering only enough medication to achieve clearance.

- Due to variability in generic formulations and the common addition of propylene glycol, a common allergen, allergic reactions from TCS can be a conundrum. If a corticosteroid allergy is suspected, desoximetasone ointment 0.05% is the treatment of choice until the allergen is confirmed. Referral to dermatology can identify specific allergens through patch testing with Thin-layer Rapid Use Epicutaneous Test (TRUE Test). This product includes the common chemicals tixocortol pivalate and budesonide, which can help identify TCS allergies. These tests are widely utilized in dermatology and allergy practices. Testing for propylene glycol, however, requires a more comprehensive patch series such as the North American Series, which is usually provided only at larger academic or occupationally focused clinics. See Section 4.2 for additional information about allergic contact dermatitis.

- Atrophy or thinning of the skin from the application of TCS can occur within a fairly short period of time with potentially permanent results. Atrophy can be manifested by fragile skin and striae (Fig. 1.4-1A,B).

- *S. aureus* folliculitis is a possible side effect of TCS, especially when using it under occlusion. If noticed early, this can sometimes be reversed by drying out the skin with aluminum acetate compresses (i.e., Dombero solution) or treated with OTC chlorhexidine 4% wash or benzoyl peroxide 4% to 10% wash. However, folliculitis may require the addition of oral antibiotics to resolve the eruption.

- Adrenal suppression is a possible side effect of the stronger TCS, especially if used on a large surface area. This side effect is generally reversible and frequently associated with long-term oral corticosteroid therapy. Infants and small children being treated with TCSs may have a higher risk of this side effect due to their large body surface area compared to their body mass. Also, patients who also take corticosteroids in different forms such as oral, inhaled intranasal, etc. are at higher risk of this uncommon side effect.

Potency

Careful selection of TCS potency is vital for optimal efficacy and minimal adverse effects. TCSs are categorized according to vasoconstriction assays that usually correlate to clinical efficacy (see inside of back cover). Body location, severity, age, and characteristics of the dermatoses should be considered when prescribing at TCS.

- *Low potency*—use on infants; body areas like axillae, face, neck, groin; thin skin; and, areas of occlusion.

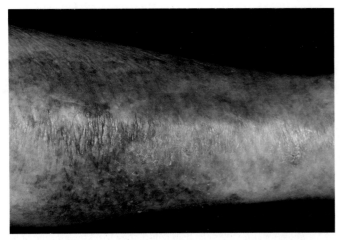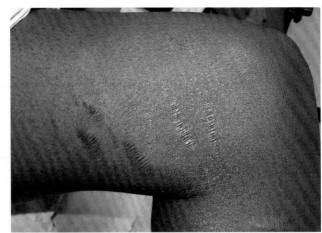

FIG. 1.4-1. **A:** Steroid atrophy. **B:** Striae on knees caused by chronic use of topical corticosteroids. (Photos courtesy of M. Bobonich.)

- *Moderate/intermediate potency*—trunk and extremities; short term; extensive dermatosis; and, not usually for infants and children.
- *High or super high potency*—use on scalp, back, palms/soles; short term for severe or recalcitrant dermatoses; thick or hyperkeratotic skin; and, not for children or infants.

Dispensing

As the cost of medications increase and health plans requirements of high deductibles and copays, it is important to order an adequate amount of medication. "Rule of hand" and fingertip unit (FTU) guidelines can aid providers in calculating the amount of drug to dispense (Table 1.4-4). The rule of hand method guides prescribers to visualize the surface area of four adult hands (both front and back, including digits) and to use this estimation of the size of the area requiring 1 g of medication per application, or 14 g for a twice-daily, 2-week course of treatment. Similarly, the FTU formula helps the provider estimate the correct quantity to prescribed topical medication that comes out of a tube with a 5-mm diameter covering the area from the distal crease of the forefinger to the ventral aspect of an adult fingertip (Fig. 1.4-2). For example, 2.5 FTUs are needed to cover the entire neck and face for one treatment, thus requiring a 35-g tube of cream for a 2-week course be prescribed. For a child ages 1 to 5 years old, one half of this amount would be needed to cover the same area. For an infant, one quarter of the adult amount would be sufficient. FTUs can be used to education about the appropriate amount of TCS for use in one application.

Occlusion

For increased penetration of very thick skin plaques or to treat a full body rash, occlusion may be used for a period of 2 hours twice daily. Medication is applied, and plastic wrap is used to cover the entire area where it is practical, such as an arm or leg. Alternatively, corticosteroid-impregnated flurandrenolide (Cordran Tape) is available as an adhesive and useful for small, thickened and stubborn to treat areas. If the entire body surface is involved, a plastic suit often called a "sauna suit," can be worn for a few hours in the day after applying the corticosteroid to all areas. This should be limited to 2 to 3 days. Occlusive plastic suits are inexpensive and can be found at most sporting goods stores.

Management and Patient Education

- Follow-up office visits for reassessment should be made for conditions being treated with TCS on a long-term basis, especially when frequent refill requests are being requested. Prescriptions given to noncompliant patients should not be refilled indefinitely,

TABLE 1.4-4	Estimated Amounts for Topical Medication	
LOCATION	**PER APPLICATION, FTUs**	**AMOUNT FOR 2 WEEKS, ADULT (g)**
Entire face and neck	2.5	35
One hand (both sides)	1	14
One entire foot	2	28
One arm (both sides)	3	42
One leg	6	84

Conversions: Adult: 30 g covers entire adult body in one application; children: $^{1}/_{2}$ of the adult amount; infants (6–12 months): only $^{1}/_{4}$ of the adult amount; 1 FTU = 0.5 g per application. FTU, fingertip unit.

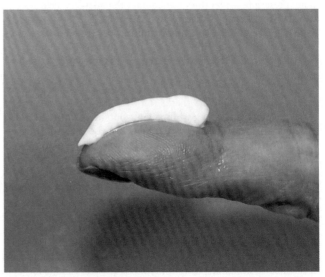

FIG. 1.4-2. Fingertip units can be used for estimation of dosage for application of topical therapies. (Photo courtesy of Gail Lenahan.)

and nonsteroidal alternatives may be a better option for some individuals.

Any patient who is not improving on TCS should be reevaluated, and the provider should consider the following:

- contact dermatitis due to the corticosteroid or preservative in the corticosteroid
- noncompliance
- tachyphylaxis (a decrease in the pharmacologic response after repeated administration of a topical agent)
- monitor for secondary infections
- consideration of an incorrect diagnosis when TCSs are not effective for contact dermatitis

Systemic Corticosteroids

Systemic corticosteroids are classified as short, intermediate, and long acting. Prednisone, which is the corticosteroid of choice in dermatology, is an intermediate-acting medication that can be delivered orally, intramuscularly and intralesional for outpatient care. Prednisone is actually the inactive form of the drug and must be converted to the active form, prednisolone, by the liver. Therefore, if the patient has decreased liver function, prednisolone is the drug of choice.

Indications

The immunosuppressive and anti-inflammatory effects of systemic prednisone are used for treatment of moderate to severe steroid-responsive dermatoses. It is often prescribed for allergic contact dermatitis, one of the most common and usually short-term dermatologic conditions treated by primary care providers. Most practitioners are comfortable managing patients on TCS. They are able to choose the proper dose, vehicle, and limit the quantity for the patient. Those same practitioners, however, are far less confident in prescribing systemic corticosteroids when they are needed due to their concern of the drug's potential side effects.

Prednisone Dosing

Oral corticosteroids may be indicated when TCSs are not feasible due to the extensive body surface area affected or the severity. Inexperienced clinicians tend to undertreat this condition with a low-dose, short-duration corticosteroid bursts. If instead a higher dose of medication for 5 to 7 days is ordered followed by halving the dose for the second week and continuing to slowly taper over 2 more weeks, it decreases the risk of rebound. Experienced clinicians find that treating an adult patient with a significant inflammatory condition with a high dose of prednisone (e.g., 40 to 60 mg daily) for 2 weeks often resolves the eruption and not requiring a taper. Patients who experience steroid side effects may benefit from a shorter taper.

Clinicians prescribing systemic corticosteroids should consider many variables when deciding on the dosage, duration, and frequency (Box 1.4-1). Evidence for tapering prednisone is lacking but suggestions. Alternatives to a Medrol Dose Pack are noted in Table 1.4-5.

- Prednisone is generally given as a single-daily oral dose in the morning because it is more synchronous with the body's natural diurnal variation. The same daily dose of prednisone split and administered twice daily has an increased effect and are generally reserved for more acute or severe conditions.
- The length of a treatment course depends entirely on the condition. In acute dermatoses such as contact dermatitis, a short 2- to 3-week tapering course or "burst" is typically prescribed.

BOX 1.4-1 Considerations for Systemic Corticosteroid Selection

Age and weight of patient
Comorbidities: diabetes mellitus, hypertension, peptic ulcer disease, osteoporosis
Systemic infections: fungal
Short term (2–3 weeks) versus long term (months)
Need for vitamin D and calcium supplementation
Bisphosphonates if on oral corticosteroids for more than 4 weeks
Known hypersensitivities
Drug interactions
Frequency of dosing: b.i.d. dosing has a more potent effect than QD dosing but should only be used for acute therapy of life-threatening illness

---

- In severe conditions which will require more than 4 weeks of treatment, a taper of alternate day dosing schedule can be used. Once the skin condition has cleared, the dose will be carefully decreased in increments until the patient maintains improvement on a minimal dose.

Adverse Effects

Clinicians commonly use short bursts of oral corticosteroids lasting between a few days to 2 weeks. Many consider steroid bursts as relatively safe especially in the nonelderly and healthy patient population. Yet the safety of this treatment is unclear. In a recent large case series study in Taiwan, Yao et al. (2020) reported a single steroid burst in 2,623,327 adults between ages of 20 and 64 years old for as short as 3 days, had a 1.8- to 2.4-fold increased risk of adverse events of GI bleeding, sepsis, and heart failure, especially days 5 to 30 following the initiation of treatment compared to the reference group. Skin disorders and respiratory tract infections were the most common indication for prescribing the steroid. The sobering reality is that while most clinicians are cautious about prescribing short steroid bursts to the elderly, the prescribing practices of short oral corticosteroid burst even younger, healthy patients or those with comorbid conditions, should be carefully weighed against the potential for serious harm.

Side effects associated with oral corticosteroid therapy are usually dose and duration dependent. Some preexisting conditions are associated with an increased risk for adverse events and include

---

TABLE 1.4-5	Prednisone Taper Suggestions (Alternative to Medrol Pack)	
DURATION OF TAPER	**DOSE AND AMOUNT**	**PATIENT INSTRUCTIONS**[a]
2 weeks in decreasing daily doses	5-mg tabs, dispense #114	Day 1: Take 14 pills (70 mg), then decrease by 1 pill each day for 14 days
3 weeks	10-mg tabs, dispense #70	Wk 1: 6 tabs QAM Wk 2: 3 tabs QAM Wk 3: 1 tab QAM
4 weeks (simplified)	10-mg tabs, dispense #70	Wk 1: 4 tabs QAM Wk 2: 3 tabs QAM Wk 3: 2 tabs QAM Wk 4: 1 tab QAM

Note: Calculations based on dosing 0.5–1 mg/kg for 150-lb (68-kg) adult.
[a]In addition to dosing, patient instructions should include: "To avoid recurrence of symptoms, do not stop taking pills without being instructed by your provider."

diabetes, hypertension, dyslipidemia, heart failure, cataracts or glaucoma, peptic ulcer disease, concurrent use of nonsteroidal anti-inflammatory drugs, presence of infection, low bone density, and osteoporosis.

Avascular necrosis (AVN) is another very rare side effect that can be caused by either topical or systemic corticosteroids. AVN has been documented with long-term use of TCS. Magnetic resonance imaging of the hip should be ordered for suspected AVN symptoms, which include pain in the groin, hip, buttock, or knee that increases with activity and is relieved with rest.

Consider the patient's risk of fracture when prescribing oral prednisone. Bone loss is a serious, potential side effects of glucocorticoid therapy and needs to be monitored closely. The glucocorticoid dose and duration of therapy should be as low as possible. Topical therapy is preferred over systemic and should be used instead whenever possible.

Prophylaxis

The 2017 American College of Rheumatology (ACR) Guideline for the Prevention and Treatment of Glucocorticoid-Induced Osteoporosis (GIOP) offers some suggestions to consider for patients that are on long-term steroid treatments in attempts to prevent future fractures. The recommendations are offered as guidelines to be followed when treating patients with long-term corticosteroids. There is no available research that can yet universally determine that the current therapies offer more benefit than harm.

The ACR recommendations for adults older than or equal to 40 years of age (men and women *not of childbearing potential*) taking more than 2.5 mg/day of glucocorticoids for greater than or equal to 3 months should have an initial fracture risk assessments and bone mineral density testing as soon as possible for all patients but at least within 6 months of long-term GC treatment start. Adults considered to be at low risk should have calcium intake of 1,000 to 1,200 mg per day and vitamin D intake of 600 to 800 IU per day through either diet (preferred) and/or supplements. All patients should be advised to eat a balanced diet, maintain a healthy weight, stop smoking, perform regular weight-bearing or resistance training exercises, and limit alcohol intake to 1 to 2 alcoholic beverages/day.

The addition of bisphosphonates should be considered based on individual risks, which include gender, age, and fracture risk, especially if the course of corticosteroids is intended for several months. The drugs teriparatide, denosumab, and raloxifene may also be considered when appropriate.

Other recommendations are made for patients with higher risk of fractures, those on high doses of glucocorticoids, adults younger than 40, women of childbearing potential, those with history of organ transplant, with low glomerular filtration rate, and children.

Patient Education and Monitoring

When prescribing systemic corticosteroids, clinicians should educate patients for achieving maximum outcomes with minimal side effects:

- Take prednisone with food.
- Bid dosing will have a more potent effect than once per day dosing but is not recommended for short-term treatment.
- Taking prednisone early in the morning helps diminish the possible side effects of hyperactivity or sleep disruption and decreases risk of adrenal suppression.
- Patients should be advised against stopping prednisone dosing abruptly and to continue medication until the entire taper course is complete to prevent rebound dermatitis.

- All patients on long-term oral corticosteroids should be monitored for elevated blood sugar, hypertension, and weight gain after 1 month and then every 2 to 3 months.
- Complaints of eye pain, blurry vision, or halos may be indicative of increased intraocular pressures, and patient suffering from these complaints should be seen by an ophthalmologist.
- Providers should use caution in prescribing oral corticosteroids to patients who have the comorbidities of hypertension, diabetes, and obesity or to those who abuse alcohol or tobacco as these patients are already at high risk for developing infections, ulcers, and glaucoma.
- Long-term oral corticosteroid use is also associated with possible gastrointestinal perforation; an upper gastrointestinal series may be ordered if the patient has a history of peptic ulcer disease.

Special Considerations

Corticosteroids in Pregnancy

Practitioners will inevitably encounter women who are pregnant in their practice and must be familiar with medication safety when providing care to this vulnerable population. Prescribing medication during pregnancy can be particularly challenging given the insufficient data and research on the safety of medications during this period. Some skin conditions of the pregnant woman will require both topical and systemic treatment (see Section 12.2).

The Food and Drug Administration (FDA) established pregnancy letter categories in 1979 to indicate a medication's potential to cause birth defects (Table 1.4-6). These categories are now being phased out and replaced by new labeling language that assists providers and patients in making informed decisions about therapies based on the benefits versus the risks. Effective June 30, 2015, the Pregnancy and Lactation Labeling Rule (PLLR) will replace the previous pregnancy categories (U.S. FDA, 2014). In addition to pregnancy and lactation,

TABLE 1.4-6	Previous FDA Pregnancy Categories
CATEGORY	**DEFINITION**
A	Adequate and well-controlled studies have failed to demonstrate a risk to the fetus in the first trimester of pregnancy, and there is no evidence of risk in later trimesters.
B	Animal reproduction studies have failed to demonstrate a risk to the fetus, and there are no adequate and well-controlled studies in pregnant women.
C	Animal reproduction studies have shown an adverse effect on the fetus, and there are no adequate and well-controlled studies in humans, but potential benefits may warrant use of the drug in pregnant women despite potential risks.
D	There is positive evidence of human fetal risk based on adverse reaction data from investigational or marketing experience or studies in humans, but potential benefits may warrant use of the drug in pregnant women despite potential risks.
X	Studies in animals or humans have demonstrated fetal abnormalities, and/or there is positive evidence of human fetal risk based on adverse reaction data from investigational or marketing experience, and the risks involved in use of the drug in pregnant women clearly outweigh potential benefits.

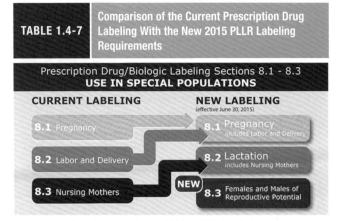

TABLE 1.4-7	Comparison of the Current Prescription Drug Labeling With the New 2015 PLLR Labeling Requirements

Taken from https://www.fda.gov/vaccines-blood-biologics/biologics-rules/pregnancy-and-lactation-labeling-final-rule

the labeling includes labeling requirements and recommendations for females and males of reproductive potential before, during, and after drug therapy (Table 1.4-7).

Topical Corticosteroids

High-quality randomized controlled trials are not available when studying the effects of medication on a fetus/infant due to the ethical issue of exposing the offspring to danger. The current available data on the safety of mild-to-moderate TCS during pregnancy do not support an association between their use by the mother and oral clefts as previously postulated. The most recent Cochrane Database of Systematic Reviews (2015) on the safety of pregnant women treated with TCS identified a probable risk of low-birth-weight babies born to women use potent/very potent TCS during pregnancy. They found no evidence of this same risk with use of mild to moderate TCS. Also, no causal relationship was found between maternal use of TCS and other pregnancy outcomes including mode of delivery, congenital abnormality preterm delivery, fetal death, or low Apgar scores.

Systemic Corticosteroids

Studies are limited on the safety and potential teratogenic effects on a fetus, because of the medical ethical principle involved in testing corticosteroids drugs in pregnancy. However, when topical agents aren't enough, the provider and patient must weigh the risk versus benefit of oral agents.

With oral glucocorticoids, there is a potential for increased risk of premature rupture of the membranes (PROM) and intrauterine growth restriction. There may also be an increased risk of pregnancy-induced hypertension, gestational diabetes, osteoporosis, and infection. They should be avoided during the first trimester when the hard palate is forming. When necessary, the lowest effective dose should be used.

Glucocorticoids are excreted in breast milk in very low amounts and are considered safe while breastfeeding. There is no need to advise mother "pump and dump" their breast milk. They simply need to wait 4 hours following a prednisone to decrease the likelihood that it to be passed on to the baby.

READINGS AND REFERENCES

Bandoli, G., Palmsten, K., Forbess Smith, C. J., & Chambers, C. D. (2017). A review of systematic corticosteroid use in pregnancy and the risk of select pregnancy and birth outcomes. *Rheumatic Diseases Clinics of North America, 43*(3), 489–502. https://doi.org/10.1016/j.rdc.2017.04.013

Chi, C. C., Wang, S. H., Wojnarowska, F., Kirtschig, G., Davies, E., & Bennett, C. (2015). Safety of topical corticosteroids in pregnancy. *Cochrane Database of Systematic Reviews,* (10), CD007346. https://doi.org/10.1002/14651858.CD007346.pub3

Chopra, R., Vakharia, P. P., Sacotte, R., & Silverberg, J. I. (2017). Efficacy of bleach baths in reducing severity of atopic dermatitis: A systematic review and meta-analysis. *Ann Allergy Asthma Immunol, 119*(5), 435–440. https://doi.org/10.1016/j.anai.2017.08.289

Das, A., & Panda, S. (2017). Use of topical corticosteroids in dermatology: An evidenced-based approach. *Indian Journal of Dermatology, 62*(3), 237–250.

Eichenfield, L. F., Tom, W. L., Berger, T. G., Krol, A., Paller, A. S., Schwarzenberger, K., Bergman, J. N., Chamlin, S. L., Cohen, D. E., Cooper, K. D., Cordoro, K. M., Davis, D. M., Feldman, S. R., Hanifin, J. M., Margolis, D. J., Silverman, R. A., Simpson, E. L., Williams, H. C., Elmets, C. A.,…, Sidbury, R. (2014). Guidelines of care for the management of atopic dermatitis: Section 2. Management and treatment of atopic dermatitis with topical therapies. *J Am Acad Dermatol, 71*(1), 116–132. https://doi.org/10.1016/j.jaad.2014.03.023

Fritz, S. A., Camins, B. C., Eisenstein, K. A., Fritz, J. M., Epplin, E. K., Burnham, C.-A., Dukes, J., & Storch, G. A. (2011). Effectiveness of measures to eradicate Staphylococcus aureus carriage in patients with community-associated skin and soft-tissue infections: A randomized trial. *Infection Control & Hospital Epidemiology, 32*(9), 872–880. https://doi.org/10.1086/661285

George, S., Karanovic, S., Harrison, D., Birnie, A., Bath-Hextall, F., Ravenscroft, J., & Williams, H. (2019). Interventions to reduce staphylococcus aureus in the management of eczema. *Cochrane Database of Systematic Reviews, 2019*(10), CD003871. https://doi.org/10.1002/146518.CD003871

Mehta, A. B., Nadkami, N. J., Patil, S. P., Godse, K. V., Gautam, M., Agarwal, S. (2016). Topical corticosteroids in dermatology. *Indian J Dermatol Venereol Leprol, 82*(4), 371–378.

Rosenberg, M. E., & Rosenberg, S. P. (2016). Changes in retail prices of prescription dermatologic drugs from 2009 to 2015. *JAMA Dermatology, 152*(2), 158–163. https://doi.org/10.1001/jamadermatol.2015.3897

U.S. Food & Drug Administration [FDA]. (2014). *Pregnancy and Lactation Final Rule.* Retrieved October 3, 2020, from https://www.fda.gov/vaccines-blood-biologics/biologics-rules/pregnancy-and-lactation-labeling-final-rule

Yao, T.-C., Huang, Y.-W., Chang, S.-M., Tsai, S.-Y., Wu, A. C., & Tsai, H.-J. (2020). Association between oral corticosteroid bursts and severe adverse events: A nationwide population-based cohort study. *Annals of Internal Medicine, 173*(5), 325–330. https://doi.org/0.77326/M20-0432

CLINICAL PEARLS

- Avoid prescribing combination corticosteroid and antifungal topicals for diaper dermatitis. The high potency of TCS in these products is not FDA approved for children and is too strong for the diaper area. Additionally, the antifungal is minimally effective.

- Labeling on the tube of a TCS rather than on the outer box (which is usually discarded) may help patients follow instructions on how much and where medication is to be applied, thereby reinforcing instructions given during the office visit.

- When prescribing a potent or ultrapotent corticosteroid, patients should not use more than one 45-g tube per week. Pharmacists will not usually refill ahead of time, so calculate correctly for best results.

- Mild- to moderate-strength TCSs appear to be safe during pregnancy for short-term use and considered the first line of therapy for inflammatory skin conditions that necessitate treatment.

- Avoid high-potency TCS if possible, especially during the first trimester. If high-potency corticosteroids are needed, as always, they should be used for the shortest amount of time.

- The popular and conveniently packaged methylprednisolone dose pack is an insufficient short-term remedy that tends to prolong patients' suffering due to rebound flaring.

- Patients who are on long-term prednisone therapy should be seen at least every 1 to 2 months for evaluation and more frequently if symptoms of possible complications arise. Close monitoring for possible side effects may be done in collaboration with the patient's dermatologist.

Photobiology, Photoprotection, and Photodermatoses

Mandy Wever

Many patients have memories that encompass time spent outdoors in the sunshine. Exposure to the sun can have a myriad of both positive and negative effects. Positive effects from time spent outdoors include an elevated mood, increased physical activity and creativity, in addition to vitamin D synthesis. However, there are also negative effects from acquiring too much sun which include acute sunburns, aging skin, and particularly the risk of developing cataracts and skin cancer.

Currently, skin cancer is the most common diagnosed cancer in the United States. Photoaging skin (e.g., wrinkling, pigmentation) increases with ultraviolet (UV) light exposure. Sunburns are a known risk factor for the development of skin cancer. The U.S. Department of Health and Human Services (USDHHS, 2019) identified that overexposure to the sun was a very common cause of patient complaints, affecting more than one in three U.S. patients. The following section will present the fundamentals of photobiology that will serve as a framework to guide best sun protection practices tailored to specific patients and populations. Following a review of photobiology, the most common photodermatoses will be reviewed.

ULTRAVIOLET LIGHT

Photobiology

In discussing the impact of the environment on skin health, ultraviolet radiation (UVR) must be at the forefront to address the favorable benefits and negative impact of exposure. The basic concepts of photobiology are fundamental when assessing both the risks and benefits and when educating patients.

- Ultraviolet light is a form of radiation, not visible to the human eye and composed of three wavelengths: UVA, UVB, and UVC. These wavelengths differ primarily in the depth to which they penetrate the skin. The effects of UVB radiation can be immediate such as in sunburn or allergic skin reaction. UVA and UVB cause more long-term effects as in photoaging and skin cancer (Fig. 1.5-1).
- UVA is the longer wavelength and is measured at 320 to 400 nm. UVA can penetrate more deeply than UVB, causing skin and eye damage. UVA is the predominant wavelength of most tanning beds and is responsible for their damaging effects. UV radiation, from the sun and from tanning beds, is classified as a human carcinogen, according to the USDHHS and the World Health Organization. UVA rays also penetrate glass and clouds increasing the risk for individuals who drive frequently for work or recreation and for those who do not use sunscreen as directed.
- UVB rays are the middle range wavelengths between 280 and 320 nm. They are found in combination with UVA in some tanning beds that contribute to the risk of this practice. Not only is UVB responsible for photoaging, sun tanning, and sunburns, but it can also cause ocular diseases such as cataracts, glaucoma, and macular degeneration.
- UVC wavelength is 100 to 280 nm, filtered by the ozone, and almost completely absorbed by atmosphere. Very little UVC reaches the earth's surface; however, it can be emitted from artificial light sources. UVC can also be utilized to purify water or kill microbes on work surfaces.

Phototherapeutics

- Specialized narrowband UVB (NBUVB) is used in many dermatology offices to treat skin conditions such as psoriasis. The short-term side effects of NBUVB include erythema and blistering. For those with a preexisting herpes simplex, an increased frequency of a herpes outbreak could occur. Long-term side effects may include photoaging and increased risk of skin cancer. However, the photocarcinogenic effects of NBUVB have not been determined to date. Therefore, based on current evidence, NBUVB is well tolerated by patients and is considered a safe treatment with no identified increased risk of skin cancer. Additional long-term studies are needed to determine the effect of NBUVB on photocarcinogenesis (Sokolova et al., 2015). While patients are undergoing NBUVB, protective measures are provided for eyes and noninvolved skin for each treatment. Patients who are receiving NBUVB for dermatologic conditions should have annual routine skin examinations.

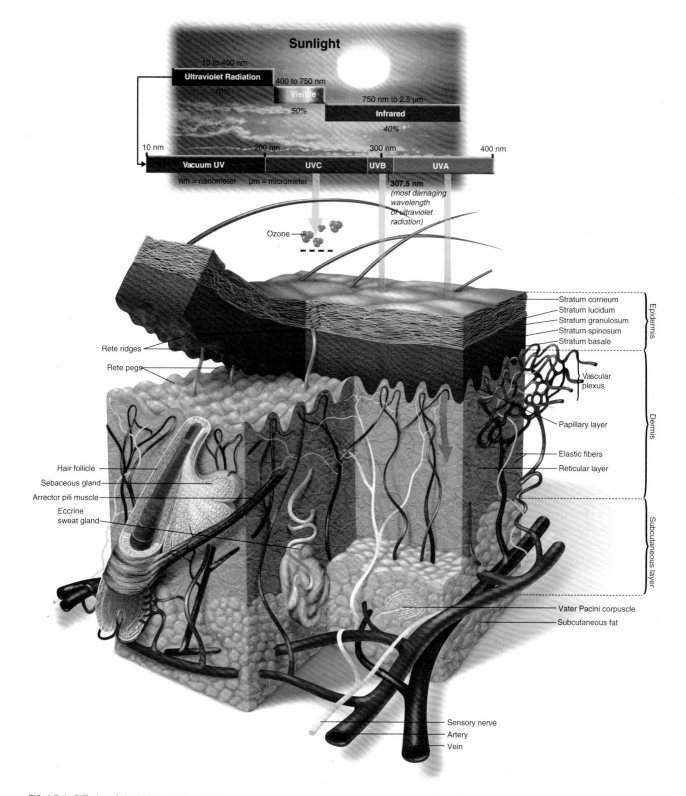

FIG. 1.5-1. Diffusion of ultraviolet radiation. UVC is completely absorbed by the ozone layer, whereas UVB is partially filtered, and UVA is without any filtration.

- Other targeted types of phototherapy are utilized by dermatology specialists and are mentioned here briefly. The detailed principles and indications are beyond the scope of this textbook. UVA1, which delivers a narrow wavelength deeper into the dermis compared to NBUVB, may be prescribed for skin diseases like atopic dermatitis, morphea (localized scleroderma), cutaneous T-cell lymphoma, pityriasis rubra pilaris, etc. Photodynamic therapy (PDT) is another therapeutic where the patient's skin is prepared with a photosensitizing agent, 5-aminolevulinic acid or methyl aminolevulinate, and then exposed to red or blue light. It is most often used for patients with large areas of actinic keratosis. Less often, it can be used for treatment of superficial basal cell skin cancers, and off-label use for acne.

UV Index

- The UV Index is a means of predicting risk of overexposure to UV radiation on a scale from 0 to 11+, with the higher number indicating higher risk. A special "UV Alert" may be issued for a particular area, if the UV Index is forecast to be higher than normal.
- The risk is calculated by taking into consideration ozone depletion, weather, geographic location, and the seasons of the year.
  - The ozone layer acts as a filter to the earth and when it is compromised living things are susceptible to damage from UVR penetration.
  - Weather conditions directly impact the ozone, as warm temperatures generally enhance ozone production, and wind and rain can limit its creation. Cloud formation is related to weather conditions and less cloud cover allows more UV penetration, whereas, in turn thick clouds can block UVR.
  - The geographic location also influences risk of overexposure for UVR. For example, people that live, visit, or work (e.g., flight crew members) in high altitudes are at a greater risk of UV radiation. With each 1,000 ft incline in elevation the UVR increases between 6% and 10% (Knezevic, 2019).
  - Finally, the seasons of the year also affect UVR, which in the United States, peak in the summer and decline in the winter.
- The National Weather Service (https://www.weather.gov) calculates the UV Index forecast for most ZIP codes across the United States, and the Environmental Protection Agency (https://www.epa.gov/sunwise/uvindex.html) publishes this information. The UV Index is then accompanied by recommendations for sun protection and is a useful tool for planning sun-safe outdoor activities (Table 1.5-1).

Sun Protection

- Public education regarding skin cancers and the photodamaging effects of the sun has led to increased use of sunscreens in many populations. Australia launched one of the earliest and most successful sun protection programs in history by educating the public about sun-protective measures through the "Slip Slop Slap Seek and Slide" campaign.
- In 2014, the USDHHS responded with the Surgeon General's call to action for skin cancer prevention to improve health outcomes for citizens by preventing skin cancer and reducing healthcare costs. This publication is updated annually and adds value to the current knowledge (https://www.cdc.gov/cancer/skin/what_cdc_is_doing/progress_report.htm). Unfortunately, skin cancer rates have continued to increase in the United States. Therefore, it is essential that as providers we deliver education to both patients and communities on specific actions to enhance positive sun protection and simultaneously minimize or eliminate recurrent episodes of skin damage.
- These efforts have encouraged an increase in preventative behaviors and community policies. Although we have made advances in educating patients regarding the use of sunscreen in the United States, more efforts are needed to encourage patients to use sun-protective clothing, sunglasses and to seek shade

TABLE 1.5-1	Sun Protective Behaviors

General Guidelines
- Avoid midday sun (10 AM–4 PM) when possible
- Avoid tanning and the use of tanning beds
- Avoid getting a sunburn
- Use extra caution with water, sand, snow, and high altitudes
- Use protective barriers including tightly woven clothing and wide-brimmed hats
- Wear UV protective glasses and sunscreen daily
- A head to toe skin exam should be performed monthly using a mirror.

Sunscreen
- Counsel patients to use a sunscreen that they like as there are numerous formulations, which include creams, lotions, gels, lip balms, sticks, or sprays (be careful to avoid inhalation and ensure rubbing in after spray) with or without tint.
- Choose a broad-spectrum chemical absorber (organic) or physical agent (inorganic) sunscreen with minimum of SPF 30 or greater with broad-spectrum coverage:
  - *Chemical absorbers (Organic)*
    - Avobenzone (Parsol 1789)
    - Benzophenones (Oxybenzone)
    - Cinnamates (Octymethyl cinnamate)
    - Ecamsule (Mexoryl SX)
    - Salicylates (Homosalate)
  - *Physical agents (Inorganic)*
    - Titanium oxide
    - Zinc oxide
- Apply sunscreen (average adult 2 tablespoons) at least 15 min prior to sun exposure.
- Reapply sunscreen every 2 hrs. Apply more frequently if swimming, exercising or sweating.
- Identify the expiration date on the sunscreen prior to purchasing and replace when needed. Discard and purchase new sunscreen if left in extreme heat.
- Use only sun avoidance and protective clothing on infants under 6 mo as they should not use sunscreen.

more often. Providing the public with outdoor tents in gathering places such as parks, pools, and beaches is one example of such an effort.

Clothing

- Loose fitting clothes and tightly woven fabrics in long pants and long-sleeved shirts offer the best source of sun protection.
- A typical cotton T-shirt offers a sun protection factor (SPF) of about 5 and a wet T-shirt offers much less protection than a dry one.
- Darker colors may add a bit more protection than lighter ones.
- Hats with wide brims are highly recommended.
- Fashionable sun-protective clothing with the minimum standard ultraviolet protection factor (UPF) of 40 to 50+ is available by several companies such as Coolibar; Radicool Australia, Sunday Afternoons, SunPrecautions, Tilley Endurables, Tuga sun protective sunwear and Wallaroo hat company.

Sunglasses

- UV damage to the eyes is cumulative just as it is for the skin.
- The eyes are specifically at an increased risk of forming cataracts and melanoma with prolonged sun exposure. Thus, it is vitally important to begin protecting your eyes by wearing sunglasses at an early age.
- Children's eyes are still developing and actually at higher risk for damage.
- Choose sunglasses that provide full protection against ultraviolet light. Consider large-framed sunglasses to diminish light sources from angles.
- The coating used for UV protection is clear so a tinted sunglass will not necessarily be more protective. Look for a label or a sticker that says one or more of the following:
  - Lenses block 99% or 100% of UVB and UVA rays.
  - Lenses meet American National Standard Institute Z80.3 blocking requirements.
  - UV 400 protection blocks light rays with wavelengths up to 400 nm, which shields the eyes from even the tiniest UV rays.

Sunscreens

- Sunscreens are topical agents that lessen the effects of ultraviolet light either by reflecting, scattering or absorbing the light (Fig. 1.5-2).
- There are two categories of sunscreens, "inorganic" or "physical" sunscreens which include zinc oxide and titanium dioxide–based products and "organic" or "chemical" sunscreens (Table 1.5-2).

Chemical sunscreens

Chemical sunscreens act to weaken ultraviolet radiation before it causes damage to DNA in the nuclei of skin cells. Chemical sunscreens absorb ultraviolet radiation within the spaces between the skin cells, convert it into specific chemicals, and release the energy as insignificant amounts of heat. The higher the SPF rating of the chemical sunscreen, the longer it takes for sunlight to damage the skin.

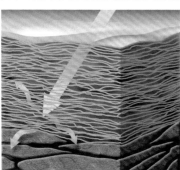

Physical sunscreens

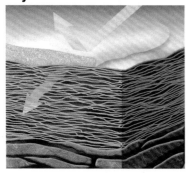

Physical sunscreens prevent ultraviolet radiation from entering the skin at all. Physical sunscreens form a thin film of inert metal particles (zinc oxide, etc.) that reflect back into the atmosphere.

FIG. 1.5-2. Illustration showing how sunscreens work.

TABLE 1.5-2	Sunscreen Ingredients		
		PROTECTION	
INGREDIENT	**UVA1**	**UVA2**	**UVB**
Physical Agents			
Titanium dioxide	•		•
Zinc oxide	•		•
Chemical Absorbers			
Aminobenzoic acid (PABA)			•
Butyl methoxydibenzoylmethane (Avobenzone)	•		
Dioxybenzone		•	•
Ecamsule (Mexoryl SX)		•	
Ethoxyethyl p-methoxycinnamate (cinoxate)			•
Homomenthyl salicylate (homosalate)	•		
Octyl methoxycinnamate (octinoxate)	•		
Oxybenzone	•	•	•
Octocrylene	•	•	•
Sulisobenzone	•	•	•
Ethoxyethyl p-methoxycinnamate (cinoxate)			•

UVA, ultraviolet A; UVB, ultraviolet B.

- Sunscreen efficacy is determined by their ability to protect against the erythema caused by both UVA and UVB. Sun Protective Factor (SPF) is the unit of measure used to describe how well a sunscreen can protect the skin from the harmful effects of the sun. It particularly measures the length of time it takes UVB rays to cause erythema of the skin when using a sunscreen versus without the product.
- The SPF for each sunscreen is determined in a laboratory by comparing an individual's response to sun with and without sunscreen use. The American Association of Dermatologists recommends patients choose sunscreen with an SPF of 30 or higher.
- The average adult should apply at least 2 tablespoons or a "shot glass full" on sun-exposed areas of the body whenever outdoors for any length of time. Sunscreen should be reapplied every 2 hours or after sweating or swimming regardless of latitude.
- The FDA regulates sunscreen as an over-the counter medication. It requires the use of the term broad spectrum (UVA and UVB coverage) to be proportional and included on any sunscreen packaging. In addition, sunscreen labels should contain water resistance to show the duration of time the product is effective and the SPF strength.
- Only broad-spectrum sunscreens with an SPF value of 15 or higher can claim to reduce the risk of skin cancer and early skin aging if used as directed with other sun-protection measures. Sunscreens with an SPF value less than 15 can only claim to help prevent sunburn.

- Manufacturers cannot label sunscreens as *waterproof* or *sweatproof*, because these claims overstate their effectiveness. Water-resistance claims on the front label must indicate whether the sunscreen remains effective for 40 minutes or 80 minutes while swimming or sweating, based on standard testing.

- Sunscreens also cannot identify their products as "sunblocks" or claim to provide sun protection for more than 2 hours without reapplication. The product's label must not claim to provide protection immediately after application.

- All sunscreens must include standard drug facts information on the back and/or side of the container. The FDA also mandates that sunscreen labels recommend reapplying sunscreen at least every 2 hours. Zinc oxide, titanium dioxide, avobenzone, or ecamsule provides adequate UVA protection and are commonly listed ingredients of broad-spectrum sunscreens. Helioplex is the name brand of a sunscreen stabilizer owned by Neutrogena, that ensures the sunscreen ingredients are more photostable, preventing chemical breakdown when exposed to the sun.

Sunscreen Allergies and Sensitivities

- Practitioners often hear from patients that they are allergic to sunscreens. The most common reactions reported with the use of sunscreens involve the skin and include irritant contact dermatitis, allergic contact dermatitis, and photoallergic contact dermatitis.

- Organic sunscreens are associated with contact dermatitis with oxybenzone, a type of benzophenone, being a frequent cause.

- Photoallergies have not been reported with inorganic sunscreens; therefore, allergy prone patients should be advised to choose these products. Examples of sunscreen brands that contain zinc and titanium dioxide as either the sole ingredient or main ingredient are Badger, Vanicream, Solbar zinc, Neutrogena Sensitive Skin, and Blue Lizard.

- Patients may also complain of acneiform eruptions with sunscreen. There are multiple oil-free sunscreen products available to patients who otherwise may not wish to use sunscreen because of fear of skin breakouts. The following oil-free products are ideal for patients prone to acne: Neutrogena, La Roche-Posay, Olay, CeraVe, and Cetaphil.

Oral Photoprotection

- *Polypodium leucotomos*, an oral carotenoid, is an extract from a species of fern grown in Central America. It has been shown to decrease UVB erythema, DNA damage, UV-induced epidermal hyperproliferation, and mast cell infiltration in humans. However, one study suggested *P. leucotomos* only provides an SPF of 3, which is insufficient for most people. This dietary supplement is sold as Heliocare.

- *Nicotinamide* 500 mg b.i.d., a water-soluble form of vitamin B_3, has been studied as an oral dietary supplement and has been shown to prevent UVR-induced immunosuppression in the skin, actinic keratoses and keratinocyte cancers (Krutmann et al., 2020).

- While there may be a potential role for supplemental oral products in patients with photoinduced conditions, it is critical to understand that these measures would be used in addition to sun-protective behaviors that include seeking shade, and using photoprotection with sunscreens, clothing, and sunglasses. These oral supplements are not currently FDA approved as studies do not provide conclusive evidence of appropriate UVR protection. Further investigation is warranted into fully recognizing the potential that nutritional supplements may play.

Sunscreen Controversies

Pre-Vacation Tan

- Many patients will advocate for their use of tanning beds or outdoor tanning as an essential "base tan" prior to going on vacation where they will have intense sun exposure.

- This myth is promulgated as valid because tanned skin has an approximate SPF 4 and yields some protection. However, any concept of protection from tanning in a booth is fallacy.

- Cosmetic tanning from a UV booth provides no photoprotection. Individuals believe they have this extra protection and extend their time in unprotected sun exposure. Although indoor tanning may still be considered fashionable it is a known human carcinogen and increases the risk of skin cancer.

Retinyl Palmitate and UV Filters

- Retinyl palmitate, an antioxidant that is used to enhance aesthetic qualities, has been accused of causing free radicals and increasing cancer risk.

- UV filters, specifically Oxybenzone and Octinoxate have been under fire recently for accusations of negative environmental impacts. The United States began legislation to ban both UV filters due to concerns of coral reef bleaching, in 2018, with Hawaii being the first state to pass the law (Narla & Lim, 2020).

- Additional sunscreen ingredient bans are following worldwide, although current studies do not prove that UV filters have a direct relationship with environmental damage.

- Of interest, both products that are banned for resale in sunscreen are used and sold commonly in other personal care products including cosmetics and fragrances.

- Sunscreens have been approved by the FDA since 1978 and now cannot be sold without extensive testing.

Systemic Absorption of Sunscreen

- The current FDA position on the safety and effectiveness of sunscreens is that zinc and titanium oxide–based sunscreens are safe and effective and that there is additional information needed to determine the safety and effectiveness of 12 other sunscreen agents.

- Some groups have claimed that oxybenzone accumulates in the body and can interfere with hormone levels. Narla and Lim (2020), reported that as to date there are no published studies proving that sunscreen or their ingredients are toxic to humans or hazardous to human health. Incidentally, a recent study involving topical application of sunscreen with UV filters was published and showed absorption by elevated plasma concentrations that surpassed FDA limits on the human test subjects. However, clinical relevance has not been determined and additional studies are needed to further explore the outcomes (Krutmann et al., 2020).

- To date what is known is the adverse risk of UV exposure and that investment in continued research and health promotion is vital to protect human life, living organisms, and the environment.

Vitamin D

- Vitamin D is an essential vitamin that has numerous effects on biologic processes including assisting with absorption of calcium in the intestines, maintaining adequate calcium/phosphate concentrations to support normal bone mineralization, reduction of inflammation, and the modulation of cell growth, glucose metabolism, and immune function.

- Sources of vitamin D include food (e.g., dairy, oily fish), sun exposure, and supplements. With the increased efficacy of sunscreen, there has been controversy regarding the impact of sunscreen causing vitamin D deficiency.

- A recent literature review concluded that vitamin D status is not compromised with daily use of broad-spectrum sunscreens in healthy patients. In fact, most individuals do not apply their sunscreen adequately or frequently enough to prevent sunburn or block the synthesis of vitamin D (Krutmann et al., 2020).

- Given the risk of DNA damage to the skin and photocarcinogenesis from overexposure to UV light, it is advised that people focus on acquiring their daily recommendation of vitamin D from food or supplements. However, patients with photosensitivity disorders should be counseled on methods to both protect skin and maintain vitamin D levels (Passeron et al., 2019).

Sunless Tanning

- There are no FDA regulations regarding sunless tanners and bronzers. These terms typically refer to products that provide a tanned appearance without exposure to the sun or other sources of ultraviolet radiation.

- Dihydroxyacetone (DHA), the most common ingredient in sunless tanners, is a color additive that darkens the skin by reacting with amino acids in the skin surface.

  - DHA is being used commonly in salons and advertised as a "spray tan" but "misting" application has not been approved for use by the FDA.

  - DHA is restricted to external application and should not be applied to the lips or any surface covered by mucous membranes.

  - When using DHA-containing products, it may be difficult to avoid exposure to the eyes, lips, or mucous membranes as well as inhalation.

  - There is no evidence of any toxicity but those using spray tanning should protect their eyes, lips, nose, mouth, and mucous membranes.

  - Previously unseen seborrheic keratoses will become more visible as the keratotic cells absorb the sunless tanning chemical.

- Bronzers are made from color additives approved by the FDA for cosmetic use. They stain the skin for a short time when applied and can be washed off with soap and water.

Tanning Pills

- Tanning pills contain canthaxanthin, a color additive similar to beta-carotene. Beta-carotene is the substance in that gives carrots their orange-like color.

- The FDA has approved some additives for coloring, but they are not approved for use in tanning agents.

- Canthaxanthin at high levels can appear in the eyes as yellow crystals, which may cause injury and impair vision. There have also been reports of liver and skin problems.

It is clear that UV radiation, skin type, altitude, time of day, tanning bed use, and sun-protection behaviors contribute to sun damage, aging skin, and skin cancer. This section reviewed education materials for best practice for skin protection (Table 1.5-1). Now more than ever, it is critical that providers and patients understand how to educate and implement these behaviors and understand the common goal is to improve overall quality of life. The following sections will explore photodermatoses causes and treatments, many of which can be avoided by minimizing sunlight and utilizing sun protection.

PHOTODERMATOSES

Photodermatoses are a group of cutaneous disorders which occur in response to ultraviolet light exposure and can be classified as immunologic, idiopathic, photosensitive (chemical- and drug-induced), inherited or photoaggravated (Nahhas et al., 2018). A light sensitivity can develop from UVA, UVB, visible light, and a wider range of radiation. UVA and UVB wavelengths have been identified as the most common culprits and can elicit a skin reaction in those with a genetic predisposition. Photodermatoses occur in males and females, all ages, and races. Environmental factors that may precipitate eruptions include seasonal variation of UVL exposure, tropical climates, increased altitudes, and outdoor hobbies or occupations. A common clue to alert the healthcare provider regarding the potential presence of a photodermatosis is the distribution of the skin eruption, which favors sun-exposed areas which include the face, ears, neck, arms, chest, and below the knee. Skin eruptions that occur as a result of sun exposure (i.e., photodermatoses) will be reviewed so that clinicians will have a working knowledge regarding the clinical presentation of photodermatoses, diagnostics available to support diagnosis, and available therapeutics to optimize outcomes, promote healing, and prevent skin damage.

POLYMORPHOUS LIGHT ERUPTION

Polymorphous light eruption (PMLE) is the most common, immunologic photodermatitis and has been estimated to have a 20% prevalence (Nahhas et al., 2018). It can occur in either sex, all ages, and all ethnicities. The outbreak commonly occurs in the second and third decades of life and affects women four times more often than men (Gruber-Wackernagel et al., 2014). It typically occurs in the springtime, following acute and intense sun exposure and is often referred to as sun poisoning. It is more common in northern climates where the sun is more intense in the spring and residents have more episodic exposure. It is less common in climates where the sun is intense all year presumably because of a type of desensitization.

PMLE has also been reported from tanning bed use, phototherapy, and also reflective light surfaces.

Pathophysiology

- PMLE is triggered by UVA in most cases, but both UVA and UVB wavelengths may incite the response.

- PMLE seems to be a delayed-type hypersensitivity reaction.

- Photoprovocation studies have shown perivascular infiltrates of CD4[+] T lymphocytes occurring within hours of UVL exposure.

- The responsible antigens have yet to be defined.

Clinical Presentation

- A complete history including physical exam with morphology of cutaneous lesions, timing of onset of symptoms, and confirmation of recent UV exposure is essential for establishing a differential diagnosis and workup plan.

Skin Findings

- The earliest symptom may be burning, itching, and erythema on sun-exposed skin.

- Areas commonly affected include:

  - Upper chest

  - Neck and shoulders

  - Arms and legs

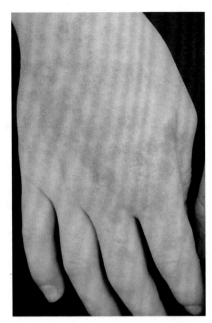

FIG. 1.5-3. Polymorphous light eruption. Thin erythematous papules coalescing into plaques on the dorsal forearms and hands. (Used with permission from Gru, A. A., & Wick, M. [2018]. *Pediatric dermatopathology and dermatology.* Wolters Kluwer Health.)

- The face and hands can be involved yet are typically spared due to hardening.
- The trunk, scalp, palms, and soles are rarely involved.
- Lesions most commonly appear within 24 hours but can appear between 2 hours and 5 days after sun exposure.
- As the name suggests, there are a variety of morphologic types. The several noted morphologies of PMLE from most to least common are:
  - Small erythematous dermal papules (papular type) appear on a patchy erythematous base (Fig. 1.5-3).
  - Urticarial plaques (plaque type) (Fig. 1.5-4).
  - Erythematous urticarial papules or plaques with vesicles (vesiculopapular type) (Fig. 1.5-5).
  - Tiny micropapular eruption (pinpoint type) with marked hyperpigmentation.

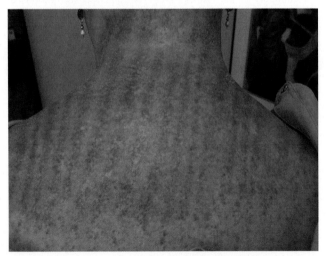

FIG. 1.5-4. Polymorphous light eruption on the upper back/neck area.

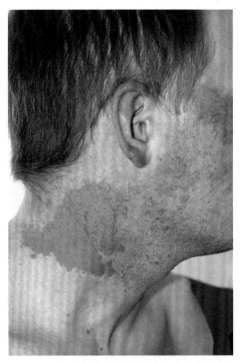

FIG. 1.5-5. Polymorphous light eruption vesiculopapular type. Pinpoint vesicles can be noted on the papules and scattered vesicles within erythematous plaques.

Non-Skin Findings

Systemic symptoms are usually absent. Very rarely, if a large amount of body surface area is affected the patient may present with or without constitutional symptoms including:

- Malaise
- Headache
- Chills
- Nausea

DIFFERENTIAL DIAGNOSIS   PMLE

- Lupus erythematous
- Phototoxic drug eruption
- Photoallergic drug reaction
- Solar urticaria
- Sunburn
- Airborne contact dermatitis
- Porphyria cutanea tarda
- Pseudoporphyria

Confirming the Diagnosis

- This diagnosis may be made clinically if one can exclude the other differential diagnoses.
- Ask about recent light exposure, new medications or topical products, other symptoms, or previous occurrences to build a differential diagnosis with the cutaneous morphology.
- The first method of workup should be performing an accurate history including if the patient had ever had a similar occurrence.
- Histopathology and laboratory tests are not specific for PMLE.

- If lupus is questioned, an antinuclear antibodies screen (ANA) should be performed. However, up to 19% of patients with PMLE may have a positive ANA (Tzaneva et al., 2008). Therefore, consider also obtaining antinuclear antibodies, SS-A, and SS-B to verify negative serologic studies. A negative result means that acute cutaneous lupus erythematosus is unlikely, but subacute and discoid lupus may still be considered. ANA screening should be interpreted with clinicopathologic correlation.

Treatment

- The goals of treatment are to decrease:
  - Cutaneous inflammation
  - Pruritus
  - Recurrent episodes

Topical

- Applying cool compresses to the skin.
- Topical corticosteroids to affected cutaneous eruption twice daily for up to 2 weeks with plan wean down to once-daily dosing for an additional week:
  - High- to mid-potency topicals to extremities or trunk.
  - Low potency for facial areas.

Systemic

- Antihistamines may be helpful for the sedation effects when treating pruritus.
- Short-term oral prednisone (0.6 to 1.0 mg/kg) for 7 to 10 days has been used for flares or prophylactically.
- Severe cases or those with chronic relapse will benefit from dermatology referral for the consideration of the following treatments:
  - Phototherapy
  - Antimalarials
  - Azathioprine
  - Thalidomide
- Prophylactic phototherapy with either NBUVB or PUVA may be used to increase the skin's tolerance to sun exposure by desensitizing the skin. It is generally administered two to three times weekly at least 1 month prior to sun exposure.

Management and Patient Education

- Many times, the rash will self-resolve within 7 to 10 days without treatment.
- For an overview of essential sun-protective behaviors to implement see Table 1.5-1.
- Dermaguard is a sun-protective film that may be applied to windows at home and in the vehicle and needs to be replaced every 5 years.
- Once the diagnosis of PMLE is made, a follow-up appointment can be made just prior to the next early spring to:
  - Review the history, new medications or products, and preventative plan of care.
  - Develop a treatment protocol for skin hardening with light therapy if indicated.
  - Discuss situations that may warrant prophylactic oral steroids and refractory care.

Special Considerations

- Consider alternative diagnoses for immediate referral if the patient has:
  - Widespread eruption
  - Fever
  - Pain
- If TCS and sun protection are not working well, refer to dermatology for consideration of phototherapy as the next desired modality of treatment.
- It is reported that up to 10% of patients with PMLE also develop lupus erythematous (O'Gorman & Murphy, 2014). Therefore, if the clinical presentation fits, additional workup should be performed.

> ### CLINICAL PEARLS
> - Photoprotection including physical interventions and behavioral modifications is a key for reduction in PMLE outbreaks.
> - Studies suggest that subsequent flares within the same patients may occur likely with the same morphology and in the same locations (Nahhas et al., 2018).

Photoallergy

Photoallergic dermatoses are true allergic reactions (type IV hypersensitivity), which require the patient's immune system to be sensitized to a particular allergen when triggered by UVL. These reactions are less common and are not related to drug concentration. It can be related to a systemic medication or a topical agent (Table 1.5-3).

Pathophysiology

- Photoallergic reactions are a cell-mediated immune response that occurs when a photosensitizing drug is activated by the sun and is transformed into a new molecule.
- This new molecule is then interpreted as foreign material by the body.
- Langerhans cells present the new material (antigen) to the T lymphocytes, which become activated and initiate an inflammatory response in the skin.

Clinical Presentation

- Photoallergic reactions are delayed and begin on sensitized patients 24 to 72 hours or even several days after the first exposure.
- A subsequent reexposure to the same allergen has a much quicker onset of eruption as the body recalls the initial insult.
- If the offending allergen is administered systemically, the reaction may be more widespread than an allergen exposed through contact.
- Lesions initially begin in photoexposed areas but may generalize to include photoprotected areas.
- Recovery is slower than with phototoxic reactions. The cutaneous eruption may be persistent even after identification and discontinuation of the offending agent.

Skin Findings
Acute Stage

- Erythematous eruption with papules or plaques with or without vesicles or scale (Fig. 1.5-6).
- Pruritus, weeping, and crusting.

TABLE 1.5-3	Oral and Topical Agents That May Induce Photoallergic Reaction
Antiarrythmics	Amiodarone, Quinidine
Antibiotics	Fluoroquinolones, Sulfonamides, Tetracyclines
Anticonvulsant	Carbamazepine
Antifungals	Azoles, Griseofulvin
Antihistamines	Diphenhydramine, Promethazine
Antimalarials	Dapsone, Hydroxychloroquine, Quinine
Antimicrobials	Isoniazid
Antipsychotics	Phenothiazines, Thioxanthenes
Antivirals	Acyclovir
Cardiovascular	Angiotensin receptor blockers, Aspirin, Calcium channel blockers, Statins
Dermatologic	5-,8-methoxypsoralen, Retinoids
Diabetic	Sulfonylureas
Diuretics	Furosemide, Thiazides
Fragrance	Methylcoumarins, Musk
NSAIDs	Celecoxib, Diclofenac, Ibuprofen, Naproxen, Ketoprofen
Oncologic	5-Fluorouracil, Dacarbazine, Flutamide, Vemurafenib
Oral Contraceptives	Ethinyl estradiols
Sunscreens	Avobenzone, Benzophenone, Cinnamates, PABA

This represents a nonexhaustive list of agents that may result in a photoallergic reaction. This table has been adapted and modified from the following sources: Hinton, A. N., & Goldminz, A. M. (2020). Feeling the burn: Phototoxicity and photoallergy. *Dermatologic Clinics, 38*(1), 165–175. Onoue, S., Seto, Y., Sato, H., Nishida, H., Hirota, M., Ashikaga, T., Api, A. M., Basketter, D., & Tokura, Y. (2017). Chemical photoallergy: Photobiochemical mechanisms, classification, and risk assessments. *Journal of Dermatological Science, 85*(1), 4–11.

Late Stage
- Lichenification
- Crusting
- Fissures

DIFFERENTIAL DIAGNOSIS   Photoallergy

- Sunburn
- Acute contact dermatitis
- Lupus erythematous
- Dermatomyositis
- Drug eruption
- Polymorphous light eruption
- Porphyria cutanea tarda

Confirming the Diagnosis

- This is generally a diagnosis made by taking a detailed history that includes:

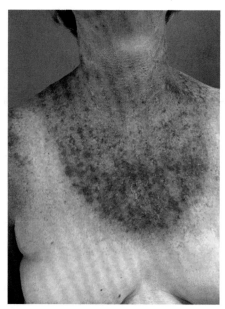

FIG. 1.5-6. Photoallergic reaction to griseofulvin. Note that the eruption is only occurring in the sun-exposed area. Upper chest involvement is common.

- Medications (including prescription and over the counter).
- Topical products.
- Sun exposure history in relationship to eruption.
- Photodistributed cutaneous findings.
- *Photopatch testing* can identify the culprit agent and is considered a gold standard for diagnosis. Patients that require patch testing should be referred to an immunologist or dermatologist who has experience in conducting photopatch testing.
- Skin biopsy typically shows nonspecific findings and is only warranted if the diagnosis is not certain.

Treatment

- Identification of the drug or allergen and sun protection are crucial.
- Even after the removal of a responsible agent, it may take a several weeks or even months before the patient has sustained relief.
- Supportive treatment includes:
  - Topical steroids may provide relief to the erupted skin:
    - High- to mid-potency topicals to extremities/trunk.
    - Low potency for facial areas.
  - Use of combined UVB/UVA sunscreens and protective clothing (Table 1.5-1).
  - Oral corticosteroids should only be used in severe cases.
  - Oral antihistamines for pruritus if indicated.

Management and Patient Education

- Patients must be counseled about the potential photosensitizing properties of medications.
- Unless sunscreens are the suspected cause of the photoallergy, they should be used.
- Educate and counsel on effects of tanning bed use if appropriate.
- The prognosis for a photoallergic reaction is good once the offending agent is discovered and removed, although the photosensitivity and lesions may take weeks to months to resolve.

- If light reactivity persists, premature aging of the skin may occur, and the risk of developing skin cancer increases.

- Hyperpigmentation does not usually result from photoallergic reactions.

CLINICAL PEARLS

- A key clue to identifying a potential photoallergic eruption is that the following areas are often spared with the initial eruption:
  - Eyelids
  - Upper cutaneous lip
  - Submental
  - Skin areas not exposed

Phototoxic Reaction

Also known as drug-induced photosensitivity, phototoxic reactions are non–immune-mediated skin reactions that occur when an individual is exposed to a light source while using a sensitizing systemic or topical agent.

Pathophysiology

- Phototoxic reactions occur when predominantly ultraviolet A transforms cosmetic, drugs, or industrial agents into photoactivated compounds (Table 1.5-4).

- The subsequent photoactivation of these compounds results in the production of reactive oxygen species that results in damage to cellular DNA, lipids, and proteins.

- In addition to ultraviolet A radiation, ultraviolet B radiation and visible light may also contribute to the development of phototoxic reactions.

TABLE 1.5-4	Agents that Cause Phototoxic Reactions

Topical Agents

5-Aminolevulinic acid (Ameluz)
Coal tar derivatives
5-Fluorouracil
Methyl-5-aminolevulinic acid (levulan)
Perfume (Bergamot)
PDT prophotosensitizers

Systemic Agents

Acitretin
Amiodarone
Fluoroquinolones
Furosemide
Hydrochlorothiazide
Isotretinoin
Itraconazole
Nonsteroidal anti-inflammatory drugs
PABA
Phenothiazines
Sulfonamide
Tetracycline
Vemurafenib
Voriconazole

Adapted from Kim, W. B., Shelley, A. J., Novice, K., Joo, J., Lim, H., & Glassman, S. J. (2018). Drug induced phototoxicity: A systemic review. *Journal of American Academy of Dermatology, 79,* 1069–1075.

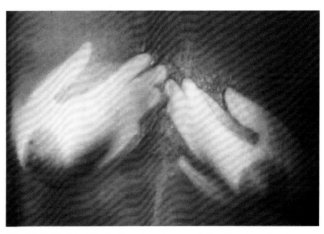

FIG. 1.5-7. Phototoxicity. Erythematous (exaggerated sunburn) reaction in a person who was taking demeclocycline (Declomycin) and fell asleep on the beach. (Used with permission from O'Connor, F. G. [2012]. *ACSM's sports medicine: A comprehensive review.* Wolters Kluwer Health.)

Clinical Presentation

Skin Findings

- Skin findings often present within minutes to hours after sun exposure.

- Erythematous patches (sunburn-like changes) with or without blisters/bulla are noted in sun-exposed areas (Fig. 1.5-7).

- May be associated with burning and pruritus.

- Upon resolution of the erythematous patches, patients may have hyperpigmented tan or brown macules or patches consistent with postinflammatory hyperpigmentation.

- Occasionally skin changes will not manifest until 24 hours after sun exposure. In these cases, the likely causative agent is psoralens.

Systemic Findings

- Any of the following signs or symptoms may be seen in severe generalized phototoxic reactions:
  - Malaise
  - Fever
  - Chills
  - Nausea
  - Headache

DIFFERENTIAL DIAGNOSIS   Phototoxic Reaction

- Photoallergic dermatitis
- Sunburn
- Porphyria cutanea tarda
- Pseudoporphyria
- Dermatomyositis
- Contact dermatitis
- Phytophotodermatitis
- Lupus erythematous

Confirming the Diagnosis

- Phototoxic reactions typically do not require additional diagnostics as the diagnosis is based upon history and physical exam.

- However, dermatology referral for diagnostic testing with photo-testing, photopatch, and patch testing can be performed if unable to discern the diagnosis.
- Punch biopsy may be considered if the eruption is widespread or involves atypical cutaneous features.
- Histopathology
  - Histopathology should reveal necrotic keratinocytes which is suggestive of phototoxicity, but not conclusive.
  - A skin biopsy may also differentiate cutaneous lupus or porphyria cutanea tarda from a phototoxic reaction.

Treatment

- First, identification and avoidance of the photosensitizing agent must be done.
- Topical corticosteroids may provide relief to the erupted skin:
  - High- to mid-potency topicals to extremities and trunk.
  - Low potency for facial areas.
- Cool compresses are helpful in relieving discomfort.
- Nonsteroidal anti-inflammatory drugs (NSAIDs) are a known photosensitizer. Although they may help decrease the acute discomfort, they are not recommended, as they may potentiate the phototoxic reaction.
- With severe reactions, early administration of systemic corticosteroids may help to reduce the inflammation.

Management and Patient Education

- Sun protection usually prevents reactions. Educate the patient about limiting UVL sources and appropriate sun protection. As phototoxic reactions are primarily triggered by UVA, patients should use sunscreens that are broad spectrum and contain UVA-protective ingredients. Individuals must be educated on photosensitizing properties of both nonprescription and prescription of oral and topical agents.
- If systemic symptoms are noted the potential for electrolyte and fluid replacement may be required and may warrant referral.
- If repeated phototoxic injury occurs, there may be chronic effects on the skin. These effects include:
  - Premature aging of the skin.
  - Increased risk of skin cancer.
  - Postinflammatory hyperpigmentation.

CLINICAL PEARLS

- A phototoxic reaction cannot occur in the absence of UVL exposure.
- A phototoxic reaction is often related to high-intensity, acute sun exposure.
- It is relevant to know that UVA is able to pass through standard windows. Therefore, assessing the frequency of light exposure, in context to the eruption is important even if recent sun exposure is not identified.
- Generally, this eruption gets worse before better and pigment takes time to fade.

Phytophotodermatitis

Phytophotodermatitis (PPD) is a phototoxic reaction that may occur when the skin comes in contact with a plant or fragrance containing *furocoumarin* and UVA. Furocoumarins are chemical compounds

BOX 1.5-1   Plants Containing Psoralen Compounds

Angelica
Bergamot orange
Carrot
Celery
Citrus fruits (lemon, lime, mango, orange, and pineapple)
Cow parsley
False bishop's weed
Fig (wild)
Hogweed
Meadow grass (agrimony)
Parsnip (wild parsnip)
Rue
Queen Anne's lace
Wildflowers

which occur naturally in a variety of plants, fruits (e.g., limes) and vegetables (e.g., celery) commonly ingested. In nature, they are used as a defense against predators and are responsible for the classic eruption known as PPD in humans. The average dose commonly ingested is unlikely to elicit this phototoxic reaction. Patients may have had an exposure to a furocoumarin-containing plant or have used a fragrance product containing oil of Bergamot (Box 1.5-1). PPD has no predilection for any ethnicity, age, or either sex. Agricultural workers, bartenders, grocers, and culinary workers are at an increased risk. Also, spending time outdoors increases the risk for exposure to both psoralen compounds and UVL. Therefore, one may be at increased risk if participating in gardening, outdoor recreation, or vacations in sunny climates.

Pathophysiology

- PPD is a type of phototoxic reaction that is characterized by a non–immune-mediated process.
- When skin exposed to furocoumarins or other photosensitizing substances is exposed to UVA, a photochemical reaction occurs that results in cellular damage through direct DNA damage and indirectly through the development of reactive oxygen species.

Clinical Presentation

Skin Findings

- Primary burning and erythema of sun-exposed skin areas within 24 to 48 hours.
- Secondary erythema, vesicles, and/or bullae may follow (Fig. 1.5-8).
- Residual brown hyperpigmentation occurs within 72 hours persists for weeks to months.
- Lesions likely will have:
  - Atypical shapes
  - Streaking
  - Linear drip marks
  - Asymmetry
- Locations may include:
  - Face
  - Neck
  - Lips
  - Shoulders
  - Thighs

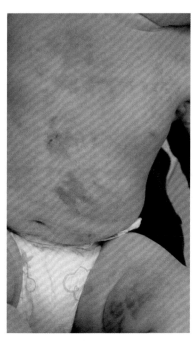

FIG. 1.5-8. Phytophotodermatitis in an infant caused by lemon juice. Note the bizarre, streak pattern of erythema and hyperpigmentation, indicating an external contactant. (Used with permission from Gru, A. A., Wick, M. [2018]. *Pediatric dermatopathology and dermatology.* Wolters Kluwer Health.)

DIFFERENTIAL DIAGNOSIS   Phytophotodermatitis

- Allergic contact dermatitis
- Autoimmune bullous disorder
- Herpes virus
- Porphyria cutanea tarda
- Phototoxic drug eruption
- Factitious dermatitis

Confirming the Diagnosis

- PPD is usually a clinical diagnosis.
- Laboratory tests are done to rule out other suspected diseases:
  - Serum porphyrin and 24-hour urine for porphyrin levels and coproporphyrin levels. Porphyrins will be elevated in porphyria cutanea tarda and negative in pseudoporphyria.
  - Consider biopsy for H&E and direct immunofluorescence. Skin biopsy (preferably punch technique) can be helpful.
  - Viral culture to rule out possible HSV.
- Photopatch testing should be done if phototoxic and photoallergic dermatitis cannot be distinguished from each other clinically.
- If the clinical picture remains unclear, skin biopsy should be helpful, as PPD has distinct histopathologic features.

Treatment

- The goal is to provide symptom management during the acute phase:
  - Cool compresses prn.
  - Topical corticosteroids:
    - High- to mid-potency topicals to extremities/trunk.
    - Low potency for facial areas.

- Nonsteroidal anti-inflammatory for pain management.
- Oral antihistamine for pruritus if needed.

Management and Patient Education

- The condition is self-limited and benign, and treatment is supportive.
- One of the primary goals of management is to prevent recurrent eruptions.
- Encourage combined sun protection and UVA/UVB sunscreens (Table 1.5-1).
- Educate patients on furocoumarin-containing compounds, so offending agent can be avoided (see Box 1.5-1).
- Teach patients to wash hands and any affected skin areas promptly if in contact with reactive agents.
- The hyperpigmentation that follows will resolve spontaneously over time. Sun avoidance will help to speed that process.

CLINICAL PEARLS

- Obtain a history that includes patient occupation, hobbies, travel, and recent UVL exposure.
- The presence of unusual geographic patterns on some exposed skin, but not all is a clue for PPD.
- A reaction may only occur on the lips or around the mouth and would likely be related to recent ingestion of psoralen-containing fruit or even lip product followed by UVL.
- The exposure to fragrance products containing oil of Bergamot usually causes the eruption to appear on the face and neck.
- Careful assessment including history and possibly biopsy is necessary to be able to delineate between PPD, physical abuse, and factitious dermatitis.

Photoaggravated Dermatoses

Photoaggravated skin disorders include a primary disease process that is naturally occurring without UVL, but that also has the potential to become exacerbated with a light source. Each disease may have a distinct UV wavelength that causes a flare. UVL is also used as a treatment in many disease processes such as psoriasis. However, although UVL generally improves the psoriatic patient, it could exacerbate a small portion of those treated.

Pathophysiology

- The exact mechanism of pathogenesis will be related to the disease state that is photoaggravated.

Confirming the Diagnosis

- It is critical to take a detailed history from the patient to be able to differentiate the primary disorder with photoaggravation from a new superimposed secondary comorbidity (Table 1.5-5).
- Refer to Dermatology if diagnosis is unknown for biopsy and further management.

Treatment

- The primary diagnosis will guide the appropriate course of treatment.

TABLE 1.5-5	Diseases Exacerbated by Ultraviolet Light

Autoimmunity	**Idiopathic**
• Bullous pemphigoid	• Actinic prurigo
• Dermatomyositis	• Solar urticaria
• Lichen planus	
• Lupus erythematous	
• Psoriasis	
Drug-induced	**Infectious**
• Pseudoporphyria	• Herpes simplex
Genodermatoses	**Acneiform**
• Darier disease	• Acne vulgaris
• Hailey–Hailey disease	• Rosacea
• Trichothiodystrophy	
• Xeroderma pigmentosum	
Miscellaneous	**Malignancy**
• Atopic dermatitis	• Cutaneous T-cell lymphoma
• Seborrheic dermatitis	• Carcinoid syndrome
• Grover disease	
• Porphyria cutanea tarda	

Management and Patient Education

- The therapeutic goal is to quiescent the disease process while simultaneously improving the quality of life.
- Photoprotective clothing and broad-spectrum sunscreen (Table 1.5-1).
- Further education and treatment should be discussed in regard to the primary disease.

CLINICAL PEARLS

- Examine the full patient in addition to body when performing a skin exam including:
  - Scalp
  - Nails
  - Mouth
  - Ask patients directly if the genital or rectal areas have been involved to take this pressure off of the patient

READINGS AND REFERENCES

Bologna, J. L., Jorizzo, J. L., & Rapini, R. P. (2008). *Dermatology* (2nd ed.). Mosby.

Gruber-Wackernagel, A., Byrne, S., & Wolf, P. (2014). Polymorphous light eruption: Clinic aspects and pathogenesis. *Dermatology for the Clinician, 32*(3), 315–334. https://doi.org/10.1016/j.det.2014.03.012

Gutierrez, D., Gaulding, J. V., Motta Beltran, A. F., Lim, H. W., & Pritchett, E. N. (2018). Photodermatoses in skin of colour. *European Academy of Dermatology and Venereology, 32*(11), 1879–1886. https//doi: 10.1111/jdv.15115

Guy, G. P., Berkowitz, Z., & Watson, M. (2017). Estimated cost of sunburn-associated visits to US Hospital Emergency Departments. *JAMA Dermatol, 153*(1), 90–92. https://doi.org/1001/jamadermatol.2016.4231

Habif, T. P. (2010). *Clinical dermatology: A color guide to diagnosis and therapy* (5th ed.). Mosby.

Habif, T. P., Campbell, J. L., Chapman, M. S., Dinulos, J. G. H., & Zug, K. A. (2011). *Skin disease diagnosis and treatment* (3rd ed.). Saunders Elsevier.

Hinton, A. N., & Goldminz, A. M. (2020). Feeling the burn: Phototoxicity and photoallergy. *Dermatology for the Clinician, 38*(1), 165–175. https://doi.org/0.1016/j.det.2019.08.010

James, W. D., Berger, T. G., & Elston, D. M. (2011). *Andrews' diseases of the skin: Clinical dermatology* (11th ed.). Saunders.

Kim, W. B., Shelley, A. J., Novice, K., Joo, J., Lim, H., & Glassman, S. J. (2018). Drug-induced phototoxicity: A systemic review. *Journal of the American Academy of Dermatology, 79*, 1069–1075. https://doi.org/10.1016/j.jaad.2018.06.061

Knezevic, J. (2019). Impact of high-altitude ultraviolet radiation on function-ability of flight crews. *Archives in Biomedical Engineering & Biotechnology, 2*(2). https://doi.org/10.33552/ABEB.2019.02.000533

Krutmann, J., Passeron, T., Gilaberte, Y., Granger, C., Leone, G., Narda, M., Schalka, S., Trullas, C., Masson P., & Lim, H. W. (2020). Photoprotection of the future: Challenges and opportunities. *Journal of the European Academy of Dermatology and Venerology, 34*(3), 447–454. https://doi.org/10.1111/jdv.16030

Nahhas, A. F., Oberlin, D. M., Braunberger, T. L., & Lim, H. W. (2018). Recent developments in the diagnosis and management of photosensitive disorders. *American Journal of Clinical Dermatology, 19*(5), 707–731. https://doi.org/10.1007/s40257-018-0365-6

Narla, S., & Lim, H. W. (2020). Sunscreen: FDA regulation, and environmental and health impact. *Photochemical and Photobiological Sciences, 19*, 66–70. https://doi.org/10.1039/c9pp00366e

O'Gorman, S. M., & Murphy, G. M. (2014). Photoaggravated disorders. *Dermatology for the Clinician, 32*(3), 385–398. https://doi.org/10.1016/j.det.2014.03.008

Onoue, W. S., Seto, Y., Sato, H., Nishida, H., Hirota, M., Ashikage, T., Api, A. M., Basketter, D., & Tokura, Y. (2017). Chemical photoallergy: Photobiochemical mechanisms, classification, and risk assessments. *Journal of Dermatological Science, 85*, 4–11. https://doi.org/10.1016/j.jdermsci.2016.08.005

Passeron, T., Bouillon, R., Callender, V., Cestari, T., Diepgen, T. L., Green, A. C., van der Pols, J. C., Bernard, B. A., Ly, F., Bernerd, F., Marrot, L., Nielsen, M., Verschoore, M., Jablonski, N. G., Young, A. R. (2019). Sunscreen photoprotection and vitamin D status. *British Journal of Dermatology, 181*(5), 916–931. https://doi.org/10.1111/bjd.17992

Rutter, K. J., Ashraf, I., Cordingley, L., & Rhodes, L. E. (2020). Quality of life and psychological impact in photodermatoses: a systematic review. *British Journal of Dermatology, 182*(5), 1092–1102. https://doi.org/10.1111/bjd.18326

Sokolova, A., Lee, A., & Smith, S. D. (2015). The safety and efficacy of narrow band ultraviolet B treatment in dermatology: A review. *American Journal of Clinical Dermatology, 16*(6), 501–531. https://doi.org/10.1007/s40257-015-0151-7

Tzaneva, S., Volc-Platzer, B., Kittler, H., Honigsmann, H., & Tanew, A. (2008). Antinuclear antibodies in patients with polymorphic light eruption: A long-term follow-up study. *British Journal of Dermatology, 158*(5), 1050–1054. https://doi.org/10.1111/j.1365-2133.2008.08500.x

U.S. Department of Health and Human Services (HSS), Centers for Disease Control and Prevention (CDC). (2019). *Skin cancer prevention progress report.* https://www.cdc.gov/cancer/skin/pdf/SkinCancerPreventionProgressReport-2019-508.pdf

United States Environmental Protection Agency (EPA). (2019). *UV index scale.* https://www.epa.gov/sunsafety/uv-index-1

Moles and Melanoma

Theodore D. Scott

In This Chapter

- Pathophysiology of Pigmented Skin Lesions
- Benign Pigmented Lesions
  - Epidermal Melanocytic Neoplasms
    - Lentigo
    - Café Au Lait Macule
    - Nevus Spilus
    - Becker Nevus (BN or Becker Melanosis)
  - Dermal Melanocytic Neoplasms
    - Mongolian Spots
    - Nevus Ota and Ito
    - Melanonychia Striata
  - Melanocytic Nevi

- Congenital Nevi
- Acquired Melanocytic Nevi
  - Spitz Nevus
  - Halo Nevus
  - Blue Nevus
- Dysplastic Nevi
- Malignant Melanoma
  - Superficial Spreading Melanoma
    - Nodular
    - Lentigo Maligna and Lentigo Maligna Melanoma
    - Acral Melanoma

Patients often seek evaluation of their nevi, or "moles," because of a concern for possible malignancy or disconcerting appearance. Primary care clinicians are strategically positioned to assess skin lesions not only when it is the patient's chief complaint but also during office visits for other health concerns. Skin examinations, integrated into patient visits, are opportunities for early recognition and treatment of skin cancer. The simple practice of having patients remove their shirt when listening to heart and lung sounds can provide visualization of their back, chest, and arms—some of the most common areas for melanoma, but should not be a substitute for an annual full-body skin exam.

The examination of a patient with numerous pigmented lesions can be challenging for both novice and experienced clinicians. There are multiple tools and common characteristics that can help health care providers discern benign lesions from those that warrant further investigation. For lesions that do suggest possible pathology, this chapter will address the various sampling techniques and initial interpretation of the pathology report.

PATHOPHYSIOLOGY OF PIGMENTED SKIN LESIONS

- Pigmented skin lesions are due to melanocytes that develop from dendritic cells in the neural crest of the embryo and migrate to the epidermis. Melanosomes, contained in the melanocytes, produce *melanin,* which provides the skin with its color. There is about one melanocyte for each 10 basal keratinocytes (Fig. 2.1-1).

- Variation in the color of skin among races is due to the size and distribution of melanosomes, not the number of melanocytes. Individuals with dark skin have larger melanocytes that are distributed more linearly along the basement membrane. Likewise, light-skinned people have clustered smaller-sized melanocytes which contain less melanin.

- Exposure to both natural and artificial ultraviolet radiation (UVR) increases the production of melanin, which results in larger melanocytes, giving lighter skin a tanned appearance. Estrogen and progesterone can also influence the production of melanin, which manifests as darkening nevi or melasma during pregnancy, hormone replacement therapy, and use of oral contraceptives.

- Melanin also has a protective function as it both absorbs and scatters UVR, which protects the keratinocytes from DNA mutations that can lead to oncogenesis. This small measure of protection (about SPF 4) does not justify the social practice of going to tanning beds to acquire a "base tan" before vacation. This creates a challenge for clinicians in teaching patients about the increased skin cancer risk from UVR for all types of skin.

BENIGN PIGMENTED LESIONS

Patients present to both primary care and dermatology providers for the evaluation of new or changing nevi. Whether a nevus has raised, developed hair, changed color, or become speckled, patients rely on the clinician's assessment for reassurance or appropriate diagnostics to rule out malignancy. Moreover, not all "brown spots" are nevi, and understanding the pathophysiology and risk for malignancy of pigmented lesions can improve the clinician's diagnostic acumen and patient outcomes.

Epidermal Melanocytic Neoplasms

Most pigmented epidermal lesions are benign and have a vast variation in clinical presentation. The characteristics of lesions are based upon the number, size, amount of melanin, and distribution of the melanocytes at the dermoepidermal junction (DEJ).

Superficial

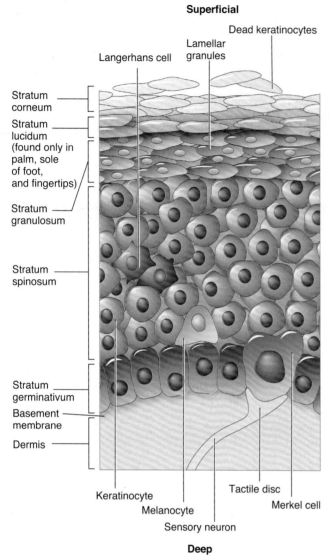

Deep

FIG. 2.1-1. Anatomy of the epidermis and location of melanocytes. (Premkumar, K. [2011]. *The massage connection: Anatomy and physiology* [3rd ed.]. Wolters Kluwer Health I Lippincott Williams & Wilkins.)

Lentigos

Lentigines (the plural of lentigo and pronounced len-tij´ĭ-nēz) present as pigmented macules that have an increased number of melanocytes or increased amount of melanin. Despite their benign pathology, patients may request treatment to minimize lesion appearance. They occur in a number of different clinical forms:

- *Ephelides*—commonly called freckles, characterized by hyperpigmented brown macules found on sun-exposed areas during childhood, usually increase with summer-sun exposure and significantly fade during the winter, caused by UVR damage which increases the size of the melanocytes, not the quantity (Fig. 2.1-2).

- *Lentigo simplex*—larger and darker than an ephelides, can also appear during childhood, but are not affected by sun exposure and therefore do not fade in the winter months, can occur anywhere as solitary, hyperpigmented brown 0.5- to 1.5-cm macule. Characterized by an increased number of melanocytes at the DEJ, these benign lesions require no treatment (Fig. 2.1-3).

- *Solar lentigines*—common response to sun exposure in fair-skinned, blue-eyed, blonde or red-haired individuals, onset

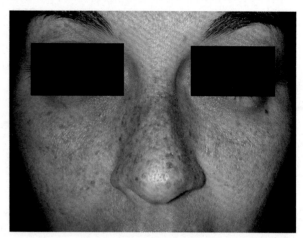

FIG. 2.1-2. Ephelides or common freckles are the result of UVR exposure and usually fade in the winter. (Photo courtesy of Theodore Scott.)

during childhood, distributed in large numbers (sometimes coalescing) on the sun-exposed face, neck, shoulders, arms, and dorsal hands (Fig. 2.1-4). Unlike ephelides, these do not fade with sun avoidance. Pigmentation is the result of increased melanin production due to prolonged UV exposure. Treatment is not necessary unless the patient is seeking cosmetic improvement, which can be difficult if they are extensive. Close examination should be performed to identify any abnormal or "ugly duckling" lesions (different from its neighbors).

- *Labial, penile, and vulvar lentigines*—pigmented macules occurring on the labia, vulva, glans penis, or mucosa of lips, solitary lesions are usually not concerning but should be monitored for any features of dysplasia or melanoma (Fig. 2.1-5). Numerous hyperpigmented brown macules on the lips, mucosal surfaces,

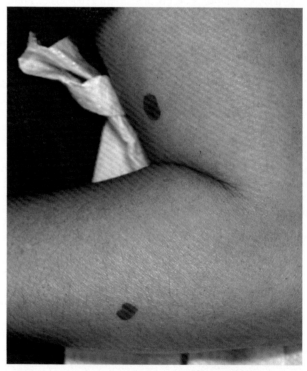

FIG. 2.1-3. Lentigo simplex. (McConnell, T. H. [2007]. *The nature of disease pathology for the health professions*. Wolters Kluwer Health I Lippincott Williams & Wilkins.)

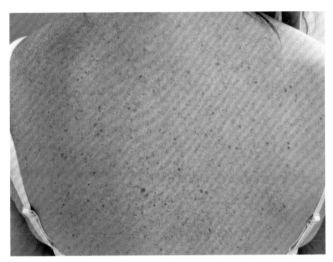

FIG. 2.1-4. Solar lentigines from sun exposure do not fade in the winter. (Courtesy Jeremy Honoker.)

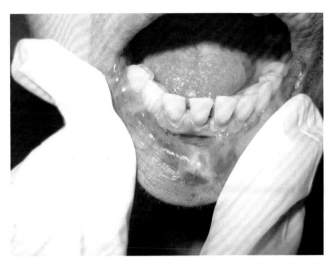

FIG. 2.1-6. Numerous orolabial gray brown macules (lentigines) suspicious for Peutz–Jeghers syndrome. (Photo courtesy of M. Bobonich.)

and genitalia, should alert the clinician for potential Peutz–Jeghers syndrome (Fig. 2.1-6). Patients diagnosed with this syndrome during childhood are at higher risk for gastrointestinal adenocarcinomas, as well as breast and ovarian cancers. These are a

proliferation of melanocytes, with an increase in the number of dendrite melanocytes, which are different from the melanocytes found in typical keratinocytes.

Café Au Lait Macule

- Uniformly pigmented, light brown macules and patches which typically appear at birth or during infancy.
- Usually flat, ovoid in shape, and lighter brown than congenital nevi (Fig. 2.1-7), these lesions are found in 20% of the general population.
- Multiple café au lait macules can be associated with the autosomal dominant genodermatoses, neurofibromatosis type 1 and type 2 (NF1 and NF2, respectively). A full-skin examination should be performed to assess for the number and size of café au lait macules/patches, presence of neurofibromas, and axillary freckling. Clinical presentations suspicious for NF1 or NF2 should be referred for neurologic and developmental evaluation. In adults, a full-skin examination should be performed for skin cancer screening.

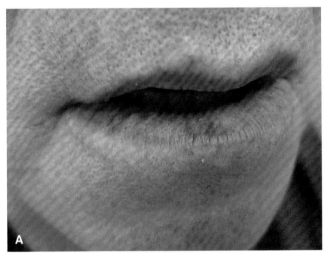

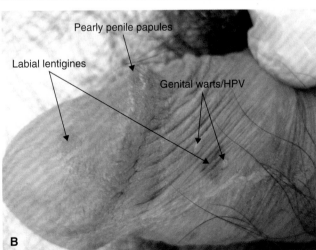

FIG. 2.1-5. **A:** Labial lentigines more common on the lower lip. **B:** Penile lentigines in addition to pearly penile papules and HPV. (Photos courtesy of M. Bobonich.)

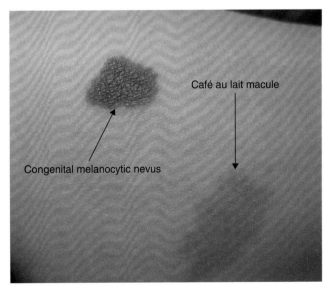

FIG. 2.1-7. Comparison of a café au lait macule on inner thigh (irregularly shaped uniform tan patch) beside a small congenital melanocytic nevus (slightly irregular dark-brown thin plaque). (Photo courtesy of M. Bobonich.)

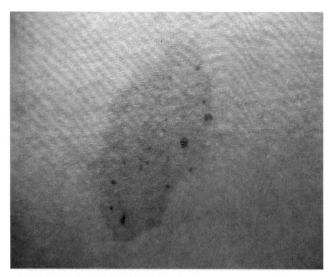

FIG. 2.1-8. Nevus spilus. Speckled brown to dark brown macules within a larger tan patch. (Photo courtesy of M. Bobonich.)

Nevus Spilus

- A congenital epidermal nevus with an appearance similar to a café au lait.
- Present in infancy as a light brown patch with darker hyperpigmented brown macules or speckles (also called speckled lentiginous nevus) within the lesion.
- Most are located on the trunk or lower extremities and are benign (Fig. 2.1-8).

Becker Nevus (BN or Becker Melanosis)

- Typically a very large, light brown to tan patch with or without an increased amount of darker hair growth. The most common location is on the shoulders, upper chest, or back, becoming more evident during adolescence, with a higher incidence in males.
- While not a true nevomelanocytic lesion, Becker nevi are cutaneous hamartomas involving keratinocytes, hair follicles, arrector pili muscles, and melanocytes.
- While there are case reports of melanoma arising within a Becker nevus, epidemiologic studies have not identified BN as a risk factor for melanoma. The risk of malignant transformation is therefore considered very rare.
- They are usually unilateral and may be associated with ipsilateral hypoplasia of breast and skeletal anomalies including scoliosis, spina bifida occulta, or ipsilateral hypoplasia of a limb (Fig. 2.1-9).

Dermal Melanocytic Neoplasms

Mongolian Spots

- Commonly located over the sacrum of infants, these dark blue-brown patches are usually found in those with dark skin tones.
- The hyperpigmented blue color is from elongated melanocytes, giving the patch the appearance of a bruise. Given the location of the lesion and bruise-like appearance, many providers have mistaken this for a sign of child abuse (Fig. 2.1-10).
- They are benign and usually fade significantly by adulthood. While uncommon, it is possible for adults to develop this type of dermal melanocytosis.

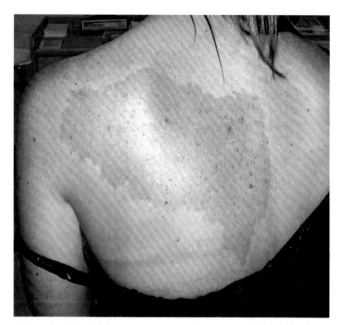

FIG. 2.1-9. Becker nevus. Large, well-defined irregularly shaped patch on the shoulder/upper back. Also commonly seen on superior shoulder or upper chest. (Photo courtesy of Theodore Scott.)

Nevus of Ota and Ito

Nevus of Ota is oculodermal melanocytosis. It is thought to be due to the failure of the melanocytes to migrate from the dermis up to the epidermis during embryonic development.

- Present with a dark/blue hyperpigmented patch, usually with a unilateral distribution along the trigeminal nerve (V1 and V2 branches). The underlying mucosa, conjunctiva, and tympanic membranes may also be pigmented and darken with age. There is an increased prevalence in women and Asian, African American, and Indian races (Fig. 2.1-11).

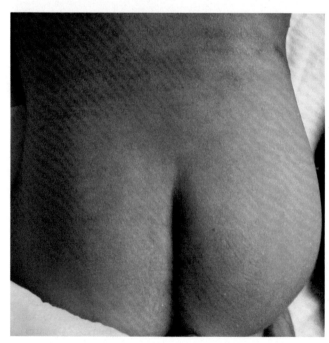

FIG. 2.1-10. Mongolian spot or dermal melanocytosis. Commonly located over the sacrum. (Photo courtesy of M. Bobonich.)

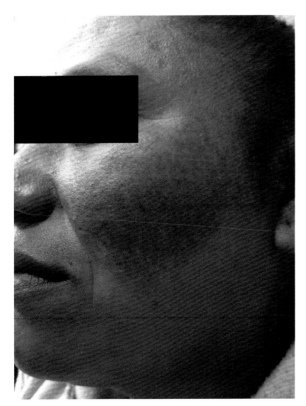

FIG. 2.1-11. Nevus of Ota. Mottled tan–blue patch on the superior cheek. (Photo courtesy of M. Bobonich.)

- Glaucoma has been associated with Nevus of Ota. Although usually benign, these lesions can have a psychological impact on the patient's body image. Camouflage makeup is often used, but topicals have no effect. Q-switched laser, requiring repeated treatments, provides the most promising cosmetic results.

The less common nevus of Ito is similar but involves the lateral supraclavicular or lateral brachial nerve distribution. Like any pigmented lesion, these should be monitored for signs and symptoms of melanoma.

Melanonychia Striata

- Thin, uniform, brown longitudinal stria (plural is striae) that occurs in the nail, but does not involve the nail folds.
- Can be a normal variant, more common in darker-skinned patients, and typically there is a consistent pattern present in several nails.
- Clinicians should carefully assess all nails for atypical features that may indicate a developing periungual melanoma and prompt a referral to a dermatologist for evaluation (Box 2.1-1).

BOX 2.1-1   Lesion Characteristics in Nails That Should Raise a Red Flag

- Location: Single digit, thumb, or great toenails
- Appearance: Fast growth, longitudinal melanonychia, bandwidth more than 3–5 mm
- Hutchinson sign: Periungual pigmentation of skin
- Nail dystrophy: Notch in free distal nail margin, surface irregularity, oozing, or bleeding lesion similar to ingrown nail

---

BOX 2.1-2   Ways to Classify Melanocytic Nevi

Onset
- Congenital: present at birth or soon thereafter
- Acquired: occurs after 6 months old

Location of Nevus Cells
- Epidermal: arising in the epidermis only
- Junctional: arising at the dermal–epidermal junction
- Dermal: nests in the dermis or subcutaneous fat only
- Compound: a combination of junctional and dermal

Type of Cells
- Melanocytic: melanocytes only
- Spindle cell: spindle-shaped cells as in Spitz nevus
- Blue pigmented cells: cellular blue nevi

Melanocytic Nevi

Pigmented nevi are composed of nevus cells (nevocytes) that are derived from melanocytes located in nests near the DEJ. Nevocytes are similar to melanocytes but are nondendritic cells and larger in size. Some nevus cells remain at the DEJ while others eventually migrate down into the dermis, accounting for some of the normal physiologic changes that can occur throughout the lifespan. Hence, since most common nevi have a very low risk for malignancy, understanding the normal characteristics and evolution of nevi can reduce the number of unnecessary biopsies on benign nevi, which can be costly, scarring, and stressful for patients. It can also help assist the clinician to recognize atypical features or suspicious symptoms indicating risk for melanoma and necessitate a biopsy.

The subtypes of nevi can be classified in several ways, including *onset* of the lesion, *location* of the nested cells, and *type* of cells (Box 2.1-2). There can be an overlap in the classification of the same lesion. For example, an *intradermal* nevus is an *acquired* nevus located in the dermis. Nonetheless, these categories can help you understand pathophysiology and clinical presentation.

Congenital Nevi

Nevomelanocytes clustered in the deeper dermis and subcutaneous that appear at birth, or within the first 6 months of infancy, are called congenital melanocytic nevi (CMN; Fig. 2.1-12; Fig. 2.1-13A,B). CMN occur in approximately 2% to 6% of newborns and have been historically categorized according to the predicted adult size (PAS). This has guided clinicians in anticipating the risk for malignancy and management options (Table 2.1-1).

Although all CMN have the risk of developing melanoma, small- and medium-sized lesions carry the lowest risk (<1%), which would most likely occur after puberty. In contrast, large (also called giant or garment) nevi have an estimated lifetime risk of up to 5%, with half of these melanomas occurring before the age of 5 years. Yet many experts argue that lesion characteristics, in addition to size, should be considered in the classification criteria and ultimately risk stratification (Krengel et al., 2013). Krengal et al., also proposed new criteria in hopes of providing a better prognostic tool to measure risk and guide care. Lesion characteristics were added to the classification system as variables influencing risk for malignancy (Box 2.1-3). The stratification of CMN sizes was also expanded to include a separate "giant size" category. Large CMN overlying the spinal column and skull have been associated with neurocutaneous melanosis (NCM) with symptoms of increased cranial pressure, vascular birthmarks, spinal cord compression, tethered spinal cord, or leptomeningeal melanoma.

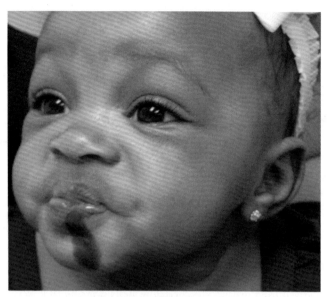

FIG. 2.1-12. Medium-sized CMN on the lip and chin of a toddler with significant cosmetic impact. (Photo courtesy of M. Bobonich.)

Clinical Presentation

- The initial presentation of small or medium CMN can be varied from pink to dark brown and with some color variation including a speckled appearance. They are usually well circumscribed and may have hypertrichosis.

- As the child ages, CMN commonly rise into a plaque.

- Large CMN may develop a cobblestone surface with color variation. Garment or bathing suit nevi may involve any area of the body and have a dermatomal distribution.

- A segmental or circumferential distribution can be associated with underlying musculoskeletal abnormalities.

- All CMN, like any pigmented lesion, should be assessed for clinical characteristics of melanoma using the classic *ABCDE* checklist (Box 2.1-4). The common variation of color and irregular borders of large and giant CMN can make this risk assessment very complex. Particular attention should be given to the development of satellite lesions, nodularity, and ulceration.

BOX 2.1-3 **Proposed Characteristics of Congenital Melanocytic Nevi That Increase Risk for Malignancy**

Size
Number of medium CMN
Location
Number of satellite nevi by 1 year of age
Heterogeneity of color
Rugosity
Hypertrichosis
Extensive nodules

Adapted from Krengel, S., Scope, A., Dusza, S. W., Vonthein, R., & Marghoob, A. A. (2013). New recommendations for the categorization of cutaneous features of congenital melanocytic nevi. *Journal of the American Academy of Dermatology, 68*(3), 441–451.

Confirming the Diagnosis

- Document the specific characteristics of any congenital nevus during the physical examination of a newborn or child. The size, number, and location of each lesion should be noted.

- CMN are usually classified according to their predicted largest diameter in adulthood, known as the "Predicted Adult Size" (or diameter), or PAS. The PAS should be estimated since the lesion grows proportionally with the patient into adulthood and stratifies the patient risk for melanoma. To calculate the PAS, multiply the diameter of the lesion (in millimeters) by 2, if it is located on the head, or 3 if it is on the trunk.

- Changes in a CMN or suspicious features indicate the need for a biopsy. However, this can be difficult since most CMN are large in size, making excisional biopsy (preferred method for any lesion suspicious for melanoma) by nonsurgical clinicians difficult.

- A punch biopsy offers little value for determining an accurate assessment of risk and management if the sample only represents a small portion of the lesion. A normal histology report may give a false sense of safety because the punch specimen does not represent the melanocytic features of the entire lesion. Therefore, there is a risk of misdiagnosing a possible melanoma with a punch biopsy. It is recommended that a deep shave (saucerization) or an excisional biopsy of the entire lesions be performed; or clinicians can refer the patient to a dermatologist or plastic surgeon when a biopsy is indicated.

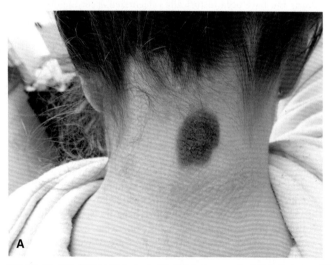

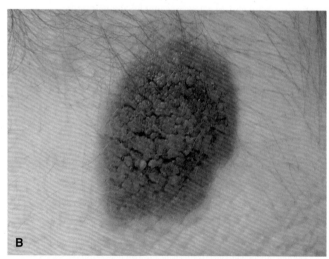

FIG. 2.1-13. **A,B:** CMN posterior neck. (Photo B is close-up view). Note that some CMN can have a cobble-stone or verrucous surface. (Courtesy Douglas DiRuggiero.)

TABLE 2.1-1	Risk Stratification Based on Size of Congenital Melanocytic Nevi	
	SIZE OF LESION	MANAGEMENT

Small	<1.5 cm diameter	Greatest risk for malignancy occurs *after* puberty
		
		If no atypical features:
		    Routine prophylaxis excision is controversial
		    Regular skin self-checks—ABCDEs
		    Annual clinical examinations or with any changes
		    Documented baseline photo of lesion, UVR avoidance and protection
		    Elective excisions can be delayed until puberty
		
		If any concern:
		    PCPs may monitor small lesions if they are confident in their skin assessment skills

Medium	≥1.5 to 10 cm diameter	Refer to a dermatologist for regular monitoring or biopsy of medium lesions, atypical symptoms, or if PCP is unsure
Large/Giant	>20 cm or ≥10% BSA	Greatest risk for malignancy occurs *before* puberty Refer immediately to dermatologist if located over head or spine due to increased risk for neurocutaneous melanosis Coordination of care with a neurologist, plastic surgeon, and other specialists Counseling patient and parents Lifelong monitoring and ultraviolet radiation avoidance

Modified from Kopf, A. W., Bart, R. S., & Hennessey, P. (1979). Congenital nevocytic nevi and malignant melanomas. *Journal of the American Academy of Dermatology, 1*(2), 123–130; Kinsler, V. A., O'Hare, P., Bulstrode, N., Calonje, J. E., Chong, W. K., Hargrave, D., Jacques, T., Lomas, D., Sebire, N. J., & Slater, O. (2017). Melanoma in congenital melanocytic naevi. *The British Journal of Dermatology, 176*(5), 1131–1143.

Treatment

- Evaluate every CMN on a case-by-case basis given the size, location, suspicious features, symptoms (if any), parents' concern for malignancy and potential disfigurement, or loss of function from surgery. Note that treatment of CMN continues to be controversial as dermatologists, dermatopathologists, and surgical specialists worldwide vary in their management approach.

- Non-dermatology providers who elect to monitor small CMN should be confident in their ability to accurately assess potential malignant changes.

- Patients with a medium-sized and large CMN should be referred to a dermatologist for evaluation, management, and monitoring.

- Referral to a dermatologist should occur early in childhood. Surgical excision of these large lesions during early childhood may have better outcomes because infants and children have greater laxity in their skin. Further, many large and giant CMN can require serial surgeries to achieve the best cosmetic outcomes (Fig. 2.1-14).

- Atypical features such as ulcerations, erosions, or nodules have become increasingly important in weighing the decision for surgical management of CMN.

- Infants born with a large CMN that are notably at risk for NCM should be referred immediately for coordinated evaluation and care with a dermatologist, neurologist, ophthalmologist,

and other specialists as appropriate. Imaging of the brain and spine is usually performed within the first few months of life, as well as neurologic and developmental assessment. Patients with evidence of CNS involvement often require neurosurgical intervention.

- Psychological assessment and counseling should be considered for patients with large or giant CMN. Whether or not the lesion is excised, CMN can be severely disfiguring or may result in a permanent loss of function. Parents should be carefully counseled about all of the risks, benefits, and complications so that they can make an informed decision for treatment.

Management and Patient Education

- Emphasize the importance of lifelong clinical skin examinations and routine (monthly) self-examinations for all patients with CMN, regardless of the size.

- Patients with a history of NCM should be diligent in maintaining routine physical examinations (including lymph nodes), age appropriate screening, and neurologic evaluations for metastasis or new primary melanoma.

- The nevus or scars from excision should always be examined closely for recurrence or any atypia.

- Patients should be strongly counseled to avoid excessive UVR and to monitor for any changes in the nevus. Employing the ABCDE skin cancer guidelines is helpful for all patients; but other symptoms that may suggest malignant transition include

BOX 2.1-4   ABCDE Checklist for Lesion Characteristics of Melanoma

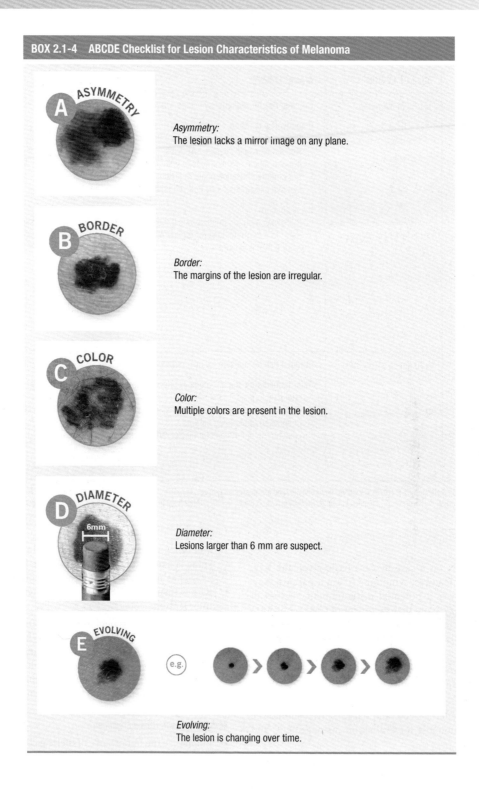

Asymmetry:
The lesion lacks a mirror image on any plane.

Border:
The margins of the lesion are irregular.

Color:
Multiple colors are present in the lesion.

Diameter:
Lesions larger than 6 mm are suspect.

Evolving:
The lesion is changing over time.

new satellite lesions, ulcerations, tenderness, and changes in surface growths like nodules.

Acquired Melanocytic Nevi

Most people have benign, acquired melanocytic nevi (AMN) or "nevi" that typically appear during childhood and can occur anywhere on the body. Patients at higher risk for developing AMN are those with a family history of multiple nevi, repeated UVR exposure (including tanning beds), male gender, and occupational exposure like truck drivers and construction workers. Common nevi are usually classified based upon the location of nevus cells in the skin (Box 2.1-2). Nevi can occur anywhere on the body but are increased in areas of sun exposure.

Clinical Presentation

- Depending on the histologic location, nevi can have a wide variation of appearance such as on the palms, soles, and scalp (Fig. 2.1-15).

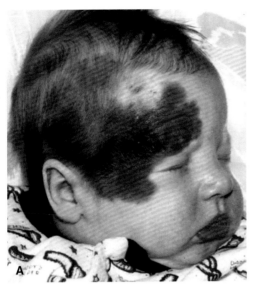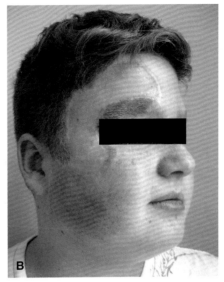

FIG. 2.1-14. **A:** Giant CMN on newborn with increased risk for neurocutaneous melanosis due to location on head. **B:** Excision of congenital nevus and appearance 10 years later. (Photos courtesy of M. Bobonich.)

- *Junctional Nevi*—nevi common in childhood, appearing as round or oval, flat brown macules usually less than 6 mm in diameter.

- *Compound Nevi*—normal changes characteristically occur during adolescence and adulthood where some (not all) of the nevus cells migrate downward into the dermis. The resulting *compound nevi* become slightly elevated and sometimes darker or with a halo effect.

- *Intradermal Nevi*—during adulthood, nevi cells may continue to migrate so that all of the nevus cells relocated in the dermis. These *intradermal nevi* are more raised and have dome or nodular appearance (Table 2.1-2).

- Benign nevi can involute or fade around the sixth or seventh decade. Geriatric patients have fewer nevi (but may have a lot

of seborrheic keratoses). Growing or symptomatic changes in a nevus on an elderly patient should elicit concern for transformation into a malignancy.

Spitz Nevus

- Derived from spindle-shaped melanocytes and clinically presented as a single pink to brown papule on the extremities or face (Fig. 2.1-16). While usually solitary, multiple lesions have been reported.

- Most appear during the first two decades of life, with 50% occurring in children under 10 years of age.

- These lesions may appear very innocuous and are commonly mistaken for a pyogenic granuloma or wart.

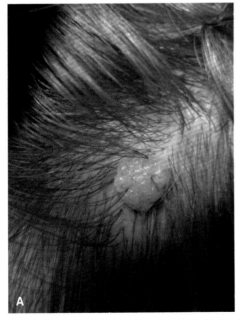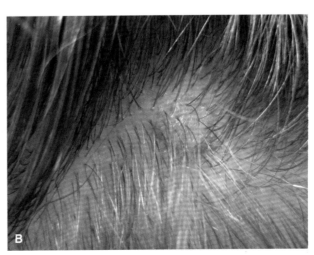

FIG. 2.1-15. **A:** Polypoid dermal nevus on scalp. **B:** Halo-type appearance of a nevus on the scalp characterized by tan–brown rim and flesh-toned to hypopigmented center. (Photos courtesy of M. Bobonich.)

TABLE 2.1-2	Characteristics of Acquired Melanocytic Nevi (Common Moles)		
TYPE OF MOLE	**FEATURES**	**EXAMPLES**	**LOCATION OF NEVUS CELLS**
Junctional nevus	Childhood Flat or slightly elevated Uniform, flesh, brown Well defined <6 mm diameter Scalp-brown halo		Dermal–epidermal junction
Compound nevus	Adolescents and adults Macule with papule/nodule Large variation Fried egg or halo look Brown or flesh Coarse hair sometimes Increasing elevation with age		Dermal–epidermal junction with some nevus cells in dermis
Dermal nevus	Adulthood Dome, verrucal, polypoid, or stalk base Flesh to brown shades Can be translucent Anywhere but frequent on head and neck Larger up to 1 cm		Nevus cells migrated into dermis

- Clinicians must include Spitz nevi as an important differential diagnosis as it can be very aggressive and impact management.

Treatment and Management

- There is some controversy as to whether they should be completely excised or simply observed, but biopsy all lesions suspicious for Spitz nevi and send for histopathologic analysis.

- Consultation with a pediatric dermatologist and dermatopathologist is highly recommended for diagnosed Spitz nevi, especially when there is a family history of melanoma or equivocal biopsy report. Clinical and histopathologic correlation is paramount for the correct diagnosis and plan of care. Diagnosed Spitzoid melanomas may prompt a sentinel lymph node biopsy (SLNB).

Halo Nevus

Also known as a Sutton nevus, halo nevus is the development of a hypopigmented halo surrounding an acquired melanocytic nevi (AMN) (Fig. 2.1-17A).

- They usually appear on the trunk during adolescence and may be associated with a concomitant vitiligo.

- The patient may have several AMN lesions developing a halo phenomenon and in different stages of transformation. Although the etiology is uncertain, many opine that it is an autoimmune response to the normal melanocytes and nevus cells that causes pigment regression.

- They often involute completely, leaving a hypopigmented macule or normal skin color (Fig. 2.1-17B).

Treatment and Management

- Most Halo nevi are benign but warrant a full-skin examination. The AMN inside the halo is the lesion that should be evaluated for atypical features using the ABCDE checklist.

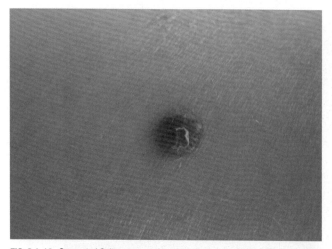

FIG. 2.1-16. Suspected Spitz nevus on the thigh of a 7-year-old boy. Often a benign-appearing, new pink or flesh-colored papule on a child or young adult. Histopathology of this lesion showed spitzoid melanoma. (Photo courtesy of M. Bobonich.)

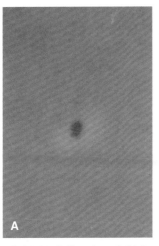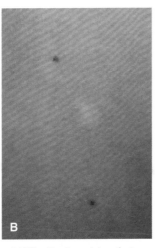

FIG. 2.1-17. **A:** Hypopigmented halo around AMN without suspicious features. If central lesion is pink, biopsy lesion to rule out non-pigmented melanoma. **B:** Complete pigment regression of halo nevus. (Photos courtesy of M. Bobonich.)

Blue Nevus

A blue nevus is an acquired or congenital melanocytic lesion which has more deeply located pigment cells, which appear bluish in color due to the scattering of light through the epidermis (a phenomenon known as Tyndall effect).

- Presents as dark blue to black (<0.5 cm) well-circumscribed papules, easily mistaken for melanoma (Fig. 2.1-18).

- Clinical signs that help differentiate a common blue nevus from a melanoma are the presence of normal skin markings, homogenous color and surface, symmetry, and well-defined border—usually not seen in melanoma, but one should have a very low threshold for biopsy.

- Cellular blue nevus, a variant type, has an increased risk for malignancy. They are typically larger (>1 cm), nodular, and found on the scalp or sacral region. Some blue nevi may have a combination of both types.

Treatment and Management

- In the presence of multiple blue nevi, patients should be referred to a dermatologist to rule out Carney complex (NAME/LAMB syndrome) with associated atrial myxomas.

DYSPLASTIC NEVI

Dysplastic nevi (DN), also called *atypical nevi*, *Clark nevi*, and *atypical melanocytic nevi*, are found in about 5% of the adult Caucasian population. There is an equal prevalence in men and women. The onset of DN can begin during adolescence and extend into the fifth and sixth decades of life. Individuals who report a frequent history of sun exposure, especially sunburns, before the age of 20 years have a higher incidence of DN. Yet there is no evidence to establish a causal relationship between UVR and DN.

DN are an independent risk factor for melanoma and considered by most as a *potential* precursor lesion. Although DN should alert clinicians to an increased risk for melanoma, it should be carefully noted that only 20% to 30% of melanomas arise in DN, compared to 70% to 80% arising de novo on normal skin (Cymerman et al., 2016). Consequently, clinicians should be cautioned not to equate risk of one or two DN with that of patients with dysplastic nevus syndrome (DNS). DN have histopathologic and clinical characteristics that differ from common benign nevi as described in the previous section and are therefore important to identify.

Pathophysiology

The pathogenesis of DN is unknown. Research is focused on genetic factors such as germline mutations and environmental factors (i.e., UVR exposure). The result is an alteration in the nevus cells in both their appearance (cellular atypia) and arrangement (architectural atypia). These changes equate to an increased risk for malignant transformation into melanoma.

- DNS, also called *atypical* or *B-K mole syndrome*, is a familial association of multiple DN and inherited melanoma attributed to a mutation of CDKN2A tumor-suppressor gene. CDKN2A mutations have been associated with increased risk for pancreatic cancers and is concerning for patients with DNS. These patients have a 500-fold increased risk for developing melanoma, typically at an earlier age onset. DNS patients often present with more than 100 pigmented nevi on their body (Fig. 2.1-19).

Clinical Presentation

- Typically present during adolescence or adulthood, not during childhood like common benign nevi—this timing can be a helpful diagnostic clue.

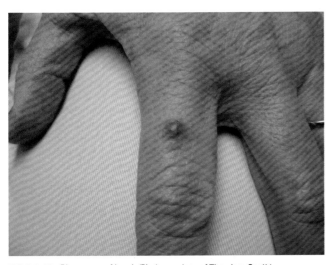

FIG. 2.1-18. Blue nevus of hand. (Photo courtesy of Theodore Scott.)

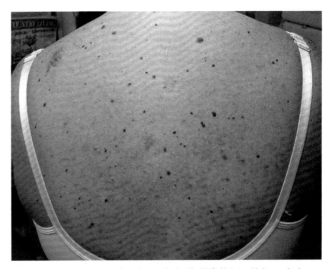

FIG. 2.1-19. Large number of nevi on patient with DNS. Note multiple surgical scars from mole removals. (Photo courtesy of Theodore Scott.)

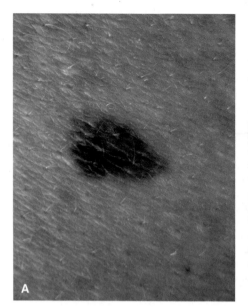 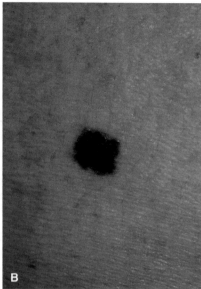 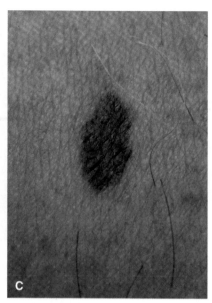

FIG. 2.1-20. A–C: Dysplastic nevi. Note color variation, border irregularity, and asymmetry in these lesions. (Photos courtesy of M. Bobonich.)

- Suspicious features include large size, asymmetry, flat, and varied color or pigmentation (Fig. 2.1-20).
- Discriminating between benign nevi and DN can be difficult for any clinician. Keeping in mind the characteristics of common nevi, a comparison between benign and atypical features can be helpful (Table 2.1-3). Use *ABCDE* for early recognition of melanoma.

Confirming the Diagnosis

- **Skin examination**—The foundation of any skin cancer screening is a full-body skin examination, especially in patients with more than 50 nevi. Patients at high risk for DN, or with a personal or family history of DN, should have a full-skin examination each year by an experienced clinician. A "peek-a-boo" examination can be incomplete and risks a missed diagnosis of DN or malignancy. A skin examination incorporated into a full physical examination can begin with a global look for any "ugly duckling" lesions that stand out "different from its neighbors," or more simply stated, don't match the color, shape, or size of a

patient's other moles. These lesions have high clinical suspicion for atypia. For clinicians who are not confident in their ability to recognize precursor or cancerous lesions, a referral to dermatology is highly recommended. Furthermore, any changes in nevi reported by the patient should be investigated and biopsied as necessary.

- **Dermoscopy** (epiluminescent microscopy) can be valuable in the assessment of pigmented lesions but is dependent on the user's knowledge, training, and experience in evaluating the suspicious characteristics of malignancy. While some dermatoscopes use nonpolarized light, most consist of a polarized light source and $10\times$ magnification, which allows the clinician to identify any suspicious lesion characteristics. Dermoscopy utilized by an experienced clinician may reduce the number of unnecessary biopsies and increase diagnostic accuracy of melanoma.

- **Biopsy**—The definitive diagnosis of a DN can only be made histologically. Pigmented lesions with suspicious features should be biopsied with a 2-mm clearance from the lesion margin. Punch biopsy is preferred for pigmented lesions, but only if the entire lesion can fit within a punch. With lesions larger in diameter, saucerization of the entire pigmented portion, with adequate depth into the reticular dermis, is now preferred by dermatopathologists—as it allows for the complete lesion to be evaluated.

- **Histopathology**—Send all mole or lesion tissue removed from a patient for histologic examination by a pathologist, preferably a dermatopathologist. The atypia of a DN is usually reported as mild, moderate, or severe; or it may be standardized into categories (I, II, or III) for coding purposes. Clinicians who biopsy a lesion should be capable of interpreting the pathology report, which determines the patient's plan of care. If there is any question or doubt about the pathology, collaborate with the dermatopathologist or an experienced dermatology clinician.

The degree of atypia and management may be categorized as:

- *Mild Atypia* (category I) has melanocytes with nuclei that are ovoid or ellipsoid-shaped, hyperchromatic, and smaller (or nonexistent) than nuclei of basal keratinocytes.
- *Moderate Atypia* (category II) includes melanocytes with large nuclei (one to two times the size of basal keratinocyte nuclei),

TABLE 2.1-3	Comparison of Benign Acquired Melanocytic Nevi and Dysplastic Nevi	
NORMAL NEVI	**DYSPLASTIC NEVI**	
Onset childhood	Onset adolescence to adulthood	
Usually <5 mm	Usually >6 mm	
Symmetrical	Asymmetrical	
Well-defined border	Poorly-defined border	
Consistent color	Variegated color	
Uniform surface	Irregular surface	
Unchanging	Changing appearance	

hyperchromatic, ellipsoid- or rhomboid-shaped, with a small nucleolus visible in the center of the nucleus.

- *Severe Atypia* (category III) is characterized as spindle- or epithelioid-shaped, hyperchromatic nuclei larger than basal keratinocytes (two or more times or greater than nuclei of basal keratinocytes), but with distinct nucleoli. There is variability in the grading of atypia among dermatopathologists, which emphasizes the difficulty in differentiating severe atypia from melanoma. A severely atypical DN is considered, by many dermatology specialists, to be analogous to a melanoma in situ (MIS).

DIFFERENTIAL DIAGNOSIS   Dysplastic Nevi

- Blue nevus
- Dermatofibroma
- Lentigo
- Melanoma
- Melanocytic nevi
- Seborrheic keratosis
- Spitz nevus

Treatment

The management of dysplastic nevi are predicated on the degree of atypia identified in the histopathology report coupled with the patient's medical history and melanoma risk factors. Additionally, the clinician should note the presence or absence (clearance) of atypia on the margins of the biopsy specimen sent for analysis. This may impact the plan of care, as well as anticipate the recurrence of a pigmented lesion at the site of biopsy.

- *Mild DN* (category I)—DN with mild cytologic atypia usually does not require reexcision even when atypical cells are present on the biopsy margins, but many well-respected dermatologists still excise these lesions, especially if the patient has a history of melanoma.
- *Moderate DN* (category II)—Unfortunately, management of these lesions is also not straight forward and is currently debated. Many dermatologists, dermatology surgeons, and dermatopathologists prefer to have moderate atypical DN reexcised with conservative margins, ensuring that all atypical cells are completely excised. The decision for reexcision may be further influenced by the patient's or family's history of DN and melanoma. Conversely, other dermatology specialists do not reexcise moderately atypical DN with clear margins in all areas, believing the specimen was fully excised based on the histopathology. Specimens collected by shave biopsy may transect the base of the lesion, leaving cells on the margin and typically require reexcision.
- *Severe DN* (category III)—There is no uncertainty about the need for reexcision of all severely atypical DN. A reexcision of 5-mm margins is usually considered adequate but should be confirmed with histopathology. Nonsurgical clinicians receiving a pathology report with a severe DN should refer the patient to a dermatologist or surgeon.

Management and Patient Education

- Patients with a history of DN should be taught to perform regular skin self-checks and follow-up with annual clinical examinations. Many dermatology practitioners follow patients with a history of severe DNs at more frequent intervals.

- Patient education about DN is the same as for a patient with melanoma. With an emphasis on sun avoidance and protection, patients should understand the risk of UVR.
- Patients with known family CDKN2A mutations should have clinical skin examinations yearly, starting at the age of 10 years (more frequently if DN or melanoma is diagnosed).

CLINICAL PEARLS

- DNs are considered possible precursor lesions to melanoma.
- Patients with a personal or family history of DN or melanoma are at higher risk for melanoma.
- Patients with DN should perform self-examinations, with particular attention to the *ABCDE* guidelines, and regular clinical skin examinations for early detection and treatment.
- Reducing UVR exposure is the single most important aspect of prevention. Hats, sunglasses, photo-protective clothing, and sunscreen of SPF 30 or higher are recommended.

MALIGNANT MELANOMA

The American Cancer Society estimates that nearly 100,000 new cases of melanoma and 7300 people will die of melanoma every year, with a lifetime melanoma risk of about 2.5% (1 in 40) for whites, 0.1% (1 in 1000) for blacks, and 0.5% (1 in 200) for Hispanics. Melanoma is the deadliest of all skin cancers, responsible for 75% of the deaths associated with skin cancer (ACS, 2019). Shockingly, melanoma is the most common cancer in 25- to 29-year-olds and the leading cause of *cancer deaths* in females aged 25 to 30. In younger populations (15- to 29-year-olds), melanoma is the second leading cancer, striking young adults in the prime of their lives!

Melanoma can occur anywhere on the body. Genitals, soles, postauricular, and oral mucosa are not typically examined by clinicians but may be affected. The highest incidence of cutaneous melanoma is on the back, chest, and arms in white males, while the most common locations for white females is on their backs, arms, and legs. Although more rare, in patients with dark skin tones, palmar, plantar, mucosal, and subungual areas are the most common locations.

All patients should be assessed for risk factors for melanoma. Intermittent sun exposure (weekends and vacations) resulting in painful sunburns during childhood and adolescence is the major predisposing risk factor for melanoma. However, other genetic and environmental risk factors can increase an individual's risk (Box 2.1-5). Individuals are also at increased risk for melanoma if they have a family history of melanoma or DNS. If a first-degree relative (parent, sibling, or offspring) has a history of diagnosed melanoma, then the risk of developing melanoma doubles for an individual and is significantly higher if there are three or more family members with a history.

BOX 2.1-5   Risk Factors for Melanoma

Unprotected UVR exposure, especially chronic, severe intermittent, or blistering sunburns
Fair complexion, blue or green eyes, blond or red hair with the tendency to freckle or burn
The presence of large number of nevi or history of DN and DNS
Large or garment CMN
Family and/or personal history of melanoma
CDKN2K, BRAF, NRAS, MC1R, and *BRCA2* mutations
Xeroderma pigmentosum
Immunosuppressed patients

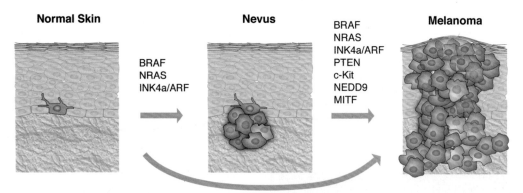

FIG. 2.1-21. Gene mutations in the development of melanoma. (DeVita, V. T., Lawrence, T. S., & Rosenberg, S. A. [2018]. *DeVita, Hellman, and Rosenberg's cancer: Principles & practice of oncology* [11th ed.]. Wolters Kluwer Health I Lippincott Williams & Wilkins.)

Pathophysiology

Melanoma is a cancer originating from the melanocytes, which are the pigment-producing cells in the epidermis. The term *malignant melanoma* is becoming obsolete because the word "malignant" is redundant as there are no benign melanomas (Fig. 2.1-21). The genomics of cutaneous melanoma are vastly expanding in search of risks and mutations that predispose individuals to cutaneous melanoma. Approximately 50% of melanomas harbor oncogenic *BRAF* (a protein kinase) mutations, which are known to increases the risk of melanoma.

Clinical Presentation

A thorough skin examination is the most low-cost, straightforward screening tool that can have a significant impact on patient outcomes. A complete skin examination should include the "not so common" areas, including the scalp, postauricular, axillae, interdigital spaces, genitals, gluteal cleft, palms, and soles. Inspection of the oral mucosa and eyes should be considered if the patient has not had a screening by their dentist and ophthalmologist. Although the *ABCDE* checklist for melanoma is helpful, caution should be used in discounting lesions that do not fit into these classic criteria (Box 2.1-4).

- Melanoma can look like anything, especially in individuals with red or blonde hair who may develop melanoma that is only lightly pigmented or amelanotic (pink or flesh-colored).

- Lesions can be macular, papular, or nodular. The surface may be smooth or rough and vary in pigmentation from pink to brown to gray, blue, or black.

- Some patients may report a sudden onset of burning, pruritus, ulceration, or tenderness of a lesion which could signify potential malignancy.

- Melanoma can arise in a previously benign lesion, like a dermal nevus or freckle that the patient has had for years. This emphasizes the importance of listening to patients with worrisome complaints about a specific changing lesion.

There are four clinical subtypes of melanoma with associated characteristics or distribution. The most common type of melanoma is superficial spreading subtype (70%), followed by nodular melanomas (10% to 15%), lentigo maligna melanoma (LMM) (5% to 10%), and acral lentiginous (7%).

Superficial Spreading Melanoma (SSM)

- Flat or slightly raised (papular) appearance, pigment is usually variegated with brown, black, blue, or pink colors. Most are asymmetrical and have irregular borders.

- SSM is commonly found on the trunk in both genders, with an onset in the fourth or fifth decade of life. Of the subtypes, SSM is most associated with a pre-existing nevus and grows very slowly.

- SSM can progress into a vertical growth phase, invading the dermis, and become an invasive melanoma (Fig. 2.1-22). *Invasive melanoma* is most commonly noted on the trunk and sun-exposed areas of the head and neck in both sexes (Fig. 2.1-23).

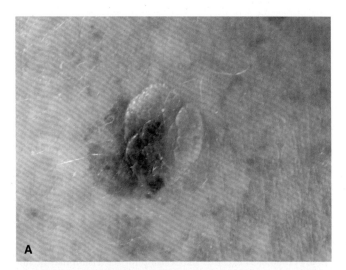

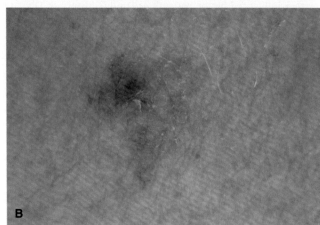

FIG. 2.1-22. A: Asymmetrical irregular black–brown discoloration (SSM) extending upward on flesh-toned papule (dermal nevus). **B:** SSM. Irregularly shaped with dark-brown, tan, and pink discoloration. SSM can also have red or blue discoloration. (Photos courtesy of M. Bobonich.)

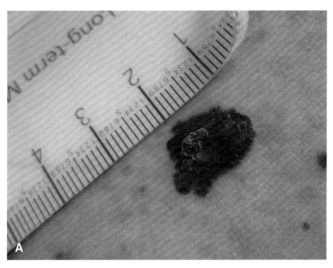
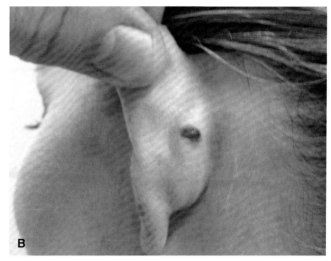

FIG. 2.1-23. **A,B:** Invasive melanoma. (Photos courtesy of M. Bobonich.)

Nodular Melanomas

- Nodular melanomas usually occur on the extremities or back.
- Typically a rapidly growing dark brown to black papule or dome-shaped nodule (can be pink), prone to ulceration with a friable surface. They can be any color, are rarely amelanotic (without pigment), and can easily be mistaken for basal cell carcinoma or squamous cell carcinoma.
- This is the most aggressive type of melanoma and more often develops *de novo* instead of from a pre-existing nevus. Nodular melanoma has usually advanced at the time of initial diagnosis (Fig. 2.1-24).

Lentigo Maligna (LM) and Lentigo Maligna Melanoma (LMM)

- Lentigo maligna (LM) and LMM appear as irregular, mottled brown macules with variegated pigment and can be hidden among solar lentigines on sun-damaged skin (Fig. 2.1-25).
- LM is synonymous with MIS (Fig. 2.1-26); while *LMM* is considered a progression toward invasive melanoma.

- These melanomas develop on the sun-exposed regions, with cheeks, nose, and temples being the most common sites, usually during the sixth and seventh decades of life.
- Notably, both of these lesions are in the radial growth phase of development and have subclinical extension beyond the visible border.

Acral Melanomas

- Acral melanoma (ALM) is a less common type of melanoma, yet it accounts for 20% of diagnosed melanomas in darker-pigmented individuals (Fitzpatrick type IV to VI) compared to 2% in Caucasians.
- Pigmented macules develop on the palms, soles, and subungual (beneath the nail plate) areas. The highest incidence is on the plantar aspect of the foot and is easily mistaken for a hematoma (Fig. 2.1-27).
- ALM is frequently misdiagnosed or delayed, resulting in a poor 5-year survival rate of 25% to 51% (Miranda et al., 2012) (Fig. 2.1-28).

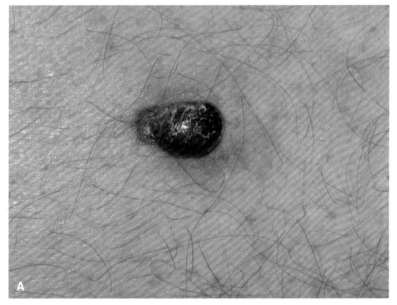
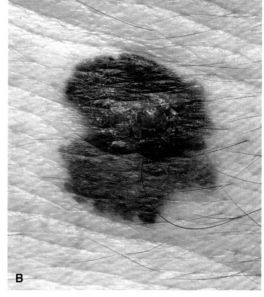

FIG. 2.1-24. **A,B:** Nodular melanoma. (Photo B is courtesy of Douglas DiRuggiero.)

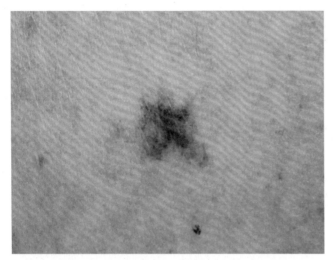

FIG. 2.1-25. Lentigo maligna (LM). (Photo courtesy of Theodore Scott.)

- Subungual lesions present with diffuse nail discoloration or longitudinal pigmentation that may extend to the proximal nail fold, commonly referred to as the *Hutchinson sign* (Fig. 2.1-29A,B). Nail findings noted on examination may be a red flag and

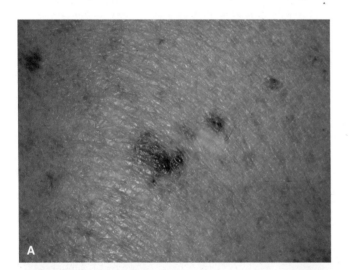

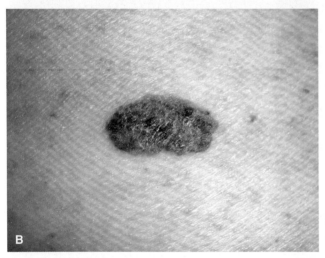

FIG. 2.1-26. **A,B:** Melanoma in situ (MIS); synonymous with LM. (Photos courtesy of M. Bobonich.)

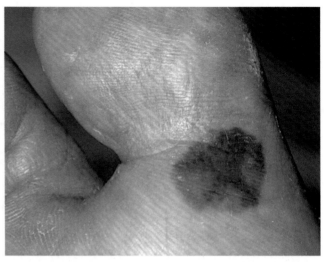

FIG. 2.1-27. Acral lentiginous melanoma. (Goodheart, H. P. [2015]. *Goodheart's photoguide of common skin disorders* [4th ed.]. Wolters Kluwer Health | Lippincott Williams & Wilkins.)

indicate the need for biopsy (Box 2.1-1). Subungual melanomas are the most commonly missed lesion on clinical examinations and account for the most frequent cause of judgments against clinicians who fail or delay diagnosis.

Confirming the Diagnosis

Biopsy

- Biopsy is essential for the diagnosis of melanoma. Excisional biopsy (excising the complete lesion with 1 to 2 mm beyond the edge and full depth of the dermis) is the recommended method of sampling. Punch biopsies are appropriate for small lesions if

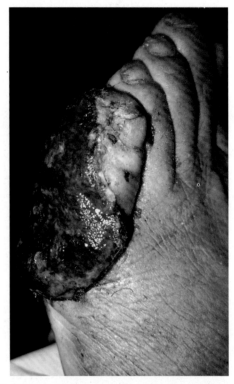

FIG. 2.1-28. Advanced acral melanoma presenting as a black, red ulcerated tumor. (Photo courtesy of M. Bobonich.)

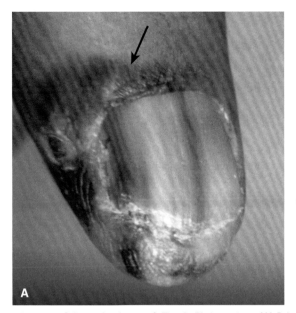
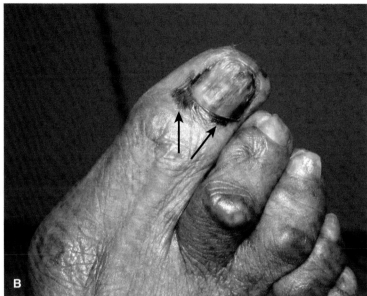

FIG. 2.1-29. Subungual melanoma. **A:** Thumb. (Photo courtesy of M. Bobonich.) **B:** Great toe. (Photo B is from Center for Disease Control PHIL #1342). Note the pigment on the surrounding cuticle (*arrows*): a positive Hutchinson sign.

you can remove the entire lesion with one punch. A deep shave (sometimes referred to as a scoop or saucerization) biopsy to the reticular dermis for small lesions is acceptable but requires much practice to perfect. An incisional biopsy may be performed for lesions that are too large to excise for biopsy. Furthermore, if the lesion is on the face or cosmetically sensitive areas, consider a referral to a Mohs or plastic surgeon—but without delay.

- It cannot be overemphasized that when a clinician is not skilled in biopsy or excision, they should collaborate with a qualified clinician who can perform the biopsy right away. The patient should not be left to wait weeks for an appointment. A phone call from provider to provider may be necessary to facilitate patient access for a prompt appointment. Developing a relationship with a local dermatologist or surgical provider who will accommodate urgent requests can be invaluable. In this scenario, we would recommend that the patient's appointment be scheduled before they leave your office and a follow-up confirmation with the patient to ensure that they have completed the biopsy and received the appropriate management from the specialist if indicated.

Histopathology

- Many histologic characteristics reported about the melanoma are key variables used to stage or classify the tumor, predict morbidity, and guide treatment. Therefore, the clinician can impact the diagnostic value of the biopsy by providing a quality specimen (discussed above) and key clinical information on the pathology request form, including the following: a photograph (if available), pertinent medical history, and complete description of the lesion. Details such as "0.8 cm blue and black variegated papule with irregular border and central ulceration located on the left upper chest at the MCL" can be helpful, while "a bump on chest" will be of little value to the dermatopathologist.

- The *depth* of the lesion will be reported in the histopathology report and is the most predictive factor in staging melanoma. Two methods are used for reporting lesion depth. *Breslow's depth* measurement (in millimeters) is the accepted standard currently used in AJCC Melanoma Tumor Classification and measures the invasion of the lesion from the top of the epidermis to the deepest

point of melanocyte proliferation (Fig. 2.1-30). You may also see some histopathology that report a *Clark's level,* but this is becoming less frequently reported.

- The histopathology report will note tumor characteristics, like the presence of microscopic ulceration, which upgrades a tumor's seriousness and can move it into a later stage. Mitotic rate (cancer cell division) has been introduced into the staging system based on recent evidence that it is also an independent factor predicting prognosis. Perineural or perivascular invasion will be noted if present. The presence of any or all of these features suggests a more aggressive disease and will impact the staging of the lesion (Amin, 2017).

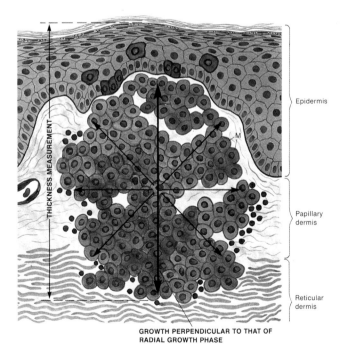

FIG. 2.1-30. Breslow's depth measurement of invasion by melanoma. (Rubin, R., Strayer, D. S., & Rubin, E. [2019]. *Rubin's pathology: Clinicopathologic foundations of medicine* [6th ed.]. Wolters Kluwer Health | Lippincott Williams & Wilkins.)

- Molecular testing on confirmed melanomas (BRAF, MEK, NF1) is becoming increasingly important to guide treatment and prognosis information. If this information is not included in the pathology report, it should be requested.

Sentinel Lymph Node Biopsy (SLNB)

- The depth of a melanoma usually guides the surgeon's decision to perform an SLNB. Lesions with a thickness of 1 mm or greater are more likely to metastasize to the lymph vessels and then regional lymph nodes. Accordingly, SLNB is usually recommended for lesions 1 to 4 mm in thickness or if the lesion is less than 1 mm and has noted ulceration. An SLNB to assess for lymph node involvement is often performed at the same time as the surgical excision of the primary melanoma. A positive SLNB indicates metastasis to lymph nodes and the possible need for further lymph node dissection of the regional basin. It may also indicate the need for further diagnostics such as serologies and positron emission tomography (PET scan) to assess for distant metastases. Negative SLNB does not rule out metastasis but has a better prognosis over time.

DIFFERENTIAL DIAGNOSIS   Melanoma

- Cherry angioma
- Junctional or compound nevi
- Kaposi sarcoma
- Pigmented basal cell carcinoma
- Pyogenic granuloma
- Seborrheic keratosis

Treatment

Staging of melanoma (or any cancer) helps clinicians classify the severity of the primary tumor and possible metastasis of the cancer patient. It is invaluable in calculating the patient's prognosis and guidelines for treatment. Other factors such as patient's health and comorbidities may influence treatment choices and plan of care.

Surgical Excision.   Surgical excision with histologically proven clear surgical margins is the gold standard of treatment for all biopsy-proven primary melanoma. While most primary care clinicians refer these patients to dermatologists or dermatology surgeons, some elect to perform the surgical excision. Providers should have competent surgical skills and current knowledge regarding the recommendations by the National Cancer Institute, which guides most dermatologists, Mohs, and oncology surgeons. The recommended surgical margins are as follows:

- MIS: 0.5-cm margin
- Melanomas <1 mm depth: 1.0-cm margin
- Melanomas 1 to 4 mm in depth: 2.0-cm margin
- Melanomas >4 mm in depth: ≥2.0-cm margin

Oncologists and surgeons may consider additional or alternative treatments such as radiation, cryotherapy, and topical immuno-modulators for a large MIS and LMM that would disfigure a patient or in a patient who is a poor surgical candidate. For these patients, referral to a dermatologist is essential. Mohs surgery can be beneficial in areas where full surgical margins are not possible or where cosmetic concerns are significant. This technique remains somewhat controversial as some experts believe that it is difficult to visualize melanoma cells in a fresh frozen specimen. The introduction of immunohistologic stains should make this a more utilized technique in the future.

Chemotherapy and Immunotherapy.   In spite of the advances in new drug therapies, these drugs do not cure metastatic melanoma. They offer only the hope of slowing the progression and extending life during advanced stages of the disease. Referral to oncology specialists is necessary for these treatments.

- *Interferon alfa-2b* was the first Food and Drug Administration (FDA)–approved adjunctive therapy for stage IIIB–IIIC melanoma with an improved survival rate and disease-free period. Yet the toxicities and side effects of the drugs, especially the high-dose regimen with the longest survival rate, can be difficult for patients to tolerate and advance beyond the 3-month induction phase of therapy.

- *Immunotherapy Vaccines* currently being studied in clinical trials offer an antigen-directed approach by stimulating an immune response to melanoma-associated tumor cells. They have reported lower toxicities but some hypersensitivity reactions. At this time, vaccine trials are numerous and promising but have not offered any significant improvement in melanoma survival rates.

- *Immunotherapy Check-point Inhibitors* nivolumab (Opdivo) and pembrolizumab (Keytruda) are protein PD-1 inhibitors and ipilimumab (Yervoy) is a monoclonal antibody which activates the immune system by targeting CTLA-4. All of these therapies are indicated for unresectable or advanced metastatic melanomas, and while hailed as a breakthrough medication, when used as monotherapy, about half of patients do not respond. However, combinations of these treatments with each other, and other traditional chemotherapies, are making an impact on melanoma survival.

Management and Patient Education

Prevention

- Education is the clinician's greatest tool in reducing the incidence of melanoma. The following teaching points are aimed at prevention and early recognition:

  - Monthly patient self-examinations are highly recommended (reinforced at each visit).

  - Frequent clinical skin examinations by a dermatology provider for patients with a history of melanoma.

  - Examination every 3 to 6 months after diagnosis is needed for the first few years; some experts recommend examinations every 6 months for life.

  - The *most* important factor is avoidance of UVR exposure, including tanning bed use.

  - Let your dentist, ophthalmologist, and gynecologist know about your history of melanoma.

  - Counsel your family (parents, siblings, and children) about their increased risk for melanoma.

  - Recommend reliable sources for patient information like the Skin Cancer Foundation.

Follow-Up

- Clinicians should emphasize the importance of clinical follow-up after diagnosis of melanoma to reduce the risk of mortality and morbidity. While there are many varied beliefs and opinions regarding the monitoring of patients diagnosed with primary cutaneous melanoma without metastasis, the American Academy of Dermatology provides an evidence-based algorithmic approach to the diagnoses, treatment, and management (Fox et al., 2013).

- During the initial 2 years following diagnosis, patients should have a total skin examination every 3 to 6 months, then 1 to 2 years thereafter.

- For patients with metastatic disease, the oncologist should recommend and guide follow-up management and monitoring in collaboration with a dermatologist.

Survival

- Melanoma is curable with early detection and treatment.

- The 5- and 10-year survival rates for melanoma are published by the ACS and based on the AJCC 8th edition Staging Manual (ACS, 2019).

- The diagnosis and surgical treatment of early melanoma (stage I) has a 97% 5-year survival rate, which means it is eminently curable; and with continued follow-up, a patient should have a normal life span.

- Moreover, the ACS emphasizes the drastic decrease in survival for patients with metastatic melanoma or advanced stages (III and IV) where the 5-year survival rate plummets to 78% and 15%, respectively.

- Additional factors that increase the risk for morbidity include diagnosis in elderly, African Americans, ALMs, and immunosuppressed patients.

CLINICAL PEARLS

Early Recognition and Diagnosis of Melanoma

- Stand back for a "five-foot view" of the patient's skin and look for the "ugly duckling."

- Not all melanomas are brown or pigmented.

- LISTEN to patients with a heightened concern about a *specific* lesion and consider biopsy even if the lesion has benign characteristics.

- Make sure to look in all the cracks and crevices and palms and soles.

- Ask about sun-protective behaviors at each office visit and teach prevention.

- Biopsy the entire suspicious lesion. A small biopsy of a large lesion can lead to a false-negative result and fatal outcome.

- Refer early and often if you have any doubts or if you are unable to biopsy.

- Photograph lesions and include images into patient's chart for future comparative evaluations. Encourage patients to photograph their own moles and save in a separate photo file for ongoing, regular self-evaluations.

READINGS AND REFERENCES

Ali, A. (2015). *Dermatology: A pictorial review* (3rd ed.). McGraw-Hill Medical.

American Cancer Society (ACS). (2019). *American cancer society facts and figures.* Retrieved on December 7, 2019, from https://www.cancer.org/content/dam/cancer-org/research/cancer-facts-and-statistics/annual-cancer-facts-and-figures/2019/cancer-facts-and-figures-2019.pdf

American Cancer Society (ACS). (2019). *Melanoma skin cancer overview.* Retrieved on December 7, 2019 from http://www.cancer.org/cancer/melanoma-skin-cancer.html

Amin, M. B., Edge, S., Greene, F., Byrd, D. R., Brookland, R. K., Washington, M. K., Gershenwald, J. E., Compton, C. C., Hess, K. R., Sullivan, D. C., Jessup, J. M., Brierley, J. D., Gaspar, L. E., Schilsky, R. L., Balch, C. M., Winchester, D. P., Asare, E. A., Madera, M., Gress, D. M., Meyer, L. R. (Eds.). (2017). *AJCC cancer staging manual* (8th ed.). Springer.

Chen, L., James, N., Barker, C., Busam, K., & Marghoob, A. (2013). Desmoplastic melanoma: A review. *Journal of the American Academy of Dermatology, 68*(5), 825–833. https://doi.org/10.1016/j.jaad.2012.10.041

Cymerman, R. M., Shao, Y., Wang, K., Zhang, Y., Murzaku, E. C., Penn, L. A., Osman, I., & Polsky, D. (2016). De novo vs nevus-associated melanomas: Differences in associations with prognostic indicators and survival. *Journal of the National Cancer Institute, 108*(10), djw121. https://doi.org/10.1093/jnci/djw121

Fox, M., Lao, C., Schwartz, J., Frohm, M., Bichakjian, C., & Johnson, T. (2013). Management options for metastatic melanoma in the era of novel therapies: A primer for the practicing dermatologist: Part I: Management of stage III disease. *Journal of the American Academy of Dermatology, 68*(1), 1.e1–e9. https://doi.org/10.1016/j.jaad.2012.09.040

Gershenwald, J. E., & Ross, M. I. (2011). Sentinel-lymph-node biopsy for cutaneous melanoma. *The New England Journal of Medicine, 364*(18), 1738–1745. https://doi.org/10.1056/NEJMct1002967

Kinsler, V. A., O'Hare, P., Bulstrode, N., Calonje, J. E., Chong, W. K., Hargrave, D., Jacques, T., Lomas, D., Sebire, N. J., & Slater, O. (2017). Melanoma in congenital melanocytic naevi. *The British Journal of Dermatology, 176*(5), 1131–1143. https://doi.org/10.1111/bjd.15301

Krengel, S., Scope, A., Dusza, S. W., Vonthein, R., & Marghoob, A. A. (2013). New recommendations for the categorization of cutaneous features of congenital melanocytic nevi. *Journal of the American Academy of Dermatology, 68*(3), 441–451.

Marghoob, A. A. (2012). *Nevogenesis: Mechanisms and clinical implications of nevus development.* Springer-Verlag. https://doi.org/10.1007/978-3-642-28397-0

Miranda, B. H., Haughton, D. N., & Fahmy, F. S. (2012). Subungual melanoma: An important tip. *Journal of Plastic, Reconstructive & Aesthetic Surgery, 65*(10), 1422–1424. https://doi.org/10.1016/j.bjps.2012.03.001

Price, H. N., & Schaffer, J. V. (2010). Congenital melanocytic nevi-when to worry and how to treat: Facts and controversies. *Clinics in Dermatology, 28*(3), 293–302.

Rapini, R. P. (2012). *Practical dermatopathology* (2nd ed.). Elsevier/Saunders.

Russak, J. E., & Rigel, D. S. (2012). *Melanoma and pigmented lesions.* Saunders.

Wong, S. L., Balch, C. M., Hurley, P., Agarwala, S. S., Akhurst, T. J., Cochran, A., Cormier, J. N., Gorman, M., Kim, T. Y., McMasters, K. M., Noyes, R. D., Schuchter, L. M., Valsecchi, M, E., Weaver, D. L., & Lyman, G. H.; American Society of Clinical Oncology; Society of Surgical Oncology (2012). Sentinel lymph node biopsy for melanoma: American Society of Clinical Oncology and Society of Surgical Oncology joint clinical practice guideline. *Journal of Clinical Oncology, 30*(23), 2912–2918. https://doi.org/10.1200/JCO.2011.40.3519

Precancerous Lesions and Nonmelanoma Skin Cancers

Victoria Lazareth

In This Chapter

- Actinic Keratosis
- Squamous Cell Carcinoma
- Basal Cell Carcinoma
- Merkel Cell Carcinoma
- Atypical Fibroxanthoma
- Dermatofibrosarcoma Protuberans

- Sebaceous Carcinoma
- Extramammary Paget Disease
- Cutaneous T-Cell Lymphoma
  - Mycosis Fungoides
  - Sezary Syndrome
- B-Cell Lymphoma

Each year, 2 million Americans develop nonmelanoma skin cancers (NMSC), costing health care nearly $500 million. Untreated or incompletely treated tumors lead to disfigurement, nerve damage, functional impairment, and even death. Advanced practice clinicians (APCs) can provide early diagnosis and treatment of NMSC, reducing patient morbidity and mortality. Additionally, APCs can provide valuable preventative education regarding sun safety and early detection of skin cancer through clinical and self-examinations. While many think of squamous cell carcinoma (SCC) and basal cell carcinoma (BCC) as the only types of NMSC, this chapter highlights several other tumors which fall into this category: Merkel cell carcinoma (MCC), atypical fibroxanthoma (AFX), dermatofibrosarcoma protuberans (DFSP), microcystic adnexal carcinoma, sebaceous carcinoma, and cutaneous T-cell and B-cell lymphoma.

PRECANCEROUS LESIONS

Actinic Keratoses

Actinic keratoses (AKs) are extremely common lesions which develop in increasing number with cumulative sun exposure and advancing age. Approximately one in five Americans will develop AKs in their lifetime. Patients who develop AKs tend to have fair skin and a history of chronic or intense, intermittent sun exposure, and often have clinical signs of photoaging, including freckles, lentigines, and pigmentary dyschromia. AKs may present years after the sun exposure. These precancerous lesions constitute one of the most common reasons for patients to present to a dermatology clinician.

While it is estimated that up to 20% of AKs may develop into SCC, there is no way to discern clinically if a given lesion will progress (Patel et al., 2011). Lesions which become large, thickened, tender, or ulcerated are worrisome for SCC. AKs may resolve spontaneously with sun-protective measures, but persistent lesions are usually treated both for symptomatic relief and to prevent their progression into skin cancer.

Pathophysiology

The epidermal layer of the skin is composed of keratinocytes, which slowly migrate from the base to the surface of the epidermis (Fig. 2.2-1). Ultraviolet radiation (UVR) damage to the keratinocytes can result in premalignant transformation. AKs are altered epidermal keratinocytes that have an increased mitotic rate and are thought to represent an intermediary step along a continuum to SCC development. If the atypical keratinocytes extend across the full extent of the epidermis, they are designated as localized or in situ SCC.

Clinical Presentation

- AKs initially present as a pink to red, rough area with a texture likened to that of sandpaper (Fig. 2.2-2).

- Lesions may develop a thick scale, which may evolve into sharp papules or plaques, which may in turn become crusted or bleed when removed.

- AKs are often better detected by feel than by sight, so a tactile examination with the fingertips over sun-exposed areas (i.e., nasal dorsum, helical rims of the ears, and dorsal hands) should be performed.

- Several variants of AK exist:

  - *Pigmented actinic keratoses (PAKs)*—identical to AKs with a brown, blue, or black hue which results from melanocytes within the lesion. More often seen in individuals with darker skin tones.

  - *Hypertrophic AKs*—lesions which have become very thick, scaly, or crusty plaques. Often large, yellow, and crusty (Fig. 2.2-3). A biopsy is often needed to exclude invasive SCC.

  - *Cutaneous horn*—hyperkeratotic papules which becomes protuberant (Fig. 2.2-4). Similar lesions may develop from benign seborrheic keratoses or warts, so a biopsy is necessary to identify SCC in situ (SCCIS).

  - *Actinic cheilitis*—designation for AKs of the lower lip (Fig. 2.2-5). These lesions are rough, scaly, fissures, or plaques which may

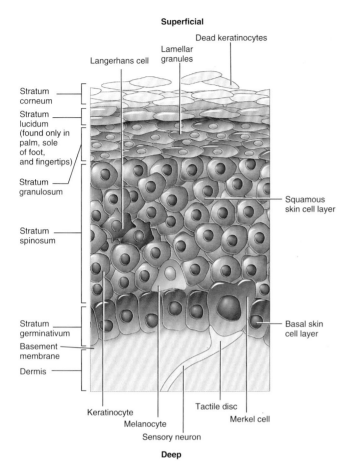

Superficial

Dead keratinocytes

Lamellar granules

Langerhans cell

Stratum corneum

Stratum lucidum (found only in palm, sole of foot, and fingertips)

Stratum granulosum

Stratum spinosum

Squamous skin cell layer

Stratum germinativum

Basement membrane

Dermis

Basal skin cell layer

Keratinocyte

Melanocyte

Sensory neuron

Tactile disc

Merkel cell

Deep

FIG. 2.2-1. Anatomy of the epidermis.

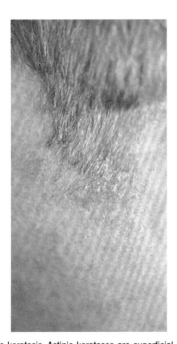

FIG. 2.2-2. Actinic keratosis. Actinic keratoses are superficial, flattened papules covered by a dry scale. Often multiple, they may be round or irregular, and are pink, tan, or grayish. They appear on sun-exposed skin of older, fair-skinned persons. Though themselves benign, these lesions may give rise to squamous cell carcinoma. (Used with permission. Source of photo: Sauer, G. C. [1985]. *Manual of skin diseases* [5th ed.]. JB Lippincott.)

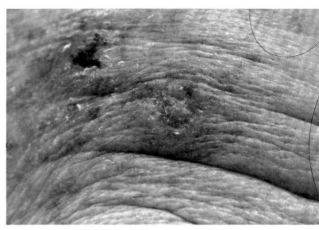

FIG. 2.2-3. AKs presenting as thin and thick scaly papules on the hand. (Photo courtesy of Victoria Lazareth.)

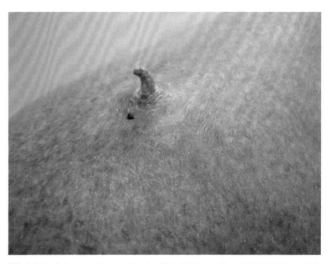

FIG. 2.2-4. Cutaneous horn on the shoulder. (Photo courtesy of Victoria Lazareth.)

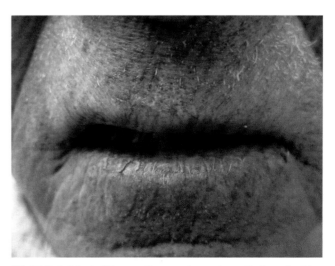

FIG. 2.2-5. Actinic cheilitis presenting as scaly macules on the lower lip. A key finding supporting actinic cheilitis is the blurring of the normally very demarcated vermillion border. (Photo courtesy of Victoria Lazareth.)

be white or hyperpigmented. It is not uncommon for them to become tender, bleed, or ulcerate. Actinic cheilitis persists longer than an HSV lesion and does not resolve with emollients typically helpful for chapped or dry lips.

DIFFERENTIAL DIAGNOSIS	Actinic Keratoses
• Squamous cell carcinoma • Lichenoid keratosis • Basal cell carcinoma • Psoriasis • Eczema • Seborrheic keratosis	• Chondrodermatitis nodularis helicis • Solar lentigo • Melanoma • Wart • Herpes simplex virus

Confirming the Diagnosis

- Lesions thought to be AKs, but do not resolve with initial therapy, as well as a cutaneous horn, should also be biopsied. AKs which are becoming larger, thicker, tender, or ulcerated are worrisome for SCC and also require histologic evaluation.

- The shave biopsy is an efficient, well-tolerated procedure that can provide a sufficient tissue sample for histology (described in Section 15). Yet, if the sample is too shallow and does not include a portion of the dermis, an invasive SCC could be misdiagnosed as an in situ lesion, risking incomplete treatment and recurrence.

Treatment

There are many treatment options for AKs, including watchful waiting with careful sun-safety measures. Consideration must be given to patient selection, efficacy, risks, side effects, psychosocial variables, cosmesis, compliance, cost, and duration of therapy in selecting the best treatment option for a given patient. Competent primary care providers often provide effective treatment for patients with a few, well-defined AKs using FDA-approved immunotherapy and cryotherapy. However, off-label treatment regimens with immunotherapy and more advanced procedures should be referred to experienced dermatology providers to avoid the risk of misdiagnosis, inadequate treatment, and/or complications.

Local Therapy

When there are a few clearly identified AKs, localized therapy can provide prompt and effective treatment. The knowledge and experience of the clinician providing treatment will impact the patient's experience and treatment outcomes.

- *Cryotherapy*—most widely used modality to treat isolated AKs. It is a quick, effective, and generally well-tolerated in-office procedure which does not require local anesthesia. The lesions are destroyed by freezing with liquid nitrogen (−196.5°C), which crystallizes the tumor cells, producing necrosis and tissue destruction. The freezing time varies from 2 to 5 seconds or more, with the "ice ball" extending 1 mm beyond the clinical margin. A single freeze-thaw cycle is adequate for thin lesions, while a double freeze-thaw cycle is required for thicker lesions. Blisters often form and dry into crusts, usually healing within 1 to 2 weeks. Potential adverse effects include pain, hypopigmentation, or scarring, which may be of concern in cosmetically sensitive areas. The advantage is that it requires one visit for treatment, and has been traditionally covered by insurers compared to prescription immunotherapies which can be more costly. The efficacy of liquid nitrogen cryotherapy has been evaluated in a limited number of randomized trials with a response rate ranging from 39% to 76% (Heppt et al., 2019).

- *Curettage*—used to debulk hypertrophic lesions immediately following a shave biopsy, which is sent for histology to exclude invasive SCC. A skin biopsy for histopathologic examination should be performed for indurated, painful, ulcerated, or bleeding lesions or hypertrophic actinic lesions which failed to resolve after standard therapy or have recurred rapidly (<3 months). The provider uses a curette to scrape off the friable, damaged keratinocytes until normal, firm dermal tissue is reached. Electrocautery is used to control any bleeding. The procedure should only be performed by clinicians trained and experienced with this technique. Disadvantages of curettage include risk of hypopigmented, atrophic and/or hypertrophic scarring.

Field Therapy

Patients may present with clinically well-defined AKs, or with multiple clinical and subclinical lesions in moderately and severely photodamaged skin. Subclinical lesions are not detected by visual inspection or palpation, and field cancerization describes the presence of genetically altered cells at risk of malignant transformation in clinically normal skin. There are medical and procedural options that can provide field-directed therapy to these areas including immunotherapy, photodynamic therapy (PDT), dermabrasion, chemical peels, and laser resurfacing.

- *Immunotherapy*—can be considered for both local and field therapy. There are several FDA-approved topical agents outlined in Table 2.2-1 with varied mechanisms of action, dosages, contraindications, side effects, and duration of therapy. First-line therapies include topical imiquimod and fluorouracil, while ingenol mebutate and diclofenac sodium are considered second-line strategies. In general, patients receiving topical therapy are advised to avoid application to the mucous membranes and UVR exposure during and immediately after therapy. Common side effects for almost all topical therapies include irritant contact dermatitis, burning, crusting, dryness, edema, erosion, erythema, hyperpigmentation, irritation, pain, soreness, and ulceration (Fig. 2.2-6A). Patients may struggle with the red, crusted appearance during treatment, but are usually pleased with the final cosmetic results. Additionally, topical immunotherapy effectively treats subclinical lesions (Fig. 2.2-6B).

- *PDT*—consists of topical application of a photosensitizer agent to the involved area, followed by exposure to a visible wavelength light source. Multiple trials and two meta-analyses have compared PDT with other therapies for AK finding it an effective therapy for patients with multiple AKs. Multiple PDT regimens have been used for treatment of AK. Depending on the topical photosensitizer used, the incubation times, light sources, and pretreatment regimens have varied across studies, making it difficult to compare outcomes. PDT is performed in dermatology offices and selectively causes destruction of the damaged cells. Many patients compare the experience to that of a severe sunburn. PDT has a better cosmetic result than cryotherapy and 5-fluorouracil (5-FU); however, the treatment itself causes significant discomfort and

TABLE 2.2-1	Topical Field Therapy Treatment for Actinic Keratosis		
DRUG AND MECHANISM OF ACTION	**GENERIC AND BRAND DOSING**	**SIDE EFFECTS**	**CLINICAL GUIDANCE**
Imiquimod[a] Immunomodulator	*Imiquimod* 5% cream; *Aldara* 5% cream: apply twice per wk at bedtime for 16 wk *Zyclara* 2.5% cream: nightly for 2 wk; off for 2 wk; then repeat for 2 more wk (*Zyclara 3.75% indicated for HPV*)	Redness, edema, scale, pruritus, erosions, crusts, burning, URI, flu-like symptoms, headache, photosensitivity	Should not use topical corticosteroids Treatment should be stopped when erosions or ulcerations develop
5-Fluorouracil[a] Antineoplastic and antimetabolite	*5-Fluorouracil 2*% and 5% cream, 2% solution; *Efudex* 5% cream; *Fluoroplex* 1% cream or solution: apply one to two times per day for 2–4 wk *Carac* 0.5% microsphere: apply once daily for up to 4 wk	Redness, edema, scale, pruritus, maculopapular rash, erosions or ulcers, N/V, diarrhea, stomatitis headache, photosensitivity	Can use topical corticosteroid to calm SE after therapy Treatment should be stopped when erosions or ulcerations develop
Diclofenac sodium 3% gel Nonsteroidal anti-inflammatory	*Solaraze* 3% gel Apply b.i.d. for 60–90 days Often used in combination with *hyaluronic acid* for increased percutaneous absorption	Redness, edema, scale, pruritus, erosions or ulcers **Hematologic:** Blood coagulation disorder, burning sensation in eyes, keratitis, lacrimal drainage, increased intraocular pressure **Contraindicated:** hypersensitivity to diclofenac or NSAIDs	Avoid concomitant use of NSAIDs Well tolerated in sensitive individuals sensitive to other treatments

[a]Imiquimod 5% and 5-fluorouracil 5% are also FDA approved for the treatment of superficial basal cell carcinoma, but require a different dosage regimen.

**Ingenol mebutate (Picato) is a cytotoxic topical agent that was used for treatment of actinic keratoses. Permanent discontinuation of manufacturing occurred in late 2020 after the European Medicines Agency (EMA) and the Food and Drug Administration (FDA) suspended the drug's license due to studies showing increased risk of skin malignancies.

burning. Patients must avoid all sun exposure for at least 3 days post treatment.

- **Dermabrasion**—an in-office procedure used occasionally for treatment of AKs. It physically removes the surface of the epidermis using a surgical sanding tool or laser therapy. The skin is red and abraded initially, but then heals with healthy keratinocytes.
- **Chemical peels** (medium depth)—using trichloroacetic acid or glycolic acid to exfoliate the stratum corneum and can be

effective in reducing actinic lesions. The skin can become very red and irritated initially, but then skin heals with a soft, smooth texture. Deep chemical peels are rarely used due to risk of systemic and cutaneous complications.

- **Laser resurfacing**—carbon dioxide or erbium:yttrium aluminum garnet (Er:YAG) lasers are used for the treatment of extensive actinic damage and epithelial dysplasia implicated in the development of aggressive skin cancer. Sustained efficacy with laser resurfacing has not been established.

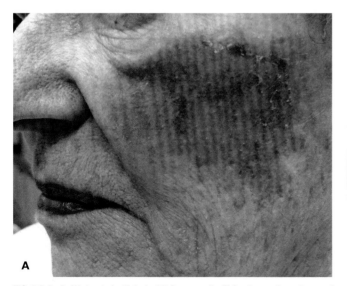

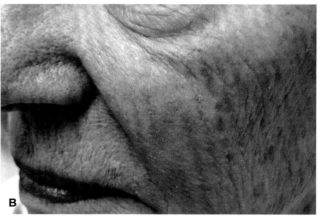

FIG. 2.2-6. A: AKs treated with topical 5-fluorouracil will develop erythematous scaly crusty patch that progressively worsens over the treatment period. **B:** One month after completed treatment, there is a mild pink patch representing postinflammatory hyperpigmentation that often fades with time.

Management and Patient Education

- Regular preventive strategies and early treatment of precancerous AKs and SCCIS are very important in immunosuppressed patients. These lesions can rapidly develop into aggressive, invasive skin cancers.

- There are few complications associated with treatment of AKs by experienced providers. Complications like scarring and systemic side effects vary with each modality. Patients may report resolution after treatment only to experience recurrence after new sun exposure. Up to 20% of AKs may progress to invasive SCC.

- Patients with an extensive number of AKs, poorly defined lesions, and those resistant to treatment should be referred to dermatology. Primary care APCs would be prudent to maintain a low threshold for referral to dermatology for management of multiple, unresponsive lesions.

- Oral nicotinamide (vitamin B3) has been found to be safe and effective in reducing the rates of new NMSC and AKs in high-risk patients (Starr, 2015).

- Patients treated for AKs must be counseled about the effectiveness, risk for recurrence, and progression.

- Recommended follow-up after completed treatment is 6 to 12 months.

CLINICAL PEARLS

- AKs are preventable with consistent, careful sun-protective and sun-safety measures. Regular application of sunscreen has been shown to actually decrease the number of AKs and thereby significantly decrease SCC development by almost 40%.

- Discerning an advancing AK from SCCIS requires histologic diagnosis made by the dermatopathologist or pathologist. Therefore, AKs with suspicious features, including sensitivity to touch or sun exposure, spontaneous bleeding, size larger than 1 cm, or location adjacent to a previously diagnosed NMSC, warrant a biopsy.

SQUAMOUS CELL CARCINOMA

While the incidence of many cancers has been on the decline, cutaneous SCC has *doubled* over the past 40 years with an estimated incidence of more than 700,000 new cases per year in the United States. This development is likely due, at least in part, to an increasing exposure of the population to UVR—especially UVB radiation. Patients who develop SCCs tend to be fair skinned with a history of chronic or intense, intermittent sun exposure and have clinical signs of solar elastosis, including freckles, lentigines, and pigmentary dyschromia.

- Historically, cutaneous SCC occurred more often in men and in older patients though female and younger patients are increasingly affected. While rare, SCC is the most common type of skin cancer that occurs in African Americans and Asian Indians.

- Melanin provides a sun protection factor (SPF) of approximately 13.4 in African-American skin, compared to 3.4 in Caucasian skin, which unfortunately creates the misconception that dark skin is invulnerable to skin cancer. SCC lesions in dark-skinned people are often diagnosed at later stages and may be more advanced and potentially fatal. The development of cutaneous SCC in these patients is often secondary to non-healing wounds or chronic inflammation.

- The metastatic rate of SCC caused by chronic UVR in Caucasians is <10%, whereas the metastatic rate of SCC caused by chronic inflammatory diseases in blacks is nearly 30% (Gloster & Neal, 2006).

- Other subsets of patients are also at increased risk for developing SCC.

  - A history of lymphoproliferative disease is an independent risk factor for SCC, which does not revert back to normal with control of the disease.

  - HIV patients are more susceptible to human papillomavirus (HPV) infections and therefore three times more likely to develop SCC than the general population.

  - The health of organ transplant recipients (OTRs) relies on immunosuppression to prevent rejection of the new organ. Unfortunately, this increases the risk of skin infections and skin cancers in this population. By 20 years post transplantation, 40% of OTRs in the United States will eventually develop skin cancers, especially SCCs which behave far more aggressively than those in immunocompetent patients.

  - Immunosuppressed patients with cutaneous SCC of the head and neck present more frequently with high-risk pathologic features and inferior outcomes (Manyam et al., 2015).

Pathophysiology

SCC is a malignant epithelial tumor arising from a proliferation of keratinocytes (squamous cells) from the epidermis. Damage to the keratinocytes results in a mutation of cellular DNA. Irregular nests of the damaged cells form a tumor which invades into the dermis.

Clinical Presentation

- Invasive SCC presents as papules, plaques, or nodules which develop in sun-exposed areas, including areas of thinning hair at the scalp and at the anterior lower extremities (Fig. 2.2-7).

- Tumors may have a smooth or hyperkeratotic surface or they may develop a cutaneous horn. The lesions grow slowly, become increasingly indurated over time, and may eventually ulcerate.

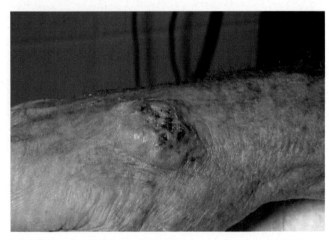

FIG. 2.2-7. SCC on the dorsal wrist presenting as a hypertrophic erythematous plaque with scale and crust. (Used with permission from Hall, J. C., Hall, B. J. [2017]. *Sauer's manual of skin diseases* [11th ed.]. Wolters Kluwer Health.)

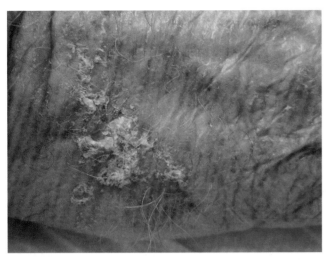

FIG. 2.2-8. SCC in situ on the hand presenting as an irregularly shaped erythematous thin plaque with thick scale.

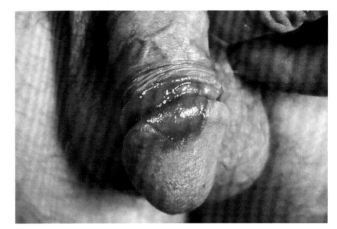

FIG. 2.2-10. Erythroplasia of Queyrat presenting as irregularly shaped erythematous smooth plaque involving the glans penis. (CDC Public Health Image Library PHIL # 17535.)

- Invasive SCC may bleed, become tender or painful.
- **Subtypes of SCC**
  - *SCCIS*—an AK which has progressed through the full thickness of the epidermis and extended into the hair follicles, which is referred to as *"follicular* or *adnexal extension."* Thicker than an AK, they have an erythematous base, can enlarge and become increasingly tender, bleed easily, or ulcerate (Fig. 2.2-8).
  - *Bowen disease*—an SCCIS which develops in hair-bearing epithelium, often in areas with limited sun exposure such as the trunk or extremities. Can look like a plaque of eczema (Fig. 2.2-9).
  - *Bowenoid papulomatosis (BP)*—Bowen disease thought to be induced by HPV. Lesions are solitary, sharply defined, red papules or plaques that ooze or crust. Usually located on the genitals and can affect both males and females. Up to 5% of BP may become invasive carcinoma.
  - *Erythroplasia of Queyrat*—an SCCIS that develops in the mucosal epithelium (glans and prepuce of the penis) often in

older, uncircumcised males. It presents as a solitary, sharply defined, shiny, red plaque which may ulcerate but is generally nontender. Up to 30% of cases may become invasive carcinoma (Fig. 2.2-10).

- *Keratoacanthoma (KA)*—a low-grade SCC variant which develops in sun-exposed areas (Fig. 2.2-11). Presents as a 1- to 2.5-cm dome-shaped, flesh-colored to red, firm nodule which can be tender. Can have central, hyperkeratotic crusting or horn, often resembling a volcano. Tumors grow very quickly and may involute within 6 months.

- *Verrucous carcinoma (VC)*—also a low-grade SCC variant developing in the genital or oral regions, but can also be found on the sole of the foot and other sites of chronic irritation and inflammation (Fig. 2.2-12). VC is an exophytic, verrucal, or fungating tumor associated with HPV. A nonaggressive tumor, however, the location of the lesions can create high morbidity for patients.

- **"High-risk" SCCs** are tumors which present a high risk for recurrence or metastasis. Lesion characteristics and patient history are

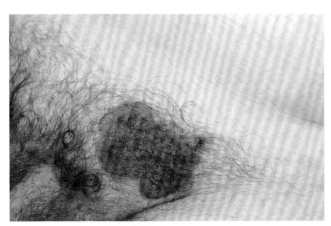

FIG. 2.2-9. Bowen disease in left pubic area presenting as a plaque-like lesion. Extramammary Paget disease and dermatitis can have similar presentations. (Used with permission from Hall, J. C., & Hall, B. J. [2017]. *Sauer's manual of skin diseases* [11th ed.]. Wolters Kluwer Health.)

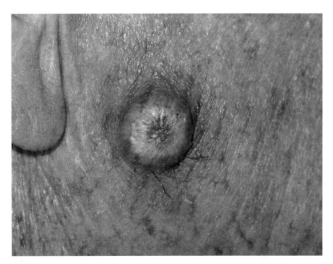

FIG. 2.2-11. Preauricular keratoacanthoma. Note marked symmetry of the lesion. (Used with permission from Hall, J. C., & Hall, B. J. [2017]. *Sauer's manual of skin diseases* [11th ed.]. Wolters Kluwer Health.)

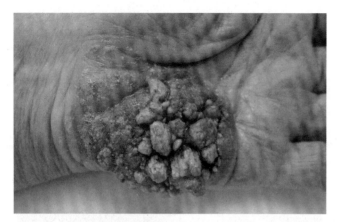

FIG. 2.2-12. Verrucous carcinoma on the palm with numerous hyperkeratotic verrucal projections from erythematous plaque.

vital for an accurate assessment of risk of recurrence of SCC. Both the National Comprehensive Cancer Network (NCCN) and the American Joint Committee on Cancer (AJCC) identify several high-risk features of cutaneous SCC which include large size, a deeply invasive lesion (>2 mm), incomplete excision, high-grade/desmoplastic lesions, perineural invasion (PNI), lymphovascular invasion, immunosuppression, and high-risk anatomic locations (Skulsky et al., 2017; Chu et al., 2014) (Fig. 2.2-13).

- *Location.* Seventy percent of SCCs develop on the head and neck and 15% on the upper extremities. SCCs which develop at the ears, lips, tongue, genitalia, and distal extremities have a much higher rate of recurrence than those that develop at other locations. The risk of nodal metastasis is fivefold greater for cutaneous SCCs on the vermilion lip compared with those on the cutaneous lip. Additionally, the scalp is increasingly being considered a high-risk location as SCC can penetrate the bony outer table of the skull (Fig. 2.2-14).

- *Size.* SCCs which are greater than 2 cm have up to three times the metastatic rate of smaller tumors.

- *Etiology.* SCCs which develop in scars, sinus tracts, chronic ulcers, and areas of previous radiation also present higher rates of recurrence (Fig. 2.2-15).

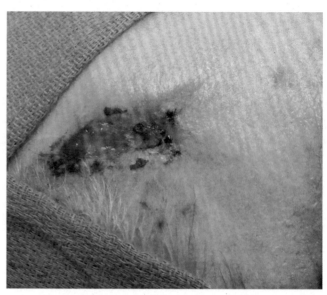

FIG. 2.2-14. Large SCC on the left parietal scalp presenting as a nonhealing wound.

- *Cellular behavior.* Certain SCC cellular subtypes may also present aggressive behavior. Those which are poorly differentiated, invade nerves (called perineural invasion or PNI), or invade blood vessels present a particularly high risk for recurrence. Patients with perineural cutaneous SCC have an increased risk of local recurrence and have a 30% risk of death compared with patients with no PNI. The presence of desmoplastic growth and tumor thickness of 6 mm or greater identify patients at high risk for tumor-specific death (Table 2.2-2).

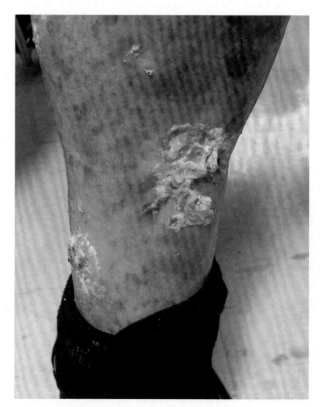

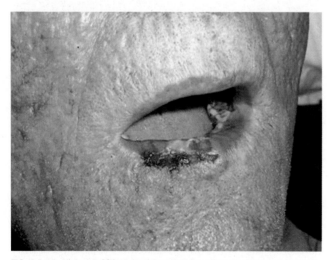

FIG. 2.2-13. High-risk SCC on the lower lip presenting on ulcerative irregularly-shaped plaque.

FIG. 2.2-15. SCC presenting as hyperkeratotic (thick) scaly irregularly shaped plaques in and around old traumatic scars on lower extremity.

TABLE 2.2-2	Risk Assessment of Nonmelanoma Skin Cancer			
TYPE OF TUMOR	**LOCATION**	**SIZE/DEPTH**	**HISTOLOGY**	**HISTORY**
Low-risk BCC	Any location including <6 mm in the H-zone (postauricular scalp, ears, preauricular cheek, temples, periorbital, eyelids, nose, lips, chin, mandible), hands and feet	<10 mm on head, forehead, cheeks, neck <20 mm on all other areas	sBCC or nodular BCC Lacks perineural invasion	Primary tumor, well defined Immunocompetent patient No history of radiation therapy at site
High-risk BCC	H-zone Hands and feet	>10 mm at the head, forehead, cheeks, neck >20 mm in all other areas	Micronodular Morpheaform Sclerosing Perineural invasion Poorly defined	Recurrent tumor Immunocompromised patient History of radiation therapy at site
Low-risk SCC	Trunk and extremities—excluding hands and feet	<20 mm Depth: epidermal: SCCIS or Bowen disease	Well differentiated	Primary tumor, well defined Immunocompetent patient No history of radiation therapy at site
High-risk SCC	Scalp, face, ears, mucosa, digits; tumors arising in scars, chronic ulcers, burns, sinus tracts, genitalia	>20 mm Invasive	Moderately differentiated Poorly differentiated Perineural invasion	Recurrent tumor, poorly defined Older age Male gender History of radiation/PUVA therapy at site Arsenic ingestion Immunocompromised patient RDEB

BCC, basal cell carcinoma; sBCC, superficial BCC; PUVA, psoralen plus ultraviolet A radiation; RDEB, recessive dystrophic epidermolysis bullosa; SCC, squamous cell carcinoma; SCCIS, squamous cell carcinoma in situ.

DIFFERENTIAL DIAGNOSIS Squamous Cell Carcinoma

- Actinic keratoses
- Basal cell carcinoma
- Seborrheic keratosis
- Psoriasis
- Eczema
- Verruca vulgaris
- Melanoma
- Extramammary Paget disease

Confirming the Diagnosis

- A shave biopsy is necessary to confirm the diagnosis of SCC. If the sample is too shallow, an invasive SCC could be misdiagnosed as in situ lesion.
- Biopsy suspicious lesions arise in highly sensitive areas, even though they may bleed profusely or heal slowly. Not doing so will risk recurrence or metastasis. Imaging studies may be indicated for clinically palpable nodes or other high-risk tumors without nodes.
- Sentinel lymph node biopsy is being considered as a new tool in staging head and neck SCC. Patients with high-risk factors (cutaneous SCC with a tumor thickness >4 mm or recurrent disease) may develop metastases within the first 2 years, despite a negative SLNB.

Treatment

SCC In Situ

- **Excision.** As SCCIS (Bowen disease) is not an invasive disease, minimization of healthy tissue excision is desirable; however,

the data show that a hypothetical reduction of the safety margin from 5 mm to 4 or 3 mm decreases the complete excision rate from 94.4% to 87% and 74.1%, respectively.

- **Electrodesiccation and Curettage (EDC).** The operative time and expense for EDC are less than those required for treatment with surgical excision.

- **Topical immunotherapy.** The available data do not support the use of topical modalities for the treatment of cutaneous SCC. The off-label use of topical imiquimod or 5-FU for the treatment of SCCIS should be reserved for use by experienced dermatology providers.

- **PDT and laser.** Available data for PDT and laser therapy do not currently support the efficacy of either modality for treatment of SCC.

Invasive SCC

- **Standard surgical excision**, with a margin of several millimeters of healthy tissue, is the gold standard for the management of most cutaneous neoplasms, including most SCCIS. Outpatient excisions offer relatively low cost, favorable patient tolerability, outpatient care, and good cosmetic results. Activity restrictions during the immediate postoperative period, and increased cost and disfigurement if flaps or grafts are required, should be considered and discussed with patients. Surgical excision offers a 5-year cure rate of over 90% for most tumors. Tissue excised during the procedure should be evaluated by pathology to assure that tissue margins are free of cancerous cells.

High-Risk Invasive SCC

- The best approach to the management of high-risk cutaneous SCC is not definitively known. Mohs micrographic surgery, surgical excision with complete circumferential peripheral and deep margin assessment (CCPDMA), radiation therapy (XRT), and immunotherapy are used in the management of these lesions.

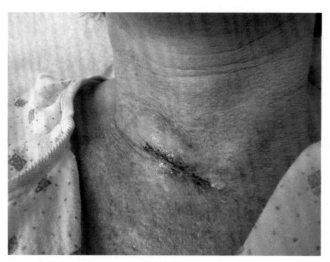

FIG. 2.2-16. Surgical excision of a cutaneous neoplasm at the anterior neck.

- Treatment modalities for SCC depend on the subtype and may include immunotherapy, standard surgical excision, Mohs micrographic surgery (MMS), XRT, or a combination. Patients with a biopsy-proven SCC should be referred to a dermatology or a Mohs surgeon for management, as these tumors can be deceptively aggressive (Fig. 2.2-16).

Mohs Micrographic Surgery (MMS)

- MMS is the standard of care for all high-risk skin cancers, high-risk patients, low-risk tumors in cosmetically sensitive areas, or those close to vital organs because of its high cure rate and tissue-sparing technique. The primary goal of MMS is to completely eradicate a tumor by examining 100% of the margins while maximally preserving normal tissue. MMS has a cure rate of 94% to 97% for primary SCC.

- MMS is typically performed in an ambulatory surgical suite. Mohs surgeons are dermatologists who go on to attend an extensive 1-year fellowship training program to establish integrated, but separate and distinct, roles as cancer surgeon, dermatopathologist, and reconstructive surgeon. The Mohs procedure entails the surgical removal of skin cancer layer by layer, then examining the tissue under a microscope while the patients wait until healthy, cancer-free tissue "clear margins" around the tumor is reached. The surgeon precisely identifies and removes the entire tumor while leaving the surrounding healthy tissue intact. Then the wound is surgically repaired (Fig. 2.2-17A–C).

- In addition to the above, advantages of MMS include the highest possible cure rate and outpatient surgical procedure. Disadvantages include the relatively limited access to Mohs surgeons nationwide, increased cost of the frozen sections performed during the procedure compared to conventional histology, and time-consuming nature of the procedure (Table 2.2-3).

Radiation Therapy (XRT)

- XRT can be successfully employed to treat NMSC and has the benefit of sparing normal, healthy tissue. The cure rate for primary NMSCs treated with XRT is over 90%, with a recurrence rate of approximately 9% (Gunaratne & Veness, 2018).

- A typical course of radiation requires multiple treatments over several weeks, with some tumors requiring up to 30 treatments. There are many potential adverse effects such as permanent

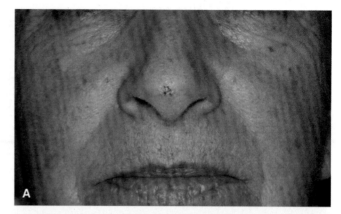

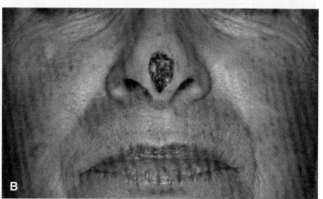

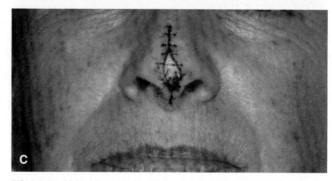

FIG. 2.2-17. Mohs micrographic surgery. **A:** Preoperative view. **B:** Postoperative view. **C:** Repair.

alopecia, chronic radiation dermatitis, and delayed radiation necrosis, which may present with initial therapy or years later.

- XRT is very expensive, does not provide margin control, can only be delivered once to a given site, and there is a small risk of developing additional skin cancers in a treated area. Radiation treatment of NMSC is usually reserved for patients who are poor surgical candidates, for adjuvant therapy for incompletely excised tumors, or for tumors that have spread to lymph nodes. XRT can be utilized for metastatic SCC to the parotid gland and adjacent lymph nodes which can be a challenging problem associated with aggressive SCCs arising in the head and neck area (Fig. 2.2-18).

Special Considerations

- Epidermal growth factor receptor inhibitors such as cetuximab or erlotinib should be considered as second-line treatment after mono- or poly-chemotherapy failure and disease progression

TABLE 2.2-3	Surgical Excision versus Mohs Micrographic Surgery
SURGICAL EXCISION	**MOHS MICROGRAPHIC SURGERY**
Description Standard for surgical management of most NMSC Removal of the entire tumor plus healthy skin margins BCC needs 3–5-mm margins SCC needs 4–6-mm margins SCC large tumor needs 10-mm margins Cure rate: small, nodular primary BCCs is 95%	**Description** Gold standard for high-risk tumors, high-risk patients, and low-risk tumors in cosmetically sensitive areas Complete removal of tumor by examining 100% of the margin, maximizing the preservation of healthy tissue
Advantages Relatively low cost Favorable patient tolerability and cosmetic result Widely accessible	**Advantages** High cure rate: primary BCC is 99%; and primary SCC is 97% Lowest rate of tumor recurrence Smaller margins create smaller surgical defects Functional and cosmetic benefit of tissue sparing at ears, eyes, lips, nose, digits, genitals
Disadvantages 1-cm margins for large SCC is equivalent to melanoma Increased cost if flaps or grafts are required Increased costs associated with tumor recurrence	**Disadvantages** Relatively limited number of Mohs surgeons Increased cost of frozen sections compared to conventional histology Time-consuming procedure Not foolproof as there may be skip areas of tumor

or within the framework of clinical trials. Among patients with advanced cutaneous squamous cell carcinoma, cemiplimab induced a response in approximately half the patients and was associated with adverse events that usually occur with immune checkpoint inhibitors.

- Organ transplant recipients (OTRs) require special consideration as the development of SCC is considered to be a sentinel event in these patients and warrants referral to a dermatology provider. Optimal patient outcomes for OTRs with SCC require collaborative efforts between the transplant team, dermatology, and primary care.

- Pretransplant skin cancer is associated with an increased risk of posttransplant skin cancer, posttransplant lymphoproliferative disorders, solid organ cancer, death, and graft failure. The development of skin cancer post transplantation portends tremendous morbidity, adversely affecting the quality of life for many transplant recipients. In the posttransplantation population, older patients, male patients, white patients, and thoracic transplant recipients had increased mortality from skin cancer.

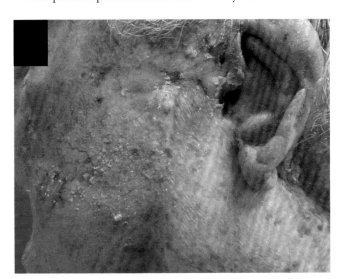

FIG. 2.2-18. Metastatic SCC at the left parotid.

- Immunosuppressed patients with cutaneous SCC of the head and neck have dramatically lower outcomes compared with immunocompetent patients, despite receiving bimodality therapy.

- Malignancy is one of the most common reasons for mortality following transplantation, and the most common of these cancers are cutaneous in origin. Recently, the incidence of these malignancies has been on the rise, partly due to the fact that recipients of these transplants are living longer as a result of improvements in surgical technique, immunosuppression, and perioperative management. Tumors classified by the Brigham & Women's Hospital as T2b/T3 identify cutaneous SCC patients who are at high risk for metastasis.

- Findings suggest that most cutaneous SCCs associated with positive sentinel lymph node biopsy findings occur in T2 lesions that are greater than 2 cm in diameter. Tumors which have the greatest potential for metastasis are those which are large (>2 cm), are located on or near the ears and lips, are poorly differentiated, or are invading nerves. Lymph node metastases from head and neck SCC tumors are associated with diminished survival rates. Moderately differentiated tumors also present an independent risk factor for lymph node metastasis.

- Additionally, patients with cutaneous SCC and chronic lymphocytic leukemia (CLL) experience higher rates of skin cancer recurrence and death than expected in an immunocompetent population.

Management and Patient Education

- SCC is generally responsive to treatment, especially when treated early. If untreated, SCC can invade the subcuticular layer, cartilage, bone, and can eventually spread to the lymphatic system leading to metastasis to solid organs, most often the lungs and the liver. Approximately 2% to 5% of cutaneous SCCs metastasize to regional lymph nodes or more distant sites.

- A patient who has had one skin cancer has an increased risk of developing another skin cancer, including melanoma. A patient who has had a first SCC has up to a 50% risk of a second SCC within 5 years. Additionally, these patients have twice the risk of developing other malignancies, such as lung, colon, and breast cancers.

- While most SCCs can be managed without significant risk for recurrence, this cancer can be deceptive as certain locations and subtypes can have small but aggressive tumors. Patients diagnosed with SCC should be referred to a dermatology provider for further evaluation of the subtype, locations, risk factors, and comorbidities, and review appropriate treatment options with the patient to establish a plan of care.

- Patients with histologically aggressive tumors or those in cosmetically or functionally sensitive locations may require comanagement with plastic surgery, oculoplastic, ENT, or radiation oncology subspecialists. Nonetheless, patients should maintain follow-up and regular monitoring with a dermatology provider.

- Patients with invasive SCC with proven regional spread are at high risk for metastatic disease and therefore require further monitoring by radiation oncology.

- There is no standardized follow-up schedule for patients with cutaneous SCC. A close follow-up plan is recommended based on risk assessment of locoregional recurrences, metastatic spread, or development of new lesions. SCC patients are generally advised to follow-up at 3- to 6-month intervals for the first year and then at 6- to 12-month intervals thereafter. It is essential to assess the effects of treatment, identify tumor recurrence, and assure early detection of any type of a new skin cancer. Lymph nodes should be carefully assessed for enlargement or tenderness.

- Patients with multiple cutaneous SCCs warrant frequent follow-up because they have an elevated risk of local recurrence and nodal metastasis. In particular, patients with 10 or more cutaneous SCCs have markedly elevated risks of recurrence and metastasis.

- The importance of skin cancer education cannot be overemphasized. In addition to the ABCDEs for early detection, patients should be counseled about sun safety. Written materials can provide helpful hints for the patient to take home (Box 2.2-1).

BASAL CELL CARCINOMA

Greater than 3 million patients in the United States have been treated for more than 5 million nonmelanoma skin cancers. Of interest, there are now equal incidence rates for BCC and SCC in the Medicare population.

- BCC is the most common human malignancy. Fair-skinned individuals are particularly susceptible at areas of sun-exposed skin, notably, the head, neck, and upper back. A long history of intense, intermittent sun exposure or of incidental blistering sunburns is common. Yet, BCC is rarely seen on the sun-exposed dorsum of the hands or lower extremities.

- Approximately 20% of BCCs arise in areas which are relatively sun protected, such as behind the ears. BCC can also develop at sites of chemical exposure or chronic trauma.

- BCC is most common in Caucasians, Asians, and light-skinned Hispanics and is rarely seen in people with dark skin color. The incidence of BCC is higher in middle-aged to older adults, with males being more affected than females.

- Approximately 40% of patients who have had a primary BCC will develop a *new* BCC within 5 years of the first and nearly 80% of *recurrent* BCCs manifest within 5 years of treatment. Patients who develop a BCC are also at increased risk of developing both SCC and melanoma (Marghoob et al., 1995).

- The risk of subsequently developing melanoma appears to be over threefold greater than the general population. Both BCC and cutaneous SCC have been associated with a modest increase in the incidence of subsequent extracutaneous malignancies.

- The development of BCC in immunosuppressed patients, especially OTRs and those with chronic lymphocytic leukemia, is particularly significant as these tumors tend to be more aggressive. There is a 10-fold increased risk of BCC in OTRs previously diagnosed with a BCC.

Pathophysiology

Basal keratinocytes are present in the epidermis and adnexal structures, which include the hair follicles. Damage to these cells is caused by radiation treatments, unprotected exposure to UVR over many years, and intense exposure to UVR from tanning beds or phototherapy. This exposure compromises the ability of the skin to repair or destroy damaged cells. It impairs the intrinsic genetic mechanisms within the DNA of epidermal cells, which should protect the cells from malignant transformation. Many years may pass before damaged cells amass into a lesion which grows slowly and invades healthy tissue.

Clinical Presentation

- Patients begin to take notice of the growth as it thickens over time and eventually ulcerates, creating the characteristic rolled borders at the periphery (Fig. 2.2-19A,B). Often the sore waxes and wanes but never fully heals, and may bleed with minimal trauma.

- BCC lesions can easily be disregarded by patients as there may be no bleeding or sensitivity initially. BCCs may exhibit periods of rapid or deeply invasive growth; however, they rarely metastasize to distant organs.

- **Subtypes of BCC**
  - ***Nodular BCCs*** (nBCCs) are the most common subtype and are at low risk for recurrence (Fig. 2.2-20). A lack of melanocytes within the tumor can give it a pearly or translucent appearance. Eventually the center erodes or ulcerates, creating rolled borders. The tumor grows larger and deeper, and small vessels known as telangiectasias can be visible within the border. The tissue is friable, leading to scarring. Occasionally, nBCCs will have flecks of pigment rendering a mottled blue or brown color. These tumors are known as pigmented BCC (pBCC) (Fig. 2.2-21) and can resemble seborrheic keratoses or melanoma. The differential diagnosis of nBCC includes angiofibroma (fibrous papule), sebaceous hyperplasia, trichoepithelioma, molluscum contagiosum, and intradermal nevus.
  - ***Superficial BCC*** (sBCC) constitutes 17% of all BCCs (Fig. 2.2-22). As the name implies, these lesions are confined to the surface of the epidermis. They present as well-defined, scaly, rough, pink to red macules, or thin plaques which often develop on the trunk and extremities. sBCCs grow slowly, but may become sensitive or bleed spontaneously. The diagnosis may be delayed because the tumor may resemble eczema, psoriasis, AKs, Bowen disease, and extramammary Paget disease (EMPD).
  - ***Micronodular BCCs*** (mnBCCs) appear similar to nBCC clinically, but behave much more aggressively. They often have significant subclinical spread, commonly referred to as "the iceberg phenomenon," and have a high risk for recurrence.

BOX 2.2-1   Sun Safety Patient Education

You don't have to avoid sunlight completely, and outdoor activity is important for good health. However, some people think about sun protection only when they spend a day at the beach, lake, or pool. Sun exposure adds up day after day, and exposure to too much sunlight can be harmful. There are some easy steps you can take to limit your exposure to UV rays.

Seek Shade. A very important way to limit your exposure to UV light is to avoid being outdoors in direct sunlight for too long, especially between the hours of 10 AM and 4 PM, even on cloudy days, when UV light is strongest. Be especially careful on the beach or in areas with sand, water, and snow as they reflect sunlight, increasing the amount of UV radiation you receive. Typical car, home, and office windows block most of the UVB rays but only a smaller portion of UVA rays; so even if you don't feel you're getting burned, your skin may still get some damage.

Wear a Hat. A hat with tightly woven fabric, a 2- to 3-in brim all around and a dark, nonreflective underside to the brim is ideal because it protects the scalp, forehead, ears, eyes, and nose, which are often exposed to intense sun. A shade cap which has about 7 in of fabric draping down the sides and back will provide more protection for the neck and can be found in sports and outdoor supply stores. (A baseball cap protects the front and top of the head but not the nose, ears, or neck where skin cancers commonly develop).

Wear Sunglasses. UV-blocking sunglasses are important for protecting the delicate skin around the eyes, as well as the eyes themselves. Research has shown that long hours in the sun without eye protection increases your chances of developing some eye diseases such as cataracts and melanoma. The ideal sunglasses should block 99% to 100% of UVA and UVB radiation. Labels that say "UV absorption up to 400 nm" or "Meets ANSI UV Requirements" mean the glasses block at least 99% of UV rays. Large-framed and wraparound sunglasses are more likely to protect your eyes from light coming in from different angles. Darker glasses are not necessarily better because UV protection comes from an invisible chemical applied to the lenses, not from the color or darkness of the lenses.

Clothing. Wear clothing to protect as much skin as possible when you are out in the sun. Long-sleeved shirts and long pants, or long skirts, cover the most skin and are the most protective. Dark colors generally provide more protection than light colors. A tightly woven fabric protects better than loosely woven clothing. Some companies such as Coolibar, L.L.Bean, and Columbia now make clothing that is lightweight, comfortable, and protects against UV exposure even when wet. Some children's swimsuits are now made from sun-protective fabric and are designed to cover the child from the neck to the knees.

Sunscreen. Sunscreen products contain one or more active drug ingredients which absorb, scatter, or reflect UV light, and which are regulated as over-the-counter (OTC) drugs by the U.S. FDA. Sunscreen can help to protect your skin against the sun's UV rays, though sunscreen should not be used as a way to prolong your time in the sun. Sunscreens are available in many forms—lotions, creams, ointments, gels, sprays, wipes, and lip balms. Sunscreens with SPF values of 30 or higher and which have broad-spectrum protection against both UVA and UVB rays are recommended. Sunscreen should be reapplied often for maximal protection. Ideally, about 1 oz of sunscreen should be reapplied at least every 2 hours and even more often if swimming or sweating.

Sunscreen products labeled "broad spectrum" provide some protection against both UVA and UVB rays, but at this time there is no standard system for measuring protection from UVA rays. Products that contain avobenzone (Parsol, 1789), ecamsule, zinc oxide, or titanium dioxide can provide some protection from most UVA rays. The sun protection factor "SPF" number is the level of protection the sunscreen provides against UVB rays; a higher number means more protection. SPF 15 sunscreens filter out about 93% of UVB rays, while SPF 30 sunscreens filter out about 97%, and SPF 50 sunscreens filter out about 98%.

Choosing a Sunscreen. Physical sunscreens (titanium dioxide, zinc oxide) act to reflect and scatter both visible and UV light, yet tend to be thick, stain clothing, and clog pores. Chemical sunscreens (PABA) absorb UV radiation, and typically have a limited spectrum of protection. Sunscreens which combine both physical and chemical agents are also available.

Avoid Tanning Beds and Sun Lamps. Tanning lamps give out UVA and usually UVB rays as well. This intense exposure to both UVA and UVB rays causes long-term skin damage which contributes to the development of skin cancer. Tanning bed use has been linked with an increased risk of melanoma, the deadliest form of skin cancer, especially if tanning is started before the age of 30. If you want a tan, consider using a sunless tanning lotion, which can provide a darker look without the danger.

Children. Children tend to spend more time outdoors than adults, can burn more easily, and may not be aware of the dangers. Caregivers should protect children from excess sun exposure by using the steps above. If you or your child burns easily, be extra careful to cover up, limit exposure, and apply sunscreen specially formulated for children. Children need smaller versions of real, protective sunglasses—not toy sunglasses. Babies younger than 6 months should be kept out of direct sunlight and should be protected from the sun by using umbrellas, hats, and protective clothing.

Vitamin D. Vitamin D is an essential nutrient that is vital for strong bones, a healthy immune system, and may help to lower the risk for some cancers. Your skin makes vitamin D naturally when you are in the sun. How much vitamin D you make depends on many things, including how old you are, how dark your skin is, and how strong the sunlight is where you live. Dermatologists recommend that vitamin D should be safely obtained from a healthy diet that includes dairy products and fish, which are naturally rich in vitamin D, milk and cereals which are fortified with vitamin D, and/or vitamin D supplements—not from UV exposure.

- *Infiltrative BCCs* may resemble a KA or SCC (Fig. 2.2-23). These tumors also behave aggressively and extend both peripherally and vertically (depth). As such, it accounts for the high risk for recurrence.

- *Morpheaform* or *sclerosing BCCs* represent only 1% of all BCCs; and are characteristically sclerotic plaques with a waxy, atrophic, white surface (Fig. 2.2-24). They are commonly asymptomatic and easily mistaken for a scar or scleroderma. Morpheaform BCCs extend far beyond the visible surface, resulting in very high rates of recurrence.

- *Nevoid basal cell syndrome* is a rare autosomal dominant disease caused by a mutation of the tumor suppressor *PTCH*

DIFFERENTIAL DIAGNOSIS   Basal Cell Carcinoma

- Angiofibroma
- Fibrous papule
- Sebaceous hyperplasia
- Trichoepithelioma
- Molluscum contagiosum
- Intradermal nevus
- Amelanotic melanoma
- Morphea

- Eczema
- Psoriasis
- Actinic keratoses
- Bowen disease
- Extramammary Paget disease
- Keratoacanthoma
- Squamous cell carcinoma

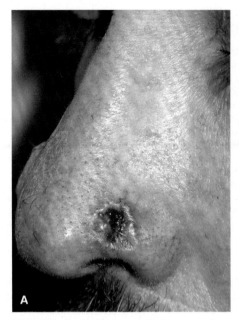

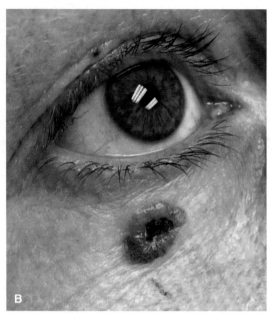

FIG. 2.2-19. Basal cell carcinoma presenting as ulcerative papules with central crusted depression, rolled border, and arborizing telangiectasias on the rim. **A:** BCC left nares. **B:** BCC lower orbital rim. (Photo A used with permission from Hall, J. C., & Hall, B. J. [2017]. *Sauer's manual of skin diseases* [11th ed.]. Wolters Kluwer Health; Photo B is courtesy of D. Diruggiero.)

gene. Multiple BCCs develop in childhood and are associated with pitted palms and soles, cysts in the jaw, calcification of falx cerebri, skeletal abnormalities, and coarse facial features.

Confirming the Diagnosis

- Once skin cancer is suspected, a skin biopsy must be obtained both to confirm the diagnosis of BCC and also to identify its subtype.
- Shave biopsy is a simple, effective means to diagnose BCC (discussed earlier under SCC). A deep shave (scoop) or complete excisional biopsy is advised if melanoma (including amelanotic melanoma) is in the differential diagnosis. This would allow for the evaluation of the depth of tumor invasion. A punch biopsy may be preferential in certain locations as the cosmetic result is often superior to that of a shave biopsy; but it is preferred by pathologists that the entire specimen be submitted (see Section 15).

Treatment

Most BCCs are curable when treated promptly; however, some have a high rate of recurrence. Treatment of BCC is indicated to prevent ulceration, gross disfigurement, and invasion into the local subcuticular layer, nerve, muscle, cartilage, and bone. When evaluating treatment options for biopsy-proven BCC, the provider must first determine the tumor subtype and risk for recurrence (Table 2.2-2). Tumor size, location, and patient history will also impact the clinician's treatment approach. A visual reminder of the "H-zone," representing high-risk locations on the head, can be helpful to clinicians (Fig. 2.2-25). The National Comprehensive Cancer Network clinical

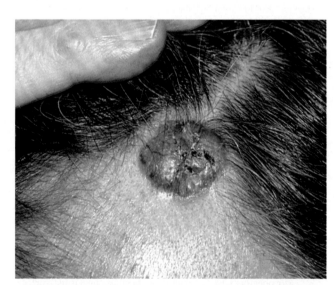

FIG. 2.2-21. Pigmented BCC on the frontal hairline presenting as an erythematous to bluish purple plaque with central ulcer. (Used with permission from Goodheart, H. P. [2003]. *Goodheart's photoguide of common skin disorders* [2nd ed.]. Lippincott Williams & Wilkins.)

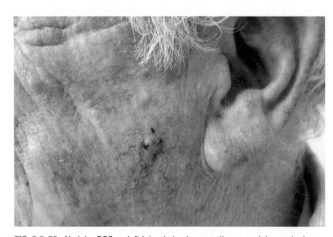

FIG. 2.2-20. Nodular BCC on left lateral cheek presenting as a pink, pearly dome-shaped papule.

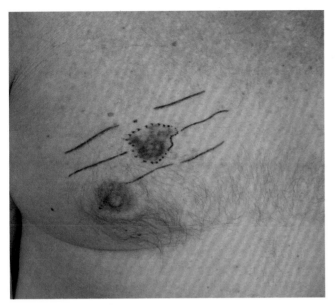

FIG. 2.2-22. Superficial BCC on the right chest presenting as erythematous patch. Superficial BCC can be mistaken as dermatitis. Note the markings preparing for Mohs surgical removal. (Used with permission from Hall, J. C., & Hall, B. J. [2017]. *Sauer's manual of skin diseases* [11th ed.]. Wolters Kluwer Health.)

practice guidelines on cutaneous BCC identify the likelihood for tumor recurrence after treatment.

- Low-risk features include:

  - Location and size: <10 mm in diameter in M areas (cheeks, forehead, scalp, neck, pretibial) and <20 mm in diameter in area L (trunk and extremities, excluding pretibia, hands, feet, nail unit, and ankles),

  - Pathology: nodular or superficial histopathologic growth pattern and lack of PNI, and

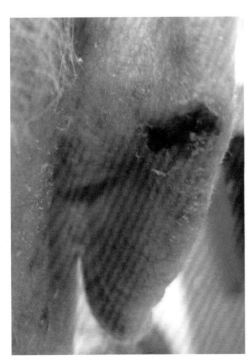

FIG. 2.2-23. Infiltrative BCC at the posterior ear.

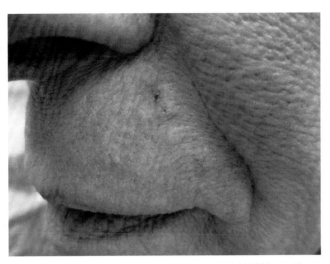

FIG. 2.2-24. Morpheaform BCC near the left superior nasolabial fold presenting as a white scar-like atrophic papule.

- Other: primary lesion (not recurrent), well-defined clinical borders, no history of XRT at the site and immunocompetent patients.

Superficial BCC

- *Topical immunotherapy* may be used alone or in combination with other treatment modalities. Prescribers should become familiar with common side effects, advantages, and disadvantages of these topical therapies or refer to a dermatology specialist experienced with these treatment modalities.

- *Fluorouracil* is an antimetabolite that inhibits DNA synth and cell proliferation, resulting in tumor necrosis. Topical fluorouracil 5% cream or solution is an FDA-approved topical treatment for superficial BCC, not for invasive lesions. It is applied twice daily for 4 to 6 weeks.

- *Imiquimod* stimulates immune responses resulting in antiviral, antitumor, and immune-regulatory properties. Topical imiquimod 5% is FDA approved for treatment of superficial BCCs with a maximum diameter of 2 cm on the neck, trunk, or extremities (excluding hands and feet). The patient applies it to the area daily at bedtime, 5 days per week for up to 12 weeks.

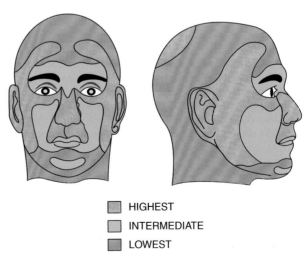

■ HIGHEST
■ INTERMEDIATE
■ LOWEST

FIG. 2.2-25. "H-zone" showing most common areas of skin cancer recurrence.

- *Photodynamic Therapy (PDT).* Although PDT has been approved in Europe, Canada, Australia, and other countries worldwide for the treatment of superficial and small nBCC, when other available therapies are not acceptable, there is a high recurrence rate. FDA approval has not been granted for the treatment of BCC with PDT.

- *Cryosurgery.* Freezing with liquid nitrogen crystallizes the tumor cells, induces localized frostbite, and produces necrosis and tissue destruction of the tumor. It can be used for the destruction of low-risk BCC; however, there is considerable risk for tumor recurrence which can develop undetected in the deep dermis. Cryosurgery is a quick, in-office, and low-cost procedure but can be painful, requires lengthy wound care, and may cause hypopigmentation or scarring. Cryosurgery should not be confused with *cryotherapy,* which is a common procedure used to treat premalignant AKs or benign warts.

- *Electrodesiccation and curettage* (ED&C or EDC) may be used to treat small, low-risk BCCs at low-risk locations (i.e., the neck, trunk, and extremities). After local anesthetics are given, friable tumor cells are easily curetted off until normal, firm dermal tissue is reached. Any remaining tissue is destroyed with electrocautery, which also controls any bleeding. The wound is then left to heal by secondary intention. Clinicians performing ED&C, especially in cosmetically sensitive areas, should be sure to discuss the risks and side effects before the procedure. Disadvantages of ED&C include slow healing, the risk for hypopigmented, atrophic and/or hypertrophic scarring, tissue contraction, and the lack of margin control. Burns and interference with cardiac defibrillators are rare but may cause serious potential adverse effects. Advantages of ED&C include the speed of the procedure and its relatively low cost. Recurrence rates are low at 3% to 6% for primary BCC <1 cm.

Low-Risk BCC

- *Surgical excision* is first-line therapy for BCC at low risk of recurrence. Surgical excision with 4 to 5 mm margins and postoperative margin assessment is recommended for primary nodular or superficial low-risk BCCs (<10 mm) located in noncritical head and neck areas (i.e., cheeks, forehead, scalp, neck) with a 5-year cure rate of 95%. Mean recurrence rates for BCCs increased incrementally when surgical margins were decreased from 5 to 2 mm. A recent literature review concluded that for BCC lesions 2 cm or smaller, with low risk, a 3-mm surgical margin can be safely utilized. (Quazi et al., 2020).

- Surgical excision with 4- to 5-mm margins is advised as first-line therapy for primary nBCCs <20 mm on trunk or extremities. C&E is an alternative option.

- **Incompletely excised lesions**. MMS is recommended for the management of incompletely excised BCCs located on the face. Standard surgical reexcision is an appropriate option for incompletely excised lesions located on the trunk or extremities. Lesions that cannot be completely removed with Mohs micrographic surgery can be treated with postoperative radiation.

High-Risk BCC

The NCCN guidelines for basal cell skin cancer include recommendations for selecting among the various surgical approaches based on patient, lesion, and disease-specific factors, as well as guidance on when to use XRT, superficial therapies, and hedgehog pathway inhibitors. In the absence of a formal staging system, the best available stratification is based on risk for recurrence. These guidelines also offer recommendations on treatment modalities

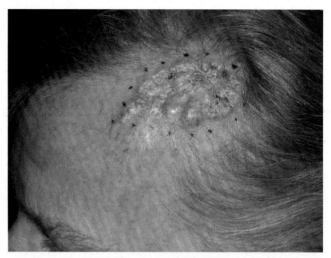

FIG. 2.2-26. High-risk large BCC on left frontal scalp.

along a broad therapeutic spectrum, ranging from topical agents and superficially destructive modalities to surgical techniques and systemic therapy.

- **Excision**—not surprisingly, the risk of recurrence increases when using simple surgical excision in the treatment of high-risk BCCs (Table 2.2-2) and is therefore not the treatment of choice for high-risk BCCs. MMS has a much higher cure rate, but simple surgical excision may be an appropriate treatment modality for some patient circumstances. Examples include lack of proximity to a Mohs surgeon or the inability of an elderly patient to tolerate a lengthy procedure. However, whenever possible, assessment of all margins is optimal for high-risk tumors.

- **Mohs micrographic surgery**—as detailed in the *Management of SCC,* is considered the gold standard for high-risk basal cell carcinoma (Fig. 2.2-26). MMS is associated with the lowest recurrence rates for primary BCC at only 1% (Table 2.2-3). Fewer recurrences occur after treatment of high-risk facial BCC with MMS compared to treatment with surgical excision. For BCC in the periocular region, MMS should be the treatment of choice for both primary and recurrent periocular BCCs.

- **Radiation therapy (XRT)**—XRT can be successfully employed to treat patients with NMSC and may be a favorable option for BCC arising on or near the eyelids, nose, ears, and lips. The procedure, advantages, and disadvantages of XRT are also discussed in *Management of SCC.* Local recurrence rates for postoperatively irradiated tumors were 3.6% for BCCs and 11.5% for SCCs (Visch et al., 2019).

- **Advanced and metastatic disease.** Hedgehog inhibitor therapy (HHIT) is a small molecule, highly potent, selective inhibitor of smoothened receptors which offers an effective systemic treatment for extensive BCCs. Vismodegib (Erivedge) is FDA approved for locally advanced and metastatic BCC. Sonidegib (Odomzo) is FDA approved for locally advanced BCC but *not* for metastatic disease. The mean response rate is 44% to 58% for advanced disease and 8% to 17% for metastatic BCC (Bichakjian et al., 2018). HHIT can decrease the morbidity of surgical treatment and increase the likelihood of curative resection. For patients with extensive BCC, a combined neoadjuvant use of HHIT and surgical treatment might be considered (Ching et al., 2015). Studies suggest that there is a clear role for Vismodegib as neoadjuvant in locally advanced periocular BCC, even in operable cases (González et al., 2019).

Special Considerations

It is not unusual for frail elders or patients who are affected by multiple comorbidities to present with BCCs. These patients and their families may question the appropriateness of treatment for BCC lesions which grow slowly and rarely metastasize. In some situations, it may be reasonable to consider less aggressive therapeutic modalities such as scoop shave excision or ED&C rather than attempting multiple XRT sessions or a lengthy MMS. Treatment decisions for BCCs in complex elderly patients with significant comorbidities should begin with a thoughtful discussion between the patient, family, and dermatology provider.

Management and Patient Education

- The procedure, advantages, and disadvantages of surgical excision are the same as discussed in *Management of SCC*.

- The prognosis for the majority of BCCs is excellent. Even large lesions and those in sensitive locations have very high cure rates with appropriate treatment, but they do have increased risk for significant local invasion if treatment is delayed or inadequate. Untreated or incompletely treated BCC can ultimately invade local soft tissue, nerves, vessels, cartilage, and bone, resulting in significant deformity and morbidity.

- Although the rate of metastasis for BCC is less than 1%, once they spread, these tumors can be extremely aggressive and result in high mortality rates. Common sites for metastasis include the regional lymph nodes, lungs, bones, skin, and liver.

- Patients may misunderstand that biopsy alone is curative. In fact, even after treatment, it is not uncommon for patients to have the misconception that BCCs are not cancerous growths. Follow-up is required to detect both local recurrences and new skin cancers and to assess posttreatment effects. Most dermatologists recommend reevaluation every 6 months for the 1 to 2 years following treatment and then annually; some recommend every 6 months for life.

- As with all skin cancers, patient morbidity from BCC will be minimized by early detection. Providers can help to prevent this common cancer by identifying patients at risk for skin cancer, detecting potentially cancerous lesions, and referring patients to dermatology as appropriate. Performing a complete skin cancer screening examination carefully and methodically with optimal tangential light will increase the likelihood of identifying even very small asymptomatic lesions.

- Patient education for skin cancer prevention and early detection is the foundation of high-quality patient care (see Box 2.2-1).

- The procedure, advantages, and disadvantages of surgical excision are the same as discussed in *Management of SCC*.

OTHER CUTANEOUS MALIGNANCIES

Merkel Cell Carcinoma (MCC)

MCC is an uncommon, aggressive neuroendocrine (sensory cell) carcinoma of the skin with a rapidly increasing rate of occurrence. The development of MCC is strongly associated with ages over 65 years, fair skin or a history of extensive sun exposure, and chronic immune suppression. Susceptible patients include older Caucasians and those with a history of organ transplantation, HIV/AIDS, leukemia, and lymphoma. In fact, MCC is 15 times more likely to develop in OTRs and at a significantly younger age than in their immunocompetent counterparts.

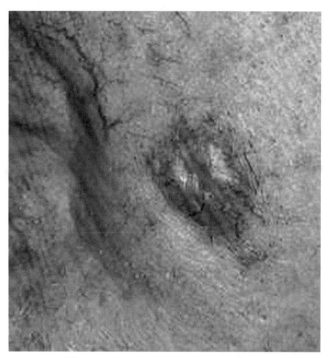

FIG. 2.2-27. MCC on the cheek presenting as dome-shaped nodule with notable arborizing telangiectasias. Similar presentation to BCC.

Pathophysiology

Merkel cells are neuroendocrine cells which reside in the epidermal basal layer and are presumably the origin of this tumor. The etiology of MCC suggests a possible infectious component associated with Merkel cell polyomavirus with a growth pattern classified as circumscribed or infiltrative. The tumors are fast growing and aggressive with a propensity for early, in-transit regional, nodal, and distant metastasis.

Clinical Presentation

- MCCs are firm, smooth, shiny, dome-shaped, flesh-colored to red, nontender nodules with telangiectasia which develop rapidly and asymptomatically over approximately 6 months.

- Lesions vary from small 2-mm to large 8-cm size nodules usually found on sun-exposed areas of the head and neck. Yet, tumors can also occur on the trunk or extremities (Fig. 2.2-27).

- MCCs have high rates of recurrence, often far from the original tumor, and have high rates of metastatic spread.

DIFFERENTIAL DIAGNOSIS   Merkel Cell Carcinoma
• Basal cell carcinoma
• Squamous cell carcinoma
• B-cell lymphoma
• Sebaceous cyst
• Cutaneous lymphoma
• Melanoma
• Cutaneous metastasis of carcinoma

Confirming the Diagnosis

A deep shave, punch biopsy, or complete elliptical excision is appropriate for diagnosis.

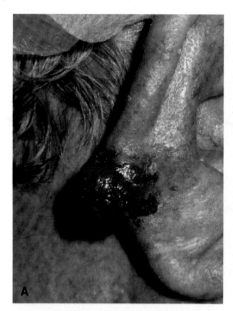
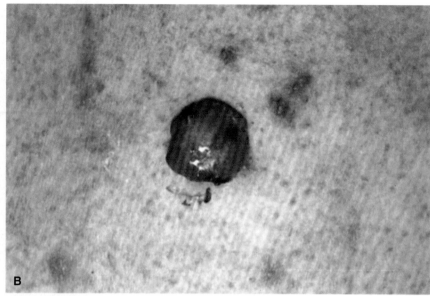

FIG. 2.2-28. Atypical fibroxanthoma (AFX), which can look like a BCC, SCC, or amelanotic nodular melanoma. **A:** AFX on the right helical rim appeared as a friable nonhealing papule. **B:** AFX as a rapidly growing symmetrical nodule on the trunk of an elderly man. (Photo A used with permission from Requena, L., & Kutzner, H. [2014]. *Cutaneous soft tissue tumors.* Wolters Kluwer Health; Photo B used with permission from Elder, D. [2020]. *Atlas of dermatopathology* [4th ed.]. Wolters Kluwer Health.)

Treatment

- Patients with MCC are at high risk for metastasis, requiring rapid consultation and management by an oncologist, Mohs surgeon, and dermatologist.
- Wide excision with concomitant sentinel lymph node biopsy is necessary. Other imaging studies may be ordered.

Management and Patient Education

- MCCs are aggressive tumors with a propensity for early, in-transit regional, nodal, and distant metastasis indicating the need for sentinel lymph node biopsy with *all* primary MCCs. Most tumors recur within 8 to 24 months. Despite surgical excision, 45% to 91% of patients develop regional node involvement, and 18% to 52% of patients develop distant metastasis. The 5-year survival rate is 40% to 75% for a primary tumor (Tarantola et al., 2013).
- Patients with a history of MCC should be followed at 3-month intervals by dermatology and oncology. Primary care clinicians should be vigilant in ensuring that the patient complete age-appropriate health screening examinations in addition to other diagnostics as indication for new complaints. Additionally, the patient's first-degree relatives should also undergo annual full-body skin cancer screening examinations.

Atypical Fibroxanthoma

Atypical fibroxanthoma (AFX) is an intradermal, spindle cell tumor of mesenchymal origin occurring most commonly on the head and neck (Fig. 2.2-28A,B). AFX has a low-to-moderate potential for metastasis. Tumor recurrence is most commonly due to incomplete excision.

Clinical Presentation

- The lesions most often present as small, firm nodules with eroded or crusted surfaces in patients with fair skin or a history of extensive sun exposure.

Treatment

- The recommended treatment is Mohs surgery.

Dermatofibrosarcoma Protuberans (DFSP)

DFSP is a relatively unusual primary cutaneous malignancy which is classified as a low-grade sarcoma. DFSP is a dermal tumor which has a propensity for deep invasion and extensive subclinical spread (Fig. 2.2-29). It has a subtle appearance and grows slowly. Lesions can invade subcutaneous tissue, muscle, fascia, and bone, but metastasis is rare.

Clinical Presentation

- One or multiple ill-defined, erythematous, firm nodules or plaques. Most lesions occur on the trunk, particularly at the

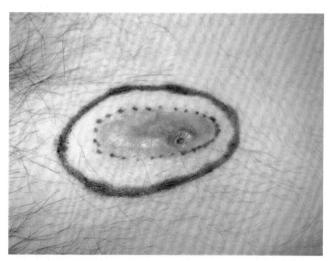

FIG. 2.2-29. Dermatofibrosarcoma protuberans at the abdomen presenting as a smooth, poorly defined flesh toned to pink–tan plaque.

shoulder or abdomen, though they can also develop at the head and neck. DFSP affects young- to middle-aged adults and may be associated with trauma.

- Tentacle-like extensions of tumor create a high incidence of local recurrence. The slow-growing, poorly defined nature of the lesions often results in delayed diagnosis, which allows tumors to become quite large.

Treatment

- Excision of DFSP with 3-cm margins, even down to the fascia, has a recurrence rate of 20%.
- MMS, with a recurrence rate of <3%, is therefore the treatment of choice.

Microcystic Adnexal Carcinoma

Microcystic adnexal carcinoma (MAC) usually presents as a poorly defined, erythematous, or hemorrhagic plaque. The tumor often invades nerves and may invade subcutaneous fat, muscle, cartilage, bone, salivary glands, and lymph nodes; and while unlikely to metastasize, tumor recurrence can occur many years following initial excision.

Clinical Presentation

- Deeply invasive, poorly defined plaque which may be red or hemorrhagic.
- Frequently located periorally, perinasally, periocularly, or on the scalp.
- Often develops in previously irradiated skin.

Treatment

- MMS

Sebaceous Carcinoma

Sebaceous carcinoma (SC) is a rare, invasive tumor which most often appears at the upper eyelids. SC is an aggressive tumor which can invade orbital structures. Approximately one in four patients experience regional lymph node metastasis, with possible distal spread to muscle, liver, spleen, viscera, and brain. It is associated with Muir–Torre syndrome.

Clinical Presentation

- Often present as a painless, yellow nodule or plaque on the upper eyelids.

Treatment

- Surgical oncologist or Mohs surgeon with experience in ocular reconstruction.

Extramammary Paget Disease

Extramammary Paget disease (EMPD) is a rare, slow-growing intraepithelial adenocarcinoma derived from keratinocytes in the epidermis which can affect anogenital skin (outside of the mammary gland). It occurs more often in older women (see also Section 11-4).

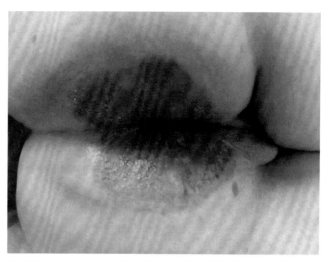

FIG. 2.2-30. Extramammary Paget disease on the perianal area presenting as an erythematous macerated eroded plaque ("strawberries & cream"). (Courtesy of Jeremy Honaker.)

Clinical Presentation

Lesions are large, eczematous, and erythematous plaques which may be asymptomatic or painful. EMPD is characteristically very pruritic (Fig. 2.2-30).

DIFFERENTIAL DIAGNOSIS   Extramammary Paget Disease
• Eczematous dermatitis
• Psoriasis
• Tinea
• Seborrheic dermatitis
• Lichen sclerosis
• Lichen planus

Confirming the Diagnosis

- Suspicious lesions should be biopsied if they do not resolve after 3–4 weeks of treatment.

Treatment

- MMS is the standard of care, but there is still a 10% to 12% rate of recurrence; and 25% of patients have a nonassociated genitourinary, rectal, or breast carcinoma (Shepherd et al., 2005).

PRIMARY CUTANEOUS LYMPHOMAS

Cutaneous T-Cell Lymphoma

Cutaneous T-cell lymphoma (CTCL) is a class of non-Hodgkin lymphoma that is not a skin cancer, but manifests its symptoms in the skin. The cause of this non-Hodgkin lymphoma is unclear. There is a higher incidence in African Americans than in Caucasians and in those over 60 years old. Males are twice as likely to develop CTCL than females. Patients with CTCL have an increased incidence of secondary cancers, especially lymphoma.

The disease presents in the skin, but can also affect the lymph nodes, blood, and internal organs.

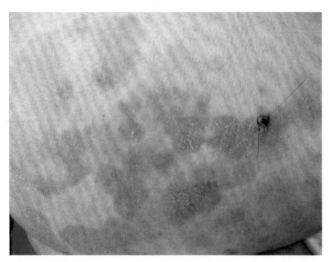

FIG. 2.2-31. CTCL at the left buttock presenting as erythematous thin patches and plaques with a fine scale.

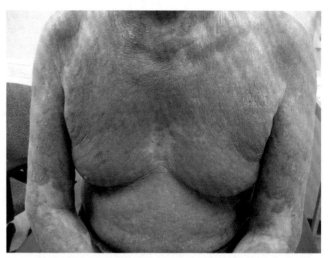

FIG. 2.2-32. Mycosis fungoides with confluent erythematous plaques covering most of the body. (Used with permission from Hall, J. C., & Hall, B. J. [2017]. *Sauer's manual of skin diseases* [11th ed.]. Wolters Kluwer Health.)

Pathophysiology

A mutation of the T cells in the immune system can result in the migration of the malignant T cells to the skin. They can cause a variety of lesions to develop and may produce erythema and itching of the skin. The most common subtypes of CTCL are mycosis fungoides (MF) and Sezary syndrome (SS).

Clinical Presentation

Mycosis Fungoides

- Patients with MF have skin lesions which are persistent and become increasingly progressive. The importance of recognizing potential MF should not be underemphasized as it can easily be misdiagnosed for common dermatoses such as psoriasis, eczema, and tinea.
- Categories of skin lesions
  - **Patches**—often large (>5 cm) and vary in size, shape, and color (Fig. 2.2-31).
  - **Plaques**—well defined and are dusky to violaceous red color.
  - **Tumor stage**—usually means a more aggressive form of MF. Tumors are red and dusky and may ulcerate. They commonly occur around the head, neck, groin, breasts, and axillary areas.
  - **Erythroderma**—advanced disease may present with erythroderma, severe scale, bright-red patches or plaques covering ≥90% BSA. It is often accompanied by intense pruritus, fever, chills, and malaise (Fig. 2.2-32).
- It is not uncommon for initial lesions to be ill-defined, scaly plaques which require repeated biopsies before the diagnosis is made.
- Eventually, the lesions present with mixed morphology and lesions from all stages and/or erythroderma which can be localized or widespread.
- The histopathologic criteria can be difficult to identify due to inflammation in the skin. A dermatology referral can be helpful in determining the diagnosis of MF.

Sezary Syndrome

- Sezary syndrome (SS) refers to systemic involvement of MF.
- The skin may appear like erythroderma or become flaky. Patients may experience feeling hot, sore, or sensitive accompanied by intense pruritus. Additional symptoms may include hyperkeratosis at the palms and soles, alopecia, onychodystrophy, and ptosis.
- SS is a chronic and advanced form of MF. Approximately 10% of patients with MF have atypical lymphocytes (Sezary cells) in their blood and erythroderma of 80% to 90% of their body surface area.
- Diffuse lymphadenopathy is often reported.

DIFFERENTIAL DIAGNOSIS   Cutaneous T-Cell Lymphoma
• Psoriasis
• Nummular eczema
• Tinea
• Drug eruption—Sezary
• Photodermatitis—Sezary

Treatment

Once suspected, MF should be referred to a dermatology provider experienced in the care of CTCL patients who can further evaluate and stage the disease. Staging, based on the primary tumor, regional lymph nodes, metastasis, and serum studies, provides treatment guidelines and prognostic value.

- **Limited cutaneous involvement**—topical corticosteroids, topical chemotherapy (nitrogen mustard), topical retinoids, local radiation, and narrow-band UVB phototherapy.
- **Systemic/Sezary syndrome**—treatment options include systemic retinoids, immunotherapies, extracorporeal photopheresis, chemotherapy, and bone marrow or stem cell transplantation.

Management

- Patients with CTCL should be immediately referred to a dermatology or oncologist provider experienced in managing the disease.

Cutaneous B-Cell Lymphoma

The disease seems to start as a hyper reactive inflammatory response related to an immunodeficiency disorder, a viral infection, or a bacterial infection.

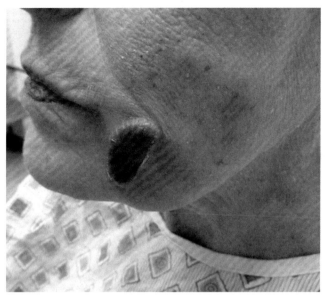

FIG. 2.2-33. Cutaneous B-cell lymphoma at the lower cheek presenting as erythematous to maroon tumor.

Pathophysiology

A mutation of the B cells of the immune system can result in the migration of the malignant B cells to the skin or lymphoproliferation.

DIFFERENTIAL DIAGNOSIS   Cutaneous B-Cell Lymphoma
• B-cell pseudolymphoma
• CTCL
• BCC

Clinical Presentation

- Solitary or multiple red nodules or plaques on the head, trunk, or extremities (Fig. 2.2-33).

Treatment

- Treatment options include surgical excision for a solitary lesion, antibiotic therapy (doxycycline or cefotaxime), or radiotherapy for multiple lesions.

- The prognosis of the most common marginal zone B-cell lymphomas (MZL) is excellent with a 5-year survival rate of greater than 90% (Fig. 2.2-33).

READINGS AND REFERENCES

Ad Hoc Task Force; Connolly, S. M., Baker, D. R., Coldiron, B. M., Fazio, M. J., Storrs, P. A., Vidimos, A. T., Zalla, M. J., Brewer, J. D., Begolka, W. S., Ratings Panel; Berger, T. G., Bigby, M., Bologna, J. L., Brodland, D. G., Collins, S., Cronin, T. A., Jr., Dahl, M. V., Grant-Kels, J. M., Hanke, W. C.,...Wisco, O. J. (2012). AAD/ACMS/ASDSA, ASMS 2012 appropriate use criteria for Mohs micrographic surgery: A report of the American Academy of Dermatology, American College of Mohs Surgery, American Society for Dermatologic Surgery Association and the American Society for Mohs Surgery. *Journal of the American Academy of Dermatology, 67*(4), 531–550.

Alam, M., Armstrong, A., Baum, C., Bordeaux, J. S., Brown, M., Busam, K. J., Eisen, D. B., Iyengar, V., Lober, C., Margolis, D. J., Messina, J., Miller, A., Miller, S., Eliot Mostow, E., Mowad, C., Nehal, K., Schmitt-Burr, K., Aleksandar Sekulic, A., . . . Phillip Rodgers, P. (2018). Guidelines of care for the management of basal cell carcinoma. *Journal of the American Academy of Dermatology, 78*(3), 540–559.

American Cancer Society (ACS). (n.d.). *Cancer facts and figures 2019.* https://www.cancer.org/research/cancer-facts-statistics/all-cancer-facts-figures/cancer-facts-figures-2019.html

Bath-Hextall, F., Ozolins, M., Armstrong, S. J., Colver, G. B., Perkins, W., Miller, P. S. J., & Williams, H. C.; Surgery versus Imiquimod for Nodular Superficial basal cell carcinoma (SINS) study group. (2014). Surgical excision versus imiquimod 5% cream for nodular and superficial basal-cell carcinoma (SINS): A multicentre, non-inferiority, randomised controlled trial. *The Lancet Oncology, 15*, 96–105.

Bichakjian, C. K., Olencki, T., Aasi, S. Z., Alam, M., Andersen, J. S., Berg, D., Bowen, G. M., Cheney, R. T., Daniels, G. A., Glass, L. F., Grekin, R. C., Grossman, A., Higgins, S. A., Ho, A. L., Lewis, K. D., Lydiatt, D. D., Nehal, K. S., Nghiem, P., Olsen, E. A.,...Engh, A. (2016). Basal cell skin cancer, version 1.2016, NCCN clinical practice guidelines in oncology. *Journal of the National Comprehensive Cancer Network, 14*(5), 574–597.

Chen, A. C., Martin, A. J., Choy, B., Fernández-Peñas, P., Dalziell, R. A., McKenzie, C. A., Scolyer, R. A., Dhillon, H. M., Vardy, J. L., Kricker, A., George, G., Chinniah, N., Halliday, G. M., & Damia, D. L. (2015). A phase 3 randomized trial of nicotinamide for skin-cancer chemoprevention. *The New England Journal of Medicine, 373*(17), 1618–1626.

Ching, J. A., Curtis, H. L., Braue, J. A., Kudchadkar, R. R., Mendoza, T. I., Messina, J. L., Cruse, C. W., Smith, D. J., Jr., & Harrington, M. A. (2015). The impact of neoadjuvant hedgehog inhibitor therapy on the surgical treatment of extensive basal cell carcinoma. *Annals of Plastic Surgery, 74*(4), S193–S197.

Chu, M. B., Slutsky, J. B., Dhandha, M., Beal, B. T., Armbrecht, E. S., Walker, R. J., Varvares, M. A., & Fosko, S. W. (2014). Evaluation of the definitions of "high-risk" cutaneous squamous cell carcinoma using the American Joint Committee on Cancer staging criteria and National Comprehensive Cancer Network guidelines. *Journal of Skin Cancer, 2014*, 154–340.

Eigentler, T. K., Leiter, U., Häfner, H. M., Garbe, C., Röcken, M., & Breuninger, H. (2017). Survival of patients with cutaneous squamous cell carcinoma: Results of a prospective cohort study. *The Journal of Investigative Dermatology, 137*(11), 2309–2315.

Garrett, G. L., Lowenstein, S. E., Singer, J. P., He, S. Y., & Arron, S. T. (2016). Trends of skin cancer mortality after transplantation in the United States: 1987 to 2013. *Journal of the American Academy of Dermatology, 75*, 106–112.

Gloster, H. M., & Neal, K. (2006). Skin cancer in skin of color. *Journal of the American Academy of Dermatology, 55*(5), 741–760.

Gogia, R., Binstock, M., Hirose, R., Boscardin, W. J., Chren, M. M., & Arron, S. T. (2013). Fitzpatrick skin phototype is an independent predictor of squamous cell carcinoma risk after solid organ transplantation. *Journal of the American Academy of Dermatology, 68*(4), 585–591.

González, A. R., Etchichury, D., Gil, M., & Del Aguila, R. (2019). Neoadjuvant vismodegib and Mohs micrographic surgery for locally advanced periocular basal cell carcinoma. *Ophthalmic Plastic and Reconstructive Surgery, 35*, 56–61.

Goon, P., Clegg, R., Yong, A. S., Lee, A. S. W., Lee, K. Y. C., Levell, N. J., Tan, E. K. H., & Shah, S. N. (2015). 5-Fluorouracil "Chemowraps" in the treatment of multiple actinic keratoses: A norwich experience. *Dermatologic and Therapy, 5*(3), 201–205.

Gunaratne, D., & Veness, M. J. (2018). Efficacy of hypofractionated radiotherapy in patients with non-melanoma skin cancer: Results of a systematic review. *Journal of Medical Imaging and Radiation Oncology, 62*(3), 401–411.

Haisma, M. S., Plaat, B. E., Bijl, H. P., Roodenburg, J. L. N., Diercks, G. F. H., Romeijn, T. R., & Terra, J. B. (2016). Multivariate analysis of potential risk factors for lymph node metastasis in patients with cutaneous squamous cell carcinoma of the head and neck. *Journal of the American Academy of Dermatology, 75*(4), 722–730.

Heppt, M., Steeb, T., Ruzicka, T., & Berking, C. (2019). Cryosurgery combined with topical interventions for actinic keratosis: A systematic review and meta-analysis. *The British Journal of Dermatology, 180*(4), 740–748.

Kagy, M. K., & Amonette, R. (2000). The use of imiquimod 5% cream for the treatment of superficial basal cell carcinomas in a basal cell nevus syndrome patient. *Dermatologic Surgery, 26*(6), 577–578.

Karia, P. S., Jambusaria-Pahlajani, A., Harrington, D. P., Murphy, G. F., Qureshi, A. A., & Schmults, C. D. (2014). Evaluation of American Joint Committee on Cancer, International Union Against Cancer, and Brigham and Women's Hospital tumor staging for cutaneous squamous cell carcinoma. *Journal of Clinical Oncology, 32*(4), 327–334.

Karia, P. S., Morgan, F. C., Califano, J. A., & Schmults, C. D. (2018). Comparison of tumor classifications for cutaneous squamous cell carcinoma of the head and neck in the 7th vs 8th edition of the AJCC cancer staging manual. *JAMA Dermatology, 154*(2), 175–181.

Karia, P. S., Morgan, F. C., Ruiz, E. S., & Schmults, C. D. (2017). Clinical and incidental perineural invasion of cutaneous squamous cell carcinoma: A systematic review and pooled analysis of outcomes data. *JAMA Dermatology, 153*(8), 781–788.

Kauvar, A. N., Arpey, C. J., Hruza, G., Olbricht, S. M., Bennett, R., & Mahmoud, B. H. (2015). Consensus for nonmelanoma skin cancer treatment, part II: Squamous cell carcinoma, including a cost analysis of treatment methods. *Dermatologic Surgery, 41*(11), 1214–1240.

Krediet, J. T., Beyer, M., Lenz, K., Ulrich, C., Lange-Asschenfeldt, B., Stockfleth, E., & Terhorst, D. (2015). Sentinel lymph node biopsy and risk factors for predicting metastasis in cutaneous squamous cell carcinoma. *The British Journal of Dermatology*, *172*(4), 1029–1036.

Levine, D. E., Karia, P. S., & Schmults, C. D. (2015). Outcomes of patients with multiple cutaneous squamous cell carcinomas: A 10-year single-institution cohort Study. *JAMA Dermatology*, *151*(11), 1220–1225.

Manyam, B. V., Garsa, A. A., Chin, R. I., Reddy, C. A., Gastman, B., Thorstad, W., Yom, S. S., Nussenbaum, B., Wang, S. J., Vidimos, A. T., & Koyfman, S. A. (2017). A multi-institutional comparison of outcomes of immunosuppressed and immunocompetent patients treated with surgery and radiation therapy for cutaneous squamous cell carcinoma of the head and neck. *Cancer*, *123*(11), 2054–2060.

Manyam, B. V., Gastman, B., Zhang, A. Y., Reddy, C. A., Burkey, B. B., Scharpf, J., Alam, D. S., Fritz, M. A., Vidimos, A. T., & Koyfman, S. A. (2015) Inferior outcomes in immunosuppressed patients with high-risk cutaneous squamous cell carcinoma of the head and neck treated with surgery and radiation therapy. *Journal of the American Academy of Dermatology*, *73*(2), 221–227.

Marghoob, A. A., Slade, J., Salopek, T. G., Alfred W. Kopf, A. W., Robert S. Bart, R. S., & Darrell S. Rige, D. S. (1995). Basal cell and squamous cell carcinomas are important risk factors for cutaneous malignant melanoma. Screening implications. *Cancer*, *75*, 707–714.

Migden, M. R., Rischin, D., Schmults, C. D., Guminski, A., Hauschild, A., Lewis, K. D., Chung, C. H., Hernandez-Aya, L., Lim, A. M., Chang, A. L. S., Rabinowits, G., Thai, A. A., Dunn, L. A., Hughes, B. G. M., Khushalani, N. I., Modi, B., Schadendorf, D., Gao, B., Seebach, F., … Fury, M. G. (2018). PD-1 blockade with cemiplimab in advanced cutaneous squamous-cell carcinoma. *The New England Journal of Medicine*, *379*(4), 341–351.

Mihalis, E. L., Wysong, A., Boscardin, W. J., Chren, M. M., & Arron, S. T. (2013). Factors affecting sunscreen use and sun avoidance in a U.S. national sample of organ transplant recipients. *British Journal of Dermatology*, *168*(2), 346–353.

Ouhib, Z., Kasper, M., Perez Calatayud, J., Rodriguez, S., Bhatnagar, A., Pai, S., & Strasswimmer, J. (2015). Aspects of dosimetry and clinical practice of skin brachytherapy: The American Brachytherapy Society working group report. *Brachytherapy*, *14*(6), 840–858.

Patel, R. V., Frankel, A., & Goldenberg, G. (2011). An Update on Nonmelanoma Skin Cancer. *J Clin Aesthet Dermatol*, *4*(2), 20–27.

Peris, K., Fargnoli, M. C., Garbe, C., Kaufmann, R., Bastholt, L., Seguin, N. B., Bataille, V., Del Marmol, V., Dummer, R., Harwood, C. A., Hauschild, A., Höller, C., Haedersdal, M., Malvehy, J., Middleton, M. R., Morton, C. A., Nagore, E., Stratigos, A. J., Szeimies, R.-M., … Grob, J. J.; European Dermatology Forum (EDF), The European Association of Dermato-Oncology (EADO), The European Organization for Research and Treatment of Cancer (EORTC). (2019). Diagnosis and treatment of basal cell carcinoma: European consensus-based interdisciplinary guidelines. *European Journal of Cancer*, *118*, 10–34.

Quazi, S. J., Aslam, N., Saleem, H., Rahman, J., & Khan, S. (2020). Surgical margin of excision in basal cell carcinoma: A systematic review of literature. *Cureus*, *12*(7), e9211. https://doi.org/10.7759/cureus.9211

Que, S. K. T., Zwald, F. O., & Schmults, C. D. (2018). Cutaneous squamous cell carcinoma: Management of advanced and high-stage tumors. *Journal of the American Academy of Dermatology*, *78*(2), 249–261.

Rigel, D. S., Robinson, J. K., Ross, M., Friedman, R. J., Cockerell, C. J., & Lim, H. W. (Eds.). (2011). *Cancer of the skin* (2nd ed.). Elsevier Saunders.

Rogers, H. W., Weinstock, M. A., Feldman, S. R., & Coldiron, B. M. (2015). Incidence estimate of nonmelanoma skin cancer (keratinocyte carcinomas) in the U.S. population, 2012. *JAMA Dermatology*, *151*(10), 1081–1086.

Roscher, I., Falk, R. S., Vos, L., Clausen, O. P. F., Helsing, P., Gjersvik, P., & Robsahm, T. E. (2018). Validating 4 staging systems for cutaneous squamous cell carcinoma using population-based data: A nested case-control study. *JAMA Dermatology*, *154*(4), 428–434.

Ruiz, E. S., Karia, P. S., Besaw, R., & Schmults, C. D. (2019). Performance of the American Joint Committee on Cancer Staging Manual, 8th edition vs the Brigham and Women's Hospital tumor classification system for cutaneous squamous cell carcinoma. *JAMA Dermatology*, *155*(7), 819–825.

Shepherd, V., Davidson, E. J., & Davies-Humphreys, J. (2005). Extramammary Paget's disease. *International Journal of Gynecology & Obstetrics*, *112*(3), 273.

Sin, C. W., Barua, A., & Cook, A. (2016). Recurrence rates of periocular basal cell carcinoma following Mohs micrographic surgery: A retrospective study. *International Journal of Dermatology*, *55*(9), 1044–1047.

Skulsky, S. L., O'Sullivan, B., McArdle, O., Leader, M., Roche, M., Conlon, P. J., & O'Neill, J. P. (2017). Review of high-risk features of cutaneous squamous cell carcinoma and discrepancies between the American Joint Committee on Cancer and NCCN clinical practice guidelines in oncology. *Head & Neck*, *39*(3), 578–594.

Starr, P. (2015). Oral nicotinamide prevents common skin cancers in high-risk patients, reduces costs. *American Health & Drug Benefits*, *8*(Spec Issue), 13–14.

Tarantola, T. I., Vallow, L. A., Halyard, M. Y., Weenig, R. H., Warschaw, K. E, Grotz, T. E., Jakub, J. W., Roenigk, R. K., Brewer, J. D., Weaver, A. L., & Otley, C. C. (2013). Prognostic factors in Merkel cell carcinoma: Analysis of 240 cases. *Journal of the American Academy of Dermatology*, *68*(3), 425–432.

Tufaro, A. P., Azoury, S., Crompton, J. G., Straughan, D. M., Reddy, S., Prasad, N. B., Shi, G., & Fischer, A. C. (2015). Rising incidence and aggressive nature of cutaneous malignancies after transplantation: An update on epidemiology, risk factors, management and surveillance. *Surgical Oncology*, *24*(4), 345–352.

van Loo, E., Mosterd, K., Krekels, G. A., Roozeboom, M. H., Ostertag, J. U., Dirksen, C. D., Steijlen, P. M., Martino Neumann, H. A., Nelemans, P. J., & Kelleners-Smeets, N. W. J. (2014). Surgical excision versus Mohs' micrographic surgery for basal cell carcinoma of the face: A randomised clinical trial with 10 year follow-up. *European Journal of Cancer*, *50*(17), 3011–3020.

Visch, M., Kreike, B., & Gerritsen, M. J. P. (2019). Long-term experience with radiotherapy for the treatment of non-melanoma skin cancer. *The Journal of Dermatological Treatment*, *31*(3), 290–295.

Wang, D. M., Kraft, S., Rohani, P., Murphy, G. F., Besaw, R. J., Karia, P. S., Morgan, F. C., & Schmults, C. D. (2015). Association of nodal metastasis and mortality with vermilion vs cutaneous lip location in cutaneous squamous cell carcinoma of the lip. *JAMA Dermatology*, *154*(6), 701–707.

Wermker, K., Kluwig, J., Schipmann, S., Klein, M., Schulze, H. J., & Hallermann, C. (2015). Prediction score for lymph node metastasis from cutaneous squamous cell carcinoma of the external ear. *European Journal of Surgical Oncology*, *41*, 128–135.

Westers-Attema, A., van den Heijkant, F., Lohman, B. G., Nelemans, P. J., Winnepenninckx, V., Kelleners-Smeets, N. W. J., & Mosterd, K. (2014) Bowen's disease: A six-year retrospective study of treatment with emphasis on resection margins. *Acta Dermato-Venereologica*, *94*(4), 431–435.

Williams, H. C., Bath-Hextall, F., Ozolins, M., Armstrong, S. J., Colver, G. B., Perkins, W., & Miller, P. S. J.; Surgery Versus Imiquimod for Nodular and Superficial Basal Cell Carcinoma (SINS) Study Group. (2017). Surgery versus 5% imiquimod for nodular and superficial basal cell carcinoma: 5-year results of the SINS Randomized Controlled Trial. *Journal of Investigative Dermatology*, *137*(3), 614–619.

Work Group, Invited Reviewers; Kim, J. Y. S., Kozlow, J. H., Mittal, B., Moyer, J., Olencki, T., & Rodgers, P. (2018). Guidelines of care for the management of basal cell carcinoma. *Journal of the American Academy of Dermatology*, *78*(3), 540–559.

Wu, S. Z., Jiang, P., DeCaro, J. E., & Bordeaux, J. S. (2016). A qualitative systematic review of the efficacy of sun protection education in organ transplant recipients. *Journal of the American Academy of Dermatology*, *75*(6), 1238–1244.e5.

Benign Lesions and Growths

Kathleen Haycraft

Primary care providers are often the first to evaluate and identify benign neoplasms. Most benign neoplasms can be evaluated and treated by a primary care provider who has been properly educated in basic dermatology. If one is not sure of the diagnosis, a biopsy should be performed and/or a dermatology referral should be made. Remember to explain the lesion(s) in layman's terms, and if treatment is requested or required, cosmetic outcomes and expected recovery should be discussed and documented. Proper evaluation of benign cutaneous lesions can help in the identification of underlying systemic disease. In short, become an expert at identifying benign neoplasms—it can reduce biopsies and expense and allow you to offer reassurance and expertise to your patients.

SEBORRHEIC KERATOSIS

Seborrheic keratosis (SK) is considered the most common benign skin lesion. These lesions are associated with both aging and genetics. Archaic terms such as "age spots," "seborrheic verruca," and "senile warts" are inaccurate and misleading to patients and therefore should be avoided. While more common in those with lighter-colored skin, most individuals will eventually develop at least one SK. The male to female ratio is the same.

Pathophysiology

- Majority of SKs are related to failure of two suppressor genes: FGFR3 and P13K. These genes are responsible for "laying down" the perfect amount of keratin for each location on the body.

- Clonal expansion results in neighboring activation of surrounding keratinocytes. Over time, these genes fail and there is currently no known way to reactivate. This is the basis for treatment and usual reoccurrence.

- Anecdotal evidence includes increase in the presence of SKs after a drug eruption, erythrodermic psoriasis, exfoliative erythroderma, and in the setting of gastrointestinal and/or genitourinary erythroderma (Leser-Trelat sign).

Clinical Presentation

- SKs can occur anywhere on the body where hair follicles are located (never seen on palms and soles); but they have a predilection for the face, chest (particularly under the breasts), back and arms (Fig. 2.3-1).

- They can present with a variety of colors, but darkly pigmented or pink SKs can be confused with melanoma or other skin cancers, thus if in doubt, refer or biopsy (or both).

- Lesions occur slowly and feel waxy and rough in texture as they mature. Gently scraping on the lesion can reinforce the concept that this lesion is just excess keratin and can be removed by a variety of techniques.

- Some lesions may be irritated and/or pruritic.

- There are subsets of SKs (Fig. 2.3-2A–H), including:

  - Dermatosis papulose nigra—more common in skin of color, smaller, tends to occur on the face, can look like skin tags.

  - Stucco keratosis—occurs on the lower extremities, especially on ankles and dorsal feet, and look like barnacles. They have some link to ultraviolet exposure and are more common in lighter skin.

  - Pigmented SKs—occur when involved keratinocytes trigger neighboring melanocytes, darker in color, can be confused with melanoma. Any dark, tender, or rapidly changing pigmented SK needs to be biopsied.

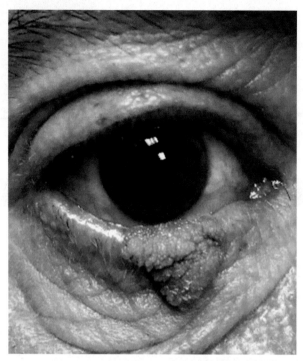

FIG. 2.3-1. Seborrheic keratosis (SK) eyelid. (Courtesy Douglas DiRuggiero.)

- Reticulated SKs—multiple colors and variable patterns; thought to occur in the keratinocytes of sunspots (lentigo).
- Cerebriform SKs—many ridges and grooves resembling the surface of the brain.
- Multiple SKs—can interfere with an accurate visual assessment of the skin as they may "hide" other lesions. It is not unusual to get a biopsy of an SK that has another lesion with it. This is referred to as a collision tumor.

DIFFERENTIAL DIAGNOSIS   Seborrheic Keratosis

- Pigmented actinic keratosis
- Pigmented basal cell carcinoma
- Squamous cell carcinoma
- Melanoma
- Wart
- Intradermal nevus
- Sebaceous nevus
- Prurigo nodularis (picker's papule)
- Acrochordon (skin tag)

Treatment

- Most do not require treatment, but many patients request treatment for irritated SKs or desire removal for cosmetic reasons.
- Conservative cryotherapy. This treatment should be performed by a provider who is well trained in this procedure and is absolutely certain the lesion is an SK. If in doubt or if not trained and skilled in various biopsy techniques, refer to a dermatology provider. Warning: cryotherapy can result in hypo or hyperpigmentation, particularly in skin of color.
- Shave excision on thick or large lesions is reasonable, but tissue must be sent for biopsy.

- Soap bars contain pumice. Patients are advised to moisturize with a thick moisturizing cream for at least 30 minutes before bathing and soaking and "scrubbing" the lesion. This process is greatly appreciated by patients as it allows them a way to keep the lesions at bay.
- Curettage.

Management and Patient Education

- The lesions can make patients very self-conscious.
- Treatment options and potential side effects need to be reviewed.
- The biggest potential complication is that a lesion can be misdiagnosed, and a malignancy may be missed.
- If an SK is very tender without signs of trauma, biopsy lesion. Squamous cell carcinoma can mimic an SK.
- Leser–Trelat sign is when patients develop sudden eruptions of numerous SKs in the presence of underlying malignancy (usually GI or GU). Providers should be aware that appropriate screening and history and physicals (H&P) should be performed (Fig. 2.3-3).
- A tender or any variation in a darkly pigmented SK should result in biopsy to rule out melanoma.

SEBACEOUS HYPERPLASIA

Sebaceous hyperplasias (SHs) are common benign lesions that are associated with middle-age adults. The sebaceous glands are enlarged and have a central dell (umbilication) with a rim of crown vessels. They are common on the face but can occur anywhere, including the genitalia. The lesions occur in the sebaceous gland and develop due to the influence of androgens (male hormones). Estrogens reduce SH. SH is associated with immune suppression.

Clinical Presentation

- Soft, somewhat yellowish, small papules usually occurring commonly on the face and other areas that have dense sebaceous glands (Fig. 2.3-4).
- Central dell (depression) with crown vessels.
- SHs involving the lips, buccal mucosa, glans penis, or clitoris are referred to as Fordyce spots.
- Enlarged sebaceous glands involving the areola are called Montgomery glands.
- Eyelid involves the meibomian glands.
- They may occur in newborns and are not a cause for alarm.

DIFFERENTIAL DIAGNOSIS   Sebaceous Hyperplasia

- Acrochordon (skin tag)
- Acne or rosacea papules
- Basal cell carcinoma
- Milia
- Wart
- Molluscum
- Sebaceous adenoma or carcinoma
- Sarcoidosis
- Syringoma
- Trichoepithelioma
- Xanthoma

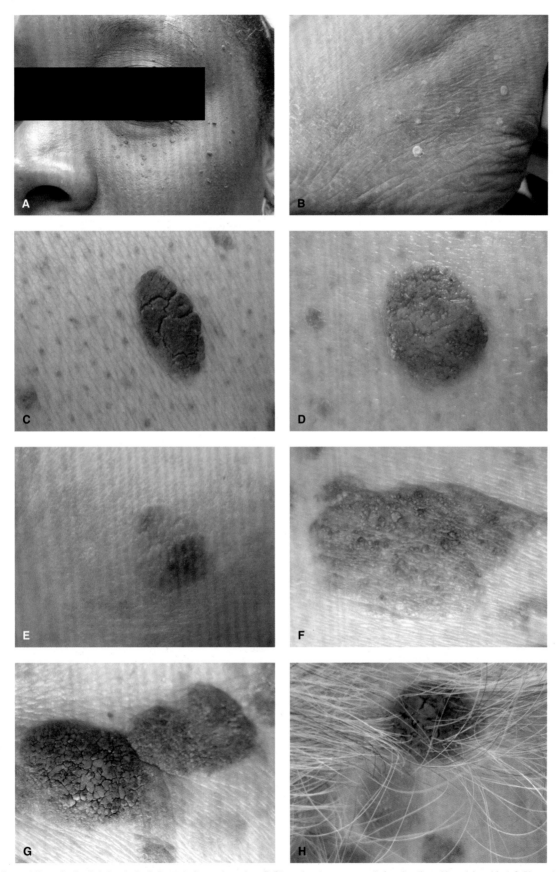

FIG. 2.3-2. Presentations of seborrheic keratosis. **A:** Dermatosis papulosa nigra. **B:** Stucco keratoses commonly found on the ankle and dorsal foot. **C:** Pigmented seborrheic keratosis. **D:** Cerebriform seborrheic keratosis. **E:** Reticulated seborrheic keratosis. **F:** Pseudocysts or horny pearls of seborrheic keratosis. **G:** Dark brown to black seborrheic keratosis often concerning patients for skin cancer. **H:** Seborrheic keratosis of the scalp can appear differently due to the hair follicles.

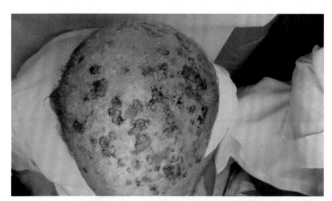

FIG. 2.3-3. Leser–Trélat sign. Sudden eruption of seborrheic keratoses in man diagnosed with genitourinary cancer. (Photo courtesy of M. Bobonich.)

Treatment

- Reassurance; usually they do not need treatment. Aggressive destructive treatment may result in more disfigurement.
- Chemical peels, micro-needling, and laser therapy are somewhat effective cosmetic treatments in well-trained hands.
- Photodynamic therapy.
- Isotretinoin in extreme or refractory cases, but only by a certified iPLEDGE prescriber.

Management and Patient Education

- SH may occasionally mimic a basal cell or sebaceous carcinoma.
- Sebaceous neoplasms in the presence of squamous cell cancer may prompt an evaluation for colorectal or genitorectal malignancies (known as Muir–Torre syndrome).

SYRINGOMA

These benign neoplasms of the eccrine sweat gland ducts are more commonly found on female preadolescents and adolescents. These papules occur most frequently around the eyes but can occur in other areas where sweat ducts are concentrated. Familial syndromes have been reported and diabetes mellitus

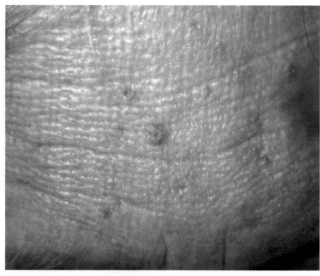

FIG. 2.3-4. Sebaceous hyperplasia grouped on forehead. Note central dell and crown of jewels outer border.

may be associated. Nearly 40% of those with Down syndrome have syringomas (Fig. 2.3-5A,B).

Clinical Presentation

- Flesh colored, translucent, or yellow papules usually very small.
- Common on eyelids, axilla, umbilicus, or vulva.
- More common in women and tend to occur at puberty.
- May be distressing cosmetically.

Treatment

- Reassurance; treatment not necessary except for cosmetic reasons.
- Destructive therapies may result in scarring and pigment changes.
- Laser therapy and chemical peels may be helpful.
- Oral isotretinoin, acitretin, and topical tretinoin are not FDA approved but may be helpful.

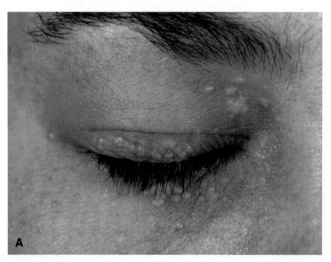

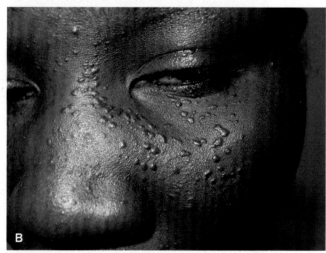

FIG. 2.3-5. **A,B:** Syringomas on face. (Figure A: Used with permission from Craft, N., Fox, L. P., Goldsmith, L. A., Papier, A., Birnbaum, R., Mercurio, M. G., Miller, D., Rajendran, P., Rosenblum, M., Taylor, E., & Tumeh, P. C. [2010]. *VisualDx: Essential adult dermatology.* Wolters Kluwer Health; Figure B: Image provided by Stedman's.)

- Basal cell cancer
- Cutaneous tuberculosis
- Sarcoidosis
- Granuloma annulare
- Microcystic adnexal carcinoma
- Milia
- SH
- Steatocystoma
- Trichoepithelioma
- Xanthelasma

Management and Patient Education

- Scalp lesions can cause scarring alopecia.
- Cosmetic appearance may affect self-esteem.
- Syringomas of the vagina may result in vaginal/vulvar pruritus.
- Syringomas may be rarely associated with severe pain upon sweating.
- Multiple lesions may be linked to Brooke–Spiegler syndrome and Down syndrome.

SKIN TAGS (ACROCHORDON)

Acrochordons include skin tags and fibroepithelial polyps. They are benign lesions but may become irritated. Very large acrochordons are fibroepithelial polyps and frequently become irritated. The plural form of acrochordon is properly stated as acrochordia. They tend to affect women more than men and have been linked to HPV types 6 and 11. These benign fibrous papules are covered with normal epidermis. They increase with age, but can rarely be found in children (more common in those with metabolic syndromes). There is some evidence for a familial pattern (Fig. 2.3-6).

Clinical Presentation

- Soft pedunculated papules.
- Flesh-colored or occasionally hyperpigmented.
- Common in axilla, neck, or groin.
- Can be large and floppy; if >1 cm, usually referred to as a fibroepithelial polyp as opposed to a "tag" (Fig. 2.3-7).

DIFFERENTIAL DIAGNOSIS   Skin Tags

- Neurofibroma
- Malignancies like melanoma may occur at the base
- Basal cell carcinoma or Pinkus tumor
- Premalignant fibroepithelial tumor
- SKs
- Verruca

Treatment

- Do not require treatment, but may be treated if irritated. Biopsy lesions if suspicious.
- Electrodessication.

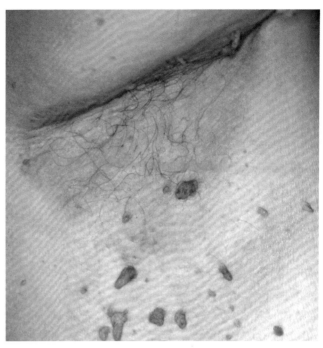

FIG. 2.3-6. Skin tags or acrochordons commonly found in areas of friction. (Used with permission from Craft, N., Fox, L. P., Goldsmith, L. A., Papier, A., Birnbaum, R., Mercurio, M. G., Miller, D., Rajendran, P., Rosenblum, M., Taylor, E., & Tumeh, P. C. [2010]. *VisualDx: Essential adult dermatology.* Wolters Kluwer Health.)

- Scissor excision (clipping).
- Ligation.
- Over-the-counter (OTC) products that contain salicylic acid, retinols, exfoliation (Fig. 2.3-8).

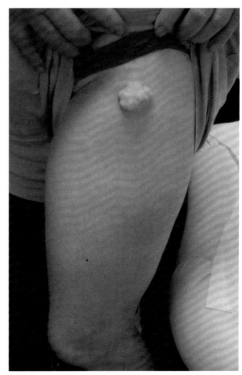

FIG. 2.3-7. A large pedunculated fibroepithelial polyp. Always send larger lesion for biopsy to rule out other pathologies. (Photo courtesy of M. Bobonich.)

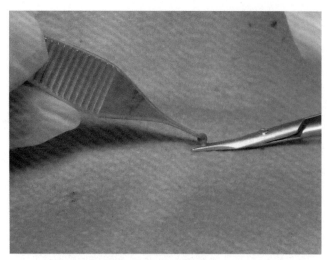

FIG. 2.3-8. Clipping skin tags at the base for removal.

Management and Patient Education

- Beware of possible misdiagnosis of melanoma, basal cell carcinoma, or Pinkus tumor; thus biopsy any deeply pigmented, unusual, or symptomatic skin tag.
- Can be associated with obesity, dyslipidemia, type 2 diabetes mellitus, insulin resistance, hypertension, and elevated C-reactive protein. Appropriate work-ups should be considered.

FIBROUS PAPULES

Harmless, 2- to 5-mm papules commonly found on central face, which are considered a variant of facial angiofibromas. May develop due to antibodies formed against specific keratinocytes. They are considered a variant of facial angiofibroma.

Clinical Presentation

- Firm, nontender papules that tend to occur on the bottom of the nose.
- Clinically they may be difficult to distinguish from an early basal cell cancer, however, most fibrous papules are much firmer to the touch and do not have the characteristic tree-like blood vessels seen in basal cell carcinomas (Fig. 2.3-9).

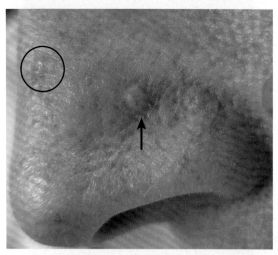

FIG. 2.3-9. Fibrous papule of the nose (*arrow*). If lesion changing, tender, or bleeds, proceed with biopsy. Note pearled lesion with central depression within the *circle*. This lesion suspicious for BCC.

DIFFERENTIAL DIAGNOSIS   Fibrous Papules

- Basal cell carcinoma
- Melanocytic nevus
- Ruptured hair follicle
- Angiofibromas, commonly found in tuberous sclerosis

Treatment

- Reassurance; treatment largely for cosmesis.
- Curettage or shave removal may be done but patients should be warned of scar and reoccurrence. Lesions should always be sent for biopsy to rule out malignancy.
- Punch excision reduces rates of recurrence.

Management and Patient Education

- Excellent prognosis.
- Multiple fibrous papules and/or angiomas in a butterfly distribution on the face may be a sign of tuberous sclerosis.
- If lesion is tender, friable, or has an unusual appearance, proceed with biopsy to rule-out malignancy.

NEUROFIBROMA

A neurofibroma (NF) is a rare benign tumor of the nerve sheath that results in unique soft bumps in the skin. They are formed when peripheral fibroblasts synthesize collagen, which then wraps around the nerves and associated Schwann cells. Extraordinarily rare for these tumors to become cancerous.

Clinical Presentation

- Soft, fleshy papules that may vary from pink to white in color.
- Button holing may be present (finger pressure may invaginate or telescope the lesion beneath the skin) (Fig. 2.3-10).

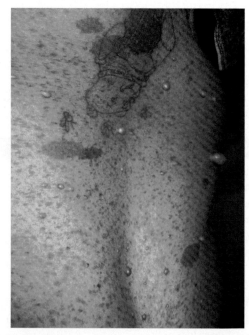

FIG. 2.3-10. Neurofibromas and café au lait patches on a patient with neurofibromatosis.

- Basal cell cancer
- Melanocytic nevus

Treatment

- Solitary lesions, they usually resolve without any significance.
- Excision may be considered if symptomatic or cosmetically undesirable.
- Shave excision should be avoided as they can result in excessive scarring.

Management and Patient Education

- Isolated lesions are not of serious concern, reassurance.
- Removal if cosmetically sensitive by punch biopsy; larger lesions may require complete excision.
- If the lesion is suspicious, a biopsy should be done to rule out malignancy.
- If more than 3 NFs, more than 6 café au laits macules, or axillary freckling, or Lisch nodules, one should be evaluated for neurofibromatosis (Fig. 2.3-10).

PRURIGO NODULARIS

(Also see Section 5: *The Itchy Patient* for more information on PN.)

Prurigo nodularis (PN) are benign lesions that can be a challenge for the clinician. It is considered to be a form of neurodermatitis with many possible underlying etiologies. It is seen frequently in pruritic conditions such as atopic dermatitis, HIV, hepatic disease, post CVA, anemia, thyroid disease, renal disease, celiac disease, stress, lymphoproliferative disease, compression of intervertebral discs, recreational drug use, malignancies, and allergic reactions to foods or medicines. Picker nodules and Hyde nodules are synonyms. It results from repeated scratching or rubbing of the skin which leads to hyperkeratosis and lichenification (thickening). These nodules are also associated with hypertrophy of the dermal nerve fibers (Fig. 2.3-11).

Clinical Presentation

- Solitary or multiple nodules usually distributed on extremities, face, or the trunk (usually where the patient can reach).
- Firm nodules that vary in size and range from red to purple.
- Over time, they may coalesce or become fissured and somewhat verrucous in appearance or may have a linear distribution.

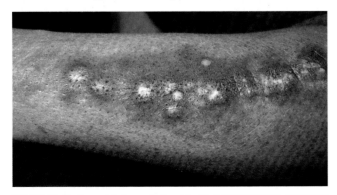

FIG. 2.3-11. Prurigo nodularis usually found on the extensor surfaces, sometimes developing a linear distribution.

- Some lesions are asymptomatic, but most are pruritic, ranging from severe to intense.

- Squamous cell carcinoma
- Basal cell carcinoma
- Melanoma
- SKs
- Warts

Treatment

- Reassurance; but a thorough H&P, as well as appropriate diagnostic workups based on H&P findings, should be performed.
- Treatment of any underlying disorders is imperative; punch biopsies are helpful.
- Moderate to high potency steroids may be applied to the elevated lesions.
- For lower-extremity lesions, moderate-strength steroid application followed by an application of an Unna boot or occlusive wraps can help tremendously.
- Injection of triamcinolone to lesions followed by cryotherapy (performed monthly) can provide much relief and may stop the scratch/itch cycle.
- Topical capsaicin or lidocaine may provide itch and pain relief.
- In cases of liver, renal, or other systemic diseases, UVB therapy with petroleum jelly can provide dramatic relief. Home units are available when the therapy has been proven to be effective. UVB light is safe, tanning beds are not.
- There are no great pharmacologic treatments for pruritus, but second- or third-generation antihistamines (usually only helpful at two to four times the standard dose) can be useful as long as there is no glaucoma or urinary retention.
- Use first-generation antihistamines with caution, there is an increased Alzheimer's risk and substantial sedation.
- Other medications (all are off label) that can be considered include gabapentin, antidepressants, naltrexone, as well as topical vitamin D3, calcipotriene, and/or TCIs such as tacrolimus or pimecrolimus.

Management and Patient Education

- Prognosis depends on the etiology of pruritus, and cases that are difficult to diagnose may require chronic treatment.
- Any patient who is persistently itchy should have an extensive workup for underlying systemic disease including: atopic dermatitis, HIV, hepatic disease, post CVA, anemia, thyroid disease, renal disease, celiac disease, stress, lymphoproliferative disease, compression of intervertebral discs, recreational drug use, malignancies, and allergies to foods or medicines.
- Do not view this as a primary psychiatric disease until the above mentioned potential diagnostic etiologies are considered and eliminated.

DERMATOFIBROMA

Dermatofibromas (DFs) are commonly found, firm nodules that are pigmented with pink to purple to brown outer pigment. They are believed to be associated with small breaks in the skin from minor

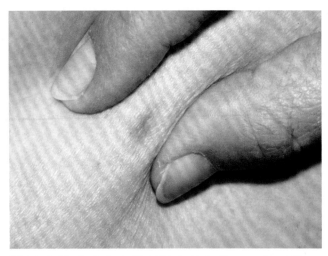

FIG. 2.3-12. The dimple sign (or Fitzpatrick sign) helps diagnose a dermatofibroma (DF). A DF can be pink, violaceous, or brown in color.

injuries, insect bites, or shaving. Also referred to as a superficial benign fibrous histiocytoma. More common in women. Histology reports typically reveal a bundle of spindle cells haphazardly extending deep into the subcutaneous tissue. It is thought that transforming growth factor-beta (TGF-beta) signals the growth of fibrin, which leads to formation of these nodules.

Clinical Presentation

- Slow-growing solitary nodule on an extremity, lower more than upper.
- Usually asymptomatic but may be slightly tender or pruritic
- Characteristic "dimpling" when lesion is pinched (called a Fitzpatrick sign) (Fig. 2.3-12).
- Have a stellate or star-like center surrounded by darker pigment.

DIFFERENTIAL DIAGNOSIS	Dermatofibroma

- Dysplastic nevus
- Basal cell carcinoma
- HIV cutaneous lesions
- Merkel cell cancer
- Keloid/Hypertrophic scar
- "Pink" melanoma
- Prurigo nodularis
- Spitz nevus

Treatment

- Reassurance; treatment generally not indicated.
- Steroid injection and/or cryotherapy may offer some success.
- Excisions are generally avoided, but biopsy if lesion is suspicious.

Management and Patient Education

- Reassurance.
- Spontaneous regression may occur.
- Avoid surgical treatment to avoid scars.
- Even though DFs are benign, there is a slightly increased risk for basal cell cancer to occur on the overlying epidermis.

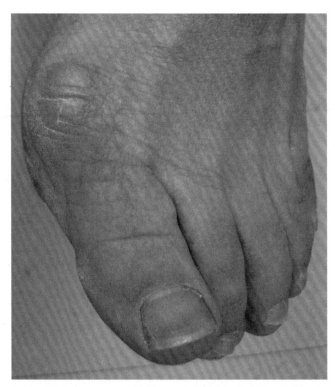

FIG. 2.3-13. Callus formation over the first metatarsal resulting from a bunion.

- Multiple DFs (more than six) have been associated with underlying diseases (systemic lupus, myasthenia, AIDS, and internal malignancies).

CORNS AND CALLUSES

Corns tend to occur on toes, feet, or hands. They are a small, usually round, papule composed of thickened dead skin. There is usually a small soft center. Calluses occur on larger areas of hands, feet, knees, and elbows. Both are usually from recurrent friction and pressure, resulting in hyperkeratosis.

Clinical Presentation

- Papules (corns) or larger patches (calluses) of thick scaly yellow or gray hyperkeratotic skin.
- They may become painful (Figs. 2.3-13 and 2.3-14).

DIFFERENTIAL DIAGNOSIS	Corns and Calluses

- Warts—but a corn will lack the black pinpoint vessels and disruption of rete ridges
- Squamous cell carcinoma
- Talon noir. If pigmented, don't miss a melanoma

Treatment

- Do not need treatment unless they create pain.
- Begin with analysis of friction source.
- Salicylic acid (OTC) can thin lesions.
- Keratolytics (OTC) like 40% urea can be effective.
- Paring the lesions, per patient request, can be helpful. Surgical excision is rarely, if ever, indicated.

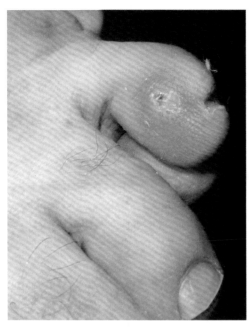

FIG. 2.3-14. Corns develop from pressure points on the feet and toes.

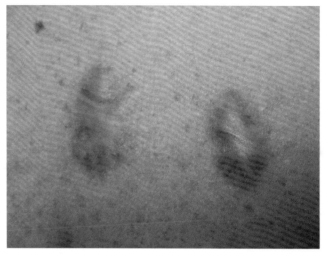

FIG. 2.3-15. Hypertrophic scars are thickened scars that do not exceed the wound border.

Management and Patient Education

- May be chronic unless source of pressure found and resolved.
- A thorough history of patient's processes at home and work may lead to causation and change in pressure points.
- Have patient bring two pairs of shoes and observe fit and stride to determine causation and change in pressure points.

KELOIDS AND HYPERTROPHIC SCARS

Both represent exuberant growth of scar-like tissue. Young adults between ages 10 and 30 have a higher risk of keloids related to tattoos, piercings, vaccination sites, and pseudofolliculitis barbae. Older adults can exhibit hypertrophic scars after extensive surgery like coronary artery bypass grafting. Darker skin color has higher keloid risk. Keloids and hypertrophic scarring have a familial tendency.

- Keloids are scars initially composed of type 3 collagen that is later replaced by the proliferation of type 1 collagen.
- Hypertrophic scars have organized collagen in packages of fibroblasts and small vessels.
- DeltaN63 overexpression and p53 underexpression have a link to keloids.

Clinical Presentation

- Often, terms are used interchangeably.
- Hypertrophic scars present as thickened scar tissue that remains within the borders of the original injury.
- Keloids appear as an exuberant amount of scar tissue extending beyond the border of the original injury.
- They may vary from fleshy to brown to reddish hyperpigmentation.
- Keloids may occur with acne and should prompt brisk treatment.
- Darker skin, Hispanics, and Asians have a higher risk of keloids (Figs. 2.3-15 and 2.3-16).

Treatment

- Injection of triamcinolone mixed with lidocaine followed by liquid nitrogen therapy (LN2) at monthly intervals can result in excellent resolution with minimal discomfort and cost.
- Surgical excision should only be used if combined with imiquimod or superficial radiation.
- Silicone gel and sheeting may be used adjunctively.
- Laser treatment have varied results.

Management and Patient Education

- History of keloids and hypertrophic scars increase risk of future scars.

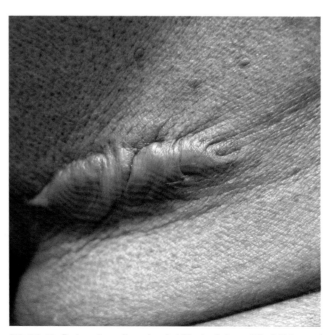

FIG. 2.3-16. Exuberant scar tissue in a keloid extends beyond the initial wound border. (Photo courtesy of M. Bobonich.)

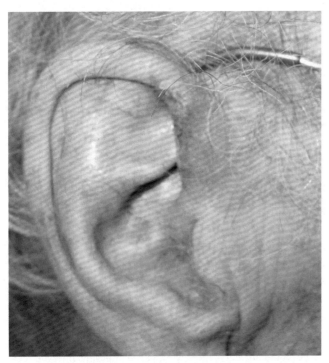

FIG. 2.3-17. Chondrodermatitis nodularis helicus (CNH) on anterior helical rim. Firmly attached crusty papule on an erythematous base usually on the same side where the patient sleeps the most. Can mimic an AK, SCC, or BCC; so biopsy often necessary. (Image provided by Stedman's.)

- Always ask about scars—are they caused by trauma, surgery, piercing, chick pox, acne, etc.? If there is no known etiology, biopsy lesion to rule sarcoidosis or malignancy masquerading as a scar.

Chondrodermatitis Nodularis Helicis

Chondrodermatitis nodularis helicis (CNH) is an inflammatory condition which affects the helical or antihelical rim of the ear. While the exact cause is still not known, modest blood supply and minimal cushioning of the ear allows several contributing factors to result in tender nodules, crusts, or shallow erosions. These contributing factors include: repeated, chronic pressure while sleeping (mostly those who sleep on one side), long-term sun or cold exposure, or trauma from headphones, mobile devices, hardhats, or other protective or occupational gear. Most commonly found on fair-skinned, older males.

Clinical Presentation

- Tender, erythematous scale or crust, with or without shallow erosion, that develops on the helix or antihelix.
- Can present as a small nodule which bleeds or produces scant drainage.
- Typically unilateral (on the sleeping side). Most commonly on the helix in men and on the antihelix in women.
- May mimic an actinic keratosis or squamous cell/basal cell carcinoma (Fig. 2.3-17).

DIFFERENTIAL DIAGNOSIS   Keloids and Hypertrophic Scars

- Actinic keratosis
- Squamous cell carcinoma
- Basal cell carcinoma
- Chondritis including polychondritis

Treatment

- Emollients to the ear before bedtime may reduce inflammation.
- Moderate-potency topical steroids may reduce inflammation.
- Change in sleep position, doughnut pillow.
- Broad-brimmed hat and sunscreen may help reduce further UV damage.
- A shave excision may be diagnostic and curative.
- Cryotherapy may also provide mild relief.

Management and Patient Education

- Can be associated with connective tissue disease (lupus erythematosus, dermatomyositis, scleroderma) and chondritis.
- Don't miss the diagnosis of squamous cell or basal cell carcinoma.
- Most respond to chronic management and/or shave excision.

EPIDERMOID CYST

Epidermoid cysts are usually present as a shallow, compressible mobile subcutaneous mass that can range from soft to firm in density. A foul-smelling thick discharge (degraded keratin) can often be expressed from the lesion. The cyst results from a keratin plug that blocks the sebaceous unit in the epidermis. They are more commonly found on males (during third to fourth decade) and have a predilection for the face, back, scalp, ears, upper arms, scrotum, and chest. Synonyms include sebaceous cyst, inclusion cyst, and infundibular cyst. The proper term is epidermoid cyst. While they can present as red and indurated, they are rarely infected (usually an inflammatory response).

Clinical Presentation

- Compressible nodule.
- Can be fleshy, yellow, or white in color.
- A central punctum may be present.
- Slow growing, may or may not be tender.
- They may spontaneously rupture.
- Sebaceous cysts that occur on the scalp are called pilar cysts or rarely "wens" (Fig. 2.3-18).

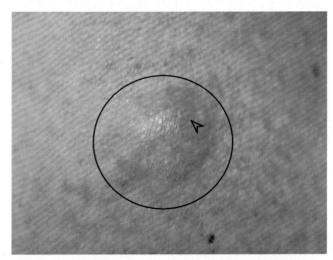

FIG. 2.3-18. Epidermoid cysts are soft, yellow to flesh tone nodules that often have a connecting pore (*arrowhead*). (Photo courtesy of M. Bobonich.)

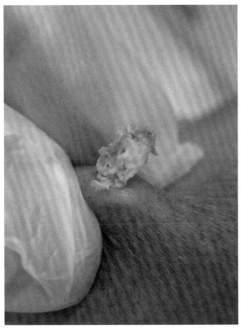

FIG. 2.3-19. A simple I&D of epidermoid cyst can reduce the size and expel odorous, thick white keratin.

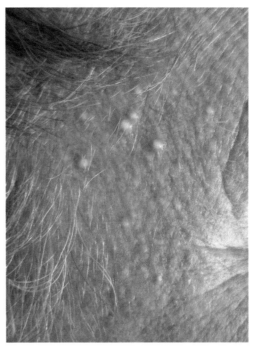

FIG. 2.3-20. Milia.

DIFFERENTIAL DIAGNOSIS   Epidermoid Cyst

- Abscess
- Lipoma
- Steatocystoma multiplex
- Lymph node
- Cystic BCC or SCC

Treatment

- Small cysts may be monitored.
- Symptomatic cysts may be excised by a punch technique or a surgical excision. Always remove the cyst wall to prevent reoccurrence.
- Avoid just an incision and drainage (I&D), as they will result in recurrence.
- If cysts have had a previous I&D, surgical excision will be needed.
- Avoid removing cysts on heavily sun-exposed skin (dermatoheliosis) of the face (Favre–Racouchot syndrome) as they are associated with extensive scarring beneath the surface (Fig. 2.3-19).

Management and Patient Education

- Some cysts may resolve.
- All excised cysts should be sent for biopsy, particularly with older patients, as concomitant squamous cell carcinoma or basal cell cancer has been reported.
- Multiple sebaceous cysts can be seen with Gardner syndrome as well as Basal cell nevus syndrome.

MILIUM/MILIA

Milia are small keratin-filled sebaceous cysts that occur commonly on the face and periorbital area. Congenital milia are common and

can also be seen on the palate (Epstein pearls). Secondary milia can occur anywhere on the body with a history of associated traumas.

Clinical Presentation

- Firm, 1- to 3-mm papules which sit right under the surface of the skin.
- They can be white, yellow, or tan in color.
- Most common on face, but can be present in other areas (Fig. 2.3-20).

DIFFERENTIAL DIAGNOSIS   Milium/Milia

- Acne (comedones)
- Syringoma
- Trichoepithelioma

Treatment

- Harmless and do not require treatment.
- If of cosmetic concern: curette, topical retinols, and retinoids.
- Hyfrecation.

Management and Patient Education

- Subtypes of milia include: neonatal, juvenile (associated with several genetic disorders), primary milia in kids and adults, multiple eruptive milia, milia en plaque, trauma-induced, and drug related with topical medications, such as corticosteroids, hydroquinone, and 5-fluorouracil cream.

Digital Myxoid Cyst

Benign shiny tumors typically found out the distal fingers or toes. It is referred to as a pseudocyst because it is not surrounded by a capsule. While usually associated with degenerative arthritis, they can be tender

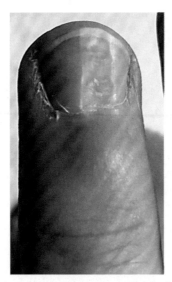

FIG. 2.3-21. Digital myxoid cyst causing a groove deformity of nail plate.

with pressure, and if near the nail plate, can cause deformity (longitudinal groove) of the nail. A sinus tract may be present communicating with the underlying joint. It is also referred to as digital ganglion cyst, a digital myxoid cyst, or a digital synovial cyst (Fig. 2.3-21).

Clinical Presentation

- Usually a solitary dome-shaped papule that is translucent or flesh colored.
- Firm but fluctuant.
- Can be tender with pressure.

Treatment

- Topical steroids may provide modest relief if lesion is small.
- If not connected to a joint, I&D will remove the gelatinous debris and relieve pressure.
- Intralesional corticosteroids, cryotherapy, and laser ablation may reduce the size of the lesion.
- Refer to hand surgeon or orthopedics for complete excision.

Management and Patient Education

- Patients are advised not to attempt draining the cyst by themselves to avoid infection.

LIPOMAS

Encapsulated adipose tissue forms a benign tumor of the subcutaneous layer of the skin. Familial lipoma syndrome can cause hundreds of lipomas in young adults.

Clinical Presentation

- Common on trunk and extremities.
- Soft mobile tumor with slippage sign.

DIFFERENTIAL DIAGNOSIS   Lipomas
• Sebaceous cyst
• Liposarcoma
• Lymph node enlargement

Treatment

- Reassurance.
- If rapidly enlarges or becomes painful, schedule for excision.

Management and Patient Education

- May occur as a result of some anti-HIV treatments.
- Lipomas on the frontalis are deep in the muscle and are difficult to remove and scar. They are best managed by a plastic surgeon.
- Lipomas over the mid-sacral region should be referred for a neurologic evaluation.
- Multiple lipomas are associated with Madelung disease, Dercum disease, and Gardner syndrome.

Xanthoma/Xanthelasma

Xanthomas can occur anywhere on the body and are more likely to be associated with elevated cholesterol. They can be associated with genetic defects in lipid metabolism and have an increased incidence in hypothyroidism, diabetes, renal failure, cirrhosis, and certain malignancies. Xanthelasma are a type of xanthoma which appear symmetrically on the upper and lower eyelids (also called xanthelasma palpebrarum).

Clinical Presentation

- Xanthelasma are sharply-demarcated, yellowish smooth plaques occurring in the periorbital region. Usually symmetrical.
- Xanthomas can present as pinhead to 1 cm-sized white to yellow papules on the skin, most often distributed on the joints (especially elbows), buttocks, hands, and feet (Fig. 2.3-22).

DIFFERENTIAL DIAGNOSIS   Xanthoma/Xanthelasma
• Amyloidosis
• Sarcoidosis
• Necrobiosis lipoidica

Management and Patient Education

- Perform H&P and evaluate lipid levels.
- Statins rarely improve cutaneous lesions.
- Surgical excisions are rarely effective, and recurrence is common.

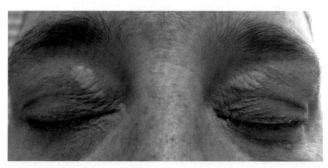

FIG. 2.3-22. Xanthelasmas are most often caused by a defect in lipid metabolism.

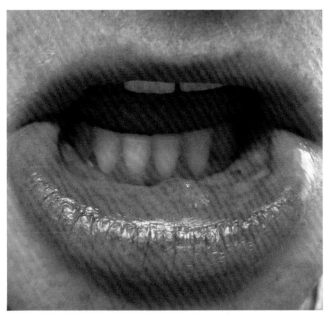

FIG. 2.3-23. Mucocele commonly found on the inside of the lower lip.

- Cosmetic treatments include laser therapy, acid peels, or electrodessication—but only in the most skilled hands.
- Can be caused by medications such as retinoids, prednisone, estrogens, tamoxifen, prednisone, and cyclosporine.

MUCOCELE

Benign mucous filled cysts of the oral mucosa caused by mild inflammation and swelling of the connective tissue. Most common location is the lower lip.

Clinical Presentation

- Palpation reveals a painless, smooth, fluctuant to firm papule.
- Due to trauma from biting or from an aphthous ulcer that preceded the papule (Fig. 2.3-23).

DIFFERENTIAL DIAGNOSIS   Mucocele
• Parotid duct cyst
• Dermoid cyst (from the floor of the mouth)
• Hemangioma

Treatment

- I&D will allow you to express the gelatinous material and confirm diagnosis.
- Surgical excision or laser therapy if recurrent.

Management and Patient Education

- Many lesions resolve on their own.

CHERRY ANGIOMA

Angiomas are the most common vascular neoplasm. Angiomas are a benign growth of blood vessels that create small macules or papules.

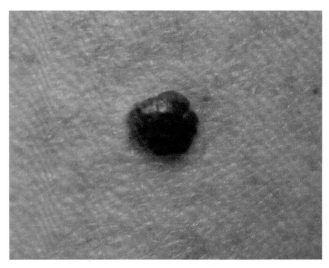

FIG. 2.3-24. Cherry angioma.

They occur commonly in pregnancy and can involute in the postpartum period. The lesions begin to proliferate during the third to fourth decade of life.

Clinical Presentation

- The lesions may be red, blue, or purple. The majority being red resulting in the common name of cherry angiomas.
- The lesions do not blanch.
- They are commonly distributed on the trunk but can occur anywhere including the scrotum and vulva.

DIFFERENTIAL DIAGNOSIS   Cherry Angioma
• Melanoma
• Insect bite
• Pyogenic granuloma

Treatment

- Focused on reassurance. Most are benign and asymptomatic.
- Many patients want cosmetic clearance. Consideration may be given to hyfrecation, laser, and curettage (Fig. 2.3-24).

Management and Patient Education

- If any suspicion of melanoma, proceed with a referral or shave biopsy.
- Multiple, eruptive cherry angiomas can rarely be associated with solid organ tumors.

VENOUS LAKE

Venous lakes are dilated venules that are caused by solar damage to the vessel and the elastic tissue in the skin.

Clinical Presentation

- Dark blue compressible macules/patches.
- Distributed on lips, face, neck, hands, and ears.
- They are more commonly found on individuals over the age of 50.
- Will collapse and blanch when compressed, slowly refill.

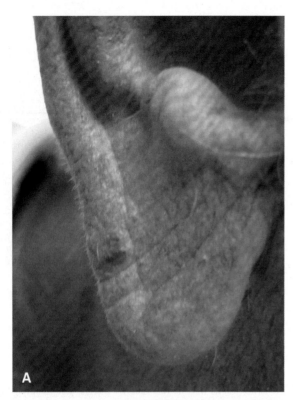

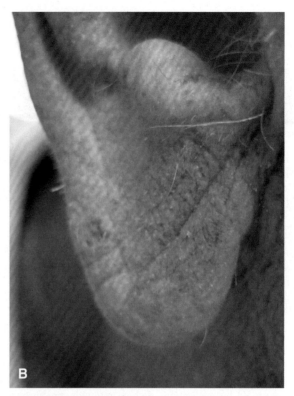

FIG. 2.3-25. **A:** Venous lake commonly found on the ears. **B:** When compressed, the lesion will blanch initially, then return to the blue-purple color within seconds.

DIFFERENTIAL DIAGNOSIS Venous Lake

The most important differential diagnosis is melanoma (if blanching does not occur) (Fig. 2.3-25A,B)

Management and Patient Education

- Focused on reassurance.
- If treatment is desired for cosmetic purposes, hyfrecation, shave excision, laser, and LN2 can be considered.

PYOGENIC GRANULOMA (PG)

Pyogenic granulomas are acquired vascular growths. These lesions usually occur from trauma with resultant inflammation and rapid vascular growth (Fig. 2.3-26).

Clinical Presentation

- Solitary rapidly growing dome-shaped lesion with a specific collar around the base of the dome referred to as a collarette.
- Common in children and young adults with a slight increase during pregnancy.

DIFFERENTIAL DIAGNOSIS Pyogenic Granuloma

- Cherry angioma
- Basal cell carcinoma
- Amelanotic melanoma
- Spitz nevus
- Glomus tumor

Treatment

- Shave biopsy with electrocautery.
- Laser therapy.

Management and Patient Education

- PGs during pregnancy can be monitored and may resolve after delivery.
- Sudden onset in childhood on face and extremities, occurring without a history of trauma may suggest Spitz nevus and referral to dermatology is recommended.

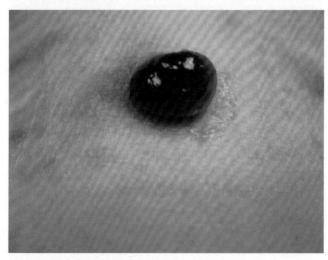

FIG. 2.3-26. Pyogenic granulomas are easily traumatized, causing bleeding. (Photo courtesy of M. Bobonich.)

CLINICAL PEARLS

- Advise the patient of healing times before elective treatments.

- All procedures have a risk of scarring, infection, and abnormal pigmentation. Make sure patients are advised and appropriate written consents are obtained.

- Do a test site in a less-visible site to check healing response before removing multiple lesions.

- Evaluate comorbidities and weigh risk and benefits (especially those that are cosmetically sensitive or difficult to heal).

- Clinicians should always send excised specimens to dermatopathology. Patients' desire to reduce cost should not drive this decision.

- Know the appropriate biopsy technique (shave vs. punch) for what you are looking for is critical. If you do not know, refer.

- Excessive hyfrecation or cryotherapy can result in scarring, changes in pigment, and damage to surrounding tissue.

READINGS AND REFERENCES

Bolognia, J. L., Schaffer, J. V., & Cerroni, L. (2018). *Dermatology* (4th ed.). Mosby Elsevier.

Habif, T. P. (2020). *Clinical dermatology: A color guide to diagnosis and therapy* (7th ed.). Mosby.

James, W. D., Elston, D., Treat, J., Rosenbach, M., & Berge, N. I. (2019). *Andrews' diseases of the skin: Clinical Dermatology* (13th ed.). Saunders.

Acne/Rosacea/Perioral Dermatitis

Dorothy A. Sullivan and Nicole Bort

In This Chapter

- Acne Vulgaris
- Rosacea
- Perioral Dermatitis

ACNE AND RELATED DISORDERS

Clinical presentations of papules, pustules, nodules, or cysts often times involve skin conditions that are frequently challenging to differentiate and even harder to treat. In this chapter, we will discuss the distinguishing features of acne vulgaris and acne-like eruptions to aid in an accurate diagnosis and optimal treatment regimens.

Acne Vulgaris

Acne vulgaris is a multifactorial chronic inflammatory disease of pilosebaceous units. There is variability in the disease presentation ranging from mild comedones to large inflamed papules, pustules, nodules, cysts, and scarring. Due to the visible nature of the condition and the potential for permanent scarring, acne is frequently associated with psychological distress, depression, anxiety, and decreased self-esteem. Acne patients "wear" their disease for all to see.

- Acne is one of the most common conditions seen by dermatologists and 13th most common seen by nondermatologists.
- It affects approximately 50 million people in the United States and 650 million people worldwide.
- The onset of acne frequently correlates with puberty and as early as 8 to 12 years old.
- Males tend to develop acne somewhat later in adolescence but have greater disease severity.
- Females tend to have less severe, but a more chronic disease course.

Pathophysiology

Acne involves a complex interplay of four key pathogenic factors (Fig. 3.1-1):

1. Follicular hyperkeratinization
2. Microbial colonization with *cutibacterium acnes* (formerly known as *propionibacterium acne*) continues to trigger inflammatory mediators throughout the active state

3. Sebum production
4. Inflammation

- Contributing factors include diet, genetics, neuroendocrine regulatory mechanisms, increased sebum production, and altered follicular differentiation.
- There is some debate about the role hormones play in acne as it is unknown whether the primary abnormality is related to the levels of circulating hormones or the actual processing of hormones.
- Acne can be exacerbated by stress, hormonal fluctuations, endocrine disorders, smoking, and ultraviolet radiation.
- Medications can potentially trigger or worsen acne and include topical and systemic corticosteroids, progesterone, testosterone, antidepressants, anti-seizure medications, isoniazid, and anti-cancer drugs, specifically the epidermal growth factor receptor (EGFR) drugs.
- While it is uncommon, the psychosocial impact of severe acne has been linked to depression including suicide ideations and attempts.
- Acne commonly occurs in individuals with endocrine disorders such as polycystic ovarian syndrome (PCOS), hypotestosteronemia, Cushing syndrome, and precocious puberty.

Clinical Presentation
Skin Findings

- Acne is a chronic inflammatory disease with the presence of open or closed comedones with or without the addition of inflammatory lesions that include papules, pustules, cysts, and nodules.
- The presentation is variable and may assume different forms, but the initial lesion is usually an open comedone (blackhead) or a closed comedone (whitehead).
- Comedones are clinically considered a noninflammatory lesion and the presence of comedones is required for the clinical diagnosis of acne vulgaris.
- Acne is typically found on the face, chest, and back, which are often the sites of greatest concentration of pilosebaceous units and sebaceous activity.

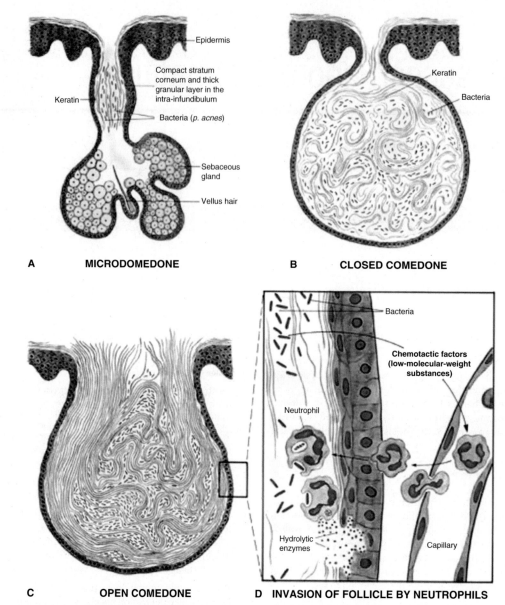

FIG. 3.1-1. Pathogenesis of acne vulgaris.

- Acne may be classified as *mild*, *moderate*, or *severe* depending upon the type and number of lesions, location, and presence/absence of scarring. The degree of disease severity should provide the basis for an evidence-based approach that is individualized for the patient (Table 3.1-1).

- Ongoing monitoring and regular reassessment are essential for early recognition of disease progression.

- Scarring is the result of prolonged inflammation and is more common with nodulocystic lesions. The presence of scarring should immediately classify the condition as *severe* acne. Early intervention is essential to diminish the formation of permanent scars.

Non-Skin Findings

- A thorough history is critical when assessing the acne patient and determining a treatment regimen that will promote adherence and optimize outcomes (Table 3.1-2).

Acne Subtypes

Acne Neonatorum

- Acne neonatorum refers to neonatal acne and infantile acne.

- Neonatal acne usually begins within the first few weeks of life and resolves by 6 months of age. The etiology is unknown but may be related to hormonal stimulation of sebaceous glands by maternal androgens.

- Open and closed comedones are most common; inflammatory papules and pustules are seen occasionally.

- When neonatal acne is associated with *Malassezia* yeast overgrowth, lesions appear more pustular.

- Neonatal acne and infantile acne resemble acne vulgaris, but usually only involve the face.

- Infantile acne occurs 5:1 males to females and starts at 6 to 12 months old. Infantile acne, which starts later, tends to be more severe and persistent than neonatal acne, and may occasionally be associated with an underlying systemic disease or hormonal abnormality.

TABLE 3.1-1	Therapeutic Approach to Acne Based on Severity

MILD ACNE
Open and closed comedones

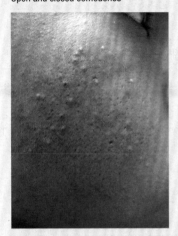

First-line topical therapies only:
- Benzoyl peroxide (BPO)
- Retinoid
- BPO and retinoid
- BPO and antimicrobial
- BPO, antimicrobial, and retinoid

Reevaluate:
- Response to tx and adherence in 6–12 wk

Consider:
- Add/change retinoid
- Add azelaic acid or dapsone

No/little response:
- Increase to moderate acne therapy, acne surgery, photodynamic therapy, chemical peels

MODERATE ACNE
Open/closed comedones, inflammatory papules and pustules, involves face, chest and/or trunk

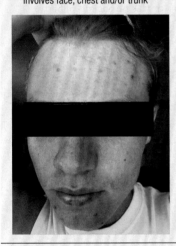

First-line therapies:
Topicals:
- Same as for mild acne

Systemics:
- Topical BPO and retinoid *plus* oral antibiotic
- Oral antibiotics should not be used as monotherapy

Reevaluate:
- Response to tx and adherence in 6–12 wk
- Oral antibiotic therapy recommended shortest duration, usually requiring 3-month trial before seeing improvement

Consider:
- Add/change topical retinoid
- Add/change topical or oral antibiotic
- Females—OCPs if appropriate and spironolactone

No/little response:
- Increase to severe acne therapy
- Assess for possible endocrine disorder

SEVERE ACNE
Open/closed comedones, inflammatory papules or pustules, cysts, nodules involving the face or trunk. Scarring.

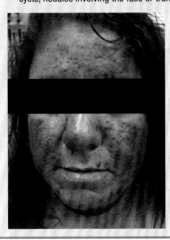

First-line therapy:
- If there is any evidence of scarring, the therapy is escalated to severe.
- Initiate therapy noted in moderate acne until the patient is seen by referral

Dermatology:
- Topical combinations and oral antibiotics
- Oral contraceptives
- Spironolactone (females only)
- Isotretinoin (only prescribed by registered iPLEDGE clinicians)

Modified from Zaenglein, A. L., Pathy, A. L., Schlosser, B. J., Alikhan, A., Baldwin, H. E., Berson, D. S., Bowe, W. P., Graber, E. M., Harper, J. C., Kang, S., Keri, J. E., Leyden, J. J., Reynolds, R. V., Silverberg, N. B., Gold, L. F. S., Tollefson, M. M., Weiss, J. S., Dolan, N. C., Sagan, A. A.,… Bhushan, R. (2016). Guidelines of care for the management of acne vulgaris. *Journal of the American Academy of Dermatology, 74*(5), 945–973. (Mild acne photo courtesy of M. Bobonich; Moderate acne photo courtesy of Nicole Bort; Severe acne photo courtesy of M. Bobonich.)

TABLE 3.1-2	Acne Health History

Onset
- Age at initial breakout

Location
- Face/neck/jawline/chest/back

Duration/Frequency
- Cyclical
- Timing related to menstruation
- Acute or chronic presentation

Alleviating or Provoking Factors
- Cosmetic products
- Stress
- Including diet high in dairy or high glycemic index

Associated or Systemic Conditions
- Endocrinopathies
- Symptoms of PCOS (Stein–Leventhal syndrome)
- Cushing's
- Behavior health/psychological disorders
- Inflammatory bowel disease

Responses to Treatments (including Dose, Vehicle, Frequency)
- Topical therapies
- Systemic therapies
- Over-the-counter products

Women's Health
- Pregnant
- Planning
- Breastfeeding
- Method of contraception
- Increased androgen-dependent hair
- Thinning of scalp hair

Family History
- Acne or other skin conditions
- Hidradenitis suppurativa

Extracurricular Activities
- Including sports

- Infantile acne in a patient with a positive family history of severe acne may be a predictor of more severe adolescent acne.

Confirming the Diagnosis

- Infantile acne is almost always a clinical diagnosis.
- Direct examination of pustule contents with KOH may identify yeast.
- A culture and sensitivity may be indicated if there is suspicion of bacterial infection.
- If acne is especially severe or persistent, serologic tests for abnormal androgen production should be considered.

Treatment

- Nearly all cases of acne neonatorum resolve spontaneously in about 1 to 2 weeks; although, treatment may hasten resolution.

- Cleansing with gentle soap and water daily can clear many cases.
- Mild inflammatory acne can be treated safely in patients of all ages. Topical antibiotics, such as erythromycin or clindamycin are not recommended as monotherapy because they take a long time to start working and are associated with high rates of bacterial resistance.
- Neonatal and infantile acne are typically self-limiting but can be treated with off-label topical retinoids that may be used in combination with benzoyl peroxide wash.
- Patients with *Malassezia* can be treated with topical antifungal creams or shampoos, like ketoconazole 2% or selenium sulfide 2.5% which are off-label.
- If severe, patients should be referred to dermatology. Refer to endocrinology if there are any signs of virilization or growth abnormalities.

Mid-Childhood Acne

- Occurs in children 18 months to 7 years old.
- It is often misidentified as keratosis pilaris, rosacea, perioral dermatitis, or *Demodex* folliculitis.
- Acne in this age range is rare and can be concerning as it may be indicative of an underlying systemic condition such as Cushing syndrome, premature adrenarche, congenital adrenal hyperplasia, gonadal/adrenal tumors, or true precocious puberty.
- Mid-childhood acne mostly presents as comedones, inflammatory papules and/or pustules.

Confirming the Diagnosis

- Patients in this age group, who present with chronic, severe, or virilizing acne require further evaluation for systemic disease.
- An appropriate evaluation would include use of pediatric growth charts, bone scans, total/free testosterone, dehydroepiandrosterone (DHEA), prolactin, LH/FSH, 17-OH progesterone levels, and androstenedione.

Treatment

- Topical therapies similar to those used in infantile acne may be recommended.
- For severe cases, oral therapies are advised with the exception of prescribed tetracycline products, which are not recommended to children age 8 years and younger.

Management and Patient Education

- Address the underlying cause and monitor for signs and symptoms of a hyperandrogenic state.

Preadolescent Acne

- Preadolescent acne occurs in children 8 to 12 years old.
- This may be an indicator of emerging puberty as it corresponds to additional sebum production and increase in the size of sebaceous follicles.
- There is some evidence to suggest that the severity and prevalence of acne in the preteen years is predictive of advanced prepubertal maturity.

Treatment

- Traditional topical therapies are advised until the individual's level of severity and potential for scarring can be accurately assessed.

TABLE 3.1-3	Acne Variants
Acne excoriee	Habitual picking, usually by young women, in a vain attempt to eradicate them. Often leaving "punch out" sores, scars, and postinflammatory inflammation (Fig. 3.1-2).
Acne mechanica	Caused by friction or chafing from chin straps, sports padding or equipment.
Chloracne	Due to occupational exposure to toxins like chlorinated or halogenated chemicals. Large comedones and pustules face, behind the ears, trunk, genitals and axillae.
Acne cosmetica	Adolescent females who wear a lot of makeup. Characteristically numerous tiny bumps across skin on face.
Pomade acne	Often presenting on the forehead as closed comedones which are caused by heavy hair products that block the pilosebaceous units.
Acne associated with endocrine abnormalities	Often accompanied by hirsutism, menstrual irregularities, and virilizing characteristics. Usually characterized by pustules, cysts, or nodules.

Adolescent Acne

- The onset during puberty occurs about 80% of the time and lasts approximately 5 years.
- Acne can present simply as comedones and a few papules, or it can progress to multiple inflammatory papules, pustules, nodules, and cysts.
- Individuals will vary with regard to lesion type, extent, location, and development of scarring.

Adult Acne

There are acne variants that can develop as the result of exogenous and endogenous factors (Table 3.1-3).

DIFFERENTIAL DIAGNOSIS Acne

- Milia—appear similar to closed comedone, but there is an absence of open comedone, papules, pustules, cysts and erythema
- Sebaceous hyperplasia—these bumps are often indented in the center
- Perioral dermatitis—location is primary around the mouth, sparing the vermillion border, and absence of comedones
- Rosacea—has an absence of comedone
- Folliculitis (gram positive and gram negative; Pityrosporum)— gram negative—monomorphic eruptive papules and pustules; gram positive appears similarly to acne, but should be considered if eruptions are acute
- Pseudofolliculitis barbae—has an absence of comedone and primary affects only hair-bearing areas
- Angiofibromas—have violaceous hue
- Keratosis pilaris—absence of comedone

Confirming the Diagnosis

- Clinical diagnosis is typically made with visual inspection.
- Additional tests to rule out differential diagnoses can include bacterial culture of a pustular lesion.
- On occasion, the onset of acne may be an indicator of a systemic process or endocrine abnormality necessitating additional diagnostics. Testing is indicated for those with clinical features of hyperandrogenism and include DHEA and free testosterone as initial screening laboratory studies to evaluate hormonal influences.

Treatment

- Treatment should be started early to prevent permanent sequelae.
- When developing an individualized treatment plan for the patient, one must consider morphology, distribution, severity, history, and patient preference and resources.
- Topical and systemic agents should be selected with the goal of targeting the pathogenic factors contributing to patients' type and severity of acne (Table 3.1-4).

TABLE 3.1-4	Acne Therapies Targeting the Pathogenic Factors of Acne			
	DECREASE SEBUM	**NORMALIZE KERATINIZATION**	**DECREASE *C. ACNES***	**DECREASE INFLAMMATION**
Topical Therapies				
Antimicrobial			X	X
Retinoids		X		X
Benzoyl peroxide		X	X	X
Azelaic acid		X	X	X
Systemic Therapies				
Oral antibiotics			X	X
Isotretinoin	X	X	X	X
Oral birth control pills	X			
Spironolactone	X			

- There are many over-the-counter therapies, like topical and oral zinc oxide, nicotinamide, probiotics, etc., that have been suggested as effective alternatives in acne care. However, there is a paucity of data and additional studies are needed to evaluate the safety and efficacy over time.

Topical Therapies

First-line therapy for most patients with acne vulgaris should be topical therapy—specifically a topical retinoid plus an antimicrobial agent. There are a vast number of agents that offer different mechanism of actions, dosing, formulation, side effects, and safety considerations (Table 3.1-5). Topical therapies are also available as combination products targeting multiple pathogenic features including several that have a synergic effect. Combination products may help with patients who have difficulties adhering to treatment but are often branded and more expensive (Table 3.1-6).

A note about retinoids

- Ideal for treatment of comedonal acne and often combined for the additional acne variants due to the fact that they are both comedolytic and anti-inflammatory.

- Most of these topical agents are available as monotherapy or combination products.

- The most common side effects include erythema, irritation, and dryness.

- There is a higher risk of photosensitivity and sunburn with retinoids, so daily sunscreen should be encouraged. Tretinoin is not photostable and should be applied in the evening.

- Topical tretinoin may be oxidized and inactivated by coadministration of benzoyl peroxide, so it is recommended that they be applied at different times of the day.

- A discussion regarding pregnancy risk is important for women of child-bearing age. Tretinoin and adapalene are Pregnancy Category C (using old system) but tazarotene is Pregnancy Category X.

Systemic Therapy

Systemic therapy is indicated for moderate to severe acne, when there is widespread involvement of face, chest, and back, or if there are cystic lesions anywhere (Table 3.1-7). Long-term systemic antimicrobials are not recommended and should always be used for the shortest duration possible. However, it usually takes at least 3 months before an optimal clinical response is observed.

- *Oral antibiotics*
  - Suppress the growth of cutaneous flora such as *C. acnes,* and some can also have an anti-inflammatory effect.
  - Oral antibiotics should not be used as a monotherapy and be used in combination with topical benzoyl peroxide. Concomitant use of maintenance topical regimens in addition to oral antibiotics cannot be overemphasized to help reduce the likelihood of bacterial resistance.

- *Hormonal therapies*
  - Combined oral contraceptive pills (COCPs)—There are currently four COCPs approved by the FDA for the treatment of acne. Treatment is ideal for acne treatment in women who also desire contraception. Patients should be assessed for contraindications and risk factors prior to starting therapy.
  - Spironolactone—there is limited data on the efficacy in acne, but it has shown to be effective in select groups. It is currently used off-label for the treatment of acne. Male should not use because they are at risk for development of gynecomastia. The best candidates for successful use of spironolactone are adult women with

acne lesions primarily distributed on the lower face and mandible when androgen-related acne is suspected. Dosing ranges from 25 to 100 mg b.i.d., with most evidence showing improvement between 50 to 100 mg daily either as monotherapy or adjunctive.

Spironolactone is a Pregnancy Category C but definitely not recommended during pregnancy or for females contemplating pregnancy. It is contraindicated in pregnancy as some animal studies have shown feminization of male fetuses. Side effects are dose related and include breakthrough bleeding or spotting, menstrual irregularities, headaches, diuresis, dizziness, fatigue, potential hyperkalemia, and breast tenderness. Laboratory monitoring for hyperkalemia is not necessary in young, healthy women with normal hepatic and renal function who are taking spironolactone for acne treatment. Monitoring should be considered in those with a history of renal disease, cardiovascular disease, or who are taking an angiotensin-converting enzyme inhibitor or an angiotensin receptor blocker.

- Low-dose prednisone—doses ranging from 5 to 15 mg have shown some efficacy in the treatment of acne and can be used for the treatment of acne fulminans or isotretinoin-induced acne fulminans-like eruptions. Long-term adverse side effects prohibit prednisone as a primary or long-term treatment modality for acne.

Oral Retinoids

- *Isotretinoin* is FDA approved for the treatment of severe nodulocystic acne that is refractory to treatment or acne that causes severe psychosocial distress.

- Isotretinoin is highly teratogenic and a Pregnancy Category X, requiring two forms of birth control methods in females of child-bearing potential.

- Patients on isotretinoin are required to participate in the FDA risk management distribution program known as iPLEDGE for the duration of their treatment. Patients should be referred to an approved dermatology provider for management.

Adjunct Treatments

Laser and light therapy

- There is still much research to be conducted regarding the best light source, dose, and frequency of use.

- Among the treatments being offered are intense pulsed light, pulsed dye laser, potassium titanyl phosphate laser, fractioned and nonfractioned infrared lasers, and photodynamic therapy with or without photosensitizing agents.

- Initial research indicates that these options are *best* used in partnership with other traditional medical therapies or for those who cannot withstand a typical regimen.

Intralesional injections

- Small amounts of triamcinolone 10 mg/mL diluted 1:1 with lidocaine or normal saline is the treatment of choice.

- It is recommended that this therapy be used by clinicians skilled in intralesional injections.

- The risks of atrophy and depigmentation should be discussed in detail prior to the procedure.

Chemical peels

- Glycolic acid peels and salicylic acid peels have been used as adjunct treatment for mild acne. Results are limited to mild improvements in noninflammatory (comedonal) acne lesions only.

TABLE 3.1-5	Topical Agents for Treatment of Acne	
AGENT	**GENERIC/BRAND**	**COMMENTS**
Cleansers	Mild cleansers (nonabrasive)	b.i.d. Preference nonsoap cleansers Antibacterial cleansers are drying
	Benzoyl peroxide wash, creamy wash, or leave-on	Daily or b.i.d. Can bleach fabrics, dryness and irritation Keratolytic, anti-inflammatory, antimicrobial Pregnancy Category C
	Salicylic acid 2%	Keratolytic/Comedolytic OTC Pregnancy Category C
Antimicrobials	BPO 2.5%–10% (OTC and Rx)	Daily wash or leave-on gel Bleaches fabrics, drying/irritating, and can leave a white haze visible on dark skin types Possible development of allergic contact dermatitis MOA incl. prevention of bacterial resistance Keratolytic, decreases free fatty acids Pregnancy Category C
	Sodium sulfacetamide (Plexion, Rosaderm, Sulfa Cleanse)	b.i.d. If sulfur combination, more drying Antimicrobial Pregnancy Category C
	Azaleic Acid 15% gel (Finacea) 20% cream (Azelex, Finevin)	b.i.d., good for skin of color Mild comedolytic, anti-inflammatory, antibacterial Some lightening effect in hyperpigmentation Pregnancy Category B
	Clindamycin 1% sol, lotion, gel (Cleocin T, Clindagel, Evoclin)	Daily or b.i.d. Rare pseudomembranous colitis Growing bacterial resistance Pregnancy Category B
	Erythromycin 2% (Akne-Mycin ointment, Ery pads, and solution)	Daily or b.i.d. Good for sensitive or dry skin Antibacterial but growing bacterial resistance Often requires refrigeration Pregnancy Category B
	Dapsone 5%, 7.5% (Aczone gel)	b.i.d., but not at same time as BPO because skin will turn orange skin-reversible Anti-inflammatory Pregnancy Category C
	Minocycline 4% foam (Amzeeq)	Severe acne patients 9 yr and older Can get discoloration skin, scars, and teeth
Retinoids	Tretinoin (Retin A 0.025%, 0.05%, 0.1%; Renova 0.02%, 0.05%; Retin A Micro 0.04%, 0.6%, 0.8%; Atralin gel 0.05%; Altreno lotion 0.05)	Retinoids have keratolytic, comedolytic, and anti-inflammatory properties. Irritating, use on dry face Apply small amount at nighttime Start twice weekly and slowly increase Use nightly as maintenance Indicated for facial acne >12 yr and older except: Altreno >9 yr and older for facial acne Trifarotene >9 yr and older facial & acne Pregnancy Category C Tazarotene 0.045% approved for >9 yr and older Pregnancy Category X
	Adapalene 0.1% (Differin lotion; generic or gel: 0.3% Cream	
	Trifarotene 0.005% (Aklief)	
	Tazarotene (Tazorac 0.1%; Arazlo 0.045% lotion)	

TABLE 3.1-6	Combination Topical Acne Agents by Age

Approved for 9 yr and older:

Epiduo	Adapalene 0.1%/BPO 2.5%

Approved for 12 yr and older:

Epiduo Forte	Adapalene 0.3%/BPO 2.5%
Benzamycin gel	Erythromycin 3% BPO 5%
Ziana, Veltin	Clindamycin 1%/tretinoin 0.025%
Acanya, BenzaClin, Duac, Onexton	Clindamycin 1–1.2%/BPO (2.5–5%)

Complementary/Alternative Therapies

Tea tree oil and herbal agents like oral ayurvedic, oral barberry extract, and gluconolactone solution are well tolerated and may have some benefits in acne. These agents, however, are not recommended as alternatives to traditional therapies.

Dietary Recommendations

Some evidence suggests a link between high glycemic diets and diets high in some dairy products (especially skim milk) as having an adverse effect on acne. There are currently no official recommendations on dietary modifications.

TABLE 3.1-7	Systemic Therapy for Management of Moderate to Severe Acne

THERAPY	DRUG/DOSE/COMMENTS
Antibiotic[a,b] First-line therapy	**TETRACYCLINE CLASS** • Antimicrobial and anti-inflammatory • Many drug interactions, do not take with calcium and GI upset, vaginal candidiasis, hypersensitivity reactions **Tetracycline** 250–500 mg • Not available **Sarecycline** 60-mg, 100-mg, 150-mg doses • Daily; weight-based dosing 1.5 mg/kg/day • First in class tetracycline derivative with narrow spectrum activity against gram-positive bacteria (including *Cutibacterium acnes*), displaying a low propensity for development of antimicrobial resistance • Indicated for >9 yr and older. Pregnancy—limited available human data **Minocycline** 50–100 mg • Daily or b.i.d. • Stevens–Johnson syndrome, lupus-like syndrome, abnormal hyperpigmentation, dizziness, and tinnitus • Pregnancy Category D **Doxycycline** 50–100 mg • Daily or b.i.d. • Similar SE as minocycline but greater photosensitivity • Pregnancy Category B **Doxycycline** 20 mg and 40 mg (Oracea) • Subantimicrobial dose (i.e., 20 mg b.i.d. or 40 mg daily) used as anti-inflammatory • Taken on empty stomach • Greater photosensitivity than minocycline • Pregnancy Category D
	MACROLIDES **Erythromycin** 250–500 mg • Higher risk of gastrointestinal upset and cardiac conduction abnormalities • Off-label use in acne • Growing bacterial resistance to *C. acnes* • Pregnancy Category
Antibiotic[a–c] Alternatives	**Sulfamethoxazole/trimethoprim** 200 mg • Daily or b.i.d. • Use cautiously for severe refractory cases • Pregnancy Category C
	Amoxicillin 250–500 mg • Daily or b.i.d. • GI symptoms, vaginal candida, hypersensitivity • Pregnancy Category B
	Cephalexin 500 mg • b.i.d. • GI upset, vaginal candida, hypersensitivity • Pregnancy Category B

THERAPY	DRUG/DOSE/COMMENTS
	Azithromycin 250 mg • 3–4 days a month • Higher risk of gastrointestinal upset and cardiac conduction abnormalities • Pregnancy Category B
Hormones	**Combined Oral Contraceptive Pills[d] (COCPs)** Reduce inflammatory and comedone lesion counts based on anti-androgenic properties. Usually takes 3 cycles before effect. Used alone or in combination with other acne therapy. FDA approved: • Ethinyl estradiol/norgestimate • Ethinyl estradiol/norethindrone acetate/ferrous fumarate • Ethinyl estradiol/drospirenone • Ethinyl estradiol/drospirenone /levomefolate COCP use is associated with CV risks and increased risk of breast cancer in some women. Therefore, careful assessment along with risks vs. benefits and contraindications should be done prior to prescribing
	Spironolactone • Off-label use for acne in females, especially those affect lower face or mandibular distribution. • Usually takes 3 cycles before effect. • Start 50 mg/day, increase to b.i.d., max 200 mg/day. • Caution and consultation if used in female with family history of breast cancer. • Avoid concomitant use with K^+ sparing diuretics, ACE inhibitors, K^+ supplements, lithium. • Can be used in combination with drospirenone (OCPs) but increased risk for hyperkalemia. • Pregnancy Category C—some studies showed feminization of male fetus. • Male patients at risk for gynecomastia.
Retinoids	**Isotretinoin** • Refer to dermatology specialist enrolled in iPledge program. • Approved for the treatment of severe nodulocystic acne, acne that has been refractory to treatment or that causes severe psychosocial distress. • Highly teratogenic, Pregnancy Category X medication, requiring two forms of birth control methods in females of childbearing potential. • Patients on isotretinoin are required to participate in the FDA risk management distribution and monitoring program known as iPledge for the duration of their treatment.
Corticosteroids	**Prednisone** • Low-dose prednisone (5–15 mg/day) has shown some efficacy in treatment of acne flares and in treatment of acne fulminans, conglobata or isotretinoin-induced flares. • Long-term side effects prohibit the use of prednisone as a primary treatment modality for acne.

[a]Antibiotics may render OCPs less effective. Back up birth control method is recommended.
[b]Use as monotherapy is not recommended; should use topical benzoyl peroxide with any topical or systemic antibiotic for acne therapy.
[c]Off-label, limited studies, alternative antibiotics should only be used when first-line agents cannot be used; routine use not recommended.
[d]FDA approved for acne treatment in females who also desire contraception.

Management and Patient Education

- Acne can be self-limiting but is often a disease of chronicity and can last throughout late adulthood with unpredictable flares, exacerbations, and scarring. Relapse is not uncommon.

- Acne regimens require at least 3 months of faithful use to see evidence of improvement.

- Wash face daily with a gentle cleanser not more than twice a day. Overwashing can lead to excess oil production and worsen acne.

- Wash face after excessive sweating.

- Apply a "pea-size" amount of medication to the entire face as prescribed. More is not better.

- Applying a gentle moisturizer daily will help with dryness and irritation often caused by topical acne medications.

- Wear sunscreen daily.

- Topical benzoyl peroxide stains clothing, towels, and bed linen.

- Consider medication reminders like texts or cell phone alarm to help remember to take medications.

- Never squeeze or pick acne lesions as this can lead to scarring or postinflammatory hyperpigmentation (Fig. 3.1-2).

- Avoid harsh exfoliants or scrubbing as this can lead to significant irritation and inflammation making acne worse.

- Use "noncomedogenic" and oil-free facial products.

- If a patient fails to respond after 3 to 6 months of therapy or has evidence of scarring, refer to a dermatologist immediately for other treatment considerations.

- Clinicians often dismiss acne as a benign, normal part of maturation, but it is important to remain cognizant of the subtle cues that may signify a deeper, significant psychological turmoil that sometimes exists.

- If there is a suspicion of precocious puberty, PCOS, or hyperandrogenism, a referral to endocrinology is appropriate.

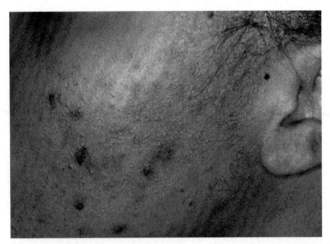

FIG. 3.1-2. Acne excoriee caused by scratching or picking which can leave scarring and postinflammatory hyperpigmentation especially in dark skin types. (Photo courtesy of M. Bobonich.)

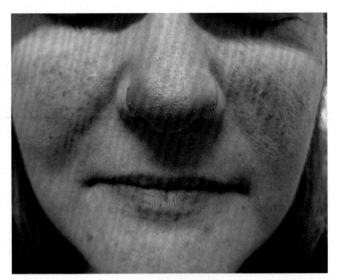

FIG. 3.1-3. Rosacea, erythematotelangiectatic type. (Photo courtesy of M. Bobonich.)

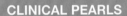

CLINICAL PEARLS

- Ongoing maintenance therapy, particularly with a topical retinoid, is the best strategy to combat the likelihood of relapse.
- Topical retinoids should be applied to entire face and not just "spot" treatment.
- The vehicle selected for topical treatment will impact the overall effect.
- It is important to remember that topically applied products are absorbed percutaneously through the body, therefore may be contraindicated in pregnancy—particularly retinoids.
- Abrupt-onset acne that is monomorphic in nature, uncommonly severe, or unresponsive to treatment should prompt further investigation, as this may indicate an endocrine disorder, drug-related onset, or another problem of a systemic nature. Referral to a dermatologist can be helpful.

ROSACEA

According to the National Rosacea Society, it is estimated that over 16 million people are affected by rosacea. The onset is most common during middle-aged (between the ages of 30 and 50 years) but has been reported in children and the elderly. Women are affected at an earlier age, but rosacea is more severe in men. The rhinophymatous subtype is almost exclusive to men. It is more often found in patients with Celtic ancestry and with an inherited predisposition. It occurs very infrequently in skin of color.

Pathophysiology

Advances in the understanding of the pathogenesis and pathophysiology of rosacea are progressing rapidly. The most recent research suggests rosacea is a multivariate disease process that underlies varied clinical manifestations of the condition.

- Suspected contributing factors include neurologic and genetic factors, autoimmune, repeated vasodilation, changes in the pilosebaceous structure, and colonization of microorganisms like *Demodex folliculorum.*
- Chronic sun exposure can prompt edema, impair lymphatic drainage, and produce the characteristic telangiectasia and skin thickening.
- There is an association, but not a causal relationship, with a growing number of underlying systemic disorders including cardiovascular, neurologic, gastrointestinal, autoimmune and certain malignancies.

- Impairment of the skin barrier function in rosacea can result in transepidermal water loss making the skin prone to sensitivity, dryness, scaling, and peeling.

Clinical Presentation

Skin Findings

- Rosacea is a chronic, relapsing inflammatory disease of the skin that causes persistent erythema, papules, pustules, facial erythema or telangiectasia, flushing/blushing and mild edema that can affect the nose, cheeks, chin, and forehead.
- Phymatous changes or thickening can occur in some cases and occasionally a disseminated violaceous hue (Figs. 3.1-3 to 3.1-6).

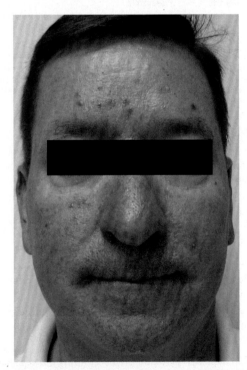

FIG. 3.1-4. Rosacea, papulopustular type. (Photo courtesy of M. Bobonich.)

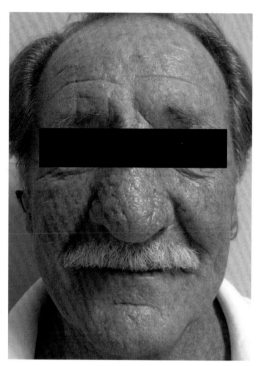

FIG. 3.1-5. Rosacea, phymatous type. (Photo courtesy of M. Bobonich.)

- Rosacea often affects the convex surfaces of the face, including the nose, centrofacial area, and forehead. The nasolabial folds are generally spared.
- Rosacea has been traditionally classified into four subtypes. Each subtype has distinct clinical features that predominate and are unique to its category, although some features may overlap (Table 3.1-8).

- A new rosacea classification has been proposed which provides a more individualized approach for the assessment according to the patient characteristics or phenotype.Recommended management should then be based on these features to optimize patient outcomes (Table 3.1-9).

Non-Skin Findings

- Assessment of patients with rosacea should involve a detailed pertinent history (Table 3.1-10).
- Rosacea can often lead to decreased self-esteem and self-confidence, which can impact social and professional relationships.
- Ocular symptoms can include dryness, irritation, burning/ stinging, or itching. While infrequent, keratitis, scleritis, and iritis can occur.

DIFFERENTIAL DIAGNOSIS   Rosacea

- Acne vulgaris—differentiated from rosacea by the presence of comedones.
- Perioral dermatitis—while they can look similar, perioral dermatitis is often not present on the malar cheeks and very often has a clear cause.
- Steroid-induced acneiform eruption—affiliated with current or recent exposure to steroids.
- Seborrheic dermatitis—the distribution of seborrheic dermatitis ranges from mild scaling to widespread involvement of scalp, ears, brows, and paranasal area.
- Polymorphous light eruption—intermittent and recurrent more often in the spring or early summer without the chronic nature of rosacea.
- Lupus erythematous—the erythema associated often has a more violaceous hue and has a more abrupt cutoff, especially at the lateral margin.

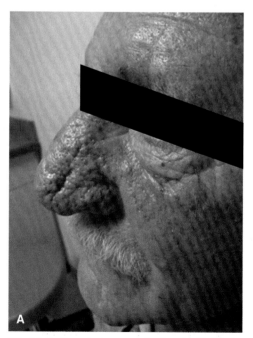

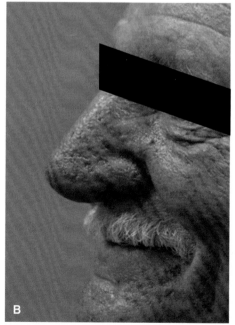

FIG. 3.1-6. Phymatous rosacea treatment with CO_2 laser. **A:** Rhinophyma before laser treatment. (Photo before, courtesy of M. Bobonich.) **B:** Rhinophyma after laser treatment. (Photo after, courtesy of Jeffery Scott, M.D. and Margaret Mann, M.D.)

TABLE 3.1-8	Rosacea Subtypes and Therapeutics

Erythro-Telangiectatic

Persistent erythema with intermittent flushing/blushing. Facial telangiectasias may be present. Burning and stinging sensations are common (Fig. 3.1-3).

- Topical alpha$_2$-agonist brimonidine 0.33% gel (Mirvaso) daily.
- Oxymetazoline (Rhofade) can be applied to reduce the appearance of redness. The direct vasoconstriction can last for up to 12 h. This does not treat associated telangiectasias.
- Adrenergic antagonists: mirtazapine (alpha blocker), propranolol (beta blocker) and carvedilol (both alpha and beta blocker) can be used to help with flushing symptoms. Use of low doses to avoid adverse side effects such as hypotension, fatigue, and bronchospasm.
- Laser or impulse light therapy can be helpful to treat refractory erythema and telangiectasia but does not treat the flushing.

Papular/Pustular

Inflammatory papules and pustules scattered on a background of central facial erythema with or without edema. Usually sparing the periocular areas and nasolabial folds. Treatment of the inflammatory papules and pustular lesions is dependent on the severity of the disease (Fig. 3.1-4).

Mild to moderate

- Topical metronidazole 0.75% or 1% cream/lotion/gel once to b.i.d.
- Topical azelaic acid 15% gel or 20% lotion once to b.i.d.
- Topical combination of 10% sodium sulfacetamide and 5% sulfur cream/lotion form b.i.d.
- Topical ivermectin 1% daily
- Topical dapsone 7.5% gel applied daily
- Topical benzoyl peroxide (completed Phase 3 Clinical Trials but not FDA approved at this time)

Moderate to severe, or recalcitrant

When first-line treatments are inadequate in mild cases or when disease is more severe at presentation, it is recommended to combine topical therapies with oral agents.

- Long term use of oral antibiotics should be avoided, and treatment should be stopped or tapered when control of the disease is achieved.
- Doxycycline 20–100 mg b.i.d. Data supports the use of low-dose doxycycline (40 mg) showed similar efficacy with less adverse effects than higher dosing. Photosensitivity is the main adverse effect. Minocycline carries an increased risk of pigmentation, liver disorders, and lupus-like syndrome.
- Erythromycin 250–500 mg once or b.i.d., if doxycycline is contraindicated.
- Azithromycin 250–500 mg two to three times weekly may be considered.
- Clarithromycin 250 mg daily can also be considered, but data is limited.
- Referral to dermatology specialist for oral isotretinoin 0.25–0.30 mg/kg/day for 12–16 wk has be reported to be effective in severe cases but should not be used in women who are pregnant or wish to become pregnant.

Phymatous

Marked thickening of the skin from chronic inflammation and edema most commonly found on the nose (rhinophyma). Sebaceous hyperplasia and enlarged pore size is often present. Men are more often affected than women (Fig. 3.1-5).

Clinically inflamed

- Topical retinoids
- Doxycycline 20–100 mg b.i.d.
- Oral isotretinoin (following guidelines for safe therapy and monitoring)

Clinically noninflamed

- Laser ablative therapy (Fig. 3.1-6)
- Surgical intervention
- Referral to dermatology

Ocular

Examination findings include conjunctivitis, blepharitis, and hyperemia. Patients often complain of dry, itchy, irritated eyes. Can occur in conjunction with or without cutaneous findings.

- Eyelid hygiene with use of warm water and artificial tears twice daily
- Doxycycline 20–100 mg b.i.d.
- Referral to an ophthalmologist to rule out additional diagnosis and prevent vision-threatening complications

Confirming the Diagnosis

- There are no definitive diagnostic tests for rosacea.
- Rosacea is a clinical diagnosis based on careful history taking and examination.
- The clinician should identify each individual patient characteristics or phenotype based on diagnostic, major, and minor features (Table 3.1-9)
- Skin scraping for demodex (Fig. 3.1-7) can be helpful in severe or recalcitrant disease and guide therapy (Fig. 3.1-8).

- A diagnostic workup is not typically required for rosacea unless the condition fails to respond to treatment or is progressively worsening despite good adherence to treatment and trigger avoidance.
- If symptoms of lightheadedness, sweating, or palpitations accompany the symptoms of flushing attributed to rosacea, then further evaluation for possible underlying systemic disease should be prompted. Underlying systemic causes may include polycythemia vera, connective tissue disorders (i.e., lupus or dermatomyositis), carcinoid syndrome, and mastocytosis.

TABLE 3.1-9	New Standard Classification System for Rosacea[a]
CLASSIFICATION	**FEATURES**
Diagnostic	Any of these features is diagnostic of rosacea • Phymatous changes usually involving the nose • Persistent erythema including ongoing centrofacial redness
Major	Two or more of these features may be considered diagnostic of rosacea • Flushing or transient erythema • Papules and/or pustules • Telangiectasias • Ocular manifestations
Minor	Consideration of these features for assessment of disease severity • Burning sensation • Stinging sensation • Dryness • Edema (localized facial edema) • Ocular manifestations

[a]Modified from Schaller, M., Almeida, L., Bewley, A., Cribier, B., Del Rosso, J., Dlova, N. C., Gallo, R. L., Granstein, R. D., Kautz, G., Mannis, M. J., Micali, G., Oon, H. H., Rajagopalan, M., Steinhoff, M., Tanghetti, E., Thiboutot, D., Troielli, P., Webster, G., Zierhut, M., van Zuuren, E. J., … Tan, J. (2020). Recommendations for rosacea diagnosis, classification and management: update from the global ROSacea COnsensus 2019 panel. *The British Journal of Dermatology, 182*(5), 1269–1276. https://doi.org/10.1111/bjd.18420

- Patients with a suspected diagnosis of rosacea should be questioned as to the presence of eye symptoms such as burning, grittiness, stinging, or itching. Ocular rosacea may exist without significant cutaneous manifestations, and a referral to ophthalmology may be warranted.

Treatment

- Rosacea is a chronic condition that commonly has episodes of remission and relapses with treatment individualized for each patient's dominant features of the disease (Table 3.1-8).
- Treatment is recommended for at least 6 weeks to assess for appropriate response.

TABLE 3.1-10	Pertinent History in Rosacea Patient

- Recent travel
- Timing: onset (sudden versus gradual), location, duration
- Characteristics: itch, tenderness, bleeding, burning
- Triggers:
  - Environmental—UVR, sun, heat, cold, wind, humidity
  - Intake—spicy food, hot beverages, caffeine, chocolate
  - Lifestyle—smoking, stress, alcohol
  - Medications: calcium channel blockers, sildenafil, nitrates, nicotinic acid, and niacin have all been associated
  - Oral hygiene products
- Associated symptoms or conditions: hypertension, anxiety disorders, gastrointestinal conditions, thyroid dysfunction, allergies, asthma, female hormonal imbalance, and metabolic diseases. However, further research is required to establish true pathophysiologic connections.
- Report of previous treatments and responses.

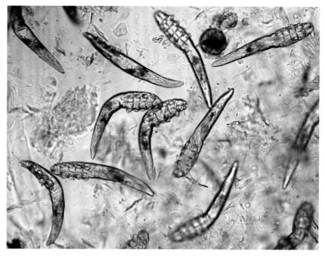

FIG. 3.1-7. *Demodex Folliculorum* from a skin scraping and then placed on a microscope slide with mineral oil. (Photo courtesy of M. Bobonich.)

- The use of topical steroids should be avoided.
- Patients should be made aware that topical therapy is generally continued after remission to reduce the risk of recurrence.

Management and Patient Education

- Rosacea is a chronic disease and requires long-term management.
- Management should include education on general management of the disease, routine skin care recommendations, trigger avoidance, and often combination therapies.
- Although there is no cure for rosacea, achieving clear or almost clear skin should be the treatment goals.
- Given the multivariant nature of rosacea, treatment is based on each individual's phenotype. Patients may require one or two treatment modalities. There is no "one size fits all" therapy for rosacea patients.

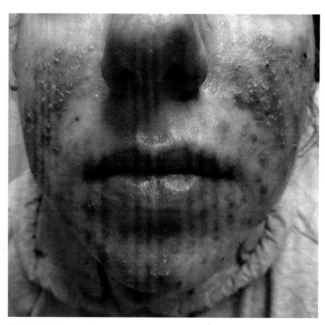

FIG. 3.1-8. Recalcitrant and severe rosacea caused by *Demodex folliculorum* can be violaceous red and often pustular. (Photo courtesy of M. Bobonich.)

General Care for All Rosacea Patients

- Daily broad-spectrum protection against ultraviolet A and ultraviolet B radiation with an SPF of at least 30.

- Use of mild moisturizers and soap-free cleansers.

- Triggers that exacerbate the condition should be identified and avoided. Since they are unique to the individual, keeping a diary to identify stimuli can be helpful. A common list of triggers includes spicy food, alcoholic or caffeinated beverages, irritant cosmetic products, emotional influences, physical exertion, and temperature- or weather-related factors.

- Avoid waterproof make-up, exfoliating scrubs, astringents, toners or products that contain alcohol, witch hazel, fragrance, menthol, camphor, peppermint, and eucalyptus oil.

- Camouflage green-based cosmetics neutralize red pigment can be helpful in reducing appearance of redness.

- It is important to provide education and support about the benign nature of the condition and also set realistic expectations. There is no cure for rosacea. The goal is for control of this chronic disease that tends to have periods of remission and relapse.

- Follow-up is important to evaluate the efficacy of the prescribed therapy, emphasis on proper skin care techniques, and to discuss identified triggers.

- Patients can find out more at National Rosacea Society: www.rosacea.org

- Referral to dermatology is appropriate for recalcitrant or difficult cases that have not improved with appropriate therapies.

- Ocular involvement should be referred to an ophthalmologist for evaluation.

- If systemic lupus is suspected, referral to rheumatology is warranted.

Special Populations

Pediatrics

- Rosacea has been observed in the pediatric population but is not common.

- Erythromycin 2% gel would be an appropriate first-line therapy.

- Tetracycline products should not be prescribed to children 8 years of age and under.

Pregnancy and Nursing

- For treatment of inflammatory lesions, metronidazole, azelaic acid, and erythromycin 2% gel can be used.

- Oral treatment, tetracyclines, and isotretinoin are absolute contraindications while oral macrolide antibiotics (erythromycin, clarithromycin, and azithromycin) are acceptable treatment alternatives.

CLINICAL PEARLS

- An important characteristic of rosacea is the absence of comedones, a hallmark sign of acne vulgaris. Although acne and rosacea can coexist, the absence of comedones is more suggestive of rosacea.

- It is of critical importance not to overlook the possibility of HIV or AIDS, which may present as a papulopustular eruption of the face in early adulthood. Rosacea is seen more frequently in the latter decades of life.

PERIORAL DERMATITIS

Perioral dermatitis (PD) is an inflammatory disorder with localized erythematous papules and pustules that involves the nasolabial folds, upper and lower lips, and the chin. It is a common problem that almost exclusively affects females between the ages of 15 to 35 years. PD can occur in men and has been identified in children between the ages of 7 months and 13 years with no favored gender.

Pathophysiology

- Initially, it was thought that PD was related to the use of topical corticosteroids on the facial skin prior to the onset of the rash. Topical steroids cause a direct vasoconstrictive effect and local immune suppression, which leads to an overgrowth of bacteria, yeast, and demodex mites within the hair follicle. When the steroid is withdrawn, the local immunity is reconstituted resulting in inflammation of the hair follicles and suppurative folliculitis accompanied by erythema, scaling, inflammatory papules, and pustules.

- In recent years, however, use of occlusive moisturizers and foundation has also been implicated in its etiology.

- Patient who uses nasal or inhaled corticosteroids may be at greater risk.

- Other suspected causes include candida, *Demodex* mites, topical or inhaled fluorinated corticosteroids, toothpaste, and lip licking.

- Granulomatous changes can also be seen.

- This disease is not infectious, nor contagious and prognosis is favorable. Some argue that PD is a subtype of rosacea or seborrheic dermatitis and there is a possible link between PD and atopy.

Clinical Presentation

Skin Findings

- Typical manifestations include a monomorphic acneiform eruption with pink discrete papules and pustules on an erythematous base accompanied with fine scale involving the nasolabial folds, upper and lower cutaneous lips, and chin (Fig. 3.1-9).

- The vermillion border is typically spared and comedones are not present.

- It can also affect the periocular and paranasal skin and is referred to as *periorificial dermatitis*.

- It is usually symmetric in distribution but can be unilateral.

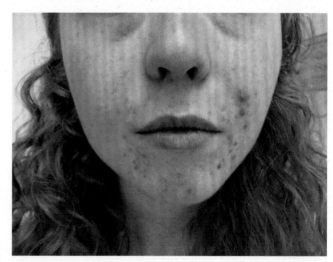

FIG. 3.1-9. Perioral dermatitis sparing the vermillion border. (Photo courtesy of M. Bobonich.)

Non-Skin Findings

- The eruption can be asymptomatic, but often accompanied by complaints of skin sensitivity, a burning sensation, or an intolerance to heat, water, or cosmetics at affected sites.
- Detailed history of symptoms include:
  - Sudden versus gradual onset
  - Location
  - Duration
  - Characteristics
  - Alleviating or provoking factors
  - Associated symptoms/systemic symptoms
  - Responses to prior treatments
  - Facial products
  - Use of oral or nasal steroid inhalers
  - Recently changed oral hygiene products or those with favors and additives
  - Symptoms like fatigue, joint pain, weight loss, or pulmonary symptoms

DIFFERENTIAL DIAGNOSIS   Perioral Dermatitis

- Acne—acneiform papules and pustules with the presence of comedones distributed on the forehead, nose, cheeks, or chin.
- Rosacea—rosacea also includes acneiform papules and pustules in the absence of comedones, however, distribution is typically on the nose, cheeks, and chin with the presence of telangiectasias.
- Seborrheic dermatitis—initiated by the overgrowth of *Pityrosporum* yeast with a distinct distribution with it commonly occurring on the scalp, eyebrows, glabellum, nasolabial folds, and external auditory canals. Acneiform lesions are not seen in this condition.
- Irritant or allergic contact dermatitis—can be caused by flavoring agents (especially cinnamon), preservatives, soaps, detergents, and harsh chemicals. Erythema, scaling, and papulovesicular eruptions are common. Acneiform lesions are not present in this condition.
- Gram-negative folliculitis—often includes monomorphic pustules in clusters on hair-bearing area.
- Angular cheilitis—erythema and burning often present, there is an absence of acneiform lesions.
- Sarcoidosis—reddish/brown papules or macules on the face and lips, but often associated with systemic symptoms.

Confirming the Diagnosis

- Clinical diagnosis is typically made with visual inspection.
- Additional tests to rule out differential diagnoses can include potassium hydroxide (KOH) for yeast, scraping for *Demodex* mites, bacterial culture and sensitivity of pustular lesions, patch testing for suspected contact allergens, and skin biopsy.

Treatment

- Discontinue any topical corticosteroids or aggravating topicals suspected.
- Oral therapy typically takes a minimum of 6 to 8 weeks and then a taper off the medications.
- Clearance is typically achieved within weeks of treatment and full resolution expected within months.

Oral Antibiotics

First-line therapy for PD are oral tetracyclines in patients 8 years and older; however, side effects can be problematic. Adverse effects such as gastrointestinal upset, diarrhea, and photosensitivity should be discussed prior to treatment.

- Doxycycline 100 mg b.i.d., but is known to cause gastrointestinal upset, esophageal irritation, and photosensitivity.
- Minocycline 100 mg b.i.d. for 4 to 8 weeks, side effects of minocycline include pseudotumor cerebri, blue–gray hyperpigmentation, vertigo, and lupus-like syndrome.
- Pregnant women and children under 8 years old will require alternative treatment.
- While there are no randomized control trials, it has been reported that oral erythromycin 250 mg b.i.d. to t.i.d. administered in conjunction with topical treatments was effective.

Topical Therapies

Topical metronidazole, erythromycin, clindamycin, tacrolimus, and pimecrolimus are also appropriate as either monotherapy or combination with oral antibiotics.

Metronidazole

- Topical metronidazole 1% b.i.d. for 8 weeks has been reported to be effective and can be used in combination with oral medications. The lower concentration of 0.75% metronidazole gel b.i.d. for 14 weeks also showed improvement.

Erythromycin/Clindamycin

- Topical erythromycin or clindamycin 1% topical can be applied b.i.d. for 7 weeks. Efficacy on use of topical clindamycin is derived from effectiveness in rosacea patients.

Pimecrolimus 1% and tacrolimus 0.1%

- Due to the fact the topical calcineurin inhibitors are nonsteroid-based creams, they are a suitable option in treatment for corticosteroid-induced dermatitis. Used off-label, they are applied b.i.d. and generally well tolerated. Burning is a common complaint upon initiation of therapy but then usually subsides after 2 weeks.

Management and Patient Education

- Some individuals have a propensity for recurrences so follow-up is necessary to ensure therapeutic response and complete resolution.
- Patients must be warned that they will likely flare or worsen before they improve, when a causative topical steroid is discontinued.
- Referral should be made to a dermatology specialist if treatment is unsuccessful or recalcitrant.

Cysts and Hidradenitis Suppurativa

Dorothy A. Sullivan and Nicole Bort

In This Chapter

- Epidermoid Cysts
- Hidradenitis Suppurativa

EPIDERMOID CYSTS

Epidermoid cysts are the most frequently occurring cyst on the skin. There is no racial predilection, but there is a male gender preference. They tend to occur in the third or fourth decade of life but may appear in adolescence. The term sebaceous cyst is often used interchangeably but is a misnomer as the content of the cyst is keratin and not sebum. Other synonyms include epidermal inclusion cyst, keratin cyst, and infundibular cyst.

Pathophysiology

- Epidermoid cysts develop from excess keratin plugging the pilosebaceous unit in the epidermis. They may develop from trauma or inflammation.
- They may result from deep penetrating injuries or follicular inflammation. They often arise in sites of previous acne flares.

Clinical Presentation

- An epidermoid cyst presents as a compressible nodule that ranges from 5 mm to 2 cm.
- They have a predilection for the face, back, scalp, ears, upper arms, scrotum, and chest.

- They can also occur on the acral sites either due to trauma or blockage of the eccrine duct.
- Epidermoid cysts can be flesh, yellow, or white in color with a smooth surface due to the outward pressure from the contents.
- A central punctum is often obvious, and the cyst is freely moveable over underlying tissue (Fig. 3.2-1).
- Since the cyst is slow growing, it is typically asymptomatic.
- Cysts may grow large, develop erythema and tenderness, and spontaneously rupture. They may evolve alone or be in groups (Fig. 3.2-2).
- Pilar cysts are a type of epidermoid cyst that occurs on the scalp. The thicker, fibrous capsule of keratin tends to be smoother and can make the excision of an intact cyst easier.

DIFFERENTIAL DIAGNOSIS   Cysts

- Abscess
- Lipoma
- Steatocystoma multiplex
- Pilar cysts

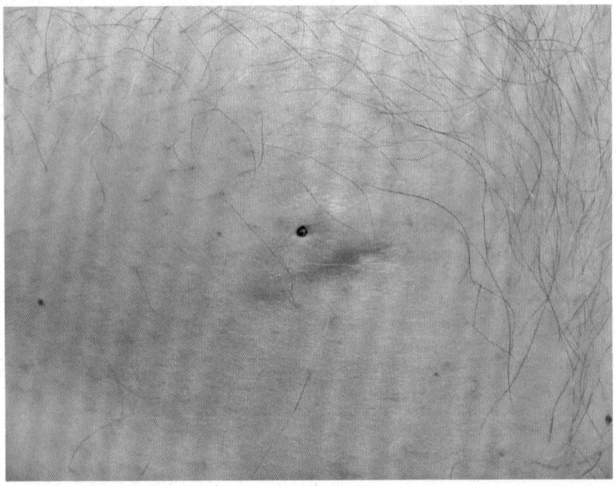

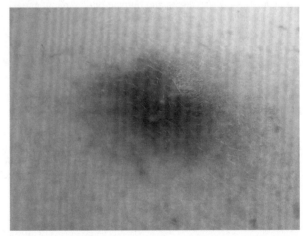

FIG. 3.2-1. Common epidermoid cyst with central open punctum. (Photo courtesy of M. Bobonich.)

FIG. 3.2-2. Enlarged and inflamed epidermoid cyst that is sterile and not infected. (Photo courtesy of M. Bobonich.)

Confirming the Diagnosis

- If there is any doubt, a simple incision and drainage (I&D) can be performed. Expression of keratin confirms the diagnosis of the cyst and aids in reducing the size and discomfort.
- Ruptured cysts are often erroneously diagnosed as infection but can be cultured.
- Biopsy is not necessary unless there is a suspicion of a co-occurring skin cancer or if you are unsure of the diagnosis.

Treatment

- Infected or cosmetically undesirable cysts can be excised or drained. Surgical treatment includes elliptical or punch excision. Care should be taken to remove the cyst wall as well as reducing the dead space with closure. Patients should be advised that there is a risk of recurrence.
- Although epidermoid cysts are typically sterile, some clinicians prefer to I&D inflamed lesion and treat with antibiotics before surgical excision.
- Pilar cysts, which are usually firmer, originate in the hair follicle but treatment is the same.
- Ruptured or inflamed cysts can be injected with intralesional triamcinolone 2 to 5 mg/mL.

Management and Patient Education

- Small epidermoid cysts do not require treatment and may even go unnoticed.
- Patients often self-treat by expressing the cyst and report a foul odor from the thick, curd-like contents.
- The epidermoid cyst can be reduced without surgical intervention with a simple I&D allowing for contents to be gently expressed. Patients should be informed that this intervention does not result in definitive removal and merely reduces the size of the lesion.
- Although erythema may be interpreted as an infected cyst, in the majority of cases, the inflammatory response is attributed to a foreign-body reaction and/or pressure which does not require an antibiotic.
- In roughly 30% of the cases, the cyst wall will suddenly burst and is entirely destroyed by the inflammatory response, which results in total eradication of the lesion.
- Secondary infection can occur especially with chronic manipulation by the patient. Procuring a wound culture and managing therapy based on results and the clinical findings provides optimum care. Naturally, removal should be deferred until the infection is resolved as to prevent wound dehiscence.
- Multiple or large epidermoid cysts can be cosmetically undesirable and may affect the patient's self-esteem.
- Scarring is the greatest risk with surgical excision, and abnormal pigmentation of the overlying skin can occur if the cyst is chronically inflamed or ruptured.
- Skin cancers rarely occur at the site of the cyst.

HIDRADENITIS SUPPURATIVA

Hidradenitis suppurativa (HS), also known as *acne inversa*, is a persistent, chronic, inflammatory disorder of the hair follicles that has a profound debilitating effect on patient's quality of life. It most commonly affects intertriginous sites causing painful inflammatory nodules and abscesses that often lead to scarring and tunneling sinus tracts. It is often unrecognized, which can lead to delays in diagnosis and puts patients at risk for the development of debilitating medical and psychosocial sequelae. This disease is not infectious, nor contagious; however, untreated can lead to significant scarring, psychological impact, and risk of several associated comorbidities.

- The incidence of HS ranges from 0.1% to 4% with varying degrees of severity.
- The onset of HS most frequently occurs after puberty with an average onset in the third and fourth decades of life. It is typically not seen in the elderly.
- Both males and females appear to be equally affected.
- Women are three times more likely to be diagnosed with HS, but men are prone to a more severe disease. A new diagnosis of HS is rare in postmenopausal women.
- It has also been linked to greater likelihood in individuals: of African descent; those who are obese; smokers; and those with a low socioeconomic status; and those with Down syndrome.

Pathophysiology

- The etiology of HS is not completely understood. It was originally thought that HS was a result of apocrine gland dysfunction, but current research has linked to series of complex events originating from follicular occlusion from excess cellular debris within the follicle. The follicle eventually ruptures, causing a cascade of inflammatory responses.
- Additional contributory factors are thought to include pathogenic organisms, smoking, obesity, glucose dysregulation, biofilms, and genetic factors.
- There have been no definitive genetic markers linked, but several are thought to be implicated. Approximately 30% to 40% of patients have a known genetic predisposition with 34% having a first-degree relative with disease.
- Hormonal involvement remains unclear, but women often report flares with menstruation.
- Environmental factors like heat, sweat, physical exertion, shaving, and friction have all been attributed to worsening the condition.

Associated Disorders

There are several disorders associated with HS. Therefore, careful screening of patients is recommended (Table 3.2-1).

- Hormonal conditions: PCOS.
- Auto-inflammatory diseases: pyoderma gangrenosum, Crohn disease, and spondyloarthritis.

TABLE 3.2-1	Routine Screening for HS Patients

- *Smoking*
- *Metabolic syndrome*
- *Type II diabetes*
- *Follicular occlusion tetrad*
- *Acne*
- *Depression/Anxiety*
- *Squamous cell carcinoma of HS affected skin*
- *Inflammatory bowel disease*
- *Arthropathies*
- *Polycystic ovarian syndrome*

- Syndromal associations: acne, psoriatic arthritis, synovitis, pustulosis, hyperostosis, and osteitis.
- Follicular occlusions: nodulocystic acne, pilonidal sinus, dissecting cellulitis, and keratosis pilaris.
- Genetics: Down Syndrome
- Cancers: buccal cancer and primary liver cancer are found to be more common in HS patients, but data is unclear if the relationship is linked to the disease itself or the high prevalence of smoking and alcohol use in this population.
- Anal fistulas are seen with perianal HS due to recurrent abscesses. Due to constant and repeated scarring, those with HS are at a four to five times greater risk of developing cutaneous squamous cell carcinoma and a 50-fold risk in general for increased malignancy, so regular skin checks and primary care monitoring is strongly encouraged.
- Psychological conditions: moderate or severe HS patients should be screened for:
  - Depression and suicide.
  - Recent research also indicates a higher prevalence of schizophrenia.
  - Higher rate of substance abuse with alcohol abuse, opioids, and cannabis among the most frequently used.
  - More likely to be victims of domestic violence.

Pertinent History
Onset—chronicity and postpubertal onset
Location
Duration
Characteristics
Alleviating or provoking factors
Associated symptoms/systemic symptoms
Responses to prior treatments

Clinical Presentation

- Characteristic lesions appear as a recurrent or cyclical tender, erythematous, indurated papules, or nodules (often referred to as "boils") with an intertriginous predominance and most often a symmetric distribution (Fig. 3.2-3).
- Lesions can present with or without sinus tract formation and scarring.
- The most frequent anatomical site for HS is the axillae, but lesions can also occur in the perineum, inframammary area, inguinal folds, medial thighs, occipital scalp, and anogenital areas. Aberrant locations can exist.
- A hallmark sign is the *double-headed* comedone arising from follicular occlusion causing the appearance of multiple blackheads within one follicle.
- Lesions often have malodorous purulent drainage or active weeping. Signs of secondary bacterial infections may be present.
- There is often variability in skin findings based on stage of disease and can include a range of symptoms from acute to chronic characteristics.
- Hurley staging provides a classification of disease severity based on clinical findings (Table 3.2-2). This staging should guide the clinician with recommended therapies for treatment.

DIFFERENTIAL DIAGNOSIS   Hidradenitis Suppurativa

- Infection (abscesses, furuncles, carbuncles, cat scratch disease, granuloma inguinale, inguinale, lymphogranuloma venereum, noduloulcerative syphilis, and tuberculous abscess)—HS patients are afebrile and clinically well. The majority of HS lesions are sterile. Infectious etiologies typically do not have a symmetric distribution limited to the intertriginous areas
- Cysts (epidermoid, dermoid, pilonidal, or Bartholin gland cyst)—while benign cysts can reoccur, they do not often have a symmetric distribution limited to the intertriginous areas
- Acne—typically distributed on the face and trunk and not intertriginous areas
- Crohn's Disease—often present with gastrointestinal symptoms, ulcerations, and an absence of comedones

Confirming the Diagnosis

- Clinical diagnosis is typically made with visual inspection.
- HS characteristics supporting the diagnosis:
  - Presence of characteristic lesions (inflammatory or noninflammatory nodules, abscess, sinus tracts, or scars).
  - Involvement of axilla, inframammary folds, perineum, groin, or gluteal area.
  - Reoccurrence of lesions more than twice in a 6-month period or persistence for more than 3 months.
  - Secondarily, a family history of HS or a negative microbiology workup may be indicative of disease presence.
- Additional tests to rule out differential diagnoses may include bacterial or fungal culture and sensitivity from a pustular or draining lesion.
- Additional laboratory testing for either underlying or associated systemic conditions.
- On occasion, the onset of HS may be an indicator of an underlying or concomitant systemic process that may necessitate additional diagnostics. In patients with a clinical signs and symptoms of hyperandrogenism, labs should include a DHEA and free testosterone as initial screening laboratory studies to evaluate hormonal influences.
- Cutaneous manifestations of inflammatory bowel disease (i.e., Crohn disease) should be considered if perianal lesions and concomitant gastrointestinal symptoms are present. A skin biopsy should be performed.

Treatment
Topical Therapies
Antibiotics—while antibiotics are a common mainstay in treatment for HS that is mild to moderate, the data is limited on its efficacy. It has been postulated to be effective through antibacterial and immunomodulatory properties.

- Clindamycin 1% (solution or gel) applied b.i.d.
- Concurrent use of benzoyl peroxide increases efficacy in addition to reducing the risk of bacterial resistance, so monotherapy is not recommended.
- For mild involvement, application of a multistep topical therapy with antimicrobial soap, warm compresses, and topical sodium fusidate ointment or gel for suspected staphylococci infections.

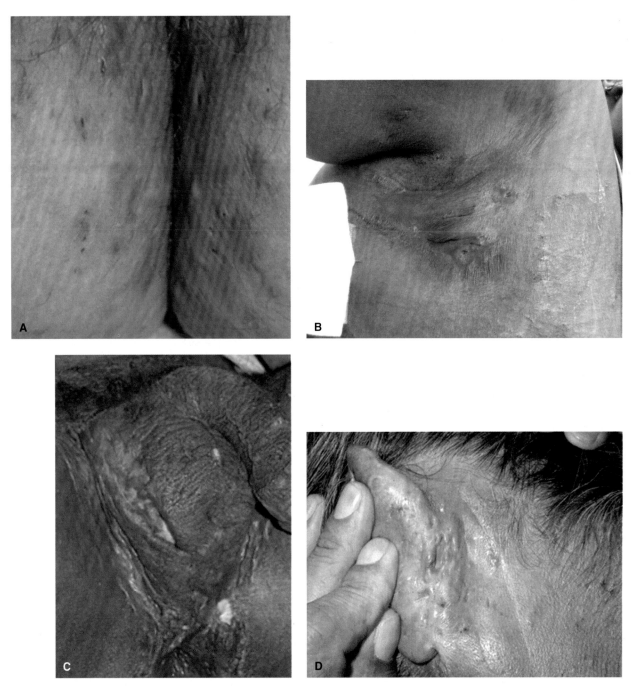

FIG. 3.2-3. **A:** Hidradenitis suppurativa, Hurley stage I. Hidradenitis suppurativa can be distinguished from furunculosis by the presence of comedones that may be subtle or marked, as well as poor response to antibiotics, and nondiagnostic cultures. **B:** Hidradenitis suppurativa, Hurley stage II, showing recurrent abscesses with sinus tracts and scarring: single or multiple widely separated lesions. **C:** Hidradenitis suppurativa, Hurley stage III, occurring in the anogenital area can be extremely difficult to manage and a poorer prognosis. It produces mutilating scarring, and the ongoing inflammation should be monitored for malignant transformation. **D:** Hidradenitis suppurativa can occur in the postauricular area.

Cleansers—there is no data that specifically delineates that one topical agent is superior to another, however, experts agree that agents that may be helpful include benzoyl peroxide, chlorhexidine, and pyrithione zinc.

Keratolytic agents—resorcinol 15% cream is both an antiseptic and keratolytic which can be efficacious when used twice daily as maintenance for Hurley stage I and II. It may cause some irritation.

Systemic Therapy
Antimicrobials

- Tetracyclines class have shown a reduction in Hurley stage I & II
- Clindamycin and rifampin combined (300 mg each b.i.d.)
- Dapsone as a long-term therapy is not recommended. A 3-month trial must be given before improvement is noted; however, flares are common after discontinuation

TABLE 3.2-2	Hidradenitis Suppurativa Classification
HURLEY STAGE	**CLINICAL FINDINGS**
Stage I Mild	Transient nonscarring inflammatory lesions/abscesses without evidence of sinus tracts or scars
Stage II Moderate	Recurrent inflammatory lesions/abscesses with sinus tracts or lesions that are distinct and widely separated by normal appearing skin
Stage III Severe	Multiple interconnected sinus tracts with scarring and inflammation or disease with diffuse coverage of an entire area

Hormonal therapy—consideration for hormonal therapy must be made on an individual patient basis.

- *Oral contraceptive pills* (OCPs)
  - Ethinyl estradiol/norgestrel or ethinyl estradiol and cyproterone acetate may be helpful.
  - Progestogen-only regimens may worsen HS in some cases, so close monitoring is recommended. Patients should be assessed for contraindications and risk factors prior to starting therapy.
  - Other forms of contraception, such as medroxyprogesterone (Depo Provera) injection or the levonorgestrel-releasing intrauterine device (Mirena), are not known to be effective.
  - *Metformin* has shown some improvement at 500 mg b.i.d. to t.i.d. in patients with a history of PCOS.
- *Spironolactone*
  - Dosing 100 to 150 mg daily has shown some improvement, especially in women with verbalized menstrual or cyclical flares. If improved, the dose may be tapered to the lowest possible dose that maintains control.
  - Common side effects include breakthrough bleeding or spotting, menstrual irregularities, headaches, diuresis, dizziness, fatigue, potential hyperkalemia, and breast tenderness.
  - Contraindicated in pregnancy, it should only be considered for nonpregnant women.
  - Spironolactone has a black-box warning as mandated by FDA because it can cause feminization of the male fetus.
- *Biologics*
  - Adalimumab, a human monoclonal antibody that inhibits TNF-α, is the only FDA-approved treatment for HS.
  - Alternative treatment for moderate to severe HS that has not been controlled with oral antibiotics, retinoids, or hormonal therapy.
- *Adjunct treatments*
  - *Zinc gluconate* has been used for its anti-inflammatory effects. In one study, 90 mg daily has showed preliminary evidence that is beneficial for mild to moderate disease. Further studies are indicated.
  - *Intralesional injections* with corticosteroids for large stubborn painful cystic lesions can give relief to the patient with use of triamcinolone 10 mg/mL (Kenalog) with doses between 0.2 and 2.0 mL into lesion. It is recommended that clinicians skilled in intralesional injections use this therapy. The risks of atrophy and depigmentation should be discussed in detail prior to the procedure.

- Treatment with neurotoxins, radiotherapy, cryotherapy, PDT, and nonablative radiofrequency has reported some improvement in limited cases.

Surgical Intervention

- Surgery is a part of the therapeutic armamentarium for HS. Conservative surgical options for milder cases can include incision and drainage, deroofing, and excision (both surgical and laser) of chronic lesions and associated sinus tracts.

Management and Patient Education

- Management should be guided by the severity of the disease.
- It is extremely important to dispel the notion that HS is the result of poor hygiene. One should also debunk the myth that HS is either contagious or an STD when neither is true.
- Avoid harsh scrubbing to affected areas and tight clothing.
- Decreased intake of dairy products and high glycemic intake has been associated with improvement.
- Smoking cessation and a reduction in BMI should be recommended for all HS patients as it can improve overall health and possibly reduce flares.
- The importance of early referral of severe HS patients to a dermatologist cannot be overemphasized.
- Aggressive treatment with a multidisciplinary approach should be instituted before extensive scarring occurs, offering the patient the highest reduction in morbidity.
- Consultation with radiation therapy and plastic surgery may be necessary in severe and recalcitrant cases.

Lifestyle Modifications

Lifestyle or behavioral modifications are beneficial for all Hurley stages.

- *Weight loss*—evidence is variable on the effects of weight loss on disease progression as the pathogenesis of HS and the effects of weight reduction are not completely understood. There is some evidence that weight loss does have a positive effect on symptom management and a reduction in the number of involved sites.
- *Smoking cessation*—the overall effect of smoking cessation has not been systematically evaluated, but there is supporting evidence that nicotine plays a role in pathogenesis of HS. Smoking cessation is strongly justified not only as a benefit to overall health, but the possibility exists that it leads to clinical improvement.
- *Clothing*—avoidance of restrictive clothing may be beneficial due to the established role of friction in the pathogenesis of HS.

Pain Management

Pain is a prominent feature of HS, thought to result from both sequelae of ongoing inflammation and the associated depression. No studies have evaluated the efficacy of different pain control regimens in HS, but lidocaine 5% ointment, diclofenac 1% gel, ice packs, anti-inflammatory drugs, acetaminophen, gabapentin, pregabalin, and the serotonin-norepinephrine reuptake inhibitor duloxetine have all been utilized with mild to moderate improvement.

Psychological Therapy

Any patient who exhibits impairment in their social, work, or sexual functioning should be screened and referred for counseling. Patients also have in-person support groups and/or online forums for accurate information and useful tips about daily management. Further information can be accessed through the Hidradenitis Suppurativa Foundation website (www.hs-foundation.org).

Acne Keloidalis Nuchae and Pseudofolliculitis Barbae

Dorothy A. Sullivan and Nicole Bort

In This Chapter

- Acne Keloidalis
- Pseudofolliculitis Barbae

ACNE KELOIDALIS NUCHAE

Acne keloidalis nuchae (AKN) is a chronic folliculitis with unknown etiology of the scalp that often results in scars, keloidal lesions, and alopecia. The misleading term *AKN* was originally used by Bazin in 1872, for an entity now known to be unrelated to the pathogenesis of acne vulgaris. AKN is not a true keloid, nor is it limited to the nuchal area.

- The patient population most affected is African-American males with a prevalence in those with 0.5% to 13.6% of that population. There has been some evidence in the literature of AKN arising in Asian and Hispanic individuals, but it is rare in Caucasians.

- It generally begins in adolescence or early adulthood and rarely begins after age 50.

- Prognosis for AKN is good if treated early. Treatment is far more difficult and less responsive once scarring occurs.

- Consequences of progressively worsening disease may include keloid formation, scarring alopecia, chronic discharge, and vulnerability to repeated episodes of secondary infection.

Pathophysiology

- Initially, AKN was postulated to be an inflammatory, follicle-based process akin to folliculitis or PFB. This theory has since been disproven and experts now classify AKN as a primary form of cicatricial alopecia causing permanent hair loss.

- Some experts believe that frequent aggravation from rough curly hairs in the skin prompts an inflammatory process and subsequent development of lesions.

- It has been observed that chronic rubbing from shirt collars, hats, helmets, and close shaving haircuts all make acne keloidalis worse.

- Other inciting factors have been proposed and include an innocuous chronic bacterial infection, frequent haircuts, curvature of the hair follicles, altered immune process, or increased mast cells in localized areas of the scalp.

- Due to the predilection for males, androgens may also play a role.

- An association of AKN with metabolic syndrome and truncal obesity has been observed in some patients, although it has yet to be proven to be a causative factor on a large scale.

- In some individuals there is an associated folliculitis decalvans, PFB, central centrifugal cicatricial alopecia, and androgenetic alopecia.

Clinical Presentation

Skin findings

- The appearance depends on the progression of disease.

- Initially, discrete and coalescing follicular papules and/or pustules on the nuchal and/or occipital region characterize AKN (Fig. 3.3-1).

- It can be asymptomatic, but often pruritic and irritating.

- Bleeding may occur and a burning sensation is sometimes described. Follicular papules transform into fibrotic, hypertrophic papules and keloidal plaques in advanced disease.

- Secondary erosions from picking or crust from secondary infections can occur.

- Comedones are typically not a feature.

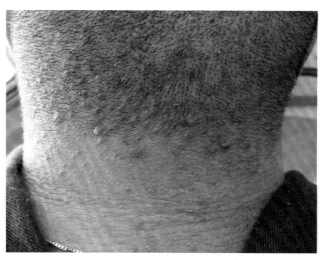

FIG. 3.3-1. Acne keloidalis nuchae commonly affecting the occipital scalp. (Photo courtesy of M. Bobonich.)

DIFFERENTIAL DIAGNOSIS Acne Keloidalis Nuchae

- *Folliculitis decalvans*—typically has redness and swelling to the hair follicles with the presence of pustular lesions.
- *Acne*—has the presence of comedones distributed on the forehead, nose, cheeks, or chin.
- *Dissecting folliculitis*—oftentimes also affects the vertex and not only the occipital area.
- *Bacterial, fungal, or viral folliculitis*—often not isolated to only the posterior scalp.
- *Tinea capitis*—typically does not affect only the occipital area.
- *HS*—most commonly affects intertriginous areas.
- *Sarcoidosis*—reddish/brown papules or macules, but often associated with systemic symptoms.

Confirming the Diagnosis

- AKN is a diagnosis that is made clinically; however, if there is a suspicion of scarring alopecia, biopsy would be recommended.
- If lesions are weeping or crusted, samples should be taken for culture and sensitivities to rule out a rare occurrence of bacterial or fungal etiology.
- Other diagnoses should be considered if lesions arise in an unexpected age range or in women.

Treatment

Topical Treatment

- High-potency topical steroids applied b.i.d. alternating every 2 weeks.
- Topical retinoid like tretinoin 0.025% can be added to the routine.
- Topical clindamycin 1% can be used b.i.d. if pustular lesions are present.
- Intralesional injections of triamcinolone acetonide at a dose of 5 to 40 mg/mL can be injected every 4 weeks. Patients should be made aware that the potential side effects include hypopigmentation and skin atrophy to injected sites.
- Cryotherapy can be useful in early lesions but can result in abnormal pigmentation.

Systemic Treatment

- Tetracycline derivatives such as doxycycline 100 mg b.i.d. or minocycline 100 mg b.i.d. can be useful for both their anti-inflammatory and antibacterial effects for more severe disease.
- Oral retinoids can be useful in patients with concurrent folliculitis decalvans.

Surgical and Other Treatments

- Typically reserved for severe disease that has not otherwise responded to medical therapies (Fig. 3.3-2).
- Laser and ultraviolet B radiation have also been used in refractory cases.

Management and Patient Education

There is a universal agreement that early treatment has the greatest likelihood of ameliorating the problem and disrupting the progression of disease, thus limiting subsequent alopecia.

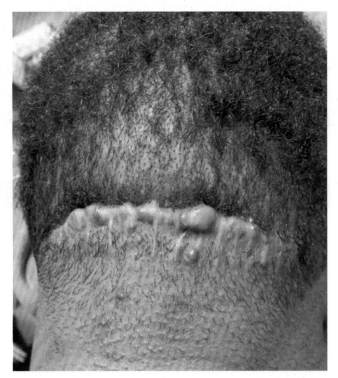

FIG. 3.3-2. Surgical treatment of acne keloidalis nuchae, which can be as cosmetically disfiguring as the skin condition itself. (Photo courtesy of M. Bobonich.)

- The goals for treatment include avoidance of exacerbating factors and triggers (discourage picking of lesions, wearing of tight-collared shirts, and avoid close shaving), arresting disease progression by treating any possible infections, and relieving symptoms.
- Permanent scarring and keloid formation may arise in those who have chronic outbreaks or in patients not appropriately treated.
- Referral to a dermatology provider should be initiated if there is evidence of scarring, progressive worsening of the condition, or infection.
- Antiseptic or tar containing shampoos can help prevent secondary bacterial infections.

Discuss with patients the importance of minimizing shaving.

PSEUDOFOLLICULITIS BARBAE

Pseudofolliculitis barbae (PFB) is a common, chronic, inflammatory follicular skin condition of the beard. While it is difficult to determine the exact incidence of the FPB, it occurs more frequently in those with tight curly hair. FPB is most commonly in African-American males with a prevalence of 40% to 80% but has also been reported in Asians, Hispanics, and Caucasians. Hirsute women of color and women who have attempted facial hair removal (especially by plucking) have been observed to develop these lesions. This disease is not infectious, nor contagious, and prognosis is favorable.

Pathophysiology

- Despite the similar clinical appearance, PFB is unrelated to the pathogenesis of acne vulgaris.

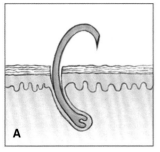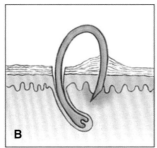

FIG. 3.3-3. **A,B:** Pathophysiology of pseudofolliculitis barbae. (Goodheart, H. P. [2015]. *Goodheart's photoguide of common skin disorders* [4th ed.]. Wolters Kluwer Health | Lippincott Williams & Wilkins.)

- It is a disorder most associated with the unique features of hair follicle curvature inherited in certain ethnicities.
- During shaving, tightly curled hair is transected in a somewhat diagonal fashion, which results in a pointed tip at the distal end. This hair then curls back as it begins to grow piercing and reentering the skin a few millimeters from the original follicular opening. That penetration causes a foreign body reaction and subsequent inflammation (Fig. 3.3-3).
- A common contributing factor is frequent shaving and improper shaving technique.

Associated Disorders

- Postinflammatory hyperpigmentation
- AKN

Clinical Presentation

Skin Findings

- Patients typically report painful lesions localized to the beard, neck, and inferior chin.
- This condition presents as skin-colored or erythematous, folliculocentric papules or pustules on the lower face, jaw, chin, and neck (Fig. 3.3-4).
- Hyperpigmentation and scarring may be present from chronic inflammation.

- Abscesses or larger clusters of pustules may arise in secondarily infected skin.
- There is a variant of PFB called pseudofolliculitis pubis, which may occur when the pubic area is shaved. This subset affects both men and women. While PFB is infrequently found in Caucasians, it is reported to be common in Caucasian renal transplant recipients.

DIFFERENTIAL DIAGNOSIS   Pseudofolliculitis Barbae

The differential diagnosis for PFB can include other conditions commonly known to cause papules and pustules on the face.

- *Traumatic folliculitis* (razor burn) can occur after a close shave, but typically resolves within 24 to 48 hours.
- *Acne*—acneiform papules and pustules with the presence of comedones distributed on the forehead, nose, cheeks, or chin with the distribution in both hair-bearing and non–hair-bearing areas.
- *Bacterial folliculitis* and impetigo are rarely scarring or chronic in nature.
- *Tinea barbae* has peripheral scale and central clearing.
- *Sarcoidosis* should be considered on individuals with dark skin, but lesions are typically larger, monomorphic, and remain unchanged for long periods of time.

Confirming the Diagnosis

- A clinical diagnosis is typically made with visual inspection.
- Any clinical findings suggestive of secondary bacterial infection should be swabbed for culture and sensitivity.
- Likewise, if a fungal etiology is among diagnostic considerations, a KOH test can be performed on the contents of a pustule.
- Hairs may also be plucked and plated for fungal culture.
- Any suspicion of sarcoidosis should be evaluated by biopsy.

Treatment

- PFB is a chronic condition whose symptoms can be remedied by discontinuation of shaving either permanently or temporarily

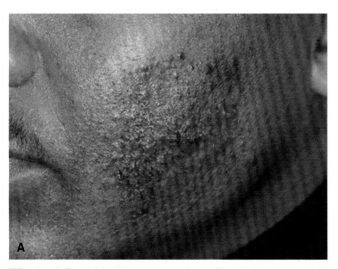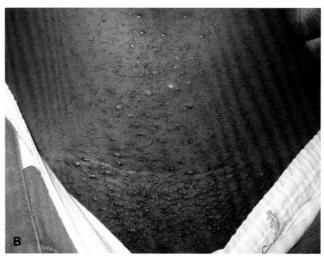

FIG. 3.3-4. **A:** Pseudofolliculitis barbae occurring locally on the face and beard with hyperpigmentation and scarring that can occur. **B:** Pseudofolliculitis barbae can occur in other hair-bearing areas, including the abdominal and pubic regions as shown. (Images provided by Stedman's.)

TABLE 3.3-1	Patient Education for Pseudofolliculitis

Principles for Shaving

- If you must shave, daily shaving has been shown to diminish the severity of pseudofolliculitis barbae.
- Prior to shaving, eliminate observable hair with electric clippers leaving a 1- to 2-mm residual stubble.
- Cleanse the affected area with a gentle acne soap and textured face cloth. If ingrown hairs are observed, use a toothbrush in a circular motion to dislodge the embedded hairs.
- Remove soap, then use face cloth and warm water to apply a compress for several minutes before shaving.
- Lather involved skin with favorite shaving cream and massage into affected site.
- Before the cream dries, begin shaving *with* the grain, *not* against it.
- Refrain from applying tension or pulling the skin.
- Use fresh, sharp razors with only one blade. Multiple blades worsen the condition.
- Shave with short brief strokes and *do not* shave the same area repeatedly.
- Rinse the area thoroughly with water. Apply an aftershave preparation or lotion which is comforting.
- Use topical corticosteroids only if directed by your provider's instructions.

until papules and pustules have resolved. If that is not possible, minimizing a close shave with use of hair clippers, electric razor, or safety razors is encouraged.

- Topical corticosteroids like hydrocortisone 1% and 2.5% are efficacious in reducing inflammation but should not be used for long periods of time on the face.

- Topical and oral antibiotics are helpful in reducing the inflammatory process and combat secondary infections if they arise, but does not address the underlying cause.

- Topical retinoids, such as tretinoin cream 0.05%, have demonstrated benefit in some early cases.

- Complete destruction of the hair follicle with laser therapy or electrolysis has shown to be effective, but affordability can be limiting.

Management and Patient Education

- Patients must utilize management strategies to reduce discomfort, inflammation, and potential infection (Table 3.3-1).

- Complete discontinuance of shaving can resolve the problem but is not feasible for many people.

- Patients who cannot be unshaven should be counseled on skin care and techniques to minimize the condition and prevent complications.

- Postinflammatory hyperpigmentation, scarring, and keloid formation may arise in those who have chronic outbreaks or in patients not appropriately treated.

- Referral should be initiated if there is any evidence of early scarring, postinflammatory hyperpigmentation, secondary infection, or keloid formation.

READINGS AND REFERENCES

Alikhan, A., Sayed, C., Alavi, A., Alhusayen, R., Brassard, A., Burkhart, C., Crowell, K., Eisen, D. B., Gottlieb, A. B., Gottlieb, A. B., Hamzavi, I., Hazen, P. G., Jaleel, T., Kimball, A. B., Kirby, J., Lowes, M. A., Micheletti, R., Miller, A., Naik, H. B.,...Poulin, Y. (2019). North American clinical management guidelines for hidradenitis suppurativa: A publication from the United States and Canada Hidradenitis Suppurativa Foundations Part I: Diagnosis, evaluation, and the use of complementary and procedural management. *Journal of the American Academy of Dermatology*, 81, 76–90. http://dx.doi.org/10.1016/j.jaad.2019.02.067

Alikhan, A., Sayed, C., Alavi, A., Alhusayen, R., Broussard, A., Burkhart, C., Crowell, K., Eisen, D. B., Gottlieb, A. B., Gottlieb, A. B., Hamzavi, I., Hazen, P. G., Jaleel, T., Kimball, A. B., Kirby, J., Lowes, M. A., Micheletti, R., Miller, A., Naik, H. B.,...Poulin, Y. (2019). North American clinical management guidelines for hidradenitis suppurativa: A publication from the United States and Canadian Hidradenitis Suppurativa Foundations Part II: Topical intralesional and systemic medical management. *Journal of the American Academy of Dermatology*, 81, 91–101. http://dx.doi.org/10.1016/j.jaad.2019.02.068

Blok, J. L., van Hattem, S., Jonkman, M. F., & Horváth, B. (2013). Systemic therapy with immunosuppressive agents and retinoids in hidradenitis suppurativa: A systematic review. *The British Journal of Dermatology*, 168(2), 243–252.

Cuda, J. D., Rangwala, S., & Taub, J. (2019). Benign epithelial tumors, hamartomas & hyperplasia. In S. Kang, M. Amagai, A. Bruckner, A. Enk, A. McMichael, J. Orringer, & D. Margolis (Eds.). *Fitzpatrick's dermatology* (9th ed., Chapter 108). [Kindle DX].

Fitzpatrick, J. E., & High, W. A. (2018). *Urgent care dermatology: symptom based diagnosis.* [Kindle version]. Retrieved from http://www.books.google.com

Garg, A., Strunk, A., Midura, M., Papagermanos, V., & Pomerantz, H. (2018). Prevalence of hidradenitis suppurativa among patients with Down syndrome: A population-based cross sectional analysis. *The British Journal of Dermatology*, 178(3), 697–703.

Gold, D. A., Reeder, V. J., Mahan, M. G., & Hamzavi, I. H. (2014). The prevalence of metabolic syndrome in patients with hidradenitis suppurativa. *Journal of the American Academy of Dermatology*, 70(4), 699–703.

Goldburg, S. R., Strober, B. E., & Payette, M. J. (2020). Hidradenitis suppurativa: Epidemiology, clinical presentation, and pathogenesis. *Journal of the American Academy of Dermatology*, 82(5), 1045–1058. https://doi.org/10.1016/j.jaad.2019.08.090

Hood, C., & Shanmugan, V. (2019). Hidradenitis suppurativa—diagnosis and management. *The Journal for Nurse Practitioners*, 15, 713–716.

James, W. D., Elston, D., Treat, J., Rosenbach, M., & Neuhaus, I. (Eds.). (2020). *Andrews' diseases of the skin: Clinical dermatology* (13th ed.). Edinburgh: Elsevier.

Johnson, S. M., Berg, A., & Barr, C. (2019). Recognizing rosacea: Tips on differential diagnosis. *Journal of Drugs in Dermatology*, 18(9), 888–894.

Kellen, R., & Silverberg, N. (2017). Pediatric periorficial dermatitis. *Cutis*, 100(6), 385–388.

Kromann, C. B., Ibler, K. S., Kristiansen, V. B., & Jemec, G. B. (2014). The influence of body weight on the prevalence and severity of hidradenitis suppurativa. *Acta Dermato-Venereologica*, 94(5), 553–557.

Lee, G., & Zirwas, M. (2015). Granulomatous rosacea and periorficial dermatitis: Controversies and review of management and treatment. *Dermatologic Clinics*, 33(3), 447–455.

Matusiak, Ł., Bieniek, A., & Szepietowski, J. C. (2014). Bacteriology of hidradenitis suppurativa-which antibiotics are the treatment of choice? *Acta Dermato-Venereologica*, 94(6), 699–702.

Miller, L. (2019). Superficial cutaneous infections and pyoderma. In S. Kang, M. Amagai, A. Bruckner, A. Enk, A. McMichael, J. Orringer & Margolis, D. (Eds.), *Fitzpatrick's dermatology* (9th ed., p. 150). McGraw-Hill.

Ogunbiyi, A. (2019). Psuedofolliculitis barbae; current treatment options. *Clinical, Cosmetics and Investigational Dermatology*, 12, 241–247. https://doi.org/10.2147/CCID.S149250

Ogunbiyi, A. (2016). Acne keloidalis nuchae: Prevalence, impact, and management challenges. *Clinical, Cosmetic and Investigative Dermatology*, 9, 483–489.

Ogunbiyi, A., & Adedokun, B. (2015). Perceived etiological factors of folliculitis keloidalis nuchae and treatment options amongst Nigerian men. *The British Journal of Dermatology*, 173, 22–25.

Olazagasti, J., Lynch, P., & Fazel, N. (2014). The great mimickers of rosacea. *Cutis*, 94(4), 39–45.

Patel, N., McKenzie, S., Harview, C., Truong, A., Shi, V., Chen, L., Grogan, T. R., Bennett, R. G., & Hsiao, J. (2019). Isotretinoin in the treatment of hidradenitis suppurativa: A retrospective study. *Journal of Dermatological Treatment*, 1–3. http://dx.doi.org/10.1080/09546634.2019.1670779

Rivero, A. L., & Whitfeld, M. (2018). An update on the treatment of rosacea. *Australian Prescriber*, 41(1), 20–24. https://doi.org/10.18773/austprescr.2018.004

Schaller, M., Almeida, L., Bewley, A., Cribier, B., Del Rosso, J., Dlova, N. C., Gallo, R. L., Granstein, R. D., Kautz, G., Mannis, M. J., Micali, G., Oon, H. H., Rajagopalan, M., Steinhoff, M., Tanghetti, E., Thiboutot, D., Troielli, P., Webster, G., Zierhut, M., van Zuuren, E. J., ... Tan, J. (2020). Recommendations for rosacea diagnosis, classification and management: update from the global ROSacea COnsensus 2019 panel. *The British Journal of Dermatology*, 182(5), 1269–1276. https://doi.org/10.1111/bjd.18420

Shanmugam, V. K., Mulani, S., McNish, S., Harris, S., Buescher, T., & Amdur, R. (2018). Longitudinal observational study of hidradenitis suppurativa: Impact of surgical intervention with adjunctive biologic therapy. *International Journal of Dermatology*, 57(1), 62–69. http://dx.doi.org/10.1111/jd.13798

Sinclair, W. (2017). Guidelines for the management of acne vulgaris. *South African Family Practice*, 59(1), 24–29. doi:https://doi.org/10.4102/safp.v59i1.4629

Sisic, M., Tan, J., & Lafreniere, K. D. (2017). Hidradenitis suppurativa, intimate partner violence, and sexual assault. *Journal of Cutaneous Medicine and Surgery, 21*(5), 383–387. http://dx.doi.org/10.1177/1203475417708167

Spell, C. A., Badon, H. R., Flischel, A., & Brodell, R. T. (2020). Acne and rosacea in pregnancy. In Tyler, K. (Ed.). *Cutaneous disorders of pregnancy*. Springer. https://doi.org/10.1007/978-3-030-49285-4_6

Taieb, A., Khemis, A., Ruzicka, T., Barańska-Rybak, W., Berth-Jones, J., Schauber, J., Briantais, P., Jacovella, J., & Passeron, T.; Ivermectin Phase III Study Group. (2016). Maintenance of remission following successful treatment of papulopustular rosacea with ivermectin 1% cream vs. metronidazole 0.75% cream: 36-week extension of the ATTRACT randomized study. *Journal of the European Academy of Dermatology and Venereology. 30*(5), 829–836.

Tchero, H., Herlin, C., Bekara, F., Fluieraru, S., & Teot, L. (2019). Hidradenitis suppurativa: A systematic review and meta-analysis of therapeutic interventions. *Indian Journal of Dermatology, Venereology and Leprology, 85*(3), 248–257.

Tempark, T., & Shwayder, T. (2014). Perioral dermatitis: A review of the condition with special attention to treatment options. *American Journal of Clinical Dermatology, 15*, 101–113.

Thiboutot, D., Anderson, R., Cook-Bolden, F., Draelos, Z., Gallo, R. L., Granstein, R. D., Kang, S., Macsai, M., Stein Gold, L., & Tan, J. (2020). Standard management options for rosacea: The 2019 update by the National Rosacea Society Expert Committee. *Journal of the American Academy of Dermatology, 82*(6), 1501–1509.

Thoracius, L., Cohen, A., Gislason, G., Jemec, G., & Egeberg, A. (2018). Increased suicide risk in patients with hidradenitis suppurativa. *Journal of Investigative Dermatology, 138*(1), 52–57.

Tilton, E. E., Bavola, C., & Helms, S. E. (2015). Rash around the mouth: What is it? *The Journal of the American Dental Association, 146*(5), 337–340.

Tzur, D. B., Berzin, D., & Cohen, A. D. (2019). Hidradenitis suppurativa and schizophrenia: A nationwide cohort study. *Journal of the European Academy of Dermatology & Venereology, 34*(3), 574–579.

Van Zuuren, E. J. (2017). Rosacea. *The New England Journal of Medicine, 377*(18), 1754–1764.

Wortsman, X. (2018). Diagnosis and treatment of hidradenitis suppurativa. *JAMA, 15*, 1617–1618.

Zaenglein, A., Pathy, A. L., Scholosser, B. J., Alikhan, A., Baldwin, H. E., Berson, D. S., Bowe, W. P., Graber, E. M., Harper, J. C., Kang, S., Keri, J. E., Leyden, J. J., Reynolds, R. V., Silverberg, N. B., Stein-Gold, L. F., Tollefson, M. M., Weiss, J. S., Dolan, N. C., Saga, A. A., … Bhushan, R. (2016). Guidelines of care for the management of acne vulgaris. *Journal of the American Academy of Dermatology, 74*(5), 945–973.

Atopic Dermatitis and Other Eczemas

CHAPTER 4.1

Susan Tofte

ECZEMA

Eczematous inflammation, commonly referred to as "eczema," is the most common of all inflammatory skin diseases. The term *eczema* comes from the Greek word "eczeo," which literally means "to effervesce or boil over." It often presents as a papulovesicular, weeping dermatitis. *Eczema* is a generic or general term used to describe a variety of eczematous disorders, including nummular eczema, contact or irritant dermatitis, xerotic (asteatotic) eczema, dyshidrotic (pompholyx), dermatophytids (Ids), or seborrheic dermatitis. Atopic dermatitis (AD) is a type of eczema, which when combined with asthma, and allergic rhinitis, is known as the atopic triad.

In the early acute phase, eczema will appear intensely erythematous, often with vesicles which can rupture, ooze, and become weepy. When secondary changes occur and eczema becomes less acute, erythema continues, but with increased scaling, excoriations, and sometimes fissures. Vesicles are usually dried at this stage. As eczema evolves into a chronic stage, the skin becomes lichenified (thickened) with accentuated skin lines, the result of rubbing and scratching. Pruritus and evidence of scratching can be present at any stage, but is most intense during the acute stage when inflammation is more extreme. The skin barrier becomes more compromised with fissures and excoriations because of scratching, making it more susceptible to infection.

Histologic changes are similar in every stage of eczema, but can vary depending on the degree of inflammation. Edema is most evident during the acute phase of eczema, revealing a high degree of spongiosis as well as increased numbers of lymphocytes. As eczema becomes chronic, histologic changes show more evidence of a thicker (lichenified) stratum corneum.

ATOPIC DERMATITIS

Many studies have looked at the prevalence of AD in infants and children by using clinical evaluations, surveys, and questionnaires. Based on studies from Northern Europe, United States, and Japan, the prevalence of AD ranges from 15% to 20%, with a higher incidence noted in children (Avena-Woods, 2017; Kowalska-Olędzka et al., 2019). Greater than 60% of AD cases develop during the first year of life; thus, it is often referred to as a childhood disease. Although rare, it can present in adulthood. Research has shown that there is a strong concordance with monozygotic twins.

Quality of Life and Cost of Care

- AD impacts not just the patient, but the entire family. Parents miss work to care for their child, affecting income and health benefits. Healthy siblings compete for attention from parents, who can find themselves focused on the arduous task of caring for the child with AD.

- Studies as far back as 1995 (Lewis-Jones & Finlay) indicate that AD has a higher impact on childhood "quality-of-life" indicators than any other childhood dermatoses, with the exception of scabies.

- AD-associated pruritus is often more intense and relentless than with other skin disorders, leading to disruptions in sleep, play, and recreational activities, as well as impacting social interactions and development.

- The economic impact of caring for a family member with AD has been compared to the cost of other chronic diseases such as emphysema or epilepsy. AD care costs in the United States are estimated to be over $300 million annually (Chung & Simpson, 2018), with emergency room visits for acute flares as the largest contributor.

Pathophysiology

- AD is an inflammatory and xerotic skin disease, thought to arise from both genetic and environmental factors.

- There is a strong genetic association with epidermal barrier defects which encompass not only eczematous skin inflammation, but also allergic rhinitis (hay fever) and asthma. This trio, a combination of AD, asthma, and allergic rhinitis, is referred to as the "atopic triad."

- An overproduction of IgE and cytokines such as IL-4, IL-10, and IL-13 contribute to the inflammatory cascade of erythema, pruritus, and edema.

- Early onset, respiratory allergy, and urban living may all be predictors of a more severe disease prognosis. Very often, children will outgrow the disease by the time they reach school age, but many carry it into adulthood, where it may become more localized to one area or region.

- Research has uncovered filaggrin as a key protein in the normal skin barrier. Mutations of this essential protein were found in the epidermis of patients with ichthyosis vulgaris as well as in patients with AD (Drislane & Irvine, 2019). These mutations represent a strong genetic predisposition for atopic eczema, asthma, and allergies.

- Loss of filaggrin means a poorly formed stratum corneum and a subsequent xerotic barrier that is prone to water loss (Palmer et al., 2006). The ability for the skin barrier to absorb and hold water is essential in AD as well as in other xerotic skin diseases. Xerosis leads to pruritus, which promotes scratching and excoriations. As the skin barrier is further disrupted by prolonged itching and scratching, it becomes vulnerable to a host of potential infections and penetration of allergens that trigger IgE production.

Clinical Presentation

- The hallmark of AD is pruritus, which is often intense and relentless, disrupting every aspect of the patient's life. The course tends to be chronic and relapsing.

- Expect varying degrees of erythema, with inflammatory excoriated papules, which coalesce into eczematous plaques and areas of weepy dermatitis.

- Often evolves into scaly, xerotic plaques; and as the disease becomes more chronic, lichenified changes become evident due to extended periods of itching and scratching.

- Morphology and distribution vary with age (Fig. 4.1-1):
  - Infants and young children—affects face (Fig. 4.1-2) and extensor arms and legs (Fig. 4.1-3A). The diaper region, where moisture tends to be retained, is often spared.
  - Older children and adults—distribution favors flexural areas, including anterior neck, antecubital fossa, and popliteal space, and can affect the breasts, nipples (Fig. 4.1-4), and trunk (Fig. 4.1-3B,C). The scalp, face, and eyelids can also be affected, and in general, the axillae and groin folds are spared at any age.

- Excoriations are nearly always evident in both acute and chronic lesions.

DIFFERENTIAL DIAGNOSIS   Atopic Dermatitis
• Tinea
• Psoriasis
• Nummular eczema
• Allergic/Irritant contact dermatitis
• Molluscum contagiosum dermatitis
• Seborrheic dermatitis
• Lichen simplex chronicus
• Cutaneous T-cell lymphoma, mycosis fungoides type

Confirming the Diagnosis

- A clinical diagnosis with common cutaneous features is often all that is needed to diagnose AD (Box 4.1-1).

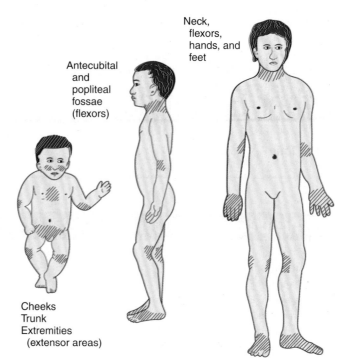

FIG. 4.1-1. Distribution of atopic dermatitis at various ages. Children have involvement of their face and neck. The extensor aspects of extremities are affected in infants, whereas the flexural aspects are more affected in older children and adults. Atopic dermatitis usually spares the axillae and groin.

- A KOH test can differentiate tinea from AD.
- Punch biopsy will identify psoriasis and other noneczematous dermatoses.

Treatment

Bathing and Moisturizing

- Patients are often confused about when and how often to bathe. Bathing is beneficial, as it hydrates the skin, allows for added penetration of topically applied therapies, and can help debride crusts and scaling. Generally, 15 to 20 minutes in a bath is ample time for

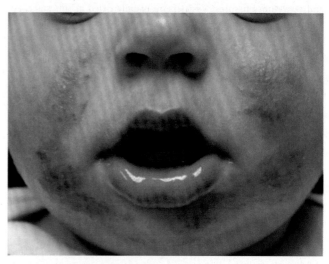

FIG. 4.1-2. Atopic dermatitis frequently affects the cheeks of infants. (Used with permission from Gru, A. A., & Wick, M. [2018]. *Pediatric dermatopathology and dermatology.* Wolters Kluwer Health.)

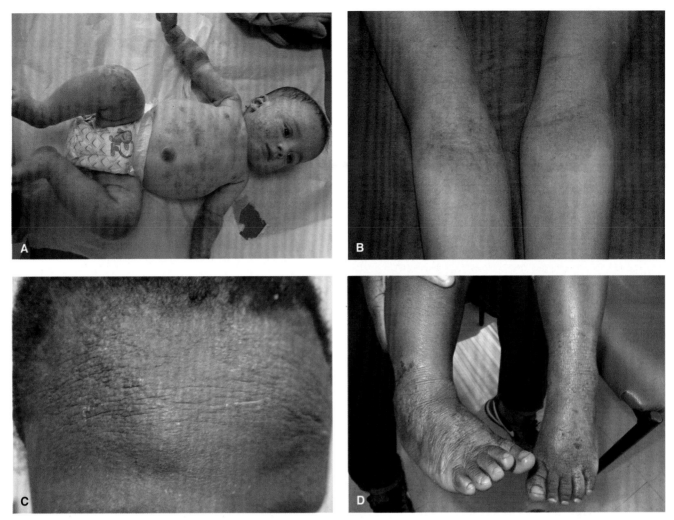

FIG. 4.1-3. A: Atopic dermatitis infant. This photo demonstrates the distribution of AD in infant involving the face, trunk, and extensor surfaces of extremities. (Photo courtesy of M. Bobonich.) **B:** Typical distribution of atopic dermatitis in the antecubital fossa as a child gets older. (Used with permission from Hall, J., & Hall, B. [2017]. *Sauer's manual of skin diseases* [11th ed.]. Wolters Kluwer.) **C:** On dark skin; it may be difficult to appreciate the erythema of scaly papules and plaques. Chronic lichenified, and hyperpigmented plaques on the forehead. (Used with permission from Gru, A. A., & Wick, M. [2018]. *Pediatric dermatopathology and dermatology.* Wolters Kluwer Health.) **D:** Atopic dermatitis in young child. This photo demonstrates the symmetrical distribution of AD. The child uses each foot to rub the dorsal surface of the other. (Photo courtesy M. Bobonich.)

the skin to become hydrated. Bathwater should be warm or cool (not hot), and patients should be ready to apply a moisturizer or topical corticosteroid (TCS) within 3 minutes of exiting the tub, when the stratum corneum is soft and supple, and penetration of the treatments is maximized. In the most severe cases, where skin involvement is extensive, wet wraps may be useful as a substitute for a soaking bath for a few days until the skin has begun to heal and getting into water is more comfortable.

- *Bleach Baths,* can be helpful if the patient develops recurrent skin infections, to decolonize the skin (one quarter cup of bleach to a full tub for pediatric patients, one half cup for adults), soaking for only 5 to 10 minutes, once a week is usually adequate.

Emollients

- The skin barrier is important to the pathogenesis of AD, and many research trials are focused on restoring skin barrier function in order to see better therapeutic outcomes with less need for prescription medications. Therefore, once AD is adequately controlled, moisturizers should be continued on a regular, daily, or several-times-daily basis to maintain control. Emollients are the cornerstone of maintenance therapy and prevention of

relapse. Greasy or creamy emollients are always recommended, and some creamy emollients with a lipid concentration may provide an even more durable barrier than other water-based creams. Lotions tend to contain increased amounts of water and alcohol and, upon evaporation, may actually cause more dryness. A helpful hint is to remind patients that creamy or greasy products are, with few exceptions, found in jars rather than in pump bottles.

Medications

- *Topical corticosteroids.* TCSs are the first-line therapy for AD and usually offer effective, swift control of a flare. There is a myriad of choices, but generally a mid- to high-potency corticosteroid (triamcinolone 0.1% ointment, fluocinonide 0.05% ointment, or betamethasone 0.05% ointment) will adequately treat flares. Creams can be used if patients insist, but ointments are always preferred. Typically, a mid-strength corticosteroid is applied twice daily for 3 to 5 days on the thinner skin areas (face, eyelids, neck, breasts, and buttocks) and twice daily for 7 days on the trunk and extremities. For practical reasons and to avoid confusion, it is best to prescribe one-strength TCS for all areas involved and to eliminate the risk of

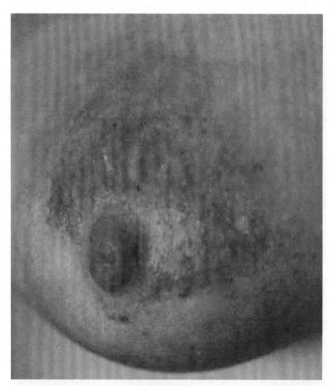

FIG. 4.1-4. Nipple eczema on patient with atopic dermatitis. (Image provided by Stedman's.)

mistakenly using a stronger corticosteroid in a thin-skinned area. A mid-strength TCS can safely be used 2 days per week for long-term control and to prevent relapse. Often topical nonsteroidal anti-inflammatory drugs (see TCIs and PDE below) are used for maintenance once a disease flare has been controlled by a TCS.

BOX 4.1-1   Clinical Criteria for a Diagnosis of Atopic Dermatitis

Essential Features (Required)[a]
Pruritus
Eczema (typical morphology and age-specific pattern)
Chronic or relapsing history

Important Features (Observed in a Majority of Cases and Add Support to Diagnosis)
Early age of onset
Atopy (personal or family history, IgE reactivity)
Xerosis

Associated Features (Suggest the Clinician Consider the Diagnosis of AD)
Atypical vascular responses (facial pallor, white dermographism, delayed blanching response)
Keratosis pilaris, Pityriasis alba, or Ichthyosis
Hyperlinear palms
Periocular (Dennie–Morgan lines) and/or perioral changes, cheilitis
Perifollicular accentuation
Lichenification/prurigo lesions

[a]AAD guidelines mandate the exclusion of other common cutaneous disorders before diagnosis, such as contact dermatitis and cutaneous lymphomas.
Adapted from Eichenfield, L. F., Ahluwalia, J., Waldman, A., Borok, J., Udkoff, J., & Boguniewicz, M. (2017). Current guidelines for the evaluation and management of atopic dermatitis: A comparison of the Joint Task Force Practice Parameter and American Academy of Dermatology guidelines. *Journal of Allergy and Clinical Immunology, 139*(4S), S49–S57.

Combination therapy of a mid-strength TCS 2 days per week and nonsteroidal anti-inflammatories 5 days per week is a practical and effective plan to induce and maintain control of atopic disease.

- *Topical Calcineurin Inhibitirs (TCIs).* There are three nonsteroidal anti-inflammatory topical medications approved for use in AD: tacrolimus ointment (Protopic) and pimecrolimus cream (Elidel). Applied to the skin, calcineurin inhibitors modulate the body's immune response to AD. Both tacrolimus 0.03% and 0.1% ointment are approved for use in adults with moderate to severe AD, only 0.03% for children aged 2 to 15 years. Pimecrolimus 0.1% cream is prescribed for ages 2 and older with mild to moderate AD. The calcineurin inhibitors are designated as second-line therapies, while TCSs remain as first-line therapy for AD. Both calcineurin inhibitors have a black box warning regarding risk of cancer, although to date, there has been no statistical evidence linking development of cancer and the use of these topical agents, and short-term data on systemic side effects for both drugs are reassuring. Long-term safety data are ongoing.

- *PDE-4 inhibitor.* Crisaborole (Eucrisa) is a topical anti-inflammatory agent that inhibits PDE-4. It is also approved for patients 2 years of age and older. Cutaneous side effects of burning, itching, and stinging can be accentuated and uncomfortable on flared skin, leading to medication noncompliance but these complaints typically subside after the first or second application of the medication.

- *Antihistamines.* Sedating antihistamines such as diphenhydramine or hydroxyzine can be helpful for their somnolent effect when taken at bedtime. They can help promote more restful sleep and help reduce scratching during the night. Nonsedating antihistamines can be helpful for patients who suffer from allergic rhinitis, but should not be prescribed as an antipruritic treatment. Topical antihistamines are generally not recommended as they can be irritating to atopic skin and have the potential to cause allergic contact dermatitis (ACD).

- *Antibiotics.* Eczematous areas can become secondarily infected with *Staphylococcus aureus* (most common) and other bacterial skin infections (Fig. 4.1-5A). Topical antibiotics such as polysporin or mupirocin can be used when infection is localized and the skin is not significantly flaring. If infection is widespread and/or flaring, oral antibiotics should be initiated. Generally, 5 days of cephalexin or dicloxacillin are adequate to treat a staph infection. Overuse of antibiotics potentially leads to multidrug-resistant *S. aureus* in AD patients and should be avoided. In patients who have frequent or recurring staph infections, addition of rifampin for 10 days or taking newer generation tetracyclines for 30 days (if age appropriate) in conjunction with topical mupirocin may help halt the chronic nature of infections. It is important for patients to recognize the signs of a skin infection and to know that it is often the reason for a flare, and if left untreated, the flare-up is likely to persist. As stated above, with recurrent skin infections, bleach baths can be helpful to decolonize the skin. Culturing for sensitivities to rule out drug-resistant bacteria is always advised if the patient does not respond to standard antibiotic therapy.

- *Approved Biologics.* Dupilumab (Dupixent) is currently the only biologic treatment approved for moderate to severe AD in pediatrics (ages 6 to 12), adolescents (ages 12 to 17), and adults who are not adequately controlled with TCSs and/or nonsteroidal anti-inflammatory treatments. Administered as a subcutaneous injection, dupilumab is a fully human anti-interleukin-4 receptor α-monoclonal antibody that is directed against interleukin IL-4 and IL-13 to inhibit signaling. IL-4 and IL-13 are key drivers of

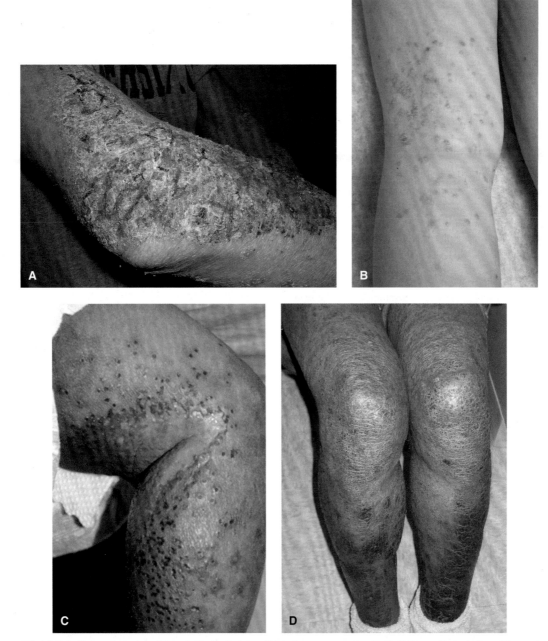

FIG. 4.1-5. **A:** Severe atopic dermatitis patient with staph impetiginization on upper extremity. **B:** Children with atopic dermatitis are at increased risk for molluscum contagiosum with the tendency to become widespread because of their tendency to scratch and spread the lesions. **C:** Eczema herpeticum featuring multiple eroded vesicles with umbilication and crusting overlying a patch of eczematous skin. **D:** Chronic scratching in AD can lead to alterations in pigmentation and lichenification. (Photos courtesy of Susan Tofte.)

type 2/Th2-mediated inflammation that causes erythema, edema, weeping, and severe pruritus associated with AD (Beck et al., 2014). Prescribers must be aware of loading doses, weight-based dosing regimens, and side effects prior to initiating therapy. The most common side effects of dupilumab observed in patients are injection site reactions and conjunctivitis, blepharitis, keratitis, or eye pruritus. Patients are advised to see their healthcare provider if these side effects are experienced. Patients should avoid the use of live vaccines while using dupilumab. Dupilumab is also approved as an adjunct maintenance treatment for moderate to severe asthma in children (>12 years old) and adults. Consultation with the patient's allergist or pulmonologist is advised before modifying an asthma treatment regimen.

- *Emerging AD Therapies.* New AD treatments in phase II or phase III trials (or pending FDA approval) include: monoclonal antibodies that target cytokine IL-13 (tralokinumab and lebrikizumab) and IL-31 (nemolizumab), monoclonal IgG antibody targeting Anti-OX40 antibody, and several small-molecule janus kinase (JAK) inhibitors (baricitinib, abrocitinib, and upadacitinib). These therapies show great promise and may become part of the AD therapy armamentarium in the near future.

Severe, Extensive Disease

- When flares are severe and extensive, oral corticosteroids may be necessary to regain control. Generally, a tapering 6- to 10-day course of prednisone is adequate with the addition of a TCS at the end of the taper.

- In recalcitrant disease, a course of cyclosporine (CSA) can be utilized. This is generally prescribed when intense topical therapy and/or courses of prednisone have not halted the AD flare. Baseline labs of chemistry panel, complete blood count, and urinalysis need to be obtained prior to starting this therapy and monitored monthly. Blood pressure is also monitored regularly. Due to the potential for renal toxicity and hypertension, it is not a therapy that can be used indefinitely, and after a 6-month course, transition to another therapy is warranted. Patients with known renal disease or uncontrolled hypertension should not take CSA. The starting dose of CSA when prescribed is usually at 5 mg/kg/day. This dose will quickly reduce both pruritus and inflammation and induce a remission, giving patients worn down by their disease a reprieve.

- Ultraviolet therapy or other systemic therapies, including methotrexate, azathioprine, mycophenolate mofetil, and interferon-γ, have shown varying levels of efficacy in severe AD patients.

- As discussed above, dupilumab is indicated for moderate to sever AD for ages 6 and above.

Complications

- *Eczema herpeticum* can result from primary outbreaks of herpes simplex virus (HSV) (Fig. 4.1-5C). Treating HSV with acyclovir 400 mg t.i.d. for 1 week is adequate; however, treatment for eczema herpeticum should include zoster doses of antivirals and could require hospitalization with IV antiviral therapy.

- *Tinea infections* can initiate and exacerbate AD flares. Checking toe web spaces, groin, and other intertriginous areas is important when looking for causes of a continued flare. Widespread fungal infections may need systemic antifungal treatment.

- Abnormal pigmentation, lichenification, scars, striae, and secondary infection with molluscum, warts, and/or bacterial impetiginization are complications from AD (Fig. 4.1-5D).

Management and Patient Education

- AD patients require long periods of time and educational dialogue in order to understand the fundamentals of how to manage flares, maintain control of the disease, and recognize signs of skin infections.

- Severe AD patients require more clinic time in order to address trigger factors, explanation of treatments, side effects, and detailed instructions regarding use of medications. Psychological factors may also need to be addressed, such as sleep disruption, anxiety, and depression.

- Erythrodermic AD patients will need inpatient hospitalization. A referral to a dermatologic professional who specializes in atopic disease is appropriate.

- The National Eczema Association (NEA) and the National Eczema Society (NES) are nonprofit patient-centered organizations for patients and their families. Both offer valuable educational information and support for families and healthcare professionals.

- Compliance to treatment plans is essential for maintenance once the skin disease is under control. Ideally, a nurse or medical assistant will be involved in the teaching and demonstration of treatments, as this can be a time-consuming process that may not automatically be built into the providers' schedule.

NUMMULAR ECZEMA

Nummular eczema (*nummular or discoid dermatitis*) is a common and chronic skin disorder characterized by its annular or round, "coin-shaped" lesions. Males are more affected than females; with the age of onset over 50 years for males and for females around 30 years of age. Nummular eczema can, and often does, overlap with AD, stasis dermatitis, and asteatotic eczema; but unlike AD, clinical signs of atopy (and a history of atopy) are not present with nummular eczema. It can also be misdiagnosed as psoriasis or as a fungal infection because of similarities in initial presentation.

Pathophysiology

- The pathogenesis of nummular eczema is not well understood. Some theorize that a microbial component plays a role, possibly due to bacterial colonization, although clear signs of infection are not always evident.

- It is evident that xerotic skin changes in elderly patients lend themselves to the development of cracking and fissuring of the stratum corneum in dry, cold winter weather and often progressing to nummular lesions.

- As the stratum corneum becomes increasingly compromised, it also becomes more damaged from scratching and manipulating due to the extreme pruritus and dryness, which is nearly always present in nummular eczema lesions. With the compromised skin barrier issue, various allergens now have a portal of entry through the skin, which may further aggravate the eczematous process (Box 4.1-2).

BOX 4.1-2 Common Allergens Associated with Eczema

Bacitracin
Balsam of Peru
Cobalt chloride
Formaldehyde
Fragrance mix
Neomycin sulfate
Nickel sulfate
Propylene glycol
Quaternium-15
Sodium gold thiosulfate
Thimerosal
Thiuram mix

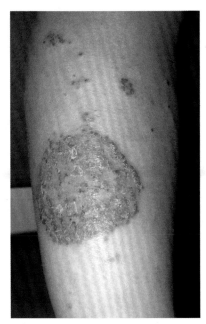

FIG. 4.1-6. Nummular eczema on the lower legs with the characteristic "coin-shaped" erythematous plaques. (Photo courtesy of M. Bobonich.)

- It is associated with contact sensitization (nickel, fragrances, chromates, balsam of Peru) (Box 4.1-2) and venous hypertension.

Clinical Presentation

- Erythematous annular plaques, and sometimes thinner scaly patches, typically distributed on the upper and lower extremities (Fig. 4.1-6).
- Lesions are typically well demarcated and start out as small papules that expand into larger plaques measuring between 1 and 3 cm.
- Acute plaques can be vesicular and weeping (Fig. 4.1-7). However, a typical nummular eczema plaque eventually becomes lichenified and hyperkeratotic, demonstrating the chronicity of the lesions.
- Excoriations due to intense pruritus are nearly always evident in both acute and chronic lesions.
- Males will show a predominance of involvement on the lower extremities and females more likely on the forearms and dorsal hands.

DIFFERENTIAL DIAGNOSIS   Nummular Eczema

- Tinea
- Psoriasis
- Contact dermatitis
- Psoriasis
- Lichen simplex chronicus
- Drug eruption
- Cutaneous T-cell lymphoma, plaque type

Confirming the Diagnosis

- The diagnosis of nummular eczema is usually a clinical one.
- Bacterial cultures or KOH prep may be performed if infection is considered.
- A punch biopsy is not usually necessary and can yield nonspecific findings of spongiotic dermatitis, which cannot differentiate it from

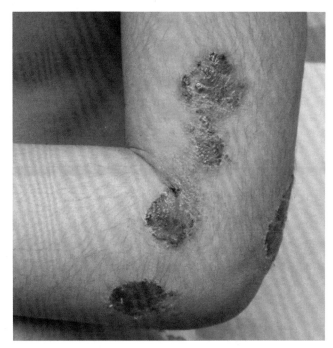

FIG. 4.1-7. Acute plaques of nummular eczema can be very vesicular and weepy erythematous, scaly annular "coin-shaped" lesions seen in nummular eczema. (Photo courtesy of Susan Tofte.)

other eczematous conditions. It would, however, help to exclude drug eruption, cutaneous T-cell lymphoma, psoriasis, and tinea.
- Patch testing may be recommended for severe or recalcitrant cases.

Treatment

Topical

- Nummular eczema generally requires a potent TCS such as clobetasol 0.05% ointment to provide adequate and effective treatment. An ointment rather than cream base is preferred, and application immediately after a shower, soaking bath, or wet compress is recommended.
- Sometimes occlusion of the lesions on the extremities for 1 week (at bedtime) will enhance penetration of the corticosteroid and accelerate healing. Occlusion of a plaque can be achieved by wrapping the extremity with plastic wrap after the application of the TCS.
- Cordran tape, an impregnated tape *with* flurandrenolide, can be applied directly to the lesion and left on for up to 12 hours. It is especially helpful with lichenified lesions.
- As with any other eczematous condition, moisturizing the skin with a creamy or greasy emollient is fundamentally essential, particularly after a bath or shower, to enhance penetration of the emollient.

Systemic

- Systemic corticosteroids may be needed in short bursts for the more severe and severely pruritic cases, but generally TCSs are adequate to bring this disease under control.
- Intralesional triamcinolone injections, phototherapy, and application of Unna boots may also be helpful.
- Recent studies have shown successful treatment of severe cases in children with methotrexate (Knöpfel et al., 2018) and in adults with dupilumab (Choi, 2020). These are non-FDA approved, off-label uses for these medications.

Management and Patient Education

- Nummular eczema is a chronic skin condition that can be challenging to control.
- Infections can develop secondary to chronic scratching and may require treatment.
- Chronic plaques can result in permanent scarring and hyperpigmentation.
- Patients should be taught good skin care measures for the prevention and treatment of nummular eczema.
- Understanding the appropriate use of TCS, including risks and benefits of long-term use, is very important.
- Patients should seek evaluation if there are any signs or symptoms of infection.

ASTEATOTIC ECZEMA

Nearly everyone after their sixth decade of life experiences some type of skin dryness (xerosis). For some, it may only be a patch or two of dryness in the winter months, but more often it involves extensive areas or the entire body. Asteatotic eczema (also called *eczema craquelé* or *desiccation dermatitis*) is severely dry skin that is inflamed and fissured. It is linked to outside influences, including drier climates, cold winter weather, and individuals who bathe, swim, or shower often without caring for their skin immediately after being out of the water. Asteatotic eczema can be seen in most any part of the world and to a slight degree affects men more than women. There are many factors which can influence and aggravate xerotic skin, including drier climates, detergents with higher alkalinity, showering or bathing excessively, malnutrition, renal insufficiency, hereditary skin conditions (ichthyosis vulgaris), and those with a history of atopy.

Pathophysiology

- Dry skin (xerosis) in an aging individual is not related to a deficiency of oil or sebum production, but rather from functional problems with the stratum corneum.
- Low levels of intercellular lipids lead to an inability to bind and retain water. The dehydrated cells shrink and become rigid, forming deep fissures in the epidermis and sometimes extending into the dermis.
- Factors that contribute to or aggravate dryness include low humidity, low ambient temperatures, chronic ultraviolet light, excessive use of soaps, habitual scrubbing, and excessive water exposure.
- Perfumed soaps and other skin cleansers may provoke the cutaneous nerve fibers, leading to a release of proinflammatory cytokines which then begins the cycle of inflammation.

Clinical Presentation

- Often presents (or worsens) during colder months and is referred to as "winter itch." Mild disease may have no symptoms, but in moderately or severely affected skin, patients are likely to complain of pruritus, burning, or stinging.
- Dry or xerotic skin appears dull, dry, and scaly. The scaling associated with general xerosis and with asteatotic eczema is described as fine, bran-like scales.
- The skin can actually demonstrate a crisscross show of superficial cracks as well as fissures in the horny layer, sometimes referred to as "crazy-paving" or "dried-river bed" cracks (Fig. 4.1-8).

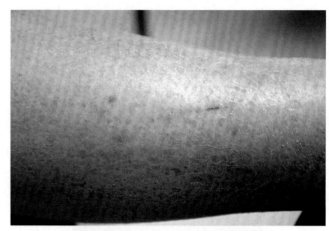

FIG. 4.1-8. Asteatotic skin typical with dried curled edges and erythema. (Photo courtesy of M. Bobonich.)

- The affected areas can appear pink or mildly erythematous. In chronic, advanced asteatotic eczema, a background of dull erythema with oozing, crusting, and excoriations can be seen.
- Vesicles and pustules are generally not seen with asteatotic eczema.

DIFFERENTIAL DIAGNOSIS Asteatotic Eczema

- Atopic dermatitis
- Allergic contact dermatitis
- Cellulitis
- Stasis dermatitis

Confirming the Diagnosis

- Laboratory studies are not indicated for the diagnosis of asteatotic eczema.
- Bacterial cultures or a fungal KOH may be indicated if there is clinical suspicion for infection.

Treatment

- Use of a mid-potency TCS ointment for 5 to 7 days is usually sufficient to clear the inflammation from asteatotic eczema and bring it under control.
- Maintenance can generally be achieved with regular use of a creamy or greasy emollient.
- Use of urea or lactic acid preparations can also be beneficial for some patients.
- Patients should be educated to continue moisturization and avoid known aggravating factors.

Management and Patient Education

- Asteatotic eczema can be an acute problem that can be resolved. Yet, recurrence is not uncommon in individuals with chronic environmental exposure or poor skin care.
- Eczema craquelé can develop when dry skin is perturbed by contact with irritating substances in topical skin preparations.

- Secondary infections and inflammation are common complications. Furthermore, scratching behavior may result in ulceration.
- A referral to a specialist is generally not indicated unless chronic wounds develop and require wound care. Patients should be educated about the signs and symptoms of infection.
- Although the elderly cannot halt the physiologic changes in the skin from aging, they can reduce the environmental triggers and actively prevent dermatitis with good skin care.

DYSHIDROTIC ECZEMA

An intensely pruritic form of eczema, dyshidrotic eczema is characterized by the appearance of vesicles on the hands and feet. It occurs twice as often in females as males. It can present at any age but most often develops in the second to fourth decade. Risk factors for dyshidrotic eczema include a history of atopic or ACD, industrial exposure to certain metals (cobalt, nickel, and chromium), and anxiety or stress.

Pathophysiology

- The etiology of dyshidrotic eczema is unknown. Unlike hyperhidrosis (excessive sweating of the palms, soles, and axillae), dyshidrotic eczema (also called *pompholyx*) is not related to sweat gland activity.
- It is thought to be associated with psychogenic factors (stress related), fungal infection, id reaction (literally an eczematous reaction to a fungal infection somewhere else on the body), drug reaction, and in many cases is idiopathic.

Clinical Presentation

- The clinical picture of dyshidrotic eczema is a vesicular eruption, appearing as clear or white small deep vesicles (described as tapioca pearls) on the palms, fingers, and soles (Fig. 4.1-9).

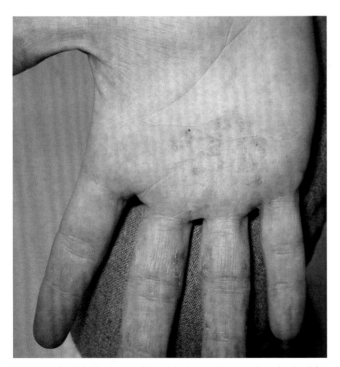

FIG. 4.1-9. Dyshidrotic eczema with vesicles and erythema on the palms involving the lateral aspects of the finger.

- It distinctly spares the dorsum of the hands or feet, but may extend to the lateral aspects of the fingers and soles. Once the vesicles dry, scale is usually the most notable symptom.
- Patients often complain of severe pruritus and sometimes burning pain.

DIFFERENTIAL DIAGNOSIS   Dyshidrotic Eczema

- Palmar–plantar pustular psoriasis
- Tinea
- Contact dermatitis
- Bullous impetigo

Confirming the Diagnosis

- Bacterial culture and sensitivity and/or a KOH can help identify bacterial or fungal pathogens.
- Skin biopsy is not necessary but can help to differentiate this condition from psoriasis or tinea. A biopsy for direct immunofluorescence (DIF) can rule out autoimmune blistering disease.

Treatment

- Treating the suspected cause (infections, drugs, stress) of dyshidrotic eczema can be curative.
- Stress and anxiety management may help reduce recurrence.
- Underlying infection, either bacterial or fungal, should be treated with the appropriate antibiotics.
- Treatment with high-potency TCS twice daily is the first-line therapy. Once controlled, tapering the TCS to milder-potency TCS or a calcineurin inhibitor can be effective.
- If the dyshidrotic eczema is severe, a short-term course of systemic corticosteroids may be indicated.
- Systemic antihistamines may be helpful for less scratching at bedtime and improved sleep quality.
- Dermatologists treating recalcitrant disease often use immunosuppressants including methotrexate, CSA, azathioprine, and PUVA (psoralen followed by UV light therapy).

Management and Patient Education

- Referral to a dermatologic specialist may be warranted if first-line therapies are not effective or the dyshidrotic eczema is severe or recurrent.
- In some cases, referral to a psychotherapist may be beneficial and appropriate in controlling stress.
- Dyshidrotic eczema can have a significant impact on an individual's daily living and essential function. It can interfere with interpersonal relationships, employment, and home life, all of which impact the general quality of life.
- Instructions to avoid contact with irritants and continue diligent daily hand care will help to maintain better control and to prevent flares.
- Reducing stress and avoiding excessive water exposure may prevent flares.
- Dietary modifications may be helpful if allergy and patch testing identifies allergens.

SEBORRHEIC DERMATITIS

Seborrheic dermatitis is a common skin disease identified by erythematous, greasy yellowish scaling or crusty plaques typically seen on the scalp, eyelids, eyebrows, glabellar forehead, nose/nasal folds, ears, periorally, and in more severe cases on the central chest, umbilicus, and axilla. It is common in infants and children where it is referred to as "cradle cap." Seborrheic dermatitis can be misdiagnosed as AD but is generally significantly less pruritic. The scaling associated with seborrheic dermatitis presents as a greasier, oilier scaling whereas the scaling associated with AD is more xerotic.

Seborrheic dermatitis is reviewed in detail later in this section (Section 4.3), as well as in the Childhood Skin Disorders (Section 13-3).

ID REACTION

An id reaction is an inflammatory dermatitis which is the body's response to an infection, inflammatory condition, or substance. It is also referred to as *autosensitization, disseminated eczema,* or *dermatophytids.* It is estimated that at least two thirds of patients with contact dermatitis develop disseminated eczema, whereas one third of the patients with a history of stasis dermatitis have developed autosensitization.

Pathophysiology

- The pathogenesis is not clearly understood but thought to be an immune-mediated response of the body to an infection, trauma, or antigens from an inflammatory process.
- Fungus is the most common pathogen seen that triggers an immunologic response, however, bacteria, mycobacteria, and viruses, such as the pox virus in molluscum, can trigger autosensitization dermatitis.
- Epidermal antigens from inflammatory skin conditions like contact dermatitis can lead to hypersensitization, resulting in an id reaction.

Clinical Presentation

- Symptoms of id reaction can vary with the stimuli causing the immune response.
- Id can be characterized by poorly demarcated eczematous patches, papules, petechiae, or vesicles may present on the extremities, face, and, occasionally, the trunk.
- The reaction may occur near the sites of infection (i.e., surrounding the molluscum papules) or remotely on distant sites not affected by the primary pathogen or inflammatory process.
- Thus, an annular plaque of tinea on a patient's face could result in an id reaction located on their hands and fingers (Fig. 4.1-10).
- Likewise, a patient with stasis dermatitis may appear to have a diffuse, papulovesicular eruption spreading to other extremities and even overlying the original stasis dermatitis of the shins.
- Autosensitization is not immediate and develops days to weeks after the onset of the initial infection or inflammatory condition. The dermatitis will continue to spread until the underlying condition is treated.

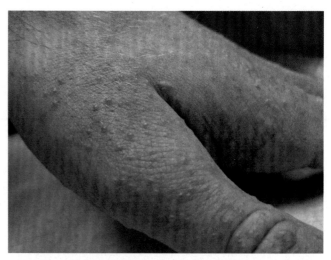

FIG. 4.1-10. Id reaction with vesicles located on the hands and fingers in a young man with tinea on his leg. (Photo courtesy of M. Bobonich.)

DIFFERENTIAL DIAGNOSIS   Id Reaction
• Contact dermatitis
• Nummular eczema
• Granuloma annulare
• Autoimmune blistering diseases
• Dyshidrotic eczema
• Viral exanthem
• Scabies
• Drug eruption

Confirming the Diagnosis

- Laboratory studies should include culture and sensitivity.
- Scraping to identify fungal hyphae, scabies mites, or scybala.
- Skin biopsy has limited diagnostic value and will only exclude eczematous dermatoses.
- Patch testing will help identify allergens.

Treatment

- The most important therapeutic intervention for id reaction is the treatment of the underlying infection with the appropriate antimicrobial or therapeutic treatment.
- Use of TCS can provide some relief from the pruritus but is somewhat controversial as some clinicians believe that corticosteroids can suppress the cutaneous immune system and allow further spread of a cutaneous infection.
- For weeping patches and plaques, wet dressings or Burow compresses (aluminum acetate available as Domeboro) can be effective.

Management and Patient Education

- An id reaction is self-limiting and will resolve spontaneously once the associated infection or inflammatory process is treated.
- Patients should be instructed to follow up for signs and symptoms of infections.

LICHEN SIMPLEX CHRONICUS (LSC)

A chronic disorder resulting from excessive scratching and rubbing of the skin, LSC or neurodermatitis is a very frustrating skin disease. Breaking the itch–scratch cycle is most important and can be quite challenging. It is more commonly seen in adults in the sixth decade of life or older. LSC in children is usually seen in adolescents. Patients with a history of AD or anxiety have a higher incidence of LSC.

Pathophysiology

- The etiology of LSC is thought to be associated with sensitization.
- LSC can develop from rubbing or scratching in response to pruritus from a primary process like contact dermatitis, insect bites, psoriasis, stress, etc.
- Perpetuation of the itch–scratch cycle may be further aggravated by psychological stress or anxiety disorders.
- Environmental factors such as heat, irritants, or sweat can contribute to the pruritus.

Clinical Presentation

- LSC lesions are identified as hyperpigmented, thick, lichenified plaques with a leathery appearance that evolve over time.
- Patients may or may not be aware of their habitual scratching and rubbing, and it may occur when the patient is asleep.
- Secondary erosions may be noted.
- LSC is located in easy to reach areas like the back of the neck and occipital scalp, extensor aspects of the arms and legs, vulva/scrotum, and perianal area (Fig. 4.1-11A,B).

DIFFERENTIAL DIAGNOSIS   Lichen Simplex Chronicus

- Hypertrophic lichen planus
- Psoriasis
- Nummular eczema
- Lichen sclerosus
- Human papillomavirus
- Tinea
- Insect/Scabies infestation

Confirming the Diagnosis

- LSC is usually a clinical diagnosis.
- Skin biopsy may help identify a primary disease or a condition which causes pruritus fundamental to the itch–scratch cycle.
- Cultures for secondary infections may be indicated.

Treatment

Topical

- Emollients can provide immediate relief of pruritus.
- High-potency TCS with or without occlusion can ease the pruritus and, equally important, provide a barrier to prevent more scratching or rubbing to affected areas.
- Flurandrenolide impregnated tape (Cordran tape) can be applied directly to LSC lesions for 8–12 hours.
- Treatment goals should also include risk reduction for secondary infections.

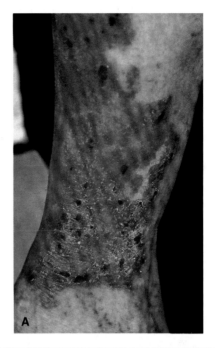

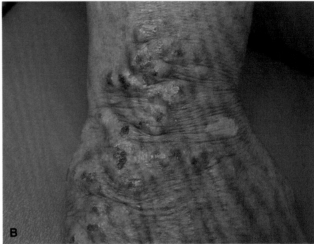

FIG. 4.1-11. A: Lichen simplex chronicus from chronic scratching on the lower leg. This is a common location. Note the lichenification and excoriations due to the marked pruritus. (Used with permission from Hall, J., & Hall, B. [2017]. *Sauer's manual of skin diseases* [11th ed.]. Wolters Kluwer.) **B:** Prurigo nodules (picker's papules) on dorsal hand; a form of LSC. (Image provided by Stedman's.)

Systemic

- Intralesional corticosteroids are effective in controlling pruritus and reducing the size of involved lesions.
- Doxepin seems to be the most effective antihistamine in helping with pruritus, but sedation is a common side effect.
- LSC has been associated with obsessive compulsive and anxiety disorders where patients treated with selective serotonin reuptake inhibitors (SSRIs) or oral doxepin have shown some improvement.

Management and Patient Education

- Counseling may be necessary and helpful to identify stressors which may cause or exacerbate rubbing and scratching behaviors.
- Secondary infection, hyperpigmentation, and scarring are the most common complications of LSC.

- Complete resolution of lesions can be achieved if the patient is successful in halting the scratching behaviors.
- Patients with LSC easily triggered by stress or unable to break the itch–scratch cycle are likely to experience recurrence.
- Prevention and awareness of rubbing or scratching behaviors is important. Patients should be educated that resolution of the symptoms will require more than pharmacologic intervention and be dependent on behavioral modification. If the patient is using TCS, follow-up with the clinician should include routine examination of the site.

KERATOSIS PILARIS

Keratosis pilaris (KP) is an autosomal dominant skin disorder of follicular keratinization commonly seen on the outer proximal arms, thighs, and cheeks. KP is frequently associated with AD, acne vulgaris, scarring alopecia, obesity, insulin-dependent diabetes, ectodermal dysplasia, and ichthyosis vulgaris (Thomas & Khopkar, 2012). With equal distribution between males, females, and all ethnic groups, KP usually appears during childhood or early adolescence. Some sources report a pediatric population prevalence as low as 2% to 12% (Del Pozzo-Magaña et al., 2012); while others report nearly 50% to 80% of all adolescents and 40% of adults are impacted (Alai & Elston, 2019).

Pathophysiology

Etiology is not fully understood but filaggrin mutations have been documented and likely produce defective keratinization of the follicular epithelium, which causes horny plugs in the keratotic infundibulum. Thomas & Khopkar (2012) challenged the histologic data of KP, and through dermoscopic evaluations, postulated that KP may not be a disorder of keratinization, but rather, is "caused by the circular hair shaft which ruptures the follicular epithelium leading to inflammation and abnormal follicular keratinization."

Clinical Presentation

- Symmetrical distribution of keratotic follicular papules with variable perifollicular erythema distributed most commonly on upper extensor arms, anterior and lateral thighs, and lateral facial cheeks (Fig. 4.1-12). It can also involve the dorsal forearms, back, and buttocks.
- Excoriations can be noted from patients picking the follicular horny plugs: usually not from pruritus. Condition is usually symptomatically benign but often cosmetically displeasing.

DIFFERENTIAL DIAGNOSIS Keratosis Pilaris
Atopic dermatitis
Acne vulgaris
Follicular eczema
Follicular lichen planus
Acneiform drug eruption
Juvenile pityriasis rubra pilaris
Ichthyosis follicularis
Perforating folliculitis
Phrynoderma

Treatments

- To diminish the bumpy appearance and improve texture, emollients containing urea or lactic acid are most commonly used, but

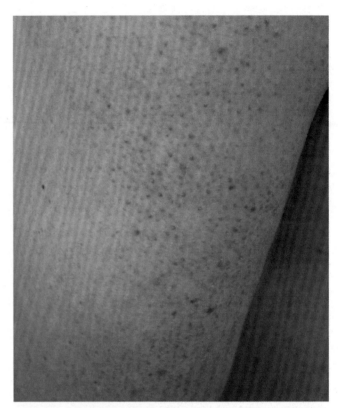

FIG. 4.1-12. Keratosis pilaris. Note the keratotic follicular papules, common on the upper arms. (Image provided by Stedman's.)

α-hydroxy acid, glycolic acid, and salicylic acid preparations can also be utilized. These topical therapies can be applied one to two times per day as monotherapies, or can be used in combination with each other or with other treatments listed below.

- Retinoid creams (tretinoin, retinol, adapalene, tazarotene) can also be applied with emollients at bedtime.
- A mid-potency TCS cream applied to affected areas at bedtime for up to 2 weeks can help improve perifollicular erythema.
- If topicals fail to offer improvement, phototherapy and laser treatments are additional modalities (Ciliberto et al., 2014).

Management and Patient Education

- For many patients, KP improves and gradually fades with time, but it should be emphasized that due to an inherited defect in filaggrin production, there is no known cure for this skin disorder.
- Mild exfoliation of the affected areas three to four times a week can help remove dead skin cells and improve texture; but aggressive and frequent scrubbing can result in irritation and increased inflammation.

READINGS AND REFERENCES

Alai, N., & Elston, D. (2019). Keratosis pilaris. *eMedicine*. Retrieved on October 18, 2020, from http://emedicine.medscape.com/article/1070651-overview

Avena-Woods, C. (2017). Overview of atopic dermatitis. *American Journal of Managed Care, 23*(8), S115–S123. https://www.ajmc.com/view/overview-of-atopic-dermatitis-article.

Beck, L., Thaçi, D., Hamilton, J., Graham, N., Bieber, T., Rocklin, R., Ming, J., Ren, H., Kao, R., Simpson, E., Ardeleanu, M., Weinstein, S., Pirozzi, G., Guttman-Yassky, E., Suárez-Fariñas, M., Hager, M. D., Stahl, N., Yancopoulos, G. D., & Radin, A. R. (2014). Dupilumab treatment in adults with moderate-to-severe atopic dermatitis. *New England Journal of Medicine, 371*(2), 130–139. https://doi.org/10.1056/NEJMoa1314768

Choi, S., Zhu, G. A., Lewis, M. A., Honari, G., Chiou, A. S., Ko, J., & Chen, J. K. (2020). Dupilumab treatment of nummular dermatitis: A retrospective cohort study. *Journal of the American Academy of Dermatology, 82*(5), 1252–1255.

Chung, J., & Simpson, E. (2018). The socioeconomics of atopic dermatitis. *Annals of Allergy, Asthma & Immunology, 76*(5), 958–972. https://doi.org/10.1016/j.anai.2018.12.017

Ciliberto, H., Farshidi, A., Berk, D., & Bayliss, S. (2014). Photopneumatic therapy for the treatment of keratosis pilaris. *Journal of Drugs in Dermatology, 12*(7), 804–806.

Del Pozzo-Magaña, B., Lazo-Langner, A., Gutiérrez-Castrellón, P., & Ruiz-Maldonado, R. (2012). Common dermatoses in children referred to a specialized Pediatric Dermatology Service in Mexico: A comparative study between two decades. *ISRN Dermatology, 2012,* 351603.

Drislane, C., & Irvine, A. (2019). The role of filaggrin in atopic dermatitis and allergic disease. *Annals of Allergy, Asthma & Immunology, 124*(1), 36–43. https://doi.org/10.1016/j.anai.2019.10.008

Eichenfield, L. F., Ahluwalia, J., Waldman, A., Borok, J., Udkoff, J., & Boguniewicz, M. (2017). Current guidelines for the evaluation and management of atopic dermatitis: A comparison of the Joint Task Force Practice Parameter and American Academy of Dermatology guidelines. *Journal of Allergy and Clinical Immunology, 139*(4S), S49–S57. https://doi.org/10.1016/j.jaci.2017.01.009

Feldman, S. R., Cox, L. S., Strowd, L. C., Gerber, R. A., Faulkner, S., Sierka, D., Smith, T. W., Cappelleri, J. C., & Levenberg, M. E. (2019). The challenge of managing atopic dermatitis in the United States. *American Health & Drug Benefits, 12*(2), 83–93.

Fishbein, A. B., Hamideh, N., Lor, J., Zhao, S., Kruse, L., Mason, M., Ariza, A., Bolanos, J., Necheles, J., & Kaye, B. (2020). Management of atopic dermatitis in children younger than two years of age by community pediatricians: A survey and chart review. *Journal of Pediatrics, 221,* 138–144.e3. https://doi.org/10.1016/j.jpeds.2020.02.015

Gruber, R., Sugarman, J. L., Crumrine, D., Hupe, M., Mauro, T. M., Mauldin, E. A., Thyssen, J. P., Brandner, J. M., Hennies, H. C., Schmuth, M., & Elias, P. M. (2015). Sebaceous gland, hair shaft, and epidermal barrier abnormalities in keratosis pilaris with and without filaggrin deficiency. *American Journal of Pathology, 185*(4), 1012–1021. https://doi.org/10.1016/j.ajpath.2014.12.012. Epub 2015 Feb 7

Hanifin, J., Gupta, A. K, & Rajagopalan, R. (2002). Intermittent dosing of fluticasone propionate cream for reducing the risk of relapse in atopic dermatitis patients. *British Journal of Dermatology, 147*(3), 528–537.

Hwang, S., & Schwartz, R. A. (2008). Keratosis pilaris: A common follicular hyperkeratosis. *Cutis; Cutaneous Medicine for the Practitioner, 82*(3), 177–180.

Knöpfel, N., Noguera-Morel, L., Hernández-Martín, A., & Torrelo, A. (2018). Methotrexate for severe nummular eczema in children: Efficacy and tolerability in a retrospective study of 28 patients. *Pediatric Dermatology, 35*(5), 611–615.

Kowalska-Olędzka, E., Czarnecka, M., & Baran, A. (2019). Epidemiology of atopic dermatitis in Europe. *Journal of Drug Assessment, 8*(1), 126–128. https://doi.org/10.1080/21556660.2019.1619570

Lugović-Mihić, L., Bukvić, I., Bulat, V., & Japundžić, I. (2019). Factors contributing to chronic urticaria/angioedema and nummular eczema resolution—which findings are crucial? *Acta Clinica Croatica, 58*(4), 595–603. https://doi.org/10.20471/acc.2019.58.04.05

Molin, S., Diepgen, T. L., Ruzicka, T., & Prinz, J. C. (2011). Diagnosing chronic hand eczema by an algorithm: A tool for classification in clinical practice. *Clinical and Experimental Dermatology, 36*(6), 595–601.

Paller, A. S., Siegfried, E. C., Vekeman, F., Gadkari, A., Kaur, M., Mallya, U. G., Héroux, J., Miao, R., & Mina-Osorio, P. (2020). Treatment patterns of pediatric patients with atopic dermatitis: A claims data analysis. *Journal of the American Academy of Dermatology, 82*(3), 651–660. https://doi.org/10.1016/j.jaad.2019.07.105. Epub 2019 Aug 7

Palmer, D. N., Irvine, A. D., Terron-Kwiatkowski, A., Zhao, Y., Liao, H., Lee, S. P., & McLean, W. H. (2006). Common loss-of-function variants of the epidermal barrier protein filaggrin are a major predisposing factor for atopic dermatitis. *Nature Genetics, 38*(4), 441–446.

Silverberg, J. I., & Hanifin, J. M. (2013). Adult eczema prevalence and associations with asthma and other health and demographic factors: A US population-based study. *Journal of Allergy and Clinical Immunology, 132*(5), 1132–1138.

Thomas, M., & Khopkar, U. (2012). Keratosis pilaris revisited: Is it more than just a follicular keratosis? *International Journal of Trichology, 4*(4), 255–258. https://doi.org/10.4103/0974-7753.111215

Yum, H. Y., Kim, H. H., Kim, H. J., Kim, W. K., Lee, S. Y., Li, K., Lee, D. H., & KAAACI Work Group on Severe/Recalcitrant Atopic Dermatitis. (2018). Current management of moderate-to-severe atopic dermatitis: A survey of allergists, pediatric allergists and dermatologists in Korea. *Allergy, Asthma & Immunology Research, 10*(3), 253–259. https://doi.org/10.4168/aair.2018.10.3.253

Contact, Allergic, and Occupational Dermatitis

A. Matthew Brunner

In This Chapter

- Irritant Contact Dermatitis
- Allergic Contact Dermatitis
- Occupational Dermatitis

Contact dermatitis is defined as an inflammatory skin disorder resulting from exposure of the skin to an external agent. There are two primary types of contact dermatitis: irritant contact dermatitis (ICD), a nonimmunologic disease resulting from an irritating substance coming in direct contact with the stratum corneum (outermost layer of the skin); and allergic contact dermatitis (ACD), an immunologic response to an external agent resulting in a type IV delayed-type hypersensitivity reaction in a previously sensitized patient (Nassau & Fonacier, 2020).

As a primary care or dermatology provider, we are not only faced with treating an acute dermatitis but we are challenged to pursue the matter if the condition does not resolve or recurs frequently. We must be keenly aware of our patient's daily routines and be mindful of hobbies, habits, and occupation. Understanding how to differentiate one dermatitis from another and how and when to refer is key to the management of these conditions.

IRRITANT CONTACT DERMATITIS

The irritants involved in ICD have a direct effect on the skin, leading to skin barrier dysfunction and resulting dermatitis (Holness, 2019). ICD is responsible for the majority (approximately 80%) of contact dermatitis seen in outpatient care. Virtually everyone in the general population is at risk for developing ICD, but patients with atopic dermatitis (AD) have a much greater risk of developing ICD (Tan et al., 2014). Both infants and the elderly can readily be affected by ICD because of a thin and more vulnerable epidermal barrier, and when affected, experience more severe dermatitis.

Pathophysiology

ICD is not due to an immunologic response as in ACD, but rather due to exposure or repeated exposures to an irritating and/or drying substance. The offending agent in ICD may be a caustic chemical or solvent, plant or flower, or abrasive product causing microtrauma. The most common of all irritants is water, sometimes called the universal solvent. When water contacts the skin and then evaporates without sealing moisture, there is potential to develop an eczematous reaction to the wet–dry cycle; repeated episodes of irritant dermatitis can occur each time the skin is exposed to water.

Strong alkaline soaps or solvents may elicit a similar or more robust irritant response. Even weak irritants with repeated contact with the skin can result in an irritant response (Tan et al., 2014). When the stratum corneum, the outermost skin layer, is compromised, nearly any substance has the potential to produce an inflammatory response, often resulting in an cytotoxic effect and subsequent ICD.

- There are several cellular components that play a role in ICD. It is presumed that inflammatory cytokines in the skin are primary mediators in T-cell inflammation.
- There are differences in cell and skin barrier disruption in acute ICD when compared to chronic ICD.

Acute ICD

- The pathogenic route in acute ICD starts with penetration through the stratum corneum and a release of inflammatory mediators, which then activate T cells. When activation has begun, this cascade continues independently from the offending antigen.

Chronic ICD

- In chronic ICD, the stratum corneum has already been altered and lipids in the stratum corneum, which normally provide barrier protection, are weakened, leading to scaling of the epidermis and transepidermal water loss (TEWL).
- As the skin works to retain hydration and repair the protective barrier, it is unable to accomplish this due to chronic exposure. The epidermal barrier demonstrates a chronic eczematoid irritant reaction.

Clinical Presentation

Acute Irritant Contact Dermatitis

- Dorsal hands are the most likely location for lesions; palms are more resilient to the development of ICD (Novak-Bilić et al., 2018).
- Erythematous patches with crusts and scales can be hemorrhagic.
- Serous vesicles and erosions are also possible.
- Tend to have sharply demarcated borders.

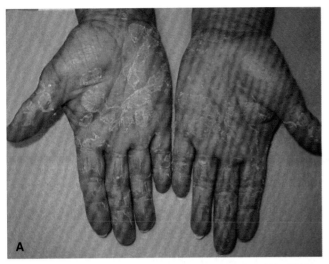
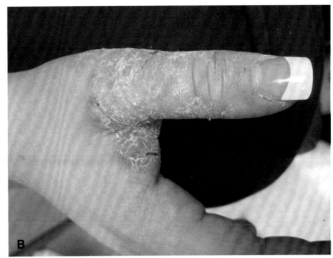

FIG. 4.2-1. Irritant contact dermatitis. **A:** Hands of a healthcare worker. (Photo courtesy of Susan Tofte.) **B:** Chronic ICD demonstrating fissuring and lichenification on the hand of a coffee barista (repeated exposure to wet cleaning clothes).

- Pruritus, burning, and/or pain are all common complaints.
- The onset of symptoms can be rapid, which improves with avoidance of the offending agent.
- The skin's reaction with acute ICD is immediate and can peak within minutes to hours after the exposure. The intensity of clinical signs and symptoms depends on the properties of the irritating substance and the degree of skin barrier impairment at the time of exposure.
- Environmental factors such as temperature, mechanical pressure on the skin, humidity, concentration of the irritating substance, pH, and contact duration can all affect the severity of ICD. Acids and alkaline solutions capable of producing chemical burns are the most common potent irritants resulting in acute ICD (Fig. 4.2-1A).

Chronic Irritant Contact Dermatitis

- Chronic ICD results from multiple subthreshold contacts when the skin does not have ample time between exposures to completely recover and restore normal skin barrier function.
- Lichenification and fissures.
- Lesions of chronic ICD contrast with those of acute ICD, in that the lesions are more likely to be seen as poorly defined, thickened, fissured, or hyperpigmented from long-standing rubbing and scratching (Novak-Bilić et al., 2018) (Fig. 4.2-1B).

DIFFERENTIAL DIAGNOSIS	Irritant Contact Dermatitis

- Allergic contact dermatitis
- Atopic dermatitis
- Scabies
- Psoriasis
- Tinea

Confirming the Diagnosis

- ICD is usually a clinical diagnosis but may require patch testing if ACD is suspected.
- Bacterial and fungal cultures can help identify infections.

- A KOH prep is a rapid, in-office test that can identify hyphae indicating a fungal infection, and a mineral prep can be used to identify scabies (see Section 15 for office procedures).
- A biopsy is helpful only in differentiating ICD from other dermatoses like psoriasis.

Treatment

- The primary treatment for the management of both ICD and ACD is the avoidance of the triggering agent.
- Regular use of emollients helps repair the skin barrier.
- Topical corticosteroids (TCSs) and topical calcineurin inhibitors (TCIs—tacrolimus and pimecrolimus) are also beneficial if the causative agent has been identified and is avoided. TCIs have been shown to be particularly beneficial for ICD of the face (Tan et al., 2014).

Management and Patient Education

- ICD can be chronic and relapsing, especially if the individual has difficulty avoiding contact with the offending agent. This can be seen when the patient's occupation results in unavoidable exposure to irritants, forcing them to make a choice between finding another occupation and dealing with chronic ICD.
- The most common complications include secondary infections, scarring, pigmentary changes, and lichen simplex chronicus (LSC).
- Severe or chronic dermatitis ICD can have a significant impact on the patient's quality of life, which should be addressed by the clinician.
- Patients with ICD should be educated about the appropriate use of TCS, side effects (long and short term), and signs and symptoms of secondary infection.
- Prevention education is important as patients are their best advocates in identifying and avoiding contact irritants.

ALLERGIC CONTACT DERMATITIS

ACD accounts for roughly 20% of contact dermatitis and is characterized as an immunologic type IV delayed hypersensitivity

BOX 4.2-1   Common Allergens

Bacitracin
Balsam of Peru
Cobalt chloride
Formaldehyde
Fragrance mix
Neomycin sulfate
Nickel sulfate
Propylene glycol
Quaternium-15
Sodium gold thiosulfate
Thimerosal
Thiuram mix

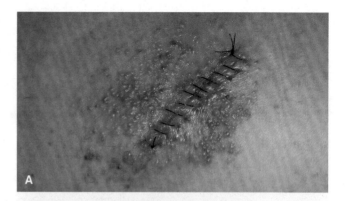

response to an agent to which the patient has been previously sensitized (Nassau & Fonacier, 2020). Examples of ACD include a very specific dermatitis that develops from wearing jewelry containing nickel, cobalt, or gold or that resulting from direct contact with poison ivy (also called *Toxicodendron* dermatitis or *Rhus* dermatitis). Identifying the allergen allows patient avoidance and subsequent dermatitis resolution. It becomes a more complicated clinical picture when ACD is chronic and when it affects hands, face, or eyelids without an obvious identifiable cause. Allergens and exposure to allergens vary from region to region, and the preservatives added to skincare products can also vary depending on government regulations in specific geographic locations.

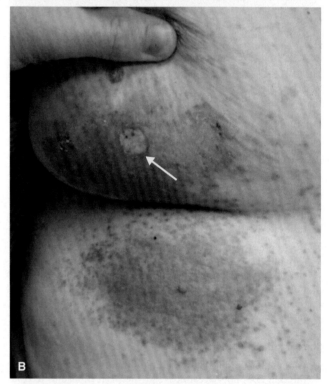

ACD affects patients of all ages, gender, and ethnicity. Occupation and hobbies play a significant role in exposures. ACD accounts for the majority of occupational skin diseases affecting the hands. Many patients with these diagnoses will find it necessary to change jobs or will have extended absences from work because of their dermatitis; some even find it necessary to leave the workforce altogether in order to avoid repeated exposures to offending agents (Box 4.2-1).

Pathophysiology

- ACD is an allergen-specific reaction caused by a type IV delayed hypersensitivity when a patient comes in contact with a specific allergen.

- When antigen-presenting Langerhans cells find and digest the antigen on the cell surface, the Langerhans cell then moves toward the closest lymph node, presenting the antigen to the T-memory cell. At this point, the now activated T lymphocytes converge back to the skin where the cascade of inflammatory events is triggered (pruritus, erythema, blistering).

- When an allergen first contacts and penetrates the skin, initial sensitization occurs. Reexposure at a later date, even in a low or minimal concentration, will lead to a release of cytokines and chemotactic factors resulting in an inflammatory, pruritic, and/or weepy dermatitis.

- This cascade of events occurs rapidly once sensitization is established, usually within 12 to 48 hours of exposure, and if vesicular, can last for days or weeks before resolution.

Clinical Presentation

- Well-demarcated, pruritic eczematous eruption, often acute, with edema and vesicles or bullae that open and can become moist and weepy (Figs. 4.2-2 to 4.2-4).

- Scaly plaques and lichenification if ACD is chronic (Fig. 4.2-5).

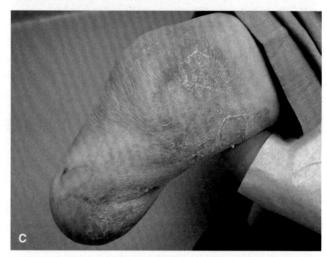

FIG. 4.2-2. Allergic contact dermatitis. **A:** Bacitracin on a surgical site. (Photo courtesy Douglas DiRuggiero.) **B:** Neosporin-induced ACD under the breast. Patient applied neosporin on and around a biopsy site (see *arrow*) and it transferred to the intertriginous portion of the upper abdomen. (Photo courtesy Douglas DiRuggiero.) **C:** ACD from rubber prosthetic sleeve. (Photo courtesy Douglas DiRuggiero.)

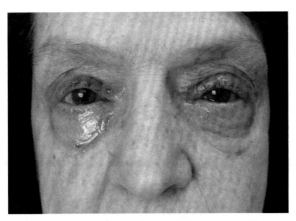

FIG. 4.2-3. Allergic contact dermatitis from medicated eye drops. (Photo courtesy of M. Bobonich.)

- The areas of involvement are typically localized to areas of exposure; however, ACD can become diffuse depending on the vehicle of the causative agent. For example, shampoos or cleansing washes which may rinse over larger areas of the body and thus affect other areas as well as the primary point of contact (Fig. 4.2-6).

DIFFERENTIAL DIAGNOSIS	Allergic Contact Dermatitis

- Tinea
- Perioral dermatitis
- Seborrheic dermatitis
- Drug eruptions
- Asteatotic eczema
- Drug-induced photosensitivity
- Irritant contact dermatitis

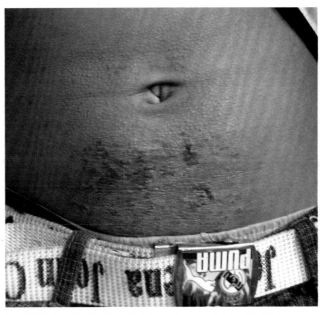

FIG. 4.2-5. Chronic allergic contact dermatitis from a belt buckle. Note hyperpigmentation and lichenification.

Confirming the Diagnosis

- The gold standard for diagnosis of ACD is patch testing.

Patch Testing

- The thin-layer rapid use epicutaneous test (TRUE test), a U.S. FDA–approved testing tool, is the most common, pre-impregnated allergen series used for quick, convenient patch testing. It

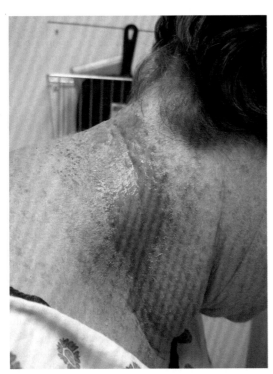

FIG. 4.2-4. Allergic contact dermatitis from necklace containing nickel. (Photo courtesy of M. Bobonich.)

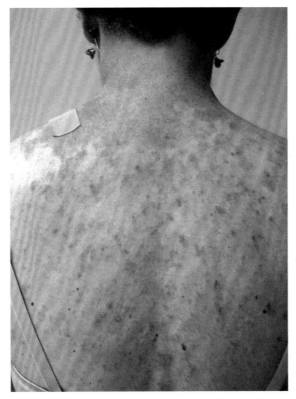

FIG. 4.2-6. Allergic contact dermatitis from shampoo resulted in eczematous papules and plaques in a washed-out pattern from the scalp. (Photo courtesy of M. Bobonich.)

consists of a three-panel system that includes 36 allergens, allergen mixes, and controls used to diagnose the majority of the most common allergens seen in ACD. Dermatology specialists typically utilize a much larger allergen panel which is individually prepared in the office and can be customized to a patient's occupation, hobbies, or suspected environmental exposures. Patients with persistent unresolved ACD can suffer for months or even years, impacting their ability to live a full and productive life. Through patch testing, causative agents can be identified and avoided, thereby improving the patient's quality of life.

- There is no consensus on interpretation, but the International Contact Dermatitis Research Group has developed a standardized scoring system often used in the evaluation of skin reactions to allergens. The noted reaction may range from a weak positive to a bullous skin reaction. These results must be interpreted in the context of the patient's clinical presentation and symptoms to determine the clinical relevance of the allergic reaction. All positive results may not be significant. A true test of clinical relevance is the resolution of ACD when the offending agent is removed.

- The process of patch testing is not complex but does require experienced clinicians in dermatology or allergy/immunology to both apply and interpret the results of the tests. Understanding how and when to patch test patients requires training and experience.

- Patch tests are generally placed on the upper back of the individual and require that the area of skin is clear of dermatitis. This is important and prevents interference from existing dermatitis.

- TCSs may be necessary to clear dermatitis on the patient's back but must be discontinued 1 week prior to the application of the patch tests. Ideally, systemic corticosteroids should be discontinued 1 month prior to patch application.

- Patients should be warned that they will not be allowed to take a shower, exercise, bend or twist their back during the testing time, which lasts for 3 to 5 days. After the initial application of the patches, patients are asked to return to the office in 48 hours for removal of the patches and the first reading. Sites of application are marked in order to identify the location of specific allergens (Fig. 4.2-7). A second reading is taken in 72 hours to 7 days after the patches were initially placed. As mentioned, the interpretation of patch test results should be done by knowledgeable and skilled clinicians.

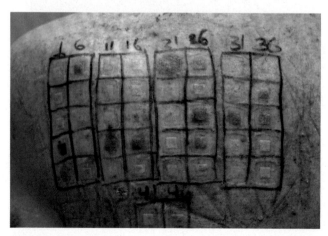

FIG. 4.2-7. Patch testing mapping and results on patient's back. (Photo courtesy of M. Bobonich.)

Management and Patient Education

- Once positive allergens are identified, avoidance is the key treatment for ACD.

- If dermatitis is present after testing is completed, the use of a TCS or systemic corticosteroid is appropriate to clear any residual dermatitis. Forewarn patients that it can take up to 6 weeks for dermatitis to completely clear once the offending agent has been removed.

- Patients should be provided detailed written information about the causative allergens identified from patch testing. The chemical name, as well as possible synonymous or brand names, should be provided along with instructions as to how to prevent future exposure.

- It is important that patients learn how to read product labels and compare them to their chemical list in order to avoid contact.

- When ACD is chronic or affecting critical areas such as hands and/or face, referral to dermatology or allergy/immunology for patch testing is crucial for diagnosis and treatment.

OCCUPATIONAL DERMATITIS

Occupational contact dermatitis (OCD) consists of both ICD and ACD and is responsible for most cases of occupational skin disorders in the western world (Nassau & Fonacier, 2020). The importance of OCD is that it can lead to a significant loss of productivity and disability for affected workers. Occupations with a higher risk for exposure to irritants and subsequent development of ICD include food catering, furniture industry workers, healthcare providers, housekeeping workers, food service workers, hair stylists, industrial workers exposed to chemical irritants, dry cleaners, metal workers, florist shop employees and designers, and warehouse employees. Similarly, workers in the following fields have higher rates of developing ACD due to their repeated work with common allergens: hair stylists, healthcare workers, food handlers, construction, and metal workers (Nassau & Fonacier, 2020). In the case of suspected OCD, an important component of the history taking involves periods of improvement and exacerbation of symptoms around the times of vacation and sick leave.

Common Causes

- Wet-work conditions, including occupations that require frequent handwashing (fast-food workers and healthcare workers) (Nassau & Fonacier, 2020).

- Nail salon technicians due to their chronic exposure to methacrylate, prior to nail treatment stabilization with UV light (Milam & Cohen, 2019).

- Beauticians and hairstylists with their exposure to fragrances.

- Beauticians, hair stylists, and tattoo artists exposure to paraphenylenediamine in hair dyes and henna tattoos.

Management and Patient Education

- Same treatments and avoidance measures as noted in ICD and ACD sections, including TCS and emollients to repair the skin barrier.

- The primary treatment for the management OCD is the avoidance of the triggering agent which may require job reassignment and/or a change in occupation if the offending agent cannot be avoided in the workplace (Fig. 4.2-8).

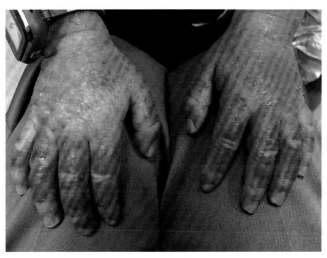

FIG. 4.2-8. Occupational contact dermatitis (OCD) on bilateral hands of a carpet mill assembly-line worker, from wearing required work gloves. (Photo courtesy Douglas DiRuggiero.)

CLINICAL PEARLS

- All patients are susceptible to ICD; but the very young, the elderly, and patients with AD are at greater risk.

- Identification of the triggering allergen via patch testing and subsequent avoidance is key to the management of ACD.

- Occupation and hobbies play a significant role, along with personal care products, in exposure to allergens.

- All forms of reactive dermatitis respond to emollients, TCS, and TCIs but only if the causative agent has been identified and avoided.

- Systemic corticosteroids can be used to clear residual, persistent dermatitis; but clearance is temporary unless allergens are identified and eliminated.

READINGS AND REFERENCES

Holness, D. L. (2019). Occupational dermatosis. *Current Allergy and Asthma Reports, 19*(9), 1–8. https://doi.org/10.1007/s11882-019-0870-6

Mcguckin, M., & Govednik, J. (2016). Irritant contact dermatitis on hands. *American Journal of Medical Quality, 32*(1), 93–99. https://doi.org/10.1177/1062860615611228

Milam, E. C., & Cohen, D. E. (2019). Contact dermatitis. *Dermatologic Clinics, 37*(1), 21–28. https://doi.org/10.1016/j.det.2018.07.00

Nassau, S., & Fonacier, L. (2020). Allergic contact dermatitis. *Medical Clinics of North America, 104*(1), 61–76. https://doi.org/10.1016/j.mcna.2019.08.012

Novak-Bilić, G., Vučić, M., Japundžić, I., Meštrović-Štefekov, J., Stanić-Duktaj, S., & Lugović-Mihić, L. (2018). Irritant and allergic contact dermatitis—skin lesion characteristics. *Acta Clinica Croatica, 57*(4), 713–720. https://doi.org/10.20471/acc.2018.57.04.13

Tan, C. H., Rasool, S., & Johnston, G. A. (2014). Contact dermatitis: Allergic and irritant. *Clinics in Dermatology, 32*(1), 116–124. https://doi.org/10.1016/j.clindermatol.2013.05.03

Seborrheic Dermatitis

Susan Tofte

In This Chapter

- Seborrheic Dermatitis

SEBORRHEIC DERMATITIS

Seborrheic dermatitis (SD) is a chronic, relapsing skin disorder that causes erythema and a waxy, yellowish scale on the scalp, ears, face, and the middle chest. SD has a distinctive pattern in different age groups and this section will focus on SD in adults (see Section 13 for pediatric SD). There is a 1% to 5% worldwide distribution with no racial predilection, but males are affected more than females. The well-known problem of *dandruff* is the mildest form of SD, but its predilection is not typically included in distribution calculations. There is an increased prevalence in individuals with Down syndrome, Parkinson disease, neurologic disorders (including epilepsy, head injury, stroke, mood disorders), alcoholism, eating disorders, acne/rosacea, and in those who are immunocompromised. One study notes that SD is also more common in those with folliculitis, onychomycosis, tinea pedis, rosacea, acne, and psoriasis (Zander et al., 2019). SD tends to be chronic, with remissions and exacerbations, often improving in the summer and worsening in the winter. Lithium, psoralens, and interferon have all been associated with the initiation and exacerbations of SD. Stress, hormone changes, and illnesses can also trigger this skin disorder.

Pathophysiology

While the pathogenesis is not fully understood, SD is associated with the lipophilic yeast *Malassezia* (specifically *M. furfur;* formerly known as *Pityrosporum ovale*), a normal inhabitant of the skin. Increased sebum levels and a proliferation of this yeast could cause a disruption in the normal microbiome resulting in an abnormal inflammatory response—but individual susceptibility can vary. Research indicates that this inflammatory response is thought to be more irritant-mediated, rather than immune-mediated (Balato et al., 2019).

Clinical Presentation

SD can have a distinctive pattern in different age groups; this section focuses on an adult presentation (see Section 13 for pediatric SD).

- Areas of erythema covered by dry or moist greasy yellowish-white scale in the sebum-rich areas of the skin (Fig. 4.3-1). Distribution is often symmetric.
- Commonly involves scalp, forehead, eyebrows, glabella, nasolabial folds, ears, and postauricular skin. Less often, the axillae, inguinal folds, and trunk (Fig. 4.3-2A,B).
- Severity waxes and wanes; skin sensitivity and mild itch are common and can be exacerbated by heat, sunlight, fever, and irritating topical therapy.

- In men, SD can erupt in the sternal area with a thin papular erythematous, scaly rash (sometimes in an annular pattern) and may be evident over the upper back.
- Hypopigmentation is seen in skin of color.
- In the scalp, can range from mild patchy scaling to widespread, thick, adherent crusts with pruritus (Fig. 4.3-3).

DIFFERENTIAL DIAGNOSIS Seborrheic Dermatitis

- Rosacea
- Psoriasis
- Lupus erythematosus
- Periorbital dermatitis
- Tinea versicolor
- Contact dermatitis (irritant or allergic)
- Atopic dermatitis
- Pityriasis rosea
- Candidiasis
- Tinea faciei, capitis, corporis
- Secondary syphilis

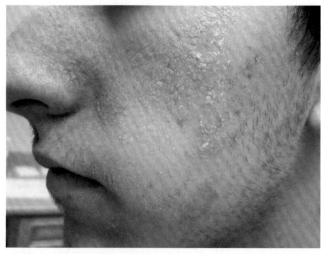

FIG. 4.3-1. Waxy scale of seborrheic dermatitis on the face. (Photo courtesy of International Psoriasis Council.)

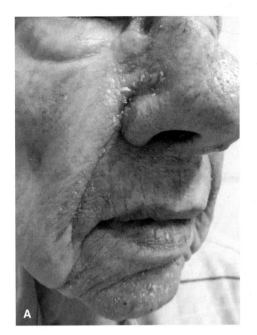

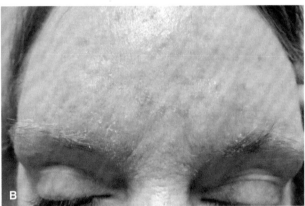

FIG. 4.3-2. **A:** Classic seborrheic dermatitis involving the nasolabial folds. **B:** Seborrheic dermatitis may also present with fine scale and erythema involving the brows, glabella, and eye lashes. (Photos courtesy of M. Bobonich.)

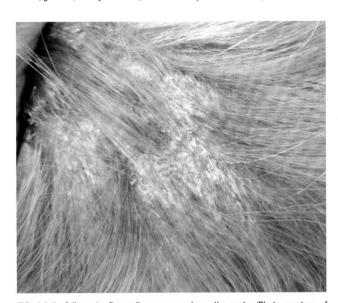

FIG. 4.3-3. Adherent, often yellow waxy scale on the scalp. (Photo courtesy of M. Bobonich.)

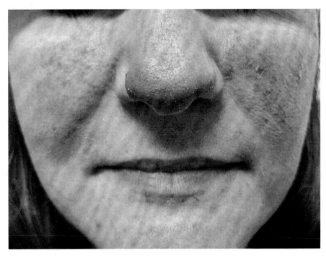

FIG. 4.3-4. Classic "butterfly" rash of systemic lupus erythematosus sparing the nasolabial folds. (Photo courtesy of M. Bobonich.)

Confirming the Diagnosis

- An erythematous eruption on the central face is characteristic of several different disorders and can be challenging to distinguish. These clinical clues may help:
  - Systemic lupus erythematosus (SLE)—the facial "butterfly" distribution spares the nasolabial and mesolabial folds (Fig. 4.3-4). The color is often a brighter red, and there is often photosensitivity.
  - Rosacea—may include redness, dilated vessels, papules, or pustules on the central face, but there is minimal scale and it spares the nasolabial folds (Fig. 4.3-5).
  - Psoriasis—it can be very difficult to differentiate SD from psoriasis and there may be an overlapping condition referred to as "sebopsoriasis." The scale associated with SD is typically not adherent compared to psoriasis, where the plaque is difficult to remove and may result in microvascular bleeding (Auspitz sign).
  - A biopsy is rarely needed but can be helpful in securing the diagnosis.

Treatment

With mild to moderate SD, Kastarinen et al. (2015) concluded that both topical azole antifungals and topical corticosteroids (TCS) achieve

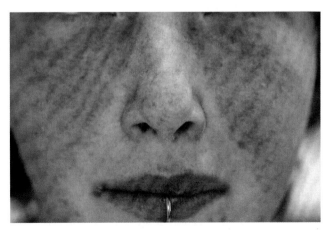

FIG. 4.3-5. Acne rosacea. Note the erythema, papules, and pustules appear across cheeks and nose yet spare the nasolabial folds. (Photo courtesy of M. Bobonich.)

TABLE 4.3-1	Treatment for Seborrheic Dermatitis			
SEVERITY[a]	SELF-CARE	SHAMPOOS	TOPICAL AGENTS	COMMENTS
Mild	Shampoo daily (once weekly for African Americans) Antifungal or dandruff shampoo, OTC, or Rx products (apply to wet scalp, lather, wait 5 min, rinse) Facial cleansing to remove oil and scale (can use antifungal shampoo as wash) Apply a moisturizing or barrier cream	Ketoconazole 1%[b] or 2% (Nizoral) Ciclopirox 1% (Lupron) Selenium sulfide 2.5% (Selsun) Zinc pyrithione 1% and 2%[b] (Head & Shoulders)	Ketoconazole 2% C, G, ciclopirox 1% C, butenafine C, G terbinafine C, G OTC Nutradeica Topical lithium salts (lithium gluconate 8% gel)	If facial rash persists, consider adding a topical calcineurin inhibitor (TCI) to the face daily to b.i.d.
Moderate	Follow measures for mild disease P&S solution (leave on overnight, wash out in the morning)	*Keratolytic shampoos:* Salicyclic acid 2% Sh, Tar Sh, P&S Sh[b]	*Scalp:* *Corticosteroids:* Clobex[c] Sh, Capex[c] Sh Fluocinolone acetate 0.01% in peanut oil (Derma-Smoothe F/S) Fluocinolone 0.05% solution Betamethasone dipropionate 0.05% Clobetasol 0.05% Sp. *Face and body:* *Topical calcineurin inhibitors (TCIs):* Tacrolimus ointment (Protopic)[b,d] 0.03% and 0.1% Pimecrolimus cream (Elidel)[b,d] *Nonsteroids:* Metronidazole cream 0.75% and 1.0% q.d. or b.i.d. Azelaic acid 15% b.i.d. Sodium sulfacetamide lotion, gel wash, shampoo (Klaron, Ovace, Mexar) Promiseb C, G, L; daily to b.i.d. Hyaluronic acid 0.2% (Bionect) C, G, Sp *Corticosteroids:* Hydrocortisone 1% and 2.5%[b], desonide 0.05%[b] cream and lotion	A combination of therapies may be most effective: antifungals with TCIs or TCSs. If there is thick, adherent scale on the scalp, use a keratolytic agent. Low- to mid-potency TCS may be applied to the scalp daily or b.i.d. for 2–3 wk. TCS on face b.i.d. for only 3–5 days, then taper.
Severe	Derma-Smoothe F/S scalp oil[c] at night with cap. Apply antifungal in AM and PM	Follow measures for mild disease	*Scalp:* If scale persists despite frequent shampooing, increase the topical corticosteroid to mid to high potency (i.e., clobetasol b.i.d.) *Face and body:* May need to combine more than two agents. Mid-potency TCS (Triamcinolone 0.5% can be used for 2–4 days only)	Reconsider diagnosis; conditions like rosacea and seborrhea often coexist. In severe or recalcitrant cases, refer to dermatologist.

Sunscreen: water-based (non-oily), noncomedogenic, immediate-absorption, broad-spectrum (UVB and UVA), high SPF sunscreen which contains hyaluronic acid.
[a]There is no accepted standard for assessing the severity of SD.
[b]Available over the counter
[c]Scalp only.
[d]Black box warning.
C, cream; F, foam; G, gel; L, lotion; Sh, shampoo; Sp, spray.

similar efficacy in short-term use (4 weeks), but topical steroids had a higher risk of long-term side effects. Table 4.3-1 provides an overview of treatment options in the management of SD.

Topical

- *Azole antifungals*—the mainstay of therapy because of their effect on the *Malassezia* organism. Ketoconazole 2% or miconazole creams b.i.d. for trunk and face. SD tends to be chronic and recurrent primarily because once the patient sees improvement, treatment is often discontinued. *Malassezia* will continue to grow slowly, and within a few weeks the symptoms recur (see Section 6-1, Table 6-1).

- *Calcineurin inhibitors* (TCIs—Elidel, Protopic)—while not FDA indicated for treatment of SD, may be beneficial, especially with frequent recurrences of facial SD, to combine an antifungal with a topical calcineurin inhibitor (TCI; should only be used in those >2 years old).

- *Low-potency TCS*—also used in combination with antifungals, but with caution and for short durations (only 3 to 5 days). Response will be faster than with TCIs alone, but rebound flaring can occur after prolonged use and an abrupt withdrawal.

- *Nonsteroidal OTC cream*—Nutradeica (containing piroctone olamine, zinc salt of L-pyrrolidone carboxylate (PCA), and hydroxyphenyl propamidobenzoic acid) shows promise as monotherapy for mild to moderate SD, or can be an adjunctive therapy (Balato et al., 2019).

- *Lithium salts* (Lithium gluconate 8% gel; Rx Lithioderm 8% gel (hard to get in the United States; more only available in Europe) improve SD by reducing the release of fatty acids and prostaglandins in the skin, without significant increase of serum lithium levels (Piquero-Casals et al., 2019).

- *Shampoos*—daily shampooing with longer lather times (5 to 10 minutes); ketoconazole 2%, ciclopirox 1%, selenium sulfide 2.5%, or zinc pyrithione shampoos tend to help the most. Prescription corticosteroid shampoos can be utilized in severe scalp cases. Medicated shampoos can be used for washing the ears, face (with caution to avoid the orbits of the eye), and chest.

- *Cleansers and moisturizers*—use nonsoap cleansers and mild, fragrance-free moisturizers. Choose topical medications with nonirritating vehicles in order to prevent concomitant irritant dermatitis.

- *Sunscreens*—sunscreens with hyaluronic acid sodium salts have demonstrated improvement of all symptoms of facial SD (Schlesinger & Powell, 2014). Ideally, patients should seek a water-based (non-oily), noncomedogenic, immediate-absorption, broad-spectrum (UVB and UVA), high SPF sunscreen which contains hyaluronic acid (Piquero-Casals et al., 2019).

Systemic

- Severe or recalcitrant cases may require oral antifungals (fluconazole, itraconazole, terbinafine), but there is limited treatment evidence and none of these are FDA indicated for treatment of SD. Oral steroids should not be used for SD. Oral ketoconazole has a black box warning and is not appropriate for treatment of superficial fungal infections.

Management and Patient Education

- With African-American hair, daily oiling of the scalp may contribute to worsening, so patients are encouraged to use the ketoconazole cream or gel in place of their oil at least several times per week. Shampooing should be encouraged at least once a week; with the shampoo massaged into all affected areas (including non–hair-bearing) and left in place for 5 to 10 minutes before rinsing.

- Patients should follow up in 6 to 8 weeks in order to assess response to therapy and adjust treatment if the condition is not improved. Patients need to be educated that the goal of management is control of the disease and not cure.

CLINICAL PEARLS

- Adult SD has a chronic relapsing course with remissions and exacerbations. Although complications are rare, erythrodermic forms can occur and may be associated with underlying HIV. Sudden onset of severe disease, or SD that is resistant to treatment, may also be a cutaneous sign of immunocompromise.

- Topical steroids should NOT be monotherapy; should only be low-potency; should be dispensed in small amounts and without refills.

- The treatment of scalp and beard SD generally involves shampooing several times a week, if not daily. African-American hair generally is not shampooed as often, so understanding individual cultural practices is important to the success of the treatment.

- Triggers include stress, illnesses, hormone changes, and medications such as lithium, interferon, and psoralens.

READINGS AND REFERENCES

American Academy of Dermatology. Seborrheic dermatitis: Overview. https://www.aad.org/public/diseases/a-z/seborrheic-dermatitis-overview

Balato, A., Caiazzo, G., Di Caprio, R., Scala, E., Fabbrocini, G., & Granger, C. (2019). Exploring anti-fungal, anti-microbial and anti-inflammatory properties of a topical non-steroidal barrier cream in face and chest seborrheic dermatitis. *Dermatologic Therapy*, 10(1), 87–98. https://doi.org/10.1007/s13555-019-00339-w

Clark, G. W., Pope, S., & Jaboori, K. (2015). Diagnosis and treatment of seborrheic dermatitis. *American Family Physician*, 91(3), 185–190.

Gupta, A. K., & Versteeg, S. (2017). Topical treatment of facial seborrheic dermatitis: A systematic review. *American Journal of Clinical Dermatology*, 18(2), 193–213. https://doi.org/10.1007/s40257-016-0232-2

Kastarinen, H., Okokon, E. O., & Verbeek, J. H. (2015). Topical anti-inflammatory agents for seborrheic dermatitis of the face or scalp: Summary of a Cochrane Review. *JAMA Dermatology*, 151(2), 221–222. https://doi.org/10.1001/jamadermatol.2014.3186

National Eczema Association. Seborrheic dermatitis. https://nationaleczema.org/eczema/types-of-eczema/seborrheic-dermatitis

Piquero-Casals, J., Doris Hexsel, D., Mir-Bonafe, J. P., & Eduardo Rozas-Muñoz, E. (2019). Topical non-pharmacological treatment for facial seborrheic dermatitis. *Dermatologic Therapy*, 9(3), 469–477.

Schlesinger, T., & Powell, C. (2014). Efficacy and safety of a low molecular weight hyaluronic acid topical gel in the treatment of facial seborrheic dermatitis final report. *The Journal of Clinical and Aesthetic Dermatology*, 7(5), 15–18.

Zander, N., Sommer, R., Schäfer, I., Reinert, R., Kirsten, N., Zyriax, B., Maul, J., & Augustin, M. (2019). Epidemiology of seborrheic dermatitis. *British Journal of Dermatology*, 181, e92–e92. https://doi.org/10.1111/bjd.18388

Psoriasis

Lakshi M. Aldredge

PSORIASIS

Psoriasis is an autoimmune skin condition that affects 2% to 5% of the world population. There is no race that is spared from this disease, although there is a lower incidence in African Americans for unknown reasons. It is equally present among males and females, and onset can occur at any age; however, it is most likely to appear between the ages of 15 and 30 years. Approximately one third of patients with psoriasis have a first-degree relative affected with the disease, and most experts agree that there is strong evidence to demonstrate a genetic family link.

Medications such as β-blockers, lithium, and antimalarials have been associated with inducing or exacerbating psoriasis. Emotional stress, streptococcal and other bacterial infections, and viral infections, such as HIV, can initiate psoriasis as well as induce flares of the disease. Environmental conditions, such as weather, can also precipitate or exacerbate psoriasis. Interestingly, psoriasis has also been triggered by surgery or trauma, with the resulting initial plaque occurring directly over the injury or incision (Koebner phenomenon).

PATHOPHYSIOLOGY

The exact cause of psoriasis and psoriatic disease is unknown. It is a chronic and systemic immune–mediated disease that can be triggered by medical, emotional, and environmental factors, although in many cases, the sudden onset of disease has no precipitating factors. Psoriasis is believed to be a primarily Th-17–mediated condition which triggers a cascade of cytokine-driven sequences, resulting in hyperproliferation of skin cells and angiogenesis. Over the past three decades, advancements in immunologic research has demonstrated that specific cytokines, such as tumor necrosis factor (TNF)-α and interleukins (ILs) 12, 17, and 23, as well as numerous other immune mediators, are key factors in the development and progression of psoriatic disease. It is now understood that these cytokines cause inflammation in numerous other organ systems.

Clinical Presentation

Cutaneous symptoms of psoriasis can occur in several forms and are subsequently named based on clinical presentation. While the classic thick, red plaques of *plaque psoriasis* affect approximately 80% to 90% of patients, it is important to be able to identify key characteristics of other psoriatic disease presentations. Plaques can vary in the amount of scale or erythema given the location of the body, stage of development/resolution, therapeutics, or patient's skin type (Fig. 4.4-1A–D).

Historically, the severity of disease was based on the amount of skin surface involved, or body surface area (BSA). Typically, psoriasis is characterized as mild (BSA 1% to 3%), moderate (BSA 4% to 10%), and severe (BSA >10%) (Fig. 4.4-2). The surface area of a patient's palmar hand, including the fingers, determines 1% BSA. However, severity of psoriasis is now also determined by the impact on the patient's quality of life (QOL) or involvement of sensitive areas (palms, soles, face, scalp, and genitals). For example, palmoplantar psoriasis, which covers a relatively small surface area, can have a significant impact on an individual's QOL due to the constant itch, pain, and impact on ability to perform activities of daily living.

Plaque Psoriasis

- *Plaque psoriasis* affects approximately 80% to 90% of patients. Plaques can range from a violaceous red to pinkish-red, which may be covered with a thin- or thick-adherent silvery scale (Fig. 4.4-3).

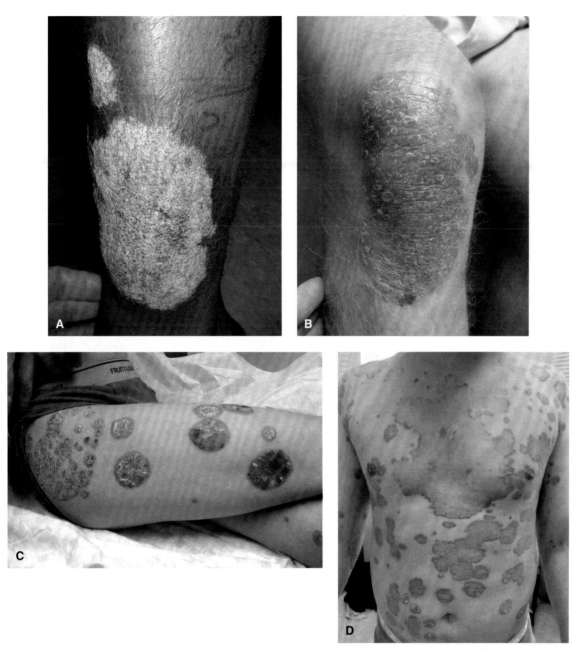

FIG. 4.4-1. Varied characteristics of scale in plaque psoriasis. **A:** Psoriasis plaque on the lower leg with thick adherent silvery scale. **B:** Thin white scale on psoriasis plaque on knees. **C:** Plaques on a 9-year-old boy's lateral thigh. **D:** Confluent plaques on an adult's trunk. (Photo "D" courtesy of M. Bobonich.)

- Lesions have well-demarcated borders and occur anywhere on the body, but typically favor the scalp and extensor surfaces of the knees and elbows (Fig. 4.4-4A,B), usually in a symmetrical pattern. This is compared to eczema, which favors flexural surfaces and is typically vaguely demarcated. It also favors area such as the umbilicus or posterior sulcus of the ears.

- Removal of scale from a psoriasis plaque will reveal punctate blood vessels that bleed (Auspitz sign) and aid in the clinical diagnosis of psoriasis.

Scalp Psoriasis

- Often appears as a "cap" of thick, silvery, adherent scale on an erythematous or violaceous base (Fig. 4.4-5A).

- Scalp psoriasis can be a particularly distressing manifestation for patients due to the visibility of the plaques, the significant pruritus, extensive scaling that sheds on clothing and hair loss (Fig. 4.4-5B).

- Can be mistaken for seborrhea or seborrheic dermatitis (SD), which has more of a yellow, waxy scale (Fig. 4.4-5C).

Palmoplantar Psoriasis

- Erythematous papules/plaques of scale on the palms, palmar and interdigital fingers, soles, and arches of feet (Fig. 4.4-6A).

- Painful fissures can form on the palms, fingers, and plantar feet; along with dystrophic nail changes.

- Palmoplantar pustular psoriasis is a variation presenting with deep-seated vesicles and pustules (Fig. 4.4-6B). While it may

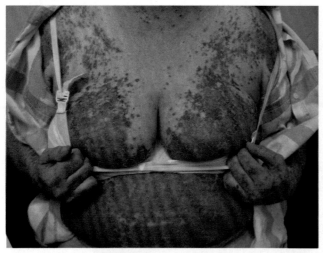

FIG. 4.4-2. Severe plaque psoriasis covering more than 10% of body surface area. (Photo courtesy of M. Bobonich.)

appear that it is a bacterial or viral infection, a culture of these sterile papules is typically negative for any microorganisms.

Guttate Psoriasis

- Characterized by round 1- to 10-mm, salmon-pink papules ("dew-drops") with a fine white scale (Fig. 4.4-7).

- Can be preceded by a *Streptococcus pyogenes* infection (strep pharyngitis) or sinus infection (and has been reported with some viral infections), however, the pathophysiologic association between the infection and disease is not clearly understood.

- Presents in only 2% of psoriatic patients, usually younger than 30 years.

Inverse Psoriasis

- Thin, erythematous, shiny patches with little to no scale that occurs in the intertriginous areas of the skin, namely the folds of

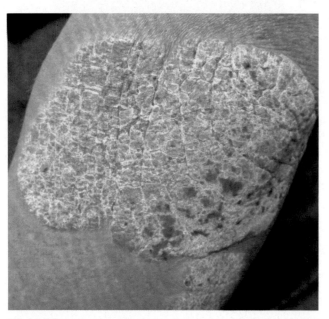

FIG. 4.4-3. Plaque psoriasis with classic white adherent scale. (Photo courtesy of M. Bobonich.)

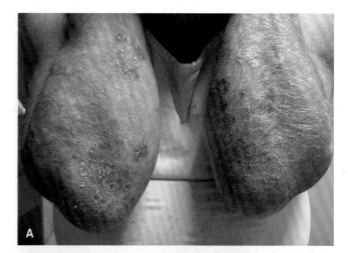

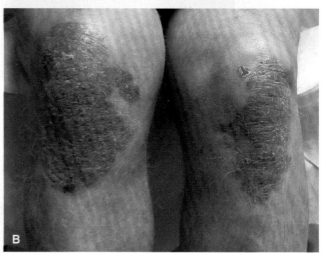

FIG. 4.4-4. **A, B:** The elbows and knees are a common location for plaque psoriasis. (Photos courtesy of M. Bobonich.)

the axillae, groin, intergluteal, inframammary, and pannus of the abdomen (Fig. 4.4-8A).

- It is not unusual for patients to be treated with topical or systemic antifungals for months before making the diagnosis of inverse psoriasis, as it is often mistaken for a fungal or candida infection (Fig. 4.4-8B).

Genital Psoriasis

- Genital psoriasis presents as of erythematous patches on the labia or penis that usually lacks the classic micaceous scale of plaque psoriasis. Genital psoriasis can be extremely itching and painful in this vulnerable location of the body (Fig. 4.4-9).

- Patients may not recognize the symptoms as a subtype of psoriasis and fear it is a sexually transmitted disease or a contagious condition. It can be especially distressing for patients and their intimate partners.

- Fissuring within the thin plaques may cause significant pain and discomfort and may become secondarily infected.

- Lastly, patients who suffer with genital involvement may have difficulty engaging in sexual relationships due to feelings of self-consciousness.

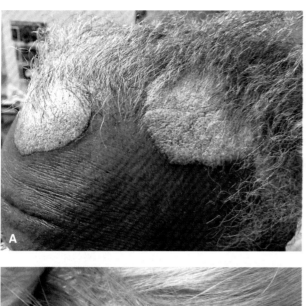

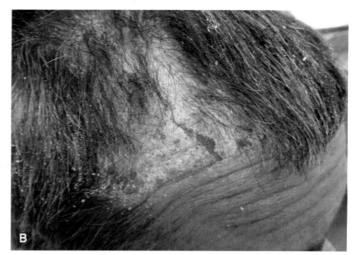

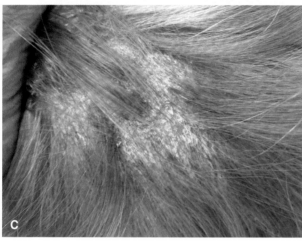

FIG. 4.4-5. A: Scalp psoriasis can present with thick, silvery adherent scale on erythematous base that can extend onto the face. **B:** Scalp psoriasis resulting in hair loss. **C:** It can be difficult to differentiate between seborrhea and scalp psoriasis. (Photos courtesy of M. Bobonich.)

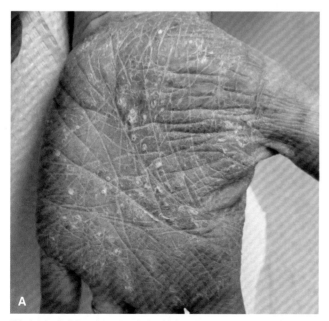

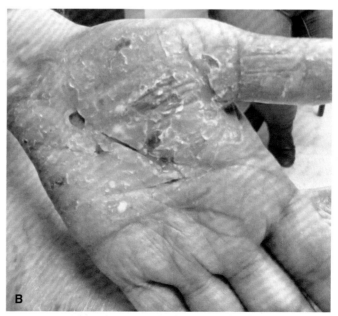

FIG. 4.4-6. A: Palmoplantar psoriasis with hyperkeratotic plaques. **B:** Palmopustular psoriasis with sterile vesicles and pustules. (Photos courtesy of M. Bobonich.)

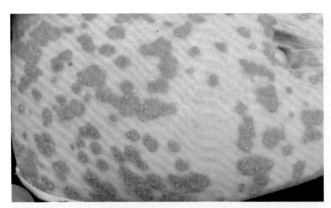

FIG. 4.4-7. Guttate psoriasis erupting after a *Group A β-hemolytic streptococcus* throat infection. (Photo courtesy of M. Bobonich.)

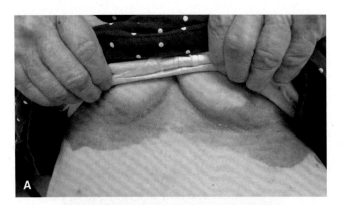

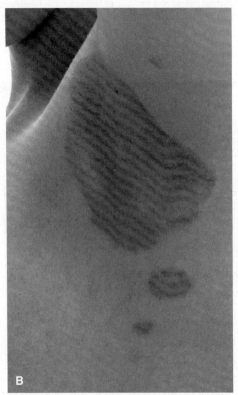

FIG. 4.4-8. **A:** Inverse psoriasis of the inframammary folds is often misdiagnosed at intertrigo or *Candidiasis* infection. **B:** Inverse psoriasis in the axilla can be mistaken for contact dermatitis. (Photos courtesy of M. Bobonich.)

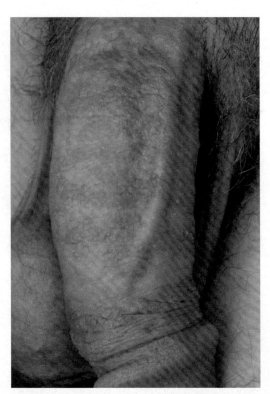

FIG. 4.4-9. Genital psoriasis often lacks classic white scaly plaques. (Photo courtesy of M. Bobonich.)

Erythrodermic Psoriasis

- This is a more severe form of psoriasis with full-body (>90% BSA) erythema and scaling. May be referred to as *erythroderma* (Fig. 4.4-10).

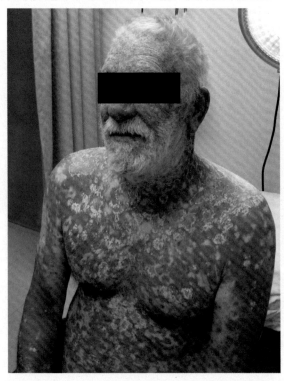

FIG. 4.4-10. Erythrodermic psoriasis involving greater than 90% BSA. (Photo courtesy of M. Bobonich.)

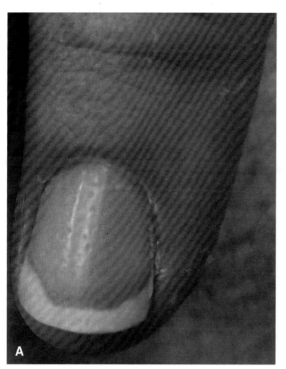
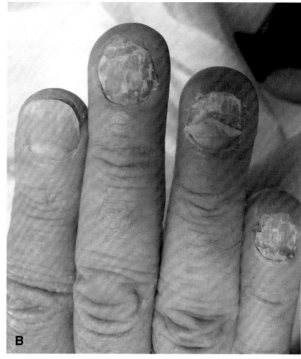

FIG. 4.4-11. A: Pitting can be a subtle clue for psoriatic disease. **B:** Psoriatic nails can present with yellow, thickened nails with debris or complete destruction of the nail plate. It is commonly misdiagnosed as a fungal nail infection (onychomycosis). (Photo B courtesy of M. Bobonich.)

- Can be triggered by environmental factors or as a response to medication.

- Patients with plaque psoriasis treated with systemic corticosteroids may show an initial remission, and then experience a severe "rebound," resulting in erythrodermic psoriasis. Most dermatology providers do not treat any form of psoriasis with systemic corticosteroids for this very reason. Patients with erythroderma often require hospitalization.

Generalized Pustular Psoriasis of von Zumbusch

- A rare, life-threatening variant of psoriasis presents with sheets of erythema topped by pinpoint, sterile yellow pustules covering most of the skin.

- The cutaneous findings are accompanied by burning, erythema, fever, malaise, and leukocytosis.

- Patients are usually hospitalized and require systemic immuno-suppressants and supportive therapies.

Pustular Psoriasis of Pregnancy

- Pustular psoriasis of pregnancy (PPP) tends to occur early in the third trimester and can occur with or without a pre-existing personal or family history of psoriasis.

- Clinically appears as erythematous patches with pustules, typically in the intertriginous areas, sparing the face and palmoplantar areas. The pustules may coalesce into larger plaques.

- Patients may experience fatigue, fever, diarrhea, and even delirium. Studies are controversial regarding fetal risk and psoriasis, although some patients may have difficulty conceiving, have higher incidences of placenta previa, ectopic pregnancy, spontaneous abortion and preterm birth (Bobotsis et al., 2016).

Nail Psoriasis

- Most patients with moderate to severe psoriatic disease will develop finger and toenail involvement.

- Nails are thickened, dystrophic, and often yellow, and may separate from the nail bed (often mistaken for fungal disease).

- Pinpoint "pitting" on the nail surface is a more subtle finding and is classically associated with psoriatic arthritis (PsA) (Fig. 4.4-11A).

- "Oil spots" are a nail finding in some patients with psoriasis and present as pink or tan round areas within the nail.

- Nail involvement can be incredibly disfiguring and painful, presenting a therapeutic challenge (Fig. 4.4-11B). Severe nail dystrophy may require removal of the entire nail and nail matrix in order to alleviate painful symptoms. Fortunately, the development of biologic therapies in psoriatic disease has provided an effective alternative in the management of psoriatic nail disease.

Psoriasis Comorbidities

Initially believed to be only a cutaneous disorder, psoriasis is now known to be a systemic immune–mediated disease which causes inflammation not only in the skin, but also in the joints, heart, brain, and other organs. Patients with more severe psoriasis have demonstrated an increased incidence of joint disease (PsA), cardiovascular disease, hypertension, obesity, diabetes, and other immune-mediated conditions such as Crohn disease (Dauden et al., 2018). Additionally, there are numerous psychological disorders that can be associated with psoriasis, including depression, increased risk of suicide, alcoholism, and social isolation. Furthermore, patients with plaque psoriasis may be self-conscious of their appearance and therefore avoid participating in exercise or social activities. The lack of physical activity may result in increased weight gain, hypertension, diabetes, and chronic pain syndromes.

Understanding that psoriasis is an immune-mediated, multiorgan inflammatory disease is critical for two reasons. First, it heightens the clinician's awareness to screen psoriasis patients for associated comorbidities as soon as psoriasis is diagnosed (Table 4.1-1). Secondly, the early detection of psoriasis comorbidities can result in the

TABLE 4.4-1	Monitoring of Comorbidities in Patients with Psoriasis[a]		
COMORBIDITY	**CLINICAL PRESENTATION AND SYMPTOMS**	**SCREENING PARAMETERS**	**PATIENT EDUCATION**
Psoriatic arthritis	Stiffness and pain in joints (hands, feet, back) upon awakening or after prolonged sitting; bony deformity of fingers/toes; sausage digits (dactylitis); enthesitis; fatigue, nail pitting, oil spots, difficulty performing activities of daily living due to joint pain (buttoning shirt, opening food cans), changes in radiographic imaging of hands/feet	X-rays of affected joints/spine; ESR, CRP; Screening tools including Psoriasis Epidemiology Screening Tool, the Toronto Psoriatic Arthritis Screen, the Psoriatic Arthritis Screening and Evaluation, and the Early Arthritis for Psoriatic Patients questionnaire	Patient education regarding the risk of developing debilitating, irreversible joint damage and the association with psoriasis; referral to rheumatology specialist if indicated
CVD	HTN, CVA, MI, angina	Height, weight, blood pressure, evaluation for pedal edema, blood glucose, hemoglobin A1c, lipid levels, abdominal circumference, and calculation of BMI	Patient education regarding risk of CVD/MACE events and psoriasis; efforts aimed at lifestyle modification (dietary changes to achieve and maintain a normal BMI, smoking cessation, exercise regimen; ensure patient has a PCP and refer to cardiology specialist if indicated
Metabolic syndrome	HTN, hyperlipidemia, obesity, hyperglycemia	Blood pressure, weight, waist circumference, fasting blood glucose and/or hemoglobin A1c, and fasting lipid levels	Patient education regarding risk of developing diabetes and hyperlipidemia; lifestyle modification to include healthy diet, exercise, smoking cessation; ensure patient has PCP and is referred to endocrinology specialist if indicated
Mental Health	Suicidal or homicidal ideations or attempts, emotional lability, relationship stability, work pattern fluctuations, alcohol and drug use, family history of depression	Quality-of-life tools such as DLQI	Patient education regarding the relationship between psoriasis and mental health conditions. Referral to mental health specialist if indicated
Nonalcoholic fatty liver disease	Elevated LFTs, abnormal liver imaging	LFTs, CBC, liver fibroscan, liver ultrasound, CT scan	Patient education regarding the increased risk of liver abnormalities and psoriasis; avoidance of alcohol and other hepatotoxic agents; lifestyle modification including healthy diet, exercise; referral to hepatology specialist if indicated
Inflammatory bowel disease (IBD)	IBD symptoms including frequent diarrhea, abdominal cramping, bloody stools	Frequent symptom review, stool guaiac tests, colonoscopy	Patient education regarding the risk of Crohn or ulcerative colitis and psoriasis; referral to GI specialist as indicated; therapeutic agent management in patients with psoriatic disease treatment-related IBD symptoms
Malignancy	New-onset symptoms not limited to weight loss, lymphadenopathy, breast pain or lump, abdominal pain, hematuria, melena, fatigue, shortness of breath, suspicious skin findings	Family history of skin cancer screening, mammography, colonoscopy, prostate screening, skin cancer screening, lymph node palpation, abdominal palpation	Patient education regarding the link between certain cancers and psoriasis; age-appropriate cancer screenings; lifestyle modification; alcohol moderation and tobacco avoidance
Chronic kidney disease	Elevated kidney function, urinalysis, HTN	Blood urea nitrogen, creatinine, urine microalbumin	Patient education regarding the risk of kidney disease and psoriasis; healthy lifestyle; avoidance of nephrotoxic medications
Sleep apnea	Sleep disturbances loud snoring, fatigue, OSA-associated risk factors including obesity, hypertension, and diabetes	Sleep study, blood pressure, weight, BMI, blood glucose and/or HgA1c	Patient education regarding the risk of sleep apnea and psoriasis; referral to sleep specialist as indicated
COPD	SOB, cough, air hunger	CXR, pulmonary functions testing	Patient education regarding the relationship between COPD and psoriasis; lifestyle modification including tobacco avoidance, exercise; referral to pulmonary specialist as indicated
Uveitis	Conjunctivitis, ocular pain, blurred vision, photosensitivity	Symptom evaluation to include photosensitivity and pain, visual inspection of external eye	Patient education regarding the association between uveitis and psoriasis; referral to ophthalmologist as indicated

[a]Elmets, C. A., Leonardi, C. L., Davi, D. M. R., Gelfand, J. M., Lichten, J., Mehtal, N. N., Armstrong, A. W., Connor, C., Cordoro, K. M., Elewski, B. E., Gordon, K. B., Gottlieb, A. B., Kaplan, D. H., Kavanaugh, A., Kivelevitch, D., Kiselia, M., Korman, N. J., Kroshinsky, D., Lebwohl, M., . . . Menter, A. (2019). Joint AAD-NPF guidelines of care for the management and treatment of psoriasis with awareness and attention to comorbidities. *Journal of the American Academy of Dermatology, 80*(4), 1073–1113.

initiation of appropriate therapy, thereby preventing further morbidity and mortality.

Cardiovascular Disease

- Additionally, the chronic inflammatory nature of psoriasis itself may lead to other inflammatory conditions such as peripheral vascular disease and atherosclerosis.

- Patients with severe psoriasis have an increased risk of vascular disease including hypertension, myocardial infarction, and stroke (Takeshita et al., 2017). Psoriasis is an independent risk factor for MI, stroke, and death due to cardiovascular disease (MACE) (Arnett et al., 2019).

- Dermatology providers should consider screening psoriasis patients for CVD (or ensure that it is being done by a primary care provider [PCP]) to include measuring height, weight, abdominal circumference, body mass index calculation, blood pressure, blood glucose, hemoglobin A1c, and lipid levels (Elmets et al., 2019).

- It is especially important to screen young patients with more severe disease for these conditions and refer to their PCP or the appropriate specialty practitioner.

Metabolic Syndrome

- Metabolic syndrome raises an individual's risk for heart disease, stroke, and diabetes. Studies have demonstrated that there is an increased risk of metabolic syndrome in patients with psoriasis (Gelfand & Yeung, 2012).

- Clinicians should assess psoriatic patients for the coexistence of obesity, hyperlipidemia, hypertension, insulin resistance, and prothrombotic and proinflammatory states.

- Younger patients with moderate to severe psoriasis and early symptoms of metabolic syndrome should be given appropriate therapies sooner than in nonpsoriatic young patients in order to prevent worsening hypertension, hyperlipidemia, diabetes, and CVD.

Depression

- Most patients with psoriasis suffer from depression throughout the course of their disease. Social isolation may contribute to increased risk of depression and anxiety, smoking, alcoholism, job instability, and financial problems.

- In addition to depression, patients with psoriatic disease often contend with low self-esteem and chronic pain issues. Patients report difficulties maintaining relationships due to fears of being ostracized due to their skin disease. Young patients often avoid participating in sports or social events as they are concerned their peers may think that their condition is "contagious."

- In a pivotal study, psoriasis patients were found to miss more days of work and change jobs more often than their nonpsoriatic counterparts. In addition to the extraneous factors that can affect depression and anxiety, the inflammatory factors that affect the skin, heart, and joints can also affect the brain, resulting in increased risk of psychological pathology (Armstrong et al., 2012).

Malignancy

- Patients with psoriasis have a significantly elevated risk of developing certain cancers and cancer-related mortality was found to be increased in more severe psoriatic disease.

- Inflammatory pathogenesis associated with psoriasis, chronic inflammation, and the use of certain immunomodulatory therapies in the treatment of psoriasis may all play a part in the increased risk of cancer.

- Although phototherapy with narrow-band ultraviolet radiation is a common treatment for skin psoriasis, it has a low but nonetheless significant risk for the development of squamous and basal cell carcinomas.

- The overall increased risk of smoking and alcohol use in patients with psoriasis may also contribute to cancer risk.

Psoriatic Arthritis (PsA)

- Approximately 10% to 30% of psoriasis patients develop joint disease referred to as PsA. The inflammatory mechanisms that form thickened skin plaques also result in bony destruction and overgrowth in joints. Patients with PsA suffer from significant joint pain and dystrophic changes, which make performing routine activities of daily living very difficult.

- Patients with more severe skin disease and nail involvement are at higher incidence for developing PsA.

- In addition to examining the skin, it is imperative that the clinician obtain a thorough history of joint pain and family history of rheumatologic diseases, as well as conduct a physical examination of hand and foot joints. Patients may have dactylitis (sausage digits), asymmetrical oligoarticular (few joints) arthritis, distal interphalangeal arthropathy, and joint deformity (Fig. 4.4-12). Axial disease is inflammatory involvement of the spine and can result in debilitating neck and back pain.

- Patients with psoriasis should be assessed at least yearly for PsA, and if suspected, should be referred to rheumatology. Early

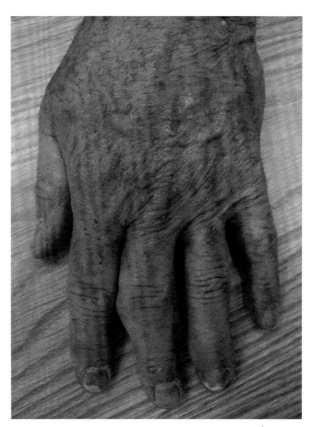

FIG. 4.4-12. Psoriatic arthritis with dactylitis ("sausage joint") and deformity.

diagnosis and aggressive treatment with systemic therapies can prevent permanent joint destruction and significantly improve the QOL for psoriatic patients.

Nonalcoholic Fatty Liver Disease

- Psoriasis patients may be at increased risk of liver disease. Evaluation of liver tissue in psoriasis patients demonstrates excessive accumulation of triglycerides in hepatocytes in the absence of significant alcohol consumption (Ogdie et al., 2017). In addition, the increase in proinflammatory cytokines seen in psoriatic disease may increase insulin resistance, resulting in hepatic lipid accumulation.

- It is important to screen patients with psoriasis for underlying liver disease. Patients with elevated liver enzymes may warrant referral to a hepatologist. In addition, underlying hepatitis disease may limit treatment options, such as methotrexate.

Inflammatory Bowel Disease

- Psoriasis patients may be at increased risk for Crohn disease, ulcerative colitis, as well as celiac disease. This risk is increased in patients with more severe psoriasis and PsA. It is important to screen patients for underlying inflammatory bowel disease symptoms as it may impact the selection of certain psoriasis biologic therapy, specifically, IL-17 inhibitors.

DIFFERENTIAL DIAGNOSIS   Psoriasis

- Atopic dermatitis
- Contact dermatitis
- Squamous cell carcinoma
- Seborrheic dermatitis
- Xerosis
- Dermatophyte infections
- Cutaneous T-cell lymphoma
- Nummular eczema
- Tinea corporis and capitis
- Pityriasis rosea
- Onychomycosis

Confirming the Diagnosis

- The diagnosis of psoriasis is largely a clinical one, achieved after conducting a detailed patient history, physical examination, and evaluation of the current prescription and over-the-counter medications.

- In more complex or atypical presentations, a punch biopsy of the affected skin can aid in the diagnosis.

- Laboratory studies are usually not helpful in diagnosing psoriasis but are critical in identifying comorbidities. Radiology studies are indicated if the patient is suspected of PsA.

Equally important in the assessment and diagnosis of a psoriasis patient is the perceived impact on their QOL. The **Dermatology Life Quality Index (DLQI)** is a 10-point questionnaire that is a validated and useful tool in documenting QOL. A clinician may diagnose the patient with mild cutaneous disease; however, it may be incredibly distressing for the patient based on location, appearance, and symptomatology. Other screening tools used for depression, anxiety, and substance abuse should be utilized when there is clinical concern in these realms.

Treatment

Unfortunately, there is no cure for psoriasis, and control of the disease is the goal of management. Once diagnosed, treatment of the psoriasis patient is focused on symptom management, disease control, reducing the risk for comorbidities, and optimizing QOL (Menter et al., 2019). Developing a plan of care for psoriasis patients should consider the type of psoriasis, location, severity and extent of disease, age, symptoms and comorbidities, response to previous treatments, pregnancy (or intent) and lactation, access to treatment facilities, economic factors related to insurance coverage and cost of care, and QOL. The severity of the disease can be a starting point for the clinician in selecting appropriate treatment options.

Treat to Target

The National Psoriasis Foundation's "Treat to Target" guidelines (Armstrong et al., 2016) provide practical treatment goals:

- Goal: reduce patient's psoriasis to 1% BSA or less within 3 months of initiating treatment.

- Acceptable response: psoriasis covers 3% BSA or less or the patient has experienced 75% improvement in BSA.

- Once the patient has reached 1%, monitor every 6 months at a minimum to ensure maintenance of response.

- If the goal has not been achieved, consider changing medication dose, or adding a new treatment or switching therapy.

Mild Psoriasis (Limited to <3% BSA)

Topical therapy is appropriate for mild or localized disease. Good skin care including emollients should be employed even before prescribing therapy.

- *Topical corticosteroids (TCSs)* are the **first-line treatment for mild disease**; however, patients should be warned about the side effects with prolonged use. Use of TCS should be avoided or limited on the face, axillae, and genitals. Reevaluate adult patients in 4 weeks and children in 2 weeks to assess their response to topical steroid therapy. If there is an inadequate response, evaluate the patient's understanding and use of TCS, consider changing the class of TCS, or add another topical agent (TCS chart on inside of back cover). There are many nuisances in optimizing the efficacy and minimizing the adverse events of TCS—See Box 4.4-1.

- *Topical calcineurin inhibitors (TCIs),* which are nonsteroidal, are often selected for treatment in sensitive areas (face, axillae, and genitals) and/or as an adjunctive therapy or step-down therapy from TCS. With only FDA indicated for treatment of atopic dermatitis, TCIs are used off-label for psoriasis.

- *Vitamin D derivatives* can be used as adjuvant topical therapy and are safe to use in steroid-sparing regions; however, they may cause some skin irritation initially.

- *Coal tar* has been used for centuries to treat psoriasis but is less common now; it decreases the rapid proliferation of skin and reduces inflammation. It can be very effective for controlling the itch associated with psoriasis, but can the unwanted side effects of "tar smell" and staining of skin and clothes.

- *Keratolytics* help thin the plaques of psoriasis and improve the penetration of TCS (Table 4.4-2).

- Management of scalp psoriasis can be frustrating for both the patient and the clinician (Fig. 4.4-5). The first-line treatment for

TABLE 4.4-2 | **Topical Therapies for Psoriasis**

CLASSIFICATION	AGENT/FORMULATION	DOSING	ADVERSE EVENTS	KEY CONSIDERATIONS
Topical corticosteroids (TCSs) *(see Section 2 and TCS chart inside back cover)*	Mild/moderate psoriasis or sensitive areas (face, eyelids, axillae, genitals): mild to moderate potency TCS Moderate/severe disease or thick skin areas: potent to very potent TCS	Apply thin film directly to lesions q.d.-b.i.d. for 2–4 wk	SE: acne, irritation, telangiectasias, xerosis, skin atrophy, striae, hypopigmentation, and rebound when discontinued. Increased risk of cataract and glaucoma if applied around the eyes Adrenal suppression if long term	Slows proliferation of keratinocytes and reduces inflammation Assess children after 1–2 wks and adults after 2–3 wks. Taper to 1–2 times a week if controlled. LIMIT the quantity and number of refills in to ensure patient follow-up Caution if using occlusion which increases potency and side effects
Topical immunomodulators (not FDA approved for tx of psoriasis)	Calcineurin inhibitors: tacrolimus (Protopic)[a] ointment FDA approved: 0.1% for >16 yr and older; 0.03% for 2–15 yr of age	Apply thin film to lesions b.i.d.	May initially cause burning and irritation, but usually subsides after 2–3 days	Anti-inflammatory Patient education regarding SE increases adherence. Can be used on face, eyelids, and flexural areas without risk of skin atrophy or telangiectasias
Vitamin D₃ analogs	Calcitriol (Vectical) Calcipotriene (Dovonex) Combination of calcipotriene and betamethasone propionate (Taclonex)	Apply thin layer q.d.–b.i.d. to affected areas for up to 8 wk Combination applied once daily	May cause irritation Can lower vitamin D levels (especially in children) Possible elevation of serum calcium level	Blocks hyperproliferation of keratinocytes and anti-inflammatory properties Safe for use on face and intertriginous areas Combination therapy (with TCS) is more effective and more expensive Mix with petrolatum to reduce irritation
Vitamin A analogs (retinoids)	0.05% and 0.1% tazarotene gel (Tazorac) Combination of halobetasol propionate and tazarotene lotion (Duobrii)	Apply at night, followed by mid- to high-potency TCS in am. Start with 0.05%, can increase to 0.1% after 4 wks Combination once daily for 8 wk	May cause scaling and irritation Pregnancy category X (not be used by women considering pregnancy, who are pregnant or nursing)	Apply zinc oxide or moisturizer to healthy skin around the plaque to prevent irritation Optimal efficacy when used as combination rather than monotherapy
Tar preparations (OTC)	Many brands	Massage into scalp and leave on for 5–10 min, then rinse	Can stain clothing, bathtubs, or skin Irritation and photosensitivity for up to 24 hr after application	Often used as adjunctive therapy Helpful for pruritus, especially the scalp
Keratolytic agents	Shampoos, lotions, creams, and gels containing salicylic acid, lactic acid, urea	Shampoos: apply to scalp, wait 5–10 min, then rinse Apply creams/lotions daily to plaques	Can cause nausea and tinnitus if used over large areas of the body Can cause atrophy of healthy skin	Softens thick plaques and removes scale Enhances penetration of other topicals EXCEPT salicylic acid Inactivates vitamin D₃ analogs, so should not be used together

[a]Black box warnings.

scalp psoriasis is the initiation of topical therapies at the first sign of erythema, scaling, or scalp pruritus. Tar preparations, salicylic acid, and oils are recommended for mild disease and are now available in easier-to-use shampoos, solutions, gels, and foams. Some are used as overnight applications for a greater effect.

Mild to moderate scalp involvement may require the addition of TCS, vitamin D analogs, or both. Patients should be advised not to pick or scratch the scale of their scalp, which puts them at increased risk for infection and koebnerization. Scalp psoriasis that is severe should be referred to a dermatologist.

BOX 4.4-1   Treatment Pearls for Topical Corticosteroids

- Evaluate response in 2 to 3 weeks (1–2 weeks for children).
- Once disease is controlled, taper to twice a week or lower potency.
- If the skin does not improve, assess the patient to determine whether medication is being used properly before switching the class of TCS or adding another topical agent.
- Ointments are preferable for thicker plaques with adherent scale.
- Solutions, gels, foams, and lotions are preferable for hair-bearing areas.
- Avoid use of potent or very potent TCS for more than 2 weeks of use on the face, genitals, intertriginous, or flexural areas due to risk of skin atrophy. Topical calcineurin inhibitors can be used (off-label) to reduce the risk of long-term side effects.
- Provide drug holidays from TCS by rotating other topicals such as vitamin D analogs or keratolytics.
- If skin symptoms worsen after use of TCS, consider superinfection with dermatophyte.
- For thicker scales, consider application of keratolytic or topical tazarotene prior to application of TCS for better absorption. Some combination topicals are available.

Moderate to Severe Psoriasis (>3% BSA, Areas of Involvement and Quality-of-Life Impact)

Moderate to severe psoriatic disease warrants a referral to a dermatology practitioner experienced in psoriasis care. The definition of "moderate to severe" has varied and complicated metrics that are used in clinical trials but are not very practical in primary care. For the purposes of this text, indications for referral are outlined in Box 4.4-2.

Phototherapy

Phototherapy can be a very effective modality for moderate or severe psoriasis including:

- Narrow-band UVB
- Home light-box therapy
- Excimer laser
- Chemophototherapy (PUVA)

- When phototherapy is not available, unaffordable, or not effective, systemic therapies must be considered. These traditional agents have been utilized in the management of psoriasis for decades; however, they do pose significant health risks, not limited to, but including liver, kidney, cardiovascular, and blood dyscrasias.

BOX 4.4-2   Referral to Dermatology for Moderate to Severe Psoriasis

Refer patient to dermatology when:
- Disease is not responding or adverse response to topical therapy
- Patients with moderate to severe disease based on >3% BSA[a]
- Disease involving the face/scalp, genitals, or palmar–plantar area
- Disease which has a major impact on patient's quality of life or psychosocial well-being
- Diagnostic uncertainty
- Nail disease
- Guttate psoriasis that may require phototherapy
- Immediate attention for erythroderma
- Children and pregnant women

[a]1% BSA is approximately the area of one palmar hand.

Conventional Oral Agents

There are several oral agents that are frequently utilized as first-line therapies for patients with moderate to severe psoriasis. Their use should be predicated by a thorough review of the patient's medical history, family planning goals, and current prescription and over-the-counter medications and supplements.

- *Methotrexate* is a disease-modifying agent that is used in the treatment of both psoriasis and PsA. Patients should be started on a low dose and gradually uptitrated as tolerated. It has several significant side effects including hepatotoxicity and pancytopenias and therefore requires frequent lab monitoring. It should be avoided in women of childbearing age due to its teratogenicity.

- *Cyclosporin* is a highly effective agent that is typically utilized as a rescue agent for patients with severe disease, such as erythroderma. It can cause significant renal complications and thus, should be used for a short period of time as a "bridge" to start a long-term therapy. It requires judicious monitoring of blood pressure and renal function.

- *Acitretin* is a synthetic retinoid that has a slow onset of efficacy but can be helpful in certain types of psoriasis such as palmoplantar psoriasis, along with phototherapy. Side effects such as dry eyes, skin and lips, and photosensitivity can be difficult for patients to tolerate. It is important to monitor liver function and triglycerides as these can be elevated with acitretin use. It should be avoided in women of childbearing age due to its teratogenicity.

Novel Oral Agents

- *Apremilast* is a novel, PDE4 inhibitor and is a novel oral agent that provides a convenient alternative for psoriasis patients that may have significant comorbidities limiting their use of other therapeutic agents. The most common side effects include diarrhea and GI upset, mood changes, and possible weight loss. There is no lab monitoring required. It is FDA approved for adults with psoriasis or active PsA.

Biologic Agents

Biologics are the newest therapeutic agents for the management of moderate to severe psoriasis and have transformed the management of plaque psoriasis and PsA. Several are also used and indicated for other autoimmune conditions. Selection of a biologic agent along with ongoing care should be individualized for every patient and based on available evidence (Menter et al., 2019).

These systemic agents directly target specific chemical mediators within the immune systemic that are associated with psoriatic disease. While biologics are usually prescribed by dermatology practitioners, the primary care practitioner should understand the basic concepts behind each class of biologic therapy used for psoriasis. This knowledge will enable the PCP to monitor psoriasis patients appropriately while on biologic therapy.

- *TNF-α inhibitors:* adalimumab, certolizumab, etanercept, and infliximab

  - First class of biologic agents utilized for psoriasis and PsA.

  - Patients should be screened for tuberculosis (TB) and hepatitis B prior to starting treatment and TB screening should be done annually thereafter,

  - Patients may be at increased risk for serious infections and certain cancers (particularly lymphomas). Patients with a history of chronic infections such as pneumonia, cellulitis, and other infections should avoid this class of biologic.

  - Patients may be at increased risk of developing demyelinating neurologic disorders such as multiple sclerosis,

Guillain-Barré, and optic neuritis. If patients have a first-line family member with a history of neurologic disorders, it is prudent to seek consultation from a neurologist in order to have baseline screening.

- TNF-α inhibitors may cause new-onset or worsening congestive heart failure (CHF). Patients should be monitored for signs and symptoms of CHF at every primary care and dermatology visit.

- Certolizumab is the preferred treatment for use during pregnancy as it has minimal drug crossing the placental barrier.

- *IL-12/23 inhibitors:* ustekinumab

  - FDA indicated for PsO and PsA and aproved for 6 years or older.

  - This class of biologic has convenient dosing at weeks 0, 4, and then every 12 weeks thereafter.

  - This dosing schedule may be useful for patients who do not wish to give themselves their own injection but would rather come to a provider's clinic to have nursing staff administer the injections.

  - Patients should have baseline TB testing prior to starting therapy.

- *IL-17A inhibitors:* brodalumab, ixekizumab, and secukinumab

  - Patients being treated with this class of biologic are at higher risk for developing fungal or candida infections.

  - Patients should be asked about a history of irritable bowel disease (IBD), as IL-17 inhibitors can initiate or worsen these conditions.

  - Some are indicated for both PsO and PsA and ixekizumab can used for those 6 years and older.

  - Brodalumab carries an increased risk of mood change and suicidal ideation based on the prescriber information data. Patients being treated with brodalumab require registration in a federal monitoring program known as the Risk Evaluation and Mitigation Strategy (REMS) program.

- *IL-23 inhibitors:* guselkumab, risankizumab, and tildrakizumab

  - These are the newest approved biologic agents for the treatment of psoriasis, therefore long-term clinical experience is needed to truly assess their long-term safety. Guselkumab recently approved for PsA.

  - Patients require baseline TB screening, but no further monitoring is required.

  - The dosing is weeks 0, 4, then every 8 to 12 weeks thereafter depending on the specific agent.

Special Considerations

Pregnancy
Psoriasis can be unpredictable during pregnancy, with remission or severe flare. Pregnant females or those trying to conceive who have mild disease can be managed with emollients, TCS, or vitamin D_3 analogs. If phototherapy is considered or second-line therapies are required for moderate to severe psoriasis, pregnant females should be managed by a dermatologist. As noted above, certolizumab is the preferred during pregnancy as minimal to no drug is transferred to the fetus (Porter et al., 2017).

Children
Approximately 1% of children are diagnosed with psoriasis. Although plaque psoriasis can present any time from infancy to advanced years, it is commonly diagnosed during adolescence. Skin manifestations of psoriasis in children differ somewhat from those in adulthood. The psoriatic plaques are usually thinner and there is usually more involvement of the scalp and face. Psoriasis in children can have a tremendous psychosocial impact.

Mild psoriasis in children may be managed with TCS as a first-line therapy (Menter et al., 2019). Children with moderate to severe disease should be referred immediately to a dermatologist, where phototherapy (depending on their age), methotrexate, biologics, or a combination may be used.

Immunodeficiency
Human immunodeficiency virus (HIV) is a risk factor for psoriasis. Patients presenting with plaque psoriasis can be treated with TCSs and may be referred to dermatology. Severe disease can be a cutaneous manifestation of poorly controlled HIV. Treatment with highly active antiretroviral therapy (HAART) by an HIV specialist for control of the infection may improve or resolve the psoriasis.

Management and Patient Education

- Psoriasis that does not have a classic presentation or respond to common treatment modalities should be referred to a dermatology provider to ensure the correct diagnosis. Furthermore, it cannot be overemphasized that patients with moderate and severe psoriasis should be referred early and managed by a dermatologist to reduce morbidity.

- Patients with signs or symptoms of joint stiffness and pain should be referred to a rheumatologist for evaluation of PsA.

- In severe cases of depression or suicidal ideation, a mental health provider should be involved in the management of care as these patients have a significantly increased risk of suicide.

- Gastroenterologists may assist patients with symptoms of IBD and hepatologists should be consulted for suspicions of new or existing liver disease. Patients with psoriasis require ongoing education and support for their chronic disease management, which can greatly impact their QOL.

- Patients with psoriasis should be reevaluated one to two times per year. With an additional focus on comorbidities and PsA related to psoriasis, both dermatologist and primary care clinicians have the opportunity to reduce mortality and morbidity through routine screening, management, and recommendations to reduce risk factors.

- Skin care and skin cancer prevention should not be forgotten especially for patients receiving phototherapy or immunosuppression. Fortunately, there are numerous tools and resources available that support psoriasis education and counseling for both patients and providers (Box 4.4-3).

BOX 4.4-3 Provider-to-Patient Discussion Points and Goals

- Patient expectations of disease course (triggers, waxing/waning nature of disease)
- Importance of compliance with treatment regimens
- Importance of regular primary care provider follow-up
- Prevention of cardiovascular disease and type II diabetes
- Smoking cessation aids
- Avoidance of alcohol and other illicit drugs
- Weight management and fitness promotion
- QOL and depression management
- Age-appropriate cancer screenings
- Vaccination protocols (especially with biologic treatment regimens)

READINGS AND REFERENCES

Armstrong, A. W., Schupp, C., Wu, J., & Bebo, B. (2012). Quality of Life and Work Productivity Impairment among Psoriasis Patients: Findings from the National Psoriasis Foundation survey data 2003–2011. *PLoSOne, 7*(12), e52935. doi: 10.1371/journal.pone.0052935.

Armstrong, A. W., Siegel, M. P., Bagel, J., Boh, E. E., Buell, M., Cooper, K. D., Duffin, K. C., Eichenfield, L. F., Garg, A., Gelfand, J. M., Gottlieb, A. B., Koo, J. Y. M., Korman, N. J., Krueger, G. G., Lebwohl, M. G., Leonardi, C. L., Mandelin, A. M., Menter, M. A., Merola, J. F., ... Van Voorhees, A. S. (2016). From the Medical Board of the National Psoriasis Foundation: Treatment targets for plaque psoriasis. *Journal of the American Academy of Dermatology, 76*(2), 290–298.

Arnett, D. K., Blumenthal, R. S., Albert, M. A., Buroker, A. B., Goldberger, Z. D., Hahn, E. J., Himmelfarb, C. D., Khera, A., Lloyd-Jones, D., McEvoy, J. W., Michos, E. D., Miedema, M. D., Muñoz, D., Smith, S. C., Jr., Virani, S. S., Williams, K. A., Sr., Yeboah, J., & Ziaeian, B. (2019). 2019 ACC/AHA Guideline on the primary prevention of cardiovascular disease: A report of the American College of Cardiology/American Heart Association Task Force on Clinical Practice Guidelines. *Circulation, 140*(11), e596–e646.

Bobotsis, R., Gulliver, W., Monaghan, K., Lynde, C., & Fleming, P. (2016). Psoriasis and adverse pregnancy outcomes: A systematic review of observational studies. *British Journal of Dermatol, 175*(3), 464–472.

Dauden, E., Blasco, A. J., Bonanad, C., Botella, R., Carrascosa, J. M., González-Parra, E., Jodar, E., Joven, B., Lázaro, P., Olveira, A., Quintero, J., & Rivera, R. (2018). Position statement for the management of psoriasis comorbidities. *Journal of the European Academy of Dermatology and Venereology, 32*(12), 2058–2073.

Elmets, C. A., Leonardi, C. L., Davi, D. M. R., Gelfand, J. M., Lichten, J., Mehtal, N. N., Armstrong, A. W., Connor, C., Cordoro, K. M., Elewski, B. E., Gordon, K. B., Gottlieb, A. B., Kaplan, D. H., Kavanaugh, A., Kivelevitch, D., Kiselia, M., Korman, N. J., Kroshinsky, D., Lebwohl, M., ... Menter, A. (2019). Joint AAD-NPF guidelines of care for the management and treatment of psoriasis with awareness and attention to comorbidities. *Journal of the American Academy of Dermatology, 80*(4), 1073–1113.

Esposito, M., Saraceno, R., Giunta, A., Maccarone, M., & Chimenti, S. (2006). An Italian study on psoriasis and depression. *Dermatology, 212*(2), 123–127.

Gelfand, J. M., Shin, D. B., Neimann, A. L., Wang, X., Margolis, D. J., & Troxel, A. B. (2006). The risk of lymphoma in patients with psoriasis. *Journal of Investigative Dermatology, 126*(10), 2194–2201.

Gelfand, J. M., & Yeung, H. (2012). Metabolic syndrome in patients with psoriatic disease. *The Journal of Rheumatology. Supplement, 89*, 24–28.

Menter, A., Cordoro, K. M., Davis, D., Kroshinsky, D., Paller, A. S., Armstrong, A. W., Connor, C., Elewski, B. E., Gelfand, J. M., Gordon, K. B., Gottlieb, A. B., Kaplan, D. H., Kavanaugh, A., Kiselica, M., Kivelevitch, D., Korman, N. J., Lebwohl, M., Leonardi, C. L., Lichten, J., ... Elmets, C. A. (2019). Joint American Academy of Dermatology-National Psoriasis Foundation guidelines of care for the management and treatment of psoriasis in pediatric patients. *Journal of the American Academy of Dermatology, 82*(1), 161–201. https://doi.org/10.1016/j.jaad.2019.08.049

Menter, A., Strober, B. E., Kaplan, D. H., Kivelevitch, D., Prater, E. F., Stoff, B., Armstrong, A. W., Connor, C., Cordoro, K. M., Davis, D., Elewski, B. E., Gelfand, J. M., Gordon, K. B., Gottlieb, A. B., Kavanaugh, A., Kiselica, M., Korman, N. J., Kroshinsky, D., Lebwohl, M., ... Elmets, C. A. (2019). Joint AAD-NPF guidelines for the management and treatment of psoriasis with biologics. *Journal of the American Academy of Dermatology, 80*(4), 1029–1072. https://doi.org/10.1016/j.jaad.2018.11.057

Ni, C., & Chiu, M. W. (2014). Psoriasis and comorbidities: Links and risks. *Clinical, Cosmetic and Investigational Dermatology, 7*, 119–132. https://doi.org/10.2147/CCID.S44843

Ogdie, A., Grewal, S., Noe, M., Shin, D., Takeshita, J., Fuxench, Z., Carr, R., & Gelfand, J. M. (2017). Risk of incident liver disease in patients with psoriasis, psoriatic arthritis, and rheumatoid arthritis: A population-based study. *Journal of Investigative Dermatology, 138*(4), 760–767. https://doi.org/10.1016/j.jid.2017.10.024

Porter, M. L., Lockwood, S. J., & Kimball, A. B. (2017). Update on biologic safety for patients with psoriasis during pregnancy. *International Journal of Women's Dermatology, 3*(1), 21–25. https://doi.org/10.1016/j.ijwd.2016.12.003

Singh, J. A., Guyatt, G., Ogdie, A., Gladman, D. D., Deal, C., Deodhar, A., Dubreuil, M., Dunham, J., Husni, M. E., Kenny, S., Kwan-Morley, J., Lin, J., Marchetta, P., Mease, P. J., Merola, J. F., Miner, J., Ritchlin, C. T., Siaton, B., Smith, B. J., ... Reston, J. (2019). 2018 American College of Rheumatology/National Psoriasis Foundation guideline for the treatment of psoriatic arthritis. *Arthritis & Rheumatology, 71*(1), 2–29.

Strober, B., Ryen, C., van de Kerkhof, P., van der Walt, J., Kimball, A., Barker, J., Blauvelt, A., & International Psoriasis Council Board Members and Councilors. (2020). Recategorization of psoriasis severity: Delphi consensus from the International Psoriasis Council. *Journal of the American Academy of Dermatology, 82*(1), 117–122.

Takeshita, J., Grewal, S., Langan, S. M., Mehta, N., Ogdie, A., Van Voorhees, A., & Gelfand, J. (2017). Psoriasis and comorbid diseases: Epidemiology. *Journal of the American Academy of Dermatology, 76*(3), 377–390.

Trafford, A., Parisi, R., Kontopantelis, E., Griffiths, C., & Ashcroft, D. (2019). Association of psoriasis with the risk of developing or dying of cancer: A systematic review and meta-analysis. *JAMA Dermatol, 155*(12), 1390–1403. https://doi.org/10.1001/jamadermatol.2019.3056

Erythroderma, Lichen Planus, Pityriasis Rosea, and Other Scaly Stuff

Douglas C. DiRuggiero

In This Chapter

- Erythroderma
- Pityriasis Rosea
- Lichen Planus

- Pityriasis Lichenoides
  - Pityriasis Lichenoides Et Varioliformis Acuta (PLEVA)
  - Pityriasis Lichenoides Chronica (PLC)
- Parapsoriasis

ERYTHRODERMA

Erythroderma is defined as a generalized redness and scaling of the skin (>80% of body surface area) associated with extensive exfoliation. While the term "Red Man Syndrome" is classically associated with a hypersensitivity reaction to the antibiotic vancomycin, full-body erythema is not a specific disease entity, but rather a manifestation of other diseases (including preexisting dermatoses such as atopic dermatitis and psoriasis), malignancies, or a reaction to multiple different drugs. The cause remains unknown (idiopathic) in approximately 30% of cases. Erythroderma, which is not due to eczema, usually develops in patients older than 40 years. It is slightly more common in males than in females. It may require hospitalization to maintain homeostasis and treat the underlying cause.

Pathophysiology

- The generalized redness is due to increased skin blood perfusion causing temperature dysregulation which results in heat loss and hypothermia. The basal metabolic rate then rises to compensate for this heat loss and high cardiac output failure may occur.
- There is also an extensive exfoliation which can contribute to hypoalbuminemia.
- Edema may be observed because of a fluid shift into the extracellular spaces.
- Immune reactions may include increased γ-globulins, serum IgE, and CD4 T-cell lymphocytopenia.

Clinical Presentation

- *Initial onset*—generalized redness (erythema) and edema of 80% or more of the skin surface; scaling (fine flakes or large sheets), typically 2 to 6 days after the onset of redness, starting on flexural skin; serous drainage, resulting in an unpleasant odor as clothes and dressings stick to skin; pruritus, severe in some cases (may be associated with excoriations); lymphadenopathy may be present (Fig. 4.5-1).
- *Chronic (>3 months)*—keratoderma, which manifests as thickening of palmar surface of hands and plantar surface of feet;

thick scale on the scalp associated with alopecia as symptoms persist. Nails may become thickened and shed overtime. Eyelid swelling/edema may result in ectropion. Pigmentary changes, resembling vitiligo, especially in individuals with skin of color. Pustules and crusting with secondary infection can develop.

- *Systemic symptoms*—may include fever, chills, hypothermia, electrolyte imbalances, and dehydration secondary to fluid loss, low serum albumin due to protein loss, and increased metabolic rate. Heart failure associated with untreated tachycardia is common in the elderly. Erythroderma with systemic symptoms constitutes a dermatologic emergency and hospitalization.

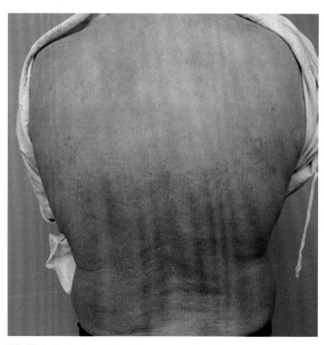

FIG. 4.5-1. Erythroderma. (Used with permission from Council, M. L., Sheinbein, D., & Cornelius, L. A. [2018]. *Manual Washington de dermatología*. Wolters Kluwer Health.)

DIFFERENTIAL DIAGNOSIS Erythroderma

- Atopic dermatitis
- Contact dermatitis
- Cutaneous T-cell lymphoma
- Stevens–Johnson syndrome (severe drug reaction)
- Staphylococcal scalded skin syndrome
- Graft-versus-host disease
- Lichen planus
- Pemphigus foliaceus
- Pityriasis rubra pilaris
- Psoriasis
- Seborrheic dermatitis

Confirming the Diagnosis

- Initially, a thorough history is needed to identify an underlying disease. Recent drug history may identify a possible drug etiology.
- Physical examination clues may help differentiate other etiologies (see DDx).
- Pemphigus foliaceous will likely have superficial blisters which may be hard to distinguish from overall crust.
- Pityriasis rubra pilaris will have characteristic "islands of sparing."
- Psoriasis requires a close look at the scalp, umbilicus, gluteal cleft, penile head, elbows, and knees for any plaque formation; look for pitting in the fingernails.
- Lichen planus may exhibit oral and nail manifestations associated with LP (see above).
- The most common histopathologic findings will reveal a subacute or chronic dermatitis (Rosenbach et al., 2010). Skin biopsy can support clinical findings and confirm diagnosis in 40% of cases.
- Repeat biopsies and hematologic studies may be necessary to detect specific conditions such as T-cell lymphoma. Immunophenotyping, flow cytometry, and B- and T-cell gene rearrangement can confirm the diagnosis of lymphoma.
- Laboratory studies may reveal an increased erythrocyte sedimentation rate, anemia, hypoalbuminemia, and hyperglobulinemia. IgE will be elevated when erythroderma is associated with atopic dermatitis.
- Peripheral blood smears and bone marrow evaluation may assist in a leukemia workup.
- Cultures may show secondary bacterial overgrowth or detect herpes virus.
- Skin scrapings may reveal hyphae of fungal infection or scabies.

Treatment

- These patients are at risk for cardiac failure and acute respiratory distress syndrome and **require hospitalization,** where management includes nutritional support (especially with elderly patients where preexisting malnutrition is not uncommon), body temperature regulation, and fluid and electrolyte replacement.
- In bed, full-body application of a midstrength TCS such as triamcinolone 0.1% cream or ointment b.i.d. under occlusion (wet dressings or sauna suit) after soaking is standard care.
- Once improved, gentle skin care should be started with the application of bland emollients.
- In drug-induced erythroderma, the offending medication must be withdrawn, and it may be prudent to discontinue all unnecessary medications initially.
- Antihistamines such as hydroxyzine 25 to 50 mg q6h (2 mg/kg/day) or cetirizine 10 mg b.i.d. may help alleviate pruritus and provide much needed sedation.
- Systemic antibiotics for signs and symptoms of secondary infection may be warranted.
- Systemic corticosteroids (prednisone 1 to 2 mg/kg/day initially) may be given and must be tapered over a 2- to 3-week period; however, this should be avoided, if possible, in patients with psoriasis and staphylococcal scalded skin syndrome (Rosenbach et al., 2010).
- Immunosuppressive systemic agents such as acitretin, cyclosporine, methotrexate, and azathioprine may be needed for psoriatic or idiopathic erythroderma (Rothe et al., 2005). Dermatology referral is highly recommended for these treatments.

Management and Patient Education

- The prognosis is dependent on the underlying etiology.
- Refer all patients with erythroderma to a dermatologist at an inpatient hospital setting.
- Educate patients on the specifics of the underlying cause of their erythroderma and the importance of diligent management of underlying disease, if any.
- Follow discharged patients on a regular outpatient basis for management of their underlying disease. For patients with idiopathic erythroderma, serial biopsies may be necessary to rule out an underlying lymphoma.

PITYRIASIS ROSEA

Pityriasis rosea (PR) is a common, self-limiting, papulosquamous dermatosis that usually affects older children and younger adults. The majority of cases affect patients between the ages of 10 and 35. While the incidence is higher in females, there is no racial predilection and the diagnosis is more common in the spring and fall (Schadt, 2018).

Pathophysiology

- Documentation of clustered cases among household members, seasonal variation, intolerance to ampicillin, and response to acyclovir at the onset of disease supports this theory. Observational studies support a viral etiology, although that has been difficult to confirm.
- Past research has greatly focused on the causal association between human herpesvirus 6 and 7 (HHV-6 and HHV-7) and PR. More recent research confirms a link between a viral etiology and PR.
- Several other factors may reflect a viral etiology: the presence of increased CD4 T-cells and Langerhans cells in the dermis may reflect an initial viral antigen pathogenesis; anti-IgM to

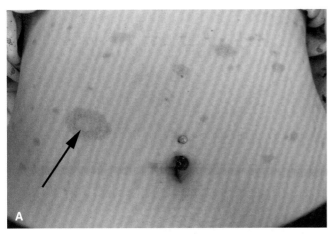
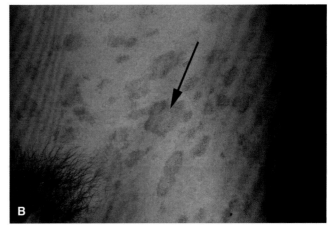

FIG. 4.5-2. **A,B:** Pityriasis Rosea. Note the "herald patch" (*arrow*). (Photo A courtesy of Victoria Lazareth; Photo B courtesy of International Psoriasis Council.)

keratinocytes has been associated with the exanthematous phase of viral infections and has been seen in patients with PR.

Clinical Presentation

- Classic PR initially presents with a "herald patch," a solitary 2- to 4-cm patch or plaque on the trunk. This can precede the typical rash by 1 to 2 weeks. Studies vary, but a herald patch is reported by only 10% to 20% of patients (Fig. 4.5-2A&B).
- The rash of PR consists of multiple pink to salmon-colored, round-to-ovoid, papules, and plaques with a fine "collarette scale" on an advancing border. Minute pustules can also be seen in this early eruptive phase.
- PR has a symmetrical distribution following the long axis of skin tension lines often resembling a Christmas or fir tree pattern on the trunk. The face is often spared, although the neck is a common occurrence. Palms and soles are usually spared.
- Approximately 25% of patients complain about pruritus, and some patients may report prodromal low-grade fever, chills, headache, fatigue, myalgias, and lymphadenopathy. The rash usually lasts for 6 to 8 weeks and then spontaneously resolves. Some cases last up to 5 months or more.
- Lymphadenopathy is a rare finding in PR. If present, it is important to rule out syphilis and obtain RPR/VDRL.

DIFFERENTIAL DIAGNOSIS   Pityriasis Rosea
• Secondary syphilis
• Tinea versicolor
• Drug eruption
• Nummular eczema
• Seborrheic dermatitis
• Guttate psoriasis
• Pityriasis lichenoides

Confirming the Diagnosis

- The diagnosis of PR is made on the basis of the characteristic clinical presentation.
- A biopsy will not be diagnostic as the histology is nonspecific, but it can assist in ruling out other differential diagnoses.

- A KOH prep can identify fungal or yeast infections to rule out infection.
- Distribution and nail involvement are key if the clinician favors a diagnosis of psoriasis.
- An RPR or VDRL should be obtained if there is a suspicion or history of high-risk sexual contact, a previous genital ulcer, or significant involvement of the palms and soles to rule out secondary syphilis.

Treatment

Topical

- PR does not typically require any treatment other than symptomatic care.
- A mild TCS lotion such as desonide 0.05% can be applied twice daily for relief of itch.

Systemic

- Pruritus may be significant and therapy with oral antihistamines, such as cetirizine or loratadine, during the day may be helpful. Hydroxyzine 25 to 50 mg or diphenhydramine 12.5 to 25 mg have sedating effects and are recommended to be taken at bedtime.
- Extensive PR with severe pruritus is uncommon but may respond to ultraviolet (UVB) light or natural sunlight.
- The use of antivirals has been debated as some clinicians believe that it is useful in patients with severe disease associated with flu-like symptoms. Acyclovir 400 to 800 mg five times daily for a week is the suggested dosage (Contreras-Ruiz et al., 2019).
- Oral erythromycin has been found to eliminate and/or reduce the severity of PR.

Special Considerations

Pregnancy

PR is associated with HHV-6 and HHV-7 infection. Premature delivery and fetal demise have been observed in pregnant patients with PR, especially if it occurs within the first 15 weeks of gestation. Referral to obstetrics is important for pregnant women with PR for a discussion about the risks of potential fetal complications and possible benefits of acyclovir (Category B) (Drago et al., 2008, 2014).

Management and Patient Education

- PR is self-limiting and has an excellent prognosis. The eruption may be cosmetically unpleasant for some patients. Some patients have reported recurrences.

- If symptoms are prolonged or not relieved by systemic or topical medications, reevaluate the patient and reconsider the diagnosis.

- Differential diagnoses such as pityriasis lichenoides, a more chronic disorder, should be considered, and referral to a dermatologist is recommended.

- Follow-up is recommended for any patients who cannot manage their symptoms or in whom the rash does not clear in several months. Patients often need reassurance about the benign nature of PR. If the patient is seen in the early phase, they should be advised that the rash may worsen and spread and that is the expected progression.

LICHEN PLANUS

Lichen planus (LP) is an inflammatory, mucocutaneous condition estimated to occur in 1% of the population. It most commonly affects middle-aged adults (highest incidence 30 to 60 years), with a slightly higher prevalence in females. Studies report a high incidence of hepatitis C virus (HCV), chronic hepatitis, and primary biliary cirrhosis in patients with LP. It has also been associated with other immune-mediated conditions involving the skin such as vitiligo, alopecia areata, lichen sclerosis, and dermatomyositis.

Pathophysiology

- LP has an unclear etiology but is known as a chronic inflammatory, autoimmune skin, nail, and oral mucosal disease (Suresh et al., 2016).

- Observations suggest that exposure to an antigen initiates T-cell-mediated damage to the basal keratinocytes of the skin, mucous membranes, hair follicles, or nails.

- Viruses, in particular HCV, medications, and contact allergens have been implicated in the development of LP.

Clinical Presentation

- Cutaneous lesions often have five classic "P" qualities: pruritic (intense), purple, planar (flat topped), polygonal (or polyangular), and papular. These lesions are present most commonly on the flexural surfaces of wrists and forearms, the dorsal hands, and anterior aspect of the lower legs (Fig. 4.5-3). Two additional "Ps" can help clinically: penile lesions (can affect glans penis) and prolonged course (≥18 months).

- Initially, lesions are small violaceous, slightly shiny papules. Overtime, they may coalesce into larger plaques.

- Characteristic fine white lines called "Wickham striae" or gray–white puncta may evolve as lesions age and are more commonly seen on oral mucosa.

- In addition to the classic characteristics described above, other morphologies can be seen, which include hypertrophic, atrophic, erosive, follicular, annular, linear, guttate, actinic, bullous, and ulcerative lesions.

- Oral LP has many forms, and may occur separately or concurrently. The reticular form is most common and appears as white plaques with a lace-like pattern affecting the buccal mucosa or lateral tongue (Fig. 4.5-4). Mucous membrane involvement may

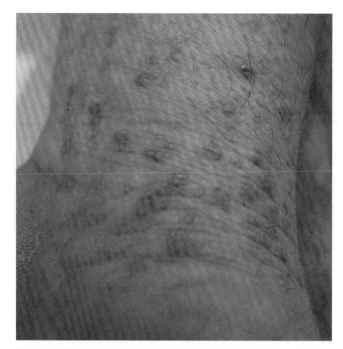

FIG. 4.5-3. Lichen planus on the wrists showing the five "P" qualities.

be severe and erosive. Lesions may be found on the conjunctiva, vulva, glans penis, anus, tonsils, larynx, and throughout the GI tract. Oral LP is highly associated with hepatitis C infection and increased incidence of oral SCC (Alaizari et al., 2016).

- LP in the genital area is further discussed in Section 11.4.

- Lichen planopilaris refers to involvement of the scalp hair and presents as erythematous, perifollicular scale, which may lead to a permanent scarring alopecia if not treated promptly. This may occur alone or in conjunction with other cutaneous involvement (Fig. 4.5-5).

- Nail changes which represent scarring are seen in approximately 10% of patients with LP. Look for lateral thinning, longitudinal ridging, thickening, and pterygium (overgrowth of the cuticle) on the proximal nail fold. See Sections 11.1 and 11.2 for discussion of hair and nail changes with LP. Linear eruptions may develop in areas of trauma/scratching (Koebner phenomenon; Fig. 4.5-6).

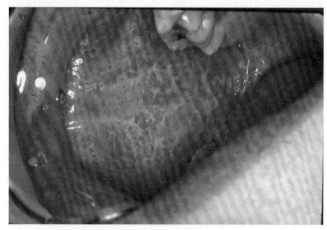

FIG. 4.5-4. Oral lichen planus. Note the white, lace-like pattern on the buccal mucosa known as "Wickham striae."

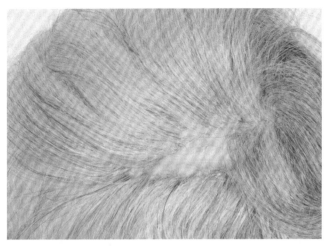

FIG. 4.5-5. Lichen planopilaris. Scale and erythema at the base of the hair. (Used with permission from Hall, J. C., & Hall, B. J. [2017]. *Sauer's manual of skin diseases* [11th ed.]. Wolters Kluwer Health.)

- A photodistribution of skin lesions may indicate drug-induced LP. In general, always consider drugs as an underlying cause of LP.
- Drug-induced LP usually occurs within months of starting the offending agent. It is important to consider that the eruption may range from 10 days to several years after starting, and multiple drugs may be considered. A lichenoid drug reaction may differ from classic LP by its generalized distribution, older mean age, photo distribution, and lack of mucosal involvement.

Confirming the Diagnosis

- LP is a clinical diagnosis most often based on the distinctive appearance and distribution of lesions. Particular attention to the oral mucosa, nail units, and scalp may support the diagnosis.
- A skin punch biopsy will confirm the diagnosis of LP. Classic pathology shows a lichenoid interface dermatitis without parakeratosis or eosinophils.

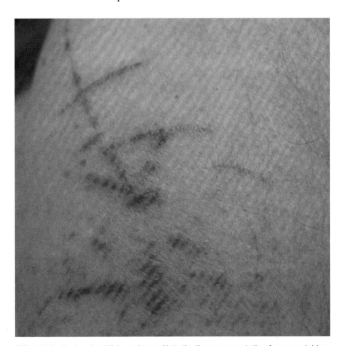

FIG. 4.5-6. Koebnerized lichen planus. Note the linear presentation from scratching.

DIFFERENTIAL DIAGNOSIS	Lichen Planus
Cutaneous Lichen Planus • Lichenoid drug eruption • Subacute lupus erythematosus • Psoriasis • Granuloma annulare • Warts • Pityriasis rosea • Tinea corporis • Mycosis fungoides • Lichen simplex chronicus • Secondary syphilis • Chronic graft-versus-host disease • Squamous cell carcinoma **Nail Lichen Planus** • Alopecia areata • Onychomycosis • Psoriasis	**Hair Lichen Planus** • Alopecia areata • Discoid lupus erythematosus • Other scarring alopecias **Mucous Membrane Lichen Planus** • Squamous cell carcinoma • Pemphigus vulgaris • Bullous pemphigoid • Benign mucous membrane • Pemphigus • Lichen sclerosus • Herpes simplex virus • Drug eruption

- A direct immunofluorescence (DIF) biopsy should reveal globular deposits of IgG, IgM, IgA, and complement and linear basement membrane deposits of fibrin and fibrinogen.
- Serologic tests for hepatitis C should be considered especially in geographic regions where LP is more commonly associated with hepatitis. High-risk regions include the Mediterranean basin and the United States.

Treatment

Although LP can resolve spontaneously, treatment is often requested because of severe pruritus.

Topical

- *Pruritus*—oral antihistamines and topical antipruritic agents are used to manage itching. Topical anesthetics may be used for itch and/or skin-pain management.
- *Localized disease*—TCS and topical immunomodulators are used to both control pruritus and promote resolution of lesions. All patients given TCS and/or oral corticosteroids should be warned that prolonged use may lead to cutaneous and systemic side effects. (See Section 2 for side effects of corticosteroid.)
- *Genital*—mid- to high-potency TCS are the first-line treatment. Steroid-sparing agents may be used for maintenance. Water-based lubricants for sexual activity.
- *Oral mucosa*—mid- to high-potency TCS are the first-line treatment; have pharmacist compound TCS into a safe oral paste (Kenalog in orabase). Intralesional Kenalog 2 to 5 mg/mL injections into refractory oral lesions can help. (Suresh et al., 2016) Meticulous dental care must be emphasized.

Systemic

- *Widespread disease*—may necessitate systemic therapy with oral antihistamines for itch, corticosteroids, or other agents, such as methotrexate, acitretin, metronidazole, cyclosporin, hydroxychloroquine, or phototherapy (Atzmony et al., 2016). Referral

TABLE 4.5-1	Treatment for Lichen Planus	
	TOPICAL	**SYSTEMIC**
Cutaneous	Topicals antipruritics Oral antihistamines Topical corticosteroids: mid to high potency (class 1 or 2); apply b.i.d. for 2–3 wk only to lesions Calcineurin inhibitors (steroid sparing)[a]	Intralesional triamcinolone (localized) Phototherapy or chemophototherapy Oral corticosteroids Dapsone Hydroxychloroquine Immunosuppressants
Genital	*Vaginal* Tacrolimus vaginal suppositories (compounded) Tacrolimus 0.1% (compounded) cream with Replens-like base *Vulvar* Super potent topical corticosteroids	Systemic corticosteroids Systemic retinoids Hydroxychloroquine Azathioprine Mycophenolate mofetil Dapsone
Oral	Topical corticosteroids[b] (mix with adhesive dental paste or triamcinolone 0.1% using a custom tray); tacrolimus 0.1% Topical retinoids Lidocaine Consider antimycotic	Systemic retinoids Cyclosporine mouthwash Cyclosporine oral Hydroxychloroquine Azathioprine Mycophenolate mofetil Photodynamic therapy

[a]Topical calcineurin inhibitors can burn, especially on inflamed skin, and long-term safety is unknown. Avoid long-term/continuous use.
[b]Consider concurrent treatment for oral candidiasis, as increased risk is associated with corticosteroid use.

to a dermatology specialist is recommended for initiation and monitoring of these treatments.

- *Drug-induced LP*—must be ruled out before starting any therapy as withdrawal of the potential offending agent will result in resolution of lesions.

Table 4.5-1 provides an overview of treatment options for management of LP.

Management and Patient Education

- The duration is dependent on the LP variant. LP may spontaneously resolve, typically after a year, or may follow a chronic, remitting course. Hypertrophic, oral, and nail LP tend to be more persistent. Ulcerative LP tends to be lifelong.
- Advise patients with genital mucosal involvement that topical treatments are available to help alleviate pain and improve sexual function.
- Oral LP requires good oral hygiene. Regular brushing and use of dental floss may prevent tooth decay and gingival damage. Regular dental cleanings are strongly recommended.
- Management of pruritus and pain may be particularly challenging and close follow-up is recommended. Ideally, patients should be seen 2 to 4 weeks after the initiation of treatment.
- Follow-up is recommended for any patient whose symptoms interfere with activities of daily living, which include eating, sleeping, the ability to engage in sexual activity, and coping with a potentially chronic skin disease.
- Refer all patients with erosive LP to a specialist (ophthalmologist, oral surgeon, gynecologist, or dermatologist) for appropriate treatment. Refer all patients with severe cutaneous LP for consideration of systemic therapy to a dermatologist.

PITYRIASIS LICHENOIDES

Pityriasis lichenoides (or Mucha–Habermann disease) is a rare skin disorder of unknown origin. It has both acute and chronic variations known as pityriasis lichenoides et varioliformis acuta (PLEVA) and pityriasis lichenoides chronica (PLC), respectively. PLEVA and PLC are two ends of a disease spectrum. There is also a rare, ulceronecrotic febrile form of PLEVA associated with high fever and constitutional symptoms. The incidence of this disease has not been established in the United States. In the pediatric population, pityriasis lichenoides has a slight male predominance. The age of onset ranges from 3 to 15 years, with a medium age of 8 years. Most cases appear before age 30, and there is no racial predilection (Zang et al., 2018).

Pathophysiology

- Pityriasis lichenoides is a T-cell lymphoproliferative disorder.
- A cell-mediated mechanism has been suggested based on a T-cell lymphocytic infiltrate which is composed of monoclonal CD8+ T lymphocytes.
- The presence of CD30+ cells is occasionally seen in pityriasis lichenoides, which leads some authors to view this as a self-healing lymphoproliferative disease.
- An infective etiology has been suggested, but no pathogen has been identified, although, an association with toxoplasmosis and PLC has been identified (Nassef & Hammam, 1997).

PLEVA

- Presents with a sudden onset of asymptomatic crops of small erythematous papules, typically affecting children and young adults (Fig. 4.5-7).

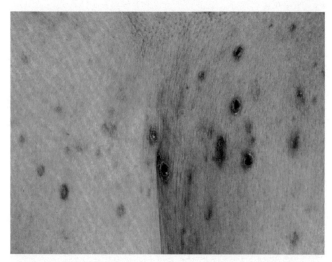

FIG. 4.5-7. Pityriasis lichenoides et varioliformis acuta (PLEVA). Note the Papular, purpuric, and ulcerative lesions.

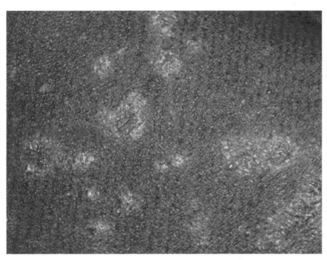

FIG. 4.5-8. Pityriasis lichenoides chronica (PLC).

- The lesions appear spontaneously, resolve within weeks, and reappear at a later date.
- The lesions typically come and go in crops so variations of individual lesions may appear concurrently as papules rapidly progressing to vesicles or pustules with crusting, necrosis, ulceration, and varicella-like scarring.
- They vary in number from a few lesions to hundreds.
- They favor the trunk, buttocks, and proximal extremities. Lesions of the scalp, face, palms, and soles are seen infrequently.
- In general, PLEVA is considered a benign disorder with spontaneous resolution of symptoms in 1 to 3 years.
- In very rare instances, progression to cutaneous T-cell lymphoma (CTCL) has been reported.

PLC

- PLC is a chronic variation of PLEVA. Typical lesions are scaly, erythematous papules which are slow to develop and take months to resolve. PLC lesions favor the lateral trunk and proximal extremities (Fig. 4.5-8).
- Patients may have ten to hundreds of lesions, but typically less than 50.
- PLC tends to last for many years, occasionally leaving hypopigmented areas which are also slow to resolve.
- PLC is also considered a benign disease. There are rare instances of patients who progress to T-cell lymphoma and therefore it is important to monitor these patients long term.

DIFFERENTIAL DIAGNOSIS   Pityriasis Lichenoides

- Lymphomatoid papulosis (LyP)
- Varicella
- Pityriasis rosea
- Lichen planus
- Guttate psoriasis
- Gianotti–Crosti syndrome
- Small-vessel vasculitis
- Arthropod reaction

Confirming the Diagnosis

- Consider biopsy of lesions that become indurated, atrophied, ulcerated, eroded, or have persistent erythema or poikiloderma (this term refers to the presence of cutaneous atrophy, telangiectasia, and hyper- and hypopigmentation).
- These clinical clues can help sort out the differential diagnosis:
  - Lymphomatoid papulosis (LyP) is typically seen in older patients, lesions are more nodular, and predominately have CD30+ cells on skin biopsy.
  - Varicella is usually accompanied by a prodrome of mild fever, malaise, and myalgia.
  - LP lesions are pruritic and may exhibit the five Ps. The presence of a "Herald Patch" may help make a diagnosis of PR.
  - Guttate psoriasis lesions are pruritic and monomorphous and rarely crusted.
  - Papular acrodermatitis of childhood typically spares the trunk, may have pruritus, and follows a viral illness.
  - Small-vessel vasculitis usually occurs on lower extremities as palpable purpura
  - Patient history and biopsy will help confirm a diagnosis of arthropod reaction.

Treatment

Therapeutic trials often group PLEVA and PLC together, so management strategies are similar. The lesions are typically not symptomatic and can resolve spontaneously without treatment, but mid-potency TCS are commonly utilized if lesions are pruritic.

Systemic

- First-line treatment for adults is phototherapy, and both narrowband UVB (NBUVB) and psoralen plus UVA (PUVA) can be used.
- In children, however, erythromycin, at a dose of 40 mg per kg in a younger child and 250 mg q.i.d. in adolescents, is recommended for 6 weeks. If children do not respond to erythromycin, phototherapy is tried as second-line therapy (Bellinato et al., 2019).
- For more severe cases, systemic antibiotics, as well as topical and systemic corticosteroids, systemic retinoids, and immunosuppressants such as cyclosporine and low-dose methotrexate may need to be utilized (Bellinato et al., 2019).

Management and Patient Education

- There is evidence to predict the outcome based on the distribution of lesions. For example, the average clinical course with lesions limited to the extremities is 33 months, and patients with wide distribution average a shorter clinical course of 11 months (Lebwohl et al., 2017b).
- Although generally considered a benign condition, PL merits awareness as there is a 1% to 2% chance of cases progressing to cutaneous lymphoma.
- The ulceronecrotic variation is more likely to progress to cutaneous lymphoma and has a mortality rate of 15% (Xing et al., 2017).
- Refer all patients with PL to a dermatologist for biopsy confirmation and/or administration of phototherapy and systemic agents.
- Patients with long-term disease or disease that is refractory to treatment should be followed by a dermatologist. If patients are receiving phototherapy, they should be followed every 6 to 8 weeks.

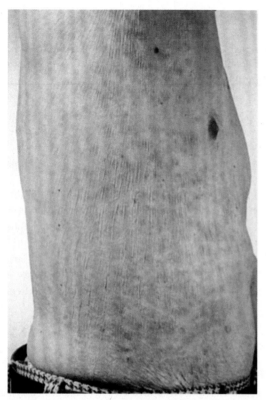

FIG. 4.5-9. Small plaque parapsoriasis, digitate pattern.

PARAPSORIASIS

Parapsoriasis refers to a group of skin disorders in the papulosquamous category. The present term refers to two specific cutaneous disorders that are characterized by T-cell predominant infiltrates of the skin and are referred to as small plaque parapsoriasis (SPP) and large plaque parapsoriasis (LPP) (Figs. 4.5-9 and 4.5-10). Both conditions are asymptomatic chronic dermatoses. Parapsoriasis is most often seen in the middle-aged to elderly individuals with a peak incidence in the fifth decade of life. It affects all races and geographic regions. There is a male predominance, greater in small plaque disease. There are no accurate statistics on incidence and frequency.

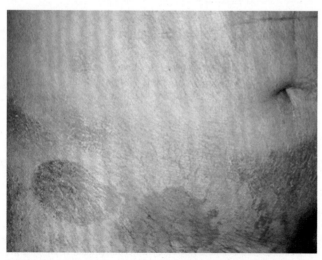

FIG. 4.5-10. Large plaque parapsoriasis. These large, scaly plaques may be evolving into cutaneous T-cell lymphoma. (Photo courtesy of International Psoriasis Council.)

Pathophysiology

- The etiology of SPP and LPP is unknown. There is a superficial dermal infiltrate composed primarily of CD4+ T cells.
- Dominant T-cell clonality is evident in many cases of LPP and only a few cases of SPP.
- It is thought that these diseases most likely signify different stages in a continuum of lymphoproliferative disorders from chronic dermatitis to a malignant state of CTCL.
- Both SPP and LPP can be regarded as forms of clonal dermatitis, with only LPP having any significant risk of transformation to overt CTCL.

Clinical Presentation

Skin Findings

In general, parapsoriasis appears as red scaly, sometimes salmon-colored patches or slightly elevated plaques that resemble psoriasis clinically.

- *SPP*—often oval to round pink, well-demarcated, minimally scaly plaques of up to 5 cm in diameter with a "cigarette paper"-like scale. Plaques may be seen over the entire body, but favor sun-protected skin such as the trunk, buttocks, and lower extremities. Lesions with a yellow hue are called xanthoerythrodermia perstans. Finger-like patches distributed symmetrically on the flank are described as digitate dermatoses. These lesions break the 5 cm rule of SPP and may elongate to 10 cm.
- *LPP*—this presents with larger (>6 cm) round or irregularly shaped, faint erythematous plaques on the trunk, buttocks, and proximal extremities. LPP frequently has a "bathing suit" distribution. The surface has minimal scale, with an atrophic "cigarette paper" quality.

DIFFERENTIAL DIAGNOSIS   Parapsoriasis

Small Plaque/Large Plaque
- Pityriasis rosea/mycosis fungoides
- Drug eruption
- Pityriasis lichenoides chronica/psoriasis
- Psoriasis/poikiloderma
- Nummular dermatitis/connective tissue disease
- Secondary syphilis
- Cutaneous T-cell lymphoma

Confirming the Diagnosis

- Initial biopsy from two distinct sites is helpful to confirm diagnosis.
- Lesions should be free of topical steroid exposure for 3 weeks prior to biopsy.
- Subsequent biopsies should be considered for any patient with an increased number of lesions, increase in lesion size >5 cm, or development of induration, atrophy, or lymphadenopathy.

Treatment

Patients with SPP should be reassured that progression to CTCL is very rare and treatment can be utilized to control symptoms. In contrast, patients with LPP should be treated despite the absence of symptoms because of the potential for progression to CTCL.

Topical

- Initial treatment may include the use of antihistamines and topical corticosteroids.
- Dry and sensitive skin care and emollients should be incorporated to reduce scaling.
- High-potency topical corticosteroids can be utilized with caution.
- Other topical agents for LPP, such as topical nitrogen mustard and topical carmustine (BCNU), can be utilized but these treatments should be initiated and followed by experienced dermatology providers.

Systemic

- PUVA is preferred for LPP and usually required for control and remission of disease

Management and Patient Education

- Patients with SPP can be reassured that this is considered a benign, chronic condition and does not progress to more significant disease. It can last from several months to years and often spontaneously resolves without treatment over time.
- LPP can remain stable for many years; however, there is potential for the disease to progress to CTCL. The 5-year survival rate remains high and is greater than 90%.
- All patients with LPP should be referred to a dermatologist. Long-term follow-up is imperative, and periodic biopsies should be performed especially if there is any change in cutaneous presentation. Close follow-up every 1 to 3 months is needed for patients undergoing treatment for LPP and then at least annually.

READINGS AND REFERENCES

Alaizari, N., Al-Maweri, S., Al-Shamiri, H., Tarakji, B., & Shugaa-Addin, B. (2016). Hepatitis C virus infections in oral lichen planus: A systematic review and meta-analysis. *Australian Dental Journal, 61*(3), 282–287. https://doi.org/10.1111/adj.12382

Atzmony, L., Reiter, O., Hodak, E., Gdalevich, M., & Mimouni, D. (2016). Treatments for cutaneous lichen planus: A systematic review and meta-analysis. *American Journal of Clinical Dermatology, 17*(1), 11–22.

Avanlowo, O., Akinkuabe, A., & Olumide, Y. (2010). The pityriasis rosea calendar: A 7-year review of seasonal variation, age and sex distribution. *Nigerian Quarterly Journal of Hospital Medicine, 20*(1), 29–31.

Bellinato. F., Maurelli, M., Gisondi, P., & Girolomoni, G. (2019). A systematic review of treatments for pityriasis lichenoides. *Journal of the European Academy of Dermatology and Venereology, 33*(11), 2039–2049.

Bhutani, T., Hong, J., & Koo, J. (2011). *Contemporary diagnosis and management of psoriasis* (5th ed.). Handbooks in Health Care Co.

Broccolo, F., Drago, F., Careddu, A. M., Foglieni, C., Turbino, L., Cocuzza, C. E., & Malnati, M. S. (2005). Additional evidence that pityriasis rosea is associated with reactivation of human herpesvirus-6 and -7. *Journal of Investigative Dermatology, 124*(6), 1234–1240.

Contreras-Ruiz, J., Peternel, S., Gutiérrez, C. J., Culav-Koscak, I., Reveiz, L., & Silbermann-Reynoso, M. (2019). Interventions for pityriasis rosea. In *Cochrane Database of Systematic Reviews.* https://doi.org/10.1002/14651858.CD005068.pub3

Drago, F., Broccolo, F., Javor, S., Drago, F., Rebora, A., & Parodi, A. (2014). Evidence of human herpesvirus-6 and -7 reactivation in miscarrying women with pityriasis rosea. *Journal of the American Academy of Dermatology, 71*(1), 198–199. https://doi.org/10.1016/j.jaad.2014.02.023

Drago, F., Brocollo, F., Zaccaria, E., Malnati, M., Cocuzza, C., Lusso, P., & Rebora, A. (2008). Pregnancy outcome in patients with pityriasis rosea. *Journal of American Academy of Dermatology, 58*(5 Suppl), S78–S83.

Gelfand, J. M., Shin, D. B., Neimann, A. L., Wang, X., Margolis, D., & Troxel, A. B. (2006). The risk of lymphoma in patients with psoriasis. *Journal of Investigative Dermatology, 126*(10), 2194–2201.

Lebwohl, M., Heyman, W., Berth-Jones, J., & Coulson, I. (2017a). Lichen planus. In *Treatment of skin disease* (5th ed.). Saunders Elsevier.

Lebwohl, M., Heyman, W., Berth-Jones, J., & Coulson, I. (2017b). Pityriasis lichenoides chronica. In *Treatment of skin disease* (5th ed.). Saunders Elsevier.

Menter, A., Korman, N. J., Elmets, C. A., Feldman, S., Gelfand, J., Gordon, K. B., Van de Kerkhof, P., & Schalkwijk, J. (2018). Psoriasis. In J. L. Bolognia, J. L. Jorizzo, & R. P. Rapini (Eds.). *Dermatology* (4th ed.). Mosby Elsevier.

Nassef, N. E., & Hammam, M. (1997). The relation between toxoplasmosis and pityriasis lichenoides chronica. *Journal of the Egyptian Society of Parasitology, 27*(1), 93–99.

Rosenbach, M., Hsu, S., Korman, N. J., Lebwohl, M. G., Young, M., Bebo, B. F., & Van Voorhees, A. S. (2010). Treatment of erythrodermic psoriasis: From the medical board of the National Psoriasis Foundation. *Journal of the American Academy of Dermatology, 62*(4), 655–662. https://doi.org/10.1016/j.jaad.2009.05.048

Rothe, M. J., Bernstein, M. L., & Grant-Kels, J. M. (2005). Life-threatening erythroderma: Diagnosing and treating the "red man." *Clinics in Dermatology, 23*(2), 206–217. https://doi.org/10.1016/j.clindermatol.2004.06.018

Schadt, C. (2018). Pityriasis rosea. *JAMA Dermatology, 154*(12), 1496. https://doi.org/10.1001/jamadermatol.2018.3290

Suresh, S., Chokshi, K., Desai S., Malu, R., & Chokshi, A. (2016). Medical management of oral lichen planus: A systematic review. *Journal of Clinical and Diagnostic Research, 10*(2), ZE10–ZE15. https://doi.org/10.7860/JCDR/2016/16715.7225

Wood, G. S., & Reizner, G. (2018). Other papulosquamous disorders. In J. L. Bolognia, J. L. Jorizzo, & R.P. Rapini (Eds.). *Dermatology* (4th ed.). Mosby Elsevier.

Xing, C., Shen, H., Xu, J., Liu, Z., Zhu, J., & Xu, A. (2017). A fatal case of febrile ulceronecrotic Mucha-Habermann disease which presenting as toxic epidermal necrolysis. *Indian Journal of Dermatology, 62*(6), 675. https://doi.org/10.4103/ijd.IJD_631_16

Zang, J., Coates, S., Huang, J., Vonderheid, E., & Cohen, B. (2018). Pityriasis lichenoides: Long-term follow-up study. *Pediatric Dermatology, 35*(2), 213–219.

Approach to the Itchy Patient

Susan T. Voss

In This Chapter

- Pruritus
- Pruritus Categories
- Approach to the Itchy Patient
- Itch without a Rash
- Pruritus Management

PRURITUS

Pruritus is defined as an unpleasant sensation of the skin leading to the desire to scratch. Itch, as a symptom, is the most common reason patients seek care in dermatology. Pruritus can either be localized (e.g., notalgia paresthetica [NP]) or generalized (e.g., renal disease) and can be acute or chronic (>6 weeks).

- Acute pruritus is often the result of an inflammatory dermatitis, whereas chronic pruritus is usually due to an underlying systemic disease.

- Chronic itch has been reported in 10% to 50% of patients with a systemic disease, but less than 1% to 8% is associated with malignancy (Fett et al., 2014). Itch may impact patients physically, mentally, and financially. Pruritic patients are estimated to spend $4,843.68 more annually in healthcare expenditures compared to their nonpruritic counterparts. Data suggest chronic pruritus is associated with $90 billion per year in health expenditures in the United States. Patients with chronic itch are some of the most challenging for a provider to manage (Tripathi et al., 2019).

Etiology of Pruritus

Although pruritus is a diagnosis, it also represents a symptom that occurs secondary to dermatologic conditions, systemic diseases, or medications. If an underlying cause of pruritus is not identified after a thorough history and physical examination, review of systems, and diagnostic evaluation, the pruritus is termed *pruritus of unknown origin*. This represents 8% of patients with chronic pruritus (Millington et al., 2018).

Pathophysiology

The pathophysiology of pruritus is complex, multifactorial, and has been debated and studied by many. Pruritic stimuli (e.g., histamines, leukotrienes, opioids, prostaglandins) cause signal transmission of itch sensation along unmyelinated C neuron fibers to the spinal cord, ascends to the spinothalamic tract, and interacts with multiple locations within the cerebral cortex. Scratching causes pain that temporarily relieves the itch sensation.

Pruritus Categories

- *Pruritus associated with primary lesions* (Table 5.1-1) suggests an underlying skin condition. The identification of the primary lesions is warranted.

- *Pruritus associated with secondary lesions* (e.g., lichenification, erosions) can be clinically misleading. The clinician must perform a thorough head to toe skin examination with the intent to identify primary lesions. In the absence of primary lesions, the secondary lesions are assumed to develop as a result of ongoing scratching due to an underlying systemic disease or pruritus of unknown origin.

- *Pruritus associated with no skin findings* indicates neither primary nor secondary lesions on examination and suggests an underlying systemic disease (Table 5.1-2) as the cause of pruritus (see Fig. 5.1-2).

- *Pruritus associated with pharmacotherapy* may present in the presence or absence of skin findings (see Table 5.1-3). Evaluation of any patient with pruritus should include a detailed history of medications including prescription, over-the-counter (OTC), and supplements. Care should be taken to also note any change in dosages, branding or generic, or formulation. When skin findings are present, the clinician should formulate a differential diagnosis for the skin eruption based upon the primary lesions (see Fig. 5.1-3).

Pruritus Distribution

- Generalized pruritus can be accompanied by primary lesions, secondary lesions, or no skin findings. If primary lesions are present, the distribution of primary lesions will assist with narrowing the differential diagnosis list (e.g., extensor surfaces and psoriasis).

- Localized pruritus may also be associated with primary lesions, secondary lesions, or no skin findings. In the absence of primary

TABLE 5.1-1	Primary Lesions of Skin Diseases Associated with Pruritus
Inflammatory Disorders Erythema, scale, papules, plaques Patches	Atopic dermatitis Contact dermatitis Drug eruptions Psoriasis Lichen planus
Infectious/Infestation Papules, pustules, crust, burrows, nits	Bacterial Viral Fungal Scabies Pediculosis Folliculitis
Autoimmune Disorders Erythema, scale Vesicles, bullae Annular erythematous patches	Bullous pemphigoid Dermatitis herpetiformis Dermatomyositis Lupus erythematosus
Genodermatoses Erythema, scale, crust, erosions	Darier disease Hailey–Hailey disease Ichthyoses
Pregnancy Papules, urticarial plaques Bullae	Polymorphic eruption of pregnancy Pemphigoid gestationis Prurigo gestationis
Malignancy Eczematous patches Red/Violaceous nodules	Cutaneous T-cell lymphoma Cutaneous B-cell lymphoma Leukemia

Adapted from Stander, S., Weisshaar, E., Mettang, T., Szepietowski, J. C., Carstens, E., Ikoma, A., & Bernhard, D. (2007). Clinical classification of itch: A position paper of the international forum for the study of itch. *Acta Dermato-Vernereologica, 87*, 291–294.

lesions, the most common causes of localized pruritus are neurologic and psychogenic.

Pruritus Characteristics

- Pruritus can be mild to severe and can be intermittent, paroxysmal, or constant.
- Consider an underlying neurologic cause when itch is associated with burning, tingling, stinging, or paresthesias.

HOW TO APPROACH A PATIENT WITH ITCH

History

- The evaluation of pruritus begins with a comprehensive personal and family history.
- A detailed review of systems can be critical in identifying underlying systemic diseases.
- A psychosocial history may reveal associated behaviors (i.e., substance abuse) or lifestyle (i.e., homeless or living group home/shelter) indicting potential causes for pruritus.
- Detailed history of prescription and nonprescription medications and skin care practices.

Physical Examination

- Patients complaining of pruritus should have a comprehensive skin examination. Often, individuals may not associate pruritus in one area of their body with skin changes in other areas.

TABLE 5.1-2	Systemic Diseases Associated with Chronic Pruritus	
SYSTEM	**DIAGNOSIS**	
Renal	Chronic kidney disease Uremic pruritus	
Hepatic	Hepatitis B Hepatitis C Chronic liver disease with or without cholestasis	
Endocrine	Hyperthyroidism Hypothyroidism Malabsorption syndrome Perimenopausal pruritus	
Neuropathic	Cerebrovascular accident Multiple sclerosis Small fiber neuropathy Brachioradial pruritus Notalgia paresthetica Postherpetic neuralgia	
Hematology	Polycythemia vera Iron deficiency anemia	
Malignancy	Lymphoma Leukemia Solid organ tumor	
Pregnancy	Pruritus gravidarum Cholestasis of pregnancy	
Infection	Human immunodeficiency syndrome with decreasing CD4 counts Parasitosis Helminthiasis	
Psychogenic	Depression Anxiety Obsessive compulsive disorder Fatigue Schizophrenia Delusions Psychosomatic	

Adapted from Millington, G. W. M., Collins, A., Lovell, C. R., Leslie, T. A., Yong, A. S. W., Morgan, J. D., Ajithkumar, T., Andrews, M. J., Rushbook, S. M., Coelho, R. R., Catten, S. J., Lee, K. Y. C., Skellett, A. M., Affleck, A. G., Exton, L. S., Mohd Mustapa, M. F., & Levell, N. J. (2018). British Association of Dermatologists' guidelines for the investigation and management of generalized pruritus in adults without an underlying dermatosis, 2018. *The British Journal of Dermatology, 178*(1), 34–60.

Diagnostic Approach

- *Is there a rash or skin findings?* Asking this important question may guide the clinician to approach the rash from two different perspectives: an itch without a rash or a rash that itches.

ITCH WITHOUT A RASH

General pruritus present for more than 6 weeks without skin lesions should be carefully evaluated.

Skin Findings

- There are no primary skin lesions.
- There may be secondary lesions, changes from chronicity, or therapies to treat the itch.

TABLE 5.1-3	**Medications Associated with Pruritus**
DRUG/ CLASSIFICATION	**AGENT(S)**
Antiarrhythmic	Amiodarone
Anticoagulant	Ticlopidine, fractionated heparin
Antidiabetic	Biguanide, sulfonylurea derivatives
Antiepileptic	Carbamazepine, oxcarbazepine, phenytoin, fosphenytoin, topiramate
Antihypertensive	Angiotensin-converting enzyme inhibitors[a], angiotensin II antagonists, adrenergic blockers, calcium-channel blockers, methyldopa
Antimicrobial, chemotherapeutic	Penicillin[a], cephalosporin, macrolides, carbapenem, quinolone, tetracycline, metronidazole, rifampin, trimethoprim/sulfamethoxazole, antimalarial (chloroquine[a,b])
Cytokines, growth factors, monoclonal antibodies	Granulocyte macrophage colony-stimulating factor, interleukin 2[a], mitumomab, lapatinib
Cytostatic	Chlorambucil, paclitaxel, tamoxifen
Erectile dysfunction	Sildenafil
Lipid lowering	Statins[a]
Plasma volume expander	Hydroxyethyl starch (HES)[a]
Psychotropic	Tricyclic antidepressants, selective serotonin reuptake inhibitors, neuroleptics
Other	Antithyroid agents, nonsteroidal anti-inflammatory drugs, corticosteroids, sex hormones, opioids[a], inhibitors of xanthine oxidase, allopurinol

[a]Most common. [b]Especially in 60% to 70% African Americans.
Adapted from Reich, A., Stander, S., & Szepietowski, J. C. (2009). Drug-induced pruritus: A review. *Acta Dermato-Venereologica, 89*, 236–244. https://doi.org/10.2340/00015555-0650.

Confirming the Diagnosis

- There is no consensus on the exact diagnostic workup for patients with severe pruritus without evidence of an underlying disease.
- An algorithmic approach to the initial diagnostics can be helpful (Fig. 5.1-1).
- A punch biopsy is of little diagnostic value if there is no primary lesion. Biopsy of secondary lesions may only show ulcerations from the trauma of scratching or picking.

Differential Diagnosis

See Table 5.1-3 for dermatologic, systemic, and medications associated with pruritus. In the absence of any positive diagnostics or ability to identify an underlying cause, it is typically classified as pruritus of unknown origin.

Treatment

- Topical therapy is the treatment of choice for pruritus without a skin eruption.

- If topical therapy fails to control the itch or if the body surface area (BSA) involved is too extensive, then the clinician may need to add or change to systemic therapy (Box 5.1-1).

Topical

- Calcineurin inhibitors (tacrolimus 0.1%, pimecrolimus 1%) b.i.d. can be beneficial in facial and anogenital pruritus.
- Topical corticosteroids (TCS medium to ultra-high potency) for a trial period of 2 to 4 weeks (see Section 1.4 for TCS guidelines).
- Doxepin 5% cream (a tricyclic antidepressant). Limit to 8 days and no more than 10% BSA. Risk of allergic contact dermatitis and toxicity from systemic absorption. Maximum 12 g per day (Millington et al., 2018). May cause drowsiness.

OTC Topicals

- Topical capsaicin in concentrations up to 0.1% four to six times daily for neuropathic/uremic pruritus.
- Pramoxine 1% or 2.5% cream three to four times daily.
- Topical anesthetics such as combination lidocaine and prilocaine 2.5% cream.
- Topical menthol provides a coolant, counter-irritant effect.

Systemic

Unfortunately, research has failed to reveal a singular effective topical or systemic therapy for pruritus. Systemic therapies for pruritus should be utilized in combination with topical therapies when the topical therapies alone are unsuccessful. When possible, the systemic treatment should be targeted at the suspected underlying cause of the itch, if identified. For example, patients with suspected chronic kidney disease (CKD) may benefit from gabapentin. The following "add-on" medications can be considered:

- Antihistamines may assist with reducing pruritus by blocking H1 receptors on afferent C nerve fibers, inhibit degranulation of pruritus mediators from mast cells, or by causing drowsiness. Antihistamines are dosed three to four times the recommended dosage, but are often of limited efficacy. While readily available, these medications should be prescribed with caution in older adults due to increased risk of anti-cholinergic adverse effects, and the following alternative systemic medications should be considered first.
- Oral glucocorticoids should be limited to controlling acute severe forms of pruritus and should not be prescribed until the underlying cause has been identified, as glucocorticoids may mask symptoms.
- Neuroactive medications—gabapentin and pregabalin—have been effective for treating pruritus caused by CKD as well as neuropathic pruritus.
- Selective serotonin reuptake inhibitors (SSRIs) such as paroxetine 10 to 20 mg daily have been reported to be beneficial for various forms of chronic pruritus. The exact mechanism by which SSRIs influence pruritus may be due to regulation of serotonin levels.
- Tetracyclic antidepressants such as Mirtazapine 15 to 30 mg may relieve nocturnal itch. The exact mechanism by which tetracyclic antidepressants influence pruritus may be due to regulation of serotonin and histamine levels.
- Tricyclic antidepressants such as amitriptyline 5 to 10 mg at bedtime may be helpful with neuropathic itch. Increase gradually to 50 to 150 mg to achieve efficacy. The exact mechanism by which

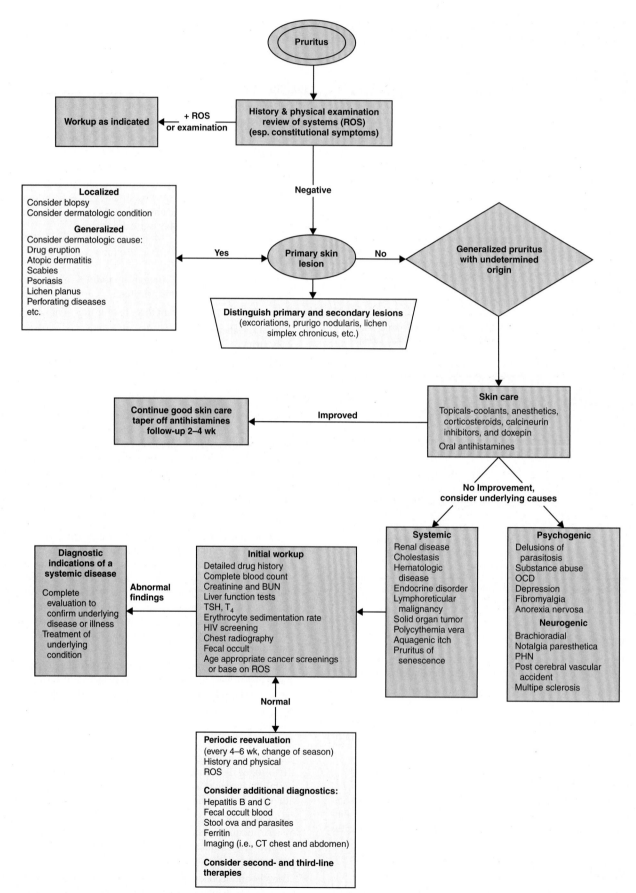

FIG. 5.1-1. Approach to assessing patients with chronic pruritus.

BOX 5.1-1 Treatment for Pruritus

First-Line Topical Therapies

Good skin care (Box 5.1-2)
Emollients—petrolatum, ceramide-based creams
Cooling agents—menthol, camphor, ice
Topical anti-inflammatory medication—corticosteroids, calcineurin inhibitors
Topical anesthetics—capsaicin, pramoxine, lidocaine/prilocaine
Predominantly nerve modulation—topical doxepin

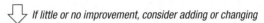 *If little or no improvement, consider adding*

Systemic: Antihistamines (AH)

Low dose—nonsedating AH daily
High dose—nonsedating AH b.i.d.–q.i.d., or combination with sedating AH at bedtime

First-Generation, Sedating	Second-Generation, Nonsedating
Hydroxyzine	Cetirizine
Diphenhydramine	Levocetirizine
	Fexofenadine
	Loratadine
	Desloratadine

If little or no improvement, consider adding or changing

Other Systemic Agents[a]

1st Choice	2nd Choice	3rd Choice
Gabapentin/Pregabalin[b]	SSRI	Naltrexone
Selective serotonin reuptake inhibitors (SSRIs)[c]	Tricyclic or tetracyclic antidepressant	Lidocaine 5% patch
Naltrexone[d]	Phototherapy: narrow-band UVR	
Aprepitant		
Dupilumab		

[a]Off-label use.
[b]Neuropathic, postherpetic, prurigo nodularis, scalp itch, genital itch, post burn itch.
[c]Paraneoplastic, polycythemia vera, or depression.
[d]Renal or liver dysfunction.
Adapted from Steinhoff, M., Cevikbas, F., Ikoma, A., & Berger, T. G. (2011). Pruritus: Management algorithms and experimental therapies. *Seminars in Cutaneous Medicine and Surgery, 30,* 127–137. https://doi.org/10.1016/j.sder.2011.05.001

tricyclic antidepressants influence pruritus may be due to regulation of serotonin and histamine levels.

- Opiate agonists and antagonist may also aid in relief of resistant chronic pruritus.

- Dupilumab, approved for atopic dermatitis (AD) is being evaluated and showing potential for treating chronic pruritus (Zhai et al., 2019).

- Acupuncture may be useful.

- Consider behavioral-modification therapy that can complement other treatment modalities.

Management and Patient Education

- Referral to a dermatology provider should be considered when the cause of the pruritus is not apparent or when basic treatments have provided no relief. Other specialists (nephrologist, hepatologist) may be consulted depending on the underlying disease.

- Prognosis depends on the possible underlying disease associated with the pruritus.

- Symptomatic relief is often the focus of treatment unless there is an identified underlying cause.

- Good skin care should be an essential part of the treatment plan for all patients with pruritus (see Box 5.1-2).

BOX 5.1-2 Basic Care of Pruritic Skin

- Keep fingernails short and smooth.
- Avoid hot water. Bathe or shower in tepid/lukewarm water for 20 minutes.
- Avoid washing with soap (especially antibacterial soaps).
- Use gentle cleansers that are moisturizing and fragrance-free when needed.
- Use mild cleansers only on the axillae, genitalia, and soles of the feet.
- Avoid abrasive products (exfoliants or scrubs) or devices (loofahs or rough sponges) on the skin during bathing.
- Apply topical emollients/moisturizers immediately after bathing to skin that has been gently patted dry.
- Moisturizers with ceramides and lipids are preferred. If cost is an issue, petrolatum (petroleum jelly) may be used.
- Moisturize an additional one to two times daily.
- Apply gently in the direction of hair growth. Caution: heavy emollients or occlusion can cause folliculitis.
- Topicals with menthol and camphor may be utilized. Refrigeration may aid in the soothing effect.
- Avoid fragrance and dyes.
- Remove tags from clothing that may exacerbate itch.
- Avoid scratching and instead try patting or tapping the skin.

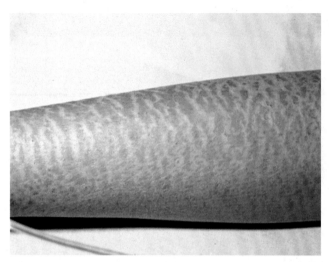

FIG. 5.1-2. Severe xerosis associated with renal failure.

- While treating the itch, it is important to monitor for signs and symptoms of secondary infection, such as impetigo, cellulitis, and herpes simplex virus, that may occur from scratching. A culture and sensitivity should be performed for diagnosis and treatment.

- Collaboration with psychiatry can be helpful in patients with psychodermatoses. The introduction of this topic should be done carefully and after the clinician has developed a relationship with the patient.

CLINICAL PEARLS

- Patients with idiopathic pruritus do not have a significant increased risk for malignant neoplasms when compared to the general population. Evaluation for an underlying malignancy should be considered if pruritus is generalized, persistent, without an identified cause, and fails to respond to conventional therapy.

- For some patients with HIV, pruritus may be from a secondary infection or process such as Norwegian scabies, candidiasis, colonization of *Staphylococcus aureus*, an overgrowth of the Demodex mite, seborrheic dermatitis, acquired ichthyosis, Kaposi sarcoma, pruritic papular eruptions, and eosinophilic folliculitis (Singh & Rudikoff, 2012).

- For patients with CKD-associated pruritus, concomitant xerosis frequently exacerbates symptoms (Fig. 5.1-2).

Itch that Rashes

Susan T. Voss

For patients presenting with the chief complaint of itch and rash, the clinician must distinguish between primary and secondary lesions.

- The identification of primary lesions (e.g., blisters, scaly plaques) will lead the clinician down the morphology based approach (see Figure 1.3-5) to diagnosing a skin lesion.

- Secondary lesions can also be associated with numerous dermatologic conditions; however, they can develop on normal skin as a result of repeated scratching or manipulation due to chronic itch.

- For patients with secondary lesions, clinicians must identify the presence or absence of primary lesions to avoid a delay in diagnosis, unnecessary testing, and inappropriate treatments.

- Three common skin conditions that present as a result of chronic itch, whether due to underlying dermatologic condition or as a result of pruritus of unknown origin are NP, lichen simplex chronicus (LSC), and prurigo nodularis (PN).

Notalgia Paresthetica

NP is an example of pruritus that is a common yet often missed diagnosis. NP is thought to be due to compression of posterior rami of the spinal nerves at the T2–T6 level and is characterized by unilateral involvement of the scapula area with associated pruritus, burning, increased sensitivity, or tenderness (Fig. 5.2-1). Skin findings are localized to the affected area and include pigmented patch, excoriations, or less often lichenification. See Section 5.1 for pruritus treatment considerations.

Lichen Simplex Chronicus

LSC is a chronic skin condition that develops from repetitive scratching and rubbing of the skin resulting in lichenification or thickening of the skin.

It is more common among women than men and does not differ in frequency among races.

LSC is more prominent in middle to older adults. It occurs more in individuals with anxiety or obsessive-compulsive disorders. AD patients may exhibit LSC due to the pruritic nature of AD.

Common Associated Conditions

- *Dermatologic*
  - AD
  - Allergic contact dermatitis
  - Seborrheic dermatitis
  - Acne keloidalis nuchae
  - Scars

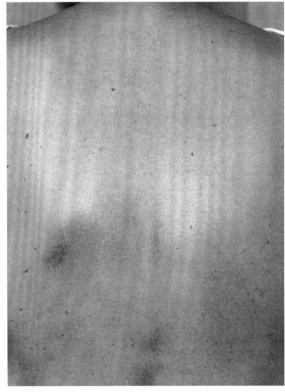

FIG. 5.2-1. Characteristics of notalgia paresthetica include hyperpigmentation from severe pruritus near the angle of the scapula.

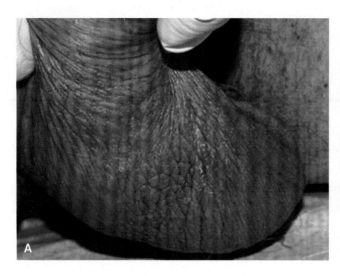
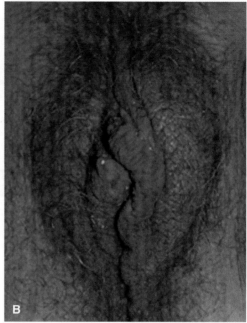

FIG. 5.2-2. **A:** Accentuated skin lines of lichen simplex of the scrotum. **B:** Even patients who are not naturally dark sometimes exhibit hyperpigmentation that obscures the inflammation of lichen simplex chronicus, as seen on this left labia majora.

- Insect bites
- Chronic pruritus
- Xerosis
- Psoriasis
- *Neurologic disorders*
  - NP
  - Brachioradialis pruritus

Psychological Factors

- Emotional tensions or anxiety disorders may play a role in inducing itch, leading to the self-perpetuating itch-scratch cycle.
  - Anxiety
  - Obsessive-compulsive disorder
  - Depression

Environmental Factors

- Environmental factors can contribute to the pruritus.
  - Heat
  - Irritants
  - Sweat

Pathophysiology

- The etiology of LSC is thought to be associated with sensitization.
- Evaluation and comparison of the histopathology features of LSC and PN provides more insight into their pathogenesis.
- LSC is characterized by epidermal hyperplasia, orthokeratosis, hypergranulosis, normal elongation of rete ridges, perivascular infiltrates of lymphocytes, and to a lesser degree macrophages. In contrast to PN, LSC does not have neural hyperplasia or increased nerve growth factor.

Clinical Presentation

Skin Findings

- Lesions present on areas easily accessible to the patient
  - Nape of the neck
  - Occipital scalp
  - Extensor surfaces of the arms and legs
  - External genitalia (Fig. 5.2-2)
  - Perianal areas
- Hyperpigmented, thick, scaly, lichenified plaques
- Exaggerated skin lines (Fig. 5.2-3)
- May evolve to a leathery texture over time
- Secondary erosions or ulcerations may be present

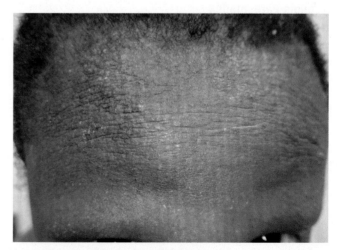

FIG. 5.2-3. Hyperpigmented scaly lichenified plaques. No exaggerated skin lines (lichenification). (Used with permission from Gru, A. A., & Wick, M. [2018]. *Pediatric dermatopathology and dermatology.* Wolters Kluwer Health.)

Non-Skin Findings

- Patient may reveal that they have a tendency to scratch or pick.
- Patients may or may not be aware of their habitual scratching and rubbing, and it may occur when the patient is asleep.
- May appear anxious or nervous during visit.
- Patient may nervously scratch or rub on skin during the visit.

DIFFERENTIAL DIAGNOSIS LSC

- Allergic dermatitis
- Atopic dermatitis
- Nummular dermatitis
- Hypertrophic lichen planus
- Psoriasis
- Lichen sclerosis
- Verruca vulgaris
- Tinea
- Acanthosis nigricans
- Notalgia paresthetica
- Acne keloidalis nuchae
- Keloid

Confirming the Diagnosis

- LSC is usually a clinical diagnosis.
- The primary focus of the clinician is to identify the underlying cause of pruritus.
- Consider skin biopsy for histopathology if:
  - underlying cause of pruritus cannot be identified.
  - clinical features suspicious for underlying malignancy (e.g., growing, bleeding).
  - failure to improve with topical therapy and considering systemic therapy.

Treatment

Goals

- Identify the underlying cause of pruritus.
- Breaking the itch–scratch cycle.
- Risk reduction for secondary infections.
- See Treatment Section 5.1 for nonpharmaceutical options for assisting with managing itch.

Topical

- Antipruritics, topical anesthetics, and emollients can provide immediate relief of pruritus (see Treatment in Section 5.1). This should be the first line when managing LSC. If desired effect is not achieved, may add in TCS.
- High-potency TCS with or without occlusion can ease the pruritus and, equally important, provide a barrier to prevent more scratching or rubbing to affected areas.
  - Clobetasol 0.05% ointment b.i.d. or daily if under occlusion.
  - Betamethasone dipropionate augmented 0.05% ointment b.i.d. or daily if under occlusion.
  - As the pruritus improves, the application of TCS can be decreased in frequency to three times weekly or switch potency to a moderate TCS (e.g., triamcinolone 0.1%).
- Upon discontinuation of TCS, a topical calcineurin inhibitor may continue to improve and maintain the LSC. Tacrolimus 0.1% ointment or pimecrolimus 1% cream twice daily to the affected area.

Systemic

- When the patient does not respond fully to topical therapies, a systemic option may provide additional relief.
- Systemic options should be added to the topical therapy, rather than abandoning the topical for systemic.
- Treatment with antihistamines, SSRIs or oral doxepin may assist with reducing pruritus.
- Intralesional corticosteroids are effective in controlling pruritus and reducing the size of involved lesions. Potency should be based on the thickness of the plaques.
  - Begin with triamcinolone 5 mg/cc taking care to stay within the lesion and avoid deep injection.
  - Very thick lesions may require triamcinolone 10 mg/cc concentration.
  - Smaller localized areas and lesions.
  - Areas not conducive to occlusion, that is, extensor surface of the elbow.

Management and Patient Education

- Patients should be educated that resolution of the symptoms will require more than pharmacologic intervention and be dependent on behavioral modification.
- Complete resolution can occur if the patient is successful in halting the scratching behaviors.
- Patients with concomitant psychological factors may be challenging to manage and may require a multidisciplinary team that includes primary care, dermatology, psychiatry, or psychologist.
- Complications of LSC include:
  - Secondary infection
  - Hyperpigmentation
  - Scarring
- Reoccurrence is more common when:
  - underlying etiology is not properly identified or treated.
  - unable to break the itch–scratch cycle.
- If the patient is using TCS, follow-up with the clinician should include routine examination of the site to evaluate efficacy and any atrophy.
- Clinicians should also monitor the patient for level of itching, improved or worsened.
- Initially when treating LSC, the patient should be evaluated every 2 weeks.
- As symptoms improve and therapy is transitioned to maintenance, the clinician can extend the follow-up to 1 to 2 months.
- If the patient is not responding to therapy or the underlying cause of LSC is not evident, the clinician should refer to dermatology.
- If the clinician is unable to distinguish LSC from other dermatologic conditions, referral to dermatology for skin biopsy may be necessary.

Special Considerations

- Anogenital LSC
  - The primary patient complaint is itch. LSC may be caused by various conditions such as allergic or irritant contact dermatitis, candidiasis, lichen sclerosus, lichen planus, psoriasis, and vulvar intraepithelial neoplasia.

- It is critical the clinician elucidate the cause in order to treat properly. If not evident, the patient may benefit from referral or consultation with dermatology, gynecology, or urology.
- Topical corticosteroids are the topical pharmacologic treatment of choice.
- The anogenital area, due to the thin epidermis and increased vascularization warrants caution when treating with TCS. Therapy should begin with low- to medium-potency TCS based on severity of lichenification (i.e., thicker lesions treat with medium-potency TCS one to two times daily for 1 to 2 weeks then wean off).
- The mucus membrane of the vulvar area is resistant to steroids and requires high-potency TCS (Thorstensen & Birnebaum, 2012). The duration of TCS should be limited to 1 to 2 weeks to prevent atrophy.

CLINICAL PEARLS

- Since LSC can occur on flexural surfaces, TCS should be used with caution in those areas. Decreasing the frequency of application by half (i.e., if usually twice daily application instead apply once daily) will help reduce chance of atrophy but still get desired result.

Prurigo Nodularis

PN is a skin condition characterized by firm papules and nodules that are extremely pruritic. PN is commonly referred to as "Picker's Nodules," affects men and women equally, occurs at any age but is more prevalent in middle-aged and older adults, and may occur in all races. One study found African Americans were 3.4 times more likely than Caucasians to have PN (Boozalis et al., 2019). Patients with PN often have a long-standing history of pruritis. They may have a medical history of dermatologic or systemic disorders (Table 5.2-1) that pruritus is a common symptom. In a recent study, patients with PN were greater than four times more likely than controls to have a malignancy diagnosis (Larson et al., 2019).

Pathophysiology

- The etiology of PN is unknown and there is no consensus among experts.

TABLE 5.2-1	Comorbidities Noted with PN Include	
DERMATOLOGIC CONDITIONS	**SYSTEMIC CONDITIONS**
• Atopic dermatitis	• Chronic kidney disease
• Insect bite reaction	• Diabetes
• Scabies	• Hepatitis C
• Stasis dermatitis	• HIV
• Allergic contact dermatitis	• Psychiatric
• Lichen planus	• Neurologic disease
• Dermatitis herpetiformis	• Postherpetic neuralgia
• Bullous pemphigoid	• Brachioradial pruritus
• Keratoacanthomas	• Primary sclerosing cholangitis
• Cutaneous lymphoma	• Primary biliary cirrhosis
	• Choledocholithiasis
	• Hepatocellular cancer

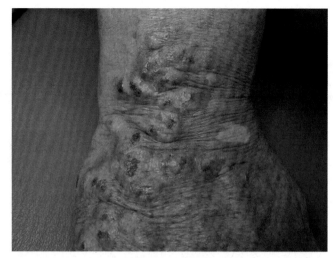

FIG. 5.2-4. Prurigo nodularis. Cluster of lichenified hypertrophic excoriated and eroded nodules on the dorsal hand. (Image provided by Stedman's.)

- Chronic repetitive friction to the skin causes epidermal hypertrophy that presents as thickening of the skin.
- Some studies indicate a neurocutaneous component with increased nerves in the papillary dermis.

Clinical Presentation

Skin Findings

- Firm discrete papules or nodules, 3 to 20 mm in diameter (Fig. 5.2-4).
- Scaly and hyperpigmented.
- Occur on areas easily reached by the patient such as:
  - Extensor surfaces of the hand, arms, and legs.
  - Upper back and to a lesser extent the trunk.

Non-Skin Findings

- Patient may reveal that they had a tendency to scratch or pick.
- Patients may or may not be aware of their habitual scratching and rubbing, and it may occur when the patient is asleep.
- Patients may appear anxious or nervous during visit.
- Patient may nervously scratch or rub on skin during the visit.

DIFFERENTIAL DIAGNOSIS   PN

- Squamous cell carcinoma, especially keratoacanthoma
- Basal cell carcinoma
- Dermatofibroma
- Lichen simplex chronicus
- Sarcoidosis
- Lichen planus
- Keloids
- Acne keloidalis nuchae
- Pseudolymphoma
- Foreign-body reaction
- Perforating folliculitis

Confirming the Diagnosis

- PN is usually a clinical diagnosis.
- The primary focus of the clinician is to identify the underlying cause of pruritus.
- Consider skin biopsy for histopathology if:
  - underlying cause of pruritus cannot be identified.
  - clinical features suspicious for underlying malignancy (e.g., growing, bleeding).
  - failure to improve with topical therapy and considering systemic therapy.

Treatment

See Section 5.1 for guidelines regarding treatment of pruritus.

Management and Patient Education

See Section 5.1 for management guidelines of pruritus.

CLINICAL PEARLS

- Since the forearms are the most common location for PN lesions, they are amenable to treatment with topical corticosteroids with occlusion.
- This can be accomplished with a liberal application of triamcinolone 0.1% ointment to the PN lesions and then occluding by applying a non-raveling gauze impregnated with zinc oxide paste (Unna boot) to the entire forearm starting at the hand.
- The wrap can be left in place for 1 week follow-up appointment. If needed, it can be reapplied.

Psychodermatoses: Self-Induced Skin Disorders

Susan T. Voss

In This Chapter

- Psychodermatoses
  - Factitious Disorder
  - Excoriation (Skin-picking) Disorder
  - Delusional Disorder Somatic Type

Many psychogenic conditions have been associated with pruritus, making diagnosis and treatment challenging. Depression, anxiety, obsessive-compulsive disorder, somatoform disorder, mania, psychosis, fatigue, and substance abuse may all be associated with an intense itch. Three psychogenic conditions that lead to self-induced skin lesions are:

- Factitious disorder (FD)
- Excoriation disorder (ED)
- Delusional disorder somatic type

Factitious Disorder

FD, also known as factitial dermatitis and dermatitis artefacta, is a psychodermatologic disorder in which the patient consciously inflicts harm to the skin in order to achieve a secondary gain (Mostaghimi et al., 2019). The patient may have an unconscious need to assume the sick role and be taken care of. Patients with FD will vehemently deny any self-trauma to the skin, unlike neurotic excoriations and delusions of parasitosis in which the patient will acknowledge picking or scratching the skin.

The exact rates of FD are unknown. Prevalence of FD at dermatology clinics varies. It is more prominent in women than men, 20:1. Although any age may be affected, onset usually is between adolescence and young adulthood (Kuhn et al., 2017).

Pathophysiology

- The pathogenesis of FD is poorly understood.
- Many patients with FD suffer from borderline personality disorder.
- Other mental issues include poor body images perhaps related to physical or sexual abuse, depression, anxiety disorder, and others.

Clinical Presentation

Skin Findings

- The lesions present on areas easily reached by the patient, the extensor surfaces of the arms, face, trunk, and upper back.
- Morphology and pattern of skin eruption varies based on the instrument or substance the patient utilizes. Morphology may include macules, patches, papules, or plaques with excoriations, erosions, or ulcers. Patterns may include angular, curved, geometric, or linear (Fig. 5.3-1).

- They may be unilateral, bilateral, asymmetrical, or symmetrical.
- The rash or lesions do not follow the typical presentation of any common dermatoses.

Non-Skin Findings

- The history of the rash is usually vague and it is difficult to get details regarding onset and aggravating factors (e.g., stressors).

DIFFERENTIAL DIAGNOSIS   Factitious Disorder

- Necrotizing vasculitis
- Bullous skin disease
- Pyoderma gangrenosum
- Vasculitis
- Collagen vascular disease
- Infestation such as scabies
- Neurotic excoriations
- Delusions of parasitosis
- Munchausen disorder
- Obsessive compulsive disorder

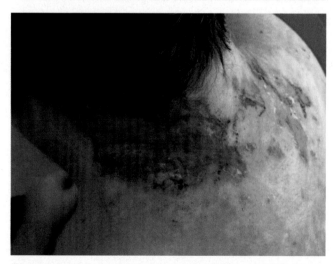

FIG. 5.3-1. Factitial dermatitis. Irregular jagged superficial ulceration to the posterior neck.

Confirming the Diagnosis

- No specific laboratory test or imaging is indicated.
- A skin punch biopsy for histology or direct immunofluorescence may help with confirming the diagnosis and eliminating other causes.

Treatment

- Referral to a mental health provider for therapy is the key. A combination of behavioral and pharmacologic therapy is often required.
- General dermatologic care should be rendered based on the lesions presented.
- Care should be taken to prevent secondary bacterial infections.

Management and Patient Education

- A complete and thorough patient and family history of physical and mental health is critical.
- Caring for the patient with FD is challenging. Establishment of a caring, empathetic, nonjudgmental relationship with the patient is important. Initially the suspected source of the lesion should not be discussed until the rapport is established.
- Care should be taken to address the stress or other symptoms that may be leading to the behavior.
- The primary care provider or dermatology provider's role is to care for the skin but referral to a mental health provider must occur.

Excoriation (Skin Picking) Disorder

ED, also referred to as neurotic excoriations, results from conscious repetitive scratching or picking of the skin that results in observable tissue injury. Exact occurrence rates for ED is unknown but is probably underreported. Some studies indicate women are more likely than men to have ED (Kuhn et al., 2017).

Triggers may be emotional or sedentary activity and boredom. The patient may have had skin pathology including pruritus initially, such as an insect bite, folliculitis, or acne. Patients may use their fingernail, tweezers, or other device to pick at the skin. Psychiatric associated disorders include trichotillomania, tic disorder, obsessive-compulsive disorder, body dysmorphic disorder, depression, and anxiety. Approximately 9% of pruritic patients have ED and 2% of all dermatology patients.

Pathophysiology

- The pathophysiology of ED is poorly understood.
- Experts believe it is a psychiatric disorder such as obsessive-compulsive disorder, that has dermatologic manifestations.

Clinical Presentation

Skin Findings

- Excoriations are limited to body areas where the patient can reach.
- The lesions tend to be on the side of the patient's nondominant hand.
- The lateral areas of the back and shoulders may be involved, while the midline back is spared ("butterfly sign") (Fig. 5.3-2).
- Lesions are also commonly found on the lateral and extensor aspects of the patient's arms and legs (Fig. 5.3-3).

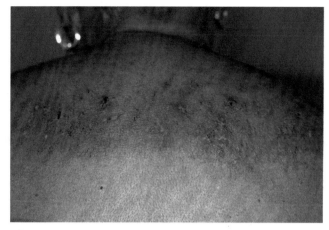

FIG. 5.3-2. Butterfly sign. Absence of lesions to areas patient cannot reach.

- Characteristic erosions have an angular or punched-out appearance from the patient picking with their nails or implements like tweezers.
- Chronic lesions may appear like prurigo nodules.
- Scarring may be present in a linear pattern and is indicative of a chronic problem.

Non-Skin Findings

- Patients are often anxious or reserved.
- Details will be vague and hard to obtain regarding the disorder.
- Patient may voice frustration with previous providers.

DIFFERENTIAL DIAGNOSIS   Excoriation Disorder

- Scabies
- Prurigo nodularis
- Delusions of parasitosis
- Dermatitis herpetiformis
- Arthropod assault
- Vasculitis

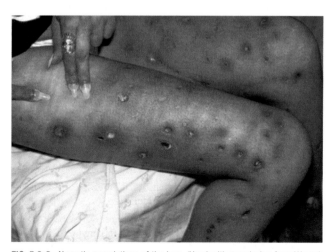

FIG. 5.3-3. Neurotic excoriations of the legs. (Used with permission from Wound, Ostomy and Continence Nurses Society®; Doughty, D. B., & McNichol, L. L. [2015]. *Wound, ostomy and continence nurses society® core curriculum: Wound management.* Wolters Kluwer Health.)

Confirming the Diagnosis

- ED is a diagnosis of exclusion and is often made on clinical appearance.
- A thorough history, including medications, is critical.
- A mineral oil prep slide can rule out scabies.
- CBC and complete chemistry panel to rule out other systemic causes, especially if the condition is generalized.
- Imaging based on any concerns gleaned from the history.
- A punch skin biopsy for histology and/or direct immunofluorescence to rule out other causes.

Treatment

Development of an empathetic nonjudgmental environment with the patient is critical. Referral to a mental health provider for cognitive-behavioral therapy (CBT) or behavior modification therapy is key.

Management and Patient Education

- Patients with ED usually acknowledge that picking is a problem but feel unable to stop.
- Referral to a mental health provider can help set the patient up for success. Emphasis should be on the options to help modify the desire to pick and not that the patient is to blame.

Delusional Disorder Somatic Type (DDST)

DDST has been referred to as delusions of parasitosis and often report a sensation of the bugs crawling under their skin. In dermatology, DDST is the most common monosymptomatic (the sole symptom/delusion experienced), hypochondriacal disorder. This is usually the only manifestation of their psychosis. The typical DDST patient is usually an older Caucasian female. Men may have DDST but are less likely (Campbell et al., 2019). Two peak age ranges exist for DDST, 20 to 30 years of age and greater than 50 years of age. Younger patients usually are of a lower socioeconomic status. In 8% to 12% of the cases, the belief is shared by a loved one, termed folie à deux (delusion for two in close association) (Wong & Koo, 2013).

Pathophysiology

The pathogenesis of DDST is unknown. It is thought to be related to neurochemical pathology.

Clinical Presentation

Skin Findings

- Physically the rash varies from mild excoriations to ulcerations.
- Common sites are areas easily accessed, such as the forearms.

Non-Skin Findings

- Patients hold firm in their belief even when presented with medical evidence that the infestation doesn't exist.
- They may become angry or frustrated when the belief is not shared by their family or the provider.
- Patients may bring in containers with pieces of skin, fiber, lint or crusts that they have removed and are convinced that they are bugs or eggs. A detailed history may be given by the patient regarding the life cycle of the bugs (Fig. 5.3-4).
- Itch or feelings of something crawling beneath the skin may be voiced.

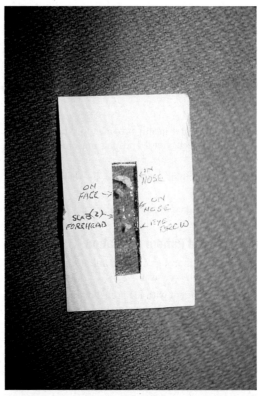

FIG. 5.3-4. Matchbox sign. Patients will bring debris, crusts, or pieces of skin in a container or display. (Used with permission from Hall, J. C., & Hall, B. J. [2017]. *Sauer's manual of skin diseases* [11th ed.]. Wolters Kluwer Health.)

DIFFERENTIAL DIAGNOSIS   Delusional Disorder

- Alzheimer's dementia
- HIV/AIDS
- Recreational use or abuse of drugs
- Side effects of therapeutic drugs
- Scabies
- Dermatitis herpetiformis

Confirming the Diagnosis

- Clinicians must do a complete examination and carefully consider the possibility of a true infestation.
- Microscopic examination of the "bugs" that the patient brings must be performed to validate their concern but also to assure the patient there is no evidence of infestation.
- Mineral oil prep for scabies.
- If pruritus is a major complaint, the appropriate pruritic workup to rule out a primary etiology is needed.
- A skin biopsy to rule out other causes of pathology.

Treatment

- Treatment for pruritus (see Section 5.1) including topical corticosteroids.
- Patients should be referred to psychiatry for treatment with psychotropic drugs. However, this is difficult and has to be broached slowly.
- Addressing proper care of the skin is important to avoid secondary infections.

Management and Patient Education

- This can be an extremely difficult patient to manage but should begin with establishing a trusting clinician–patient relationship.
- Even when there is no identified cause, the clinician should acknowledge the strong physical and psychological stress that the patient is reporting.
- The clinician should acknowledge how frustrating it must be for the patient that an infestation cannot be confirmed.
- Many patients with DDST will isolate themselves in an attempt to limit contaminating family and friends.
- On a follow-up visit, the clinician should introduce the idea of psychological counseling, not because the patient is "crazy," but because this condition is causing the patient so much anxiety and emotional upset.
- Referral to dermatology should be made to evaluate, diagnose, and treat the skin.

Special Considerations

Morgellons disease (MD) was once considered synonymous with delusions of parasitosis. However, MD differs from delusions of parasitosis in that patients believe there are fibers or filaments that lie under, protrude, or are attached to the skin.

CLINICAL PEARLS

- No matter the disorder, the importance of developing a trusting patient–clinician relationship is imperative.
- Without it, the patient will become frustrated and likely will not return for further care, leaving the condition to worsen.

READINGS AND REFERENCES

Beach, S. R., Kroshinsky, D., & Kontos, N. (2014). Case records of the Massachusetts General Hospital. Case 37-2014: A 35-year-old woman with suspected mite infestation. *The New England Journal of Medicine, 371*(22), 2115–2123.

Beck, K., Yang, E., Sekhon, S., Bhutani, T., & Liao, W. (2019). Dupilumab treatment for generalized prurigo nodularis. *JAMA Dermatology, 155*(1), 118–120.

Berger, T., & Steinhoff, M. (2011). Pruritus and renal failure. *Seminars in Cutaneous Medicine and Surgery, 30*(2), 99–100.

Boozalis, E., Tang, O., Patel, S., Semenov, Y., Pereira, M., Stander, S., Kang, S., & Kwatra, S. (2019). Ethnic differences and comorbidities of 909 prurigo nodularis patients. *Journal of the American Academy of Dermatology, 79*(4), 714–719.

Campbell, E., Elston, D., Hawthorne, J., & Beckert, D. (2019). Diagnosis and management of delusional parasitosis. *Journal of the American Academy of Dermatology, 80*(5), 1428–1434.

Elmariah, S., & Lerner, E. (2011). Topical therapies for pruritus. *Seminars in Cutaneous Medicine and Surgery, 30*(2), 118–126.

Fett, N., Haynes, K., Propert, K. J., & Margolis, D. J. (2014). Five-year malignancy incidence in patients with chronic pruritus: A population-based cohort study aimed at limiting unnecessary screening practices. *Journal of the American Academy of Dermatology, 70*(4), 651–658.

Gobbi, P., Attardo-Parrinello, G., Lattanzio, G., Rizzo, S., & Ascari, E. (1983). Severe pruritus should be a B-symptom in Hodgkin's disease. *Cancer, 51*(10), 1934–1936.

He, A., Alhariri, J., Sweren, R., Kwatra, M., & Kwatra, S. (2017). Aprepitant for the treatment of chronic refractory pruritus. *BioMed Research International, 2017*, 4790810.

Kini, S., DeLong, L., Veledar, E., McKenzie-Brown, A., Schaufele, M., & Chen, S. (2011). The impact of pruritus on quality of life. *JAMA Dermatology, 147*(10), 1153–1156.

Kowalski, E., Kneiber, D., Valdebran, M., Patel, U., & Amber, K. (2019). Treatment-resistant prurigo nodularis: Challenges and solutions. *Clinical, Cosmetic and Investigational Dermatology, 12*, 163–172.

Kuhn, H., Mennella, C., Magid, M., Stamu-O'Brien, C., & Kroumpouzos, G. (2017). Psychocutaneous disease: Clinical perspectives. *Journal of the American Academy of Dermatology, 76*(5), 779–791.

Kumar, S. S., Kuruvilla, M., Pai, G. S., & Dinesh, M. (2003). Cutaneous manifestations of non-Hodgkin's lymphoma. *Indian Journal Dermatology Venereology and Leprology, 69*(1), 12–15.

Larson, V. A., Tang, O., Stander, S., Miller, L. S., Kang, S., & Kwatra, S. G. (2019). Association between prurigo nodularis and malignancy in middle-aged adults. *Journal of the American Academy of Dermatology, 81*(5), 1198–1201. https://doi.org/10.1016/j.jaad.2019.03.083

Locala, J. (2009). Current concepts in psychodermatology. *Current Psychiatry Reports, 11*(3), 211–218.

Lotti, T., Buggiani, G., & Prignano, F. (2008). Prurigo nodularis and lichen simplex chronicus. *Dermatologic Therapy, 21*(1), 42–46.

Millington, G., Collins, A., Lovell, C., Leslie, T., Yong, A., Morgan, J., Ajithkumar, T., Andrews, M. J., Rushbook, S. M., Coelho, R. R., Catten, S. J., Lee, K. Y. C, Skellett, A. M., Affleck, A. G., Exton, L. S., Mohd Mustapa, M. F., & Levell, N. (2018). British Association of Dermatologists' guidelines for the investigation and management of generalized pruritus in adults without an underlying dermatosis. *The British Journal of Dermatology, 178*(1), 34–60.

Mostaghimi, L., Jafferany, M., & Tausk, F. (2019). Psychocutaneous diseases: In search of a common language. *International Journal of Dermatology, 59*(6), e195–e199.

Singh, F., & Rudikoff, D. (2012). HIV-associated pruritus: Etiology and management. *American Journal of Clinical Dermatology, 4*(3), 177–188.

Stander, S., Weisshaar, E., Mettang, T., Szepietowski, J. C., Carstens, E., Ikoma, A., Bergasa, N. V., Gieler, U., Misery, L., Wallengren, J., Darsow, U., Streit, M., Metze, D., Luger, T. A., Greaves, M. W., Schmelz, M., Yosipovitch, G., & Bernhard, D. (2007). Clinical classification of itch: A position paper of the International Forum for the Study of Itch. *Acta Dermato-Venereologica, 87*(4), 291–294.

Steinhoff, M., Cevikbas, F., Ikoma, A., & Berger, T. G. (2011). Pruritus: Management algorithms and experimental therapies. *Seminars in Cutaneous Medicine and Surgery, 30*(2), 127–137.

Tan, E., Tan, A., & Tey, H. (2015). Effective treatment of scrotal lichen simplex chronicus with 0.1% tacrolimus ointment: An observational study. *Journal of the European Academy of Dermatology & Venereology, 29*(7), 1448–1449.

Thiers, B. H., Sahn, R. E., & Callen, J. P. (2009). Cutaneous manifestations of internal malignancy. *CA: A Cancer Journal for Clinicians, 59*(2), 73–98.

Thorstensen, K. A., & Birnebaum, D. L. (2012). Recognition and management of vulvar dermatologic conditions: Lichen sclerosus, lichen planus, and lichen simplex chronicus. *Journal of Midwifery & Women's Health, 57*(3), 260–275.

Tripathi, R., Knusel, K. D., Ezaldein, H. H., Bordeaux, J. S., & Scott, J. F. (2019). The cost of an itch. *Journal of the American Academy of Dermatology, 80*(3), 811–813.

Tsianakas, A., Zeidler, C., Riepe, C., Borowski, M., Forner, C., Gerss, J., Metz, M., Staubach, P., Raap, U., Kaatz, M., Urban, M., Luger, T. A., & Ständer, S. (2019). Aprepitant in anti-histamine-refractory chronic nodular prurigo: A multicentre, randomized, double-blind, placebo-controlled, cross-over, Phase-II trial (APREPRU). *Acta dermato-venereologica, 99*(4), 379–385.

Wong, J. W., & Koo, J. Y. (2013). Delusions of parasitosis. *Indian Journal of Dermatology, 58*(1), 49–52.

Yosipovitch, G. (2010). Chronic pruritus: A paraneoplastic sign. *Dermatologic Therapy, 23*(6), 590–596.

Zhai, L., Savage, K., Qiu, C., Jin, A., Valdes-Rodriguez, R., & Mollanazar, N. (2019). Chronic pruritus responding to dupilumab—A case series. *Medicines, 6*(3), 1–15.

Superficial Fungal Infections

Douglas C. DiRuggiero

In This Chapter

- Diagnostics
- Antifungal Agents
- Dermatophytosis
- Tinea Incognito
- ID Reaction

- Candidiasis
- Tinea Versicolor
- Pityrosporum Folliculitis
- Nail Infections
- Special Considerations

Too often, patients assume that every round, scaly skin eruption is a "ringworm." It's a shame that this archaic term misleads many into thinking that fungal infections are always round and are caused by "worms." In truth, mycoses (fungal) infections can be cutaneous, subcutaneous, or systemic and are often tricky to diagnose and difficult to treat. Cutaneous fungal infections are commonly categorized as either dermatophytes, *Candida*, or other endogenous yeasts. Superficial infections involve the stratum corneum of skin as well as hair, nails, and mucous membranes; whereas deeper fungal infections involve the dermis and subcutaneous tissue. The clinical presentation of fungal infections varies depending on the type of fungus, location, and the immunologic response of the host. While most mycoses seen in primary care and dermatology settings are superficial infections, if left untreated, they can become debilitating, develop secondary bacterial infections, and spread to other parts of the body or to close contacts.

This chapter will present the varied presentations of cutaneous mycoses diseases, discuss clinical clues and diagnostic tests to help with accurate diagnoses, and review safe and effective treatment therapies.

Clinicians should be vigilant in developing a differential diagnosis, selecting appropriate diagnostic tests, and considering safe and effective therapies. The old medical adage, "The correct diagnosis leads to successful treatments" is never truer than when treating skin rashes. Therefore, knowing that fungal infections can mimic many other inflammatory and infectious skin conditions, knowledge and utilization of diagnostic tests is critical to avoid misdiagnosis and subsequent delayed proper treatments.

CONFIRMING THE DIAGNOSIS

Clinical presentation, along with laboratory findings, should be used to accurately diagnose tinea. Selection of the diagnostic test is based on access, cost, time, and value of pathogen identification. It should be noted, however, that the value of any fungal examination is only as good as the quality of the specimen submitted for analysis.

The appropriate sampling techniques, advantages, and disadvantages of available fungal tests are provided in Section 15.

- *Direct microscopy with potassium hydroxide (KOH) preparation—* the easiest and most cost-effective test available to clinicians

regardless of the practice setting. Scrapings are obtained from the skin, hair, or nails to confirm the presence or absence of hyphae or spores. KOH does not identify the species of dermatophyte. See Section 15 for KOH procedure details (see Figs. 15-13, 14).

- *Fungal culture—*currently the gold standard but can take 2 to 6 weeks for final results. Culture identifies specific genus and species of organisms to help differentiate nondermatophyte molds and *Candida* species from similarly appearing dermatophytes. Utilize test for recurrent or recalcitrant infections.

- *Quantitative PCR and ribosomal DNA sequencing of tissue and nail samples—*this will likely become the new gold standard (Joyce et al., 2019).

- *Dermatopathology—*a punch biopsy specimen is helpful if the KOH preparation and/or culture fails to confirm the diagnosis or if considering other etiologies. A Periodic acid–Schiff (PAS) stain should be requested with histology to confirm fungal elements. Distal nail clippings can also be sent for histology.

Hair samples and scrapings from affected areas can also be submitted to pathology labs for culture or KOH visualization to confirm tinea capitis.

- *Wood's light examination—*can help when evaluating specific fungal and bacterial infections. In tinea capitis, hair infected by *Microsporum canis* or *Microsporum audouinii* will fluoresce blue-green, compared with *Trichophyton tonsurans* and other species that do not fluoresce.

False negative results are high with this examination test, so treat if other clinical suspicions exist.

In tinea versicolor, the affected skin will appear yellow-green; while bacterial infections such as erythrasma, caused by *Corynebacterium minutissimum*, fluoresce a bright coral red. Patients must be evaluated in a completely dark environment to differentiate these subtle clinical findings (Fig. 15-16). See Section 15 for details.

- *Dermatophyte test medium* (DTM)—a convenient and low-cost, in-office test in which clinicians inoculate media with a sample of the skin, hair, or nails. After 7 to 14 days of incubation at room temperature, dermatophytes cause a change in the pH and indicate their presence by changing the medium to a red color. DTM does not identify the species and can have false positives from contaminated samples (some molds, yeasts, and bacteria) or media left for more than 14 days. It is rarely utilized in dermatology clinics due to its low-test sensitivity and specificity (see Fig. 15-15).

- Bacteriologic swab taken from pustular areas can be submitted for bacterial and fungal cultures.

ANTIFUNGAL AGENTS

Topical

Topical antifungals are effective first-line therapies for most superficial fungal infections, and because they have very little systemic absorption, there is a low risk for adverse events or drug interactions. The most common side effects reported are symptoms of irritant or allergic contact dermatitis. Selection of the most appropriate agent should be based on the suspected (or cultured) causative organism, severity, body surface area, comorbidities, cost, location(s) of infection, and potential for secondary infection. Severe or recalcitrant dermatophyte infections may require systemic treatment, with associated increased risk for side effects, drug interactions, and complications.

In general, *fungistatic drugs inhibit growth, whereas fungicidal drugs kill fungal pathogens.*

Topical antifungals used for the treatment of mucocutaneous infections belong to one of four classes: polyenes, imidazoles, allylamines/benzylamines, and others (Table 6.1-1).

- *Polyenes*—fungistatic agents effective against *Candida*, but not dermatophytes or *Pityrosporum*.
- *Azoles*—fungistatic but possess antibacterial as well as anti-inflammatory properties, and are used for dermatophyte, *Candida*, endogenous yeast, and secondary bacterial infections.
- *Allylamine/benzylamine*—broader spectrum of antifungal activity and can be both fungistatic and fungicidal. They are the

TABLE 6.1-1	Comparing Effectiveness of Topical Antifungals on Types of Organisms						
	PREGNANCY CATEGORY	DERMATOPHYTE	YEAST	GRAM + BACTERIA	GRAM − BACTERIA	ANTI-INFLAMMATORY	ADVANTAGES
POLYENES fungistatic							
Nystatin	CA (pastilles)	**0**	++++				
AZOLES fungistatic							
Miconazole 2%	C	++	+++				
Clotrimazole 1%	B	++	+++				
Ketoconazole 2%	C	++	+++	++		++	Anti-inflammatory effect in seb derm comparable to hydrocortisone
Oxiconazole 1%	B	++	+++				Vehicle great for hyperkeratotic soles and interdigital infections
Econazole 1%	C	++	+++	++	++	++	
Sertaconazole 2%	C	++	+++	++			
ALLYLAMINES fungistatic and fungicidal							
Naftifine 1%	B	++	++			+++	
Terbinafine 1%	B	+++	++			+++	
BENZYLAMINE fungicidal							
Butenafine 1%	B	++++	++			+++	
OTHER AGENTS							
Ciclopirox 1%	B	++	++++ (*C. albicans*)	+++	+++	+++	Penetrates nail plate
Selenium sulfide 2.5%	C		+++ (only *Pityrosporum*)				Effective in follicular epithelium

0, no effect or activity against specific organism; +, mildly effective activity; ++, moderately effective; +++, strongly effective; ++++, most effective.

drug of choice for dermatophytes, but relatively weak against *Candida.*

- Ciclopirox—this has a unique mode of action and structure and is fungistatic, fungicidal, and anti-inflammatory. It is effective against tinea pedis, tinea corporis, tinea versicolor, and candidiasis. Ciclopirox nail lacquer 8% (Penlac) and tavaborole (Kerydin, Jublia) are the only FDA-approved topical treatments for onychomycosis (Jinna & Finch, 2015).

- *Morpholine drug class*—includes topical amorolfine, but is currently not available in the United States. It is not included in subsequent tables and charts.

Systemic

Griseofulvin was the first systemic antifungal used for the treatment of superficial fungal infections of the hair, skin, and nails. Although effective, newer agents have improved bioavailability and absorption, resulting in greater efficacy and shorter duration of therapy.

- The most common oral antifungals include terbinafine (Lamisil) from the allylamine group, and fluconazole (Diflucan) and itraconazole (Sporanox), both from the azole group. These newer antifungals reach the layers of the stratum corneum faster and are retained longer, resulting in higher cure rates, compared with that of griseofulvin.

- Itraconazole can be detected in the eccrine sweat glands within 24 hours and is excreted into sebum, which explains why it is commonly used off-label for tinea versicolor.

- Systemic treatment for onychomycosis is also advantageous as terbinafine stays in the nail for 6 to 8 months after therapy, while fluconazole (off-label) and itraconazole remain for 6 and 12 months, respectively. Therefore, once therapy is completed, prolonged residual drug levels improve mycotic cure rate.

- A careful review of the patient's comorbidities and medications is critical when considering oral antifungal therapy. Metabolism of antifungals occurs through the cytochrome P450 system and therefore can affect the metabolism of the antifungal or other medications. Patients with liver or renal disease and the elderly may not be good candidates for oral antifungal therapy.

- Alcohol avoidance and the need for blood monitoring need to be discussed prior to initiating therapy. The risk of interactions, adverse events, monitoring, and contraindications are listed in Table 6.1-2.

- Ketoconazole: This text will not review the systemic use of ketoconazole (azole) as its use in dermatology has become very limited. Historically, oral ketoconazole (Nizoral) has been used off-label for treatment of benign mucocutaneous infections such as tinea versicolor. In 2013, the FDA warned that oral ketoconazole should not be used for dermatophyte infections or as first-line treatment for any mycotic infection in view of the risk of liver injury, adrenal problems, and drug interactions. Thus far, these risks have not been associated with topical ketoconazole, which continues to be FDA indicated for treatment of dandruff, candidiasis of the skin, tinea versicolor or pityrosporum folliculitis, seborrheic dermatitis, and tinea infections.

DERMATOPHYTES

Dermatophytes are a group of fungi comprising three genera: *Trichophyton*, *Microsporum*, and *Epidermophyton*. Dermatophyte infections are commonly called *tinea* or *ringworm*, given their annular or serpiginous borders. Some patients misunderstand and

BOX 6.1-1 Nomenclature for Tinea by Body Site	
Tinea pedis—foot	Tinea barbae—beard
Tinea cruris—groin	Tinea capitis—scalp
Tinea corporis—body	Tinea unguium—nails
Tinea manuum—hand	Tinea incognito—disguised, steroid
Tinea faciei—face	cream exacerbated

worry that there may actually be worms in their skin; so it is advantageous to teach patients about the true etiology. Unlike *Candida*, dermatophytes can survive only in the stratum corneum (top layer) of the skin, hair, and nails, and not on mucosal surfaces such as the mouth or vaginal mucosa. Subtypes of tinea are classified by the area of the body infected or the pathogen responsible for the infection (Box 6.1-1).

Pathophysiology

- The majority of tinea infections are caused by *Trichophyton rubrum*, with the exception of tinea capitis. *T. tonsurans* is the most common causative organism of capitis in the United States, while *M. canis* is the most common worldwide. Transmission occurs from direct contact with an infected host, which may be human to human (anthropophilic), animal to human (zoophilic), or soil to human (geophilic).

- Dermatophytes can survive on exfoliated skin or hair, and live on moist surfaces in showers or pools, bedding, clothing, combs, and hats for 12 to 15 months. Once exposed, the incubation time to symptoms is usually 1 to 2 weeks. Clinicians should keep this in mind when dealing with community outbreaks of tinea.

- Tinea is more common in adolescent and adult populations, except for tinea capitis which is seen mostly in children between the ages of 3 and 7 years.

- People on topical and systemic corticosteroids or with suppressed immune systems are more susceptible. Crowded living conditions, poor hygiene, high humidity, athletes in contact sports (i.e., wrestling), or close contact with infected persons, animals, or soil can increase one's risk for infection. Studies suggest that individuals may have a genetic predisposition to particular strains of dermatophytes among members of the same household.

Subtypes of Tinea

Tinea Pedis

Athlete's foot, or tinea pedis, is the most common disease affecting the feet and toes. It can present with a variety of symptoms depending on the causative organism and may include pruritus, inflammation, scale, vesicles, bullae, or may sometimes be asymptomatic. The most common pathogens are *T. rubrum*, *Trichophyton mentagrophytes*, and *Epidermophyton floccosum*.

Clinical Presentation

There are four types of tinea pedis affecting the feet and toes:

- *Moccasin* type involves one or both heels, soles, and lateral borders of the foot, presenting with well-demarcated hyperkeratosis, fine white scale, and erythema (Fig. 6.1-1). The pathogens are commonly *T. rubrum* or *E. floccosum*. This type is chronic and very recalcitrant to therapy.

| TABLE 6.1-2 | Systemic Antifungal Agents for Treatment of Superficial Cutaneous Fungal Infections |

DRUG	INDICATIONS	SIDE EFFECTS	INTERACTIONS AND MONITORING	CONTRAINDICATION AND CAUTION
Griseofulvin (Pregnancy Category C)	Adults: 500 mg daily (except tinea pedis and onychomycosis, 1 g daily)	Usually well tolerated but may have: rash, hives, headache, fatigue, GI upset, diarrhea, photosensitivity	CYP3A4 inducer (decrease levels): OCPs, warfarin, and cyclosporine increases alcohol levels	Pregnancy (or intent) Avoid: alcohol use
	Peds: Microsize: 10–15 mg/kg/day given daily or b.i.d. or 125–250 mg for 30–50 lb and 250–500 mg for >50 lb Ultramicrosize: 3–5 mg/kg/day given daily or b.i.d. or 125–187.5 mg for 35–60 lb and 187.5–375 for >60 lb Off-label use by experts: commonly use micro-size at 20–25 mg/kg/day and ultramicrosize at 10–15 mg/kg/day Improved absorption with fatty meal Duration: Capitis: 4–6 wk; corporis: 2–4 wk; pedis: 4–8 wk; cruris and barbae: till clear; fingernail: 4 mo; and toenails: 6 mo		Monitor: baseline CBC, BUN/Cr, LFTs Repeat 6 wk	Contraindicated in liver failure or porphyria
Terbinafine (Pregnancy Category B)	Adults: 250 mg daily Onychomycosis: fingernails for 6 wk and toenails for 12 wk Off-label use: tinea corporis, pedis, capitis, barbae, and candidiasis	Headache, GI upset, visual disturbance, rash, hives, elevated LFTs	Inhibits metabolism of drugs using CYP2D6	Caution with hepatic and renal disease
	Peds: Lamisil granules for capitis (>4 yr old): 125 mg/day for <25 kg; 187.5 mg/day for 25–35 kg; and 250 mg/day for >35 lb for 2–4 wk		Drug interactions: TCAs, anti-depressants, SSRIs, β-blockers, warfarin, cyclosporine, rifampin, cimetidine, caffeine, theophylline	Avoid if history of lupus
			Monitor: baseline LFTs, CBC, BUN, creatinine; repeat in 6 wk; more often if symptoms or immunosuppressed	
Fluconazole (Pregnancy Category C)	Adults: 150–200 mg Vulvovaginal candidiasis: 150 mg as a single dose only. If recurrent, 150 mg weekly Oropharyngeal candidiasis: 200 mg. Take 2 orally on the first day, then one daily for 2 wk	Headache, GI upset, abdominal pain, rash, diarrhea	Inhibits metabolism of drugs using CYP2C9	Caution if renal or hepatic disease QT prolongation Arrhythmic condition
	Peds: Oropharyngeal candidiasis (6 mo and older): 6 mg/kg/day orally on day one, followed by 3 mg/kg/day for 2 wk		Monitor: baseline LFTs Repeat in 1 mo	Contraindicated in severe liver disease
Itraconazole (Pregnancy Category C)	Adults Onychomycosis: Toenails and/or fingernails—continuous 200 mg daily for 12 wk Fingernails only—*pulsed therapy*, take 200 mg b.i.d. for 1 wk, then off 3 wk. Repeat 1–2 times	GI upset, abdominal pain, diarrhea, constipation, decreased appetite, rash, pruritus, headache, dizziness, elevated LFTs	Inhibits metabolism of drugs using CYP3A4	Patients with ventricular dysfunction or congestive heart failure
	Peds: Off-label use only Improved absorption with food, especially acidic foods		Caution: use H$_2$-blockers and PPIs, calcium channel blockers, lovastatin, simvastatin, ergot alkaloids	Contraindicated in chronic renal failure
			Monitor: baseline LFTs Repeat in 1 month Less risk of elevated LFTs with pulse therapy	

Note: In 2013, the FDA advised limited use of systemic ketoconazole in view of liver injury, adrenal gland problems, and drug interactions. Oral ketoconazole should not be used for mucocutaneous infections or first-line treatment for any mycotic infection unless it is life-threatening or alternative therapy is not tolerated or available. There are many off-label uses of systemic antifungals that can be safe and effective treatments for dermatophyte and yeast infections. Primary care providers should understand the risks, benefits, and efficacy of off-labeled prescribing, or refer recalcitrant or severe cases to dermatology.

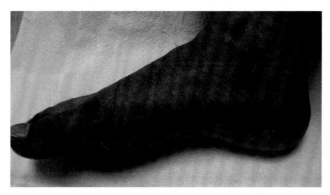

FIG. 6.1-1. Mocassin-type tinea pedis. (Photo courtesy of M. Bobonich.)

- *Interdigital* type involves infection of the web spaces and can cause very different symptoms of erythema and scaliness, or maceration and fissures. The third and fourth web spaces are most commonly involved and are at risk to develop a secondary bacterial infection (Fig. 6.1-2). Obtaining a KOH from the macerated area can be difficult and may require cultures. The causative organisms are usually *T. rubrum*, *T. mentagrophytes*, and *E. floccosum*.

- *Inflammatory/Vesicular* type involves a vesicular or bullous eruption often caused by *T. mentagrophytes* and involves the medial aspect of the foot (Fig. 6.1-3).

- *Ulcerative* type presents with erosions or ulcers in the web spaces. *T. rubrum*, *T. mentagrophytes*, and *E. floccosum* are common pathogens, with frequent secondary bacterial infections in diabetic or immunocompromised patients.

DIFFERENTIAL DIAGNOSIS   Tinea Pedis

- Psoriasis
- Dermatitis (contact and dyshidrotic eczema)
- Pitted keratolysis
- Bacterial infections
- Erythrasma
- Bullous disease

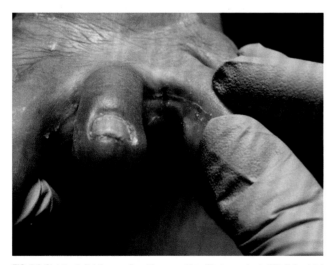

FIG. 6.1-2. Interdigital tinea pedis with maceration. (Photo courtesy of M. Bobonich.)

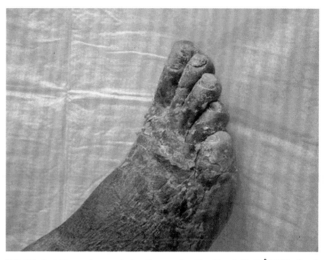

FIG. 6.1-3. Inflammatory vesicular tinea pedis. (Goodheart, H. P. [2015]. *Goodheart's photoguide of common skin disorders* [4th ed.]. Wolters Kluwer Health | Lippincott Williams & Wilkins.)

Treatment

- Hyperkeratosis, abnormal thickening of the outer layer of the skin, may accompany tinea pedis and should be treated with a keratolytic agent, which softens and thins the keratin layer and allows for better antifungal penetration.

- Topical preparations of lactic acid, ammonium lactate, or salicylic acid are available in a variety of formulations as both prescription and over-the-counter treatment.

- If vesicles are present, Burow's solution (13% aluminum acetate) can be used for anti-itch, astringent, and antibacterial properties. It is available over-the-counter, both as *Domeboro* or generic, and is applied as wet compresses four times daily.

- Topical antifungals should be applied immediately following the compresses for maximum penetration.

- Interdigital maceration can be treated with aluminum chloride hexahydrate 20% (Drysol, Hypercare) twice daily to provide an antibacterial and drying effect. Moisture-wicking socks or a change in socks or shoes midday can help decrease prolonged periods of moisture of the feet.

- The broad-spectrum activity of a topical azole, especially econazole and sertaconazole, is a good choice for interdigital maceration, as it often involves a secondary bacterial infection. Topical treatments should be continued for 1 to 2 weeks after the infection appears clinically cleared.

- Systemic antifungals are often necessary for extensive moccasin-type tinea pedis or when topical treatments have failed. Terbinafine and itraconazole are more effective than griseofulvin in the treatment of tinea pedis.

- Precautions should be taken to prevent the recurrence of tinea pedis: wash your feet daily and dry them well (especially between the toes), avoid tight footwear, wear sandals or shoes that breathe in warm weather, apply absorbent powder such as Zeasorb to feet, and wear cotton or synthetic socks and change them when they become moist.

Tinea Cruris

Often referred to as "jock itch," tinea cruris is a dermatophyte infection of the groin but may also affect inner thighs and buttocks. Clinicians should also inspect the feet of patients diagnosed with cruris as spores can be transmitted when patients are putting on

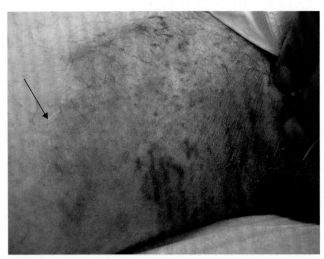

FIG. 6.1-4. Tinea cruris. Advancing border with scale (*arrow*). (Photo courtesy of M. Bobonich.)

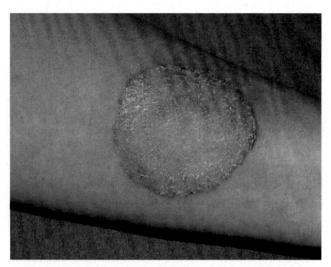

FIG. 6.1-5. Tinea corporis. The scaly border is potassium hydroxide positive. (Goodheart, H. P. [2015]. *Goodheart's photoguide of common skin disorders* [4th ed.]. Wolters Kluwer Health | Lippincott Williams & Wilkins.)

their underwear. It is helpful to have patients put on their socks first before putting on their underwear.

Clinical Presentation

- Well-demarcated erythematous or tan plaques with raised scaly borders or advancing edge (Fig. 6.1-4)
- Vesicles may present on the border with severe inflammation and pruritus as a complaint

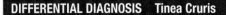

DIFFERENTIAL DIAGNOSIS Tinea Cruris
• Erythrasma
• Inverse psoriasis
• Seborrheic dermatitis
• Intertrigo
• Candidiasis
• Hailey–Hailey disease

Treatment

- Usually responds to any of the topical antifungals, but allylamines are most effective
- Apply for 2 to 4 weeks until clear, and then 1 week longer
- With a culture proven tinea, if not resolved within expected time period, change to another class of topical antifungal or to a systemic agent
- Biopsy if rash not responding to multiple topicals and/or systemic therapy

Tinea Corporis

Ringworm, or tinea corporis, is a dermatophyte infection (*T. rubrum* most common pathogen) involving areas of the trunk and extremities, not including the groin, feet, palms, face, or scalp.

Clinical Presentation

- Pruritic, erythematous, scaly macules or papules that expand outward to form classic annular or arciform lesions with a raised and sometimes a vesicular advancing border (Fig. 6.1-5)

- Central area flattens and turns from red to brown as the border broadens
- Lesions may fuse, producing large gyrate patterns, covering large body surface areas (Figs. 6.1-6 and 6.1-7)
- A clinical variant is Majocchi granuloma (Fig. 6.1-8) involves invasion of dermatophytes into the hair follicles, presents with erythematous, perifollicular papules and pustules, common on the legs of women from shaving, but can be seen in men and children in other hair-bearing areas
- Immunocompromised patients may have a more nodular presentation

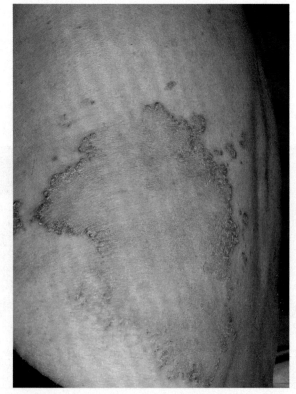

FIG. 6.1-6. Tinea corporis with gyrate lesions forming. (Photo courtesy of M. Bobonich.)

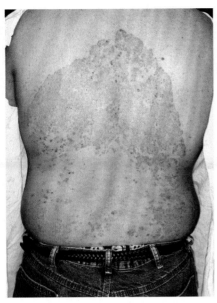

FIG. 6.1-7. Tinea corporis. Large, diffuse areas. Includes differential diagnosis eczema, CTCL mycosis fungoides, dermatomyositis, and psoriasis.

DIFFERENTIAL DIAGNOSIS Tinea Corporis	
• Dermatitis (nummular, atopic, contact, etc.)	• Annular erythemas
• Psoriasis	• Subacute lupus erythematosus
• Pityriasis rosea	• Granuloma annulare
• Tinea versicolor	• Mycosis fungoides

Treatment

- Small body surface areas usually respond quickly to topical therapy, especially from the newer agents in the allylamine and benzylamine groups.
- Systemic antifungals should be considered if the patient is immunocompromised, eruption involves large body surface areas, tinea is not responsive to topical therapy, or dermatophyte infection is Majocchi granuloma.

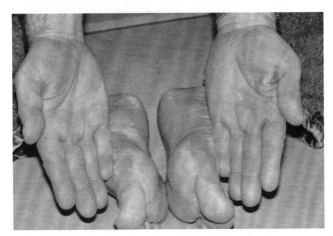

FIG. 6.1-8. "Two feet-one hand" variant of tinea pedis. The scale is present on one hand only.

- Terbinafine is a good agent for systemic therapy and is well tolerated by both children and adults. A topical antifungal may be used in conjunction with oral therapy.
- Skin eruptions diagnosed as tinea corporis that do not respond to antifungals, or are recurrent, should be biopsied.

Tinea Manuum

Tinea manuum is a dermatophyte infection of the hand, palm, or interdigital spaces. Patients often think their hand is just very dry and have no idea it is an infection. You may find patients with "two feet-one hand" syndrome, with tinea presenting in both feet and one hand—usually the hand/fingers that pick their feet or toenail fissures (Fig. 6.1-8). For this reason, it is important to examine the dorsum of the hands and feet, as well as the nails that may be involved. Because of the lack of sebaceous glands on the palm, it can have two different clinical presentations.

Clinical Presentation

- Palmar involvement—symptoms similar to moccasin-type tinea pedis, with erythema, hyperkeratosis, and fine scaling in palmar creases.
- Dorsum of hand—annular presentation similar to tinea corporis.

DIFFERENTIAL DIAGNOSIS Tinea Manuum
• Dermatitis
• Dyshidrotic eczema
• Psoriasis
• Scabies
• Lichen simplex chronicus
• Allergic or contact dermatitis

Treatment

- Topicals alone may be less effective due to the thickness of the stratum corneum, but allylamines should be utilized.
- Systemic antifungals should be considered for recurrent or non-responsive infections; follow treatment recommendations for tinea pedis using terbinafine and itraconazole.

Tinea Faciei and Tinea Barbae

Dermatophyte infections of the glabrous (non–hair-bearing) skin of the face are called tinea faciei. If tinea affects the hair follicles of the beard and mustache area, it is referred to as tinea barbae. These infections occur mostly in adolescents and men and may be the result of autoinoculation from the patient's tinea pedis or corporis. A KOH test and/or biopsy is often required to differentiate these infections from multiple other conditions.

Clinical Presentation

Tinea Faciei

- Mild erythema with some fine scales can be photosensitive.
- If treated with topical corticosteroids, it can be transformed into tinea incognito.

Tinea Barbae

- If superficial, can present as classic annular plaques, but typically barbae is more severe and inflammatory.

- Deep follicular tinea barbae is less common, often acquired from zoophilic dermatophytes such as *Trichophyton verrucosum* and *T. mentagrophytes*; and occurs in farmers who have contact with the hide of cattle.
- Alopecia and regional lymphadenopathy can be present.

DIFFERENTIAL DIAGNOSIS	T. Faciei and T. Barbae
Tinea faciei	*Tinea barbae*
• Cutaneous lupus	• Bacterial folliculitis
• Eczema	• Furuncle
• Seborrheic dermatitis	• HSV/VZV
• Polymorphic light eruption	• Acne
• Psoriasis	• Rosacea

Treatment

- Tinea faciei responds well to topical antifungals, allylamines.
- Tinea barbae usually requires oral antifungals for 2 to 4 weeks. Terbinafine is the drug of choice along with topical antifungals (azoles). Shaving could cause the spread of the dermatophytes.

Tinea Capitis

Tinea capitis is a fungal infection of the scalp and hair, and commonly occurs in children in low socioeconomic and crowded living conditions. Spores can be transmitted by hairbrushes, combs, hats, and furniture. Tinea capitis is classified as either endothrix (90% to 95% of cases in the United States) or ectothrix infections that manifest with a variety of symptoms. *T. tonsurans* is usually the causative organism with endothrix, while *M. canis* is usually found with ectothrix.

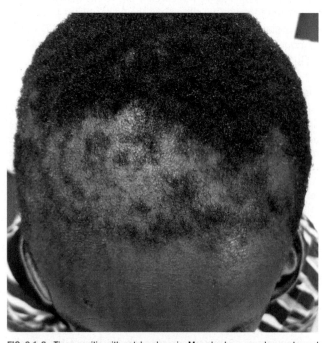

FIG. 6.1-9. Tinea capitis with patchy alopecia. May also have papules, scale, and erythema.

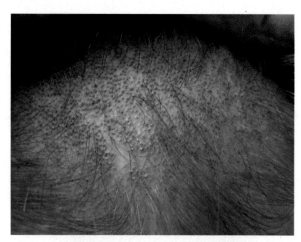

FIG. 6.1-10. Tinea capitis "black dot" characteristic presentation with *T. tonsurans.* (Photo courtesy of M. Bobonich.)

Clinical Presentation

Most tinea capitis present with alopecia, but may have scale, pruritus, papules, and pustules (Fig. 6.1-9). When these symptoms are presented along with tender lymphadenopathy, the clinician should have a high index of suspicion for tinea capitis. Inflammation may be mild to severe and depends on the pathogen, host's immune system, partial treatment, and possible secondary bacterial infections.

- Endothrix (infection on the inside of hair shaft)—also called "black dot" tinea, causes patchy alopecia with noninflammatory scaliness and black dots where hair is broken off at the follicular orifice (Fig. 6.1-10).
- Ectothrix (infection on the outside of the hair shaft)—called "gray patch" tinea capitis, presents as partial alopecia with short broken-off hairs close to the surface of the scalp (Fig. 6.1-11).
- Kerion—one third of children develop a tender boggy plaque, with pustules that sometimes form a serum crust (Fig. 6.1-12). Easy to mistake it as a bacterial infection. Conversely, the kerion is a host's exuberant immune response to the fungus and is often accompanied by cervical and/or occipital lymphadenopathy. Other symptoms can include low-grade fever, malaise, and

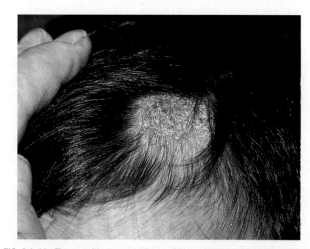

FIG. 6.1-11. Tinea capitis "gray patch type." Note alopecia with broken-off hairs close to scalp surface. *Microsporum canis* was found on culture, and the area fluoresced green with a Wood's lamp. (Goodheart, H. P. [2015]. *Goodheart's photoguide of common skin disorders* [4th ed.]. Wolters Kluwer Health | Lippincott Williams & Wilkins.)

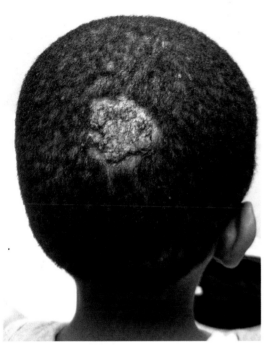

FIG. 6.1-12. Kerion in patient with tinea capitis. (Photo courtesy of M. Bobonich.)

alopecia. Sequelae such as scarring and permanent hair loss may occur in severe infections.

DIFFERENTIAL DIAGNOSIS **Tinea Capitis**

- Bacterial infection
- Seborrheic dermatitis
- Psoriasis
- Dermatitis
- Pyoderma
- Folliculitis decalvans
- Trichotillomania
- Alopecia areata
- Discoid lupus

Treatment

Tinea capitis requires treatment with systemic antifungals. Selection of the antifungal should be based on the causative organism, tolerability, availability and cost, and side effects.

- Griseofulvin has been the gold standard for tinea capitis and is inexpensive and well tolerated, with few side effects. A 6-week course of griseofulvin is the most effective antifungal treatment against tinea caused by *Microsporum* species. However, treatment duration should continue for two additional weeks after the symptoms have resolved. Infections from *M. canis* typically require a longer treatment period than do those from *T. tonsurans*.

- Studies show that off-label use of terbinafine therapy for *Trichophyton* species has a better cure rate and shorter duration of therapy. Table 6.1-2 shows dosages and duration of treatment of tinea capitis with oral antifungals. Off-label use of terbinafine, fluconazole, and itraconazole in dermatology has been safe and effective.

- Although there are no studies to support it, oral prednisone (0.05 to 1 mg/kg/day) for 7 to 10 days to help reduce the inflammatory response and pain has been utilized and reported in dermatology literature.

Management and Patient Education

- Transmission of tinea can be human to human, animal to human, or soil to human. Moreover, dermatophytes can survive on showers or pool surfaces, bedding, clothing, combs, and hats for over a year. Patients should inspect other contacts and pets for skin rashes and disinfect high-contagion areas.

- Tinea pedis is transmitted by direct contact with contaminated shoes or socks, showers, locker rooms, and pool surfaces, where the organism can thrive. It is very contagious and can lead to household outbreaks or recurrence of the infection.

- Chronic tinea pedis can lead to fungal infections of the toenails, secondary bacterial infections, or entry of organisms that can cause cellulitis of the lower legs. These disease complications are important to consider in the management of diabetic, immunocompromised, and elderly patients.

- Inspect feet of patients diagnosed with tinea cruris as spores can be transferred when patients are putting on their underwear. Have patients put on socks prior to putting on underwear.

- Management of patients with kerions should also include a bacterial culture and consideration of antibiotics as appropriate.

- Household members of patients with tinea capitis should be screened for dermatophytes in an effort to reduce the risk of transmission and reinfection. Off-label use of ketoconazole 2%, selenium sulfide 2.5%, and ciclopirox 1% shampoos are common adjunctive treatments to reduce spores in the patient's household members.

- With all tinea infections, patients should return in 2 to 4 weeks to evaluate response to treatments. If not responding, additional or repeated diagnostics should be performed.

- In general, patient should continue topical treatments for 7 to 14 days after the rash has disappeared. For chronic or recurrent cases, consider repeat culture or test for cure after symptoms are resolved.

- Clinicians should refer patients with severe or recalcitrant cases to dermatology.

ASSOCIATED SKIN FINDINGS

Id Reaction

An *id* reaction, also called auto-eczematization and dermatophytids, is an acute cutaneous reaction to a dermatophyte. Manifestations include a disseminated, erythematous maculopapular or vesicular eruption which may be pruritic. It occurs 1 to 2 weeks following the primary infection. It appears distant to the tinea and can involve the arms, legs, and trunk. The eruption will clear when the tinea has been treated, although topical steroids may help relieve some of the symptoms.

Tinea Incognito

This is a confusing diagnosis that occurs when a dermatophyte is misdiagnosed as eczema or dermatitis and is treated with a topical corticosteroid. Tinea, when treated with corticosteroids, may lose its characteristic scaly annular and defined border. Instead it may have diffuse erythema with or without scale, papules, or pustules. If you suspect a tinea incognito, have the patient stop the corticosteroid. Scale should recur within a week and a KOH test can be performed. If positive, treat accordingly.

CANDIDIASIS INFECTION

Candida albicans is the most virulent of the yeasts and is responsible for most mucocutaneous infections. This organism is a normal component

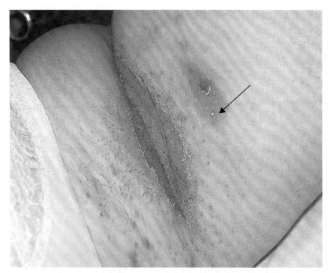

FIG. 6.1-13. Cutaneous candidiasis of the axillae. This patient has diabetes. Note the satellite pustules. (Goodheart, H. P. [2015]. *Goodheart's photoguide of common skin disorders* [4th ed.]. Wolters Kluwer Health | Lippincott Williams & Wilkins.)

of flora in the mouth, gastrointestinal tract, and vaginal mucosa. A variety of factors such as skin maceration, antibiotics, oral contraceptives, diabetes, and immunosuppression may alter the local environment and cause the proliferation of *C. albicans* sufficient to become pathogenic. Candidiasis is a fungal infection caused by a *Candida* species. It is typically diagnosed based on clinical presentation (Fig. 6.1-13).

Oral Candidiasis

- Oral candidiasis, or thrush, occurs mostly in infants, but patients who are immunocompromised, diabetic, or on antibiotic or corticosteroid therapy (i.e., asthma inhalers) are at greater risk. Also seen more commonly in those who wear dentures.

- Symptoms may include burning and pain with eating, diminished taste, erythema, and erosions.

- The yeast may extend to the corners of the patient's mouth (*angular cheilitis* or *perlèche*), causing fissures and erythema, and increasing the risk for secondary bacterial infection usually by a staphylococcal species (Fig. 6.1-14).

- Perlèche may occur independent of oral thrush and is seen in patients with poor-fitting dentures, excessive drooling or

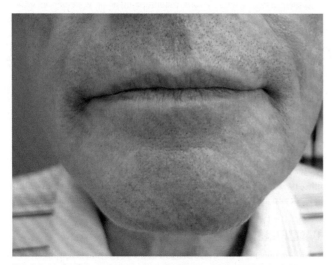

FIG. 6.1-14. Perlèche in corners of mouth. (Photo courtesy of M. Bobonich.)

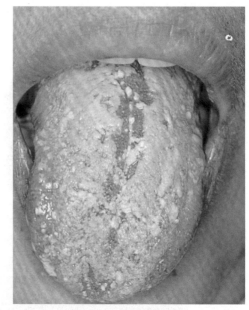

FIG. 6.1-15. Thrush, oral candidiasis with white plaques easily removed with gauze. (Goodheart, H. P. [2015]. *Goodheart's photoguide of common skin disorders* [4th ed.]. Wolters Kluwer Health | Lippincott Williams & Wilkins.)

salivation, thumb sucking, or lip licking. Deep marionette lines extending down the chin may also become inflamed and eroded.

Clinical Presentation

- Thrush—white plaques on the tongue, buccal mucosa, soft palate, and pharynx. Adherent plaques can be scraped off with a tongue blade to reveal a bright red mucosal surface (Fig. 6.1-15)

- Angular cheilitis—fissures and erythema in the corners of the mouth

DIFFERENTIAL DIAGNOSIS   Oral Candidiasis
• Oral hairy leukoplakia
• Geographic or hairy tongue
• Lichen planus
• Stomatitis
• Vitamin B$_5$ deficiency

Confirming the Diagnosis

- Diagnosis is based largely on history and clinical findings.

- Candida can be scraped from tongue, buccal mucosa, and roof of mouth with a tongue blade and evaluated microscopically with a KOH preparation. Note: fixed white lesions like leukoplakia, oral lichen planus, and hairy tongue can NOT be scraped off (see Section 11.3).

- Culture from corners of mouth, oral cavity, or throat may be helpful to confirm bacterial or fungal etiology.

Treatment

Topical

- Nystatin suspension, commonly prescribed as a "swish and swallow" is more effective in infants than in adults. The suspension can be easily administered with a dropper in the infant's mouth between the buccal mucosa and tongue.

- Clotrimazole troches (medicinal lozenges that dissolve slowly in the mouth) are very effective in adults.
- Perlèche is treated with topical azole creams and antibacterials as appropriate.

Systemic

- Fluconazole is the most commonly used systemic for severe cases or recurrent infections, but requires caution by the prescriber in view of the numerous drug interactions (Table 6.1-2).
- Systemic antifungals such as itraconazole, voriconazole, posaconazole, and amphotericin B may be necessary for immunosuppressed patients. Consultation with infectious disease experts may be necessary.

Management and Patient Education

- Management of oral candidiasis should begin by identifying the predisposing factors and correcting them. Good oral hygiene and mouth rinses after using steroid inhalers can reduce the recurrence.
- Immunosuppressed and chemotherapy patients on cancer treatment may need prophylaxis for chronic infections.
- Reinfection can be reduced by sanitizing infected surfaces of infant's bottles and nipples and treating infected nipples of breastfeeding mothers.

INTERTRIGINOUS (SKIN FOLDS) CANDIDIASIS

Clinical Presentation

- Erythematous moist plaques with satellite pustules and papules in inframammary, axilla, groin, perineum, and gluteal folds (Fig. 6.1-16).
- Interdigital involvement of the fingers and toes usually has more maceration, erythema, and erosion.
- *Intertrigo* should be mentioned here, as it can often mimic fungal infections. Intertrigo is a chronic inflammatory dermatosis with fine fissures and erythema involving the inframammary, axillary, umbilical, gluteal, and inguinal folds. It is not an infection but is due to chronic, friction, and moisture usually in obese patients.

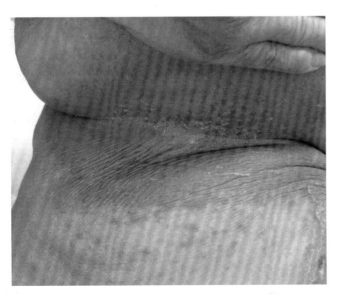

FIG. 6.1-16. Inframammary candidiasis with red satellite papules. (Photo courtesy of M. Bobonich.)

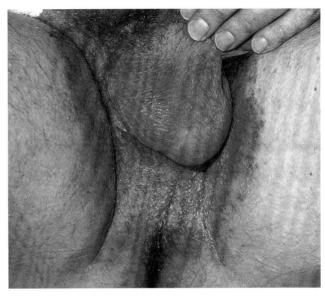

FIG. 6.1-17. Candida Intertrigo. Note the active pustular border on the left thigh. (Used with permission from Edwards, L. [2004]. *Genital dermatology atlas*. Wolters Kluwer Health.)

Conversely, intertriginous candidiasis presents with erythematous, well-demarcated plaques, which may progress to maceration, oozing and erosions, and fissures (Fig. 6.1-17).

DIFFERENTIAL DIAGNOSIS Intertriginous Candidiasis
• Intertrigo
• Inverse psoriasis
• Erythrasma
• Tinea
• Streptococcal infection
• Folliculitis
• Contact dermatitis

Confirming the Diagnosis

- KOH prep if positive, will confirm diagnosis.
- Cultures may be necessary to differentiate candidiasis from other dermatoses, but key clinical findings may provide helpful clues for differential diagnoses.
- Tinea cruris is not typically macerated and usually has bilateral involvement of the inguinal folds, but not the scrotum.
- The erythema from intertrigo usually extends equally onto the thigh and groin and includes fissures; compared with candidiasis, which usually has extensive involvement, including the scrotum, and has satellite papules and pustules.
- Inverse psoriasis is thin, red, shiny, and nonscaly with a sharply demarcated border which will commonly affect more than one intertriginous area such as the axillae, inframammary folds, gluteal folds, inguinal folds, and umbilicus.

Treatment

Topical

- Topical azole antifungals are effective but must be accompanied by treatment to keep the areas dry.

- Application of Burow's solution compresses to moist areas for 20 minutes prior to applying the antifungal can be helpful.
- Creams should be rubbed in well to prevent excess moisture, or the use of a lotion may be preferred. Patients should be instructed to carefully dry skin folds after showering.
- The goal of therapy for intertrigo is to keep the area dry, which is a difficult task. Patients should be instructed to carefully dry skin folds after showering especially under the breast and inguinal folds.
- After gently washing with a cleanser and patting the skin dry, barrier products such as zinc oxide can reduce friction and "seal" the skin from excessive moisture.
- Newer products, such as fabric impregnated with silver (InterDry), reduce the friction and odor, along with absorbing moisture and suppressing yeast, fungal, and bacterial growth.

Systemic

- If unresponsive to topical antifungals, oral itraconazole or fluconazole should be used to clear the infection and then maintained with topicals.

Management and Patient Education

- Patients should be instructed to carefully dry skin folds after showering.
- Use of a hair dryer can be helpful, especially when the skin is macerated, and can also reduce transmission of spores with a contaminated bath towel.

Candida Balanitis

Balanitis occurs most often in older uncircumcised men. The cause of candida balanitis is usually poor hygiene, and the infection occurs more frequently in men who have had vaginal or anal intercourse with an infected partner. Recurrent infections can lead to phimosis or the inability to retract the foreskin due to scarring and edema.

Clinical Presentation

- Erythema, tender papules or pustules, white exudate, and edema on the glans penis (Fig. 6.1-18).

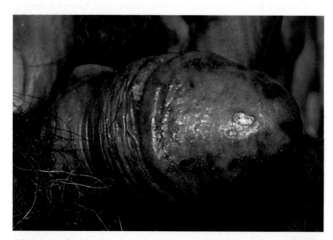

FIG. 6.1-18. Candida balanitis. (Goodheart, H. P. [2015]. *Goodheart's photoguide of common skin disorders* [4th ed.]. Wolters Kluwer Health | Lippincott Williams & Wilkins.)

DIFFERENTIAL DIAGNOSIS Candida Balanitis
• Eczema
• Psoriasis
• Lichen planus
• Lichen sclerosis

Confirming the Diagnosis

- KOH prep if positive, will confirm diagnosis
- Bacterial culture or biopsy can evaluate for other etiologies

Treatment

- Good hygiene is necessary for resolution of balanitis, cleaning with a gentle cleanser and drying thoroughly.
- Treatment should include a topical azole cream twice daily until the infection is cleared or a one-time dose of fluconazole (150 mg) along with prevention of reinfection.
- If bacterial infection suspected (or confirmed with culture), start treatment with topical bacitracin or mupirocin.

Management and Patient Education

- Most infections resolve completely with circumcision.
- For elective circumcision, or if phimosis or meatal stenosis occurs, consult a urologist.
- A sexual partner with untreated vulvovaginal candidiasis (VVC) could be the cause of recurrent candida balanitis.

Vulvovaginal Candidiasis

Most women, at some time in their lives, have experienced this unpleasant infection. More than 90% of the infections are caused by *C. albicans*, which is an opportunistic pathogen that occurs when the normal flora of the vagina is disrupted. The imbalance and infection can be triggered by recent antibiotic therapy, diabetes, a sexual partner with infection, change in hormones (HRT, tamoxifen therapy, pregnancy, and possibly oral contraceptives), tight-fitting or synthetic clothing, and immunosuppression.

Clinical Presentation

Skin Findings

- Erythema, edema, and sometimes satellite papules and vesicles that can extend from the vagina and surrounding area.

Non-Skin Findings

- Patients can complain of intense pruritus, burning, dysuria, dyspareunia, and vaginal discharge.

DIFFERENTIAL DIAGNOSIS	VVC
• Eczema/Atopic dermatitis	• Lichen planus
• Allergic contact dermatitis	• Lichen sclerosis
• Vaginal foreign object	• Sexually transmitted infections
• Psoriasis	• *Neisseria gonorrhea*
	• Chlamydia
	• *Trichomonas vaginalis*

TABLE 6.1-3	Classification and Treatment of Vulvovaginal Candidiasis	
	UNCOMPLICATED VCC	**COMPLICATED VCC**
Classification	Sporadic/Infrequent occurrence Mild-to-moderate symptoms Likely pathogen *C. albicans* Immunocompetent	Recurrent (more than 4 times/yr) Severe symptoms Not likely *C. albicans* Immunocompromised
Treatment	*Intravaginal*[a] Azoles for 1–7 days Butoconazole 2% cream for 4 days Clotrimazole 1% cream for 7 days Miconazole 2% cream for 7 days Miconazole vaginal suppositories 100 mg for 7 days 200 mg for 3 days 1,200 mg for 1 day Terconazole 0.4% cream for 7 days	*Intravaginal*[a] Azoles for 7–14 days Clotrimazole 1% cream for 14 days Miconazole 2% cream for 17 days Terconazole cream for 7–14 days *Oral* Fluconazole 150 mg—two doses 72 h apart **For azole-resistant** *Candida* Terconazole vaginal cream 7–14 days Boric acid vaginal tablets[b] 600 mg for 14 days Terconazole 0.8% cream for 3 days Terconazole suppository for 3 days Nystatin vaginal tablet for 14 days *Oral* Diflucan 150 mg PO one time only

[a]Vaginal tablets and creams applied each night before bedtime.
[b]Boric acid vaginal tablets are toxic if ingested.

Confirming the Diagnosis

- A KOH slide from the vaginal secretions will confirm diagnosis but must be obtained more than one week after any vaginal antifungal treatments.
- Fungal and bacterial cultures can be utilized to confirm etiology.

Treatment

The Centers for Disease Control and Prevention recommends the classification and treatment of VVC as simple or complicated (Table 6.1-3).

Topical

- Topical antifungal creams and vaginal tablets or suppositories are very safe and effective. Several imidazoles—miconazole, clotrimazole, and butoconazole—are available over-the-counter and may be used for 1 day to 1 week
- Prescription terconazole 0.4% intravaginal cream (Terazol) is available in 3- to 7-day doses, as well as a 80 mg vaginal suppository

Systemic
See Table 6.1-3.

Management and Patient Education

- With the availability of low-cost, over-the-counter yeast treatments, many women self-treat before even seeing their primary care provider. This can be convenient in resolving the problem, but can also delay the diagnosis and treatment of sexually transmitted infections, resistant yeast other than *C. albicans*, or recurrent VVC that needs a different therapy.

- Pruritus can be relieved with cool compresses to the perineum and use of topical antifungals on the outside of the vagina.
- Patients with severe or recurrent infections that do not resolve should be evaluated for underlying disease.

Diaper candidiasis—see Common Childhood Infections, Section 13.2.

PITYROSPORUM

The endogenous yeast *Pityrosporum orbiculare*, previously called *Malassezia furfur*, is a normal component of skin flora and is most prevalent in areas of the body with increased sebaceous activity. An overgrowth of *Pityrosporum* is responsible for both tinea versicolor and pityrosporum folliculitis, yet because it is an overgrowth of normal flora, these infections are not contagious to others. Exogenous factors such as excess heat and humidity, hyperhidrosis, pregnancy, oral contraceptives, systemic steroids, immunosuppression, or genetic predisposition can promote proliferation of the organism in the stratum corneum.

Tinea Versicolor

Tinea versicolor can be chronic and last for years because of genetic predisposition, recurrences, or inadequate treatment. This eruption is usually asymptomatic but sometimes can be mildly pruritic.

Clinical Presentation

- Sharply marginated, round macules and plaques with a fine scale on the upper trunk and neck. Usually symmetrical (Figs. 6.1-19 and 6.1-20).
- Lesions may appear pink/brown in Caucasians, while it can appear as hypopigmented or hyperpigmented in patients with darker skin—hence, various (or versi) colors.

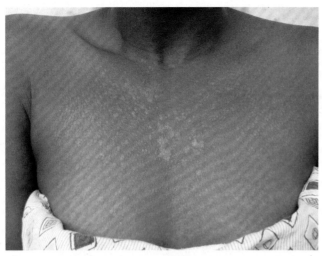

FIG. 6.1-19. Tinea versicolor with hypopigmented papules, fine scale. (Photo courtesy of M. Bobonich.)

- More evident in the summer as affected skin does not tan and creates a more obvious color contrast (dichromic appearance).

DIFFERENTIAL DIAGNOSIS   Tinea Versicolor

- Vitiligo
- Pityriasis alba
- Guttate psoriasis
- Hypopigmented mycosis fungoides
- Pityriasis rosea
- Eczema

Confirming the Diagnosis

- Diagnosis is usually made on clinical presentation alone, but a KOH prep will show budding fungal spores and short hyphae (often called "spaghetti and meatballs") (see Fig. 15-12B)
- Consider a skin biopsy for infections unresponsive to treatment

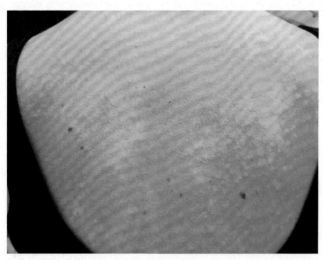

FIG. 6.1-20. Tinea versicolor with hypopigmented patches, fine scale. (Photo courtesy of M. Bobonich.)

Treatment

There are several treatment options based on the extent and location of rash. Recurrences are common so maintenance therapy is recommended.

Topical

- Topical antifungal (azoles and ciclopirox have best activity against yeasts) creams or lotions are used if small reachable areas are involved, and should be applied b.i.d. for at least 2 weeks. It can take weeks to months for the abnormal pigmentation to resolve after the yeast has been treated.
- Ketoconazole shampoo 2% applied like a lotion to wet skin is highly effective when used for 3 to 14 consecutive days. Apply the shampoo from the neck to the thighs and allow it to dry and remain for up to 4 hours, then rinse off in the shower. Selenium sulfide lotion 2.5% can be used in the same manner but for 7 to 14 consecutive days.
- To prevent recurrences, the shampoo or lotion should be used once a week as maintenance therapy during summer and once a month during winter.

Systemic

- Systemic antifungals are used off-label for cases that are extensive, unresponsive to topicals, or show frequent recurrences. Treatment can be with fluconazole (300 mg), given once a week for 1 to 4 weeks; or with itraconazole 200 mg, once daily for 5 to 7 days; or alternate dosing of 100 mg daily for 2 weeks. Azoles are highly excreted in sweat, so inducing a sweat 30 to 45 minutes after ingestion of oral treatments can increase efficacy.
- Griseofulvin and oral terbinafine are not effective. Historically, oral ketoconazole has been effective. In spite of this, clinicians should heed caution, with recent FDA warnings against the use of oral ketoconazole for most mucocutaneous fungal infections (Table 6.1-2).

Pityrosporum Folliculitis

Pityrosporum folliculitis is due to an infection of the hair follicle and causes inflammation.

It is often seen in young women and is easily misdiagnosed as acne. Key predisposing factors include occlusion, oily skin, humidity, diabetes mellitus, and recent treatment with systemic broad-spectrum antibiotics or corticosteroids.

Clinical Presentation

- Erythematous and sometimes pruritic perifollicular papules and pustules on upper back, chest, upper arms, and neck (Fig. 6.1-21)

DIFFERENTIAL DIAGNOSIS   Pityrosporum Folliculitis

- Acne
- Grover disease
- Sterile or bacterial folliculitis
- Eosinophilic folliculitis

Confirming the Diagnosis

- KOH prep can help clinicians differentiate acne from pityrosporum folliculitis and help determine management.
- If KOH is negative, a culture may confirm presence of pityrosporum.

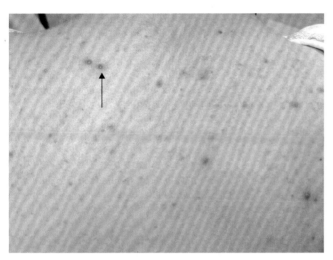

FIG. 6.1-21. Pityrosporum folliculitis with erythematous, perifollicular papules, and pustules (*arrow*). (Photo courtesy of M. Bobonich.)

Treatment

Topical

- Responds well to treatment with topical antifungals such as selenium sulfide 2.5% or ketoconazole 2% shampoo two or three times a week as a body wash to the affected areas.

Systemic

- Oral antifungals can also be used; use same oral treatments and dosing regimen for *Tinea versicolor*.

NAIL INFECTIONS

Infections of the nails are commonly caused by dermatophytes, but may also be caused by yeast and/or molds, and bacteria. Toenails have a higher rate of infection than do fingernails, and infections occur in both adults and children. Predisposing factors include trauma to the nail bed or fold (hangnails, injuries, trimming cuticles during manicure), increased age, peripheral vascular disease, immunocompromised and diabetic patients, and concomitant tinea infection of the skin. Since most dystrophic nails are often mistaken for fungal infections, diagnosis should be confirmed with direct microscopy or fungal culture.

DERMATOPHYTES

Clinical Presentation

Infections of the nails caused by dermatophytes are called onychomycosis or tinea unguium. There are three subtypes that correlate with the anatomical nail involvement.

- **Distal/lateral subungual onychomycosis (DLSO)**
  DLSO is the most common nail infection, the majority of which is caused by *T. rubrum*. Dermatophytes invade the distal area of the nail bed, causing a yellow or white nail that thickens and lifts at the distal nail bed. Subungual debris can collect and the nail can crumble or chip off (Fig. 6.1-22).
- **Superficial white onychomycosis (SO)**
  SO is a superficial invasion of the dorsal surface with *T. mentagrophytes* and *Trichophyton interdigitale* as the common pathogens. Often occurs in conjunction with bullous tinea pedis. Characteristics include a powdery white dry nail surface that stays attached to the nail bed (Fig. 6.1-23).

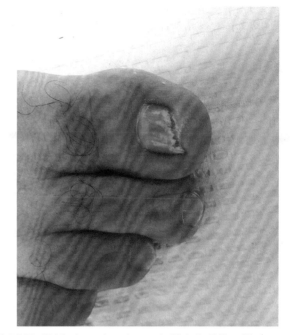

FIG. 6.1-22. Distal subungual onychomycosis. (© Janice T. Chussil.)

- **Proximal subungual onychomycosis (PSO)**
  PSO starts at the proximal nail fold area and migrates to the underlying matrix and nail plate, causing separation from the nail plate. Hyperkeratotic white debris accumulates in the proximal nail plate and obscures the lunula. *T. rubrum* and *Fusarium* species are usually the causative pathogens.
- Patients with PSO should be evaluated for a compromised immune system, specifically HIV disease.

DIFFERENTIAL DIAGNOSIS   Onychomycosis
• Psoriasis
• Eczema
• Lichen planus
• Congenital nail dystrophy
• Traumatic or chemical injury

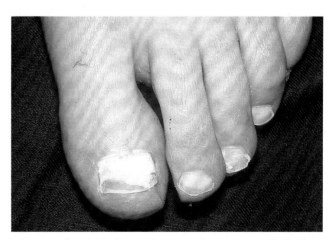

FIG. 6.1-23. Superficial white onychomycosis. (Goodheart, H. P. [2015]. *Goodheart's photoguide of common skin disorders* [4th ed.]. Wolters Kluwer Health | Lippincott Williams & Wilkins.)

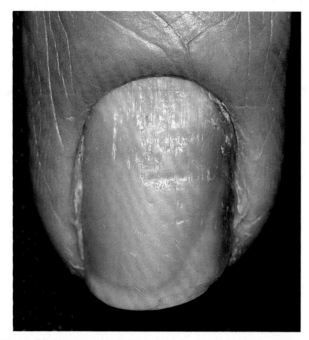

FIG. 6.1-24. Chronic paronychia. Note the swelling of the proximal nail fold, the loss of the cuticle, and the dystrophy of the nail plate. (Goodheart, H. P. [2015]. *Goodheart's photoguide of common skin disorders* [4th ed.]. Wolters Kluwer Health | Lippincott Williams & Wilkins.)

Candida Nail Infection

Candida infections of the nails are associated with chronic paronychia (infection of the nail fold or cuticle) or excessive water exposure.

Clinical Presentation

- Nails may have a varied appearance of green, yellow, black, or white with transverse ridging.
- Distal or lateral onycholysis (separation of the nail plate and bed) with yellow or white color can occur.
- Nail plate involvement occurs only in immunocompromised states.
- In chronic candida paronychia, there is separation of the cuticle from the nail plate together with edema, erythema, and tenderness of the proximal nail fold (Fig. 6.1-24).

DIFFERENTIAL DIAGNOSIS *Candida* Infection of Nail
• Tinea unguium
• Psoriasis
• Lichen planus
• Bacterial paronychia

Confirming the Diagnosis

- KOH prep from nail clippings or scrapings (see Section 15)
- Nail clippings can also be sent for histopathology. Place clippings in formalin and request PAS stain
- Fungal culture and PCR may be helpful

Treatment

The management approach to nail infections may include topical therapies, systemic antifungals, or both. Although systemic antifungals have the highest cure rates for dermatophyte and *Candida* infections, the choice of treatment will depend on the age of the patient, comorbidities, extent of nail involvement, and the patient's current medications. Topical methods should be considered first choice with limited nail involvement (only 1 to 5 nails), if patient has no risk of (or history of) liver disease, or if patient on medications that may interact with systemic antifungals. When several nails are infected or there are moderate-to-severe nail changes, systemic antifungals are preferred if circumstances are appropriate.

Topical

- Ciclopirox nail lacquer 8% (Penlac), tavaborole (Kerydin), and efinaconazole (Jublia) are the only FDA-approved topical treatments for adults and children older than 12 years for onychomycosis. (Jinna & Finch, 2015).
- Use of a keratolytic agent on thick nails before initiating therapy will aid in the absorption of the lacquer.
- It is helpful to warn patients that the treatment is a slow process (especially toenails) that takes months.
- *Recurrence prevention*—once nail infection has cleared, nail lacquers or antifungal gels or creams can be applied to the nails two to three times a week for an additional 2 to 3 months.

Systemic

- Oral terbinafine has fewer drug interactions, higher cure rate, and longer time for relapse than does itraconazole, which affects the levels of several drugs in the blood. Recommended dosage and duration of therapy using oral antifungals are detailed in Table 6.1-2.
- *Laser treatment*—there is limited evidence for the growing popularity of laser treatments for toenail fungus. It provides an alternative for patients who do not want to take or apply medications. Treatments require two to four sessions, are not covered by insurance, and can be very expensive. Recurrence rates are high so preventative measures will still need to be taken.

Management and Patient Education

- It is helpful to warn patients that the treatment is a slow process (especially toenails) that takes months. Realistic expectations of resolution of fingernails is 6 months; 9 months for toenails.
- To prevent recurrences after the nail infection has cleared, ciclopirox nail lacquer 8% or antifungal gels or creams can be applied to the nails two to three times a week.
- If you are unsure of the diagnosis or if the patient is not responding to treatment, consider repeat KOH test, fungal and bacterial cultures, a skin biopsy, and/or referral to dermatology.
- Podiatry is helpful in maintaining nail growth and foot health, especially in diabetics.
- When using systemic antifungals, clinicians should monitor serum hepatic studies, as indicated in Table 6.1-2.

SPECIAL TREATMENT CONSIDERATIONS
Pediatrics

- Griseofulvin is the only FDA-approved systemic treatment for onychomycosis in kids, but requires an extended therapy of 4 to 6 months, with limited effectiveness. Parents can crush griseofulvin tablets or use oral suspension (shaken well before administering); both should be given with a high-fat meal for better absorption. Furthermore, because griseofulvin is derived from a species of *Penicillium*, the possibility of cross sensitivity with penicillin exists, but is rare.

- *Off-label* use of other agents like fluconazole, terbinafine, and itraconazole because of their shorter duration of treatment and greater efficacy (Buck, 2006), have been reported safe in clinical trials and more than two dozen studies.

- Terbinafine is available in tablets that can be crushed and Lamisil granules (packets) are available for mixture.

- In pediatric studies, **off-label** dosing of terbinafine is a single daily dose of 62.5 mg for children 10 to 20 kg, 125 mg for children 20 to 40 kg, and 250 mg for children greater than 40 kg. A weight-based dose of 4 to 5 mg/kg/day has been suggested as an alternative (Gupta et al., 2003; Gupta & Drummond-Main, 2013). Treatment duration varies from 4 to 12 weeks.

- Ciclopirox nail lacquer can be used in children 12 years and older and offers a good alternative to systemics.

- Consider referring patients with severe or recalcitrant nail infections to dermatology.

Pregnancy

- Oral Terbinafine is FDA Pregnancy Category B (old rating system) and is the preferred drug of choice *if* the patient must be treated with a systemic antifungal before delivery.

- Diagnosis and management options should be discussed with the patient's OB/GYN before instituting an oral therapy.

- Other systemic antifungals—itraconazole, fluconazole, and griseofulvin—are category C, and are therefore contraindicated during pregnancy. Additionally, women of childbearing age treated with griseofulvin should use a backup birth control method if they are also taking oral contraceptives, as it may lower the efficacy.

- Ciclopirox nail lacquer 8% (Penlac) was designated as a category B treatment; but both tavaborole (Kerydin) and efinaconazole (Jublia) lacquers have a category C rating. Refer to Table 6.1-1 for safety ratings of topical creams and gels.

Geriatrics

- Elderly patients who have thick nails or who cannot take systemic antifungals because of drug interactions should have their nails trimmed regularly and thinned by podiatry.

- Thick nails can cause pressure and pain and impede ambulation.

- Ciclopirox nail lacquer offers a relatively safe therapy for nail infections caused by dermatophytes.

- If systemic antifungals are used, clinicians may need to consider appropriate dosage adjustments and possible lab monitoring.

CLINICAL PEARLS

- If one class of antifungals is not effective in a culture-proven mycosis, switch to another class or consider a systemic antifungal.

- Select the appropriate vehicle for application of topical antifungals. Use creams in dry areas, gels, powders, or sprays in moist areas, and lotions or gels for hairy or large areas.

- Avoid combination antifungal/steroid creams; they contain high-potency steroids, which are *not* recommended for children and can cause striae.

- If feet and nails are infected, both must be treated to avoid reinfection.

- Tinea pedis is commonly transmitted to the groin so both areas should be examined. To prevent tinea pedis from spreading to the groin, instruct the patient to put on their socks before underwear.

- Have the patient apply the topicals until the skin is clear and then for at least 1 week longer. Remind patients that fungal infections have a high rate of recurrence and may need a prescribed maintenance plan.

READINGS AND REFERENCES

Baran, R., Feuilhade, M., Combernale, P., Datry, A., Goettmann, S., Pietrini, P., Viguie, C., Badillet, G., Larnier, C., & Czernielewski, J. (2000). A randomized trial of amorolfine 5% solution nail lacquer combined with oral terbinafine compared with terbinafine alone in the treatment of dermatophytic toenail onychomycoses affecting the matrix region. *The British Journal of Dermatology, 142*(6), 1177–1183.

Bell-Syer, S. E. M., Khan, S. M., & Torgerson, D. J. (2012). Oral treatments for fungal infections of the skin of the foot. *The Cochrane Database of Systematic Reviews, 10*(10), CD003584.

Bolognia, J. L., Schaffer, J. V., & Cerroni, L. (2018). *Dermatology* (4th ed.). Mosby Elsevier.

Buck, M. (2006). Use of oral terbinafine in children. *Ped Pharmacotherapy,* University of Virginia Press, *12,* 7.

Crawford, F., & Hollis, S. (2009). Topical treatments for fungal infections of the skin and nails of the foot. (Review) Copyright © 2009. The Cochrane Collaboration. Published by John Wiley & Sons, Ltd.

González, U., Seaton, T., Bergus, G., Jacobson, J., & Martínez-Monzón, C. (2007). Systemic antifungal therapy for tinea capitis in children. *The Cochrane Database of Systematic Reviews,* (4), CD004685.

Gupta, A. K., & Drummond-Main, C. (2013). Meta-analysis of randomized, controlled trials comparing particular doses of griseofulvin and terbinafine for the treatment of tinea capitis. *Pediatric Dermatology, 30*(1), 1–6.

Gupta, A. K., Cooper, E., & Lunde C. W. (2003). The efficacy and safety of terbinafine in children. *Dermatologic Clinics, 21*(3), 511–20.

Habif, T. P. (2020). *Clinical dermatology: A color guide to diagnosis and therapy* (7th ed.). Mosby.

Jinna, S., & Finch, J. (2015). Spotlight on tavaborole for the treatment of onychomycosis. *Drug Design, Development and Therapy, 9,* 6185–6190. https://doi.org/10.2147/DDDT.S81944

Joyce, A., Gupta, A., Koenig, L., Wolcott, R., & Carviel, J. (2019). Fungal diversity and onychomycosis: An analysis of 8,816 toenail samples using quantitative PCR and next-generation sequencing. *Journal of the American Podiatric Medical Association, 109*(1), 57–63.

Paller, A. S., & Mancini, A. J. (2015). *Hurwitz clinical pediatric dermatology* (5th ed.). Elsevier.

Scott, T. D. (2011). Procedure primer: The potassium hydroxide preparation. *Journal of the Dermatology Nurses' Association, 3*(5), 304–305.

Wolverton, S. E. (2020). *Comprehensive dermatologic drug therapy* (4th ed.). Elsevier.

Superficial Bacterial Infections

Mary E. Nolen

The normal skin of a healthy individual is naturally resistant to infection. The normal skin flora, or skin microbiome, actually protects us from invasion of other organisms which vary by anatomic location. *Staphylococcus aureus*, a gram-positive organism, is usually found on the surface of exposed skin while *Pseudomonas aeruginosa*, a gram-negative bacteria, occurs on the moist areas of axilla, groin, and web spaces. Despite this frontline host protection, skin and soft tissue infections (SSTIs) are a very common cause of patient encounters in Primary Care Clinics and Emergency Departments and comprise nearly 20% of patient visits to dermatology.

There are therefore several elements which can upset the host–bacteria relationship and transform the status quo into an infectious state. The elements in play are the virulence of the organism, the portal of entry, and the ability of the host to defend and respond to the presence of the organism. Typically, it is a combination of these elements that places an individual at risk.

Bacterial infections of the skin can manifest either as a primary cutaneous process, such as impetigo, or as a manifestation of a systemic infection such as Toxic Shock Syndrome (TSS). This chapter will address the recognition and treatment of the most common SSTIs including those infections that have systemic involvement. Alternative treatments will be suggested when possible to minimize the frequency of drug resistance.

Treatment for bacterial infections often requires the use of antibiotics and other antimicrobial drugs topically or systemically. Therefore, the clinician's ability to recognize and treat infections of the skin early in the course of the disease will ensure that patients receive optimal antimicrobial therapy when indicated. Likewise, the ability to distinguish true infection from other inflammatory conditions will spare patients the risk and expense of unnecessary medicines.

ANTIMICROBIAL SELECTION

Antibiotic selection is pivotal to the treatment of any bacterial infection and the optimum choice is based on many factors. The individual pathogen and its susceptibility profile will largely determine the most appropriate antimicrobial and often vary with geographic location. The mechanism of action will determine whether the drug is bacteriostatic or bactericidal. In other words, you need to choose the best drug for the specific bug. In addition, drug interactions and adverse effects must be considered along with the patient's immune status, age, pregnancy, and genetic predisposition. A history of drug allergy is essential when deciding treatment; however, many patients confuse true allergy with side effect especially if they were advised to discontinue the drug. The degree of a penicillin allergy, for example, may not prohibit the use of cephalosporins if needed, so a careful and probing history is sometimes required.

The increase in drug resistance in this country will also influence the choice of medicines. Misuse of antibiotics is a significant contributing factor in resistance. Patients are often prescribed antibiotics for colds and viral infections inappropriately because of patient demand. Drugs are prescribed in improper doses and without bacteriologic information to support their use. Systemic medications can sometimes be eliminated altogether if other interventions such as Incision and Drainage (I&D) and supportive measures are instituted. On occasion, topical therapy may be sufficient and systemic products excessive. It is important to remember the old rule when prescribing medication: "Right Drug, Right Dose, Right Duration, Right Patient, and Right Time" (Dryden et al., 2011). The responsibility of prescribing medication for our patients should not be misused. These decisions demand that we as clinicians possess a thorough understanding of the available classes of drugs, their mechanism of action and effectiveness in various conditions, as well as special circumstances in which they should not be used.

Antimicrobial Resistance

The development of antibiotics, once seen as revolutionary progress in the fight against infection, has backfired on the medical community and general public and now represents one of the largest public health threats today. Overprescribing and incorrect prescribing of these medications has resulted in the development of resistance to the very drugs meant to cure and has become a worldwide health problem.

According to the CDC (2019) Antibiotic Resistance Report, more than 2.8 million antibiotic-resistant infections occur in the United States each year, and more than 35,000 people die as a result. The six most common pathogens responsible for these drug-resistant infections have been named ESKAPE pathogens as an acronym for the actual organisms: (*Enterococcus faecium, S. aureus, Klebsiella pneumoniae, Acinetobacter baumannii, P. aeruginosa,* and *Enterobacter* spp.). By far the ones encountered most commonly in the practice of dermatology are *S. aureus (MRSA)* and *P. aeruginosa.*

It is incumbent on the prescriber as well as the patient to recognize this threat and to take necessary steps to safeguard against this problem.

Antibiotic Stewardship

Antibiotic stewardship is defined by CDC (2013) as "the effort to measure and improve how antibiotics are prescribed by clinicians and used by patients. Improving antibiotic prescribing involves implementing effective strategies to modify prescribing practices to align them with evidence-based recommendations for diagnosis and management.

The ultimate goal of antibiotic stewardship is to maximize the benefit of antibiotic treatment while minimizing harm both to individual persons and to communities."

Antibiotic stewardship for Outpatient clinicians and facilities was developed by Sanchez et al. (2016) and augments the previous work by CDC in 2014 and 2015, respectively, for Stewardship programs in Hospitals and Nursing Homes (Box 6.2-1).

GRAM-POSITIVE BACTERIAL INFECTIONS

Staphylococcal and Streptococcal Infections

The two bacteria that most commonly cause skin infections are *S. aureus* and group A β-hemolytic streptococcus (GAS). *S. aureus* is present on all skin surfaces and is considered a normal part of skin flora. Streptococci however are secondary invaders and attack skin that is already traumatized causing infections such as cellulitis. Infections caused by both of these organisms can range from superficial skin to systemic, multiorgan involvement.

BOX 6.2-1   Antibiotic Stewardship

The following recommendations are intended for all outpatient clinicians and facilities:
- Use evidence-based diagnostic criteria and treatment recommendations.
- Use delayed prescribing practices or watchful waiting, when appropriate.
- Document drug, dose, indication, and duration.
- Self-evaluate antibiotic prescribing practices. Reevaluate after 48 hr to determine: If the infection will respond to an antibiotic, is this the right drug for the diagnosis or is there a more targeted therapeutic option, and what is the most effective duration of therapy
- Participate in continuing medical education and quality improvement activities to track and improve antibiotic prescribing.
- Provide education to patients about the potential harms of antibiotic treatment

Adapted from Sanchez, G. V., Fleming-Dutra, K. E., Roberts, R. M., Hicks, L. A. (2016). Core elements of outpatient antibiotic stewardship. *MMWR. Recommendations and Reports: Morbidity and Mortality Weekly Report. Recommendations and Reports, 65*(6), 1–12.

Impetigo

Perhaps the most familiar and widely known infection of the skin is impetigo. This is a highly contagious, superficial skin infection usually found in children. Adults can acquire it due to direct skin to skin contact. It can be seen in two forms: nonbullous and bullous type. Nonbullous is more common and occurs primarily in children on the face (nose and mouth) and extremities. Bullous is less common and tends to occur in neonates and younger children and because of the presence of blisters, it is considered to be a localized form of Staphylococcal Scalded Skin Syndrome (SSSS)—Refer to Section 13 for details.

Pathophysiology

- *Nonbullous impetigo* was caused by GAS almost exclusively in the past, but today most cases are caused by *S. aureus* alone or in combination with GAS.
- *Bullous impetigo* is caused by strains of *S. aureus* that produce a toxin which results in the formation of blisters in the epidermis.

Clinical Presentation

Nonbullous Impetigo

- More common type and occurs primarily in children on the face (nose and mouth) and extremities.

Skin Findings

- It usually begins as 2- to 4-mm erythematous macules that evolve into vesicles or pustules. Later these lesions erode with a typical honey-colored crust and surrounding erythema.
- Usually asymptomatic but itching and soreness may be mild (Fig. 6.2-1).

Bullous Impetigo

- Often begin as small vesicles that later develop into large bullae.
- Blisters are flaccid with contents that may be clear or cloudy (Fig. 6.2-2A).

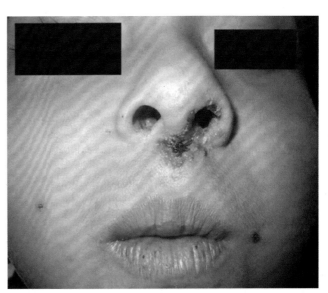

FIG. 6.2-1. Nonbullous impetigo. Clinical image of honey-crusted impetigo. (Courtesy of Dr. Karina Feria.)

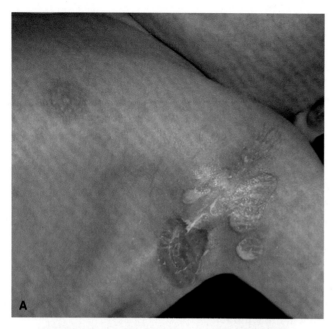

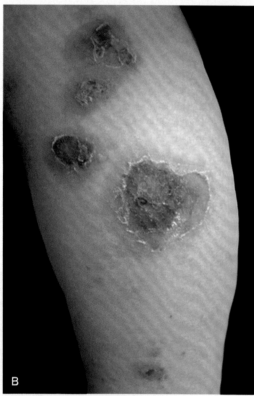

FIG. 6.2-2. A: Bullous impetigo. Clinical image of bullous impetigo in a neonate. (Courtesy of Dr. Karina Feria.) **B:** Bullous impetigo after the blisters have broken. Bullous impetigo: Remnants of the roof of the blisters are seen at the lesional edges, giving the lesions an annular appearance. (Courtesy of Dr. Rosa Ines Castro.)

- Blisters break easily and develop a perimeter of scale which may measure up to 5 cm, but no crust or surrounding erythema is seen (Fig. 6.2-2B).
- A crust may form which, if removed, will reveal a moist, red base.

- There may be few or numerous lesions and they may occur on any surface but typical infections occur on the face, trunk, buttocks, and perineum.
- Systemic symptoms rarely occur but lymphadenopathy and fever may be present in severe cases of either type.

Confirming the Diagnosis

- Impetigo is often diagnosed clinically but if the diagnosis is in question, a culture may be obtained from beneath the crust or from the fluid of an intact blister.
- Gram stain and culture of the pus or exudate from skin lesions of impetigo are recommended to help identify whether *S. aureus* and/or a β-hemolytic streptococcus is the cause, but treatment without these studies is reasonable in typical cases.
- Viral culture should be done if HSV is suspected.
- Documenting a positive culture for streptococcus may be useful in patients who are later suspected of poststreptococcal nephritis.

DIFFERENTIAL DIAGNOSIS Impetigo		
Nonbullous Type	*Bullous Type*	*Uncommon*
• HSV (viral culture may distinguish) • Insect bites • Eczema or contact dermatitis • Tinea (potassium hydroxide [KOH] can support or rule out) • Scabies • Varicella	• Allergic contact dermatitis • Bullous insect bites • Thermal burn • HSV	• Autoimmune bullous dermatosis • Bullous pemphigoid • Bullous erythema multiforme • Stevens–Johnson syndrome

Treatment

Topical

- Impetigo is often treated successfully with topical, 2% mupirocin (Bactroban, Centany) Ointment applied TID until all lesions have cleared. Ozenoxacin cream b.i.d. × 5 days is approved for patients 2 months and older for infections attributed to *S. aureus* or *Streptococcus pyogenes*. It may resolve spontaneously and clear without scarring.
- Topical retapamulin (Altabax) is also approved for uncomplicated skin infections caused by *S. aureus*. It is less effective and **not approved for MRSA**.
- Careful washing of the area with an antibacterial cleanser such as chlorhexidine (Hibiclens) may be used but **hydrogen peroxide is not recommended**. In most cases, washing with plain soap and water is adequate. Antibacterial cleansers which contain triclosan are not recommended.
- Organism is thought to be harbored in the nose and then transmitted to skin; therefore, if infections are recurrent, then patients should be evaluated for nasal carriage and mupirocin ointment 1% may be indicated for use in the nose b.i.d. for 6 months to 1 year.

Systemic

- Oral antibiotics may be needed for patients with numerous lesions, systemic symptoms such as fever, or in outbreaks affecting several people to help decrease transmission of infection.

- Because *S. aureus* isolates from impetigo are usually methicillin susceptible, a 5- to 10-day course of dicloxacillin, amoxicillin clavulanate, or a cephalosporin such as cephalexin or cefadroxil should result in rapid clearing.
- Erythromycin is less effective and penicillin V is not indicated unless cultures yield streptococci alone.

Management and Patient Education

- Failure to clear despite treatment may indicate a resistant strain of organism and needs to be seen and cultured.
- Since most impetigo occurs at the site of minor trauma, it is recommended that careful washing with antibacterial cleanser be performed at all new sites to prevent infection.
- Follow-up is not indicated if all lesions resolve.

Special Considerations

- *Athletes* engaged in a wide variety of sports are at greater risk of developing and spreading superficial bacterial infections including MRSA.

- Proper care of equipment and mats is necessary and strict personal hygiene is necessary.
- Athletes must be removed from competition until cleared or occlusive dressings must be worn during play.
- Atopic patients should be monitored carefully for occurrence of impetigo as secondary infection. Eczema and impetigo must be treated aggressively to minimize spread of infection (Table 6.2-1).

CLINICAL PEARLS

- Poststreptococcal nephritis may occur 1 to 3 weeks after an acute streptococcal impetigo. It occurs most commonly between the ages of 6 and 10 and is often asymptomatic.
- All strep infections can also trigger a guttate form of psoriasis. This may in fact be the presenting sign and the initial episode of the condition.

Folliculitis

Folliculitis is an inflammation of the hair follicle which can be caused by infection, irritation, or physical injury. It may involve the

TABLE 6.2-1	Guidelines for Treatment of Skin Infections and Return to Play	
CONDITION	**NCAA GUIDELINES**	**NFHS GUIDELINES**
Bacterial Infections		
Community-Acquired MRSA	No new lesions >48 hr	No new lesions >48 hr
Furuncles	Oral antibiotics >72 hr	Oral antibiotics >72 hr
Carbuncles	No moist, exudative, or draining lesions	No draining or oozing lesions
Impetigo	No moist, exudative, or draining lesions	No draining or oozing lesions
Cellulitis	Active infections may not be covered by participants	All lesions must be scabbed
Folliculitis	Site may be covered after infection becomes inactive and patient meets criteria to participate	All lesions must be scabbed
Infestations		
Pediculosis	Complete treatment Reexamination shows no evidence of infestation	24 hr posttreatment No evidence of infestation
Scabies	Complete treatment Negative results of mineral oil preparation	24 hr posttreatment No evidence of infestation

			MEDICATION AND DOSAGE	
HERPES INFECTIONS	**TREATMENT PURPOSE**	**ACYCLOVIR**	**FAMCICLOVIR**	**VALACYCLOVIR**
H Gladiatorum	Primary (14-day treatment)	400 mg 5 times daily	500 mg 3 times daily	1000 mg 2–3 times daily
H Zoster	Recurrent (5-day treatment)	400 mg 3 times daily	125 mg 2 times daily	1000 mg 2 times daily
H Labialis	Chronic (daily suppression)	400 mg 2 times daily	250 mg 2 times daily	<10 episodes/yr: 500 mg daily; ≥10 episodes/yr or <2-yr history of infection: 1 g daily
H Whitlow				

Adapted from Sports-Related Skin Infections Position Statement and Guidelines: National Federation of State High School Associations (NFHS), Sports Medicine Advisory Committee (SMAC). (2018).

superficial portion of the hair follicle or it may be a deeper process. This section will address bacterial folliculitis caused by common gram-positive organisms. Please see the gram-negative section for additional types.

Pathophysiology

- Many infectious agents may be responsible including bacteria, fungus, and yeast.
- A noninfectious process may also occur from shaving, secondary to certain drugs such as systemic steroids or the long-term use antibiotics for acne.
- Diabetes or immunosuppression are important risk factors for folliculitis.

Clinical Presentation

Skin Findings

- Superficial folliculitis is usually caused by *S. aureus* and appears as an erythematous papule or pustule surrounding the hair.
- A deeper process may present initially as a red, tender nodule which may eventually develop a point in center (Fig. 6.2-3A,B).

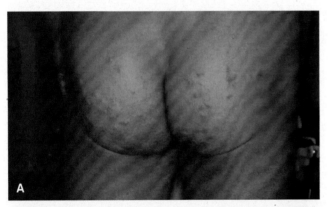

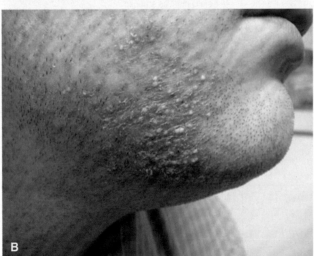

FIG. 6.2-3. A: Buttock folliculitis. A child with erythematous papules over the posterior buttocks consistent with folliculitis. (Courtesy of Jan Edwin Drutz, MD.) **B:** Folliculitis beard. (Used with permission from Goodheart, H. P. [2010]. *Goodheart's same-site differential diagnosis: A rapid method of diagnosing and treating common skin disorders.* Wolters Kluwer.)

DIFFERENTIAL DIAGNOSIS	Folliculitis (Varies with Location)
Impetigo	Steroid acne (trunk)
Fungal infection	Keratosis pilaris (extremities)
Candida folliculitis	Perioral dermatitis (face)
HSV	Scabies
Pseudofolliculitis barbae (face)	Insect bites

Confirming the Diagnosis

- It may be important to know the specific cause of the folliculitis so that appropriate treatment can be rendered.
- Bacterial culture and sensitivities should be done if there is a fresh pustule.
- The most effective way to culture is to nick the pustule with a #11 blade to expose the contents and transfer them to a culture swab.
- Removing the pustule with a #15 blade and depositing the material on the culture swab can also be done to eliminate contamination of the culture by contacting the surrounding skin.
- Potassium hydroxide (KOH) prep could also be done on the contents of a pustule to rule out fungus or yeast.

Treatment

- Superficial infection may be treated successfully with antibacterial cleansers such as chlorhexidine (Hibiclens) and topical antibiotics such as 1% clindamycin solution or gel applied b.i.d. after washing.
- Bleach Body Wash such as CLn BodyWash can be effective if used in addition several times a week for *S. aureus* infection.
- Systemic antibiotics may be needed if there is little response to topicals but should be prescribed based on the culture and sensitivities.

Management and Patient Education

- It is important that patients understand the prevention of bacterial infections is largely dependent on good personal hygiene. Patients should be advised to avoid sharing personal items such as razors and towels.
- Athletes must make sure they are following the NCAA Guidelines for play.
- Most superficial infections resolve without scarring.
- Some postinflammatory discoloration may persist for some time.

Cellulitis and Erysipelas

Cellulitis is an infection of the deep dermis and subcutaneous tissue and is often accompanied by lymphangitis. Erysipelas involves the upper dermis and superficial lymphatics. Both of these conditions are common infections that result from invasion of bacteria at the site of trauma or surgical wound. Maceration of web spaces and cracks in the skin from tinea pedis create a very common portal of entry.

Pathophysiology

- Cellulitis is generally seen in adults and caused by *GAS or S. aureus.* Cellulitis that is diffuse or unassociated with a defined portal is most commonly caused by streptococcal species and cellulitis associated with furuncles, carbuncles, or abscesses is usually caused by *S. aureus*. Important clinical clues to other causes include physical activities, trauma, water contact, and animal, insect, or human bites.

- Erysipelas also known as St. Anthony's fire is a specific variant of cellulitis usually caused by GAS and occurs in the young, the aged, and the immunocompromised. It is often on the face or extremities and the buttock is also a frequent site.

Clinical Presentation

Skin Findings

- Both cellulitis and erysipelas are characterized by erythema, warmth, pain, swelling, and tenderness.
- Cellulitis is often preceded by fever, chills, and malaise, and produces an ill-defined area of tender, erythematous induration most often on lower extremities and may be accompanied by purulent drainage or abscess formation (Fig. 6.2-4A).
- Severe infections may present with vesicles, bulla, lymphangitis, and involvement of regional lymph nodes.

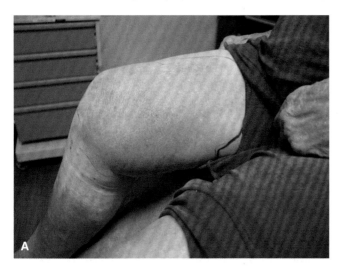

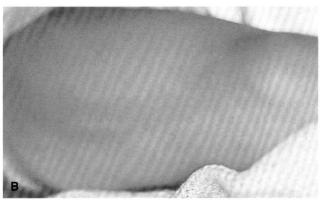

FIG. 6.2-4. **A:** Cellulitis of the knee. Cellulitis in this patient developed at the site of a minor wound. The child presented with fever and lymphangitic streaking. (Fleisher, G. R., Ludwig, W., & Baskin, M. N. [2004]. *Atlas of pediatric emergency medicine.* Wolters Kluwer Health | Lippincott Williams & Wilkins.) **B:** Cellulitis thigh. Bacterial infection involving the skin of knee and thigh. Leg is swollen, red, warm, and tender to touch. (Photos courtesy of Kimberly LeBlanc & Jeffrey A. Niezgoda.) Note the lower leg is covered with a drainage-filled bandage from chronic stasis dermatitis. (Used with permission from Baranoski, S., & Ayello, E. A. [2020]. *Wound care essentials* [5th ed.]. Wolters Kluwer.)

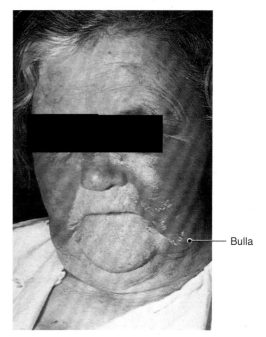

FIG. 6.2-5. Erysipelas. This patient has large, confluent erythematous plaques. A bulla is present near the angle of her jaw. (McConnell, T. H. [2007]. *The nature of disease pathology for the health professions.* Wolters Kluwer Health | Lippincott Williams & Wilkins.)

- Lymphangitis occurs as a linear area of erythema extending from the infection site to the regional lymph node (Fig. 6.2-4B).
- Erysipelas in contrast, produces a fiery-red, well-demarcated, raised plaque, with a *peau d'orange* appearance. The borders are palpable and often occur on the central face or extremities. The buttock is also a frequent site (Fig. 6.2-5).

Non-Skin Findings

- Regional lymphadenopathy is often present.
- Systemic symptoms including fever, chills, may be present in both conditions.
- The onset of erysipelas is acute, spread is rapid, and may be accompanied by pain, a burning sensation, fever, and chills.

Differential Diagnosis

Multiple inflammatory conditions, particularly, if they present on lower extremities are often misdiagnosed as cellulitis and treated inappropriately with antibiotics. These are often referred to as "pseudocellulitis" because of the presence of erythema and edema. Examples are listed as DDx of Noninfectious causes of Cellulitis and Erysipelas.

Confirming the Diagnosis

The diagnosis of cellulitis and erysipelas is generally made clinically. Diagnostics may be considered if the cellulitis is extensive, has purulent drainage, or MRSA is suspected. If the patient is immunocompromised, the infection occurs in an unusual location, or is accompanied by signs and symptoms of systemic infection then the following tests are recommended:

Laboratory

- Wound culture and drug susceptibility tests if there is drainage or the portal of entry is clinically involved

- Blood culture, complete blood cell count with differential, creatinine, bicarbonate, creatine phosphokinase, ASO titer, CRP, culture of needle aspiration
- Punch biopsy specimen is rarely indicated

DIFFERENTIAL DIAGNOSIS	Cellulitis and Erysipelas
Adults	
Infectious	*Noninfectious (Pseudocellulitis)*
Erythema migrans	Gout
Toxic shock syndrome	Contact dermatitis
Necrotizing fasciitis	Stasis dermatitis
Gas gangrene	Bursitis
Herpes zoster	Insect bites
Tinea	DVT
	Drug reactions
	Erythema nodosum
	Lymphedema
	Lipodermatosclerosis
	Granuloma faciale
Children	
Erythema migrans	Contact dermatitis
Toxic shock syndrome	Insect bites
Necrotizing fasciitis	Drug reaction
Tinea	

Hospitalization

- If patients exhibit hypotension and/or an elevated creatinine level, low serum bicarbonate level, elevated creatine phosphokinase (CPK) two to three times the upper limit and C-reactive protein level >13 mg/L, hospitalization should be considered.
- Surgical consultation for inspection, exploration, and/or drainage may be needed.

Radiology

- X-ray is performed if osteomyelitis is suspected.
- MRI or CT scan is done to determine if deeper infection to muscle or fascia is present.
- Ultrasound can help to identify abscesses.

Treatment

- Numerous studies have been performed over the years to identify the optimal choice of antibiotics, most effective dose, route of administration, and duration of treatment for cellulitis and erysipelas. A recent review of 43 studies and almost 6,000 participants (Brindle et al., 2019) revealed that no strong evidence was found to support one antibiotic over another. Trials of 5 and 10 days were also reviewed and seemed to be equally effective as was intravenous versus oral administration.
- Cellulitis which is not associated with abscess is usually treated with systemic antimicrobials against GAS or *S. aureus* for 7 to 10 days (Box 6.2-2).

Management and Patient Education

- For patients who show signs of systemic illness, have facial edema, or do not respond to oral therapy, consultation with dermatology or infectious disease is recommended.

BOX 6.2-2 Management of Uncomplicated Cellulitis

Uncomplicated Cellulitis is Defined as:
Nonpurulent cellulitis
No exudates or abscess
No fever
No immunosuppression

Empiric Antimicrobial Treatment for β-Hemolytic Streptococci[a]
Cephalexin 250–500 mg q.i.d.
Dicloxacillin 500 mg q.i.d.
Clindamycin[b] 300–450 mg t.i.d.
Linezolid[b] 600 mg b.i.d.

---

[a]Cellulitis and erysipelas are usually caused by group A β-hemolytic streptococcus.
[b]Also has activity against CA-MRSA.
Adapted from LAMBERT, M. (2011). IDSA guidelines on the treatment of MRSA infections in adults and children. *American Family Physician, 84*(4), 455–463..

- Cellulitis may be recurrent and each episode may cause lymphatic inflammation and lead to lymphedema. Identification and treatment of the portal of entry is essential to prevent recurrences.
- Patients placed on a regimen of systemic and topical antibiotic therapy should be reevaluated in 24 to 48 hours to assess their clinical response. Progression of infection, despite antibiotic therapy, could be due to an infection with resistant microbes or a deeper, more extensive process.
- Recurrent infections may also signify inadequate dosing of the antibiotic.
- It is important to explain to patients that cellulitis generally occurs where there is a break in the skin barrier. Therefore, treating an underlying infection such as tinea pedis is paramount to prevent recurrences.
- Lower leg skin care including elevation, compression, and emollients should be performed.

CLINICAL PEARL

- The presentation of cellulitis is almost always unilateral. If there is bilateral involvement, or if it does not respond to antibiotic therapy, consider an alternative diagnosis such as stasis or contact dermatitis.

Special Considerations

Periorbital Cellulitis

Cellulitis around the eye or involving the eyelid and periorbital area should be carefully investigated. Periorbital erythema and edema may be seen in both preseptal and true orbital cellulitis and the clinician should be aware of the difference.

- *Periorbital cellulitis*—Often related to trauma to the eyelid, may result in inflammation or infection and may involve the soft tissues around the eye. Although the swelling may be significant, the patient should not experience pain or limited movement of the eye. Periorbital cellulitis is generally treated adequately with antibiotics.
- *Orbital cellulitis*—Often the progression of an upper respiratory infection or sinusitis. The infection spreads beyond the orbital septum and may be the result of a tumor on the optic

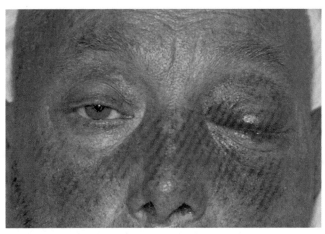

FIG. 6.2-6. Orbital cellulitis. Left orbital cellulitis with marked periorbital edema, erythema, and proptosis.

nerve. Orbital cellulitis is characterized by swelling of the conjunctiva, pain, limited eye movement and the pupil will often have a very sluggish reaction to light (afferent pupil). This condition has a high morbidity and generally, necessitates emergent recognition, intravenous antibiotics, and/or surgical intervention (Fig. 6.2-6).

ABSCESSES, FURUNCLES, CARBUNCLES, AND EPIDERMOID CYSTS

Pathophysiology

- An abscess is a walled-off collection of pus that may be sterile or the result of infection that can occur in any organ or tissue.

Sterile abscesses can arise as a response to a foreign body, an inflamed sebaceous cyst, or even an odontogenic sinus.

- A furuncle begins in a hair follicle, and therefore presents on hair-bearing areas. It is commonly associated with *S. aureus*, extends deeper into subcutaneous tissue, and may develop into an abscess.

- A carbuncle represents involvement of multiple inflamed abscesses arising in contiguous follicles and sinus tracts, forming a single mass.

- An epidermoid or epidermal cyst is the most common cyst on the skin and is derived from the upper portion of the hair follicle (infundibulum). It can be induced by trauma or follicular inflammation such as acne and can occur at any age.

- Risk factors for the above include contact with someone who has an infection caused by staphylococcus species, diabetes, and any other skin condition which may alter the skin barrier such as eczema and immunosuppression (Fig. 6.2-7).

Clinical Presentation

Skin Findings

- An abscess begins as a tender, red/erythematous nodule that eventually becomes fluctuant in the center with a prominent point (Fig. 6.2-8).

- Spontaneous rupture and drainage can occur especially with pressure or friction. Once opened, the patient becomes at increased risk for infection usually by *S. aureus.*

- Furuncles favor hair-bearing locations and tend to occur on the neck, axillae, and buttocks (Fig. 6.2-9).

- Carbuncles are larger nodules and painful masses comprised of multiple furuncles with several sinus openings (Fig. 6.2-10).

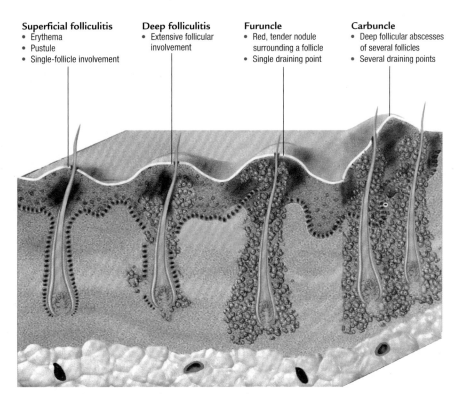

Superficial folliculitis
- Erythema
- Pustule
- Single-follicle involvement

Deep folliculitis
- Extensive follicular involvement

Furuncle
- Red, tender nodule surrounding a follicle
- Single draining point

Carbuncle
- Deep follicular abscesses of several follicles
- Several draining points

FIG. 6.2-7. Distinguishing folliculitis, furuncles, and carbuncles.

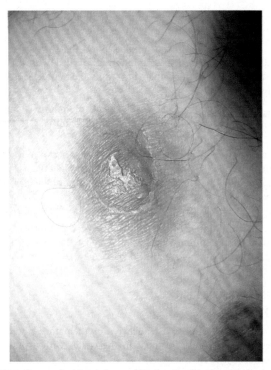

FIG. 6.2-8. Abscess. Peripheral abscess: Note the shiny thin skin. This abscess was treated by incision and drainage with resolution. (Used with permission from Harris, J. R., Lippman, M. E., Morrow, M., & Osborne, C. K. [2014]. *Diseases of the breast* [5th ed.]. Wolters Kluwer.)

- Epidermoid cysts can be solitary or multiple. They are skin-colored nodules which may have a central keratin-filled punctum on the surface through which a white, foul-smelling cheese-like substance can be expressed. Once ruptured, there may be inflammation, pain, redness, and increasing size (Fig. 6.2-11A,B).

Non-Skin Findings

- Abscesses extending into the subcutaneous area may not have an obvious point, and may be accompanied by fever, chills, fatigue, and lymphadenopathy may be present.

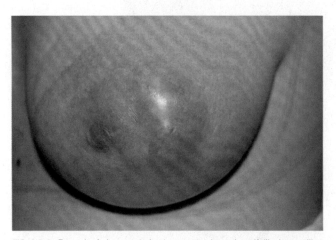

FIG. 6.2-9. Furuncle. A deep-seated cutaneous tender, red, perifollicular swelling with a superficial scale, which may terminate in the discharge of pus. (Image courtesy of R. Lee.)

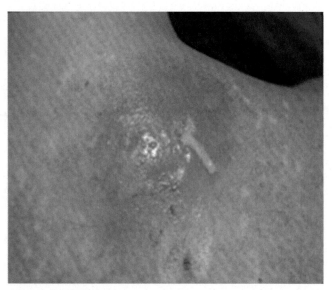

FIG. 6.2-10. Carbuncle.

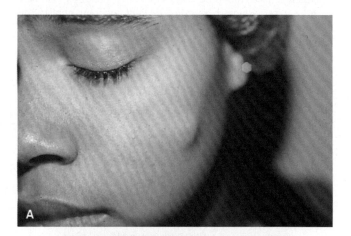

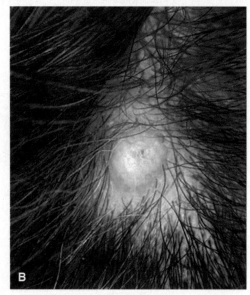

FIG. 6.2-11. A: Epidermoid cyst. (Used with permission from Weber, J., & Kelley, J. [2003]. Health assessment in nursing [2nd ed.]. Lippincott Williams & Wilkins.) **B:** A pilar inclusion cyst ("wen") is seen in the scalp of this adolescent girl. (Used with permission from Gru, A. A., & Wick, M. [2018]. *Pediatric dermatopathology and dermatology.* Wolters Kluwer.)

DIFFERENTIAL DIAGNOSIS	Abscess, Furuncles, Carbuncles, Epidermoid Cysts
• Ruptured epidermoid, pilar cyst • Cystic acne • Hidradenitis suppurativa	• Atypical mycobacterial infection • Primary and secondary immunodeficiency disease

Confirming the Diagnosis

- Gram stain and culture of pus from carbuncles and abscesses is recommended, but treatment without these studies is reasonable in typical cases.
- Gram stain and culture of pus from inflamed epidermoid cysts is not recommended.
- A central punctum is a pathognomonic sign of an epidermoid cyst.

Treatment

- In the absence of a culture-proven infection, the role of systemic antibiotics has been debated.
- The decision to administer antibiotics directed against *S. aureus* as an adjunct to I&D should be made based on presence or absence of systemic symptoms such as temperature >38°C or <36°C, tachypnea >24 breaths/min, tachycardia >90 beats/min, or white blood cell count >12,000 or <400 cells.
- An antibiotic active against MRSA is recommended for patients with carbuncles or abscesses who have failed initial antibiotic treatment or have markedly impaired host defenses or in patients with Systemic Inflammatory Response Syndrome (SIRS) and hypotension.
- I&D is the recommended treatment for inflamed epidermoid cysts, carbuncles, abscesses, and large furuncles, and is the CDC's treatment of choice for suspected community-acquired MRSA infections.
- It is recommended that topical mupirocin be applied to the anterior nares daily for the first 5 days of every month for proven MRSA infection. Frequent handwashing with antibacterial cleansers such as chlorhexidine (Hibiclens) and bleach baths (see Section 1.5) are helpful to reduce the overall bacterial colonization.

Management and Patient Education

- If the wound is deep, a drain or gauze wick may be placed to keep the wound open and allow for continued drainage.
- Warm compresses will aid in healing and will help facilitate drainage.
- A reculture after 3 months can assess the effectiveness. It is unclear whether the use of systemic antibiotics reduces the risk of reinfection. If all simple abscesses are treated with systemic antibiotics, it is feared that there will be increased resistance to the drugs most needed to treat MRSA.
- Furuncles, and especially carbuncles, can be slow to heal and result in scarring.
- A consult with infectious disease may be important for recurrent infections or for immunosuppressed individuals.

Special Consideration

Abscesses that develop on the central face, around the eyes and nose, are at increased risk for cavernous sinus thrombosis (CST) which is associated with staphylococcal or streptococcal infections. Symptoms of CST include decrease or loss of vision, chemosis (the swelling of the conjunctiva), exophthalmos, headaches, and paralysis of the cranial nerves, which course through the cavernous sinus. This infection is life-threatening and requires immediate treatment, which usually includes antibiotics and sometimes surgical intervention.

Methicillin-Resistant *Staphylococcus aureus* (MRSA)

Management of complicated skin and soft tissue infection involves the presumption that MRSA may be the causative organism. This section will primarily discuss the community-acquired infection (CA-MRSA). MRSA indicates that the oxacillin minimum inhibitory concentration (mic) is >4 mcg/mL and therefore not able to suppress the growth of the organism. The prevalence of MRSA has been increasing rapidly in both the hospital and community. It is relevant to this discussion because MRSA is the most common identifiable cause of SSTIs. Risk factors for MRSA include an underlying medical condition, recent use of antibiotics, recent trauma to the skin, foreign bodies that could be embedded in skin, exposure to contacts with the infection, and a past history of MRSA infection. *S. aureus* is very common in children and adults and lives in the nose and on the skin. It is usually spread through skin to skin contact with an infected individual's skin or personal items such as razors or towels. The most common sources of infection include schools, dormitories, and athletic facilities.

Clinical Presentation

Skin Findings

- Clinical presentations may range from superficial pustules seen in folliculitis, to large fluctuant abscesses.
- Cellulitis with or without drainage or abscess formation may be apparent (see section on abscess, furuncles, and carbuncles for further details) (Fig. 6.2-12).

Non-Skin Findings

The patient's general appearance is an important part of the presentation. The overall appearance of illness with fever, hypotension, and tachycardia as well as larger than usual areas of involvement should alert the clinician to the possibility of this type of infection.

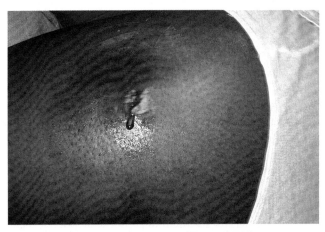

FIG. 6.2-12. MRSA infection. (Photo courtesy of Thomas P. Habif.)

DIFFERENTIAL DIAGNOSIS CA-MRSA

- SSTI
- Cellulitis
- Spider bites
- Impetigo
- Sepsis

Confirming the Diagnosis

Laboratory

- The diagnostic procedures are the same as those indicated for cellulitis. In most cases there is drainage, so wound culture must be done. Immunocompromised patients, who have failed previous treatment or who have had multiple recurrences, should be cultured with sensitivities.
- Gram stain and culture of pus from carbuncles and abscesses are recommended, but treatment without these studies is reasonable in typical cases.
- Blood cultures are done if the patient is systemically ill with fever, hypotension, tachycardia.

Treatment

- Treatment should always consider local susceptibility patterns (ISDA, 2014).
- Mild, superficial infections may be treated with topical agents alone.
- I&D is recommended if there is a collection of purulent material. If the infection is localized, I&D may be sufficient treatment as long as the patient is a healthy individual with uncomplicated skin lesions (<5 cm).
- The IDSA (2014) recommends the following options for purulent cellulitis: empiric treatment for CA-MRSA in an adult.

Management and Patient Education

- The management options for suspected MRSA in SSTI include drainage, antimicrobial therapy, wound care, patient education, and follow-up (Fig. 6.2-13).
- Adjunct antimicrobial therapy is recommended if the skin lesions are severe or extensive, there are signs of systemic infection, it is associated with chronic illness, immunosuppression, extremes of age and involvement of the hands, face, or perineum (difficult to drain areas), and those patients who failed to respond to I&D alone.
- Empiric coverage for MRSA with oral antibiotics may not necessarily improve the outcome; however, it is thought to prevent recurrences.
- If the infection is severe, hospitalization and parenteral antibiotics such as vancomycin or clindamycin are indicated.
- Preventing recurrences is a priority when dealing with MRSA infections and it requires the cooperation of the patient and family. It involves personal hygiene, which means covering wounds and eliminating exposure to others; environmental hygiene which requires cleaning high-touch areas in the home including all areas that are touched by bare hands such as doorknobs, toilet seats, and bathtubs. In some cases, if these

TABLE 6.2-2	Management of Recurrent MRSA Infection		
PERSONAL HYGIENE	**ENVIRONMENTAL**	**DECOLONIZATION**
Wound Care Cover draining wounds Hand hygiene after touching infected skin Avoid reusing/sharing personal items if active infection	Hygiene Clean high-touch surfaces	Mupirocin twice daily × 5–10 days Consider dilute bleach baths: ¼ cup per ¼ tub (13 gallons) of water for 15 min, 2×/wk × 3 mo

Adapted from LAMBERT, M. (2011). IDSA guidelines on the treatment of MRSA infections in adults and children. *American Family Physician, 84*(4), 455–463.

two measures fail, eradication of the persistent organism may require decolonization.

- CA-MRSA can be difficult to eradicate if all members of the household do not cooperate. Repeated infections should be referred to infectious disease for consideration of decolonization (Table 6.2-2).
- MRSA infection is a reportable disease in some states.

Special Considerations

Pediatrics

When MRSA is suspected in children, similar principles of treatment apply. If the lesion is fluctuant, I&D may be sufficient. If the child is ill-appearing, or febrile, adjuvant systemic therapy is recommended and includes clindamycin, TMP-SMX, and doxycycline if appropriate for children 8 years old and older.

CLINICAL PEARL

- *Recurrent furunculosis* is a hallmark of MRSA infection and the most common presentation, therefore care must be taken to minimize autoinoculation and spread of infection to others.

Perineal Streptococcal Infections

Streptococcal infection in the intertriginous areas in children can often coexist with strep pharyngitis. It is most commonly caused by group A β-hemolytic streptococcus or *S. pyogenes*.

Clinical Presentation

Skin Findings

- In young males the infection is often in perianal area and less often periurethral.
- It occurs more in the perivaginal area of young females.
- A well-demarcated area of erythema surrounds the anal opening or vaginal area for up to 3 cm (Clegg et al., 2015).

Non-Skin Findings

- There may be associated itching or burning.
- There may be pain on defecation or urination.
- Pharyngitis may occur simultaneously.

Outpatient† management of skin and soft tissue infections in the era of community-associated MRSA‡

Patient presents with signs/ symptoms of skin infection:

- Redness
- Swelling
- Warmth
- Pain/tenderness
- Complaint of "spider bite"

YES ▶

Is the lesion purulent (i.e., are <u>any</u> of the following signs present)?

- Fluctuance—palpable fluid-filled cavity, movable, compressible
- Yellow or white center
- Central point or "head"
- Draining pus
- Possible to aspirate pus with needle and syringe

NO ▶

Possible cellulitis without abscess:

- Provide antimicrobial therapy with coverage for *Streptococcus* spp. and/or other suspected pathogens
- Maintain close follow-up
- Consider adding coverage for MRSA (if not provided initially), if patient does not respond

YES

† For severe infections requiring inpatient management, consider consulting an infectious disease specialist.

‡ Visit ***www.cdc.gov/mrsa*** for more information.

1. Drain the lesion
2. Send wound drainage for culture and susceptibility testing
3. Advise patient on wound care and hygiene
4. Discuss follow-up plan with patient

Abbreviations:
I&D—incision and drainage
MRSA—methicillin-resistant *S. aureus*
SSTI—skin and soft tissue infection

If systemic symptoms, severe local symptoms, immunosuppression, or failure to respond to I&D, consider antimicrobial therapy with coverage for MRSA in addition to I&D. (See below for options)

Options for empiric outpatient antimicrobial treatment of SSTIs when MRSA is a consideration*

Drug name	Considerations	Precautions**
Clindamycin	■ FDA-approved to treat serious infections due to *S. aureus* ■ D-zone test should be performed to identify inducible clindamycin resistance in erythromycin-resistant isolates	■ *Clostridium difficile*-associated disease, while uncommon, may occur more frequently in association with clindamycin compared to other agents.
Tetracyclines ■ Doxycycline ■ Minocycline	■ Doxycycline is FDA-approved to treat *S. aureus* skin infections.	■ Not recommended during pregnancy. ■ Not recommended for children under the age of 8. ■ Activity against group A streptococcus, a common cause of cellulitis, unknown.
Trimethoprim-Sulfamethoxazole	■ Not FDA-approved to treat any staphylococcal infection	■ May not provide coverage for group A streptococcus, a common cause of cellulitis ■ Not recommended for women in the third trimester of pregnancy. ■ Not recommended for infants less than 2 months.
Rifampin	■ Use only in combination with other agents.	■ Drug–drug interaction are common.
Linezolid	■ Consultation with an infectious disease specialist is suggested. ■ FDA-approved to treat complicated skin infections, including those caused by MRSA.	■ Has been associated with myelosuppression, neuropathy and lactic acidosis during prolonged therapy.

- MRSA is resistant to all currently available beta-lactam agents (penicillins and cephalosporins)
- Fluoroquinolones (e.g., ciprofloxacin, levofloxacin) and macrolides (erythromycin, clarithromycin, azithromycine) are not optimal for treatment of MRSA SSTIs because resistance is common or may develop rapidly.

* Data from controlled clinical trials are needed to establish the comparative efficacy of these agents in treating MRSA SSTIs. Patients with signs and symptoms of severe illness should be treated as inpatients.
** Consult product labeling for a complete list of potential adverse effects associated with each agent.

Role of decolonization

Regimens intended to eliminate MRSA colonization should not be used in patients with active infections. Decolonization regimens may have a role in preventing recurrent infections, but more data are needed to establish their efficacy and to identify optimal regimens for use in community settings. *After treating active infections and reinforcing hygiene and appropriate wound care*, consider consultation with an infectious disease specialist regarding use of decolonization when there are recurrent infections in an individual patient or members of a household.

FIG. 6.2-13. Outpatient management of SSTI in the era of CA-MRSA.

DIFFERENTIAL DIAGNOSIS	Perineal Strep Infections
• Contact dermatitis (irritant or allergic) • *S. aureus* infection • Candidiasis • Seborrheic dermatitis • Pinworm infestation	• Inflammatory bowel disease • Lichen sclerosus • Child abuse • The early phase of Kawasaki disease

Confirming the Diagnosis

- Perineal streptococcal infection can be diagnosed with skin culture or group A streptococcal rapid testing, although the latter may be less specific.

Treatment

- Oral penicillin for 14 days is usually prescribed. Amoxicillin and clarithromycin are alternatives.
- Meury et al. (2008) found a 7-day course of cefuroxime was more effective than a 10-day course of penicillin in the treatment of perianal streptococcal disease.
- A repeat course of antibiotics is sometimes required.

Management and Patient Education

- Being alert to the coexistence of perineal infection and strep pharyngitis will lead to early diagnosis.
- KOH to look for yeast infection will be negative.
- Empiric treatment with antifungals will fail.

> **CLINICAL PEARL**
>
> ■ A strep infection of any kind can trigger an episode of guttate psoriasis in a predisposed individual. In the absence of throat infection, examine these other areas for signs of possible strep infection if a patient presents with guttate psoriasis and is otherwise asymptomatic.

Toxic Shock Syndrome

TSS is a systemic, multiorgan disease which can involve the kidney, liver, muscles, CNS as well as skin and mucous membranes. Originally described in 1978 in a pediatric population, TSS gained the attention of the public and the medical community in 1980, when multiple cases were linked to the use of tampons in menstruating women. Most of the cases involved young Caucasian women ages 15 to 19 years. Over time, the proportion of cases related to tampon use decreased significantly, largely because superabsorbent products, and products containing synthetic materials, were removed from the market (Gottlieb et al., 2018).

Pathophysiology

- The causative organism identified originally was a specific strain of *S. aureus* that produces a toxin. Almost 90% of the cases isolated this toxin known as Toxic Shock Syndrome Toxin-1 (TSST-1). Today, most cases are a nonmenstruating type and may be related to other toxins produced by *S. aureus*, such as staph enterotoxins A, B, C, and D. These enterotoxins behave like superantigens and stimulate the T cells to release massive amounts of cytokines such as TNF α and β, interleukins 1 and 2, and interferon γ. These cytokines are responsible for inflammation and cause fever, rash, tissue injury, and shock.

- The individuals most often at risk for developing TSS have been found to lack the antibody to TSST-1. In the general population, 70% to 80% of people possess the antibody present from birth to 6 months and 90% to 95% of people have the antibody by age 40. Patients with clinical TSS are deficient in the TSST-1 antibody. This failure to produce the antibody may explain why some individuals relapse after the first episode.

- *Group A strep (GAS)* can also produce a toxic shock-like syndrome and has several of the same clinical signs. The average age is a bit older in streptococcal TSS (20 to 50). A skin and soft tissue infection is more common in streptococcal TSS and the presence of a recent surgical wound is common.

- *Streptococcus suis* is a newer pathogen identified in Asia, which results from animal to human spread. Raw or undercooked pork is the main risk factor and *Streptococcus suis* is the pathogen that has high mortality rate.

Clinical Presentations

Skin Findings

- Staphylococcal TSS produces a diffuse erythematous eruption which begins on trunk and spreads toward extremities.
- Streptococcal TSS tends to have a soft tissue infection with erythema surrounding the wound.
- Erythema of mucous membranes (strawberry tongue and conjunctival hyperemia).
- Desquamation of palms and soles occurs 1 to 2 weeks after the development of the rash.

Non-Skin Findings

- The signs and symptoms of TSS occur rapidly in an otherwise healthy individual and may vary depending on the organ involved and the causative organism.
- Both conditions are marked by fever, headache, pharyngitis, vomiting, diarrhea, and hypotension.
- Unlike staphylococcal TSS, streptococcal infection is usually accompanied by severe pain at site of wound.
- Renal involvement is common in both and usually presents with an elevated BUN.

DIFFERENTIAL DIAGNOSIS	Toxic Shock Syndrome
• Streptococcus-like TSS (usually presents with severe pain and tenderness at a surgical site or site of trauma) • Staphylococcus TSS presents with diffuse erythema • Drug eruption • Erysipelas	• Kawasaki Disease • Scarlet Fever • Viral exanthems • SSSS • Toxic epidermal necrolysis (TEN) • Erythroderma from psoriasis, atopic dermatitis, or cutaneous T cell lymphoma (CTCL) • Contact dermatitis

Confirming the Diagnosis

- Diagnosis is based on clinical presentation using the CDC criteria (Box 6.2-3).

- Cultures should be obtained from mucosal and wound sites when possible.
- Blood cultures have very low yield for the presence of *S. aureus*, but may confirm the presence of other gram-positive or gram-negative organisms.
- Blood cultures are positive in strep TSS almost 50% of the time. Strep TSS has a much higher mortality rate.
- CBC, electrolytes, LFTs, U/A.
- Serology to R/O measles, syphilis, RMSF, hepatitis, Epstein–Barr virus.

Treatment

- Patients with suspected TSS—Clindamycin 600 mg intravenous (IV) every 8 hours plus vancomycin 30 mg/kg divided twice daily.
- Patients with confirmed methicillin-susceptible *S. aureus*—Clindamycin 600 mg IV every 8 hours plus either oxacillin IV or nafcillin IV (2 g every 4 hours).
- Patients with confirmed MRSA or penicillin allergy—Clindamycin 600 mg IV every 8 hours plus either vancomycin 30 mg/kg/day IV divided twice daily or linezolid 600 mg IV or by mouth every 12 hours. Continue antibiotics for a total of 10 to 14 days.
- Immune globulin (400 mg/kg over 2 to 3 hours) contains antibody to TSS and may be used for patients with refractory foci of infection.

Management and Patient Education

Universal Recommendations (Box 6.2-4)

- Patients suspected of TSS will likely be hospitalized. Consultation with Infectious Disease and Dermatology is indicated.
- Women using tampons are cautioned to change them regularly or every 8 hours. Alternate use of tampons and sanitary pads. Avoid the use of superabsorbent tampons.
- If using sponge, cervical cap or diaphragms, never leave one in longer than 24 hours and wash with warm soapy water after each use.
- Promptly remove tampon or any vaginal insert at the first sign of fever or illness.

CLINICAL PEARLS

- "Seven Rs of Managing and Treating TSS": Recognition, Resuscitation, Removal of source of infection, Rational choice of antibiotics, Role of adjunctive treatment (clindamycin and intravenous immunoglobulin), Review of progress, and Reduce risk of secondary cases in close contacts (Wilkins et al., 2017).
- Providers are cautioned to include TSS in the differential diagnosis *of fever and rash* even if all categories of symptoms are not present.

Necrotizing Fasciitis

Necrotizing fasciitis (NF) is a very deep, life-threatening infection which not only affects the skin and soft tissue but rapidly spreads to involve the fascia and muscle. The lay public has coined it the "Flesh-Eating Bacteria." Individuals at greater risk for contracting this infection include those with diabetes, hepatitis C infection, HIV infection and immunosuppression, alcoholism, history of injectable drug use, and recent surgical or traumatic wounds from burns or lacerations from childbirth and peripheral vascular disease. A recent history of varicella is considered a predisposing factor for NF. The use of NSAIDs has been implicated as well, because of the inhibition of neutrophil function which leads to increased cytokine production and further development of inflammation. The disease is found in all age groups and affects men and women equally.

Pathophysiology

- NF can be caused by either a mixture of organisms or one predominant organism.
- *Type 1 NF* is a mixed infection of aerobes and anaerobes, and is often associated with surgery of the abdomen and bowel.
- *Type 2 NF* is generally *GAS* alone or in combination with other *β-hemolytic strep. GAS* and *S. aureus* may occur simultaneously.
- In communities with a high prevalence of CA-MRSA, this may also be a cause of NF. The toxins released by these microbes cause occlusion of the blood vessels which quickly progresses to necrosis of the involved tissue.

Clinical Presentation

Skin Findings

- This infection usually begins as a simple skin abrasion or insect bite most commonly on the lower extremity of adults and the trunk of children.

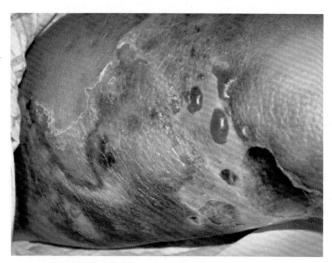

FIG. 6.2-14. Necrotizing fasciitis (NF). A clinical clue to the diagnosis may be anesthesia of the affected area.

- Progressive erythema, edema, cellulitis, and fever may be mistaken for simple cellulitis.
- The area of redness expands rapidly and develops a dusky bluish coloration centrally.
- As the infection progresses, the skin becomes insensate from thrombosis of superficial blood vessels and destruction of superficial nerves.
- There may be diffuse swelling and hemorrhagic blisters may form due to the occlusion of vessels.
- Crepitus in the tissue, caused by formation of gases from mixed bacteria, is pathognomonic and an ominous sign (Fig. 6.2-14).

Non-Skin Findings

- The pain is often exquisite and constant in the early phase, and is disproportionate to the appearance of the lesion, a hallmark characteristic.
- Systemic symptoms develop with fever, nausea, anorexia, elevated WBC, confusion, and hypotension.
- Patients may present with a mixed picture of toxic shock and NF (Box 6.2-5).

DIFFERENTIAL DIAGNOSIS	Necrotizing Fasciitis
• Cellulitis or other soft tissue infections	• Warfarin necrosis
• Deep vein thrombosis	• Brown recluse spider bite
• Septic arthritis	• Toxic shock syndrome

BOX 6.2-5   Ominous Signs of Deep Soft Tissue Infection

Constitutional symptoms
Crepitus
Necrosis
Purpura
Pain disproportionate to the clinical signs
Rapid progression

Confirming the Diagnosis

- Radiographic imaging can be useful in determining the depth of infection.
- Ultrasound may detect abscesses.
- Soft tissue x-ray, CT scan, and MRI may be helpful at visualizing gas formation along the fascial plane.
- Surgical exploration is necessary when the diagnosis is uncertain, infection is not responding to antibiotics, the local wound shows signs of necrosis, or there is a presence of gas in the tissue.
- Gram stain and culture of tissue should aid in determining antibiotic choice.

Treatment

- Antibiotic therapy is empiric initially but modified based on the culture and Gram stain. Broad-spectrum drugs effective against gram-positive, gram-negative, and anaerobic organisms are used.
- Carbapenems are used in conjunction with clindamycin for their antitoxin effect as well as agents against MRSA such as vancomycin, daptomycin, and linezolid.
- Patients with sensitivity to these drugs may be given fluoroquinolones plus metronidazole.
- IVIG may be helpful in severe GAS infections.

Management and Patient Education

- Early and aggressive surgical intervention to debride all necrotic tissue in addition to broad-spectrum antibiotic therapy is the standard treatment.
- Debridement is continued until all healthy tissue is visible. This generally results in multiple surgical procedures over the course of several days.
- Skin grafting is often necessary if the wounds are extensive (Misiakos et al., 2014).
- NF has a high degree of mortality and is most closely associated with the development of Streptococcal TSS. The hospital course and rehabilitation can take weeks and months.
- The loss of limb or amputation is very common and organ failure is possible.
- Patients often are left with significant cosmetic disfigurement and disability due to the amount of muscle, soft tissue, and bones that is removed.
- Suspicion of NF is **a true dermatology emergency** requiring patients be immediately transported to the nearest medical center. Immediate consultation with the surgeon is imperative (Misiakos et al., 2014).
- After surviving an episode of NF, patients must be prepared for a long and extensive recovery. Care must be taken to avoid future trauma, maintain meticulous personal hygiene, and to promptly treat any open wounds to avoid infection.

CLINICAL PEARLS

- The amount of pain is out of proportion to the apparent skin findings and while the pain is intense initially, the skin later becomes anesthetic.
- Watch for crepitus, rapidly progressing erythema, and the development of dusky color and hemorrhagic bullae centrally.
- Any suspicion for NF demands an emergency consult with surgery.

CORYNEBACTERIAL INFECTIONS

Erythrasma

Erythrasma is a common, superficial, bacterial skin eruption which generally occurs in the skin folds, particularly, the axilla, groin, and inguinal folds. It is often misdiagnosed as tinea cruris and can be a chronic problem for individuals. Risk factors may include obesity, hyperhidrosis, and severe cases may raise a suspicion of diabetes.

Pathophysiology

The warmth, moisture, and darkness of intertriginous areas encourage the growth of the causative organism, *Corynebacterium minutissimum*. Mixed flora may also be present.

Clinical Presentation

Skin Findings

- It can present as pink to brown, well-defined macules or patches with minimal scale and is usually bilateral.
- It is commonly seen in the groin, axilla, inframammary area and toe-web spaces where maceration is common.
- It is often mistaken for tinea or candidiasis; however, there is no inflammation or advancing border (Fig. 6.2-15A).
- Erythrasma may be asymptomatic or pruritic depending on location.

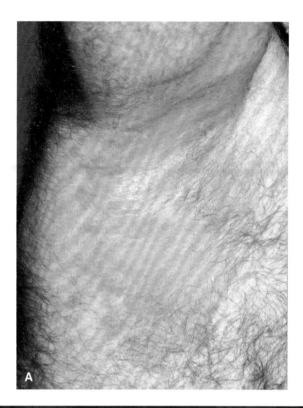

DIFFERENTIAL DIAGNOSIS	Erythrasma
• Tinea cruris or pedis	• Seborrheic dermatitis
• Inverse psoriasis	• Contact dermatitis
• Atopic dermatitis	• Tinea versicolor

Confirming the Diagnosis

- The diagnosis of erythrasma is a clinical one but can be confirmed by observing a coral red fluorescence on Wood's light examination. The fluorescence is the result of porphyrins which are produced by the bacteria (Fig. 6.2-15B) (see Skills section for details on Wood's light examination). Note that bathing prior to the test may result in removing the superficially deposited fluorescing coproporphyrins and can result in a false-negative Wood's light examination.
- KOH preparations of skin scrapings should be performed to evaluate for concomitant yeast/fungal infection but will likely be negative. It is often difficult to obtain scale for examination because of the intertriginous location (see Skills section for details on KOH preparation).
- A Gram stain will show chains of the gram-positive rods.
- In contrast to dermatophyte or candida infection, there is no inflammation and no advancing border. The color is more brown than red.

Treatment

- Washing with benzoyl peroxide followed by application of a topical antibiotic such as erythromycin solution 2%, or topical clindamycin solution 2%, applied b.i.d. for 2 weeks.
- Topical imidazole creams such as econazole cream applied to affected areas b.i.d. for 2 weeks may be useful for their antibacterial properties and in the presence of mixed infection.
- In severe cases, oral erythromycin, 250 mg q.i.d. for 2 weeks may result in clearing.

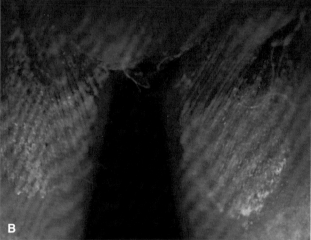

FIG. 6.2-15. **A:** Erythrasma. **B:** Coral-red fluorescence with Wood's light shows erythrasma in the groin. (Berg, D., & Worzala, K. [2006]. *Atlas of adult physical diagnosis.* Wolters Kluwer Health | Lippincott Williams & Wilkins.)

Management and Patient Education

- Erythrasma is often mistreated first as a dermatophyte infection so erythrasma should always be considered when topical antifungals fail to improve the condition.
- Treatment should be complete after 4 weeks. If not, the patient should return for reevaluation and consideration of a different diagnosis or presence of coinfection.
- Aluminum chloride solution 20% can help reduce moisture in these areas by minimizing sweating. Applying aluminum chloride solution 20% to the affected areas daily after showering will help prevent recurrences.
- In extensive cases, consider screening the patient for diabetes mellitus with a fasting glucose test and hemoglobin $A1_C$.

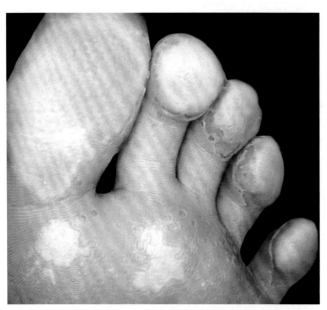

FIG. 6.2-16. Pitted keratolysis. Pitted keratolysis showing lesions ranging from small pits to large depressed areas. The pits become accentuated after immersion in water. (Used with permission from Gru, A. A., & Wick, M. [2018]. *Pediatric dermatopathology and dermatology*. Wolters Kluwer.)

Pitted Keratolysis

This is a superficial bacterial infection that is confined to the stratum corneum. It presents as a bizarre pattern which is often most apparent when the skin is wet such as after a bath or shower.

Pathophysiology

At least two organisms have been identified to be responsible: *Kytococcus sedentarius,* and *Dermatophilus congolensis,* both of which produce an enzyme that degrades the keratin and results in pitting of the stratum corneum.

Clinical Presentation

Skin Findings

- It is most common on the weight-bearing areas of the feet and is often associated with hyperhidrosis.
- There are numerous small punched out depressions on the heel, the plantar surface of the toes, and over the metatarsal heads.
- There is no inflammation and it is asymptomatic (Fig. 6.2-16).

Non-Skin Findings

- Patients often complain of a foul smell.
- Pruritus, pain, or burning may be present.

Differential Diagnosis

- This eruption is quite unique however it is often mistaken for warts.

Confirming the Diagnosis

- These organisms are difficult to culture and the diagnosis is generally made clinically.

- Immerse the affected foot in water for 15 minutes to accentuate the findings.
- A superficial shave biopsy of the skin would reveal the filamentous organisms with a regular hematoxylin and eosin stain but is rarely needed.

Treatment

- Topical erythromycin 2% (gel or lotion), clindamycin 1% (gel, lotion, solution, or swabs), mupirocin or fusidic acid ointment or benzoyl peroxide (gel, cream) can be applied b.i.d. for 2 to 4 weeks.
- Aluminum chloride 20% (Drysol) can be applied at bedtime with occlusion nightly until the sweating stops and then periodically for maintenance.

Management and Patient Education

- Controlling the sweating is again a large part of the treatment and can be applied on a regular basis.
- Advise patients to treat early if the symptoms recur.

Trichomycosis Axillaris, Pubis

This is another superficial bacterial infection that afflicts the hairs of the axilla and less commonly the pubic hairs. It is frequently undiagnosed and often patients are unaware of its presence.

Pathophysiology

- Although the name implies a fungal origin, the infection is the result of several species of Corynebacteria (*Corynebacterium tenuis, Corynebacterium propinquum, Corynebacterium flavescens*) and *Serratia marcescens.*

Clinical Presentation

Skin Findings

- Yellow, red, or even black concretions which are tightly packed bundles of bacteria are affixed to the hair.
- Malodor may be present.
- Hyperhidrosis is usually apparent.

Confirming the Diagnosis

- Dermoscopic examination reveals the presence of the encrusted hairs.
- No laboratory study is needed.
- This may be present along with other corynebacterial infections such as erythrasma or pitted keratolysis.

Treatment

- Bathing with antimicrobial cleansers or benzoyl peroxide wash and shaving the affected areas will successfully treat the condition.
- Aluminum chloride 20% can be used to minimize sweating.
- Topical antibiotics such as erythromycin 2% and clindamycin 1% may also be effective.

Management and Patient Education

- The first step in treatment is accomplished simply by shaving the involved areas, then applying antiperspirant.
- Antibacterial cleansers may help prevent recurrence.

GRAM-NEGATIVE BACTERIAL INFECTIONS

Gram-negative bacteria tend to live where the skin is warm and moist such as the axilla and groin and include such organisms as *P. aeruginosa*.

Pseudomonas Folliculitis

The most common of the gram-negative infections is *P. aeruginosa* folliculitis, also known as "hot tub" folliculitis. Outbreaks occur after exposure to a contaminated spa, hot tub, or pool and can also be associated with use of objects such as loofah sponges or swimming pool inflatables.

Pathophysiology

P. aeruginosa is an intestinal gram-negative rod commonly found in the anogenital and axillary region. This bacterium thrives in warm, moist environments and feeds off the dead skin cells shed during the bath. Chlorine or bromine are generally added to the tub or pool water to kill the bacteria. If the chemical composition of the water is not correctly balanced, the bacteria will flourish and produce an annoying and uncomfortable eruption in most individuals.

Clinical Presentation

Skin Findings

- Red, urticarial papules and plaques, often with a pustular center, may appear on all skin surfaces except the head in as little as 8 hours after exposure to a contaminated water source.
- The eruption can be widespread, tender, or pruritic and resolves after 7 to 10 days often with residual brownish discoloration (Fig. 6.2-17).

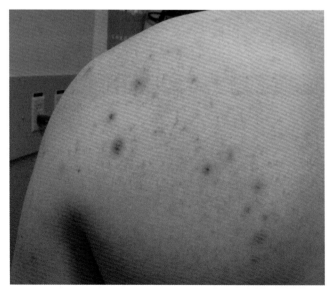

FIG. 6.2-17. Hot tub folliculitis: Back.

Non-Skin Findings

- This is often accompanied by a burning sensation and tends to be worse in the areas beneath the bathing suit.

DIFFERENTIAL DIAGNOSIS	Pseudomonas Folliculitis
• Gram-positive folliculitis	• Sea Bathers' eruption
• Acne	• Insect bites
• Candidiasis	• Impetigo
• Miliaria	

Confirming the Diagnosis

- Diagnosis is usually a clinical one supported by a history of recent exposure to hot tubs or pools.
- Spontaneous resolution generally confirms the diagnosis.

Treatment

- Often no treatment other than showering and removing the wet suit is needed.
- Topical clindamycin can be prescribed twice daily. If it is resistant to topical treatment, ciprofloxacin 500 mg can be given b.i.d. for 7 days or less if the rash resolves.

Management and Patient Education

- Complete cleaning of the tub is part of the treatment and involves draining the water completely, cleaning the tub itself, and then making sure the proper ratio of chemicals is added to the fresh water.
- Be sure to notify the hotel or owner of the tub that this problem exists.

GRAM-NEGATIVE TOE-WEB INFECTION

This is usually a mixed infection that often begins as tinea pedis. It is often associated with use of closed toe shoes (especially steel-toe) and is seen frequently in individuals who spend a lot of time engaged in physical activities, either occupationally or recreationally.

Initially, a dermatophyte infection may alter the continuity of the stratum corneum and allow for the invasion of multiple microbes. It is often associated with hyperhidrosis which provides the perfect environment for gram-negative infection with *P. aeruginosa*, one of the common pathogens.

Clinical Presentation

Skin Findings

- Peeling and cracking of the toe-web spaces may be the presenting sign.
- Foul smelling odor, erythema, erosions, and purulence.
- Increased moisture will lead to maceration and sometimes the peeling extends to the plantar surface of the toes extending down to the metatarsal heads.
- If *P. aeruginosa* is involved, you may begin to see a yellow-greenish coloration to the skin of the web spaces (Fig. 6.2-18).

Non-Skin Findings

- It is often accompanied by burning and pain rather than itch.

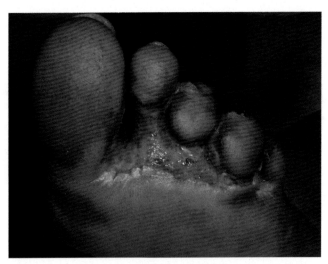

FIG. 6.2-18. Gram-negative toe-web infection (GNTWI).

DIFFERENTIAL DIAGNOSIS GNTWI	
• Tinea pedis	• Impetigo
• Erythrasma	• Candida infection
• Intertrigo	• Hyperhidrosis

Confirming the Diagnosis

- Identification of the various organisms that may be present is necessary to achieve complete resolution.
- KOH is helpful in identifying the presence of dermatophyte or yeast. A fungal culture will provide the specific organism.
- A bacterial culture should also be done to aid in the identification of organisms and selection of antimicrobials.
- A Wood's light examination will help rule out erythrasma if there is no coral fluorescence.
- If the patient's immune status is in question, a complete blood count with differential should be ordered along with a blood glucose.

Treatment

- Antiperspirant products such as aluminum chloride 20% should be recommended to minimize moisture applied nightly with occlusion until the sweating is diminished and then continued on a regular basis to maintain control.
- A broad-spectrum topical antifungal such as econazole nitrate cream 1% or OTC butenafine cream should be prescribed for b.i.d. application.
- 1% acetic acid soaks may be helpful to dry the area.
- Gentian violet can be applied daily.
- If *P. aeruginosa* persists, systemic antibiotics may be helpful.

Management and Patient Education

- In this condition, the presence of excessive sweating is a major contributing factor.
- Advise patients to be aware of new or recurrent infections such as tinea pedis and encourage early interventions.
- Regular use of antibacterial soaps is not recommended. Regular washing with plain soap and water is sufficient.

- It is recommended to see the patient back in 2 to 4 weeks. You may need to contact the patient before then to report on culture results if a change in treatment is needed, otherwise a follow-up visit in 4 weeks is reasonable.

Catscratch Disease

Catscratch disease (CSD), also known as catscratch fever, is typically a self-limiting, benign, infectious disease caused by bacteria *Bartonella henselae*. Adults rarely exhibit symptoms of the disease; children and immunocompromised patients are most often affected. Manifestations are most commonly seen 1 to 2 weeks following a cat bite or scratch. Transmission has rarely been associated without known trauma and most cases occur during the fall or winter.

Pathophysiology

- *B. henselae* is a gram-negative bacillus carried by otherwise healthy cats. Cats typically contract the disease from other affected cats via the cat flea.
- A small portion of domestic cats and up to half of all stray cats carry the bacterium in their blood.
- Cats under the age of 1 are generally at higher risk of carrying the bacterium due to flea infestation.

Clinical Presentation

Skin Findings

- In classic CSD, patients will present with a nonpruritic, red papule appearing at the site of inoculation approximately 3 to 5 days to weeks after a cat bite or scratch. Scratches most often occur on the upper extremities or face.
- This lesion evolves over the course of a few days into a vesicle, then dries into a crust.
- Skin manifestations may go unnoticed, and upon resolution, the lesion typically heals leaving a depressed scar, much like a chicken pox scar.

Non-Skin Findings

- Approximately 1 to 2 weeks following exposure, regional lymphadenopathy develops, and in some patients, flu-like symptoms including: fever, chills, headaches, fatigue, anorexia, backache, and/or abdominal pain (Fig. 6.2-19).
- CSD is often a self-limiting condition, but lymphadenopathy may persist for several months.

DIFFERENTIAL DIAGNOSES Catscratch Disease		
Infectious	*Noninfectious*	*Malignant Neoplasms*
Viral (e.g., cytomegalovirus or Epstein–Barr virus	Sarcoidosis Pyogenic granuloma	Kaposi sarcoma
Bacterial (Nocardia, LGV)		
Fungal (sporotrichosis, coccidioidomycosis)		

Confirming the Diagnosis

- Diagnosis is typically suspected after the patient presents with a primary cutaneous granulomatous lesion with regional lymphadenopathy, and exposure to a cat within the past 1 to 2 weeks.

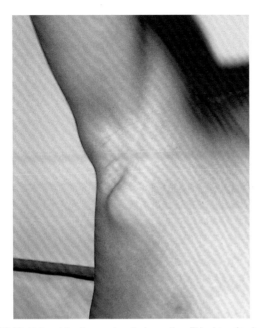

FIG. 6.2-19. Catscratch disease lymphadenopathy. This boy developed an enlarged, epitrochlear lymph node on the medial aspect of his upper extremity and axillary involvement without erythema or tenderness. (Used with permission from Fleisher, G. R., Ludwig, W., & Baskin, M. N. [2004]. *Atlas of pediatric emergency medicine.* Lippincott Williams & Wilkins.)

- Serum indirect fluorescence assay (IFA) and enzyme-linked immunoassay (ELISA) testing may be performed to detect serum antibodies to *B. henselae.*

- Skin or lymph node biopsy may be performed, but is not routinely suggested.

Treatment

- Because CSD is often self-limited, it generally requires no treatment.

- Antibiotic treatment should be considered in immunocompetent patients with systemic illness, or immunosuppressed patients, and comanagement with an infectious disease specialist is strongly recommended.

- Antibiotic treatment is aimed at gram-negative bacterial coverage, and various options include doxycycline + rifampin, ciprofloxacin, gentamicin, or trimethoprim/sulfamethoxazole.

Management and Patient Education

- Antipyretic treatment is recommended in febrile patients.

- Antibiotics are considered to be effective in decreasing lymph node size, but do not alter the duration of the disease.

- CSD generally has a favorable prognosis, and resolves spontaneously most of the time.

- Complications and morbidity occur most frequently in immunocompromised patients and include neurologic complications, vascular skin lesions (bacillary angiomatosis), ocular manifestations (Parinaud's oculoglandular syndrome), and vascular hepatitis (bacillary peliosis).

- Patients should be educated that pet quarantine or euthanasia is not necessary since the transmissibility of the organism from cats is transient.

- Teaching children to handle pets gently to avoid scratches or bites may reduce transmission.

- Avoidance of stray cats and regular flea treatments administered by their pet's veterinarian may reduce infection rates.

- Infected cats may be treated by their veterinarian with doxycycline; however, this may not decrease risk of transmission to humans.

- Follow-up is generally not necessary as this is often a self-limiting disease. Patients with systemic complications or immunosuppression should be followed closely until disease is successfully treated.

- Referral or consultation should be considered in immunocompetent patients manifesting complications, in all immunosuppressed patients, or in instances of diagnostic uncertainty.

- Referrals are most often made to an infectious disease specialist, but consultation with an ophthalmologist or neurologist may be indicated based on disease manifestations.

Special Consideration

- *Pediatrics*—Children are more often affected by CSD than healthy adults, but still generally have favorable outcomes. Treatment with doxycycline should be avoided in children <8 years old.

- *Pregnancy*—During pregnancy, azithromycin is used as a first-line treatment option for CSD.

- *Immunocompromised*—Patients have the highest risk of developing systemic manifestations with a poor prognostic outcome after infection with CSD. Multiple complications may occur. Aggressive antibiotic therapy is indicated to reduce morbidity and mortality, and consultation with an infectious disease specialist is strongly recommended.

READINGS AND REFERENCES

CDC. (2013). Antibiotic resistance threats in the United States, 2013 [Internet]. U.S. Department of Health and Human Services.

CDC. (2019). Antibiotic resistance threats in the United States. Atlanta, GA: U.S. Department of Health and Human Services.

Brindle, R., Williams, O. M., Barton, E., & Featherstone, P. (2019). Assessment of antibiotic treatment of cellulitis and erysipelas: A systematic review and meta-analysis. *JAMA Dermatology, 155*(9), 1033–1040.

Clegg, H. W., Giftos, P. M., Anderson, W. E., Kaplan, E. L., & Johnson, D. R. (2015). Clinical perineal streptococcal infection in children: Epidemiologic features, low symptomatic recurrence rate after treatment, and risk factors for recurrence. *Journal of Pediatrics, 167*(3), 503–505.

Dryden, M., Johnson, A. P., Ashiru-Oredope, D., & Sharland, M. (2011). Using antibiotics responsibly: Right drug, right time, right dose, right duration. *Journal of Antimicrobial Chemotherapy, 66*(11), 2441–2443.

Gottlieb, M., Long, B., & Koyfman, A. (2018). The evaluation and management of toxic shock syndrome in the emergency department: A review of the literature. *The Journal of Emergency Medicine, 54*(6), 807–814.

LAMBERT, M. (2011). IDSA guidelines on the treatment of MRSA infections in adults and children. *American Family Physician, 84*(4), 455–463.

Meury, S. N., Erb, T., Schaad, U. B., & Heininger, U. (2008). Randomized, comparative efficacy trial of oral penicillin versus cefuroxime for perianal streptococcal dermatitis in children. *Journal of Pediatrics, 153*(6), 799–802.

Misiakos, E. P., Bagias, G., Patapis, P., Sotiropoulos, D., Kanavidis, P., & Machairas, A. (2014). Current concepts in the management of necrotizing fasciitis. *Frontiers in surgery, 1*, 36.

Sanchez, G. V., Fleming-Dutra, K. E., Roberts, R. M., & Hicks, L. A. (2016). Core elements of outpatient antibiotic stewardship. *MMWR. Recommendations and Reports: Morbidity and Mortality Weekly Report. Recommendations and Reports, 65*(6), 1–12.

Sports-Related Skin Infections Position Statement and Guidelines: National Federation of State High School Associations (NFHS), Sports Medicine Advisory Committee (SMAC). (2018).

Stevens, D., Bisno, A., Chambers, H., Patchen Dellinger, E., Goldstein, E., Gorbach, S., Hirschmann, J., Kaplan, S., Montoya, J., & Wade, J. (2014). Practice guidelines for the diagnosis and management of skin and soft tissue infections. *Clinical Infectious Diseases, 59*(2), e10–e52.

Stevens, D. L., Bisno, A. L., Chambers, H. F., Dellinger, E. P., Goldstein, E. J. C., Gorbach, S. L., Hirschmann, J. V., Kaplan, S. L., Montoya, J. G., & Wade, J. C; Infectious Diseases Society of America. (2014). Practice guidelines for the diagnosis and management of skin and soft tissue infections: 2014 update by the Infectious Diseases Society of America. *Clinical Infectious Diseases, 59*(2), 147–159.

Wilkins, A. L., Steer, A. C., Smeesters, P. R., & Curtis, N. (2017). Toxic shock syndrome—the seven Rs of management and treatment. *The Journal of Infection, (74 Suppl 1),* S147–S152.

Viral Infections

Mark A. Hyde

In This Chapter

- Warts (Nongenital)
- Molluscum Contagiosum
- Herpes Simplex
- Herpes Zoster
- Shingles Vaccine

While patients frequently present to primary care with viral infections, they can be challenging to diagnose because of their various clinical presentations. Viruses are a large group of submicroscopic infective agents separated into two main groups, the DNA and RNA virus types. Viruses can also be classified by their mode of transmission, for example, airborne viruses. Structurally, viral particles (virion) contain a central core of genetic material (RNA or DNA) within a protein coat (capsid). Some viruses have an outer membrane, known as the envelope, which enables the virus to identify and bind to the host membrane. Viruses require living cells to grow and multiply. Infections occur when the virus introduces its own genetic material into the nucleus of a cell within the host. The host cell will then reproduce normally and subsequently reproduce the newly introduced viral particles. These particles are then spread throughout the host and infection ensues. Treatment of viral infections depends on the structure of the virus and is aimed at stopping reproduction, not killing the virus, as is often seen in antibacterial therapy. This chapter will cover a broad range of viral skin diseases; however, the viral exanthems will be discussed in Section 13, Childhood Skin Disorders.

WARTS

Warts, or verrucae, are one of the most common viral infections seen in primary care and affect approximately 7% to 10% of the population. They are small, benign growths caused by the human papilloma virus (HPV). They are frustrating for both patients and providers as treatment is often tedious and long term.

Pathophysiology

- They are double-stranded, naked (nonenveloped) DNA viruses characterized by slow growth.
- HPV infects the epithelia of the skin or mucosa and spreads through direct person-to-person skin contact or indirectly through contaminated surfaces and objects (e.g., swimming pools, showers).
- Autoinoculation of the virus from an existing lesion to adjacent skin is commonly seen on the hands, in the interdigital, and periungual areas.
- Hundred subtypes of HPV exist and are categorized as:
  - anogenital lesions (condyloma acuminatum or genital warts, discussed in Section 11.4),
  - nongenital lesions (common warts or verruca).

- The risk of infections depends on the immune status of the exposed individual, the amount of virus present, and the nature of the contact.
- While warts themselves are not cancerous, some strains of HPV may be oncogenic.

Clinical Presentation

Common Warts (Verruca Vulgaris)

- Usually occur in patients between the ages of 5 and 20 years and less commonly occur after the age of 35 years.
- They are predominantly found on the hands, particularly the fingers and palms, but can form anywhere on the body.
- Frequent immersion of hands in water is a major risk factor (frequently seen in food handlers).
- Range in size from <1 mm to >1 cm, with the average size being around 5 mm.
- Typically appear as a rough, skin-colored papule with a grayish surface that interrupts normal skin lines.
- The clinical presentation is so characteristic that "verrucous" is used as an adjective to describe the morphologic features of other dermatologic conditions with a similar appearance, such as a seborrheic keratosis.
- Periungual warts, typically seen at the proximal and lateral nail folds, are often seen in patients who bite their nails (Fig. 6.3-1).
- Warts may be seen in or around the mouth in these patients as well.
- Digitate or filiform warts, small (usually 1 to 3 mm) pedunculated skin-colored papules with multiple, small finger-like projections, can be seen on the face and scalp (Fig. 6.3-2).

Flat Warts (Verruca Plana)

- Affect children and young adults and generally appear in crops on the face, neck, dorsal hands, wrists, elbows, or knees (Fig. 6.3-3).
- Typically present as multiple 2- to 4-mm flat-topped papules and range from slightly erythematous or pink, or tan/brown on lighter skin, to darker brown or hyperpigmented on darker skin.
- They have the highest rate of spontaneous remission of all HPV subtypes.

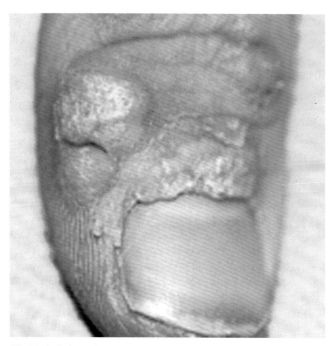

FIG. 6.3-1. Periungual warts.

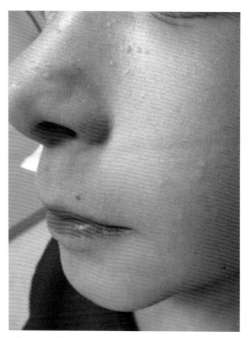

FIG. 6.3-3. Flat warts. (Photo courtesy of M. Bobonich.)

- Men who shave their faces, and women who shave their legs or underarms, can spread the virus and develop numerous flat warts at the site.

- They are frequently seen in atopic patients and can spread from scratching. The distribution is usually more linear.

Plantar Warts (Verruca Plantaris)

- Typically present as hyperkeratotic, flesh-colored verrucous papules or plaques ranging from <1 mm to >1 cm and multiple lesions present at the same time.

- May be mistaken for either a callus or a corn, due to their tendency to occur on the pressure points on the ball of the foot, particularly at the midmetatarsal area.

- Calluses, in contrast, are circumscribed areas of superficial hyperkeratosis, caused by repeated friction or pressure. If a callus is pared down, it will reveal normal-appearing skin underneath.

- A corn, or clavus, is a circumscribed thickening of the skin with a central translucent, hornlike core, also caused by repeated

friction or pressure. If a corn is pared down, it will reveal a clear, horny core. This can be useful in determining diagnosis and treatment.

Anogenital Warts and Condylomata Acuminata

- Genital warts are the most common sexually transmitted infection.

- The estimated lifetime risk for infection in sexually active adults can be as high as 80%.

- Genital HPV is closely linked with cancer of the cervix, glans penis, anus, and vulvo-vaginal area.

See Section 11.4 Genital Dermatoses for a full discussion.

DIFFERENTIAL DIAGNOSIS Warts

- *Seborrheic keratoses* can have a very verrucous appearance, and are often pigmented.

- The presence of pseudohorn cysts (keratin deposits within the thickened surface) on close examination can help to differentiate them from warts.

- *Acrochordons* (skin tags) are soft, fleshy, pedunculated skin-colored papules that can have a clinical appearance similar to filiform wart, but will lack the characteristic finger-like projections on close examination.

- Clavus (corn) typically occurs between the fourth and fifth toe with soft hyperkeratotic skin, may interrupt normal skin lines, but will not have the capillary dots when pared and will reveal a hard, central plug.

- A callus is thickened skin usually over a bony prominence with normal skin lines.

- Molluscum contagiosum (MC) are small, smooth papules with central umbilication.

- Squamous cell carcinoma, should be suspected if lesions are very resistant to various treatments or continue to recur.

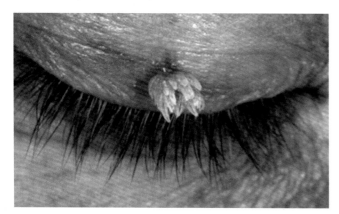

FIG. 6.3-2. Filiform warts. (Courtesy T. Habif.)

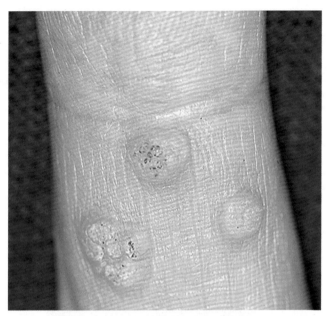

FIG. 6.3-4. Interrupted dermatoglyphics of warts. (Goodheart, H. P. [2015]. *Goodheart's photoguide of common skin disorders* [4th ed.]. Wolters Kluwer Health | Lippincott Williams & Wilkins.)

Confirming the Diagnosis

- Diagnosis is made on clinical appearance. Warts will always interrupt normal skin lines (Fig. 6.3-4), and usually, thrombosed capillaries can be seen (Fig. 6.3-5). If not immediately apparent, a scalpel blade can be used to lightly pare away hyperkeratotic debris from the surface of the lesion. When this is done, pinpoint black to red dots, which represent the thrombosed capillaries, will be revealed. This is considered a diagnostic sign and is not seen in other skin lesions with a similar clinical appearance.

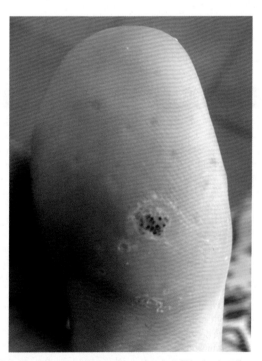

FIG. 6.3-5. Thrombosed capillaries after paring wart. This sign is pathognomonic for wart. (Used with permission from Gru, A. A., & Wick, M. [2018]. *Pediatric dermatopathology and dermatology.* Wolters Kluwer Health.)

- Biopsy is not typically necessary but may be done to rule out squamous cell carcinoma when lesions are resistant to treatment.

Treatment

Warts are benign skin conditions which spontaneously resolve in up to two thirds of patients, without treatment, within 1 to 2 years. Despite this, warts are a frequent reason for office visits and dermatology referrals. See Table 6.3-1.

- Clinicians should remember that verrucae do not necessarily need to be treated. Monitoring or not treating is an acceptable option for the patient.
- Most warts can be successfully treated in the primary care setting or even by the patient at home.
- The plan of care should be based on the clinical appearance, location, age, and the immune status of the patient.
- Treatment is indicated if the lesions are painful or interfere with function and should be pursued before they multiply and while they are still small.
- Even if the treated area appears normal, the virus may exist in the remaining tissues, and the wart may recur. All existing warts should be treated at the same time, if possible.
- The goal of therapy is to remove the wart without leaving a scar. Current therapies are not wart specific, and the mechanisms of action are either destructive or immune-based.
- Over-the-counter (OTC) and in-office therapies may take several weeks or months and recurrence is common. A Cochrane review (2012) showed that salicylic acid and cryotherapy are the two preferred treatment methods. See Table 6.3-1.

Destructive Therapies

- *Salicylic acid* is frequently the first-line prescription/OTC therapy and is available in liquid form, topical plasters, or patches and is appropriate for adults and children. It should be avoided in patients with peripheral neuropathy as the extent of tissue damage can go unnoticed. If treatment is performed in the office, a scalpel blade should be used by the clinician to pare down the thick keratotic layer prior to treatment in order to allow the medication to effectively penetrate the infected tissue and potentially shorten the course of treatment.
- *Cryotherapy,* using liquid nitrogen, is the most common in-office treatment of warts. This is useful in older children and adults, but poorly tolerated in young children. Multiple treatments spaced about 2 to 4 weeks apart are typically required. Patients may also be instructed to use salicylic acid between treatments after the blister has resolved to aid in resolution.
- *Duct tape* is a commonly used household remedy for warts; however, there is conflicting evidence to support its effectiveness. If desired, the silver brand of duct tape that is sticky enough to adhere to the skin is recommended. The goal is to keep the wart occluded with the duct tape as much of the time as possible and can be used in combination with salicylic acid for enhanced benefit.
- *Cantharidin* is a topical destructive agent that is used in the office setting. Also known as Cantharone, cantharidin is an extract of a blistering insect. It is a more tolerable treatment approach for children since the application process is pain-free. The patient can, however, develop pain when the treated sites blister. Cantharidin is not currently approved by the U.S. Food and Drug Administration (FDA), however, it is on the FDA's proposed bulk

TABLE 6.3-1	First- and Second-Line Treatment Options for Warts			
THERAPY	**ADVANTAGES**	**DISADVANTAGES**	**CONTRAINDICATIONS**	**COMMENTS**
First-Line				
Salicylic acid (keratolytic)	Available over the counter, inexpensive, easy application, effective, including plantar warts or thick lesions, nonscarring	Macerates any skin where it is applied, reapply if it gets wet, requires multiple applications, can cause tenderness	Peripheral neuropathy, peripheral artery disease, nonintact skin or erosions, pregnancy	Can be used in conjunction with cryotherapy
Cryotherapy (thermal destruction)	Effective in older children and adults, anesthesia is not necessary, great for warts on hands, safe in pregnancy and breastfeeding, fast, can treat multiple lesions and thick lesions	Painful, can result in hyper- or hypopigmentation especially on dark skin tones, caution should be used in the treatment of facial warts, requires multiple in-office treatment by clinician, which can be expensive and inconvenient	Cryoglobulinemia, cold agglutinins, cold urticaria	Treatment on fingers and toes (especially with freeze–thaw–freeze cycle) may cause hemorrhagic bullae which are benign, use caution on the digits and near nerves (severe pain and neuropathy), cautioned use in dark skin tones, treatment of periungual warts may result in nail deformity; see Section 15 for instructions on use
No intervention	No cost or risk of pain or scarring, two thirds of warts spontaneously resolve within 1–2 yr	Warts may grow or spread on self or transmission to others, psychosocial burden, pain, and bleeding especially on the hands and feet		Patient education regarding transmission and prevention of autoinoculation
Second-Line (Limited Evidence)				
Duct tape (occlusive)	Inexpensive, easy to do at home, easy for children, pain-free	Can be difficult to keep tape on, effectiveness is uncertain		Cover with duct tape, leave on for 6 days, then soak and pare; leave uncovered overnight; then repeat cycle until resolved
Cimetidine (systemic immune modulator)	Available over the counter	Many possible drug interactions	See FDA recommendations	Mostly anecdotal reports
Cantharidin (blistering agent)	Painless at time of application, useful for multiple lesions and in young children, no scarring	In-office treatment only, blisters can cause discomfort, response varies, may need additional treatment with same or other modalities	Face or genital mucosa	Caution with use on digits, severe blistering can occur if applied incorrectly; see Section 15 for instructions on use
Third-line: If no improvement with above therapies repeated over several months, consider referral to dermatology for more aggressive treatment				

substances list, which allows preparations containing cantharidin to be administered by providers in the office (see Box 6.3-1).

- Canthacur PS is a combination of cantharidin, podophyllin 5%, and salicylic acid 30%. This is a good choice for patients with multiple, thick plantar warts where deeper penetration is needed. Repeating treatments every 3 to 4 weeks may be required.

Immune-Based Therapies

- *Cimetidine:* There have been reports of the off-label use of oral cimetidine given in doses of 30 to 40 mg/kg/day being effective in the treatment of warts. This is thought to be due to its systemic immunomodulatory effects. Although this medication is generally safe, well tolerated and available over the counter, caution should be used when recommending this treatment as

there are multiple potential drug interactions associated with its use.

- Additional immune-based therapies, including topical agents and intralesional treatments, may be available for use by an experienced practitioner in a specialty setting.

Advanced Therapies (Off Label)

- Sometimes warts can be recalcitrant to common therapies. Advanced treatments are available, but should be administered by an experienced dermatology provider.
- Other off-label, topical therapies include: imiquimod cream, 5-fluorouracil, and squaric acid dibutylester. Surgical excision, ablative laser, curettage and desiccation, and shave removal can be performed depending on patient circumstances and office settings.

BOX 6.3-1   How to Apply Salicylic Acid

- Soak the area in warm water to help soften the skin and allow for better penetration
- Pare the wart down with a nail file or pumice stone
- Petrolatum can be applied around the area to be treated
- Apply salicylic acid solution or gel to the affected area and a few millimeters of surrounding skin
- If using plasters or patches, affix to clean skin and keep dry for 2 to 3 days
- After removing the patch, repeat the process until the wart has resolved
- Any implement used to pare down the warts should be dedicated only for this purpose and should not be used elsewhere on the body, or by other members of the household to minimize autoinoculation or spreading of warts

Salicylic Acid Options

- The liquid form comes in two strengths: 17% (Occlusal HP, Duoplant, Compound W, Duofilm, and Wart-Off) and 27.5% (Virasal). These are effective for children and on thinner warts in adults and allow easy application to multiple areas.
- When treating thick or plantar warts more potent preparations containing 40% salicylic acid in plaster form (Mediplast or Duofilm patch) may be necessary.

- Recurrence rates are high if these are not combined with some other therapy.
- Some dermatology specialists use intralesional immunotherapy with candida antigen or cytotoxic bleomycin.
- These more aggressive therapies have higher risks for infection, scarring, and side effects, which should be discussed with the patient in advance.
- Patients with recurrent, recalcitrant, or clinically atypical lesions should be referred to a dermatologist for evaluation and treatment and consideration of biopsy.

Special Considerations

Immunosuppression: In general, warts of all types are more common and more difficult to treat in immunosuppressed patients. The clinical presentation may be different, making correct diagnosis challenging. A referral to a dermatologist is recommended.

Pediatrics: Treatment should be aimed at using the least painful methods and lowest potential for scarring and dyschromia. More aggressive methods should be reserved for the most difficult cases where scarring is not a concern.

Pregnancy: Salicylic acid is a pregnancy category C medication and should not be used in pregnant patients due to the possibility of associated premature closure of the ductus arteriosus. Cryotherapy is the treatment of choice in pregnancy.

Management and Patient Education

- Emphasis should be placed on understanding that warts may take months to resolve so that patients do not become discouraged and stop treatment prematurely.
- Use an electric shaver (not a razor) near warts on hair-bearing areas.
- With plantar warts, avoid going barefoot through the house and disinfect the shower base with a diluted bleach solution after bathing. Wear sandals or shower shoes in public facilities or pools.
- Follow-up is individualized and depends on the patient, the extent of the disease, and the treatment being utilized. If a wart is being treated in the office setting, reasonable follow-up is every 2 to 4 weeks.

MOLLUSCUM CONTAGIOSUM

MC is a self-limiting viral skin infection commonly seen in primary care. Significant psychosocial impacts may drive patients to seek treatment which can be frustrating to all involved. Although MC is a common infection of childhood, it can occur in adolescents and adults. In adults, genital lesions are usually sexually transmitted.

Anogenital lesions in children are usually spread through autoinoculation. Immunosuppressed populations like those with atopic dermatitis have a higher incidence of MC.

Pathophysiology

- MC is a large double-stranded DNA virus that consists of four closely related members of the poxvirus group.
- Contains unique genes that encode proteins and impair the host's immune response.
- Localized, subacute viral infection of the epithelium that is spread by direct skin-to-skin contact, especially with wet or disrupted skin surfaces.
- Swimming or bathing with an infected person increases the risk of transmission.
- MC may also be spread by autoinoculation, sexual contact, shared clothing, and towel.
- Incubation period ranges from 1 to 7 weeks.

Clinical Presentation

- MC typically presents as 2- to 5-mm firm, skin-colored to pink, pearly dome-shaped papules with a central dell or umbilication (Fig. 6.3-6). The dell may not be obvious, but a soft white central core may be present.
- In children, the distribution may be generalized and can range from a few to more than 100 lesions.
- Common areas of involvement include the face, trunk, and extremities.
- Genital lesions can occur in up to 10% of childhood cases with widespread involvement. If the genitals are the only area affected the possibility of sexual abuse should be considered.

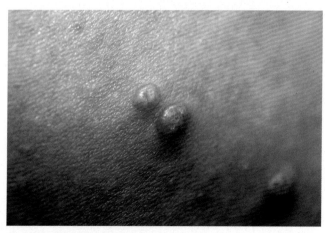

FIG. 6.3-6. Classic molluscum lesion.

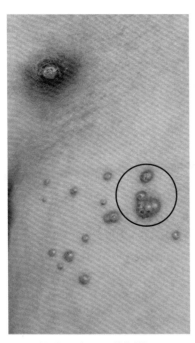

FIG. 6.3-7. Molluscum BOTE Sign. (Courtesy T. Habif.)

- Adults typically have fewer than 20 lesions, commonly seen on the lower abdomen, upper thighs, and the penile shaft in men.
- Mucosal involvement is very uncommon; however, sexually transmitted lesions will occur in the anogenital region or pubis.
- In atopic patients, lesions will commonly occur in areas of dermatitis.
- Lesions on immunocompromised patients may be large, up to 1.5 cm (known as *giant molluscum*) or may be widespread with hundreds of lesions.
- MC can spontaneously resolve in immunocompetent patients within about 2 months, and infection usually clears completely in several months.
- Lesions can become erythematous and swollen, which many believe is a sign of impending clinical resolution or the beginning of the end (BOTE) (Butala et al., 2013) (Fig. 6.3-7).
- Lesions may be pruritic or sometimes pustular.
- Molluscum dermatitis, a common phenomenon, is characterized by the development of eczematous patches or plaques surrounding the lesions. The dermatitis has been attributed to the localized reaction to the virus.

DIFFERENTIAL DIAGNOSIS   Molluscum Contagiosum

- *Genital warts* will lack the umbilicated center
- *Folliculitis lesions* may be pustular and around a hair
- *Keratosis pilaris* is also follicular with a keratotic center and usually on the upper arms or anterior thighs
- *Basal cell carcinoma* may be translucent but will have arborizing vessels in sun-exposed areas
- Infectious processes such as cryptococcosis or histoplasmosis

---

Confirming the Diagnosis

- Diagnosis is clinically made by the characteristic appearance of the lesions.

- MC lacks the verrucous appearance of warts and presents as discrete lesions, whereas warts often coalesce into larger lesions.
- Solitary lesions or a giant molluscum that occurs on the face can be differentiated from basal cell carcinomas that typically present as a translucent skin-colored papule with telangiectasias and rolled borders.
- Biopsy is not necessary but may be performed to confirm the diagnosis, especially in the case of large lesions, extensive involvement, or other atypical presentations.
- Extensive involvement should also raise the suspicion of immunosuppression, namely HIV infection.
- The virus itself cannot be cultured; however, bacterial culture may be needed if there is concern for secondary infection.
- If the central umbilication or dell is not obvious, a dermatoscope or magnifying lens may help identify the central core.
- Confirmation can also be made in the office by gently curetting the white, central core from the lesion, placing it between two slides with a drop of potassium hydroxide (KOH). The slide is gently heated and then crushed with firm, twisting pressure. The contents from the central core contain most of the viral cells and can be directly examined with microscopy. *Molluscum bodies* appear as dark, round cells that disperse easily with slight pressure (Fig. 6.3-8). Normal epithelial cells are flat, varied rectangular shapes, and tend to remain stuck together in sheets.

Treatment

MC can ultimately resolve without any treatment. Therefore, the plan of care should be individualized to the patient. Consideration should be given to the patient's age, location of lesions, number of lesions, risk for scarring, risk for hyper- or hypopigmentation, and immune status. Treatment may be provided in order to prevent lesions from spreading to other areas on the body or transmission to others. All sexually transmitted lesions should be treated along with screening for other sexually transmitted infections. Further treatment indications include pruritus, secondary infection, surrounding dermatitis, or scarring.

- Prior to treating MC, a full skin examination should be performed to identify any other lesions on the body. Incomplete treatment can result in autoinoculation and treatment failure.

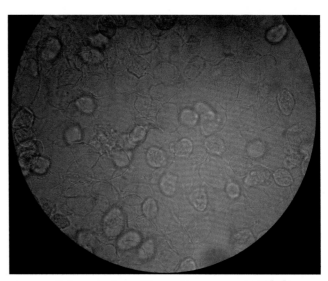

FIG. 6.3-8. Molluscum bodies on KOH prep. (Photo courtesy of M. Bobonich.)

In cases where there is associated dermatitis or pruritus, the provider may consider treating the patient with a topical agent such as Tacrolimus or Pimecrolimus that will help to repair and maintain the epidermal barrier. These products usually contain ceramides and/or essential fatty acids.

- There are many additional treatment options available; however, a 2017 Cochrane review concluded that there is no evidence showing that one method is convincingly more effective than the others.

- Topical treatment is common and includes the use of cantharidin, as discussed previously in the treatment of verruca. Since the application is painless, children are more cooperative, but painful blisters may follow application. Clinicians should consider testing two to three lesions initially to ensure that the patient does not have sensitivity to it.

- Cryotherapy is a destructive method that can be used in primary care but has limitations due to the discomfort of the procedure, especially in children.

- Curettage is a successful method used by experienced clinicians for treatment in children or adults with a limited number of lesions—geared toward removing the viral core of the MC. Topical anesthetic cream (EMLA) can be applied 30 to 60 minutes prior to treatment to minimize the discomfort associated with the procedure. This method may also cause a small scar so the treatment site should be chosen carefully.

- Nicking the lesion with a no. 11 blade and sterile needle allows the removal of the central core and can be effective.

- Less invasive approaches include application of surgical or duct tape daily (after bathing) for 16 weeks, which can lead to complete resolution. Strong adhesives may cause a contact dermatitis.

- In recalcitrant cases, generalized widespread lesions, or where immunosuppression is suspected or confirmed, referral to a dermatologist would be recommended. Treatment modalities that may be utilized in a dermatology setting include imiquimod, podophyllotoxin 0.5%, laser therapy, topical retinoids, trichloroacetic acid, and cidofovir.

- Lesions located in the periocular region should be referred to an ophthalmologist for management.

Special Considerations

Immunosuppression: Patients may be referred to an infectious disease specialist for consideration of antiretroviral (ARV) therapy. Patients with extensive lesions should be tested for human immunodeficiency virus (HIV) and the possibility of other immune deficiency disorders should be considered.

Genital lesions: Should raise suspicion for other sexually transmitted infections.

Pregnancy: Curettage, cryotherapy, and incision with expression of the central core are all safe treatment options to use during pregnancy. *Podophyllin, podofilox, and imiquimod are all teratogenic and are contraindicated during pregnancy.*

Management and Patient Education

- MC is generally self-limiting and is not associated with malignancy. Complications include secondary infection and scarring as a result of treatment. In immunosuppressed patients, MC can be difficult to treat and may recur for years.

- Patients dend parents of infected children should be educated on transmission-reducing methods.

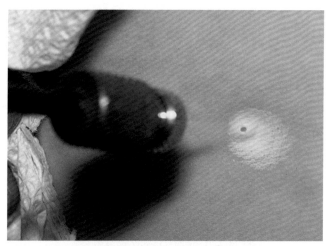

FIG. 6.3-9. Frozen molluscum. The central dell becomes apparent with light cryotherapy. (Goodheart, H. P. [2015]. *Goodheart's photoguide of common skin disorders* [4th ed.]. Wolters Kluwer Health | Lippincott Williams & Wilkins.)

- Children with MC should NOT be prevented from attending school or daycare.

- Lesions in areas that are likely to come in contact with others, such as those on the arms or legs, should be covered with clothing or a watertight bandage.

- Patient should be instructed to avoid scratching to prevent autoinoculation. Infected children should not bathe with others, and towels should not be shared.

- Sexual activity with affected individuals should be avoided until lesions are resolved (condoms will not provide a barrier from areas commonly affected with MC).

- Patients with atopic dermatitis and a history of molluscum and/or flat warts can benefit from regular moisturizing with a preparation containing ceramides to protect the normal skin barrier and help prevent autoinoculation; the use of topical corticosteroids in these patients is controversial.

- Follow-up and monitoring of patients with MC is dependent on the treatment modality used and the number of lesions on individual patients.

CLINICAL PEARL

- The central umbilication may not always be visible on clinical examination. Lightly spraying or touching the surface of the lesion with liquid nitrogen will often reveal this distinctive finding. The umbilication will appear against the frozen white background (Fig. 6.3-9).

HERPES SIMPLEX VIRUS

Herpes simplex virus (HSV) is one of the most prevalent infections worldwide. It is estimated that about 90% of adults in the United States have HSV-1 antibodies. HSV infections are caused by two different human herpes virus types. HSV-1 is more prevalent than HSV-2 and is typically associated with oral herpes simplex infections (cold sores). HSV-2 is typically associated with genital herpes simplex infections. However, HSV-1 has been found in genital infections and HSV-2 in oral infections, presumably as a result of oral genital sexual contact, or autoinoculation. Genital HSV infections are discussed in Section 11.4.

Pathophysiology

- HSV is a double-stranded, linear DNA, neurotropic virus that can be transmitted through respiratory droplets, direct contact with an active lesion, or contact with virus-containing fluid such as saliva or cervical secretions in patients with no evidence of active disease.

- It replicates at the site of inoculation and then travels along the dorsal root ganglion where it becomes dormant until reactivation.

- All persons infected with HSV-1 and HSV-2 infection are potentially infectious even if they have no clinical signs or symptoms.

- It is estimated that up to 20% of adults may be shedding HSV at any given time.

- Individuals infected with one subtype of HSV can contract the other subtype.

- HSV infections which result in open sores will increase the risk of other infections, including HIV and sexually transmitted diseases.

- HSV infection has two phases, the primary infection and the secondary phase. Most patients have no lesions or findings during the primary infection with HSV, when disease can only be detected by an elevated IgG antibody titer.

- During the primary infection, the virus becomes established in a nerve ganglion. When the patient has his/her first clinical lesion, this is usually a recurrence and represents the secondary phase.

- The risk of recurrence varies based on the virus type and site of infection. Various triggers can reactivate the virus including, but not limited to, sun exposure, stress, and physical trauma.

Clinical Presentation

- Classically characterized by grouped, uniform-appearing vesicles on an erythematous base.

- Vesicles turn into pustules, umbilicate, and subsequently dry and form crusts on the skin, or exudate on mucous membranes.

- Immunosuppression may result in an atypical presentation. Clinical hallmarks may include an active vesicular border and scalloped periphery. Early vesicles are not always noticed, and lesions may appear as erosions or crusts, and presentation is often atypical in this population.

- The repeated appearance of a lesion at the same location should make the clinician suspicious for HSV.

- Pain along a dermatome may be present and can vary with anatomic location.

- Regional lymphadenopathy may also be present.

Orolabial Herpes

Although most patients have no lesions or findings during the primary infection with HSV-1, approximately 1% of patients will develop herpes gingivostomatitis.

- This presents as herpetic lesions on the oral mucosa, tongue, and tonsils, accompanied by flu-like symptoms.

- Oral lesions have an aphthous appearance with white or yellow exudate on a red base (Fig. 6.3-10).

- Painful lesions can cause dehydration as a common complication.

- Patients can be acutely ill, and in severe cases may require treatment with intravenous antiviral therapy.

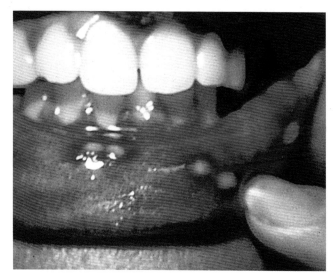

FIG. 6.3-10. Primary HSV infection. This patient has multiple erosions and gingivostomatitis. (Goodheart, H. P. [2015]. *Goodheart's photoguide of common skin disorders* [4th ed.]. Wolters Kluwer Health | Lippincott Williams & Wilkins.)

- If left untreated, symptoms can last approximately 1 to 2 weeks.

- Primary infection is usually associated with more constitutional symptoms, longer duration, and prolonged viral shedding when compared to recurrent episodes.

- Recurrent orolabial herpes is primarily caused by HSV-1 (commonly referred to as "fever blisters" or "cold sores").

- In many cases, there is a prodrome of tingling, itching, or burning that occurs 12 to 24 hours before cutaneous lesions appear.

- Clinical presentation consists of grouped vesicles over an erythematous base on the lips, commonly at the vermillion border (Fig. 6.3-11).

- Lesions can also occur wherever the virus was inoculated or proliferated during the initial episode, such as inside the mouth, cheeks, eyelids, or earlobes.

- Vesicles evolve to form crusts within a few days.

- Other associated clinical symptoms can include local discomfort, headache, nasal congestion, and mild flu-like symptoms, including fever. Lymphadenopathy is frequent.

- Common triggers for orolabial herpes include UV exposure (especially UVB), surgical and dental procedures of the lips (including braces), stress, and other systemic viral infections.

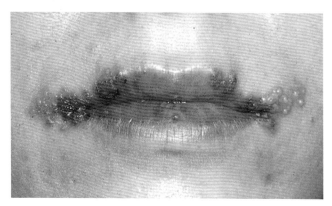

FIG. 6.3-11. Orolabial herpes. (Neville, B. W., Damm, D., White, D., & Waldron, C. [1991]. *Color atlas of clinical oral pathology.* Lea & Febiger.)

Herpes Gladiatorum

* Results from direct skin-to-skin exposure through contact sports.
* Wrestlers are especially at increased risk, and the condition can be a major problem during school tournaments and sports camps.
* It is estimated that up to one third of wrestlers will become infected after a single match with an infected individual.
* Lesions will appear approximately 4 to 11 days after exposure and may be preceded by a 24-hour prodrome.
* Common sites of infection include the lateral neck, side of the face, forearm, and ocular region.

Herpetic Whitlow

* Whitlow is the term used for lesions that develop on the fingers and periungual area.
* It was a common clinical presentation in health care workers and dentists prior to the introduction of universal precautions.
* Still seen in children with orolabial herpes who auto-inoculate by sucking their thumbs or biting their nails.
* Initial symptoms include tenderness and erythema of the nail fold or palmar surface with the development of deep-seated vesicles 24 to 48 hours after the prodrome (Fig. 6.3-12).
* Presentation can vary from no visible vesicles to classic, grouped vesicles that may or may not form erosions.

Herpetic Keratoconjunctivitis (HSV of the Eye)

* Presentation can include unilateral conjunctivitis, blepharitis with vesicles on the lid, or punctate or marginal keratitis.
* Regional lymphadenopathy can also be seen.
* Recurrences are common and can lead to ocular ulcerations and corneal blindness.
* Patients should be immediately referred to an ophthalmologist.

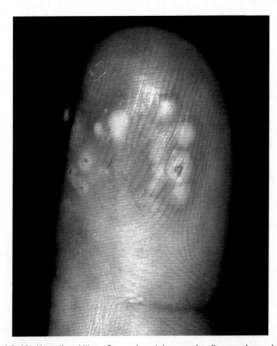

FIG. 6.3-12. Herpetic whitlow. Grouped pustules may be diagnosed as a bacterial infection. Recurrence at the same location is a clue to the diagnosis of HSV. (Courtesy T. Habif.)

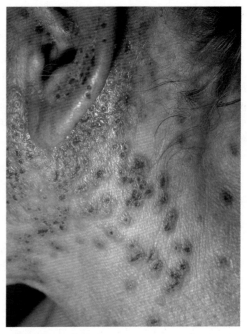

FIG. 6.3-13. Eczema herpeticum.

Genital Herpes

* Genital herpes can be caused by either type of HSV, but primarily by HSV-2.

Refer to Section 11.4 for more detailed information on this topic.

Eczema Herpeticum

* Acute development of herpetic lesions in sites of recent or active atopic dermatitis, occurring approximately 10 days after an exposure (Fig. 6.3-13).
* Associated with lymphadenopathy and high fever.
* Secondary staphylococcal infection is common.
* Eczema herpeticum typically presents as a primary HSV infection and recurrences are uncommon.
* Clinical course can range in presentation from mild to severe.
* Recurrent episodes are usually milder with fewer constitutional symptoms.

DIFFERENTIAL DIAGNOSIS   Herpes Simplex Virus

* *Impetigo*, especially in children, may be mistaken for HSV. Vesicles appear straw colored and then crust in impetigo, and in HSV they follow a classic evolution from vesicles to umbilicated pustules to discrete crusts over an erythematous base. There is no prodrome of burning or tingling associated with impetigo
* *Aphthous ulcers* may be confused with HSV but typically appear on the anterior mouth and appear grayish in color. HSV typically manifests on the hard palate and attached gingiva, and is more erythematous
* *Herpes zoster* is usually distinguished from HSV by the unilateral and dermatomal distribution
* *Bacterial infections* are commonly confused with Herpetic whitlow because of the pustular appearance, but Herpetic whitlow is very localized
* *Autoimmune blistering diseases* are not confined to one localized area

Confirming the Diagnosis

Diagnosis can usually be made with a thorough history and physical examination.

- Viral culture can be performed preferably from early vesicular, crusted, eroded, or ulcerative lesions. It is considered a very specific and relatively rapid test. Positive results are often available in 48 to 72 hours. Sensitivity, however, may be as low as 25% to 50%. Only half of the true positives are available in 2 days. The rest may take 6 days or longer to be positive.

- Polymerase chain reaction (PCR) is also listed by the Centers for Disease Control and Prevention (CDC) as the preferred way to test for HSV infection as the assays are much more sensitive.

- A biopsy may also be done and can detect viral changes and specific HSV antibodies.

- Serologic testing for diagnosis is generally not recommended.

Treatment

Treatment of HSV in the immunocompetent host is based on several factors, including the severity of the patient's symptoms, the presence of a primary or recurrent infection, site of the infection, and frequency with which the patient experiences recurrences. Careful consideration should be given to the patient's occupation, hobbies, and the cost of treatment.

Antiviral therapy is aimed at inhibiting DNA synthesis and includes acyclovir, valacyclovir, and famciclovir. There are some differences between the medications.

Acyclovir (Zovirax) is the most commonly used antiviral therapy in the world.

- It is the only FDA-approved drug in the treatment of HSV that can be used orally, topically, or intravenously.

- It has historically been labeled as a pregnancy category B drug, is generally well tolerated, and only contraindicated in patients with a hypersensitivity to the drug or any component of its formulation.

- It is not metabolized through the cytochrome P-450 pathway and therefore has very few interactions with other medications.

- Rare adverse effects include headache, nausea, and diarrhea. Acyclovir has the greatest in vitro activity against HSV-1 and HSV-2. However, it does not reduce the risk of recurrences over time.

- A new mucoadhesive buccal tablet (MBT) Sitavig, for use in immunocompetent individuals was approved by FDA in 2013. It contains 50 mg of acyclovir, is indicated for recurrent orolabial herpes, and is a single-dose method. It should be used within 1 hour of the prodromal symptoms and before the appearance of clinical signs. The tablet is applied to the canine fossa, the area of the gum right above the incisor tooth, and will adhere to the gum. Please see package insert for complete instructions.

Valacyclovir (Valtrex) and Famciclovir (Famvir)

- Valacyclovir is a prodrug of acyclovir, and famciclovir is a prodrug of penciclovir. Because of this, they have greater bioavailability and are dosed less frequently. The disadvantage is that they are also more expensive than acyclovir.

- Both drugs were historically labeled pregnancy category B and have similar mechanism of action, pharmacokinetics, safety, and side effect profile as acyclovir.

- Indications for treatment in immunocompetent hosts are summarized according to clinical scenario. Table 6.3-2 lists specific dosing for antiviral medications for treatment of uncomplicated HSV in immunocompetent individuals 12 years of age and over.

TABLE 6.3-2	Oral Therapy for HSV Infections in Immunocompetent Patients
HSV—primary infection	**Acyclovir:** 400 mg t.i.d. for 10 days; OR 200 mg 5 times daily for 10 days **Valacyclovir:** 1,000 mg b.i.d. for 10 days **Famciclovir:** 250 mg OR 500 mg t.i.d. for 10 days
HSV—initial recurrence	**Acyclovir:** 400 mg t.i.d. for 5 days **Valacyclovir:** 500 mg b.i.d. for 3 days **Famciclovir:** 125 mg b.i.d. for 5 days
HSV—chronic suppression	**Acyclovir:** 400 mg b.i.d. **Valacyclovir:** 500 mg daily for <10 episodes/yr; OR 1,000 mg daily >10 HSV episodes/yr **Famciclovir:** 250 mg b.i.d.
HSV—episodic	**Acyclovir:** 200 mg OR 400 mg taken 5 times daily for 5 days **Valacyclovir:** 2 g twice daily for 1 day **Famciclovir:** 750 mg twice daily for 1 day; OR 1,500 mg one single dose
Orolabial/herpes labialis	**Acyclovir (MBT):** 50 mg single dose, use w/i 1 h of prodrome **Topicals:** Docosonal 10% (Abreva); penciclovir 1% (Denavir): acyclovir 1% (Zovirax): acyclovir 5% and hydrocortisone 1% (Xerese) **Oral:** famciclovir for recurrence: 1,500 mg as single dose **Oral:** valacyclovir: 2 g and repeat in 12 h

Primary or Initial Infection

A symptomatic primary infection can have a duration of up to 2 weeks in untreated patients and can be complicated by systemic symptoms such as pharyngitis and odynophagia, which can result in dehydration.

- Treatment with oral antiviral therapy at the early stages of infection can help to shorten the duration of lesions, decrease the duration of odynophagia, reduce viral shedding, and lead to earlier cessation of fever.

- Initiation of antivirals should be within 72 hours of clinical presentation in order to obtain the maximum benefit. Therapy can still be considered when the patient is beyond the target 72-hour period but is continuing to develop new lesions or experiencing pain.

TABLE 6.3-3	Oral Therapy Mucocutaneous HSV—Immunocompetent Pediatric Patient

3 months to 11 years: acyclovir 40–80 mg/kg/day by mouth divided every 6–8 hours (maximum dose 1 g/day) for 5–10 days
≥12 years and <40 kg: see above
≥12 years and ≥40 kg: see adult summary

Suppression dosing (for patients who suffer from frequent recurrences, daily dosing may be necessary):
    <12 years: acyclovir 80 mg/kg/day divided every 6–8 hours (maximum dose 1 g/day)
    ≥12 years and <40 kg: see above
    ≥12 years and ≥40 kg: see adult summary

Valacyclovir is approved for use in children over the age of 12.
Famciclovir is not approved for use in children.

- Additionally, topical analgesics such as viscous lidocaine, benzocaine, and combination products may be used for painful lesions along with preparations that coat and protect lesions from irritants causing discomfort.

Recurrent Infection

Patients will often have a recurrent infection that is minimally symptomatic and short in duration, making no treatment an acceptable option in this setting. The patient and clinician can decide on treatment of recurrences based on the individual frequency, severity, and associated clinical symptoms.

- There are multiple treatment strategies including chronic suppression or episodic therapy.
- Episodic treatment can be particularly helpful in patients who have infrequent recurrences and those who experience a distinct prodrome.
- Oral antiviral therapy is started at the immediate onset of symptoms in order to reduce the duration and severity of outbreaks.
- Episodic treatment may also be used by patients prophylactically before planned exposure to a known trigger. Examples include patients who are about to undergo facial surgery, or those with anticipated exposure to UV light (i.e., photodynamic therapy or natural sunlight).
- Topical antiviral therapy, including topical acyclovir or penciclovir (Denavir), can be used for episodic care. They are of modest benefit and require frequent application (up to five times per day). A combination product containing 5% acyclovir and 1% hydrocortisone (Xerese), applied five times a day for 5 days at the onset of symptoms, has been shown to be safe and effective in the treatment of early recurrent orolabial HSV. It reduces the frequency of both ulcerative and nonulcerative recurrences, and shortens the healing time when compared to topical acyclovir alone.
- Other topicals, including benzalkonium chloride (Viroxyn) and docosanol (Abreva), may help shorten healing time and duration of symptoms.
- Chronic suppression therapy is useful for patients who have frequent recurrences (six or more outbreaks per year) that are associated with systemic symptoms (erythema multiforme [discussed below], eczema herpeticum, or aseptic meningitis). Suppression therapy can also be used in patients who do not have specific prodromes and cannot accurately predict outbreaks. Although there are no specific guidelines on how long suppression therapy should be continued, the CDC recommends reassessing the need for ongoing therapy on a yearly basis.
- In many cases, the frequency of outbreaks decreases over time, and chronic suppression is eventually unnecessary. When discontinuing therapy, caution the patient that there may be a risk of worsening outbreaks. Safety and efficacy have been documented among patients receiving chronic suppression therapy with acyclovir for as long as 6 years and with valacyclovir or famciclovir for 1 year.

Special Considerations

- *Athletes* participating in contact sports, especially wrestlers, with a history of confirmed orolabial herpes should be on antiviral suppression therapy to decrease the risk of transmission to others. According to the NCAA rules, return to play requires all of the following:
  - Oral antiviral medication (acyclovir, valacyclovir) for at least 5 days
  - No new blisters or lesions for 72 hours
  - Visible lesions must be covered with an impermeable dressing

- *Women* frequently present with lesions of HSV on the buttocks. Assumption of recurrent episodes can be made if there is evidence of scarring or postinflammatory hyperpigmentation seen in the general area.
- *Pregnant women* can generally use acyclovir which was historically classified as pregnancy category B and is recommended first line.
- *Immunocompromised and the elderly* may have atypical presentations and be more severe, persistent, symptomatic, and resistant to therapy. Prophylactic systemic antiviral therapy is sometimes required in immunocompromised patients; however, antiviral resistance with prophylactic therapy can be a potential complication. The elderly may also be at increased risk of infection and of substantial associated morbidity or mortality.
- *Neonates* who are exposed at birth or who later show signs of HSV infection, as well as patients with *eczema herpeticum,* are considered medical emergencies and require hospitalization and IV antiviral therapy.

Management and Patient Education

- In healthy immunocompetent patients, primary HSV is typically a self-limiting condition and usually resolves within 2 weeks. Recurrent episodes respond well to treatment, but can vary in duration.
- Approximately 50% of cases of erythema multiforme are associated with a preceding HSV-1 or HSV-2 infection (Fig. 6.3-14).
- Eczema herpeticum can be fatal in severe cases with associated *Staphylococcus aureus* septicemia, or viremia with infection of the internal organs. Other possible complications include herpes encephalitis, herpes pneumonia, aseptic meningitis, and herpes viremia.
- Herpes simplex infection has also been associated with Bell palsy.
- Patients should be reassured and educated about: the high prevalence of HSV and the chronicity of the infection to help reduce associated stigma.
- Prevention of disease transmission includes frequent hand washing and avoiding contact with immunocompromised individuals when they have active lesions.
- Patients with recurrent orolabial herpes should be educated about potential triggers, the effects of UV light, and the importance of sun protection to prevent outbreaks.
- For primary infections and complicated cases, patients should be followed to insure resolution of lesions and systemic symptoms.

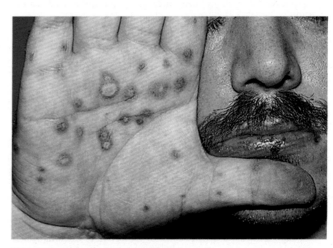

FIG. 6.3-14. HSV with erythema multiforme.

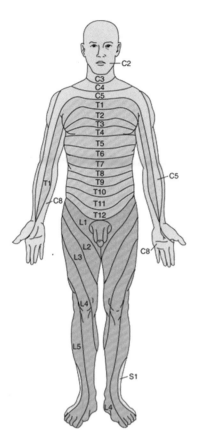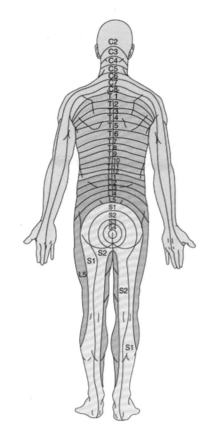

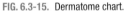
FIG. 6.3-15. Dermatome chart.

- In patients with uncomplicated recurrent disease, follow-up is on an as-needed basis.

HERPES ZOSTER

One out of three Americans will develop herpes zoster (VZV) or "shingles" during their lifetime. The unexpected skin eruption may be accompanied by severe pain, burning, itching, and vesicles and often prompts patients to seek care from their primary care provider. Recognizing the signs and symptoms (when present) and starting treatment early are vital to reduce duration, pain, and complications from the infection. The incidence of VZV, as well as associated postherpetic neuralgia (PHN) increases with age. According to the CDC, the overall rate in the United States is 4 per 1,000 people per year. When looking at those 60 and older, the rate is 2.5 times higher at 10 per 1,000 people per year (CDC, 2020).

Pathophysiology

- VZV is caused by reactivation of the virus in patients previously infected with chicken pox. The varicella virus enters the individual's dorsal root ganglia, where it remains latent. When reactivated, the virus travels down the sensory nerve into the skin causing a rash within the associated dermatome (Fig. 6.3-15).

- VZV acquired from a patient with active varicella or zoster is rare. Zoster lesions do, however, contain high concentrations of the VZV that can be spread, presumably by the airborne route, and cause primary varicella in susceptible individuals.

- Localized zoster is only contagious after the rash erupts and until the lesions crust. In general, zoster is less contagious than varicella. It is thought that various factors may play a role in the reactivation of the virus. These include immunosuppression, medications, lymphoma, fatigue, stress, spinal surgery, radiation, and chemotherapy. Virus reactivation usually occurs only once in an individual's lifetime and the incidence of a second reactivation in the same person is less than 5%.

Clinical Presentation

- Cutaneous symptoms of VZV include a prodrome described as pain, itching, or tingling for several days prior to the rash.

- Typically, a single dermatome is affected, but involvement may be seen in as many as three. Some patients may have up to 20 lesions outside the affected dermatome (Fig. 6.3-16).

- The thoracic and lumbar dermatomes are the most frequently affected in VZV.

- VZV characteristically presents as a unilateral group of vesicles, in a dermatomal distribution that does not cross the midline.

- Lesions continue to erupt for several days, and may become pustular, hemorrhagic, necrotic, or bullous.

- After approximately 7 to 10 days, the lesions crust and are no longer considered infectious. The duration is dependent on the

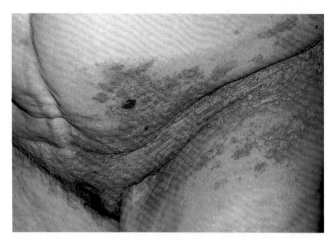

FIG. 6.3-16. Classic herpes zoster with fewer than 20 satellite lesions. (Used with permission from Edwards, L. [2004]. *Genital dermatology atlas*. Wolters Kluwer Health.)

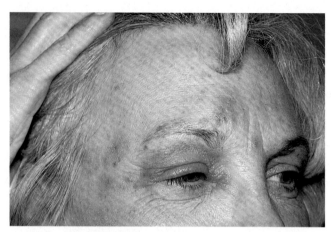

FIG. 6.3-18. Herpes zoster ophthalmicus (HZO). (Used with permission from Goodheart, H. P. [2003]. *Goodheart's photoguide of common skin disorders* [2nd ed.]. Lippincott Williams & Wilkins.)

patient's age, severity of the eruption, and the presence of underlying immunosuppression.

- In rare cases, the patient may have pain in a dermatomal distribution, but no associated skin lesions ("zoster sine herpete").
- In elderly patients, lesions may take up to 6 weeks or more to heal.

Disseminated Herpes Zoster

Disseminated VZV occurs when there are more than 20 lesions outside the affected dermatome. This phenomenon occurs chiefly in elderly, immunosuppressed, or debilitated individuals.

- The dermatomal lesions are sometimes hemorrhagic or gangrenous, and the outlying vesicles or bullae, which are usually not grouped, resemble varicella, and are often umbilicated or hemorrhagic (Fig. 6.3-17).
- Involvement of the lungs and central nervous system may occur in the setting of disseminated zoster. Hospital admission should be initiated if this is suspected.

Ophthalmic Herpes Zoster

VZV of the ophthalmic branch (V_1) of the trigeminal nerve (the fifth cranial nerve) is referred to as *ocular herpes zoster* or *herpes zoster ophthalmicus (HZO)*, and is a serious, sight-threatening condition.

- A prodrome of headache, malaise, and fever typically precedes a unilateral vesicular eruption along the trigeminal dermatome.
- HZO should be suspected in patients who develop vesicular lesions on the side and tip of the nose. This finding is known as the Hutchinson sign, and is associated with a high risk of HZO (Figs. 6.3-18 and 6.3-19).
- Patients may also experience hyperemic conjunctivitis, episcleritis, and lid ptosis. Patients with suspected HZO require immediate evaluation by an ophthalmologist and treatment with systemic antiviral therapy.
- Approximately 50% of patients with HZO develop inflammation inside the eye or *uveitis*, which has an increased risk of blindness, glaucoma, optic neuritis, encephalitis, hemiplegia, and acute retinal necrosis. Symptoms of uveitis include photosensitivity, pain, redness, and visual changes that occur about 1 to 3 weeks after the rash appears.
- The complications of HZO can be reduced from 50% to 20% to 30% with effective antiviral therapy started in the earliest stages. Ocular lesions of zoster and their complications tend to recur, sometimes as long as 10 years after the zoster episode

---

DIFFERENTIAL DIAGNOSIS   Herpes Zoster

- *Herpes simplex* is usually a distinct group of papules or vesicles that do not extend along a dermatome. Tingling and burning may be present but pain is not common
- *Contact dermatitis* may appear in numerous areas and have a more linear presentation that does not follow a dermatome. Itching may be a prominent symptom
- *Conjunctivitis* viral or bacterial may exist. Hutchinson sign would not be present however

---

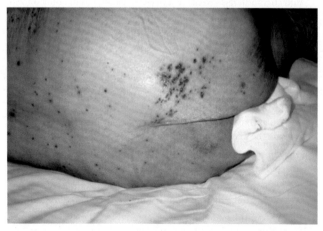

FIG. 6.3-17. Disseminated herpes zoster. Disseminated herpes zoster with more than 20 ungrouped satellite lesions. Note the initial dermatomal involvement on the buttock. (Photo courtesy of Herbert A. Hochman.)

Confirming the Diagnosis

Diagnosis is typically made based on the clinical appearance.

- The unilateral and dermatomal distribution of VZV can help distinguish it from HSV.
- HSV lesions tend to be more uniform, and vesicles associated with shingles tend to vary in size.
- HSV is a recurrent condition, and VZV typically only occurs once.
- Careful history taking can help to differentiate between the two.

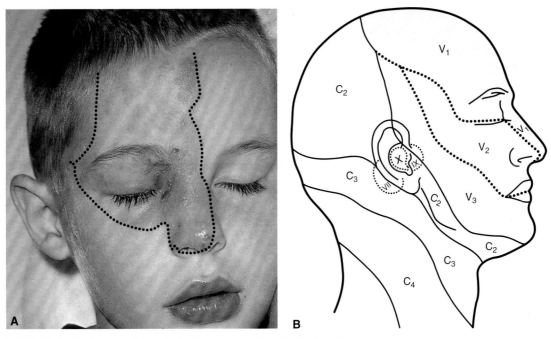

FIG. 6.3-19. **A:** Hutchinson sign. **B:** Note the involvement of the V1 branch of the trigeminal nerve.

- VZV of the hand can be particularly confusing and misdiagnosed as a contact dermatitis (e.g., poison ivy).
- Viral culture may be sent in circumstances where patients have an atypical presentation or diagnostic confirmation is required.
- PCR can be used to detect VZV DNA rapidly and sensitively in properly collected skin lesion specimens. However, PCR testing for VZV is not available in all settings.
- Direct fluorescent antibody (DFA) staining is performed on a scraping from the base of the lesion. This test is rapid, and specific, but less sensitive, than PCR.

Treatment

The goal in the treatment of VZV is aimed at lessening the severity and duration of pain associated with the acute infection, promoting rapid healing of skin lesions, preventing new lesion formation, decreasing viral shedding, and preventing the long-term complication of PHN.

- Oral antiviral therapy should be prescribed at the onset of symptoms and has been proven to decrease the duration of skin lesions, reduce acute pain, and decrease the incidence of PHN.
- Antivirals approved for the treatment of acute VZV infection include oral acyclovir, valacyclovir, and famciclovir.
- Oral antiviral treatment includes acyclovir 800 mg five times daily for 7 to 10 days; valacyclovir 1,000 mg t.i.d. for 7 to 10 days; and famciclovir 500 mg t.i.d. for 7 days.
- Valacyclovir has proven to be more effective than acyclovir at decreasing the incidence of PHN and zoster-associated acute neuritis.
- Primary care clinicians should collaborate with ophthalmologist to manage HZO. In addition to antivirals, the use of topical or systemic steroid therapy may be indicated.

Special Considerations

The vast majority of patients have no underlying illnesses; however, for patients who experience one or more recurrences, or those who

have a longer than expected duration of symptoms, immunosuppression should be suspected. There is an increased incidence of VZV and PHN in the geriatric population. It occurs less frequently in children and may occur during pregnancy.

Pregnancy. Although pregnant women with maternal varicella are at risk for having babies with congenital varicella, maternal VZV infection has not been associated with this complication. Transmission of VZV to the fetus during pregnancy is rare. All of the aforementioned antivirals used in the treatment of VZV are historically labeled pregnancy category B and considered safe for use.

Pregnant women who have not been previously infected or vaccinated for chicken pox should be cautioned that exposure to someone with VZV could cause a varicella infection. Susceptible women are at risk for developing a severe illness with varicella infection during pregnancy, and 10% to 20% of those may develop varicella pneumonia, which can be associated with significant maternal morbidity and mortality.

Also, women who experience maternal varicella infection may have increased risk of fetal abnormalities and babies who develop VZV during infancy. Women without evidence of immunity to varicella who have been exposed to the virus are advised to receive varicella-zoster immune globulin (VZIG) preferably within 72 to 96 hours after exposure.

Postherpetic neuralgia (PHN) can affect approximately 10% to 15% of patients with VZV and is one of the most common complications. It is characterized by persistent pain lasting 4 or more months beyond the initial onset of cutaneous lesions. PHN can be divided into three different types:

- Constant, monotonous, usually burning or deep, aching pain
- Shooting, lancinating, or neuritic pain
- Triggered pain which is manifested as allodynia or hyperalgesia (increased sensitivity to pain)

PHN can be difficult to control especially in patients over 60 years old, who account for approximately 50% of the cases. Severe acute neuritis, severe rash, or history of prodromal symptoms can

| TABLE 6.3-4 | Herpes Zoster Vaccine Comparison Between RZV and ZVL |

SHINGRIX/RZV (INTRODUCED IN 2018)	ZOSTAVAX/ZVL (INTRODUCED IN 2011)
Recombinant zoster virus	Live attenuated virus
Approved for adults 50 and older	Approved for adults 60 and older
May be given to patients who had varicella vaccine	Not recommended for those who have had the varicella vaccine
Two injections, second shot should be 2–6 mo after the first	One injection
Can be given to those who received ZVL	—
Contraindication: • Allergic reaction to prior dose of zoster vaccine • Has not been studied in immunocompromised persons • No data in pregnancy—not recommended in the age group of women who are likely to become pregnant • Moderate to severe acute illness (true for all vaccines)	Contraindication: • Allergic reaction to prior dose of zoster vaccine • Persons with primary or acquired immunodeficiency including AIDS, CD4 count less than 200 per mm^3, leukemia, lymphoma, or other malignancies of the marrow or lymphatic system • High dose steroid use (>20 mg per day for 2 or more weeks) • No data in pregnancy—not recommended in the age group of women who are likely to become pregnant • Moderate to severe acute illness (true for all vaccines) • Not recommended for persons with untreated active TB

also increase the risk for development of PHN. Symptoms can range in severity from trivial to debilitating.

- Tricyclic antidepressants (TCA) such as amitriptyline 25 mg can be given at bedtime and are considered first-line therapy in the treatment of PHN.
- Lidoderm patch, gabapentin, and long-acting opiates may also be used. In some cases, symptoms are so severe that patients require referral to a pain clinic. Early intervention is the best way to minimize risk.
- Scarring and postinflammatory hyper- or hypopigmentation are more common in elderly and immunosuppressed patients and correlate with the severity of the initial eruption.
- Other complications, including uveitis and keratitis, meningitis, motor neuropathy, and herpes zoster oticus (Ramsay Hunt syndrome—triad of ipsilateral facial paralysis, ear pain, and vesicles in the auditory canal and auricle), have also been reported.
- The immunocompetent patients should experience complete resolution within 14 to 21 days.

Management and Patient Education

There are now two zoster vaccines. Shingrix is an adjuvanted, non-live, recombinant vaccine and is the preferred vaccine by the CDC's Advisory Committee on Immunization Practices. Zostavax, is a live attenuated virus vaccine that is also available. See Table 6.3-4 for a summary of both.

Zoster vaccination is not recommended for persons of any age who have received varicella vaccine. There is no specific time that you must wait after having shingles before receiving the shingles vaccine. The decision on when to get vaccinated should be made with your health care provider. In general, a person should make sure that the shingles rash has disappeared before getting vaccinated.

- Patients should be educated about disease transmission and instructed to avoid contact with susceptible persons at high risk for developing severe varicella in the household and occupational settings, until lesions are crusted.

- In addition, patients who are at high risk for developing VZV, especially the elderly, should be informed about how to recognize the signs and symptoms to aid with early detection and treatment.
- It is the provider's responsibility to counsel patients about the indications and encourage them to get the vaccine.
- Follow-up is based on the duration and severity of symptoms and should be individualized for each patient.

READINGS AND REFERENCES

Bolognia, J. L., Jorizzo, J. L., & Rapini, R. P. (2017). Cutaneous manifestations of HIV, human papillomaviruses, human herpesvirus and other viral diseases. In Bolognia, J., Schaffer, J., & Cerroni, L. (Eds.). *Dermatology* (4th ed.). Elsevier Saunders.

Butala, N., Siegfried, E., & Weissler, A. (2013). Molluscum BOTE sign: A predictor of imminent resolution. *Pediatrics, 131*(5), e1650–e1653.

Catron, T., & Hern, H. G. (2008). Herpes zoster ophthalmicus. *Western Journal of Emergency Medicine, 9*(3), 174–176.

CDC. (2020). Shingles (Herpes Zoster). https://www.cdc.gov/shingles/hcp/clinical-overview.html

Gershon, A. A., Breuer, J., Cohen, J. I., Cohrs, R. J., Gershon, M. D., Gilden, D., Grose, C., Hambleton, S., Kennedy, P. G., Oxman, M. N., Seward, J. F., & Yamanishi, K. (2015). Varicella zoster virus infection. *Nature Reviews Disease Primers, 1*, 15016. https://doi.org/10.1038/nrdp.2015.16

Habif, T. P. (2018). *Warts, herpes simplex, and other viral infections. Clinical dermatology: A color guide to diagnosis and therapy* (4th ed.). Mosby Elsevier.

Hull, C. M., & Brunton, S. (2010). The role of topical 5% acyclovir and 1% hydrocortisone cream (Xerese™) in the treatment of recurrent herpes simplex labialis. *Journal of Postgraduate Medicine, 122*(5), 1–6.

James, W. D., Berger, T. G., & Elston, D. M. (2018). *Viral diseases. Andrews' diseases of the skin: Clinical dermatology* (13th ed.). Mosby Elsevier.

Johnston, C., & Corey, L. (2016). Current concepts for genital herpes simplex virus infection: Diagnostics and pathogenesis of genital tract shedding. *Clinical Microbiology Reviews, 29*(1), 149–161. https://doi.org/10.1128/CMR.00043-15

Kwok, C. S., Gibbs, S., Bennett, C., Holland, R., & Abbott, R. (2012). Topical treatments for skin warts. *The Cochrane Database of Systematic Reviews*, (9), CD001781..

Lamont, R. F., Sobel, J. D., Carrington, D., Mazaki-Tovi, S., Kusanovic, J. P., Vaisbuch, E., & Romero, R. (2011). Varicella-zoster virus (chickenpox) infection in pregnancy. *BJOG: An International Journal of Obstetrics and Gynaecology, 118*(10), 1155–1162. https://doi.org/10.1111/j.1471-0528.2011.02983.x

Stulberg, D. L., & Hutchinson, A. G. (2003). Molluscum contagiosum and warts. *American Family Physician, 67*(6), 1233–1240.

van der Wouden, J. C., van der Sande, R., van Suijlekom-Smit, L. W., Berger, M., Butler, C. C., & Koning, S. (2009). Interventions for cutaneous molluscum contagiosum. *The Cochrane Database of Systematic Reviews*, (4), CD004767. https://doi.org/10.1002/14651858.CD004767.pub3

Wolverton, S. E. (2012). *Comprehensive dermatologic drug therapy* (4th ed.). Saunders Elsevier.

Sexually Transmitted Diseases

Elizabeth Drumm and Jeffrey Viveiros

In This Chapter

- Syphilis
- Gonorrhea
- Chancroid
- Lymphogranuloma Venereum
- Granuloma Inguinale

Sexually transmitted diseases (STDs), also known as sexually transmitted infections (STIs), are very common, with millions of new infections occurring in the United States every year. STIs are transmitted from one person to another through sexual activity including vaginal, oral, and anal sex. They can also be passed through intimate physical contact.

In addition, the CDC 2018 STD Surveillance Report highlights alarming threat of syphilis in newborn. In 2018, 94 newborns died from syphilis; a 22% increase from 2017.

STIs are frequently asymptomatic and can lead to various complications. The immediate goal of screening for STIs is to identify and treat infected persons before they develop complications and to identify, test, and treat their sex partners to prevent transmission and reinfection.

SYPHILIS

Syphilis is a sexually transmitted, previously referred to as a venereal, disease that is caused by the spirochete *Treponema pallidum*. The chronic infection progresses over years to involve multiple organ systems and, therefore, a wide range of manifestations. Early detection is key to prevent serious complications from untreated disease. Furthermore, untreated syphilis can lead to higher rates of transmission of HIV, as well as infant death in 40% of cases from untreated mothers (CDC, 2018c).

The large studies of Oslo (1890–1910) and, the highly unethical, Tuskegee experiment (1932), provided insight to the natural course of disease. Syphilis is divided into stages including *primary, secondary, latency, and tertiary disease*. Early syphilis *includes primary, secondary, and early latency*. Late syphilis includes *late latency through tertiary stage* (Bolognia et al., 2018). This section will discuss primary, secondary, tertiary, ocular and congenital infections.

Epidemiology

Although most cases occur in low-income countries, syphilis is a worldwide infection. The rates have dropped since the introduction of treatment with penicillin. However, according to the Center for

Disease Control and Prevention, in 2018 the total reported cases of syphilis were at its highest since 1991 with rate of 10.8 cases per 100,000. This is a 14.9% increase since 2017.

As noted in prior years, the rate of syphilis in men remained much higher than women in 2018 with 18.7 cases per 100,000 men and 3.0 cases per 100,000 women (CDC). The primary and secondary syphilis rates have increased consistently every year in men. The cases in women, however, have fluctuated for years, with a substantial increase in women since 2013. The most recent 2017–2018 rates in women show a primary and secondary syphilis increase of 30.4% (CDC, 2018c).

Pathophysiology

- *T. pallidum* is transmitted by direct contact of infected individuals to another during vaginal, anal, or oral sex.
- Mucosal surfaces and abraded skin allow for inoculation and penetration of the organism, which then attaches to host cells and multiplies.
- These bacteria, enter the regional lymph nodes quickly and disseminate via the bloodstream to internal organs (Bolognia et al., 2018).

Clinical Presentation

See Table 6.4-1.

Associated Disorders/Pertinent HPI

Syphilis and HIV

- There is a higher risk of acquiring HIV in those with STIs, such as syphilis, when there is a lack of epithelial barrier due to an ulcer.
- The immune-mediated macrophages and T cells have receptors for HIV and therefore increase risk of transmission.
- The clinical presentation of syphilis may be altered in those with HIV.

TABLE 6.4-1	Syphilis Stages and Clinical Presentation		
	PATHOGENESIS	**SKIN FINDINGS**	**NON-SKIN FINDINGS**
Primary	Approximately 21 days (10–90 days) after infection Microorganism is identified by cells of Th1-predominant cellular response	A painless firm papule initially, develops into a painless ulcer, known as a chancre (Fig. 6.4-1) Heals spontaneously	Lymphadenopathy
Secondary	Occurs with healing or up to 6 mo after healing of primary lesion Microorganism dissemination and multiplication to different tissues Risk of transplacental transmission to fetus	Generalized nonpruritic papulosquamous and maculopapular eruption which includes palms and soles (Fig. 6.4-2) Localized "moth-eaten" hair loss (Fig. 6.4-3) Mucosal ulcers mouth Skin lesions resolve even if untreated	Low-grade fever, malaise, sore throat, adenopathy, weight loss, muscle aches, headaches, uveitis (red and painful eyes) photophobia, and visual changes
Latency	A period of early (1 yr or less) or late (>1 yr) asymptomatic time between healed lesions and late manifestations 70% untreated cases remain in this stage for life Still risk of transmission to others including in utero	Symptoms spontaneously resolve and remain asymptomatic during this stage	Asymptomatic
Tertiary	Occurs months to years after initial infection The result of the presence of a small number of residual organisms and high cellular immune reactivity against the organisms (Bolognia et al., 2018) Microorganisms invade organs skin, CNS, cardiovascular system, producing gummas in skin	Grouped red nodules with central scarring Gummas: solitary lesion with ulceration and necrosis and secondary scarring	Range of systemic manifestations, including: Bone cardiovascular neurologic

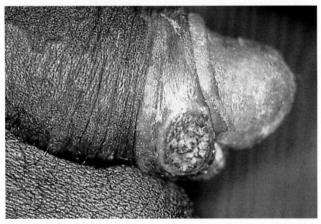

FIG. 6.4-1. Chancre syphilis.

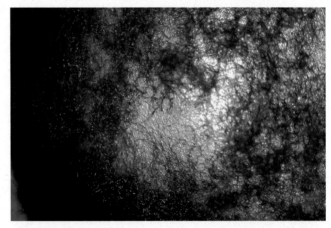

FIG. 6.4-3. Moth-eaten hair loss secondary syphilis. This photograph depicts a close view of a 13-year-old boy's scalp, which exhibited areas of alopecia, that had been attributed to a case of secondary-staged syphilis, described as "moth-eaten hair loss." (Courtesy Center for Disease Control and Prevention. Phil #17887.)

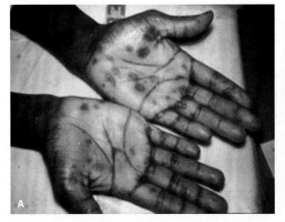

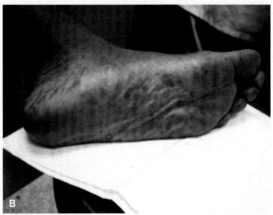

FIG. 6.4-2. **A** and **B.** Palmar–plantar rash secondary syphilis. (Source: Cincinnati STD/HIV Prevention Training Center. Department of Health and Human Services. Centers for Disease Control Prevention Atlanta, Georgia, 30333.)

DIFFERENTIAL DIAGNOSIS Syphilis		
Primary Syphilis	*Secondary Syphilis*	*Tertiary Syphilis*
• Herpes simplex virus • Chancroid • Lymphogranuloma venereum • Granuloma inguinale • Ecthyma gangrenosum • Amebiasis • Fixed drug eruption • Behçet disease • Balanitis	• Pityriasis rosea • Pityriasis rubra pilaris • Guttate psoriasis • Lichen planus • Drug eruption • Scabies • Tinea corporis	• Granuloma annulare • Sarcoidosis • Mycosis fungoides • Discoid lupus • Stasis ulcer

Confirming the Diagnosis

The options for tests to confirm the diagnosis in syphilis include direct detection and serologic tests.

Direct Detection Testing

Direct detection methods are samples obtained directly from the chancre in primary syphilis or from a localized rash in secondary syphilis. Therefore, direct detection should be performed when exudate or an adequate lesion is available.

The direct detection methods include:

- **Dark field microscopy** (see Fig. 6.4-5): Used to directly detect and visualize *T. pallidum* using a dark field microscope with trained staff.
  - Sample taken directly from chancre in primary syphilis or a localized rash in secondary syphilis
  - Positive with direct visualization of *T. pallidum* in primary or secondary syphilis. These tests may provide a diagnosis prior to the serologic response.
- **Polymerase chain reaction (PCR)**
  - Direct detection of bacterial DNA via PCR
  - Positive with detection
  - Useful in genital ulcerations
- **Direct fluorescent antibody testing for T. pallidum**
  - Direct examination, from lesion tissue or exudate, of the antigen. This does not require motile treponemes to be present. Easier to perform than dark-field microscopy
  - Histologic examination of tissue
    - Majority of skin biopsies of secondary syphilis rash will show spirochetes
    - Presence of spirochetes is a positive result

Serologic Testing

Nontreponemal tests, are ordered initially as a screening test. If this nontreponemal test is reactive, treponemal tests are ordered as confirmation of infection. The serologic testing will not indicate the syphilis stage; it will signify the presence of a past or current infection. It is important to note that nontreponemal tests may not be reactive for 3 to 6 weeks after infection. Nonreactive tests should

be repeated in 1 to 12 weeks if there is clinical concern and empirical therapy is recommended with high suspicion. See Figure 6.4-6: Syphilis testing algorithm.

Serologic tests include:

- **Nontreponemal tests** which include rapid plasma reagin (RPR) and venereal disease research laboratory (VDRL)
  - Serologic test to detect antibodies directed to treponeme-induced lipoidal antigens. Results may show false nonreactivity initially in primary syphilis
  - Usually positive in tertiary syphilis
  - Titers decline over time and become undetectable after treatment
- **Treponemal tests**
  - Serologic test to detect antibody to *T. pallidum*
  - Treponemal specific tests are performed when nontreponemal tests are reactive
  - Reactive results confirm infection however this does not identify if this is a prior, recent, treated, or untreated infection
  - False positives may occur in other infections or inflammatory diseases (such as HIV infection, autoimmune diseases, and other treponeme and spirochete family infections) and remain reactive for life, even after adequate treatment
- Specific treponemal tests are:
  - Fluorescent treponemal antibody absorbed (FTA-ABS) test
  - Microhemagglutination assay for *T. pallidum* (MHA-TP)
  - *T. pallidum* hemagglutination assay (TPHA) and Chemiluminescence immunoassays and enzyme immunoassays that detect treponemal antibodies

Confirming the Diagnosis Latent Syphilis

Diagnosis can be made based on clinical history of chancre and secondary manifestations.

- One third of individuals:
  - RPR nonreactive
  - Treponemal-specific antibody assays remain positive
  - Remain clinically asymptomatic without signs of reactivation for remainder of life
- One third of individuals:
  - RPR and VDRL remain reactive
  - Treponemal-specific antibody assays remain positive
  - Remain clinically asymptomatic without signs of reactivation for remainder of life
- One third of individuals:
  - Progress to clinical symptoms of tertiary syphilis

CONGENITAL SYPHILIS

There are risks and potentially fatal consequences in mother-to-child transmission of syphilis in utero or perinatally. There is nearly 100% risk for transmission if untreated mother is infected from conception to month 7 of pregnancy and 50% risk for transmission if untreated mother is infected 2 years prior to pregnancy.

Clinical Presentation

Early Congenital Syphilis

- Occurs in children before 2 years of age
  - Infants typically present within 3 months of life
- *Skin findings*
  - Similar to those in acquired secondary syphilis
  - Lesions are more bullous and erosive
  - Perioral and perianal fissures
- *Non-skin findings*
  - Bloody or purulent mucosal drainage known as "snuffles"
  - Skeletal involvement with reduced movement due to pain
  - Anemia and thrombocytopenia
  - Syphilitic pneumonitis
  - Hepatitis
  - Nephropathy

Late Congenital Syphilis

- Early detection (during early phase) is key to prevent detrimental effects to the child.
- In late syphilis, manifestations appear after 2 years of age and are analogous to tertiary syphilis in the adult (see Table 6.4-2).

Confirming the Diagnosis

Early Congenital Syphilis

- Dark field microscope of skin lesions/body fluids, such as nasal discharge
- Pathology review of placenta or umbilical cord

Late Congenital Syphilis

- *T. pallidum* is present in this stage therefore nontreponemal (VDRL, RPR) and treponemal tests (FTA-ABS, TPHA) should be performed

OCULAR SYPHILIS

- Less common manifestation of syphilis infection, although very serious
- All structures of eye can be affected (and devastated) by *T. pallidum* infection
- Can occur in congenital and acquired syphilis

TABLE 6.4-2	Clinical Presentation: Late Congenital Syphilis
• Rhogades: scars at site of prior skin fissures	• Interstitial keratitis with eye redness, pain, tearing, photophobia
• Hutchinson teeth: peg-shaped teeth	• Clutton joints: painless swelling of joints
• Mulberry molars	• Saber shins: bowing of anterior tibia
• Saddle nose: flat nasal bridge	• Higoumenakis sign: Clavicle thickening, can be unilateral
• Frontal bossing	• Eighth nerve deafness: vertigo and initial high-frequency hearing loss
• High palatal arch	
• Short or small maxilla (which makes normal mandible appear protruding)	

Clinical Presentation

- Conjunctivitis
- Keratitis
- Glaucoma
- Ptosis
- Pupil changes
- Uveitis
- Optic atrophy
- Blurred vision
- Pain
- Redness
- Photophobia
- Floaters

Confirming the Diagnosis

Slit lamp examination which may show evidence of old or active uveitis, and ghost vessels.

Treatment Syphilis

- Aqueous penicillin G 2.4 million units IM single dose is the treatment of choice in all stages.
- There are different recommended regimens depending on stage and manifestations.
- Doxycycline 100 mg b.i.d. × 14 days is second-line if penicillin cannot be given.
- Azithromycin 2 g single dose can be used if penicillin cannot be given.
- Treatment guidelines and additional information are provided by the Center for Disease Control and Prevention (CDC) (www.cdc.gov).

Management and Patient Education

- Nontreponemal tests (VDRL and RPR) should be performed at 1, 2, 3, 6 months and then every 6 months for 2 years after antibiotic therapy
- More frequent monitoring in HIV patients
- Monitor for late syphilis every 6 months for 3 years
- Evaluation of neurosyphilis with CSF is recommended every 6 months until cell counts are normal
- Evaluation of sexual partners is mandatory in many countries
- Reporting is mandatory in many countries

GONORRHEA

Gonorrhea (GC) is the second most commonly reported communicable disease in the United States. CDC estimates that approximately 1.14 million new gonococcal infections occur in the United States each year, and as many as half occur among young people aged 15 to 24. In 2018, 583,405 cases of GC were reported to the CDC. Any sexually active person can be infected with GC. In the United States, the highest reported rates of infection are among sexually active teenagers, young adults, and African Americans (CDC, 2019). There appears to be a higher rate of gonorrheal infection in women than men.

GC is highly contagious and primarily spread through sexual contact with the penis, vagina, mouth, or anus of an infected partner. Ejaculation does not have to occur for GC to be transmitted or acquired. It can also be passed to the fetus from a pregnant woman during childbirth or via indirect contact through sharing of contaminated objects (CDC, 2019).

The incubation period of *Neisseria gonorrhoeae* is short. The average time from infection to symptom onset is approximately 2 to 7 days.

Pathophysiology

GC is caused by infection with the *N. gonorrhoeae* bacterium. *N. gonorrhoeae,* a gram-negative intracellular diplococcus that can infect the mucous membranes of the reproductive tract, including the cervix, uterus, and fallopian tubes in women, and the urethra in women and men. *N. gonorrhoeae* can also infect the mucous membranes of the mouth, throat, eyes, and rectum.

Risk factors for acquiring *N. gonorrhoeae* include: a new sexual partner, more than one sex partner (or a sex partner with concurrent partners), and a history of STIs (or a sex partner with a history of STIs). Other risk factors include inconsistent condom use (if not in a mutually monogamous relationship), young age, and substance abuse. Some subgroups of men who have sex with men (MSM) are at higher risk as well (CDC, 2019). People who have had GC and received treatment may be reinfected if they have sexual contact with a person infected with GC.

Clinical Presentation

Skin Findings/Female

- The endocervical canal is the most common site of infection.

- Erythematous and edematous vulva with copious mucopurulent vaginal discharge.

- Examination of the vaginal vault will usually show purulent material at or around the cervical os, with edema and erythema of the cervix.

- Inflammation of the Bartholin glands may lead to acute edema of the labia with discharge of purulent material upon gentle pressure applied to the glands.

- Disseminated GC can present with pustules on a purpuric base, papules, petechiae, and/or areas of necrosis. There are typically a countable number of lesions (see Fig. 6.4-4).

Non-Skin Findings/Female

- Dysuria

- Vaginal bleeding

- Menstrual pain

- With involvement of the upper genital tract in women, there may be abdominal or adnexal tenderness with or without peritoneal signs, fever, and cervical motion tenderness (chandelier sign)

- Pelvic inflammatory disease (PID) occurs in 20% of patients as a result of ascending endocervical infection. Clinical features of PID include lower abdominal and adnexal pain, fever, and leukocytosis

- Rarely, PID can cause further peritoneal and hepatic inflammation, leading to right upper quadrant pain and gonorrheic perihepatitis (Fitz-Hugh–Curtis syndrome)

- Chronic untreated PID may lead to tubal scarring with resultant infertility or ectopic pregnancy

- Rectal involvement causes discharge, bleeding, tenesmus, constipation, and anal pruritus

- Pharyngeal GC may cause pharyngitis however it is usually asymptomatic and spontaneously resolves in a few weeks

- Systemic symptoms including fever, arthritis, tenosynovitis of large joints which occurs in less than 1% of patients. Invasive infections with *N. gonorrhoeae*, including disseminated gonococcal infection, endocarditis, and meningitis, are uncommon but can result in serious morbidity

- Risk factors for dissemination include menstruation and complement deficiency

Skin Findings/Male

- Purulent, yellow, thick urethral discharge, that usually appears 1 to 14 days after infection (see Fig. 6.4-5).

- Balanitis (inflammation of the glans of the penis) may be present and can then cause paraphimosis (inability or difficulty retracting the foreskin of the penis of uncircumcised males).

Non-Skin Findings/Male

- Dysuria from the anterior urethritis is the most common presentation.

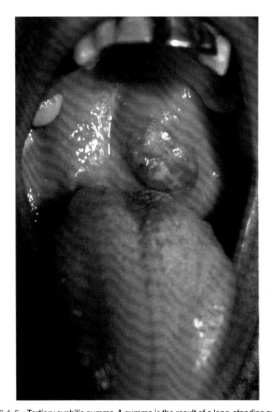

FIG. 6.4-5. Tertiary syphilis gumma. A gumma is the result of a long-standing syphilis infection, and emerges as a soft, tumor-like growth of the tissues, also known as a granuloma. (Courtesy Center for Disease Control and Prevention. Phil # 16762.)

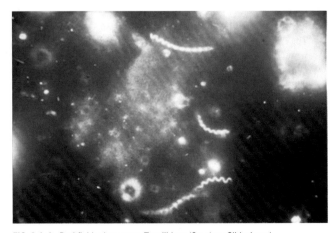

FIG. 6.4-4. Darkfield microscopy *T. pallidum*. (Courtesy Slideshare.)

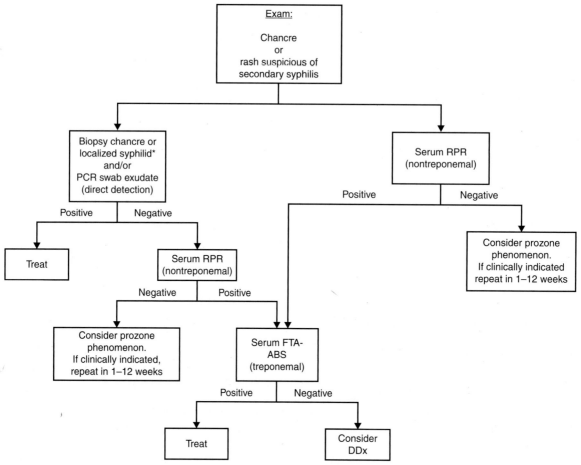

FIG. 6.4-6. Syphilis testing algorithm.

- Complications include epididymitis, vesiculitis, and prostatitis, which occur via local extension. With progression of the infection to the epididymis, patients may present with unilateral testicular edema and pain.

DIFFERENTIAL DIAGNOSIS	Gonorrhea
Men	*Women*
• Chlamydia trachomatis infection	• Trichomoniasis
• Genital herpes infection	• Vaginal candidiasis
• Other forms of urethritis	• Chlamydia trachomatis infection
• Syphilis	• Urinary tract infection
	• Bacterial vaginosis
	• Genital herpes infection
	• Human papillomavirus infection
	• Syphilis

Confirming the Diagnosis

Microbiologic diagnosis is required and is based on identifying various strains of *N. gonorrhoeae* in secretions from infected mucous membranes (see Table 6.4-3).

Treatment

See Table 6.4-4.

Management and Patient Education

- *Persistent symptoms*
- Ensure appropriate therapy with good adherence and lack of re-exposure has occurred.
- Antibiotic-resistant GC should be suspected and tested for with culture and antimicrobial susceptibility testing as the preferred diagnostic modality with or without nucleic acid amplification testing (NAAT) performed at the same time.
- Any sexually active person can be infected with GC. Anyone with genital symptoms such as discharge, burning during urination, unusual sores, or rash should be encouraged to see a health care provider immediately.
- The CDC recommends yearly GC screening for all sexually active women younger than 25 years, as well as older women with risk factors such as new or multiple sex partners, or a sex partner who has a sexually transmitted infection (CDC, 2019).
- People who have GC should also be tested for other STIs.
- If a person has been diagnosed and treated for GC, he or she should notify all sex partners within 60 days before the onset of symptoms or diagnosis, so they can see a health provider and be treated (CDC, 2019). Doing so will reduce the risk of the sex partner developing serious complications from GC, and will also reduce the person's risk of becoming re-infected.
- A person with GC and all of his or her sex partners must avoid having sex until they have completed their treatment for GC and until they no longer have symptoms.

TABLE 6.4-3	Confirming the Diagnosis: Gonorrhea		
DIAGNOSTICS	**TEST**	**USE**	**RESULT INTERPRETATION**
Laboratory	**Nucleic acid amplification tests (NAATs)** Standard recommended test Available for use with vaginal, endocervical, oropharyngeal, urethral, and rectal swabs, as well as urine specimens	**In women:** Vaginal swabs are preferred over cervical swabs **In men:** First-catch urine is the recommended specimen type • Collect approximately 20–30 mL of the initial urinary stream, without precleansing of the genital areas Urethral swab acceptable for NAAT With s/s of proctitis +/– self-reported anal sexual exposure: • Rectal swab, which can be collected by the patient, is the preferred diagnostic test • With s/s of pharyngitis plus a history of unprotected oral sex: pharyngeal swab, which can be collected by the patient, is the preferred diagnostic test	Microbiologic diagnosis is required and is based on identifying various strains of *N. gonorrhoeae* in secretions from infected mucous membranes
	Culture • Obtained on chocolate agar	**In women:** • Endocervical swabs **In men:** • Urethral swabs	Culture may be necessary for evaluating suspected cases of treatment failure or antibiotic resistance

Special Considerations

Asymptomatic Patients

- Routine screening with NAAT should be offered to sexually active patients at high risk of infection and complications from GC who present to care for other reasons. These include (Workowski et al., 2015; Aberg et al., 2014):
  - HIV-infected men and women
  - Sexually active women <25 years old
  - Individuals with new or many sexual partners
  - MSM
  - Sexually active individuals living in areas of high *N. gonorrhoeae* prevalence
  - Individuals with a history of other sexually transmitted infection(s)
  - Women ≤35 years old and men ≤30 years old entering correctional facilities, at every initial intake

Recent Exposure

If a patient presents within 1 to 2 weeks of a potential or known exposure to GC, they should be treated empirically (Workowski et al., 2015). Diagnostic testing should not be used to inform the decision to treat.

Pregnancy

- Urogenital gonococcal infections have been associated with chorioamnionitis, premature rupture of membranes, preterm birth, low birth weight or small for gestational age infants, and spontaneous abortions in pregnant women.
- If a pregnant woman has GC, she may give the infection to her baby as the baby passes through the birth canal during delivery.
- Transmission of *N. gonorrhoeae* from an untreated infected mother to her baby may occur in 30% to 50% of cases (Laga et al., 1989) and can cause blindness, joint infection, or a life-threatening blood infection in the baby.

TABLE 6.4-4	Treatment: Gonorrhea	
SITE OF INFECTION	**RECOMMENDED REGIMEN**	**ALTERNATIVE REGIMENS**
Uncomplicated Gonococcal infections of the cervix, urethra, rectum, and pharynx	**Ceftriaxone** 250 mg IM in a single dose + **Azithromycin** 1 g in a single dose	If ceftriaxone is not available: **Cefixime** 400 mg in a single dose + **Azithromycin** 1 g in a single dose
Gonorrhea and HIV infection	Persons who have gonorrhea and HIV infection should receive the same treatment regimen as those who are HIV negative	
Pregnancy	**Ceftriaxone** 250 mg IM in a single dose + **azithromycin** 1 g in a single dose	For patients allergic to cephalosporins or azithromycin, consultation with an infectious-disease specialist is recommended
For patients allergic to azithromycin For patients allergic to Cephalosporins	Ceftriaxone 250 mg IM in a single dose + doxycycline 100 mg b.i.d. for 7 days Azithromycin 2 g + either gentamicin 240 mg IM once or gemifloxacin 320 mg orally once	

CDC 2015 STD Treatment Guidelines.

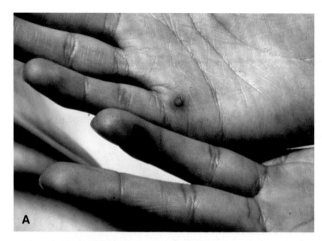

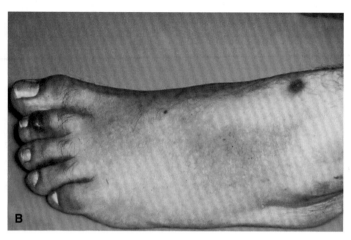

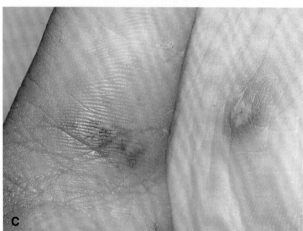

FIG. 6.4-7. Disseminated gonorrhea. **A:** Disseminated gonococcemia. This is an example of septic vasculitis. Note the two palpable purpuric hemorrhagic vesicles. (Used with permission from Goodheart, H. P. [2003]. *Goodheart's photoguide of common skin disorders* [2nd ed.]. Lippincott Williams & Wilkins.) **B:** Disseminated gonorrhea: pustule with hemorrhagic base and necrotic center. (Used with permission from Sweet, R. L., & Gibbs, R. S. [2005]. *Atlas of infectious diseases of the female genital tract.* Lippincott Williams & Wilkins.) **C:** Neisseria gonorrhoeae may disseminate from mucosal surfaces via the bloodstream and produce arthritis/arthralgia and a rash. The most characteristic lesion is the hemorrhagic vesicopustule seen in the web space of the teenage girl's hand. There is a pustule on the sole of her foot. (Used with permission from Fleisher, G. R., Ludwig, W., & Baskin, M. N. [2004]. *Atlas of pediatric emergency medicine.* Lippincott Williams & Wilkins.)

CHANCROID

Chancroid is a sexually transmitted infection that almost always occurs after sexual contact with an infected woman with genital ulcers. Untreated women remain infectious to others while lesions are present, which can be up to 45 days (Bolognia et al., 2018). Chancroid is more common in developing and low-income countries. In the United States, it is not commonly seen and had a peak in reported cases in 1947. After 1957, potentially due to an increase in antibiotics, there was a rapid decrease in disease (CDC, 2019). In 1981 to 1990, there were localized outbreaks in areas of commercial sex work. Since that time, there has again been a significant decline with less than 20 U.S. cases reported in 2011 and only 3 U.S. cases reported in 2018 (CDC, 2019).

Pathophysiology

The infection is caused by the gram-negative bacteria *Haemophilus ducreyi* which spreads via microabrasions in the epidermis of the host. A local inflammatory reaction and skin ulcer are the result of both pyogenic inflammation and inflammation related to the Th1 cell–mediated immune response (Bolognia et al., 2018).

Clinical Presentation

Skin Findings: Women

- Typically located within the introital area and sometimes on cervix, vaginal wall, or perianal area (see Fig. 6.4-8)

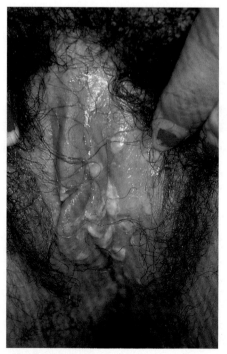

FIG. 6.4-8. Chancroid female. Multiple shaggy ulcerations with copious exudate. (Used with permission from Edwards, L., & Lynch, P. [2017]. *Genital dermatology atlas and manual.* Wolters Kluwer Health.)

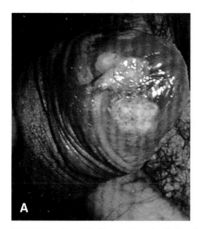 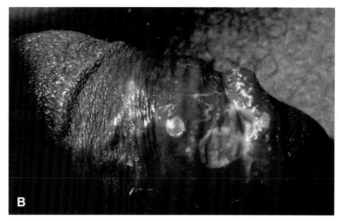

FIG. 6.4-9. **A** and **B.** Chancroid male. (**A:** Used with permission from Goodheart, H. P. [2003]. *Goodheart's photoguide of common skin disorders* [2nd ed.]. Lippincott Williams & Wilkins; **B:** Used with permission from Elder, D. [2020]. *Atlas of dermatopathology* [4th ed.]. Wolters Kluwer Health.)

- Multiple papules and ulcers
- Lesions may be only mildly symptomatic

Skin Findings: Men

- Typically located on internal or external surface of the prepuce, coronal sulcus, or around frenulum
- Painful erythematous papule progresses to pustule and then to a well-demarcated ulcer with undermined borders (see Fig. 6.4-9).
- Several ulcers may appear and can coalesce

Non-Skin Findings: Women and Men

- Painful inguinal lymphadenitis, usually unilateral
- Enlarged lymph nodes with formation of abscess (suppurative bubo)

DIFFERENTIAL DIAGNOSIS	Chancroid
• Syphilis	• Behçet syndrome
• Granuloma inguinale	• Squamous cell carcinoma
• Herpes simplex virus	• Fixed drug eruption
• Lymphogranuloma venereum	

Confirming the Diagnosis

- Diagnosis is usually clinical.
- Gram stain in a smear of exudate is nonspecific similar to other bacteria.
- Culture: sensitivity is between 60% and 80% depending on the handling of specimen.
- PCR testing is available in some countries. In the United States, there are no FDA-cleared NAATs (e.g., PCR) for *H. ducreyi*. Testing can be performed by commercial laboratories that have developed their own PCR or other NAAT, if the performance of the test has been verified with a CLIA validation study.
- HIV and syphilis testing should be done at time of diagnosis to rule out disease. If negative HIV, it should be repeated in 3 months (see Table 6.4-5).

Management and Patient Education

- The ulcers will resolve without treatment within 1 to 3 months, risking progression to lymphadenitis, buboes, and scarring.
- If treatment is successful, symptoms will improve within 3 days and ulcers should improve in 7 days. Complete resolution of ulcer depends on size as some large ulcers may require greater than 2 weeks.
- Those also infected with HIV may require longer treatment courses due to treatment failure.
- There have been no reported adverse effects of chancroid in pregnancy.
- Any sexual partner with contact during the 10 days preceding the onset of symptoms should be treated, regardless of symptoms.

CLINICAL PEARLS

- The ulcers associated with chancroid are **painful**
- The chancre of syphilis is **painless**
- Untreated women remain infectious to others while lesions are present, which can be up to 45 days

LYMPHOGRANULOMA VENEREUM

Lymphogranuloma venereum (LGV) is an uncommon ulcerating genital disease found most frequently in tropical and subtropical areas of the world, but can occur worldwide. Large outbreaks have been reported in Western Europe and North America, primarily in

TABLE 6.4-5	Treatment: Chancroid

- Treat if there is clinical concern and with exclusion of other causes for ulcer (see DDx Genital ulcers in Section 11.4)
- Azithromycin 1 g orally in single dose
- Ceftriaxone 250 mg IM in single dose
- Ciprofloxacin 500 mg b.i.d. × 3 days
- Erythromycin base 500 mg t.i.d. × 7 days

Centers for Disease Control and Prevention Treatment guidelines (CDC, 2019).

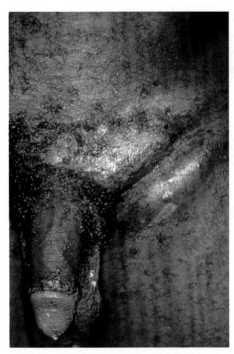

FIG. 6.4-10. Lymphogranuloma venereum. Painful lymph nodes or Buboes may form and then become fluctuant and rupture.

MSM (Nieuwenhuis et al., 2004). Two of the largest outbreaks in MSM occurred in New York City and the United Kingdom (Blank et al., 2005; Ward et al., 2007). Prior to the outbreaks in MSM, LGV was primarily endemic in heterosexuals in areas of East and West Africa, India, parts of Southeast Asia, and the Caribbean.

DIFFERENTIAL DIAGNOSIS   Lymphogranuloma Venereum

- Cellulitis
- Abscess
- Herpes simplex virus (HSV)
- Herpes zoster
- Chancroid
- Granuloma inguinale
- Carcinoma (squamous cell, basal cell)
- Behçet syndrome
- Syphilis
- Fournier or gas gangrene
- Hidradenitis suppurativa
- Pyoderma gangrenosum
- Ecthyma gangrenosum

Pathophysiology

LGV is caused by three variants or serovars of the *Chlamydia trachomatis* bacteria. The *C. trachomatis* species is divided into 15 prototypic serovars of the major outer membrane protein (Stark et al., 2007). This infection mainly affects lymphatic tissue. In mucosal chlamydial infections, inflammation is largely limited to the initial site of infection. However, in LGV the serovars induce a lymphoproliferative reaction. This occurs through direct extension from the primary infection site to the draining lymph nodes. The incubation period is 3 to 21 days (Mabey & Peeling, 2002; Habif, 2016).

Clinical Presentation

See Table 6.4-6.

Confirming the Diagnosis

According to the CDC, diagnosis is based on clinical suspicion, epidemiologic information, and the exclusion of other etiologies

TABLE 6.4-6	Clinical Presentation: Lymphogranuloma Venereum		
STAGE	**PATHOGENESIS**	**SKIN FINDINGS**	**NON-SKIN FINDINGS**
Primary	Lesions spontaneously heal within a few days to 1 wk, without scarring	Small painless papule or pustule on the genitals, that may erode to form an ulcer Occurs at the site of inoculation	Not present

Secondary	Begins 2–6 wk after the primary lesion		Fever, chills, and malaise
			• Inguinal syndrome:
			  • An inflammatory reaction in the superficial and deep inguinal nodes, causing the characteristic *"groove sign"*
			  • May form buboes (painful lymph nodes), that become fluctuant and rupture (Fig. 6.4-10)
			  • Uncommon in women, as the vagina and cervical lymph nodes drain predominantly to retroperitoneal nodes
			• Anorectal s/s may include proctocolitis, rectal discharge, rectal bleeding, anal pain, constipation, tenesmus, and hyperplasia of intestinal and perirectal lymphatic tissue
			  • An inflammatory mass present in the rectum and retroperitoneum
			  • Complications include chronic colorectal fistulas and strictures
			  • Rare cases of oropharyngeal LGV affecting cervical lymph nodes have been reported

Late			Patients initially present with proctocolitis, followed by perirectal abscesses, strictures, fistulas, and rectal stenosis Late complications include genital elephantiasis, frozen pelvis, infertility, and possibly a widespread destruction of the external genitalia, typically seen in women

for proctocolitis, inguinal lymphadenopathy, or genital or rectal ulcers (2019).

- A definitive diagnosis of LGV can be made by isolating the organism on culture, however this generally occurs less than 30% of the time.

  NAAT has improved sensitivity and specificity for diagnosis compared with other types of testing and can be used to test genital lesions, as well as rectal, pharyngeal, and lymph node specimens (lesion swab or bubo aspirate) for *C. trachomatis.* NAAT performed on rectal specimens is the preferred approach to testing (CDC, 2019).

- PCR can help differentiate LGV from non-LGV serotypes of Chlamydia. Results may take several weeks and it is not routinely available in many countries.

- Anoscopy may be helpful in patients with proctitis

  - Findings suggestive of LGV include perianal or mucosal ulcers and/or a bloody rectal discharge.

  - Pathologic findings include microscopic disease with inflammation in the lamina propria and neutrophilic infiltration of crypts when anal biopsy is performed.

- MSM presenting with proctocolitis should be tested for chlamydia. These patients should also be evaluated for *N. gonorrhoeae,* herpes simplex virus, and syphilis.

Treatment

See Table 6.4-7.

Management and Patient Education

- Treatment will cure the infection and prevent ongoing tissue damage (including scarring).

- Buboes might require aspiration through intact skin or incision and drainage to prevent the formation of inguinal or femoral ulcerations.

- Consider screening patients for other STIs, such as GC, syphilis, human immunodeficiency virus (HIV), hepatitis, and chlamydia.

- Patients should be followed clinically until signs and symptoms resolve.

- Persons with genital and colorectal LGV lesions can also develop secondary bacterial infection or can be coinfected with other sexually and nonsexually transmitted pathogens (CDC, 2019).

GRANULOMA INGUINALE

Granuloma inguinale (GI) is a chronic, superficial, ulcerating, sexually transmitted infection of the genital, inguinal, and perianal areas (Habif, 2016, p. 408). It is rare in the United States, but is endemic in certain tropical and semitropical regions, including Brazil, New Guinea, Australia, the Caribbean, India, and South Africa (CDC, 2015c).

Pathophysiology

GI is caused by the intracellular gram-negative bacterium *Klebsiella granulomatis* (formerly known as *Calymmatobacterium granulomatis*).

The incubation period is unknown, but 14 to 50 days is suspected and is mildly contagious. The rate of infection between conjugal partners varies from 0.4% to 52%. Subcutaneous nodules develop at inoculation sites that later erode. The manifestations depend on the host's tissue response, resulting in localized or extensive forms of the disease or in visceral lesions by hematogenous dissemination (Habif, 2016, p. 408).

GI predisposes individuals to transmission of human immunodeficiency virus (O'Farrell, 2002).

TABLE 6.4-7	Treatment: Lymphogranuloma Venereum and Granuloma Inguinale		
CDC TREATMENT GUIDELINES	**LYMPHOGRANULOMA VENEREUM**	**GRANULOMA INGUINALE**	**SPECIAL CONSIDERATIONS**
Recommended Regimen	Doxycycline 100 mg b.i.d. for 21 days	Azithromycin 1 g once per wk or 500 mg daily for at least 3 wk	Patients with granuloma inguinale should be treated until all lesions have completely healed
Alternative Regimen (choose one)	Erythromycin base 500 mg q.i.d. for 21 days Azithromycin 1 g once weekly for 3 wk Fluoroquinolone-based treatments might also be effective, but the optimal duration of treatment has not been evaluated	Doxycycline 100 mg b.i.d. for at least 3 wk Ciprofloxacin 750 mg b.i.d. for at least 3 wk Erythromycin base 500 mg q.i.d. for at least 3 wk Trimethoprim-sulfamethoxazole 1 double-strength (160 mg/800 mg) tablet orally b.i.d. for at least 3 wk	
Pregnancy	Pregnant and lactating women should be treated with erythromycin Azithromycin might prove useful for treatment of LGV in pregnancy, but no published data are available regarding an effective dose and duration of treatment	Treatment of choice is macrolide's (erythromycin or azithromycin) Ciprofloxacin presents a low risk to the fetus during pregnancy	Doxycycline should be avoided in the second and third trimester of pregnancy because of the risk for discoloration of teeth and bones, but is compatible with breastfeeding Sulfonamides are associated with rare but serious kernicterus in those with *G6PD* deficiency and should be avoided in third trimester and during breastfeeding
HIV Infection	Same regimens as those who are HIV negative Prolonged therapy might be required, and delay in resolution of symptoms might occur	Same regimens as those who are HIV negative	

CDC 2015 STD Treatment Guidelines.

TABLE 6.4-8	Differential Diagnosis: Genital Ulcers	
DISEASE	**CLINICAL LESION**	**ORGANISM**
Genital herpes	Eroded, "punched out," irregularly bordered ulcers; painful	Herpes simplex virus type 1 (HSV-1) and herpes simplex virus type 2 (HSV-2)
Primary syphilis	Painless, firm ulcer; usually single; nonpurulent	*Treponema pallidum*
Lymphogranuloma venereum	Painless ulcer; heals within days to 1 wk	*Chlamydia trachomatis* serovars L1, L2, and L3
Granuloma Inguinale	Superficial ulcer; raised, rolled margin, with granulation tissue–like base raised above the skin surface; beefy red	*Klebsiella granulomatis* (formerly known as *Calymmatobacterium granulomatis*)
Chancroid	Painful, well demarcated, purulent ulcer with undermined borders; often multiple ulcers	*Haemophlis ducreyi*

Clinical Presentation

Skin Findings

- Begins with single or multiple papules, nodules, or ulcers on the genitals.
- Evolves into broad, superficial ulcers with a distinct, raised, rolled margin, with granulation tissue–like base raised above the skin surface (Fig. 6.4-9).
- Slowly progressive ulcerative lesions on the genitals or perineum without regional lymphadenopathy.
- Lesions are highly vascular (beefy red appearance) and bleed.
- Autoinoculation is a common feature, producing the so-called "kissing lesions" on adjacent skin.
- Subcutaneous granulomas occur in the inguinal area that mimic lymphadenopathy (the so-called pseudo-buboes). If left untreated, can result in lymphatic obstruction leading to genital lymphedema and distortion.

Non-Skin Findings

- Lesions are usually painless, but may be accompanied by mild pain or discomfort
- Constitutional symptoms are notably absent
- Extragenital infection can occur with extension of infection to the pelvis, or it can disseminate to intra-abdominal organs, bones, or the mouth
- Secondary bacterial infection can develop and coexist with other sexually transmitted pathogen

Confirming the Diagnosis

- The causative organism of GI is difficult to culture.
- No FDA-cleared molecular tests for the detection of *K. granulomatis* DNA exist.
- Tissue biopsy: Tissue from the ulcer base is stained using Wright or Giemsa stain to identify the bipolar-staining intracytoplasmic inclusion bodies (Donovan bodies) within granulation tissue histiocytes.
- See Table 6.4-8 for differential diagnosis of genital ulcers.

Management and Patient Education

- Without treatment, GI will damage tissues.
- According to the CDC, persons who have had sexual contact with a patient who has GI within the 60 days before onset of the patient's symptoms should be examined and offered therapy.
- Screening for other STIs such as GC, syphilis, HIV, hepatitis, and Chlamydia should be considered.
- Persons should be followed clinically until signs and symptoms have resolved.

CLINICAL PEARL

- STDs are preventable, and patients should be encouraged to protect themselves and their sexual partner(s) from STIs. Having any STD also predisposes one to other diseases specifically HIV disease. Many of these STDs present initially with genital ulcers and it behooves us to think about the differential diagnoses of these lesions.

DIFFERENTIAL DIAGNOSIS   Granuloma Inguinale

- Cellulitis
- Chancroid
- Lymphogranuloma venereum
- Syphilis
- Amebiasis
- Tuberculous chancre
- Condyloma acuminate
- Buschke–Lowenstein tumor
- Fournier or gas gangrene
- Herpes simplex virus (HSV)
- Behçet syndrome
- Pyoderma gangrenosum
- Crohn disease
- Ecthyma gangrenosum
- Carcinoma (squamous cell, basal cell, melanoma)

Prophylactic measures are available now more than ever before to prevent these infections and should be discussed with and offered to our at-risk population of patients.

READINGS AND REFERENCES

Aberg, J. A., Gallant, J. E., Ghanem, K. G., Emmanuel, P., Zingman, B. S., & Horberg, M. A.; Infectious Diseases Society of America. (2014). Primary care guidelines for the management of persons infected with HIV: 2013 update by the HIV medicine association of the Infectious Diseases Society of America. *Clinical Infectious Diseases, 58*(1), 1–10.

Blank, S., Schillinger, J. A., & Harbatkin, D. (2005). Lymphogranuloma venereum in the industrialised world. *Lancet, 365*(9471), 1607–1608.

Bolognia, J., Schaffer, J. V., & Cerroni, L. (2018). *Dermatology* (4th ed., Vol. 2). Elsevier.

Bolognia, J., Schaffer, J. V., Duncan, K. O., & Ko, C. (2014). *Dermatology essentials* (p. 689). Saunders, Elsevier.

Centers for Disease Control and Prevention (CDC). (2015a). Chancroid—2015 STD treatment guidelines. https://www.cdc.gov/std/tg2015/chancroid.htm.

Centers for Disease Control and Prevention (CDC). (2015b). *Congenital syphilis—2018 sexually transmitted diseases surveillance*. https://www.cdc.gov/std/tg2015/congenital.htm

Center for Disease Control and Prevention (CDC). (2015c). Granuloma inguinale (donovanosis). https://www.cdc.gov/std/tg2015/donovanosis.htm

Center for Disease Control and Prevention (CDC). (2015d). Lymphogranuloma venereum (LGV). https://www.cdc.gov/std/tg2015/lgv.htm

Centers for Disease Control and Prevention (CDC). (2015e). *Mmwr: Recommendations and Reports*, 64(RR-03), 1.

Centers for Disease Control and Prevention (CDC). (2018a). Other sexually transmitted diseases—2018 sexually transmitted diseases surveillance. https://www.cdc.gov/std/stats18/other.htm#chancroid

Centers for Disease Control and Prevention (CDC). (2018b). *Sexually transmitted disease surveillance, 2018*. https://www.cdc.gov/std/stats18/default.htm

Centers for Disease Control and Prevention (CDC). (2018c). *Syphilis—2018 sexually transmitted diseases surveillance*. https://www.cdc.gov/std/stats18/syphilis.htm

Centers for Disease Control and Prevention (CDC). (2019). Gonorrhea—CDC fact sheet (DetailedVersion). https://www.cdc.gov/std/gonorrhea/stdfact-gonorrhea-detailed.htm

Galeano-Valle, F., Pérez-Latorre, L., Díez-Romero, C., Fanciulli, C., Aldamiz-Echeverria-Lois, T., & Tejerina-Picado, F. (2019). Cervical and oropharyngeal lymphogranuloma venereum: Case report and literature review. *Sexually Transmitted Diseases, 46*(10), 689–692.

Habif, T. (2016). *Clinical dermatology: A color guide to diagnosis and therapy* (6th ed.). Mosby, Elsevier.

Henao-Martínez, A. F., & Johnson, S. C. (2014). Diagnostic tests for syphilis: New tests and new algorithms. https://www.ncbi.nlm.nih.gov/pmc/articles/PMC4999316/?report=printable

Laga, M., Meheus, A., & Piot, P. (1989). Epidemiology and control of gonococcal ophthalmia neonatorum. *Bulletin of the World Health Organization, 67*(5), 471–477.

Lewis, D. A. (2003). Chancroid: Clinical manifestations, diagnosis, and management. *Sexually Transmitted Infections, 79*(1), 68–71.

Mabey, D., & Peeling, R. W. (2002). Lymphogranuloma venereum. *Sexually Transmitted Infections, 78*(2), 90–92.

Nieuwenhuis, R .F., Ossewaarde, J. M., Götz, H. M., Dees, J., Thio, H. B., Thomeer, M. G., den Hollander, J. C., Neumann, M. H., & van der Meijden, W. I. (2004). Resurgence of lymphogranuloma venereum in Western Europe: an outbreak of Chlamydia trachomatis serovar l2 proctitis in The Netherlands among men who have sex with men. *Clinical Infectious Diseases, 39*(7), 996–1003.

O'Farrell, N. (2002). Donovanosis. *Sexually Transmitted Infections, 78*(6), 452–457.

Patton, M. E., Su, J. R., Nelson, R., Weinstock, H.; Centers for Disease Control and Prevention (CDC). (2014). Primary and secondary syphilis—United States, 2005–2013. *Mmwr Morbidity and Mortality Weekly Report, 63*(18), 402–406.

Ratnam, S. (2005). The laboratory diagnosis of syphilis. *The Canadian Journal of Infectious Diseases and Medical Microbiology, 16*(1), 45–51. https://doi.org/10.1155/2005/597580

Sidana, R., Mangala, H., Murugesh, S., & Ravindra, K. (2011). Prozone phenomenon in secondary syphilis. *Indian Journal of Sexually Transmitted Diseases and AIDS, 32*(1), 47–49. https://doi.org/10.4103/0253-7184.81256

Stark, D., van Hal, S., Hillman, R., Harkness, J., & Marriott, D. (2007). Lymphogranuloma venereum in Australia: Anorectal *chlamydia trachomatis* serovar L2b in men who have sex with men. *Journal of Clinical Microbiology, 45*(3), 1029–1031.

Ward, H., Martin, I., Macdonald, N., Alexander, S., Simms, I., Fenton, K., French, P., Dean, G., & Ison, C. (2007). Lymphogranuloma venereum in the United Kingdom. *Clinical Infectious Diseases, 44*(1), 26–32.

Workowski, K. A. & Bolan, G. A. (2015). Sexually transmitted diseases treatment guidelines, 2015. *Morbidity and Mortality Weekly Report, 64*(RR-03), 1–137.

Zoltan, E. (2007). Sexually transmitted disease. In *Penn clinical manual of urology* (pp. 743–767). Elsevier.

HIV and the Skin

Mary E. Nolen

It is over 40 years since the first emergence and recognition of this deadly virus in the United States. Unlike other viruses, the human body is unable to eradicate it completely even with treatment. It is transmitted through certain bodily fluids and attacks one's immune system, which overtime renders one incapable of defending against infection and other diseases. Without treatment, HIV reduces the number of immune cells (T cells) specifically CD4 cells necessary to combat infection which results in acute immune deficiency syndrome (AIDS). No effective cure currently exists but over time the medical community has learned to control the disease with proper and continuous treatment and if the viral load becomes undetectable and remains undetectable, people can live long healthy lives. Transmission of the disease is the greatest public health threat and prevention is one of the largest disease prevention campaigns of the CDC.

HUMAN IMMUNODEFICIENCY VIRUS (HIV)

Epidemiology

The virus is thought to have originated in West Africa and transmitted from chimpanzees to humans who consumed the infected animals in mid- to late-70s. HIV continues to disproportionately affect countries with limited resources. Globally, sub-Saharan Africa accounts for 70% of people living with AIDS and 65% of all new cases. Gay, bisexual, and other men who have sex with men (MSM) including African American and Hispanic/Latino men are the population most affected by HIV in the United States.

Incidence

HIV can affect anyone regardless of sexual orientation, race, ethnicity, gender, or age. However, certain groups are at higher risk for HIV transmission. Socioeconomic factors in the United States can also play a role increasing risk for disease. Limited access to quality health care, lower income and educational levels, and higher rates of unemployment and incarceration may place some gay and bisexual men at higher risk for HIV (CDC, 2019).

- At the end of 2016, 1.1 million people aged 13 and older had HIV in the United States including 162,000 (14%) who remain undiagnosed (CDC, 2019).

- There were 38,968 new cases of HIV diagnosis in the United States and dependent areas in 2018.*

- The largest number of new cases in the United States, occurs in the 25- to 29-year old age group followed by 20- to 24, 30- to 34, and 40- to 44-year old age group. The smallest number of new cases occurs in 13- to 14-year old age group.

Lesbian, Gay, Transgender, Bisexual, Queer (LGTBQ)

- In 2018, 69% of the 38,968 new HIV cases diagnosed in the United States, were among adult and adolescent gay and bisexual men (24,933 MSM and 1,372 MSM who also inject drugs) (CDC, 2018). Gay, bisexual, and other MSM including African American and Hispanic/Latino men are the population most affected by HIV in the United States.

- Transgender women in the United States are disproportionately affected by HIV infection because of multiple factors, including stigma related to gender identity, unstable housing, limited employment options, and high-risk behaviors, such as sex work, unprotected receptive anal intercourse, and injection drug. In 2018, among all adults and adolescents, diagnoses of HIV infection among transgender persons accounted for approximately 2% of diagnoses of HIV infections in the United States. In 2018, among transgender adults and adolescents, the largest percentage (92%) of diagnoses of HIV infections was for transgender Male to Female (MTF) (CDC, 2018).

Persons Who Inject Drugs

Persons who inject drugs (PWIDs) are at high risk for HIV if they use and share needles, syringes, or other drug injection equipment (e.g., cookers) that someone with HIV has used. PWIDs account for about 1 in 15 HIV diagnoses in the United States. In recent years, the opioid (including prescription and synthetic opioids) and heroin crisis has led to increased numbers of PWID. HIV diagnoses among PWID have increased in the 50 states and District of Columbia.

---

*Unless otherwise noted, the term United States (U.S.) includes the 50 states, the District of Columbia, and the 6 dependent areas of American Samoa, Guam, the Northern Mariana Islands, Puerto Rico, the Republic of Palau, and the U.S. Virgin Islands.

Women

HIV diagnoses among women have declined in recent years, however, more than 7,000 women received an HIV diagnosis in the United States in 2018. Most new cases are related to heterosexual contact. One in nine women with HIV is unaware they are infected. Some women may be unaware of their male partner's risk factors for HIV (such as injection drug use or having sex with men), therefore, they may not use condoms or take preventive measures. Additionally, HIV testing rates are lower among women who engage in high-risk sexual behavior. Black/African American female adults and adolescents accounted for the largest numbers of diagnoses of HIV infection between 2014 and 2018 each year although the number decreased from 4,573 in 2014 to 4,097 in 2018. White and Hispanic/Latino female adults and adolescents had similar numbers of diagnoses of HIV infection each year. In 2018, 1,491 diagnoses of HIV infection were among white females, 1,269 among Hispanic/Latino females, 194 among females of multiple races, 104 among Asian females, 30 among American Indian/Alaska native females, and 5 among native Hawaiian/other Pacific Islander females.

Perinatal

Perinatal HIV transmission (also known as mother-to-child transmission) can happen at any time during pregnancy, childbirth, and breastfeeding. In 2017, 73 children under the age of 13 were diagnosed with perinatally acquired HIV. Between 2012 and 2016 perinatal transmission decreased 41%. Today there are effective interventions for preventing perinatal HIV transmission, and the number of infants with HIV in the United States has declined dramatically.

Pathophysiology

- HIV is a retrovirus and therefore carries a positive-stranded RNA and a DNA polymerase enzyme called reverse transcriptase.
- Once the virus attaches to the protein receptor site on the CD4$^+$ T lymphocyte, reverse transcriptase converts the viral RNA to DNA and becomes part of the host genome. New viral particles are then produced during normal cellular division, and the CD4$^+$ T lymphocytes are destroyed. A repetitive cycle of immune activation and reinfection leads to the progressive immunodeficiency that we know as autoimmune deficiency syndrome (AIDS) (Fig. 6.5-1).

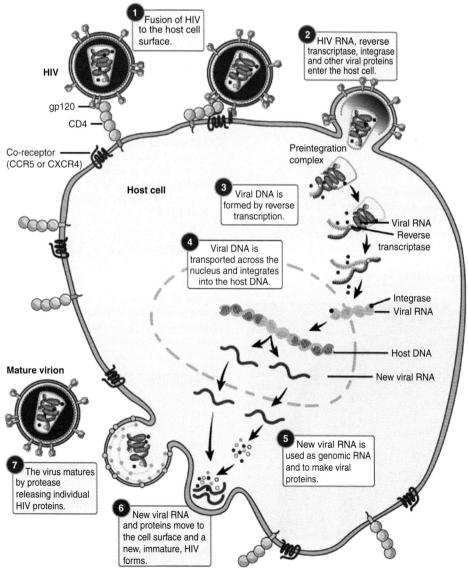

FIG. 6.5-1. HIV virus replication cycle. (NIH National Library of Medicine.)

TABLE 6.5-1	HIV Transmission		
MOST COMMON	**LESS COMMON**	**UNCOMMON**	**NO TRANSMISSION**
The following body fluids may transmit HIV when coming into contact with mucus membranes or damaged tissue, or directly injected into the bloodstream: blood, semen, preseminal fluid, rectal fluids, vaginal fluids, and breast milk.	Mother to child during pregnancy, birth or breastfeeding when mother is treated with anti-retroviral medications. HIV-contaminated needle or other sharp object.	Oral sex Receiving blood transfusions, blood products, or organ/tissue transplants that are contaminated with HIV. Eating food that has been prechewed or deep, open mouth kissing (contamination of blood from mouth erosions/bleeding gums). Being bitten by a person with HIV. Contact between broken skin, wounds, or mucous membranes with HIV-infected body fluids.	Air Water Saliva Sweat Tears Closed mouth kissing Insects Pets Sharing toilets, food, drink

Adapted from CDC HIV Transmission (2020).

Transmission

Among these high-risk groups, certain behaviors have been identified and have become the focus of all prevention campaigns (see Table 6.5-1).

- In the United States, HIV is spread mainly by:
  - Having anal or vaginal sex with someone who has HIV without using a condom or taking medicines to prevent or treat HIV. See CDC transmission for details.
  - Sharing needles or syringes, rinse water, or other equipment used to prepare drugs for injection with someone who has HIV.
  - HIV can live in a used needle up to 42 days depending on temperature and other factors.

CLINICAL PRESENTATION

Acute Primary Infection

HIV infection can present differently at various stages but generally presents with the Primary infection or acute retroviral syndrome (see Fig. 6.5-2 and Table 6.5-2). When people acquire HIV and don't receive treatment, they will typically progress through three stages of disease. Medicine to treat HIV, known as antiretroviral therapy (ART), helps people at all stages of the disease if taken as prescribed. Treatment can slow or prevent progression from one stage to the next.

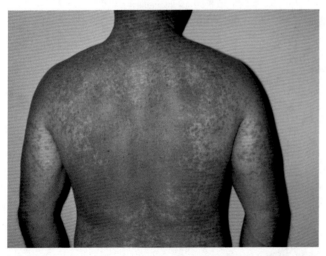

FIG. 6.5-2. Primary HIV infection. (Goodheart, H. P. [2015]. *Goodheart's photoguide of common skin disorders* [4th ed.]. Wolters Kluwer Health | Lippincott Williams & Wilkins.)

DIFFERENTIAL DIAGNOSIS	Primary Acute Retroviral Syndrome
• Acute drug reaction • Viral exanthem • Secondary syphilis	• Erythema multiforme • Pityriasis rosea • Guttate psoriasis • Urticaria

CONFIRMING THE DIAGNOSIS

- The goal of HIV testing is the early identification of individuals in the highly infectious phase of acute HIV infection to minimize transmission.
- Laboratories should conduct initial testing for HIV with an FDA-approved antigen/antibody combination (fourth generation) immunoassay to screen for established infection with HIV-1 or HIV-2 and for acute HIV-1 infection followed by a confirmatory test such as indirect immunofluorescence assay (IFA) or HIV 1 NAT (see Fig. 6.5-4).

TREATMENT

The gold standard of treatment for HIV infection remains antiretroviral therapy, which when taken consistently as prescribed will decrease the viral load to undetectable in many cases. This can lead to long healthy lives with no risk for viral transmission to an HIV negative partner. Please see below for details regarding treatment https://www.cdc.gov/hiv/clinicians/treatment/index.html

MANAGEMENT AND PATIENT EDUCATION

- At present, more than 150,000 Americans have HIV, but don't know it and would benefit from increased testing (Fig. 6.5-4).
- Patients infected with HIV should also be educated about the importance of monitoring for any signs and symptoms of disease progression or associated complications and instructed to seek prompt care as necessary.
- Patient monitoring and follow-up should be determined based on the patient's clinical status.
- Regular health screening every 3 to 4 months should include a thorough physical examination, complete review of systems, age-appropriate screening examinations, CD4 counts, and viral load evaluation.

TABLE 6.5-2	Primary Acute Retroviral Syndrome
Stage 1 Acute HIV Infection	• 2–4 Weeks after infection with HIV, people may experience a flu-like illness, which may last for a few weeks includes fever, myalgias, arthralgia, pharyngitis acute retroviral syndrome (ARS) • When people have acute HIV infection, they have a large amount of virus in their blood and are very contagious • But people with acute infection are often unaware that they're infected because they may not feel sick right away or at all • To know whether someone has acute infection, either an antigen/antibody test or a nucleic acid test (NAT) is necessary • If you think you have been exposed to HIV through sex or drug use and you have flu-like symptoms, seek medical care and ask for a test to diagnose acute infection
Skin Eruption	• Diffuse, polymorphic, erythematous, maculopapular on trunk (50–70%) • Roseola-like or morbilliform rash upper body face • Papulosquamous lesions palms and soles • Mucocutaneous lesions resembling large aphthae
Stage 2 Clinical Latency HIV Inactivity Dormancy	• Asymptomatic HIV infection or chronic HIV infection • HIV is still active but reproduces at very low levels. People may not have any symptoms or get sick during this time • For people who aren't taking medicine to treat HIV, this period can last a decade or longer • People who are taking medicine to treat HIV (ART) as prescribed may be in this stage for several decades • It's important to remember that people can still transmit HIV to others during this phase • However, people who take HIV medicine as prescribed and get and keep an undetectable viral load (or stay virally suppressed) have effectively no risk of transmitting HIV to their HIV-negative sexual partners • At the end of this phase, a person's viral load starts to go up and the CD4 cell count begins to go down
Skin Eruption	• Atypical presentations of inflammatory conditions, psoriasis, seborrheic dermatitis • Recurrent varicella zoster, numerous hyperkeratotic warts, and oral hairy leukoplakia • Kaposi sarcoma may be present before immunosuppression (see Fig. 6.5-3)
Stage 3	• AIDS is the most severe phase of HIV infection. • People with AIDS have such badly damaged immune systems that they get an increasing number of severe illnesses, called opportunistic illnesses. • Without treatment, people with AIDS typically survive about 3 years. • Common symptoms of AIDS include chills, fever, sweats, swollen lymph glands, weakness, and weight loss. • People are diagnosed with AIDS when their CD4 cell count drops below 200 cells/mm³ or if they develop certain opportunistic illnesses. • People with AIDS can have a high viral load and be very infectious.
Skin Eruption	• In presence of immunosuppression chronic herpes simplex virus, molluscum contagiosum, candidiasis, other opportunistic infections.

Adapted from CDC 2015.

- Diagnosis of an STD in an HIV-infected person indicates ongoing or recurrent high-risk behavior and should prompt referral for counseling.
- Management of infants, children, and adolescents who are known or suspected to be infected with HIV requires referral to physicians familiar with the manifestations and treatment of pediatric HIV infection.

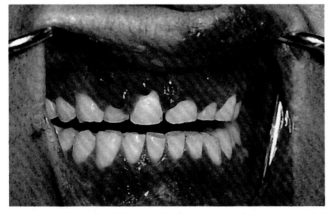

FIG. 6.5-3. Kaposi sarcoma. (Weber, J., & Kelley, J. [2017]. *Health assessment in nursing* [6th ed.]. Wolters Kluwer Health I Lippincott Williams & Wilkins.)

Prevention

- The prevention of HIV, remains one of the most universally important health care initiatives (see Fig. 6.5-5).
- Traditional practices of abstinence, regular and correct use of condoms as well as limiting the number of sexual partners remain as important and effective measures.
- Nonjudgmental prevention counseling and a review of methods and behaviors that lead to transmission should be initiated in any at-risk individual or persons seeking HIV testing.
- Today, however newer prevention medications exist for those at risk of getting infection (see Table 6.5-3).
- If already infected, the best way to stay healthy and prevent spread is to take your medicine as prescribed to keep an undetectable viral load and therefore have no risk for transmission.

SPECIAL CONSIDERATIONS

Pregnancy

- According to the NIH, women in the United States should be tested for HIV infection as early during pregnancy as possible.
- A second test during the third trimester, preferably at <36 weeks of gestation, should be considered, and is recommended for women known to be at high risk for acquiring HIV.

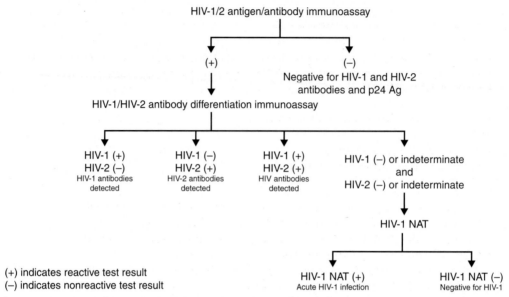

CDC Recommended Laboratory HIV Testing Algorithm for Serum or Plasma Samples

FIG. 6.5-4. HIV testing. (Centers for Disease Control and Prevention. ClinicalOptions.com.)

- Rapid HIV antibody testing at the time of labor or delivery should be performed on women with undocumented HIV status, and intrapartum ARV prophylaxis should be initiated in those who test positive.
- Breastfeeding should be avoided until results are available.

HIV-RELATED SKIN DISORDERS

The cutaneous manifestations of HIV have been recognized for decades. In the early years, Kaposi sarcoma (KS) became an AIDS-specific sign. At the same time, immune suppression led to over-whelming infections both cutaneous and visceral. Now, since millions of people are living with HIV, even after decades of ART, we are seeing a wide range of dermatoses associated with this disease. Malignancies such as KS have been a hallmark of this infection but

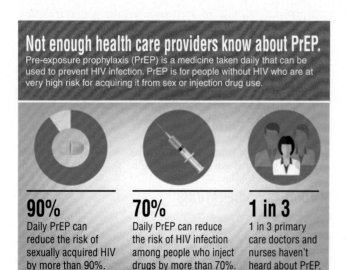

FIG. 6.5-5. HIV prevention. (Centers for Disease Control and Prevention.)

TABLE 6.5-3	HIV Prevention

Pre-Exposure Prevention (PrEP)

- Pre-exposure prophylaxis (or PrEP) when taken daily, is highly effective for preventing HIV. Studies have shown that PrEP reduces the risk of getting HIV from sex by about 99% when taken daily (CDC, 2019).
- Among people who inject drugs, PrEP reduces the risk of getting HIV by at least 74% when taken daily. PrEP is much less effective if it is not taken consistently (CDC, 2019).
- Condoms are also an important prevention strategy if PrEP is not taken consistently. PrEP should be considered part of a comprehensive prevention plan that includes a discussion about adherence to PrEP, condom use, other sexually transmitted infections (STIs), and other risk reduction methods.

(US Public Health Service Preexposure Prophylaxis for the Prevention of HIV Infection in the United States—2017 Update a Clinical Practice Guideline www.cdc.gov/prescribeHIVprevention)

- Male circumcision
- HIV treatment as prevention a person with HIV who takes HIV medicine as prescribed and gets and stays virally suppressed or undetectable has effectively no risk of sexually transmitting HIV to HIV-negative partners (CDC, 2019).

Post-Exposure Prevention (nPEP)

- The most effective methods for preventing human immunodeficiency virus (HIV) infection are those that protect against exposure to HIV. However, evidence from animal studies and human observational studies demonstrate that nPEP administered within 48–72 hours and continued for 28 days might reduce the risk for acquiring HIV infection after mucosal and other nonoccupational exposures.
- The sooner nPEP is administered after exposure, the more likely it is to interrupt transmission (CDC, 2019).
- The new nPEP recommendations also include considerations and resources for specific groups, such as pregnant women, victims of sexual assault (including children), and patients without health insurance, as well as a suggested procedure for transitioning patients between PEP and HIV pre-exposure prophylaxis (PrEP) as appropriate. www.cdc.gov/hiv/guidelines/index.html

nonmelanoma skin cancers (NMSCs) are also occurring, perhaps because people are living longer. Inflammatory skin diseases such as psoriasis and atopic dermatitis, may be more severe and recalcitrant in those people living with HIV disease. Lastly, recurrent and chronic infections with HPV and herpes virus as well as other opportunistic infections are common. In this section we will discuss some of the more common conditions in each category.

MALIGNANCIES

Many viruses common to all individuals possess oncogenic potential if they are chronic and unchecked by normal immune systems. Human herpes virus 8 (HHV-8) is thought to be responsible for the most common cutaneous malignancy associated with HIV infection, KS.

Kaposi Sarcoma

The acquired immunodeficiency syndrome (AIDS) results in a sharp increase in the risk of Kaposi sarcoma a low-grade vascular tumor. Although not as common now due to the introduction of highly active antiretroviral therapy (HAART), it was once considered a harbinger of HIV/AIDS. In the United States, MSM and persons with HIV infection are at increased risk for HHV-8 infection. Injection drug use may also be a risk factor for HHV-8 seropositivity.

CLINICAL PRESENTATION

Skin Findings

- KS manifestations vary widely, but most patients have nontender, hyperpigmented, violaceous, or reddish-brown macules or nodules on the skin.
- It may involve the face, trunk, palms, soles, and penis (Fig. 6.5-6).
- Oral lesions, gingiva, palate, and buccal mucosa occur in approximately one third of patients and may represent a less favorable treatment outcome (Fig. 6.5-7A,B).
- Lymphatic involvement is also common and may lead to debilitating lower extremity edema commonly seen in sub-Saharan Africa.
- Another more classic form of KS is typically seen in elderly Mediterranean men (especially Italian and Jewish descent) and has different clinical features. In classic KS, asymptomatic pink macules grow to become red to brown papules but is not associated with HIV disease.

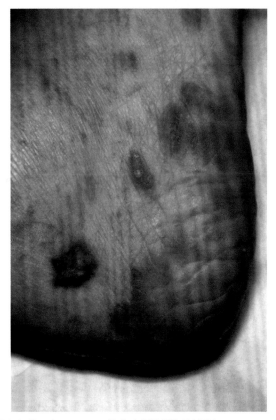

FIG. 6.5-6. Kaposi sarcoma on skin foot. (CDC PHIL #14430.)

Non-Skin Finding

- KS can metastasize to other organs such as the lungs or gastrointestinal tract. Not all patients with KS have HIV infections.

DIFFERENTIAL DIAGNOSIS	Kaposi Sarcoma
• Dermatofibroma	• Purpura
• Dermatofibrosarcoma protuberans	• Pyogenic granuloma
	• Insect bites
• Bacillary angiomatosis	• Nevi

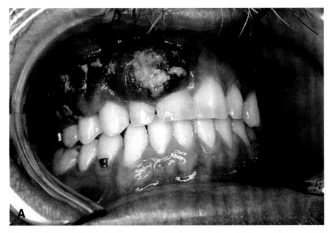

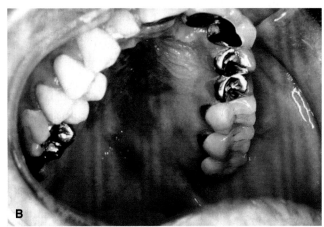

FIG. 6.5-7. **A** and **B**. Kaposi sarcoma oral lesions. (Centers for Disease Control and Prevention.)

CONFIRMING THE DIAGNOSIS

Biopsy

- Pathology may vary from increase in vessels to nodular proliferations of Spindle cells.
- HHV 8 can be detected in endothelial cells by immunohistochemistry

TREATMENT

- Treatment of KS is not curative, but can provide resolution of symptoms in most patients.
- The initiation of HAART has resulted in the involution of the lesions within 6 months in 50% of cases.
- This should be the initial management in most patients with mild-to-moderate disease (fewer than 50 lesions, and fewer than 10 new lesions/month).
- Other modalities of treatment are dependent on the CD4 cell count, as well as the number and extent of the lesions.
- Chemotherapy may be used intralesionally or systemically.
- Radiation, laser, and cryotherapy have all been used effectively, but the patient should be cautioned that the lesions may return.

MANAGEMENT AND PATIENT EDUCATION

- The initiation of HAART has resulted in the involution of Kaposi lesions within 6 months in 50% of cases. The overall prognosis of KS largely depends on the initial clinical presentation, the presence or absence of nodal involvement, and histologic pattern.
- In both the immunosuppressed and classic type of KS, the malignancy is slow growing and usually stays localized but does have a risk for metastases.

Anal Intraepithelial Neoplasia/Anal Carcinoma/Cervical Carcinoma

Papilloma virus, for example, can cause common warts or in immune suppressed patients can be responsible for cervical, and anal cancers. Anal intraepithelial neoplasia (AIN) is a premalignant lesion for anal cancer and is more commonly found in high-risk patients (e.g., human papilloma virus (HPV) HIV infections, postorgan transplantation patients, and MSM). Development is driven by HPV infection. There is little debate that AIN and cervical dysplasia can develop into anal and cervical cancer, and the main rationale for treatment is to delay the progression. The incidence of AIN is difficult to estimate, but is heavily skewed by pre-existing conditions, particularly in high-risk populations.

According to Bacik and Chung (2018), "the incidence of precursor lesions and their subsequent progression to cancer is markedly higher in HIV-positive men and women compared with HIV-negative counterparts. The relative risk for developing anal carcinoma is 37 times greater among HIV-positive MSM than the general population."

CLINICAL MANIFESTATIONS

- HPV starts as verrucous papules and plaques that can then coalesce into giant condyloma on vulva, anal, and perianal area (Fig. 6.5-8).

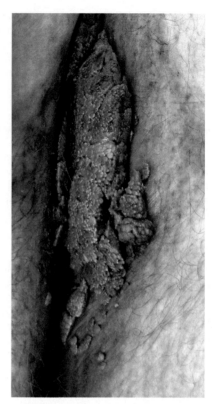

FIG. 6.5-8. Giant condyloma.

Please see Section 11.4 for discussion of Genital HPV infection and treatment.

CONFIRMING THE DIAGNOSIS

- Tissue confirmation cytology or biopsy specimens can be obtained during routine examinations. A pathologist reviews and classifies cells as low or high grade which will better predict progression from AIN to anal cancer.

TREATMENT

- Management options are separated into surveillance (watchful waiting) and interventional strategies.
- Emerging data suggest that close patient follow-up with a combination of ablative treatment (excision, fulguration, and laser therapy) and topical treatments such as imiquimod (Aldara) may offer the greatest benefit.
- HPV vaccination offers a unique treatment prior to HPV infection and the subsequent development of AIN, but its use after the development of AIN is limited.
- CDC now recommends all 11- to 12-year olds receive two doses of HPV vaccine rather than the previously recommended three doses to protect against cancers caused by HPV (MMWR December 16, 2016).
- Vaccination is recommended through age 21 if not previously vaccinated and through age 26 for males who have sex with men (MSM) and men who are immunocompromised (including those with HIV).
- HPV vaccine is not routinely recommended in adults aged 27 to 45 years due to decreasing exposure with age, however, it

is recommended that there be shared patient-provider clinical decision making to vaccinate those in this age group with a high risk for exposure (Meites et al., 2019).

Melanoma

There is little data to confirm a true association with HIV and the incidence of melanoma however, there is some evidence to suggest that HIV patients with melanoma, have a shorter disease-free period and decreased overall survival (Coghill et al., 2015).

Nonmelanoma Skin Cancer

Squamous cell carcinoma (SCC) has long been associated with immunosuppression most notably in organ transplant individuals. People with HIV have a two-fold increase in the development of Non-Aids Defining Cancers (NADC) than the general population (Vaccher et al., 2014). SCC includes oral pharyngeal, anogenital, and penile cancers. Basal cell cancers are common though not increasing in incidence in the HIV-infected population (Changa et al., 2017). As the HIV population ages, clinicians must be aware of the increased risk factors these patients possess. Also, as they age, increased sun exposure compounds the risk of developing NMSC.

See Section 2.2 NMSC for details.

PRURITUS-RELATED DISORDERS

Pruritus alone can be a presenting sign of HIV but is typically associated with a papular eruption which may be follicular or nonfollicular. Severe pruritus, resistant to treatment is relatively common and may be related to increased viral load. Patients with HIV infection may also have other causes of pruritus, such as chronic kidney disease, liver disease, and non-Hodgkin lymphoma. The most common pruritic eruptions are detailed below.

Eosinophilic Folliculitis

Eosinophilic folliculitis (EF) is the most common pruritic follicular eruption seen in HIV however, since the introduction of HAART, it has become less common. EF has a characteristic presentation of intense, intractable pruritus. The eruption has varying degrees of severity, and may spontaneously clear, only to flare unpredictably. It typically manifests in patients with a helper T-cell count below 250 cells per mL.

CLINICAL MANIFESTATIONS
Skin Findings

- Patients present with urticarial, follicular papules on the upper trunk, face, scalp, neck, which extend down the midline of the back to the lumbar region.
- Lesions typically occur in areas where there are a large number of sebaceous glands.
- Pustular lesions are rare since the pruritus is so severe that lesions become excoriated before they can progress to form pustules.

Non-Skin Findings

- A peripheral eosinophilia may be present and the serum IgE level may be elevated in about 25% to 50% of patients with HIV-associated EF.

- Biopsy—the term EF arises from the presence of mononuclear cells and eosinophils around the upper portion of the hair follicle at the level of the sebaceous gland and seen on histology.

Hypersensitivity Reactions

Hypersensitivity reactions are typical nonfollicular eruptions resulting from insect bites or arthropod assaults. These are commonly seen in temperate areas where insect bites are more common, such as in sub-Saharan Africa. Enhanced hypersensitivity reactions are simply a more exuberant response than those seen in immunocompetent patients.

CLINICAL MANIFESTATIONS

- This extreme reaction can be seen with scabies, insect bites, transient acantholytic dermatosis, granuloma annulare, and prurigo nodularis.
- Patients may have multiple eruptions simultaneously.
- Eczematous eruptions include atopic-like dermatitis, seborrheic dermatitis, nummular eczema, xerotic eczema, photodermatitis, and drug eruptions.
- Clinical presentation in this population may be much more dramatic than in an immunocompetent patient.

INFLAMMATORY DISORDERS
Psoriasis, Seborrheic Dermatitis, Eczematous Dermatitis

Extreme worsening of eczematous dermatitis or sudden development of severe seborrheic dermatitis or psoriasis may be a presenting sign of HIV infection. The diagnosis of HIV should be suspected in any at-risk individual with the correct constellation of symptoms, prolonged or recalcitrant skin disorders or the development of new onset disease.

See Sections 4.1, 4.3, and 4.4 Eczema, Seborrheic Dermatitis, and Psoriasis for details.

OPPORTUNISTIC INFECTIONS

Over time, people infected with HIV may experience fluctuations in their viral load for various reasons, particularly because of nonadherence to medication regimen. Because of a weakened immune status, various infections may emerge. These opportunistic infections take advantage of the damaged host and develop into much more exuberant and resistant infections than those typically seen in an immunocompetent individual. The infections are common but the expression in HIV-infected individuals is often much more severe and should raise the suspicion of HIV. Papilloma virus for example can cause common warts or in immune-suppressed patients can be responsible for cervical, and anal cancers as discussed above. Disorders such as KS, alone, should always raise suspicion that HIV is present.

Where treatment in an immunocompetent individual may be topical as in superficial fungal infections, in an immunocompromised individual, sustained and systemic alternatives may be needed. Treatment is individualized to specific infection and can be viewed in detail in other sections.

See Table 6.5-4 for common opportunistic infections and clinical presentations.

TABLE 6.5-4	Common Opportunistic Infections in HIV-Infected Persons

VIRAL INFECTIONS	CLINICAL PRESENTATION	
[a]Herpes simplex (common)	Persistent erosions and ulcerations chronic oral, genital Widely disseminated Resembles other infections Intractable perirectal ulcerations Regional lymphadenopathy Synergistic effect with HIV	 FIG. 6.5-9. **A** and **B**. HSV. (Figure "B": Used with permission from Edwards, L. [2004]. *Genital dermatology atlas*. Wolters Kluwer Health.)
[a]Herpes zoster/ shingles (common sign of AIDS)	Shingles may be severe, resulting in deep scarring Multiple dermatomes Persistent disseminated lesions Intractable herpetic pain	 FIG. 6.5-10. Herpes zoster. (Used with permission from Edwards, L. [2004]. *Genital dermatology atlas*. Wolters Kluwer Health.)
[a]Molluscum contagiosum	Clusters of white, umbilicated papules Persistent on face, groin numerous and large Cutaneous cryptococcus can mimic molluscum contagiosum	 FIG. 6.5-11. Molluscum contagiosum. Numerous "pearly" white- or flesh-colored papules that are smooth surfaced and dome shaped with central umbilication consistent with molluscum infection in an immunosuppressed patient. (Used with permission from Gru, A. A., & Wick, M. [2018]. *Pediatric dermatopathology and dermatology*. Wolters Kluwer Health.)

VIRAL INFECTIONS	CLINICAL PRESENTATION	
Warts/condyloma (common) Human papillomavirus (HPV)	[a]Common warts— extensive and persistent particularly genital Recalcitrant to Tx increased prevalence, number, size Cervical, anal squamous cell carcinoma (HPV types 16, 18)	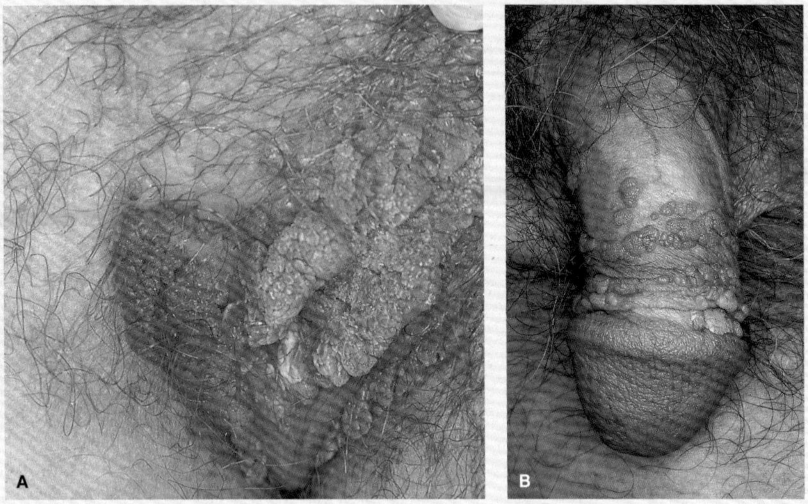 FIG. 6.5-12. Extensive HPV. **A:** Vulva. **B:** Penis. (Both images used with permission from Edwards, L. [2004]. *Genital dermatology atlas*. Wolters Kluwer Health.)
[a]Hairy leukoplakia (Epstein–Barr virus) (common)	Whitish, **nonremovable** verrucous hairy plaques on sides of tongue May resemble candida tongue infections **(removable plaques)**	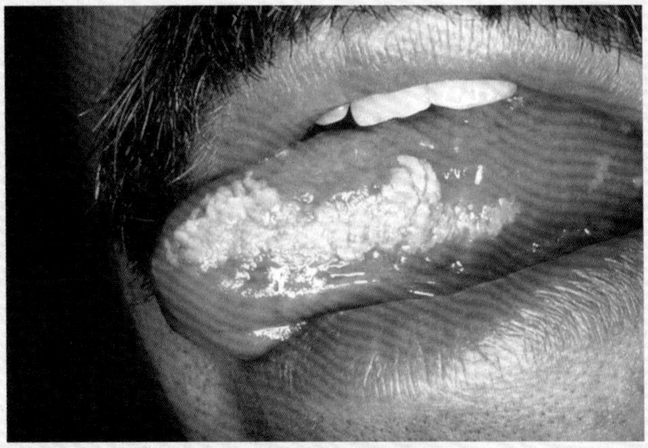 FIG. 6.5-13. Hairy leukoplakia. (Photo courtesy of M. Bobonich.)
Yeast Infection	See details in Section 6.1	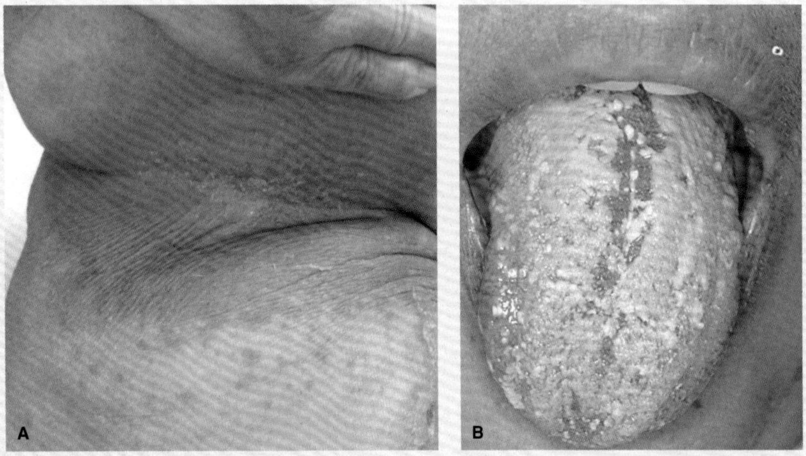
[a]*Candida albicans* (very common)	White plaques on cheeks, tongue Sore throat, dysphagia Deep tongue erosions, thick plaques on back of throat Esophageal infection Intractable vaginal infection *Candida* nail infection *Candida* intertrigo	FIG. 6.5-14. Candidiasis. Immunosuppressed patients are likely to develop mixed infections. A microscopic fungal preparation revealed. *Candida albicans* infection, but a concomitant herpes virus infection must be suspected, diagnosed, and treated for the patient to improve significantly. **A:** Inframammary candidiasis. **B:** Oral candidiasis. (*continued*)

(continued)

TABLE 6.5-4	Common Opportunistic Infections in HIV-Infected Persons (*Continued*)

YEAST INFECTIONS	CLINICAL PRESENTATION	
		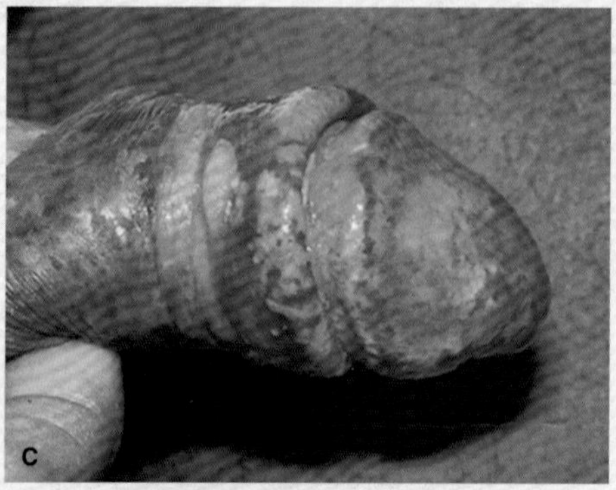 FIG. 6.5-14. (*Continued*) **C:** Genital candida. (Figure "C": Used with permission from Edwards, L. [2004]. *Genital dermatology atlas.* Wolters Kluwer Health.)
Tinea versicolor (common)	Common early and late in HIV infection Thick, scaly hypopigmented or light-brown plaques on trunk	FIG. 6.5-15. Tinea versicolor. This patient has large confluent tan scaly macules against a background of normal skin which appears hypopigmented by comparison. (Image provided by Stedman's.)
Fungal Infection Dermatophytes Tinea corporis Tinea pedis Tinea cruris Onychomycoses (common)	[a]Extensive involvement, especially groin and feet [a]Proximal subungual onychomycosis	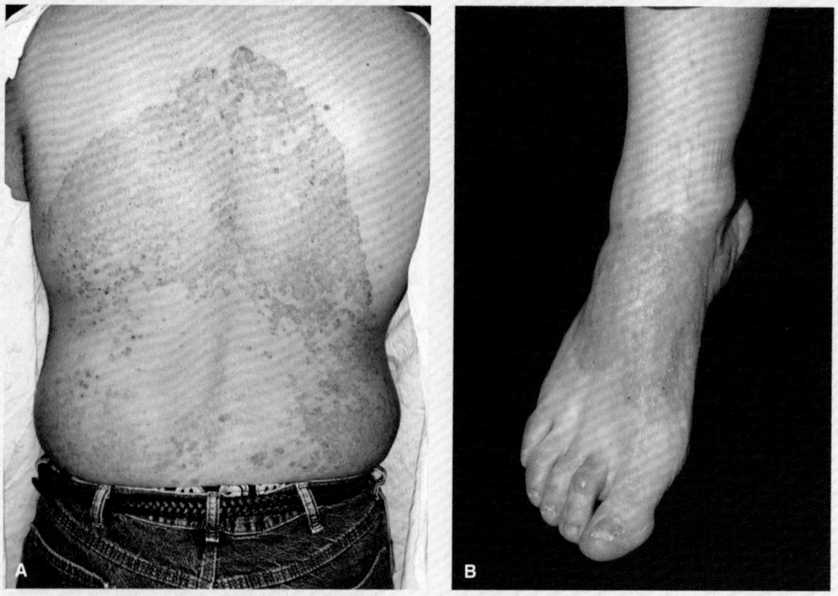 FIG. 6.5-16. Extensive dermatophyte infections. **A:** Trunk. **B:** Foot. (Photos courtesy of M. Bobonich.)

FUNGAL INFECTIONS	CLINICAL PRESENTATION	
Onychmycosis Nails	Thickened nails with subungual debris and loss of cuticles	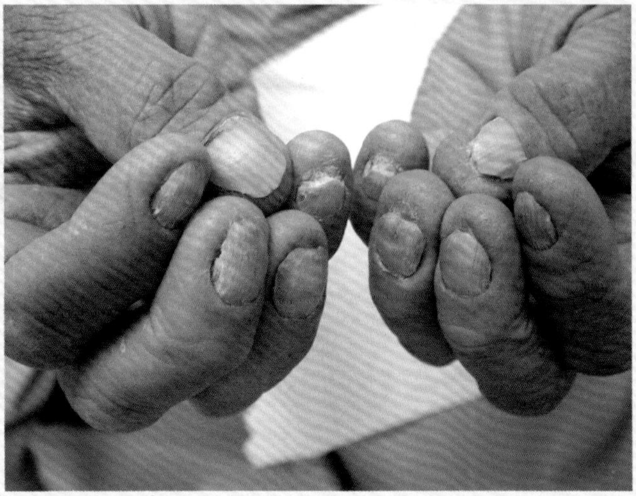 FIG. 6.5-17. Onychomycosis. Nails. (Photo courtesy of M. Bobonich.)
Histoplasma capsulatum (rare)	Multiple papules, nodules, macules, and oral and skin ulcers on arms, face, trunk Travel history (South America)	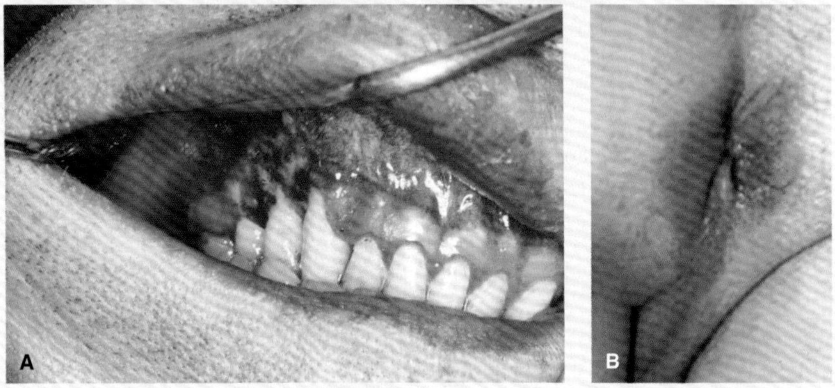 FIG. 6.5-18. Histoplasmosis. **A:** Oral (CDC Public Health Image #15363). **B:** Perianal histoplasmosis (CDC Public Health Image #20339).
Bacterial Infections	See details in Section 6.4	
[a]Syphilis (uncommon)	Primary chancre	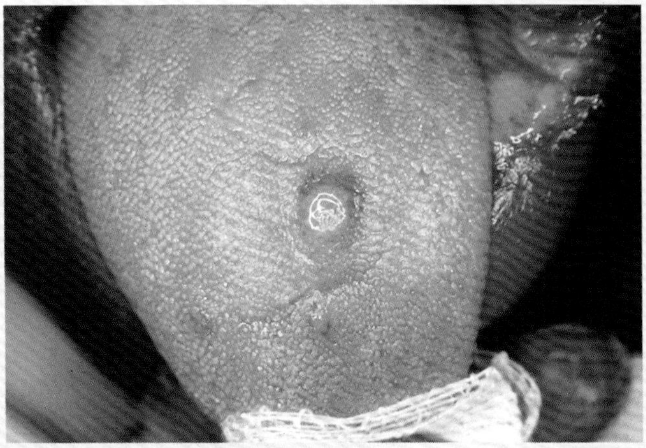 FIG. 6.5-19. Primary chancre syphilis. (Centers for Disease Control and Prevention.)

(continued)

| TABLE 6.5-4 | Common Opportunistic Infections in HIV-Infected Persons (*Continued*) |

BACTERIAL INFECTIONS	CLINICAL PRESENTATION	
Secondary syphilis	Generalized papulosquamous papules and plaques especially on palms and soles Can mimic almost any inflammatory cutaneous disorder Incubation period for neurosyphilis may be very brief (months)	 FIG. 6.5-20. Secondary syphilis. **A:** Hands and feet (Centers for Disease Control and Prevention). **B:** Oral lesions of secondary syphilis (Centers for Disease Control and Prevention).
[a]Bacillary angiomatosis (rare)	Solitary or multiple dome-shaped friable, bright-red granulation tissue-like papules and subcutaneous nodules (1 mm–2 cm) of face, trunk, extremities Visceral angiomatosis Cat bite or scratch	 FIG. 6.5-21. Bacillary angiomatosis.
Infestation	See details in Section 7	
[a]Scabies	Generalized crusted papules Scabies—generalized hyperkeratotic eruption	 FIG. 6.5-22. Crusted scabies. (Goodheart, H. P. [2015]. *Goodheart's photoguide of common skin disorders* [4th ed.]. Wolters Kluwer Health I Lippincott Williams & Wilkins.)

[a]Alone raise the possibility of HIV.

READINGS AND REFERENCES

Bacik, L., Chung, C. (2018). Human papillomavirus-associated cutaneous disease burden in human immunodeficiency virus (HIV)-positive patients: the role of human papillomavirus vaccination and a review of the literature. *International Journal of Dermatology, 57*(6), 627–634.

Bolognia, J. L., Jorizzo, J. L., & Rapini, R. P. (2017). Cutaneous manifestations of HIV, human papillomaviruses, human herpesvirus and other viral diseases. In *Dermatology* (4th ed.). Elsevier Saunders.

Centers for Disease Control and Prevention (CDC). (2010). Sexually transmitted diseases treatment guidelines. *Morbidity and Mortality Weekly Report Recommendations and Reports, 59*(12).

Centers for Disease Control and Prevention (CDC). (2013). HIV testing and risk behaviors among gay, bisexual, and other men who have sex with men—US. *Morbidity and Mortality Weekly Report Recommendations and Reports, 62*(47), 958–962.

Centers for Disease Control and Prevention (CDC). (2019). HIV surveillance supplemental report, 24(1).

Centers for Disease Control and Prevention (CDC). (2020a). HIV basics. https://cdc.gov/hiv/guidelines/index.html

Centers for Disease Control and Prevention (CDC). (2020b). HIV surveillance report, 2018 (Updated). http://www.cdc.gov/hiv/library/reports/hiv-surveillance.html

Centers for Disease Control and Prevention (CDC). (2020c). Vital signs. https://www.cdc.gov/vitalsigns/test-treat-prevent.

Changa, A., Doironb, P., & Maurer, T. (2017). Cutaneous malignancies in HIV. *Current Opinion in HIV and AIDS, 12*(1), 57–62. https://doi.org/10.1097/COH.00000000000003381746-630X

Chua, S. R., Amerson, E., Leslie, K., & Maurer, T. (2015). Papular pruritic eruption of human immunodeficiency virus (HIV) infection over 2 years of antiretroviral therapy. *Journal of the American Academy of Dermatology, 72*(5). https://doi.org/10.1016/j.jaad.2015.02.236

Coghill, A., Shiels, M., Suneja, G., & Engels, E. (2015). Elevated cancer specific mortality among HIV-infected patients in the United States. *Journal of Clinical Oncology, 33*(21), 2376–2383.

Meites, E., Szilagyi, P. G., Chesson, H. W., Unger, E. R., Romero, J. R., & Markowitz, L. E. (2019). Human papilloma virus vaccination for adults: updated recommendations of the Advisory Committee on Immunization Practices. *The Morbidity and Mortality Weekly Report, 68*(32), 698–702.

Mohamad, S., & Mutch, M. G. (2019). Anorectal disorders in the immunocompromised. *Seminars in Colon and Rectal Surgery, 30*(3). https://doi.org/10.1016/j.scrs.2019.100687

Schwartz, R., & Erdal, E., (2020). Cutaneous manifestations of HIV. https://emedicine.medscape.com/article/1133746-overview.

Silverberg, M. J., Lau, B., Achenbach, C. J., Jing, Y., Althoff, K. N., D'Souza, G., Engels, E. A., Hessol, N. A., Brooks, J. T., Burchell, A. N., Gill, M. J., Goedert, J. J., Hogg, R., Horberg, M. A., Kirk, G. D., Kitahata, M. M., Korthuis, P. T., Mathews, W. C., Mayor, A., … Dubrow, R.; North American AIDS Cohort Collaboration on Research and Design of the International Epidemiologic Databases to Evaluate AIDS. (2015). Cumulative incidence of cancer among persons with HIV in North America: A cohort study. *Annals of Internal Medicine, 163*(7), 507–518.

Tobin, N., & Aldrovandi, G., (2013). Immunology of pediatric HIV infection. *Immunological Reviews, 254*(1), 143–169. https://doi.org/10.1111/imr.12074

Vaccher, E., Serraino, D., Carbone, A., de Paoli, P. (2014). The evolving scenario of Non AIDS defining cancers: Challenges and opportunities of care. *The Oncologist, 19*(8), 860–867.

Infestations

Melissa E. Cyr

CHAPTER

7.1

In This Chapter

- Scabies (common, crusted)
- Pediculosis
- Bedbugs

Insect infestations, stings, and bites are prevalent throughout the world. Indoor-dwelling insects of those living in temperate climates can cause bites year-round and may produce an array of clinical manifestations. Although animal and human bites occur less frequently, they still have the potential to produce significant morbidity and mortality. With increased world travel, it is important to possess a broader clinical awareness of commonly encountered foreign cutaneous conditions, including those that are marine acquired.

INFESTATIONS

Scabies

Scabies is a highly contagious, common parasitic infection characterized by intense itching and superficial burrows, inflammatory nodules, and evidence of excoriation. Scabies affects both males and females of all socioeconomic and ethnic groups.

Crusted scabies (also called hyperkeratotic or Norwegian) is more severe but less common than general scabies infection. At-risk patients include the immunocompromised, elderly, and mentally or physically disabled. Compromised immunity and decreased itch sensation lead to the proliferation of hundreds to millions of mites.

PATHOPHYSIOLOGY

- The infection is caused by the microscopic mite *Sarcoptes scabiei.*
- Transmission most often occurs through direct skin-to-skin contact, with a higher incidence occurring through prolonged exposure within households or neighborhoods. For this reason, outbreaks are more common in extended-care facilities, prisons, child care facilities, and schools.
- Less frequently, the mite is transmitted by indirect contact through fomites (e.g., bedding, brushes) and can live up to 3 days on these inanimate objects.
- The adult mite that affects humans is female, approximately 0.3 to 0.4 mm long, and has a flattened, oval body with four pairs of legs (Fig. 7.1-1).

- The infestation begins when the fertilized female mite burrows into the skin and moves linearly beneath the most superficial layer of the epidermis (stratum corneum), depositing eggs and fecal pellets (scybala) along the way. These deposited eggs hatch, and within several weeks, larvae grow into adult mites, capable of reproducing and perpetuating the infestation cycle.
- After approximately 1 month, an allergic reaction (delayed-type IV hypersensitivity reaction) occurs in response to the mites, eggs, and scybala, transforming the initial, minor, localized itching into severe and widespread pruritus.
- Subsequent scabies infections in a sensitized individual can produce generalized pruritus more rapidly because of this hypersensitivity response.
- Mites involved in crusted scabies are not more virulent than those found in traditional scabies infection, but rather present in greater numbers. Individuals infected are highly contagious and therefore require quick and aggressive medical treatment.

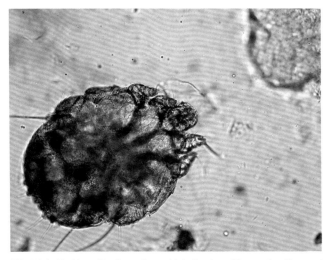

FIG. 7.1-1. Scabies mite. *Sarcoptes scabiei* mites in a skin scraping. Eggs and feces also seen. (Courtesy of T. Habif.)

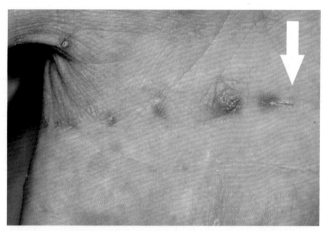

FIG. 7.1-2. Scabies linear rash. (Goodheart, H. P. [2015]. *Goodheart's photoguide of common skin disorders* [4th ed.]. Wolters Kluwer Health | Lippincott Williams & Wilkins.)

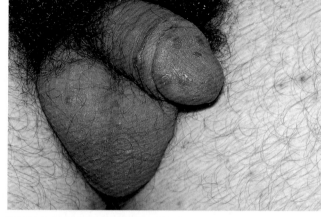

FIG. 7.1-4. Scabetic nodules scrotum. Note the papules and nodules on glans and scrotum. (Goodheart, H. P. [2015]. *Goodheart's photoguide of common skin disorders* [4th ed.]. Wolters Kluwer Health | Lippincott Williams & Wilkins.)

CLINICAL PRESENTATION

Skin Findings

- Clinical presentation varies based on lesion type and location. Symptoms begin insidiously and are often mistaken for other skin conditions (e.g., dermatitis). Light pink curved or linear burrows, occasionally seen with a black dot on one end representing the mite are pathognomonic, but not always seen (Fig. 7.1-2).
- Scratching the area can destroy burrows (Fig. 7.1-3), displace mites, and promote the spread of mites to other locations on the body.
- Older children and adults commonly present with red papules and vesicles involving the finger webs, wrists, lateral aspects of feet and hands, waist, axillae, buttocks, penis, and

scrotum. Infants and small children may develop pustules on the palms and soles, and in some cases, the head and neck (Fig. 7.1-4).

- Nodules on the trunk and axillae may erupt as a result of the host's exuberant immune response to scabies.

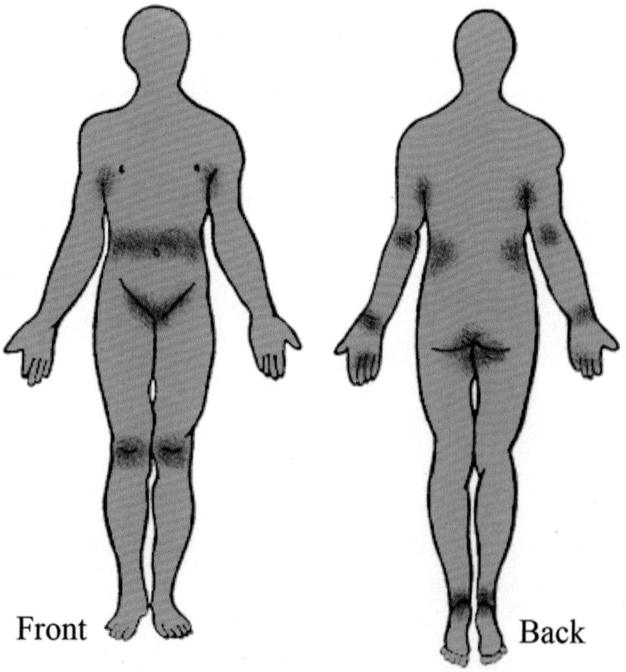

Crusted Scabies

- These patients classically present with asymptomatic, hyperkeratotic crusting on the palms and soles, thickened (dystrophic) nails, thick crusts and gray scales on the trunk and extremities, and verrucous (wartlike) growths in areas of trauma (Fig. 7.1-5).
- Hair loss also may be present. Mites involved in crusted scabies are not more virulent than those found in traditional scabies infection, but rather present in greater numbers. Individuals infected are highly contagious and therefore require quick and aggressive medical treatment.

Non-Skin Finding

- Widespread pruritus is common, and severe nocturnal pruritus is the hallmark characteristic of scabies infection.

Front   Back

FIG. 7.1-3. Scabies distribution. (Goodheart, H. P. [2015]. *Goodheart's photoguide of common skin disorders* [4th ed.]. Wolters Kluwer Health | Lippincott Williams & Wilkins.)

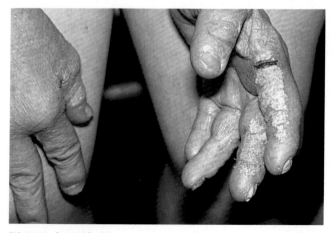

FIG. 7.1-5. Crusted Scabies.

DIFFERENTIAL DIAGNOSIS   Scabies

- Pruritus (generalized or prolonged)
- Dermatitis
- ID reaction
- Folliculitis
- Psoriasis (crusted scabies)
- Arthropod bites (i.e., bedbugs)
- Dermatitis herpetiformis
- Varicella
- Bullous pemphigoid (urticarial phase)

CONFIRMING THE DIAGNOSIS

Laboratory

- While scabies diagnosis may be established based on clinical suspicion, a definitive diagnosis is made through the identification of mites, feces (scybala), eggs, or egg casings under microscopy by performing a mineral oil mount (see Section 15).

TREATMENT

- Management requires both pharmacologic treatment and environmental eradication.
- *Warning:* Lindane 1% topical application is FDA approved for use only in adults who failed or are intolerant of other approved therapies, and is not available in all states due to the high toxicity risk.
- Oral antihistamines (e.g., cetirizine, loratadine, or hydroxyzine) and topical corticosteroids are used to manage pruritus.
- Short courses of oral corticosteroids are reserved for severe and intractable cases.

- A skin biopsy may be attained if the diagnosis is questionable or no response to treatment.

See Table 7.1-1.

MANAGEMENT AND PATIENT EDUCATION

- Bathe before topical scabicide application, which generally is recommended at bedtime.
- Apply topical scabicide to all skin from the neck down, unless the head and neck are involved ensuring all skin folds are treated, including finger and toe webs, under the trimmed fingernails, axillae, umbilicus, and the anal and vaginal clefts; inadequate coverage is the primary cause of treatment failure.
- Members of the same household, including intimate contacts, should be treated empirically with topical scabicides at the same time as the infected patient.
- All clothing, bedding, and towels in contact with infected skin must be washed and dried on the hottest possible settings. Items unable to be washed may be sealed in a plastic bag for at least 1 week.
- Crusted scabies is more challenging to treat because of the thick, hyperkeratotic scale; thus, combination therapy with topical permethrin and oral ivermectin is used frequently.
- Pruritus associated with hypersensitivity to mites may last up to 4 weeks after effective treatment and does not indicate treatment failure.

SPECIAL CONSIDERATIONS

- *Pregnancy:* There are no adverse effects of scabies in pregnancy. Permethrin is generally safe for use during pregnancy and second-line ivermectin may be used with caution.

TABLE 7.1-1	Prescribed Medications for Scabies Treatment				
MEDICATION	**ADULT NONCRUSTED**	**ADULT CRUSTED**	**PEDIATRIC NONCRUSTED**	**PEDIATRIC CRUSTED**	**SPECIAL INFORMATION**
Permethrin 5% cream (Rx) **Treatment of choice**	Apply ×1, may repeat in 14 days if live mites still present; rinse after 12 h	Apply q.d. × 7 days, then 2×/wk until cured; rinse after 12 h (recommend use w/ oral ivermectin)	≥2 mo: Apply ×1, may repeat in 14 days if live mites still present; rinse after 8–12 h	≥2 mo: Apply q.d. ×7 days, then 2×/wk until cured	• May use during pregnancy • May use while breastfeeding • Resistance has been documented • Apply neck down, w/ special attention to the nails and umbilicus
Ivermectin 3-mg tablets (Rx)	0.2 mg/kg × 1 (may repeat in 2 wk if symptoms persist)	0.2 mg/kg ×1 on days 1, 2, 8, 9, 15 (may also give on days 22 and 29 for severe cases; use with topical scabicide)	≥10 yr: 0.2 mg/kg × 1 (may repeat in 2 wk if symptoms persist)	Not FDA approved	• Caution advised during pregnancy • May use while breastfeeding • Give with food ***Use with topical scabicide***
Crotamiton 10% lotion OR cream	Apply ×1; repeat application in 24 h	Not FDA approved	≥3 mo: Apply ×1; repeat application in 24 h	Not FDA approved	• Do not apply to inflamed or raw skin • Frequent treatment failure has been reported
Sulfur 5–10% ointment	6%: Apply q.h.s. for three consecutive nights	Not FDA approved	6%: Apply q.h.s. for three consecutive nights	Not FDA approved	• 6% preferred • High rates of resistance • Safe in infants, children, and pregnant women

Source: Centers for Disease Control and Prevention (2019), retrieved from: https://www.cdc.gov/parasites/scabies/health_professionals/meds.html

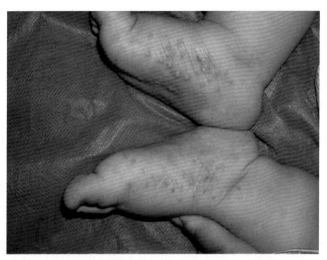

FIG. 7.1-6. Acropustulosis of infancy. Acropustulosis of infancy: pustules, erythematous papules, and crusts on the medial aspect of both feet. (Used with permission from Gru, A. A., & Wick, M. [2018]. *Pediatric dermatopathology and dermatology*. Wolters Kluwer Health.)

- *Geriatrics and immunosuppression:* The initial presentation of scabies in the elderly or immunosuppressed patient very often yields fewer cutaneous lesions than younger or otherwise healthy adults, and is more consistent with nonspecific dry, scaly skin that may have several nodules. Severe pruritus, however, is often still observed.

  More commonly, the face and scalp also may be involved with Norwegian or crusted scabies presentation in these populations. As scabies transmission is greatest in those living in close contact, and through sharing clothing and bedding, assisted care personnel or facility administration should be notified so that other residents may be screened, and measures are taken to avoid an outbreak.

- Acropustulosis of infancy (API) represents an allergic response post scabies infection and is characterized by itchy vesicles or pustules on the palms and soles in children ≤3 years old (Fig. 7.1-6). Although there are no burrows seen in API, it often is misdiagnosed as a reoccurrence. However, clinicians should perform a mineral prep to ensure the child has not been reinfected. Specific treatment is often not warranted unless lesions are extremely pruritic.

CLINICAL PEARLS

■ Pruritic papules/nodules on the scrotum or penis (diaper area for children) or nipple region in women are *highly suspicious for scabies* and should be proven otherwise.

■ Suggestive findings of crusted scabies in at-risk population include asymptomatic, hyperkeratotic crusting on the palms and soles, thickened (dystrophic) nails, thick crusts and gray scales on the trunk and extremities, and verrucous (wartlike) growths in areas of trauma.

■ Infants and children may present with more scaly papules and vesicles, especially in occluded areas such as the axillae and diaper region. Face and scalp (especially the occipital area) involvement are seen more frequently in children than in adults.

PEDICULOSIS

Pediculosis, commonly known as lice, is a contagious type of parasite that feeds on human blood. Infestation occurs through close personal contact, as well as through inanimate objects, such as brushes, combs, hats, clothing, and bedding. Lice infestations have become an increasing problem throughout the world and usually occur with crowded living conditions or poor hygiene. In endemic areas, body lice are capable of transmitting infectious diseases such as typhus, relapsing fever, and trench fever.

PATHOPHYSIOLOGY

- Lice are small (<2 mm or about the size of a sesame seed), flat, wingless insects that crawl and do not hop or fly.
- They live on the human host's skin and feed on their blood by piercing the skin and injecting saliva, causing a pruritic response.
- Without feeding, adult lice can live off of a human host for approximately 10 days or up to 3 weeks as eggs or nits.
- Pets cannot transmit human lice.

HEAD LICE

Pediculus humanus capitis, or head lice infestation, can affect any part of the scalp, with accompanied dermatitis commonly seen on the occipital scalp, neck, or behind the ears.

- Pediatric patients and their caregivers or household members have the highest prevalence of head lice, with girls affected more than boys. Infestation is seen across all ethnicities, but notably less in African Americans (Fig. 7.1-7).
- Nits are attached to the base of the hair with a glue-like substance secreted by the louse, within approximately 3 to 4 mm of the scalp (Fig. 7.1-8).
- Occasionally, eyelash involvement occurs, presenting with redness and localized eyelid edema.

BODY LICE

Caused by *Pediculus corporis,* body lice are an uncommon parasitic infestation associated with poor hygiene and the spread of infectious diseases. The louse does not live directly on the body; rather, it resides and lays its eggs on clothing seams and returns to the skin surface only to feed, making direct visualization for diagnosis difficult (Fig. 7.1-9).

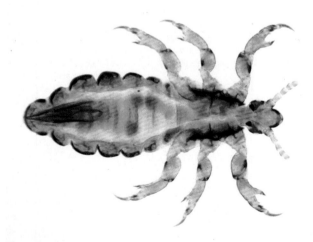

FIG. 7.1-7. Head louse. (From Wikimedia Commons.)

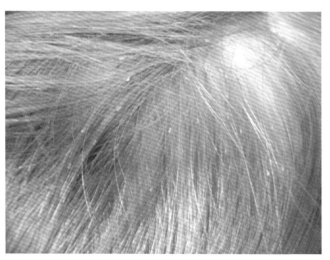

FIG. 7.1-8. Nits attached to hair.

PUBIC LICE

Pediculus pubis or pubic louse received its nickname "crabs" based on its short, broad body with large front claws resembling a crab (Fig. 7.1-10).

- Pubic lice are highly contagious, and sexual exposure with an infected partner yields a high rate of transmission.

- These patients are more likely to be at increased risk for co-infection with other sexually transmitted diseases. Pubic hair is the most common site of infestation; however, greater infestation may occur in the perianal, proximal thigh, abdominal, axillae, and facial hair.

- Eyelash involvement is usually related to pubic lice.

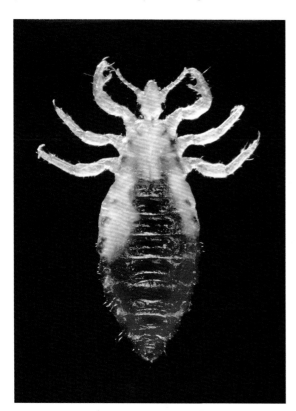

FIG. 7.1-9. Body louse. (From Wikimedia Commons.)

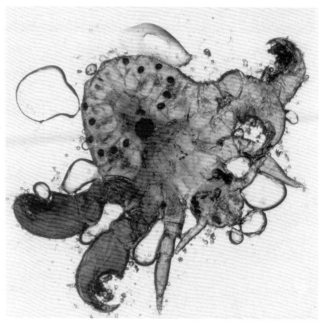

FIG. 7.1-10. Pubic louse. The nickname "crabs" comes from the obvious resemblance to the crustacean.

CLINICAL PRESENTATIONS

Skin Findings

- Inflammation, excoriation, pustules, and crusting. May occur on scalp, pubic area, or body secondary to scratching and may represent secondary infection.

Non-Skin Findings

- Lice or nits may involve eyelashes, with potential localized eyelid erythema usually related to pubic lice and less often head lice.

- Pruritus is common along with a crawling sensation in affected areas.

- Lice sensitization can occur over time, causing inflammation and regional adenopathy.

DIFFERENTIAL DIAGNOSIS Pediculosis
• Psoriasis
• Dermatophyte infection
• Seborrheic dermatitis
• Contact dermatitis
• Folliculitis
• Drug reactions
• Delusions of parasitosis
• Arthropod bites or other parasitic infestations, such as scabies
• Systemic causes of generalized pruritus

CONFIRMING THE DIAGNOSIS

- The American Academy of Pediatrics states the gold standard diagnosis is observing a live, moving louse on the scalp or pubic area; however, this is difficult as it moves quickly and tries to avoid light (Devore et al., 2015). A magnifying glass or Wood lamp may be helpful.

- A fine-toothed "nit" comb may be utilized to aid in visualization.

TABLE 7.1-2	Medication Options for Pediculosis Capitis and Pubis			
MEDICATION	**CAPITIS (DAYS 1 AND 8)**	**PUBIS (DAYS 1 AND 8)**	**SPECIAL INFORMATION**	**EFFICACY**
Permethrin 1% cream/lotion (OTC)	Topical application for 10 min to clean, dry hair	Topical application for 10 min to clean, dry hair	None	*Capitis:* Poor-fair *Pubis:* Fair
Permethrin 5% cream (Rx)	Topical overnight application to clean, dry hair	Topical application for 8–12 h	Approved for use ≥2 mo of age Pregnancy category: B	*Capitis:* Poor-fair *Pubis:* Good
Lindane 1% shampoo (Rx)	Topical application for 4 min to clean, dry hair, then add water to lather and rinse	Topical application for 4 min to clean, dry hair, then add water to lather and rinse	Potential CNS toxicity Not recommended for infants or breastfeeding Pregnancy category: C	*Capitis:* Poor-fair *Pubis:* Poor
Spinosad 0.9% cream (Rx)	Topical application for 10 min to dry hair	Not FDA approved	Approved for use ≥4 yr of age Pregnancy category: B	*Capitis:* Poor-fair
Benzyl 5% alcohol lotion (Rx)	Topical application for 10 min to dry hair	Not FDA approved	Approved for use ≥6 mo of age Pregnancy category: B	*Capitis:* Poor-fair
Ivermectin 0.5% lotion (Rx)	Topical application for 10 min to dry hair	Not FDA approved	Approved for use ≥6 mo of age Pregnancy category: C	Not available
Ivermectin 3-mg tablets (Rx)	Adults: 0.2 mg/kg PO Q10 days × 2 doses Pediatric: Not FDA approved for lice	Adults: 0.25 mg/kg PO Q10 days × 2 doses Pediatric: Not FDA approved for lice	Give on an empty stomach Potential CNS toxicity Not recommended in breastfeeding Pregnancy category: C	*Capitis:* Poor-fair *Pubis:* Excellent

Adapted from Bolognia, J. L., Jorizzo, J. L., & Schaffer, J. V. (2012). *Dermatology* (3rd ed.). Elsevier Saunders.

- In general, the closer the nits are to the scalp, the more recent the infection, but may be retained on the shafts of hair for months after successful treatment.

TREATMENT

- Treatment for head and pubic lice is similar (see Table 7.1-2).
- The Centers for Disease Control and Prevention (CDC) recommends environmental treatment measures for cases of body lice, which include removing infested clothing and laundering with hot water (at least 130°F). Carpeting, mattresses, car seat, and furniture should be vacuumed. Bedding and clothing, including hats, should be laundered on a weekly basis. Brushes and combs should be washed in hot water (>130°F) or thrown away.
- Clinicians should consider prophylactic treatment of household contacts, including sexual contacts.

MANAGEMENT AND PATIENT EDUCATION

- The application of a dilute white vinegar solution to soften the "cemented" nit on hair shafts has been reported to make nit removal easier.
- During outbreaks at schools and daycare, many parents apply a thick, occlusive substance (petrolatum, mayonnaise, olive oil) to children's hair to smother the nit and prevent adherence to the hair shaft.
- Wet combing may be performed at home using a high-quality, commercially available nit comb as an alternative to or in conjunction with topical pesticide medications.
- More drastic measures include shaving or cutting their children's hair in an effort to eradicate the lice infestation but are not recommended due to associated psychological climpications, especially in young girls.

- Prognosis is excellent since symptoms should completely resolve with successful treatment.
- Potential complications may include secondary bacterial infection from scratching or hypersensitivity reaction.
- Large, live, moving lice suggest reinfestation, whereas lice of different sizes suggest treatment resistance and patients should be reevaluated for correct diagnosis.
- Patients who are immunosuppressed or have disseminated symptoms may be referred to a dermatologist or infectious disease specialist.
- Follow-up is not generally warranted unless the patient experiences continued symptoms despite adequate treatment.
- Treatment failure is common and typically due to inadequate treatment (patient and contacts), drug resistance, or environmental control.

SPECIAL CONSIDERATIONS

Pediatrics: According to the American Academy of Pediatrics and the National Association of School Nurses, children diagnosed with active head lice pose little risk to other students from infestation and are encouraged to attend classes, but maintain distance from peers until adequately treated (Devore et al., 2015).

- The presence of pubic lice on eyelashes or eyebrows may be a sign of possible sexual abuse.

Pregnancy: During pregnancy, pharmacologic treatment options are limited. Special attention should be made when selecting an appropriate treatment. Table 7.1-2 lists treatment options available during pregnancy; other nonpharmacologic methods may also be utilized, as described under Therapeutics.

Geriatrics: There are no special considerations for elderly patients.

Stings and Bites

Melissa E. Cyr

BEDBUGS

Bedbugs are parasitic insects found worldwide, whose presence has been documented for thousands of years. Although both feed on human blood, the *Cimex lectularius* subtype is found primarily in temperate climates, and *Cimex hemipterus* in warmer climates. Higher rates of infestation occur in homeless shelters and refugee camps. Incidence rates in developed countries have increased dramatically over the past decade due to increased international travel, immigration from developing countries, and resistance to and bans on particular insecticides.

PATHOPHYSIOLOGY

- Bedbugs are thought to be vectors for certain infectious diseases, such as hepatitis B and Chagas disease.
- These parasites primarily are nocturnal and have an affinity for warm areas, particularly near or around beds or bedding.
- Bedbugs are reddish-brown insects with a flattened, oval-shaped body with a segmented abdomen, and a retroverted mouthpiece optimized for sucking blood (Fig. 7.2-1).
- They measure 5 to 7 mm in size, and have a very short life cycle, reaching adulthood and capable of reproducing in only 3 weeks.
- A history of travel, new furniture, visitors, or other means of exposure generally precedes symptom development.

CLINICAL PRESENTATION

- Bites occur due to a hypersensitivity response to the salivary proteins injected during feedings. The degree of response to the bites, as well as clinical appearance, is highly individualized and depends on one's degree of sensitization and reaction to saliva proteins. Reaction to bites may take several days to weeks to manifest.

Skin Findings

- Edematous and erythematous papules, which are often quite pruritic.

- Occasionally, bites are vesicular or urticarial, and a central, hemorrhagic punctum may be observed.
- Bites classically appear in a "breakfast, lunch, and dinner" pattern, which represents the linear journey of the bug through the night (Fig. 7.2-2). Bites also may be observed in a scattered distribution and are generally located on areas exposed during sleep, such as the arms, legs, waist, head, neck, and shoulders.
- Reaction to bites may take several days to weeks to manifest. Complications include possible secondary bacterial infections from scratching and hypersensitivity reactions.

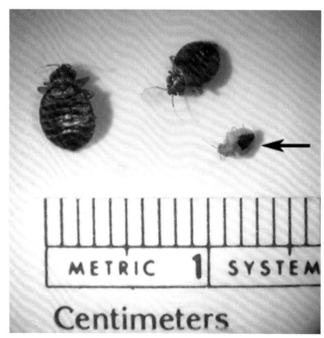

FIG. 7.2-1. Bedbugs. (Courtesy of Centers for Disease Control and Prevention.)

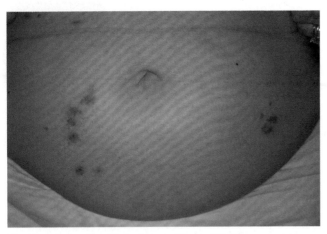

FIG. 7.2-2. Bedbug bites. (Photo courtesy of Thomas P. Habif.)

Non-Skin Findings

- Bedbugs generally hide in seams and folds of luggage, sheets, mattresses, clothing, and furniture (Fig. 7.2-3), and emerge from hiding at night to feed.
- Patients may exhibit considerable emotional stress.

> **DIFFERENTIAL DIAGNOSIS   Bedbugs**
>
> - Drug eruptions
> - Dermatitis herpetiformis
> - Other insect bites (i.e., scabies)
> - Delusions of parasitosis

CONFIRMING THE DIAGNOSIS

- The diagnosis is primarily achieved through a detailed history and clinical findings.

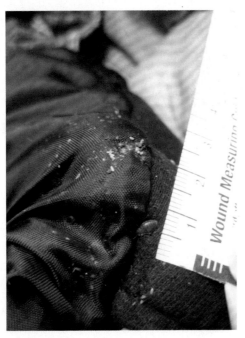

FIG. 7.2-3. Bedbugs in seams. (Photo courtesy of M. Bobonich.)

- Patients will often seek medical attention for unexplained pruritic lesions.
- Consider screening for hepatitis B or bacterial culture for suspected secondary infection.
- A skin biopsy may direct the diagnosis toward an arthropod bite, but would not specifically identify the offending insect.

TREATMENT

- Management of clinical symptoms varies based on the extent of involvement and degree of severity.
- Pruritus may be treated with topical or oral corticosteroids, or with antihistamines (e.g., cetirizine, loratadine, or hydroxyzine).
- Secondary infection may be treated with antibiotics.
- Patients with a history of asthma may experience an exacerbation of symptoms thought to be associated with bedbug excrement. Severe cases may require administration of epinephrine.

MANAGEMENT AND PATIENT EDUCATION

- The U.S. Environmental Protection Agency (EPA, 2018) has compiled its top 10 treatment and eradication tips for bedbugs (Box 7.2-1).
- Eradication has been accomplished with insecticides such as permethrin or dichlorvos.
- Other recommendations include removal by mechanical means such as vacuums or high heat (130°F) eradication.
- Cracks and crevices in headboards and walls around sleeping areas should also be inspected and treated appropriately.
- Prevention should be emphasized. The eradication of bedbugs is difficult, often requiring the assistance of professional exterminators experienced in bedbug termination. Their small bodies and ability to go without feeding for long periods of time make them easily transportable in the seams and folds of luggage, bedding, clothing, and furniture.
- Regular inspection of these items for signs of infestation, including the presence of bedbugs or their exoskeletons in the folds of mattresses or bedding, is key.
- The smell of a sweet, musty odor, or rusty-colored blood spots on mattresses and bedding from blood-filled excrements are also indications of infestation.

> **BOX 7.2-1   Top 10 Bedbug Tips**
>
> 1. Make sure you really have bedbugs, not fleas, ticks, or other insects.
> 2. Don't panic!
> 3. Think through your treatment options—don't immediately reach for the spray can.
> 4. Reduce the number of hiding places—clean up the clutter.
> 5. Regularly wash and heat-dry your bed sheets, blankets, bedspreads, and any clothing that touches the floor.
> 6. Do-it-yourself freezing may not be a reliable method for bedbug control.
> 7. Kill bedbugs with heat, but be very careful.
> 8. Don't pass your bedbugs on to others.
> 9. Reduce the number of bedbugs to reduce bites.
> 10. Turn to the professionals, if needed.
>
> *Note.* Reprinted from "Top ten tips to prevent or control bed bugs," United States Environmental Protection Agency, 2018, from https://www.epa.gov/bedbugs/top-ten-tips-prevent-or-control-bed-bugs

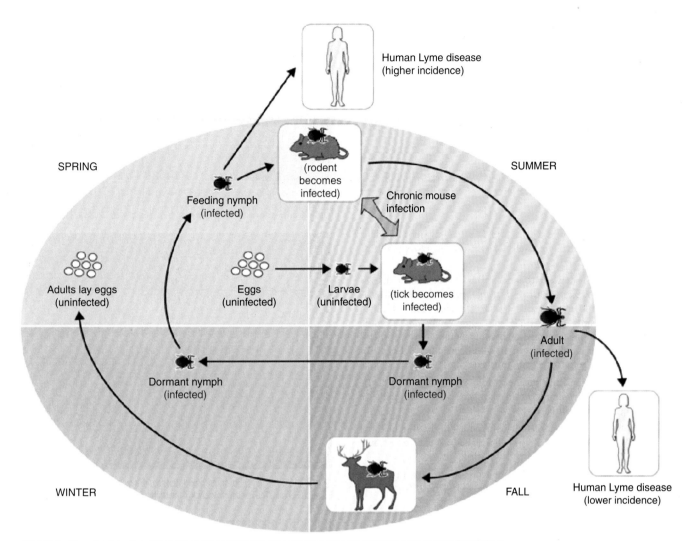

FIG. 7.2-4. Life cycle of *Ixodes scapularis* (deer tick). (Adapted with permission from the American Lyme Disease Foundation.)

CLINICAL PEARLS

- Immunosuppressed patients may have a slightly increased risk of contracting hepatitis B or Chagas disease with exposure.
- Although bedbug bites are rarely fatal, death may occur due to anaphylaxis.

BITES

Tick Bites

Ticks are nonvenomous, bloodsucking, external parasites that can harbor various infectious diseases. There are two distinct classifications of ticks: soft-bodied ticks (Argasidae) and hard-bodied ticks (Ixodidae). Hard-bodied ticks are vectors for more serious infectious diseases; they feed on their hosts much longer (up to 10 days) and are generally much more difficult to remove. Ticks feed by first using their curved, sharp mouthparts to bite, then secrete a glue-like substance to help adhere to their host. The bite itself is often painless and may go unnoticed, especially if it occurs in an inconspicuous body area. Ticks generally wait on bushes and tall grass for a host to pass by or are brought into the home by pets. Lyme disease and Rocky Mountain spotted fever (RMSF) are the two most common tick-borne infectious diseases in the United States.

Lyme Disease

Lyme disease is the most common tick-borne disease in the United States. White-tailed deer, white-footed mice, as well as other mammals and birds are important disease reservoir hosts on which these ticks feed during their 2-year life cycle (Fig. 7.2-4). Blacklegged ticks in the United States are also responsible for the transmission of several other infections, including at least three different species of *Borrelia*, babesiosis, anaplasmosis, and Powassan virus (CDC, 2018).

Although Lyme disease has been reported all across the country, there is a higher incidence throughout the Northeast, Upper Midwest, and Mid-Atlantic (CDC, 2018b). While infection may occur at any time of year, the summer or early fall is riskiest due to increased tick exposure. Aside from living in endemic areas, individuals who have outdoor hobbies (e.g., hiking or camping), an outdoor occupation (e.g., forest rangers), or children due to increased outdoor activity, are at the highest risk. Tick size and appearance may provide helpful clinical clues for the experienced clinician to distinguish this from another arthropod or tick bite (see Table 7.2-1).

PATHOPHYSIOLOGY

- LD is a bacterial spirochete infection caused by *Borrelia burgdorferi* and transmitted through the blacklegged tick (*Ixodes scapularis* or Western variant, *Ixodes pacificus* (Fig. 7.2-5).

TABLE 7.2-1	Physical Characteristics of *Ixodes Scapularis*
Nymph	Tiny and round Often compared to a poppy seed in size and appearance
Adult	Approximately 3 mm in length Four pairs of legs Color ranging from primarily black to orange reddish depending on sex
Engorged	Large, globular-shaped abdomen The abdomen will be a light grayish-blue color

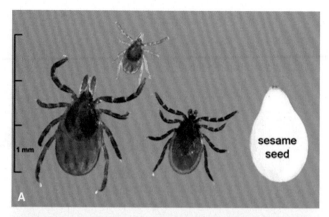

- The deer ticks' life cycle evolves from larvae, to nymphs, to adulthood. Both nymphal and adult ticks are capable of transmitting infection (see Table 7.2-1).

- Figure 7.2-6A,B shows hard ticks capable of transmitting disease in the United States, including *I. scapularis,* associated with the transmission of Lyme disease; *Dermacentor variabilis,* associated with the transmission of RMSF; and *Amblyomma americanum,* associated with the transmission of human granulocytic ehrlichiosis, tularemia, and Southern tick–associated rash illness, or STARI, which is not covered in this text.

- Feeding ticks are firmly attached to the skin (Fig. 7.2-7). If the tick is small and walking on the skin surface, it is incapable of transmitting Lyme disease.

- The presence of an engorged tick embedded in the skin or those already detached after feeding yield a higher risk of disease transmission.

- Transmission of the disease rarely occurs within the first 24 to 48 hours of attachment in nonengorged ticks (Hu, 2016).

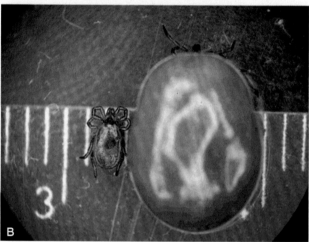

FIG. 7.2-6. **A, B:** Hard ticks that spread disease. (Bauer, S. [2009]. The Agricultural Research Service, The Research Agency of the United States Department of Agriculture.)

CLINICAL PRESENTATIONS

Skin Findings

The classic rash of Lyme disease, erythema migrans (Fig. 7.2-8), only occurs in the early stage of the disease and is described in Table 7.2-2.

Non-Skin Findings

- Symptoms can be very subtle and often attributed to a brief viral illness, never suspecting a tick-borne illness.

- Multiple organ involvement occurs in advanced cases and may affect the joints, heart, and nervous system.

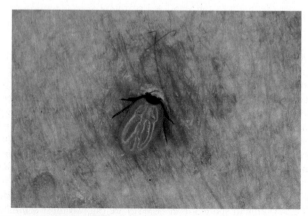

FIG. 7.2-7. Embedded, engorged deer tick.

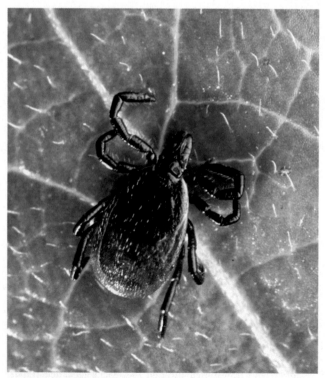

FIG. 7.2-5. Adult deer tick.

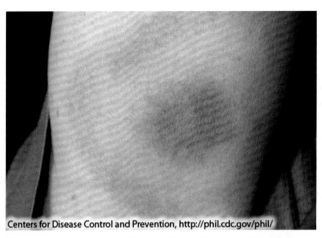

Centers for Disease Control and Prevention, http://phil.cdc.gov/phil/

FIG. 7.2-8. Erythema migrans. (Centers for Disease Control and Prevention.)

TABLE 7.2-2	Stages of Lyme Disease and Clinical Presentation	
STAGE	**ONSET**	**CLINICAL MANIFESTATIONS**
Early localized infection	3–30 days after bite	Initially erythematous papule with central punctum Erythema migrans (EM): ring-shaped, migrating, flat erythematous rash (Fig. 7.2-8) may spread beyond site of bite EM not always present Rash fades in 3–4 wk Flu-like symptoms may be experienced Excellent prognosis with treatment
Early disseminated infection	1–9 mo after tick bite	Includes cardiac, neurologic, and musculoskeletal manifestations Cardiac manifestations: pericarditis, AV node block, and mild left ventricular dysfunction Neurologic disease: meningitis, facial palsy, mild encephalitis with confusion, radiculoneuritis, mononeuritis multiplex, ataxia, and myelitis Good prognosis with appropriate treatment
Persistent/late infection	Months to years after the bite	Arthritis > neurologic manifestations Arthritic joint involvement: intermittent and persistent arthritis Chronic neuroborreliosis (Lyme-associated neurologic manifestations): rare Neurologic findings: cognitive changes, spinal pain, and distal paresthesias Post–Lyme disease syndrome: small subset of patients who experience subjective symptoms despite treatment

TABLE 7.2-3	Diagnostics in Lyme Disease
Serologic testing (Fig. 13.14)	IgM antibodies to *Borrelia burgdorferi* typically appear within 1–2 wk following clinical manifestations IgG antibodies typically appear 2–6 wk following clinical manifestations There is no indication to perform serum testing at time of bite False-positive ELISA titer levels may occur in the presence of other disease (e.g., infectious mononucleosis, RMSF, and syphilis). Prior subclinical Lyme infections may also produce false-positive results
Tick PCR testing	Routine testing of ticks for *B. burgdorferi* is not recommended since results should not direct clinical management If the tick was not attached >36 h, prophylaxis is not indicated, even if the tick tests positive for disease If the tick was attached >36 h, prophylaxis should be given as soon as possible, without awaiting results of PCR testing

Adapted from Hu, L. (2013). Evaluation of a tick bite for possible Lyme disease. In J. Mitty (Ed.), *UpToDate*.

DIFFERENTIAL DIAGNOSIS	Lyme Disease
• Other tick-borne diseases • Meningitis • Joint disorders • Dementia or delirium • Chronic fatigue syndrome or fibromyalgia	• Cellulitis • Contact dermatitis • Granuloma annulare • Heart block • Systemic lupus erythematosus

CONFIRMING THE DIAGNOSIS

Laboratory

- Laboratory testing becomes important to aid in the diagnosis of Lyme disease, especially in patients who do not present with erythema migrans, or when there is no clear history of tick bite. If serologic testing is performed, it is recommended to wait 4 to 6 weeks after the tick bite to avoid false-negative or false-positive results. Treatment should not be delayed while waiting for laboratory testing if clinical disease is suspected (see Table 7.2-3 and Fig. 7.2-9).

TREATMENT

- The pharmacologic treatment of Lyme disease depends on staging and clinical manifestations (see Table 7.2-4).
- Prophylaxis should be considered if the patient meets all the appropriate criteria described in Box 7.2-2.
- Involvement with an appropriate specialist (e.g., cardiologist, neurologist, rheumatologist, or infectious disease specialist) is recommended once the disease advances and is affecting other organ systems.
- A subset of patients may experience transient, usually self-limiting worsening during the first 24 hours of treatment, and many experience flu-like symptoms, such as fever, chills, myalgias, headache, tachycardia, or hyperventilation, described as the Jarisch–Herxheimer reaction.

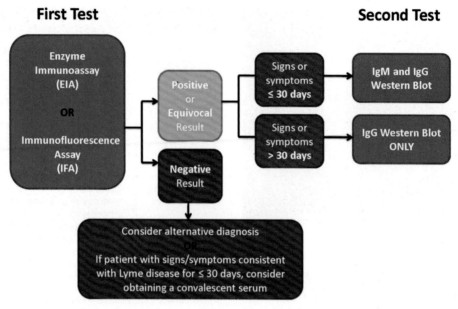

FIG. 7.2-9. Two-tiered testing for Lyme disease. (Centers for Disease Control and Prevention.)

- *Pediatrics:* Children are at increased risk for contracting Lyme disease due to increased outdoor exposure. After playing outdoors, especially in endemic areas, parents should examine children for any ticks and remove them promptly. Doxycycline, which is primarily used to treat Lyme disease, is only appropriate for use in children older than 8 years.

- *Pregnancy:* Doxycycline is not appropriate for use during pregnancy or breastfeeding. Pregnant women who contract Lyme disease should be treated promptly and thoroughly using appropriate medications, such as amoxicillin, to reduce the risk of transplacental migration of *B. burgdorferi* spirochetes to the fetus.

- *Geriatrics:* Some of the clinical manifestations of early disseminated and late/persistent infection may mimic age-related changes, such as ataxia, mild cognitive declining, or arthritis, resulting in delayed diagnosis and treatment.

MANAGEMENT AND PATIENT EDUCATION

- *Tick removal:* To avoid touching the tick, use tweezers, forceps, or gloved fingers to grasp the tick as close to the skin surface as possible, then apply constant, steady pressure pulling straight up, without twisting or jerking for 3 to 4 minutes until the tick slowly backs out (Fig. 7.2-9). Take care not to squeeze, puncture, or crush the tick. If mouthparts remain embedded, do not attempt to retrieve them; they are typically expelled spontaneously. Consumer devices are available, which safely remove ticks (e.g., tick off or tick nipper).

- Other methods of tick removal tried include petroleum jelly, dish soap, nail polish, a flame or heat source, or isopropyl alcohol; however, these methods are not generally successful. The CDC offers further patient information on their website.

TABLE 7.2-4	Pharmacologic Treatment of Early Lyme Disease

Criteria:
- Identification of deer tick (nymphal or adult)
- Tick attached ≥36 h (if time unavailable, if engorged)
- Resides in or traveled to endemic area
- It is within 72 h of tick removal
- Doxycycline is not contraindicated[a]

Early Lyme Disease

Adults: Doxycycline[a] 100 mg PO b.i.d. × 14–21 days; or amoxicillin-clavulanate 500 mg PO t.i.d. × 14–21 days; or cefuroxime axetil 500 mg PO b.i.d. × 14–21 days

Children ≥8 yr: Doxycycline 1–2 mg/kg b.i.d. × 14–21 days; amoxicillin-clavulanate 50 mg/kg PO divided t.i.d. × 14–21 days; cefuroxime axetil 30 mg/kg PO divided b.i.d. × 14–21 days

[a]Doxycycline is a relative contraindication in pregnant women and children under 8 years. The clinician should carefully weigh the risks.
Adapted from Wormser, G. P., Dattwyler, R. J., Shapiro, E. D., Halperin, J. J., Steere, A. C., Klempner, M. S., & Nadelman, R. B. (2006). IDSA Guidelines: The clinical assessment, treatment, and prevention of Lyme disease, human granulocytic anaplasmosis, and babesiosis: Clinical practice guidelines by the Infectious Diseases Society of America. *Clinical Infectious Diseases*, *43*(1), 1089–1134.

BOX 7.2-2	Prophylaxis Lyme Disease

Criteria for Prophylaxis
Identification of deer tick (nymphal or adult *Ixodes scapularis* tick)
Tick attached ≥36 hours (if time unavailable, if engorged)
Resides in or traveled to endemic area
It is within 72 hours of tick removal
Doxycycline is not contraindicated*

Prophylaxis—if all of the above criteria are met
Adults: Doxycycline* 200 mg × 1
Children >8 years: 4 mg/kg × 1 (to maximum dose of 200 mg)

*Doxycycline is contraindicated in pregnant women and children under 8 years.
Adapted from Wormser, G. P., Dattwyler, R. J., Shapiro, E. D., Halperin, J. J., Steere, A. C., Klempner, M. S., & Nadelman, R. B. (2006). IDSA guidelines: The clinical assessment, treatment, and prevention of Lyme disease, human granulocytic anaplasmosis, and babesiosis: Clinical practice guidelines by the Infectious Diseases Society of America. *Clinical Infectious Diseases*, *43*(9), 1089–1134. https://doi.org/10.1086/508667

- Adequate treatment of early Lyme disease is generally quite effective, with rare complications and overall good prognosis.

- The potential for multisystem involvement and subsequent higher risk of morbidity are associated with late-stage disease. Complications in later stages include acute and late neurologic complications, arthritic joint complications, cardiac complications, and post–Lyme disease syndrome.

- Despite appropriate treatment, patients with persistent symptoms should be considered for consultation with the appropriate specialist based on their continued symptoms (e.g., rheumatology, neurology, or cardiology).

- Discuss the general signs and symptoms of Lyme disease with patients who have experienced a tick bite, especially those in endemic areas, with instructions to notify their provider immediately with any signs or symptoms of early disease.

- Patients should be educated on disease prevention. Tick repellents (e.g., *N,N*-diethyl-meta-toluamide [DEET]) and protective clothing (e.g., long sleeves and pants tucked into socks) help prevent tick bites when outdoors. After spending time outdoors, patients should be educated to examine their skin, including the scalp, to detect and remove ticks as soon as possible (Fig. 7.2-10).

SPECIAL CONSIDERATIONS

- *Pediatrics:* Children are at increased risk for contracting Lyme disease due to increased outdoor exposure. After playing outdoors, especially in endemic areas, parents should examine children for any ticks and remove them promptly. Doxycycline, which is primarily used to treat Lyme disease, is only appropriate for use in children older than 8 years.

- *Pregnancy:* Doxycycline is not appropriate for use during pregnancy or breastfeeding. Pregnant women who contract Lyme disease should be treated promptly and thoroughly using appropriate medications, such as amoxicillin, to reduce the risk of transplacental migration of *B. burgdorferi* spirochetes to the fetus.

- *Geriatrics:* Some of the clinical manifestations of early disseminated and late/persistent infection may mimic age-related changes, such as ataxia, mild cognitive declining, or arthritis, resulting in delayed diagnosis and treatment.

CLINICAL PEARLS

- Lyme disease is an important differential diagnosis for patients presenting in the summer with flu-like symptoms and no cough.
- Lyme disease vaccine is no longer available.

ROCKY MOUNTAIN SPOTTED FEVER

RMSF is a rickettsial infection and is primarily spread by the American dog tick, Rocky Mountain wood tick, or the brown dog tick (Fig. 7.2-11). Although RMSF first got its name because of its observation in Montana, it has been reported in many areas of the United States, Canada, Central and South America. Five states account for over 60% of reported infections: Oklahoma, Tennessee, North Carolina, Arkansas, and Missouri (CDC, 2018). The highest incidence of RMSF infection occurs between late spring and early fall, when the *Dermacentor* species ticks are most active. Ticks are both a reservoir and vector for the disease, and primarily transmit the organism to their hosts through saliva while blood feeding.

PATHOPHYSIOLOGY

- RMSF is caused by *Rickettsia rickettsii*.

- Ticks must be attached for approximately 24 hours to transmit the bacteria.

- Adult ticks prefer to feed off medium-sized mammals, including pets, helping bring infected ticks into close contact with humans.

- Larvae and nymphal ticks generally prefer to feed on smaller mammals, such as rodents. Symptoms start abruptly sometime between 3 and 21 days after the bite. The classic clinical triad associated with RMSF is rash, fever, and a history of tick bite.

CLINICAL PRESENTATION
Skin Findings

- Several days after a vague fever and other nonspecific symptoms present, subtle, nonpruritic, pink macules develop on the extremities, often including the palms and soles, before moving inward toward the trunk (Fig. 7.2-12). Over the next several days, the rash may become papular, petechial, nonblanching, and red. Rocky Mountain spotless fever occurs less frequently and refers to a subset of patients who never develop the rash.

Non-Skin Findings

- Fever is a vague symptom, and because a tick bite may go unnoticed, RMSF is often a diagnostic challenge during initial disease. The earliest symptoms often are nonspecific and include headache, fever, myalgias, nausea, vomiting, and anorexia.

DIFFERENTIAL DIAGNOSIS	Rocky Mountain Spotted Fever
• Nonspecific viral or bacterial infection	• Measles (rubella or rubeola)
• Other rickettsial infections	• Dengue fever or malaria
• Meningitis	• Hepatitis
• Vasculitis and purpuric conditions	• Infectious mononucleosis
• Syphilis	• Kawasaki disease
• Bronchitis or pneumonia	

CONFIRMING THE DIAGNOSIS
Laboratory

- According to the CDC (2018), the gold standard for serologic testing at this time is the indirect immunofluorescence assay (IFA) with *R. rickettsii* antigen.

- It is important to remember that IgG and IgM levels may remain elevated for months after infection.

- Other serum laboratory testing includes complete blood count (CBC) and complete metabolic panel (CMP).

- Expected laboratory findings in RMSF include normal to low leukocytes, low platelets, elevated AST/ALT, low sodium, and elevated BUN. Clinicians living in endemic areas should possess a high degree of clinical suspicion when evaluating patients.

TREATMENT

- Treatment should be initiated immediately once the diagnosis is clinically suspected. Doxycycline is the drug of choice for the treatment of RMSF in all ages and is often trialed in patients with a suspected diagnosis of RMSF.

Tick Bite: What to Do

Ticks bites can make people sick. Below are some steps that you can take after a tick bite to reduce your chances of getting sick and how to get treatment promptly if you do get sick.

Remove the tick as soon as possible

1. Use fine-tipped tweezers to grasp the tick as close to the skin as you can.

2. Pull upward with steady, even pressure. Don't twist or jerk the tick.

3. After removing the tick, clean the bite area and your hands with rubbing alcohol or soap and water.

4. Dispose of the tick by flushing it down the toilet. If you would like to bring the tick to your healthcare provider for identification, put it in rubbing alcohol or place it in a sealed bag/container.

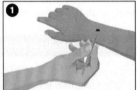 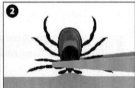 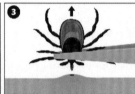 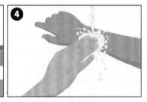

Consider calling your healthcare provider

In general, CDC does not recommend taking antibiotics after tick bites to prevent tickborne diseases. However, in certain circumstances, a single dose of doxycycline after a tick bite may lower your risk of Lyme disease. Consider talking to your healthcare provider if you live in an area where Lyme disease is common.

Watch for symptoms for 30 days

Call your healthcare provider if you get any of the following:

- Rash
- Fever
- Fatigue
- Headache
- Muscle pain
- Joint swelling and pain

Treatment for tickborne diseases should be based on symptoms, history of exposure to ticks, and in some cases, blood test results. Most tickborne diseases can be treated with a short course of antibiotics.

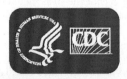

U.S. Department of
Health and Human Services
Centers for Disease
Control and Prevention

CS310465-A   August 29, 2019

FIG. 7.2-10. Tick bite: What to do: Tick check. (Centers for Disease Control and Prevention, National Center for Emerging and Zoonotic Infectious Diseases [NCEZID], Division of Vector-Borne Diseases [DVBD].)

Common questions after a tick bite

Should I get my tick tested for germs?

Some companies offer to test ticks for specific germs. CDC strongly discourages using results from these tests when deciding whether to use antibiotics after a tick bite.

- Results may not be reliable. Laboratories that test ticks are not required to meet the same quality standards as laboratories used by clinics or hospitals for patient care.

- Positive results can be misleading. Even if a tick contains a germ, it does not mean that you have been infected by that germ.

- Negative results can also be misleading. You might have been bitten unknowingly by a different infected tick.

Can I get sick from a tick that is crawling on me but has not yet attached?

Ticks must bite you to spread their germs. Once they attach to you, they will feed on your blood and can spread germs. A tick that is crawling on you but not attached could not have spread germs. However, if you have found a tick crawling on you, it's a sign there may be others: do a careful tick check.

How long does a tick need to be attached before it can spread infection?

Depending on the type of tick and germ, a tick needs to be attached to you for different amounts of time (minutes to days) to infect you with that germ.

Your risk for Lyme disease is very low if a tick has been attached for fewer than 36 hours. Check for ticks daily and remove them as soon as possible.

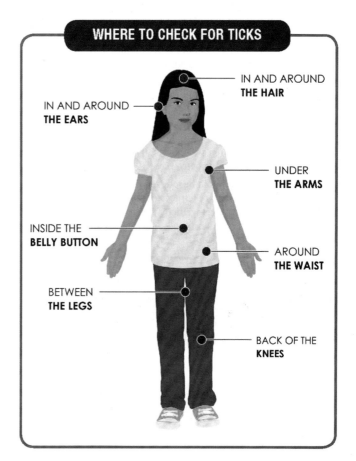

WHERE TO CHECK FOR TICKS

IN AND AROUND **THE HAIR**

IN AND AROUND **THE EARS**

UNDER **THE ARMS**

INSIDE THE **BELLY BUTTON**

AROUND **THE WAIST**

BETWEEN **THE LEGS**

BACK OF THE **KNEES**

www.cdc.gov/ticks/

FIG. 7.2-10. (*Continued*)

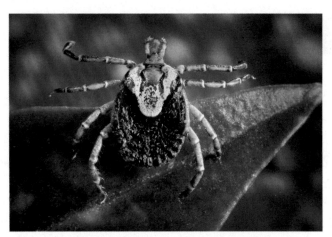

FIG. 7.2-11. Female cayenne tick, known vector for *R. rickettsia*.

- Failure to respond to therapy indicates a less likely diagnosis. Adults (except in pregnancy or lactation) should be treated with doxycycline 100 mg b.i.d. until there is no fever plus 2 to 3 additional days.
- Therapy usually takes approximately 1 week or up to 2 weeks in critically ill patients. Doxycycline may be administered intravenously for more critically ill patients unable to take oral preparation.
- *Pediatrics:* Children aged 5 to 9 years have the highest incidence of disease and develop the associated rash more rapidly than adults. Although tetracyclines are generally avoided in children under 8 years of age because of the risk of tooth staining, doxycycline remains the drug of choice for RMSF given the risks versus benefits consideration. Dosing in children weighing <100 lb (45.4 kg) is 2.2 mg/kg per dose PO or IV b.i.d. (not to exceed 100 mg per dose).
- *Pregnancy:* Pregnant patients should be referred and managed by an infectious disease specialist since tetracyclines are contraindicated during pregnancy due to teratogenicity. If considering rickettsial testing, a false-positive result may occur during pregnancy, especially during the third trimester.
- *Geriatrics:* Advanced age is a risk factor associated with increased morbidity and mortality in RMSF infection.

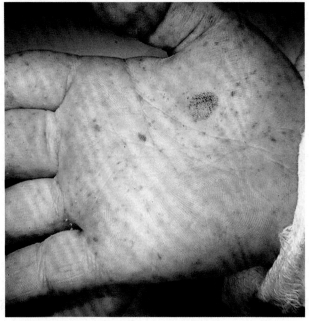

FIG. 7.2-12. RMSF palmar rash.

MANAGEMENT AND PATIENT EDUCATION

- African Americans have been linked with higher morbidity rates due to difficulty detecting the rash on darker skin, delaying diagnosis and treatment.
- Complications of RMSF are similar to other severe diseases requiring prolonged hospitalizations, including paralysis, hearing loss, movement disorders, speech disorders, bowel and bladder incontinence, amputations, and death.
- Tick bite prevention and removal information. See "Management and patient education" under Lyme Disease.

CLINICAL PEARLS

- Consider RMSF in endemic geographical areas when a patient presents with viral symptoms during summer months.
- RMSF can lead to death within 5 days if untreated; thus, early treatment (doxycycline is the drug of choice) is critical to improving health outcomes.

SPIDER BITES

Spiders are not generally aggressive arthropods and bite only in self-defense. They are carnivorous with short fangs that are often too short to penetrate human skin. Spider bites are frequently overdiagnosed by clinicians as patients present with similar appearing conditions describing a recent spider bite (e.g., methicillin-resistant *Staphylococcus aureus* infection). However, spider bites are not often noticed at the time of occurrence, making a precise diagnosis more difficult. Of all the spiders in the United States, only the black widow and brown recluse spiders are capable of producing more severe physical reactions (see Box 7.2-3).

BLACK WIDOW SPIDER

The black widow spider, or *Latrodectus mactans,* is a female spider that attained its name because it attacks and consumes male partners after mating. Although there are several other widow spiders throughout the world, this section will focus on the black widow spider as it is the most common one seen in the United States.

- Black widow spiders are black, shiny, and have a fat abdomen that resembles a grape.

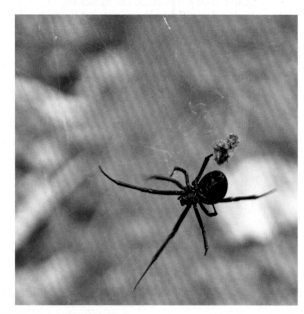

FIG. 7.2-13. Black widow spider.

BOX 7.2-3 How to Rule Out a Brown Recluse Spider Bite Diagnosis

- There is typically a single bite, **not multiples.**
- **No history** of the spider being disturbed, such as cleaning out boxes in an attic, makes diagnosis unlikely.
- Bites occur during the April to October time frame (in the United States), **not in other months.**
- Central lesion of brown recluse bite is usually white, purple, or black, **not red.**
- Lesions are flat, or even depressed, **not elevated.**
- Most bites are healed by 3 months, **not chronic.**
- Most bites are less than 10 cm, **not larger** (any larger ulcerated lesion suggests the diagnosis of pyoderma gangrenosum).
- Ulceration occurs after 7–14 days, **not earlier.**
- Bites do not lead to edema, except above the neck and on the feet; **no swelling.**
- A small vesicle may be seen at site of bite; **not purulent.**

Adapted from Stoecker, W. V., Vetter, R. S., & Dyer, J. A. (2017). NOT RECLUSE-A mnemonic device to avoid false diagnoses of brown recluse spider bites. *JAMA Dermatology, 153*(5), 377–378.

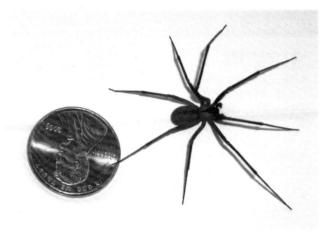

FIG. 7.2-14. Brown recluse spider.

- They have red hourglass-shaped markings ranging from one to two red triangles, spots, or irregular blotches on the ventral surface of their abdomen (Fig. 7.2-13).
- Adult females can grow up to 3 to 4 cm long and contain powerful neurotoxic venom.
- Although more prevalent in the South, black widows can be found throughout the United States and generally dwell in garages, barns, or outdoors around homes in garden equipment, tools, or woodpiles. They generally only migrate indoors during cold weather or if attracted by other insect infestations in the home.
- Venom from the black widow spider contains some of the most potent neurotoxins. Each individual reacts to the toxin differently from localized to a severe systemic reaction.

BROWN RECLUSE SPIDER

Brown recluse spiders, or *Loxosceles reclusa,* are typically difficult to identify. Common nicknames of the brown recluse include the fiddle-back spider or violin spider, because of the violin-patterned markings found on the dorsum of some. They range from cream colored to dark brown or blackish gray and from 6 to 20 mm in size (Fig. 7.2-14).

- Generally limited to the Midwestern, Southern, and Western United States, they often are encountered in homes since they populate and thrive around humans.
- Brown recluse spiders often inhabit dark, dry, and undisturbed areas such as closets, garages, woodpiles, and sheds. Human contact generally occurs when these areas are disturbed or the spiders feel threatened by someone putting on clothing where the spider is hiding.
- The brown recluse spider venom contains enzymes that cause localized tissue necrosis. It also triggers immune responses that can either be localized or, in some cases, result in anaphylaxis.
- Patients present reporting a recent history of doing yard work, spending time outdoors, cleaning their garage, or other activities which may account for their exposure.
- The diagnosis is often made clinically and is only considered definitive if the patient observed a spider inflicting the bite, and that spider was collected and identified by an expert

entomologist (Vetter, 2018). Differential diagnoses should always be entertained in the absence of definitive observation.

DIFFERENTIAL DIAGNOSIS	Black Widow and Brown Recluse Spider Bites
Black Widow Spider Bite	*Brown Recluse Spider Bite*
• Rabies	• Trauma
• Tetanus	• Infection (strep, staphl, or fungal)
• Myocardial ischemia or infarction	• CA-MRSA
• Acute surgical abdomen	• Other spider or insect bites
• Necrotizing fasciitis	• Pyoderma gangrenosum
	• Ulcers associated with arterial or venous insufficiency

CLINICAL PRESENTATION

See Table 7.2-5.

CONFIRMING THE DIAGNOSIS

Laboratory testing is nonspecific and yields little assistance in formulating the diagnosis. Abnormal laboratory results may include abnormal liver enzymes, elevated white blood cell count, increased serum creatine phosphokinase, and glucose levels (Vetter, 2018).

Biopsy

- If a skin biopsy or hair sample is attained at the site of the bite up to 3 to 4 days after the bite, the *Loxosceles* venom may be detected through various methods of testing not widely available at this time (Isbister & Fan, 2011).

TREATMENT

- Any patient experiencing systemic manifestations should be evaluated in an emergency department setting and may require intravenous hydration, steroids, and hospitalization.
- Oral analgesics may be administered to help control pain.
- Administer a tetanus booster vaccination if indicated.

MANAGEMENT AND PATIENT EDUCATION

- Conservative treatment generally is recommended for all spider bites as most are mild and rarely progress to systemic involvement.

TABLE 7.2-5	Clinical Presentation Black Widow and Brown Recluse Spider Bites
Black Widow Spider *Skin Findings:* • Bites can range from asymptomatic to a sharp, stinging sensation and typically occur on the extremities, most often the lower extremities. • Blanched, circular macules with a central punctum. • Peripheral erythema, whereas other bites present with more edema and induration (Fig. 7.2-15). • Unlike bites of the brown recluse, these bites do not become necrotic and rarely develop secondary infections. *Systemic Manifestations* • Between 20 min and 2 h after the bite, systemic manifestations begin to develop. • Symptoms are often pronounced and may include headache, nausea, anxiety, tachypnea, localized or extensive diaphoresis, painful muscle spasms, and severe abdominal pain with abdominal wall rigidity. • Systemic progression of black widow spider bites will require hospitalization.	**Brown Recluse Spider** *Skin Findings:* • Minor, erythematous plaque occasionally with two puncture marks on the trunk, upper extremities, or thighs, and rarely on the face and hands (Fig. 7.2-13). • Central pallor develops in more severe bites after several hours along with itchiness and pain. • After a few days, the bite expands to an enlarging, necrotic ulcer with eschar measuring several centimeters. • Sloughing of tissue typically stops after 10 days and tends to heal by secondary intention with rare scarring (Fig. 7.2-16). *Systemic Manifestations* • Generalized symptoms develop over several days. • Nausea and vomiting, rash, fever, myalgias, and arthralgias may occur. Rarely hemolysis, disseminated intravascular coagulation, thrombocytopenia, and even death can result. • Systemic progression of brown recluse spider bites will require hospital evaluation.

- Localized wound care and first-aid treatment are important including irrigation, ice, elevation, and immobilization.
- Cold compresses intermittently for 72 hours.
- Bites should be monitored for the development of necrosis and secondary bacterial infection.

BLACK WIDOW SPIDER BITE

- Black widow antivenins are available in endemic areas. Indications to use antivenin may include patients' age, pregnancy, underlying cardiac disease, severe pain, and muscle spasms despite other treatment, hemodynamic instability, or respiratory distress.
- Complications of the black widow bite may include secondary bacterial infection, hematuria, compartment syndrome, rhabdomyolysis, toxic epidermal necrolysis, cardiomyopathy, pulmonary edema, priapism, and intestinal ileus. Death is uncommon.

  See Fig. 7.2-15.

BROWN RECLUSE BITE

- Oral antibiotics are often used initially but may not be effective unless there is suspicion of cellulitis (see Section 6.2).

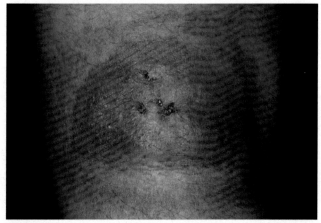

FIG. 7.2-15. Black widow spider bite.

- Dapsone is an antileukocytic antibiotic sometimes administered in brown recluse bites to prevent or decrease necrosis in wounds with a progressing, dusky center. This is not FDA approved. Check G6PD before administering.
- Antivenin is not widely available in the United States, but often prescribed for more severe variants of recluse spider bites found in South America.
- Surgical debridement should be considered once the eschar is clearly demarcated (leathery black tissue), to hasten wound healing. This occurs in 2 to 4 weeks. Consultation with a plastic surgeon or wound specialist may be necessary since patients with large, complicated wounds or delayed wound healing may require skin grafting or other interventions.
- Any patient experiencing systemic manifestations should be evaluated in an emergency department setting and may require intravenous hydration, steroids, and hospitalization.
- Patients should be followed daily after the brown recluse spider bite for wound checks until the wound has stabilized and begins to improve.
- Wound care instructions should be provided to any patient with these spider bites. The signs and symptoms of secondary wound infection and progressive skin necrosis should also be discussed. Patients who have received antivenin should be informed of the signs of serum sickness, which may develop several weeks after administration, and include rash, malaise, fever, and arthralgias.
- Bite prevention includes insecticides and traps administered by pest control services, shaking out clothing and shoes before use, wearing gloves and long sleeves while working outdoors.
- Brown recluse bites occurring during pregnancy are not associated with increased adverse risks to the mother or fetus.

  See Fig. 7.2-16.

> **CLINICAL PEARL**
>
> ▪ Brown recluse bites are painful, with localized lymphangitis, necrosis, and cellulitis, whereas black widow bites do not become necrotic and rarely develop secondary infection. They typically appear as blanched, circular macules with a central punctum and peripheral erythema.

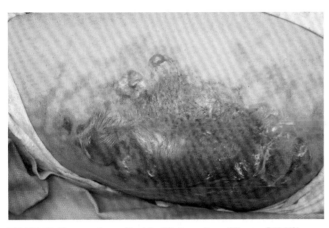

FIG. 7.2-16. Brown recluse spider bite. (Photo courtesy of Thomas P. Habif.)

DOG, CAT, AND HUMAN BITES

The most commonly encountered bite injuries are from dogs and cats. Dog bites account for 80% to 90% of all animal bites, followed by cat bites (5% to 15%) and human bites (4% to 23%) (Aziz et al., 2015). Although human bites occur less frequently than animal bites, they often harbor more pathogens than do animals and have a higher incidence of serious infections and complications.

- *Low-risk wounds* are shallow, nonpuncture wounds and generally can be monitored for the development of infection. Minor-appearing superficial bites may occlude crush or deep-seated injuries, such as lacerated tendons or vasculature, osseous or joint involvement, or organ injuries therefore careful examination is imperative.
- *Higher-risk wounds* such as cat bites, massive crush injuries, bites involving the hand, deep wounds, or those occurring in immunosuppressed individuals should be evaluated and treated. See Treatment below.

PATHOPHYSIOLOGY

Both aerobic and anaerobic bacteria are involved in dog and cat bites, in addition to a patient's own skin flora. The most common pathogen involved in both dog and cat bites is *Pasteurella* species, followed by *Staphylococci* and *Streptococci* (Aziz et al., 2015). Rabies infection in dogs is common in underdeveloped nations, but generally is not problematic in the United States due to strict vaccination laws. Because of their long, sharp, and deeply piercing teeth, cat bites are more frequently associated with anaerobic bacteria, such as *Fusobacterium, Porphyromonas, Prevotella,* and *Bacteroides.*

Aerobic and anaerobic bacteria also infect human bite wounds and are typically pathogens found in oral and skin flora, including *Eikenella corrodens* (gram-negative anaerobe), group A *Streptococcus* (aerobic gram-positive cocci), and *Haemophilus* species.

CLINICAL PRESENTATION
Dog Bites
Skin Findings

- Crush and avulsion injuries are the most commonly seen injuries associated with dog bites, due to their strong jaws and rounded teeth.
- The head and neck are common sites of injury in infants and young children.

- Extremities, particularly the dominant hand, are the most frequent sites in adults.

Non-Skin Findings

- Dog bites may range from minor wounds to quite severe and potentially fatal injuries.
- Fatalities, although rare, typically involve uncontrolled infection in deep lacerated and puncture wounds, and internal organ crush injuries affecting deeper structures such as nerves, tendons, bone, muscles, and vasculature.

Cat Bites
Skin Findings

- The upper extremities are the primary location of cat bites.
- The anatomical design of a cat's sharp and slender teeth frequently produces deep puncture wounds.
- For information on cat scratches, please refer to Section 6.3 "cat-scratch fever."

Non-Skin Findings

- Due to the nature of cat bites, damage to underlying structures can occur, including bone or joint infection.

Human Bites
Skin Findings

- The most common human bites observed are clenched-fist injuries or "fight bites."
- Bites involving the hand are at particularly high risk for developing cellulitis.
- Other bites seen are chomping injuries, which tend to be closed injuries; bites involving the ears or nose, which may involve loss of tissue and structure; and puncture wounds.
- Often an erythematous arcuate or oval-shaped area with or without bruising is observed at the site of injury.

Non-Skin Findings

- Human bites involving the hand are at greater risk for joint sepsis or osteomyelitis because of the proximity to underlying structures.

DIFFERENTIAL DIAGNOSIS   Bites

- Patients are often able to provide an appropriate history.
- Varying causative bacterial agents/infections should be considered when providing empirical prophylaxis or treating subsequent bacterial infection.

CONFIRMING THE DIAGNOSIS
Laboratory

- Cultures are generally of limited value after acute injury, but may help if the patient is not responding to treatment with broad-spectrum antibiotics after several days to weeks.
- Radiographic evaluation should be considered, especially in bites involving underlying joints or bones, to ensure there are no fractures or joint space penetration.
- CT scans may be necessary for more severe bites that may involve underlying organs, such as those occurring in young children.

TREATMENT

- Cleaning the site with high-pressure saline irrigation after injury greatly reduces bacterial count and is the cornerstone of wound management. Irrigation can be achieved by using a 10-mL syringe with an 18-G angiocatheter attached, taking care to avoid further trauma from accidental injection.

- Debridement of devitalized tissue and clots also may help prevent infection and promote quicker healing, taking care not to debride healthy underlying tissue.

- Surgical wound closure after an acute bite is controversial (Aziz et al., 2015).

- Primary wound closure is not recommended when:

  - wounds are high-risk (i.e., immunocompromised or asplenic; deep injuries extending to bone, joint, or tendons; facial, hand, or genital involvement; or moderate to severe puncture wounds) and

  - greater than 8 to 12 hours since injury;

  - signs of infection are present;

  - or hand wounds (should seek hand surgeon consult) (Bula-Rudas & Olcott, 2018).

Antibiotics

- Prophylactic administration of broad-spectrum antibiotics is controversial. Low-risk wounds do not warrant prophylactic antibiotic administration and can be monitored for the development of infection.

- Higher-risk wounds (cat bites, massive crush injuries, bites involving the hand, deep wounds, or those occurring in immunosuppressed individuals, should receive broad-spectrum antibiotic prophylaxis. If the patient still presents with an infected wound after 3 to 5 days of prophylactic antibiotics, a full 10-day course (or longer) of antibiotics is indicated (see Table 7.2-6).

- First-line therapy for a human bite wound also is amoxicillin-clavulanate. Wound cultures generally are not performed in acute bite wounds as they do not yield helpful treatment information;

however, cultures should be considered if patients do not respond to prescribed antibiotic therapy.

Immunization

- Tetanus immunoglobulin or vaccine booster should be considered based on the patient's vaccination history. Antirabies treatment may still be considered if the animal's rabies status cannot be confirmed. This treatment is generally reserved for wild animals such as bats, raccoons, or skunks, and done in consultation with the local Department of Public Health.

MANAGEMENT AND PATIENT EDUCATION

- A thorough examination, including a motor-sensory evaluation, is a vital step in the management of bite victims to determine the extent of the injury, appropriate diagnostics, and subsequent management must be tailored for each situation.

- High-risk wounds such as deep puncture wounds, underlying fractures or nerve damage, loss of tissue, or cosmetically sensitive areas necessitate specialty referral.

- Bite wounds involving the hand resulting in decreased or loss function will require evaluation by a hand surgeon.

- Minor wounds managed in the primary care setting should be evaluated again 24 to 48 hours after the initial injury.

- Patients should be instructed to perform general wound care and monitor for signs and symptoms of infection, including erythema, edema, fluctuance, and purulent drainage; development of these should be reported promptly to initiate appropriate antibiotic treatment.

- Local public health departments should be notified of all animal bites when there is a question of rabies exposure for guidance with prophylaxis. Law enforcement and animal control may also become involved for safety.

SPECIAL CONSIDERATIONS

- *Pediatrics:* Animal bites resulting in death are more prevalent in infants and small children. Dog bites account for 20 to 35 people annually in the United States, with nearly 29% attributed to pit bull breeds (Aziz et al., 2015). Young children often and unknowingly may provoke the animal with their uninhibited behavior, resulting in bites.

- *Pregnancy:* There are no special considerations aside from limited antibiotic treatment options during pregnancy.

- *Geriatrics and Immunocompromise:* Immunocompromised patients, such as those with HIV, asplenia, kidney or hepatic disease, or the elderly, are at higher risk for serious, life-threatening infection after an animal bite due to compromised immunity.

- Hepatitis B and HIV prophylaxis should be considered when treating human bite wounds.

TABLE 7.2-6	Treatment Recommendations for Dog, Cat and Human Bites	
TYPE OF BITE	**FIRST-LINE TREATMENT**	**ALTERNATIVES**
Dog bites	Amoxicillin-clavulanate §B	Doxycycline (§D/±) Clindamycin + fluoroquinolones (§C) Clindamycin + trimethoprim-sulfamethoxazole (§D)
Cat bites	Amoxicillin-clavulanate §B	Doxycycline (§D/±) Clindamycin + trimethoprim-sulfamethoxazole (§D) Cefuroxime (§B)
Human bites	Amoxicillin-clavulanate §B	Clindamycin + fluoroquinolones (§C) Clindamycin + trimethoprim-sulfamethoxazole (§D) Penicillin + first-generation cephalosporin (§B)

§B, pregnancy category B; §C, pregnancy category C; §D, pregnancy category D; ±, not appropriate in pediatrics under age 8.

CLINICAL PEARLS

- Dog bites often do not require prophylaxis, whereas cat bites often do. All immunocompromised patients should receive prophylaxis.
- Hand bites have high risk of septic arthritis and osteomyelitis.
- It is imperative to ensure that there is no underlying anatomical structural damage, which may require surgery.

Aquatic Dermatoses

Melissa E. Cyr

In This Chapter

- Jellyfish Stings
- Coral Stings
- Sea Urchin Stings
- Seabather's Eruption
- Swimmer's Itch
- Cutaneous Larva Migrans

Jellyfish Stings

Jellyfish have a bell-shaped body with long tentacles that grow up to 100 ft. There are over 10,000 species, of which about 100 are dangerous to humans, most notably the Australian box (Northern Australia), Portuguese man of war (Pacific, Atlantic, and Indian Oceans), and Irukandji jellyfish (Australia) (Cegolon et al., 2013). Although jellyfish are found worldwide, they more often reside in warm calm seawater, harbors, or sandy beaches and result in an estimated 150 million stings annually (Cegolon et al., 2013). Stings occur when contact with the tentacles occur, releasing nematocysts that discharge proteinaceous neurotoxins into the skin.

CLINICAL PRESENTATIONS

Skin Findings

- Clinical findings vary based on jellyfish type and sting severity.
- Erythematous, urticarial, or hemorrhagic streaks in whiplike patterns (Fig. 7.3-1).
- Pruritus, wheals, red papules and patches, and edema may develop in the affected area.
- Later, bullous formation may occur followed by wound necrosis and scarring.

Non-Skin Findings

- Paresthesias and severe pain accompanies the injury, which is sometimes so extreme that it leads to loss of consciousness in the victim and their inability to return safely to the shore.
- Sweating, agitation, myalgias, muscle cramping and spasms, nausea, and vomiting may occur, but generally subside within a few hours following treatment.
- Symptoms may progress to ventricular arrhythmias, cardiac arrest, neurogenic shock, respiratory arrest, and death. Children are more vulnerable to the effects of certain jellyfish venoms.

DIFFERENTIAL DIAGNOSIS   Jellyfish Stings

- Stingray injury
- Venomous fish injury (e.g., sea urchins, lionfish, cone shells)
- Shellfish poisoning
- Swimmer's itch
- Coral sting
- Seabather's eruptions
- Bites (e.g., alligator, crocodile, shark)

CONFIRMING THE DIAGNOSIS

- Diagnosis is primarily established based on one's history and clinical findings.

TREATMENT

- Topical steroids or oral antihistamines may be beneficial for associated pruritus.
- To reduce the spread of the toxic venom, apply ice to the site and avoid moving or rubbing the affected area immediately post injury.
- Some authors suggest pain relief with vinegar rinses, urinating on or rinsing the affected area with fresh water or alcohol, but conflicting reports state this may further release nematocyst toxins into the surrounding tissue after certain jellyfish stings (Cegolon et al., 2013).
- Severe associated pain may be treated with opioids (fentanyl or morphine) and lidocaine. Hospital management of other symptoms may be indicated (e.g., muscle spasms, respiratory arrest, etc.).
- Portuguese man-of-war stings necessitate saltwater rinses, while Australian box jellyfish stings should be rinsed liberally with saltwater, saline, or hot water.

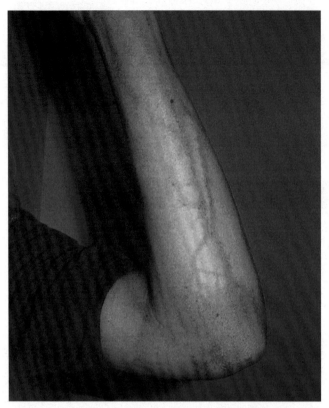

FIG. 7.3-1. Portuguese man 'o' war sting. Note the linear shape of the lesions. The sting of the Portuguese man of war is more painful than a common jellyfish sting. (Used with permission from Goodheart, H. P. [2015]. *Goodheart's photoguide of common skin disorders* [4th ed.]. Wolters Kluwer Health.)

MANAGEMENT AND PATIENT EDUCATION

- Seek immediate emergency medical attention; early treatment reduces morbidity and mortality risk. Antivenin injections are available in endemic areas for box jellyfish stings.

- Nematocysts and tentacles should be removed from the skin using gloves, forceps, and razor blades.

- Severe associated pain may be treated with opioids (fentanyl or morphine) and lidocaine. Hospital management of other symptoms may be indicated (e.g., muscle spasms, respiratory arrest, etc.).

CLINICAL PEARLS

- Consider the geographic area and endemic species where injury took place.
- Cross-hatched "tentacle prints" suggest a box jellyfish sting, whereas systemic manifestations such as hypertension, myalgias, and vomiting suggest Irukandji syndrome (Hornbeak & Auerbach, 2017).

CORAL STINGS

Coral injuries are common and may result in cutaneous cuts, abrasions, or stings. Like jellyfish or sea urchins, fire coral subtypes contain nematocysts that result in painful stings and envenomation that may lead to systemic manifestations. Fire corals are similar to hard coral and are located in shallow tropical oceans.

Soft corals also have stinging tentacles that may contain more potent toxins.

CLINICAL PRESENTATIONS

Skin Findings

- Coral abrasions or scratches on exposed skin are at risk for secondary infection. Fire coral exposure results in sharp, immediate pain and urticaria that may develop into petechial or ulcerated lesions (Hornbeak & Auerbach, 2017).

- Soft coral also results in a sharp, painful lesion with central pallor, erythema, and petechial changes that may progress to bulla formation and necrosis.

Non-Skin Findings

- Systemic manifestations of fire coral envenomation may occur and include headache, fever, chills, nausea, vomiting, malaise, conjunctivitis, and uveitis, while soft coral systemic symptoms are similar, excluding ocular symptoms, and may instead include syncope and muscle spasms (Hornbeak & Auerbach, 2017).

- Fire coral pain begins to subside after about 90 minutes, whereas soft coral envenomation symptoms generally last up to 48 hours.

DIFFERENTIAL DIAGNOSIS   Coral Stings

- Trauma from sharp rocks
- Stingray injury
- Venomous fish injury (e.g., lionfish, cone shells)
- Other marine stings (e.g., jellyfish, sea cucumber, or starfish)

CONFIRMING THE DIAGNOSIS

- Diagnosis is primarily established based on history and clinical findings.

TREATMENT

- Topical steroids or oral antihistamines may be administered for associated pruritus as needed. More severe reactions may warrant a taper with oral corticosteroids.

- If signs of infection develop, treat with topical or oral antibiotics as indicated.

- A tetanus booster should be administered if indicated.

MANAGEMENT AND PATIENT EDUCATION

- Coral injuries should be cleaned thoroughly to ensure the removal of all debris and remove any nematocysts. Current literature supports rinsing the wound with seawater (or saline) followed by prolonged rinsing with hot water (113°F or 45°C) (Hornbeak & Auerbach, 2017).

- Avoid vinegar or urine treatments as these may worsen the toxin release.

- Monitor wound for and report any signs of infection during healing.

- Consider the geographic area and what may be endemic to where the injury took place.

SEA URCHIN STINGS

Sea urchins are nonaggressive echinoderms found in saltwater around the world. Stings are common and commonly result when the sea urchin inadvertently is stepped on.

Skin irritation results from an immune response to the embedded hollow spines that contain venomous poisons, with greater mortality based on dose–response (>15 spines having poorer outcomes) and longer time until treatment receipt (Schwartz et al., 2019). Those at greatest risk for injury include snorkelers, divers, and fishermen.

CLINICAL PRESENTATIONS

Skin Findings

- Findings include localized pain, erythema, edema, and a temporary blue-black skin staining.
- Cutaneous granulomas occur in 40% to 50% of patients with retained spines, develop roughly 2 weeks post injury, and present as firm hypopigmented to pink nodules on the involved area (Schwartz et al., 2019) (Fig. 7.3-2).
- Rarely, the injured skin will develop a secondary infection.

Non-Skin Findings

- Acutely, myalgias or paresthesias may occur in response to toxin exposure. Late complications of retained sea urchin spines include degenerative arthritis, synovitis or tenosynovitis, and osteomyelitis.
- The development of systemic manifestations varies based on the subtype, toxin exposure dose, and time until treatment, but severe reactions may include hypotension, syncope, respiratory distress, and death.

DIFFERENTIAL DIAGNOSIS Sea Urchin Stings
• Trauma from sharp rocks
• Stingray injury
• Venomous fish injury (e.g., lionfish, cone shells)
• Other marine stings (e.g., jellyfish, sea cucumber, or starfish)
• Shellfish poisoning
• Other rheumatologic or infectious diseases (e.g., sarcoidosis, septic arthritis)

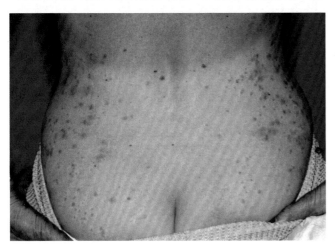

FIG. 7.3-2. Seabather's eruption. Usually occurs beneath the bathing or dive suit. (Used with permission from Goodheart, H. P. [2015]. *Goodheart's photoguide of common skin disorders* [4th ed.]. Wolters Kluwer Health.)

CONFIRMING THE DIAGNOSIS

Laboratory

- Systemic signs of infection would warrant a CBC and blood cultures.
- If bone or joint involvement is suspected, imaging studies to identify retained spines are warranted (acutely: x-ray and ultrasound, delayed: magnetic resonance imaging [MRI]).

TREATMENT

- A tetanus booster should be considered when indicated. Monitor the injured area for signs of secondary infection and treat accordingly with appropriate antibiotics should this develop.
- Immediate management includes surgical spine removal, irrigation of the affected area with hot water (110° to 115°F or 43° to 46°C), then a prolonged hot water immersion for as long as tolerable (30 to 90 minutes) to inactivate the toxins (Schwartz et al., 2019).

MANAGEMENT AND PATIENT EDUCATION

- Any signs of systemic involvement would necessitate immediate transfer to the hospital.
- Patients should be advised to watch for signs of retained spines which may not appear for several weeks.

> **CLINICAL PEARL**
>
> ■ Multiple erratic puncture wounds with or without blue-black discoloration suggest sea urchin sting (Hornbeak & Auerbach, 2017).

SEABATHER'S ERUPTION

Seabather's eruption is a *bathing suit–distributed* hypersensitivity reaction. First discovered in Florida where it was nicknamed "pica-pica" (Spanish for itchy-itchy stinging). Snorkelers, surfers, swimmers, children, or scuba divers are more likely to be affected, and it is more often encountered during warm summer months, or in tropical or subtropical geographic areas.

PATHOPHYSIOLOGY

Seabather's eruption is caused by tiny larval nematocysts of certain jellyfish and sea anemones.

The larvae become trapped under the bathing suit where pressure from the suit or rinsing with hypotonic fresh water after swimming results in toxin release into the skin and subsequent dermatitis (Rademaker, 2014). Stinging may continue up to weeks after exposure.

CLINICAL PRESENTATIONS

Skin Findings

- A tingling sensation often is experienced while still in the water; over several hours, this progresses into severe and sometimes painful pruritus and dermatitis in a bathing suit distribution that may last several weeks. Small, red papules consistent with bug bites develop in affected areas (Fig. 7.3-2).

Non-Skin Findings

- A subset of patients will experience systemic manifestations, such as headache, malaise, fever, chills, burning eyes, dysuria, nausea, or vomiting.

- Swimmer's itch
- Seaweed dermatitis
- Sand fly bites
- Allergic contact dermatitis
- Folliculitis
- Arthropod bites
- Coral dermatitis

CONFIRMING THE DIAGNOSIS

- Diagnosis is primarily established based on history and clinical findings.

TREATMENT

- A 14-day oral corticosteroid taper should be considered for the treatment of severe systemic manifestations.
- Topical steroids should be applied two to three times daily for 14 days.
- Other supportive treatments include ice packs or nonsteroidal anti-inflammatories for discomfort; calamine, lidocaine, or menthol-containing lotions to soothe skin; and oral antihistamines to reduce pruritus and the systemic reaction to toxins.

MANAGEMENT AND PATIENT EDUCATION

- Remove bathing suit and rinse affected areas with seawater or hypertonic saline. Diluted vinegar or rubbing alcohol may help neutralize toxins.
- Although tight wetsuits may provide some skin barrier, avoidance of infested ocean water is the only true means of prevention. If exposure is suspected, remove the bathing suit as soon as able and rinse affected areas with seawater or hypertonic saline. Avoid mechanical pressure or rubbing affected areas as these will promote toxin release.
- Machine wash affected clothing using hot water and machine dry to remove larvae.

SWIMMER'S ITCH

Swimmer's itch, sometimes referred to as "cercarial dermatitis," "duck itch," or "sea lice" is contracted in fresh water (see Figs. 7.3-3 and 7.3-4).

PATHOPHYSIOLOGY

- This is a reaction to an aquatic parasite infestation caused by infected birds, aquatic snails, or mammals (e.g., beavers) (CDC, 2018a) (see Table 7.3-1).
- Infestation may occur after exposure in fresh or seawater, particularly lakes, ponds, or lagoons.
- After larvae or flatworms dry on the affected skin, cercariae penetrate the human host's epidermis then die, causing a reactive dermatitis.
- It is more common during summer months when warmer temperatures encourage snail breeding, migratory birds are present, and people more often are swimming.

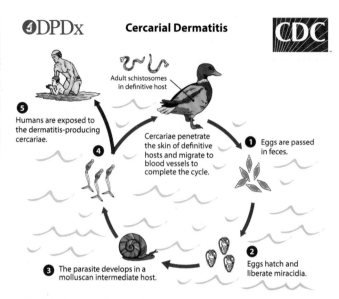

FIG. 7.3-3. Cercarial life cycle. (Centers for Disease Control and Prevention.)

CLINICAL PRESENTATIONS

Skin Findings

- Similar to seabather's eruption, a tingling sensation will develop in affected areas, which will progress into intense pruritus, burning, and bug bite–like red papules. Wheals and vesicles may develop 24 to 48 hours post exposure and then transition into a papular dermatitis that may last weeks.

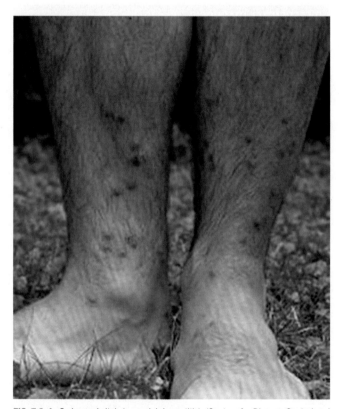

FIG. 7.3-4. Swimmer's itch (cercarial dermatitis). (Centers for Disease Control and Prevention.)

TABLE 7.3-1	Swimmer's Itch Versus Seabather's Eruption	
SEABATHER'S ERUPTION		**SWIMMER'S ITCH**
Saltwater		Freshwater
Swimsuit/diving suit distribution		Uncovered skin
Mexico, Caribbean, Eastern US coastline		Northern US and Canada
Caused by larval jellyfish and sea anemone nematocysts		Caused by aquatic parasite schistosomes from birds, snails, and aquatic mammals (e.g., beavers)

Adapted from Habif, T. (2015). Clinical dermatology: A color guide to diagnosis and therapy.

DIFFERENTIAL DIAGNOSIS   Swimmer's Itch

- Seabather's eruption
- Seaweed dermatitis
- Sand fly bites
- Allergic contact dermatitis
- Coral dermatitis

CONFIRMING THE DIAGNOSIS

- Diagnosis is primarily established based on history and clinical findings.

TREATMENT

- Most cases of swimmer's itch do not require medical attention. After exposure, ensure to rinse the affected area with isopropyl alcohol.
- Topical steroids may be applied as needed
- Consider an oral corticosteroid taper with an expansive or robust rash.
- Other supportive treatments include cool compresses; calamine, lidocaine, or menthol-containing lotions or oatmeal baths to soothe skin; and oral antihistamines to reduce pruritus.
- Secondary infections may develop from scratching and can be treated accordingly with appropriate antibiotics.

MANAGEMENT AND PATIENT EDUCATION

- Similar to a plant contact allergy, one's first exposure to cercariae may not elicit a cutaneous reaction, but a mounting immune response will result in dermatitis with subsequent exposures.
- Cercariae more often are found in shallow water.
- Discourage feeding birds near areas where people are swimming.

CUTANEOUS LARVA MIGRANS

Cutaneous larva migrans (CLM), also known as "creeping eruption," is a common parasitic infection. Incidence rates are greater in tropical or subtropical geographic areas.

PATHOPHYSIOLOGY

- This condition is caused by varying forms of hookworms that inhabit dogs, cats, and other animals, and is transmitted via animal feces.

- Although patients of all ages, sexes, and races can be affected, certain groups who have exposure to warm, damp, infected soil are at higher risk (e.g., beachgoers, farmers, gardeners, and children who play in sandpits).
- Humans become infected with the larvae after walking barefoot on soil or sandy beaches contaminated with parasitic hookworm eggs.
- The initial site of penetration generally goes unnoticed, or the patient may experience a tingling sensation. These larvae then migrate under the skin's surface, and after a few days to months, result in red, serpiginous, subepidermal lines.

CLINICAL PRESENTATION

Skin Findings

- Affected areas will have a 2- to 3-mm wide, red, serpiginous, linear skin-colored to pink raised tracks that advance a few millimeters daily, and may stretch up to 3 to 4 cm from the penetration site (Fig. 7.3-5).

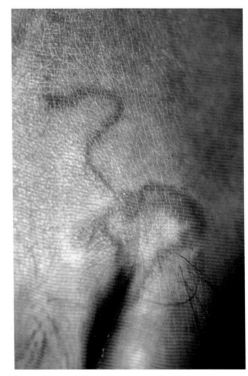

FIG. 7.3-5. Cutaneous larva migrans. This hookworm winds a serpiginous trail on the dorsal foot.

- Commonly involved areas include the feet, knees, hands, thighs, and buttocks, and infected skin is intensely pruritic.

Non-Skin Findings

- Transient elevated liver function tests (LFTs), headaches.

DIFFERENTIAL DIAGNOSIS   Cutaneous Larva Migrans

- Scabies
- Allergic contact dermatitis
- Other larva infections (larva currens)
- Phytophotodermatitis
- Erythema chronicum migrans
- Dermatophyte infection

CONFIRMING THE DIAGNOSIS

Laboratory

Biopsy

- CLM is diagnosed primarily on history and clinical presentation; rarely will the parasite be seen on pathology.

TREATMENT

- Albendazole 200 mg b.i.d. × 7 days has been reported effective (Veraldi et al., 2012).
- Several other oral antihelminthic agents also are available (e.g., ivermectin, thiabendazole) with varying degrees of treatment success (Kincaid et al., 2015).
- Topical antihelminthic agents, particularly topical thiabendazole, are effective for localized disease (applied t.i.d. for at least 10 days).
- Liquid nitrogen cryotherapy may also be used as a nonpharmacologic therapy option.
- Topical corticosteroids or antihistamines may be used if necessary for interim relief of pruritus.

MANAGEMENT AND PATIENT EDUCATION

- CLM often is a self-limiting condition; in most cases, hookworm larvae die without treatment in 4 to 8 weeks.
- Travel history is important when faced with a history of exposure in the presence of a serpiginous, pruritic rash. Patients in the United States often contract CLM through tropical overseas travel.
- Prevention is key to avoiding or decreasing exposure (e.g., wearing sandals/protective footwear, reducing contact with moist soil and sand).

READINGS AND REFERENCES

Arenas, R., Torres-Guerrero, E., Quintanilla-Cedillo, M. R., & Ruiz-Esmenjaud, J. (2017). Leishmaniasis: A review. *F1000Research*, 6(750), 1–15. https://doi.org/10.12688/f1000research.11120.1

Aziz, H., Rhee, P., Pandit, V., Tang, A., Gries, L., & Joseph, B. (2015). The current concepts in management of animal (dog, cat, snake, scorpion) and human bite wounds. *Journal of Trauma and Acute Care Surgery*, 78(3), 641–648. https://doi.org/10.1097/TA.0000000000000531

Bula-Rudas, F. J., & Olcott, J. L. (2018). Human and animal bites. *Pediatrics in Review*, 39(10), 490–500. https://doi.org/10.1542/pir.2017-0212

Cegolon, L., Heymann, W. C., Lange, J. H., & Mastrangelo, G. (2013). Jellyfish stings and their management: A review. *Marine Drugs*, 11(2), 523–550. https://doi.org/10.3390/md11020523

Centers for Disease Control and Prevention (CDC). (2018a). Parasites—Cercarial dermatitis (also known as swimmer's itch). Retrieved January 3, 2020, from https://www.cdc.gov/parasites/swimmersitch

Centers for Disease Control and Prevention (CDC). (2018b). *Tickborne diseases of the United States: A reference manual for healthcare providers*. U.S. Department of Health and Human Services (5th ed.). https://doi.org/10.1097/00006454-199404000-00032

Devore, C. D., & Schutze, G. E.; Council on School Health and Committee on Infectious Diseases, American Academy of Pediatrics. (2015). Head lice. *Pediatrics*, 135(5), e1355–e1365. https://doi.org/10.1542/peds.2015-0746

Ellis, R., & Ellis, C. (2014). Dog and cat bites. *American Family Physician*, 90(4), 239–243. https://doi.org/https://www.aafp.org/afp/2014/0815/p239.html

Habif, T. P. (2015). *Clinical dermatology: A color guide to diagnosis and therapy* (6th ed.). Elsevier.

Hornbeak, K. B., & Auerbach, P. S. (2017). Marine envenomation. *Emergency Medicine Clinics of North America*, 35(2), 321–337. https://doi.org/10.1016/j.emc.2016.12.004

Hu, L. T. (2016). Lyme disease. *Annals of Internal Medicine*, 164(9), ITC65–ITC80. https://doi.org/10.7326/AITC201605030

Isbister, G. K., & Fan, H. W. (2011). Spider bite. *The Lancet*, 378(9808), 2039–2047. https://doi.org/10.1016/S0140-6736(10)62230-1

Kincaid, L., Klowak, M., Klowak, S., & Boggild, A. K. (2015). Management of imported cutaneous larva migrans: A case series and mini-review. *Travel Medicine and Infectious Disease*, 13(5), 382–387. https://doi.org/10.1016/j.tmaid.2015.07.007

Klotz, S., Ianas, V., & Elliott, S. (2011). Cat-scratch disease. *American Academy of Family Physicians*, 83(2), 152–155.

Mead, P., Petersen, J., & Hinckley, A. (2019). Updated CDC recommendation for serologic diagnosis of Lyme disease. *MMWR. Morbidity and Mortality Weekly Report*, 68(32), 703. https://doi.org/10.15585/mmwr.mm6832a4

Rademaker, M. (2014). Sea bather's eruption. Retrieved January 3, 2020, from https://dermnetnz.org/topics/sea-bathers-eruption

Schwartz, Z., Cohen, M., & Lipner, S. R. (2019). Sea urchin injuries: A review and clinical approach algorithm. *Journal of Dermatological Treatment*, 1–7. https://doi.org/10.1080/09546634.2019.1638884

Stoecker, W., Vetter, R., & Dyer, J. (2017). NOT RECLUSE-A mnemonic device to avoid false diagnoses of brown recluse spider bites. *JAMA Dermatology*, 153(5), 377–378.

United States Environmental Protection Agency (EPA). (2018). Top ten tips to prevent or control bed bugs. Retrieved December 20, 2019, from https://www.epa.gov/bedbugs/top-ten-tips-prevent-or-control-bed-bugs

Veraldi, S., Bottini, S., Rizzitelli, G., & Persico, M. C. (2012). One-week therapy with oral albendazole in hookworm-related cutaneous larva migrans: A retrospective study on 78 patients. *Journal of Dermatological Treatment*, 23(3), 189–191. https://doi.org/10.3109/09546634.2010.544707

Vetter, R. S. (2018). Clinical consequences of toxic envenomation by spiders. *Toxicon*, 152, 65–70. https://doi.org/10.1016/j.toxicon.2018.07.021

Drugs and Rash

CHAPTER
8.1

Joe R. Monroe

In This Chapter

- Adverse Cutaneous Drug Eruptions
- Approach to Patient Suspected with Drug Eruption
- Exanthematous Eruptions
- Fixed Drug Eruptions
- SJS/TEN

- Erythema Multiforme
- Drug-Induced Lupus
- Corticosteroid-Induced Acne
- Drug-Induced Dyspigmentation
- Toxic Erythema of Chemotherapy

Medications are commonly prescribed by health care providers as part of the management of patient illness and wellness. Many individuals, especially the elderly, have multiple chronic diseases accompanied by a long list of drugs prescribed by various clinicians. Adverse reactions to such medications are quite common and can range from mild exanthematous eruptions to potentially life-threatening conditions. The term "reaction" is generic, comprising all drug reactions, regardless of etiology. Nearly 100,000 deaths are attributed to all adverse drug reactions (ADRs) each year in the United States (Lazarou et al., 1998). The cutaneous manifestations frequently associated with these ADR can provide clinical clues for early diagnosis and prompt management. Clinicians must therefore always consider the possibility of an ADR or side effect (SE) in patients presenting with skin eruptions.

ADVERSE CUTANEOUS DRUG ERUPTIONS

An adverse cutaneous drug eruption (ACDR) is, by definition, an unintended toxic response to a drug given for the purposes of prevention, diagnosis, or therapeutics. An ACDR is considered serious if it results in death, disability, birth defect, or requires medical or surgical intervention. In contrast, an SE is a predictable and less toxic adverse effect that occurs more frequently. SEs are often dose related, and include such things as unwanted sedation, dry mouth, or problems urinating.

Pertinent History

- The diagnosis of an ACDR is based on clinical suspicion, presentation, chronology, and probability.
- The most important factor in the diagnosis of an ACDR is the history and timing of the intake of the suspected drug.
- The chronology is critical to identifying the causative agent of an ACDR, including date of initiation, dosage, and first sign of the reaction.

- A *detailed* history of all prescription, nonprescription, and recreational drugs taken by the patient must be collected; however, it can be a lengthy process especially in the elderly where polypharmacy is common.
- Any family history of ACDRs should be noted.
- It can also be helpful to inquire about all *routes* of administration when accounting for their medications (Box 8.1-1).

Risk Factors

Multiple factors place an individual at increased risk for developing an ACDR, especially in patients receiving medications known to have a high risk for ACDRs. The largest number of drug-related cutaneous eruptions is caused by aminopenicillins, sulfonamides, and nonsteroidal anti-inflammatory drugs (NSAIDs). Other risk factors include the following:

- *Host.* Elderly patients are at greater risk for ACDRs, often due to polypharmacy, but which can be due to changes in drug metabolism and/or excretion related to aging. Children are also at higher risk due to their smaller body size. Presumably because of differences in pharmacokinetics, immunologic status, and increased numbers of drugs taken. Females are affected more than males by

---

BOX 8.1-1   Seven "I"s for History of Patient Medications

- Instill (eye, ear drops, contact lens solution)
- Ingest (capsules, tabs, gels, liquids)
- Inhale (corticosteroids)
- Inject (IM, IV, SC)
- Insert (suppositories)
- In secret (sharing among elders or teens)
- Intermittent (not taken every day)

a ratio of 1.5 to 1.7 (Rademaker, 2001). All patients with a history of an ACDR have an increased risk of developing a reaction to another medication.

- *Immune status.* Patients whose immune systems are depressed, or who have malignancies such as lymphoma, have an increased risk for ACDR. The degree of ACDR severity may correlate with the severity of their disease state (Lavan & Gallagher, 2016).
- *Genetics.* There is an association with HLA types present in identified races that predispose them to an ACDR induced by a specific drug like phenytoin, carbamazepine, allopurinol, sulfamethoxazole, and abacavir. Patients with a history of an ACDR may have family members who may not be able to metabolize that drug or tolerate its metabolite.
- *Medications.* The drug itself may possess factors that increase the risk for an ACDR, including the class of drug, dose, route of administration, and drug–drug interactions.
- *Infection.* Patients are at greater risk of developing a hypersensitivity reaction during viral illnesses. The most well-known example is an ampicillin-induced rash in patients with Epstein–Barr virus (EBV) or a trimethoprim-sulfamethoxazole–induced rash in patients with HIV. Drugs can also trigger latent viral infections, typically because of immune suppression.

Pathophysiology

ACDRs are classified as immunologic, nonimmunologic, or idiosyncratic. It is helpful to recognize the type so that appropriate treatment may be initiated and future reactions avoided.

Immune-Mediated Drug Reactions

Most ADRs are an immunologic response to a drug and considered a hypersensitivity reaction. Cutaneous ACDRs can be classified as type I to IV hypersensitivity reaction patterns:

- *Type I* (immediate): IgE mediated, occurs within minutes of ingesting medication. ACDRs include urticaria, angioedema, and anaphylaxis.
- *Type II*: IgG mediated and cytotoxic. Examples would include drug-induced hemolytic anemia or pemphigus.
- *Type III*: Antigen–antibody complexes deposited in skin and vessels. The onset is minutes to days after ingestion. ACDRs include serum sickness and urticarial vasculitis.
- *Type IV* (delayed): Sensitized T cells with four subtypes. This is the most common type of ACDR and typically occurs 1 to 2 weeks after initiation of the suspected culprit drug. Type IV hypersensitivity ACDRs include Stevens–Johnson syndrome/toxic epidermal necrolysis (SJS/TEN), drug reaction with eosinophilia and systemic symptoms (DRESS), contact dermatitis, and acute generalized exanthematous pustulosis (AGEP).

Nonimmunologic Drug Reactions

- High drug doses or overdosage, as well as undesirable drug SEs (i.e., chemotherapy), can elicit non–immune-mediated cutaneous reactions. Extended therapy on a medication may result in cumulative toxicity to the drug or its metabolites which may be an immediate (i.e., amiodarone) or delayed (i.e., arsenic) reaction.
- Drug–drug interactions can also occur via numerous mechanisms including the displacement of medication from binding proteins or receptor sites (i.e., tetracycline and calcium).

- As mentioned, drugs can alter the metabolism of other drugs or metabolic changes within the body.
- Lastly, drugs can exacerbate a disease or trigger a latent disease process (i.e., lithium and psoriasis).

Idiosyncratic Reactions

- When an ACDR cannot be attributed to immunologic or non-immunologic causation, it is considered idiosyncratic, that is, a reaction of uncertain causation peculiar to that individual.

Clinical Presentation

The spectrum of ACDR clinical presentations is broad and will be discussed in detail with each specific reaction. Multiple factors should be considered:

- ACDRs often mimic other skin disorders and may occur days or even years after beginning drug therapy, making diagnosis challenging.
- An important variable that impacts the quality of the physical assessment is a complete examination of all areas, including those which appear to be unaffected. Patients often perceive their eruption to be independent of any other symptoms or lesions occurring on other parts of their body.
- The *distribution* of lesions and/or cutaneous symptoms: for example, are the lesions confined to a particular area such as the trunk, hands, face, or intertriginous areas? The areas which are spared are often equally significant, for example non–sun-exposed skin, or areas the patient cannot reach.
- Clinicians should always consider drug eruption in the differential diagnosis in patients presenting with *pruritic*, *bilateral*, *symmetrical*, and *generalized* skin rashes.
- Lesion *configuration* (e.g., linear, annular, grouped).
- *Nonblanching* with red rashes (inability to turn white with digital pressure) suggests the possibility of vasculitis.
- Oral or genital involvement.
- Vital signs should be taken to assess signs of a possible life-threatening ACDR.
- Intercurrent illnesses can be caused by a drug, but are frequently misdiagnosed, which is why the provider needs to know about other providers—especially specialists—the patient is seeing.

See Table 8.1-1 for Morphology of ACDR and associated differential diagnoses.

Confirming the Diagnosis

Most ACDRs are diagnosed based on history and physical findings and do not require additional diagnostics. However, further testing may be considered if the condition is persistent or severe to confirm clinician suspicion or to rule out other disease processes.

- Skin biopsy for histopathology:
  - Patients and clinicians must understand that even if histology supports the diagnosis of an ACDR, it cannot identify the offending agent. Patients should understand this before a biopsy is performed.
- Skin biopsy for direct immunofluorescence (DIF) testing:
  - Performed when a connective tissue disease or autoimmune blistering disease is suspected.

TABLE 8.1-1	Morphology of ACDR and Associated Differential Diagnoses
MORPHOLOGY	**DIAGNOSES**
Red scaly macules/patches	Eczematous drug eruption Photosensitive drug reaction Psoriasis Drug-induced lupus
Diffuse erythema	Erythroderma Red man syndrome Photosensitive drug reaction
Red macules and papules	Exanthematous drug eruption
Urticarial papules/plaques	Urticarial drug eruption Bullous pemphigoid (early stage)
Flat topped scaly red to purple papules/plaques	Lichenoid drug eruption Lichen planus
Palpable purpura	Vasculitis
Pustules	Corticosteroid-induced acne Acute generalized exanthematous pustulosis
Blisters/Bulla	Bullous pemphigoid Stevens–Johnsons syndrome Fixed drug eruption Photosensitive drug reaction
Targetoid red papules/plaques	Erythema multiforme Fixed drug eruption Stevens–Johnsons syndrome
Hyperpigmented macules/patches	Drug-induced hyperpigmentation Fixed drug eruption
Nodules	Erythema nodosum Drug-induced lupus

- DIF must be submitted in Michels solution and promptly submitted to the laboratory.
- Avoid tissue contact with formalin during the collection process. Ideally, these should be done by dermatology providers.
- Laboratory studies are indicated in patients with systemic symptoms (Box 8.1-2):
  - Complete blood count with a manual differential.
  - Comprehensive metabolic panel.
  - Antinuclear antibodies (ANA) screening.

BOX 8.1-2	Red-Flag Symptoms for Systemic Involvement in Adverse Drug Reaction
Fever	Facial edema
Purpura	Lymphadenopathy
Erosions/Blisters of mucosal membranes	Chest pain or dyspnea
Angioedema	Meningism
Erythroderma	Arthralgia
Blisters (especially positive Nikolsky sign) or necrosis	

- Antihistone antibodies may support a diagnosis of drug-induced lupus (DIL).
- Blood cultures, bacterial cultures, viral cultures, urinalysis, and stool guaiac will help to rule out infection and vasculitis.
- Provocation testing is only considered in specific circumstances and is generally performed in carefully controlled settings, *after the eruption has cleared.*

Treatment

- The topical and systemic management of drug eruptions varies according to diagnosis as well as the severity of associated symptoms.
- SJS/TEN patients often require hospitalization and treatment similar to burn patients. These patients also often require consultation with related specialists such as ophthalmology, infectious disease, as well as dermatology.
- For many ACDRs, no treatment is required, except for discontinuation of the offending medication, as the situation resolves over time.
- For the most part, treatment is intended to ameliorate associated symptoms of itching and burning, usually with topical and/or systemic corticosteroid use.
- Please see each section below for specific treatment.

Management and Patient Education

- Management of an ACDR is relative to the specific drug and reaction type which will be discussed in this chapter. However, the first and universal approach to all ACDRs is *discontinuation of the offending drug* (Box 8.1-3).
- Regardless of the type of drug eruption, any patient diagnosed with an ACDR must be educated about lifelong avoidance of the offending drug, medications in the same drug class, or other classes that may have potential cross-reactivity.
- Good communication between the patient and health care team should ensure that all personal health records and medic-alert identifiers reflect the patient's history of serious ACDRs.
- Most importantly, patients with an ACDR should be instructed to notify their health care provider if any of the following occur:
  - Rash recurs or worsens, indicating a possible severe hypersensitivity reaction.
  - Fever
  - Redness that starts to spread over the body.
  - Blisters, ulcerations, or sores on any mucous membrane.
  - New onset of pain.
  - Stridor, tongue swelling, or shortness of breath.
- In the event the provider is unavailable, the patient should be referred to a dermatologist, or in especially severe cases, to the emergency room if systemic involvement in considered (Box 8.1-2).
- There are several valuable resources and online databases available, such as *Litt's Drug Eruption and Reaction Manual*, 27th edition (2020), which can enable clinicians to view specific drug information, reaction, and incidence. It also provides content regarding the most common drug eruptions and patterns that can aid in predicting, diagnosing, and managing the patients with suspected ACDRs.

EXANTHEMATOUS DRUG REACTIONS

As the name implies, exanthematous eruptions are maculopapular or morbilliform (measles-like in appearance). Exanthematous drug eruptions account for about 95% of all drug reactions. Often difficult to distinguish from viral exanthems such as EBV, enterovirus, adenovirus, acute HIV, HHV-6, parvovirus.

Pathophysiology

The exact mechanism of these reactions is unknown, but it is believed to represent a type IV hypersensitivity reaction characterized by a T-cell–mediated response that causes direct cellular damage.

Clinical Presentation

The onset of exanthematous ACDRs usually occurs within hours to weeks after initiation of the drug.

Skin Findings

- They generally present as bright red, pruritic macules and papules that symmetrically appear on the trunk but may coalesce and spread to the extremities (Fig. 8.1-1A).
- In adults, it usually spares the face.
- In children, it may be limited to the face and extremities.
- Confluent lesions may develop bilaterally (Fig. 8.1-1B) and in the intertriginous areas.
- Palms, soles, and mucous membranes can be involved.

Non-Skin Findings

- The associated pruritus often disturbs sleep
- A low-grade fever and/or chills may be present compared to the high-grade fever associated with a hypersensitivity syndrome reaction
- Headache
- Myalgia/Joint pain
- Conjunctivitis
- Malaise

DIFFERENTIAL DIAGNOSIS	Exanthematous Drug Reaction
• Viral exanthema	• Secondary syphilis
• Scarlet fever	• Systemic juvenile arthritis (Still disease)
• Acute graft-versus-host disease	• Sarcoidosis
• Kawasaki disease	• Disseminated allergic contact dermatitis
• Acute generalized exanthematous pustulosis	• Urticaria

Confirming the Diagnosis

An exanthematous drug eruption is usually a clinical diagnosis that correlates with a history of drug administration obviating the necessity to perform a skin biopsy except when the diagnosis is in question or to rule out other causes.

- Skin biopsy—histopathology typically shows spongiosis with a perivascular infiltrate of lymphocytes and eosinophils, though these findings require clinicopathologic correlation.
- Further diagnostics should be considered if the patient develops additional primary morphologies (blisters, pustules, etc.), fever, chills, lymphadenopathy, edema of the face, eyelids, or mouth (angioedema).
- Additional diagnostics to be considered to rule out disease states are listed in the differential diagnosis list:
  - Chest x-ray (e.g., sarcoid)
  - RPR, VDRL, Syphilis IgG (e.g., syphilis)
  - ASO titre, pharynx bacterial culture (e.g., strep infection)
  - Complete blood count (if infection is suspected)
  - Estimated sedimentation rate, C reactive protein (to assess the level of inflammation)

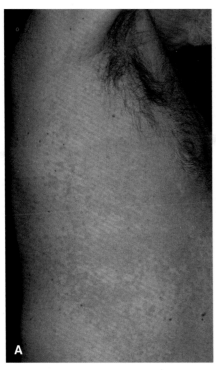
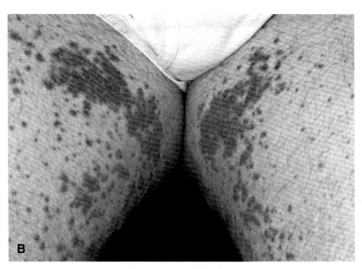

FIG. 8.1-1. **A:** Exanthematous eruption. **B:** Exanthematous eruption coalescing plaques. (Photos courtesy of Thomas P. Habif.)

- Comprehensive metabolic panel (to rule out end-organ damage, e.g., to liver or kidneys, as we might see with a hypersensitivity reaction to a medication such as an NSAID)
- In the absence of drug history, additional diagnostics should be performed based on history of foreign travel, hobbies, occupation, and sexual history.

Treatment

In addition to discontinuing the suspected drug, symptomatic treatment is usually all that is needed for a mild or moderate exanthematous drug eruption.

Topical

- Mid- to high-potency topical corticosteroid topicals may be used during the acute phase, if necessary. Since this eruption is often widespread, the steroids should be prescribed in a large enough quantity (1-lb jar), for twice daily application, though it should be used with caution on the face, skin folds, and (see Section 1.4) genitals.
- Application of cool compresses, fragrance-free moisturizing creams, and OTC anti-itch lotions can be helpful in controlling discomfort.

Systemic

- Since these reactions are not histamine-mediated, antihistamines cannot reduce pruritus, though some (e.g., hydroxyzine) help by means of sedation.
- In the rare instance in which the offending drug cannot be discontinued or the patient has a severe eruption, a short course of prednisone may be prescribed at a dose of 1 to 2 mg/kg/day for 7 to 21 days to provide symptomatic relief and induce rapid remission. (Keep in mind the usual precautions, e.g., diabetes, CHF, peptic ulcer disease, dementia, and others.)

- Occasionally, ACDRs are serious enough to require immediate "rescue" drug treatment (high doses of prednisone, mycophenolate mofetil, cyclosporine) pending evaluation by the appropriate specialist. These medications should only be prescribed by providers experienced in their use.

Management and Patient Education

- An exanthematous drug rash typically lasts for 1 to 2 weeks and then fades. Resolving lesions have hues of tan and purple, with desquamation.
- Clinicians should use great caution when patients with a morbilliform rash progress to develop fever, mucositis, erythroderma, facial edema, or blisters. Expedited referral to dermatology should be considered in such cases.

CLINICAL PEARLS

- The most common manifestation of ordinary ACDRs is the widespread blanchable exanthematous eruption most often caused by antibiotics and NSAIDs.
- The finding of *nonblanchable rashes* suggests the possibility of a vasculitic process and should be referred to dermatology (see Section 9.3 Vasculitis).
- Patients should be told that biopsy results, while essential to a thorough workup, cannot identify the offending drug.

FIXED DRUG ERUPTIONS

A fixed drug eruption (FDE) is a localized adverse skin reaction to an ingested substance (Box 8.1-4). The hallmark of FDE is the appearance of the same type of lesion(s) on the same location(s) with subsequent exposure, a feature virtually pathognomonic for FDE.

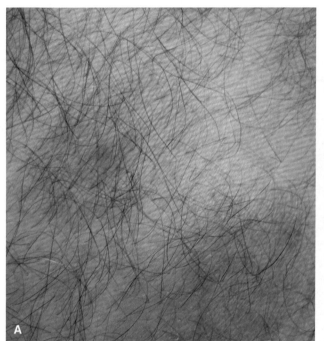
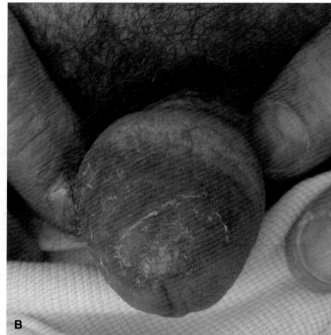

FIG. 8.1-2. Fixed drug eruption. **A:** An early lesion will present with an erythematous border and dusky center. **B:** The glans penis is a common location, especially with reaction to tetracyclines. (Photos courtesy of M. Bobonich.)

The specific location may be a clue as to the drug. Tetracyclines, for example, often produce lesions on the glans penis.

Pathophysiology

- FDE is a cell-mediated process involving CD8⁺ T cells which are increased in the lesions of FDE and apparently play a dual role in the skin.
- Normally, these intraepidermal T cells have a protective function but when there is overactivation by an antigen as with FDE, they may actually be responsible for tissue injury.

Clinical Presentation

Skin Findings

- FDE typically takes a few days to appear after initiation of the culprit drug, unless the patient has been previously sensitized to the drug, in which case lesions can develop within minutes of taking a single dose.
- Lesions usually recur in the same localized areas as the initial eruptions, but patients may develop lesions in new areas as well.
- FDE has a distinct appearance of well-demarcated, round/oval, dusky-red patches or plaques which may be solitary or multiple.

BOX 8.1-4 Medications Commonly Associated with FDE

- NSAIDs
- Antibiotics (e.g., tetracyclines, sulfonamides, penicillins, quinolones)
- Barbiturates
- Allopurinol
- Propranolol
- Phenolphthalein-containing laxatives
- Some food dyes

The lesions can become edematous and form a central vesicle/bulla, giving the lesion a target-like appearance, often leaving residual postinflammatory hyperpigmentation.

- In darker-skinned patients, the hyperpigmentation may persist for weeks to months before finally fading.
- FDE can occur anywhere on the body but favors the dorsal and palmar hands, glans penis, groin, periorbital, perioral, or oral mucosa (Fig. 8.1-2A).
- In males presenting with penile lesions, FDE should always be near the top of the differential diagnosis (Fig. 8.1-2B).

Non-Skin Findings

- Symptoms are typically mild to absent despite their appearance.

DIFFERENTIAL DIAGNOSIS Fixed Drug Eruption

- Erythema annulare centrifugum
- Acute urticaria
- Herpes simplex (genital lesion)
- Erythema multiforme
- Lichen planus
- Aphthous stomatitis

Confirming the Diagnosis

- FDE is generally a clinical diagnosis, substantiated by drug history though patients are often unaware of the connection between the medication and the outbreaks.
- Patients with occasional urinary tract infections (UTIs) for which trimethoprim-sulfamethoxazole is given are common examples of this phenomenon.

- Biopsy is rarely necessary, but shows hydropic degeneration of epidermal basal cells, pigmentary incontinence, interface dermatitis, and vacuolar changes.

Treatment

- Treatment is usually unnecessary for lack of symptoms and self-limited nature.
- Class III or IV topical corticosteroid cream may be prescribed for burning and itching.
- When the surface is erosive (rare), use aluminum acetate wet compresses to dry the surface and promote healing (see Section 1.4 for detailed instructions).

Management and Patient Education

- Skin lesions typically persist for as long as the medication is taken and may take weeks to resolve after the drug is discontinued.
- The initially erythematous lesions fade to a dark brown-purple area of hyperpigmentation, especially in skin of color.
- Educate FDE patients with dark skin to expect the hyperpigmentation to take months or even years to resolve.
- Hydroquinone cream can help to speed resolution of the hyperpigmentation.

CLINICAL PEARLS

- Recurrence of targetoid lesions in the same locations strongly suggests FDE.
- Tetracyclines and trimethoprim-sulfamethoxazole often produce lesions on the glans penis.
- Lips, arms, neck, and face are also commonly affected.
- Some food dyes can trigger FDE, especially tartrazine-containing colors (e.g., yellow, blue). Other food/drink additives (e.g., cashews, licorice) can also trigger fixed "drug" eruptions identical to those caused by drugs (Tattersall & Reddy, 2016).

ACUTE GENERALIZED EXANTHEMATOUS PUSTULOSIS (AGEP)

AGEP is a rare cutaneous pustular eruption that occurs at a rate of one to five cases per million per year. AGEP generally develops after taking certain medications, especially calcium channel blockers, NSAIDs, anticonvulsants, enalapril, griseofulvin, itraconazole, aminopenicillins, macrolides, and quinolones. Viral infections have been known to also trigger AGEP.

Pathophysiology

While the pathophysiologic mechanism is not yet understood, a genetic hypersensitivity or a type IV allergic reaction is suggested.

Clinical Presentation

Skin Findings

- AGEP has an acute onset and typically takes 1 to 3 weeks to develop in nonsensitized individuals.
- It is characterized by numerous pinpoint sterile pustules surrounded by bright-red erythema and edema.
- They are not perifollicular and can be either grouped or irregularly dispersed.

- Initially, lesions erupt on the face (Fig. 8.1-3A) and intertriginous areas, especially the neck, axillae, and inguinal folds (Fig. 8.1-3B).
- Pustules rapidly expand to cover the entire trunk (Fig. 8.1-3C).
- Facial edema may develop.

Non-Skin Findings

- High fever and leukocytosis are common from the outset.
- Nonviral hepatitis may develop.

DIFFERENTIAL DIAGNOSIS   AGEP

- Pustular psoriasis
- Sweet syndrome
- Stevens–Johnson syndrome/toxic epidermal necrolysis
- Drug reaction with eosinophilia and systemic symptoms
- Subcorneal pustulosis (Sneddon–Wilkinson syndrome)
- Bullous impetigo

Confirming the Diagnosis

- A CBC with differential typically reveals a marked leukocytosis with very elevated neutrophils and mild eosinophilia.
- Serum BUN, creatinine, and 24-hour urine may reflect a transient reduction in creatinine clearance.
- Liver function studies are usually normal.
- AGEP histology has spongiform subcorneal and/or intraepidermal pustules, vasculitis, and marked edema of the papillary dermis.

Treatment

- Resolution of this condition is spontaneous; however, patients may require hospitalization depending on the extent and severity of pustulosis or organ dysfunction.
- Treatment modalities include systemic corticosteroids, intravenous hydration, moisturizing creams, and emollients.
- Oral antihistamines and analgesics may be indicated.

Management and Patient Education

- Skin lesions typically persist for as long as the medication is taken and may take weeks to resolve after the drug is discontinued.
- The initially erythematous lesions fade to a dark brown-purple area of hyperpigmentation, especially in skin of color.
- Hospitalization for supportive care and monitoring is not uncommon for patients with AGEP. The prognosis for full recovery is excellent once the drug has been identified and discontinued.
- Consultation with dermatology can be helpful for the reassurance that this will likely resolve with just supportive measures when the offending drug is discontinued. A referral to other specialists may be indicated if there are complications.
- The pustules spontaneously resolve in about 2 weeks, and a generalized desquamation occurs.
- Complications are rare but may include hepatitis; so careful monitoring of liver function tests is important until all symptoms and adverse reactions have resolved (Table 8.1-2).

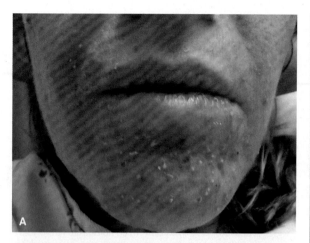

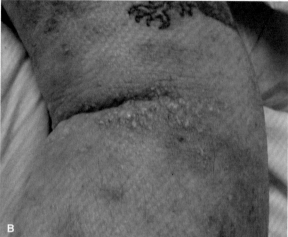

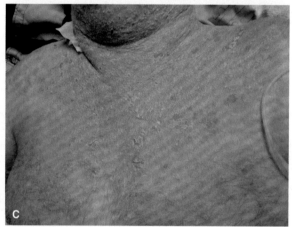

FIG. 8.1-3. Acute generalized exanthematous pustulosis. **A:** Eruption beginning on the face. **B:** Sheets of pustules in an intertriginous area. **C:** The entire trunk is involved and beginning to desquamate. (Photos courtesy of Basil Mahmoud.)

TABLE 8.1-2	Comparison of Common Adverse Drug Reaction Patterns		
	EXANTHEMATOUS (95% OF ADRS)	**FIXED DRUG ERUPTION**	**ACUTE GENERALIZED EXANTHEMATOUS PUSTULOSIS**
Onset	Insidious, 1–4 wk after initiation of drug	Rapid, hours to days	1–4 wk after initiation of drug
Etiology[a]	Drugs—sulfonamides, aminopenicillins, anticonvulsants, cephalosporins, antiretrovirals (see Box 8.1-5 for full list) IM or CMV + PCN HIV + sulfonamides Allopurinol + PCNs	Drugs—ASA, NSAIDs, sulfonamides, aminopenicillins, tetracyclines, TMP/SMX, phenolphthalein, barbiturates	Drugs: β-lactam and macrolide antibiotics, tetracyclines, calcium channel blockers, antifungals, NSAIDs, anticonvulsants Enterovirus, Epstein–Barr virus
Systemic	If present, including fever, consider *hypersensitivity syndrome reaction*	Typically none	Fever and leukocytosis, rare liver involvement (hepatitis) Watch LFTs
Morphology and Distribution	Morbilliform (papules and macules). *No blisters or pustules* Symmetrical, starts on trunk, then to extremities Favors pressure bearing areas Children: face and extremities Very similar presentation to viral exanthem	Discrete, solitary or multiple, red/dusky macules, papules, or plaques Edematous, ± *bullae* Lips, extremities, glans penis, lesions often recur in same location if offending agent reintroduced	Nonfollicular *pustules* with erythematous base Face and intertriginous areas, spreading quickly to trunk
Prognosis	Lesions fade with discontinuation, ± desquamation 1–2 wk	Lesions resolve with discontinuation, ± hyperpigmentation	Lesions resolve with discontinuation, desquamation 1–2 wk

[a]Most common cause or groups, not inclusive.
↓ Direction of spread.
CMV, cytomegalovirus; IM, infectious mononucleosis; PCN, aminopenicillins; TMP/SMX, trimethoprim/sulfamethoxazole; NSAID, nonsteroidal anti-inflammatory drug.

BOX 8.1-5	Drugs Frequently Implicated in Exanthematous Drug Reactions

Allopurinol	Glyburide
Amoxicillin	Isoniazid
Ampicillin	Lithium
Barbiturates	Naproxen
Cephalosporins	Penicillin
Captopril	Phenothiazines
Carbamazepine	Phenylbutazone
Chlorpromazine	Phenytoin
Diflunisal	Piroxicam
Enalapril	Quinidine
Gentamycin	Sulfonamides
Gold	Thiazides
Glipizide	Thiouracil
	TMP/SMX

Adapted from Dinulos, J. G. H. (2021). Exanthems and drug eruptions. In *Habif's clinical dermatology* (7th ed., pp. 525–570).

STEVENS–JOHNSON SYNDROME AND TOXIC EPIDERMAL NECROLYSIS (SJS/TEN)

While rare, SJS and TEN are true medical emergencies, presenting acutely with systemic signs and symptoms which primary care clinicians must be able to recognize and emergently manage because of their associated high mortality and morbidity. The incidence of SJS/TEN is estimated to range from 2 to 8 persons per million per year depending on geographic location and the offending drug or agent (Harr & French, 2010). The peak occurrence of SJS/TEN is during

BOX 8.1-6	Common Causes of SJS/TEN	
	Medications	**Infections**
Most Common	Sulfonamides	Herpes simplex
	Antiepileptics	Cocksackie virus
	NSAIDs	Mumps
		Mycoplasma
Less Common	Cephalosporins	Streptococcus
	Macrolides	Epstein–Barr
	Benzodiazepines	Cytomegalovirus
	H$_1$ antihistamines	
	Mucolytic agents	

summer and early spring season and occurs more often in children and young adults (Box 8.1-6).

These rare, potentially life-threatening ACDRs are characterized by full-thickness denudation of the cutaneous and mucosal surfaces. It is important to understand that SJS and TEN are part of a continuum involving similar pathophysiologic processes differentiated primarily by the percentage of body surface area (BSA) involved (Fig. 8.1-4):

- SJS involves less than 10% BSA
- TEN involves greater than 30% BSA
- SJS/TEN overlap is characterized by 10% to 30% of BSA

Medications are more often implicated in TEN compared to SJS, independent of dosage. TEN may be associated with an inherited defect in the detoxification of drug metabolites. TEN has been shown to be triggered by several of the biologics (Adler et al., 2017).

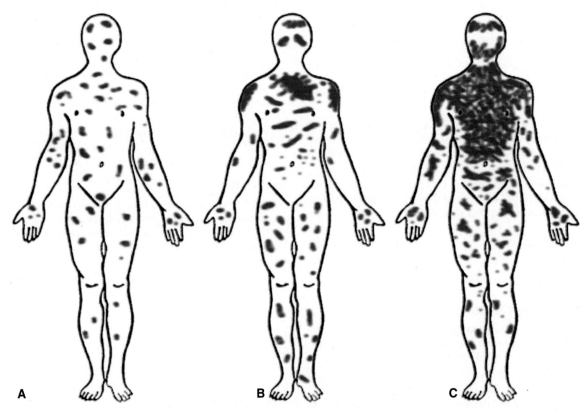

FIG. 8.1-4. Body surface area involvement of SJS/TEN. **A:** SJS: <10%. **B:** SJS/TEN: 10% to 30%. **C:** TEN: >30%.

TABLE 8.1-3	Comparison of Erythema Multiforme, Stevens–Johnson Syndrome, and Toxic Epidermal Necrolysis		
	ERYTHEMA MULTIFORME (EM)	**STEVENS–JOHNSON SYNDROME (SJS) (%BSA)**	**TOXIC EPIDERMAL NECROLYSIS (%BSA)**
Onset	Acute onset, spring and fall Adolescents	Children and young adults Slightly higher F > M	
Etiology[a]	Common: HSV infection Sometimes: *Mycoplasma pneumoniae*, drugs, other infections	Common: Drugs—antibiotics (sulfonamides, quinolones, aminopenicillins, etc.), anticonvulsants, NSAIDs Uncommon: *M. pneumoniae*, viruses, immunizations, CMV	
Systemic	*Mild, if any*	*Sick* appearance	*Toxic* appearance
Prodrome	Abrupt onset Usually no illness	High fever, malaise, ST, influenza-like symptoms, starts as macular rash aphthous ulcers	Same as SJS Increasing systemic symptoms, pulmonary involvement 25%
Morphology and Distribution	*Targetoid* (3 zones) Red with darker center *Raised* Targetoid lesions expand and may develop erosions Symmetric, acral extremities favors the extensors, palms, and soles	*Atypical* targetoid (2 zones) or typical targetoid, red *Flat* Central *vesicle* Starts on trunk, usually involves palms and soles Pruritic Negative Nikolsky sign	Papules/Plaques, dusky, diffuse/increasing BSA Flaccid *bullae* *Full-thickness* desquamation >30% BSA and increasing Extracutaneous symptoms Painful Positive Nikolsky sign
Mucus Membranes	*Few* or no oral lesions	*Usually* oral Conjunctivitis is uncommon Hemorrhagic crusts	*Always* (before the rash) Usually more than one area *Conjunctival edema*
Prognosis	Self-limiting Lesions resolve in 1 mo Usually no sequelae	5–15% mortality Heals without scarring Usually dyspigmentation	30–40% mortality Late withdrawal of drug leads to increased mortality

[a]High-risk causes or groups, not inclusive.
HSV, herpes simplex virus; CMV, cytomegalovirus; BSA, body surface area.
Adapted from James, W. D. (2020). Contact dermatitis and drug reactions. In *Andrews' diseases of the skin: Clinical dermatology* (13th ed., p. 117). Elsevier.

Pathophysiology

- Most experts consider SJS/TEN to be an idiosyncratic delayed hypersensitivity reaction to a drug. However, other causes have also been implicated (Table 8.1-3). In this reaction:
  - Cytotoxic T lymphocytes (drug specific CD8[+] cells), along with natural killer T cells, trigger keratinocyte destruction (programed cell death), resulting in a separation of the epidermis from the dermis.
- Data support a strong association between genetic susceptibility associated with HLA subtypes and the lack of ability to process specific drug metabolites (Fan et al., 2017).

Clinical Presentation

Skin Findings

- In SJS, grouped erythematous targetoid (2 zones) or atypical (3 zones) lesions erupt, some with a central vesicle (Fig. 8.1-5A).
- Palms and soles can be the first site of cutaneous eruption.
- Purpuric macules develop on the trunk and can spread to the face, neck, and extremities, developing into flaccid blisters, erosions, and detachment of the epidermis.
- The oral mucosa is almost always involved, often developing hemorrhagic crusts on the lips. Other mucous membranes like the conjunctiva, oral and nasal mucosa, as well as anogenital and vulvovaginal areas can be involved (Fig. 8.1-5B).

- TEN can present initially as SJS that rapidly progresses to involve more than 30% BSA with full-thickness desquamation of the epidermis. Yet clinicians should be cautioned that all TEN does not occur in this "linear" progression (Table 8.1-3). About half the cases of TEN develop rapidly from diffuse erythema to necrosis and epidermal detachment.
- The slightest pressure or friction on the skin near the bullae can result in a shearing off (positive Nikolsky sign) of sheets of the epidermis, exposing an erythematous, oozing dermis (Fig. 8.1-6).

Non-Skin Findings

- Patients with TEN have a toxic appearance with high fever, cardiovascular compromise, metabolic imbalances, and severe pain. Organ involvement ensues rapidly with associated ocular, pulmonary, cardiovascular, neurologic, gastrointestinal, hematologic, and renal symptoms.
- SJS is often preceded by a prodrome of symptoms occurring 1 to 3 days prior to mucocutaneous manifestation:
  - High fever
  - Sore throat
  - Cough
  - Malaise
  - Arthralgia
  - Stinging eyes
  - Upper respiratory tract infection

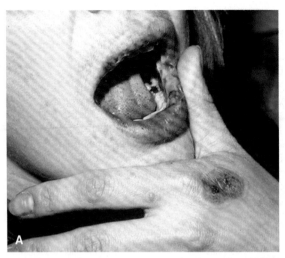
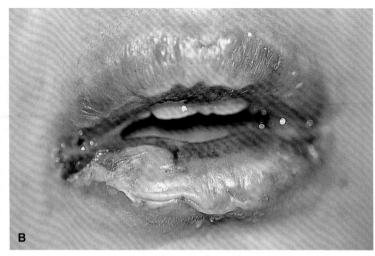

FIG. 8.1-5. Stevens–Johnson syndrome. **A:** Bullae and crusts are noted on the lips, and targetoid lesions are seen on the hand. **B:** Mucous membrane involvement.

DIFFERENTIAL DIAGNOSIS   SJS/TEN

- Exanthematous drug eruption
- Other drug eruptions AGEP, DRESS
- Fixed drug eruption
- Erythema multiforme major
- Scarlet fever
- Phototoxic eruptions
- Toxic shock syndrome
- Acute graft-versus-host disease
- Staphylococcal scalded skin syndrome
- Thermal burns
- Exfoliative dermatitis
- Generalized morbilliform eruption
- Drug-induced linear IgA bullous dermatosis
- Erythroderma

Confirming the Diagnosis

The diagnosis of SJS/TEN is based on clinical, historical, and histologic findings.

- Positive Nikolsky sign: represents the shearing away of surrounding epidermis with lateral pressure near the bullae. This can also be positive in pemphigus and staphylococcal scalded skin syndrome.

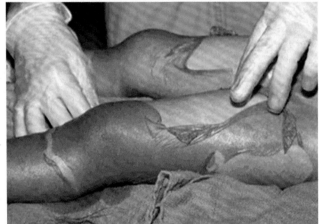

FIG. 8.1-6. Toxic epidermal necrolysis with sloughing epidermis (Nikolsky sign). (Used with permission from Wound, Ostomy and Continence Nurses Society®; Doughty, D. B., & McNichol, L. L. [2015]. *Wound, ostomy and continence nurses society® core curriculum: Wound management.* Wolters Kluwer Health.)

- Positive Asboe-Hansen sign: lateral extension of the blister to adjacent skin with application of pressure to the top of a bulla.
- Histopathology
  - Biopsy for H&E: Skin punch biopsy of perilesional skin around an early lesion is preferred. Will show epidermal necrosis and detachment with marked apoptosis, along with a lymphohistiocytic infiltrate.
  - Biopsy for DIF: Shows no changes specific to TEN, but does help to differentiate SJS/TEN from other autoimmune blistering disease such as pemphigus or bullous pemphigoid.
- Laboratory assessment of systemic end organ involvement is essential and includes:
  - Complete metabolic profile, especially renal and hepatic function
  - Complete blood count
  - Blood Cultures
- When it is unclear which drug is the offending agent in a patient with SJS/TEN, a carefully monitored provocation test or patch testing may be considered, but only long after the acute disease has resolved.

Treatment

- Discontinue the suspected drug and admit any patient with suspected SJS/TEN to the hospital, preferably one with a burn unit, to be co-managed by dermatology and other specialists as indicated.
- Aggressive management of fluid and electrolytes and wound care are priorities.
- The primary goal of treatment is to protect the dermis and promote reepithelialization while minimizing the risk of infection.

Topicals

- Skin care during the acute phases is similar to the treatment for burn patients, using moist, nonadhering dressings (e.g., petroleum-based gauze).
- Surgical debridement is not recommended.
- Sometimes bullae are gently ruptured by piercing them with a sterile needle and allowing the roof to act as a biologic dressing.

Systemics

- Treatment with high-dose parenteral corticosteroids, intravenously administered immunoglobulin, biologics, and cyclosporine have been used, but there are no proven therapies to be recommended.

- Pain management is critical and similar to that of a burn patient although this disease also includes extremely painful lesions in the mouth, nose, and eyes.
- Parenteral therapy is often needed for hydration and nutritional support. These lesions can last for weeks or months.

Management and Patient Education

- Due to significant epidermal loss, patients are at high risk for secondary infections and need intensive monitoring and supportive therapy. *This is a true dermatologic emergency.*
- Patients suspected to have SJS/TEN should be referred to a tertiary care center (i.e., hospital) for immediate care. The management of SJS/TEN requires a multidisciplinary team of burn specialist, intensivist, dermatologist, wound specialist, ophthalmology, and infectious disease.
- The overall mortality for SJS/TEN is estimated to be 10% to 30%.
- Ocular sequelae are the most common complication and can occur with either SJS or TEN. Ocular complications can range from severe corneal ulcerations, symblepharon, and blindness to dry eyes or trichiasis (eyelashes growing inward toward the eye).
- Long-term sequelae can include genitourinary, pulmonary, and cardiovascular disease, along with kidney failure requiring dialysis. These can persist for months or even years after the worst of the eruptions has resolved, often requiring ongoing surveillance by several different specialist-consultants (Lee et al., 2017).
- Long-term cutaneous sequela also includes scarring, dyspigmentation, strictures, or adhesions.
- Systemic complications include sepsis and organ failure which can be fatal or result in extensive morbidity.
- Patients with a personal history or family history of SJS/TEN must avoid the potential causative agent and any cross-reacting agents in the drug class.

Special Considerations

Patient populations from East Asian and European descent should be tested for the specific HLA subtypes before starting on oxicam, sulfamethoxazole, carbamazepine, lamotrigine, oxcarbazepine, phenytoin, abacavir, and allopurinol. The elderly, HIV-infected individuals, and those with autoimmune diseases (i.e., inflammatory bowel disease or systemic lupus erythematosus [SLE]) are at higher risk.

CLINICAL PEARLS

- The FDA recommends that patients who have Asian or South Asian ancestry and are being considered for treatment with the antiepileptic carbamazepine be screened for HLA-B*1502 as this population is at increased risk for SJS/TEN.
- The combination of mucocutaneous involvement, a blistering and/or targetoid rash, fever, and malaise is unusual and should prompt consideration of SJS/TEN.
- SJS/TEN is rare (1 to 2 cases per million) but quite dangerous if missed. SJS is fatal for 10% to 15% of victims, while TEN kills 30% to 40%.
- The vast majority of SJS/TEN cases are caused by drugs, and less commonly by certain infections, such as *Mycoplasma* and *Cytomegalovirus*.
- SJS/TEN can be triggered by at least two different biologics, rituximab and cetuximab.
- SJS/TEN can affect the following organ systems during the acute phase of the illness and for many months afterwards: eyes, kidneys, GI system, and lungs.
- SJS/TEN can be triggered by vaccination (Su et al., 2020).

ERYTHEMA MULTIFORME

Erythema multiforme (EM) was, until 1993, considered to be part of the SJS/TEN spectrum, but, for a variety of reasons, is considered to be a separate spectrum of hypersensitivity syndrome unto itself, which includes EM minor and major. In contrast to SJS/TEN, EM is generally an acute, self-limited, inflammatory skin disease associated with infectious agents in approximately 90% of cases, and less commonly medications. EM is most commonly linked to a preceding herpes simplex virus (HSV) infection and less commonly to EBV, bacteria (i.e., *Mycoplasma pneumoniae*), or dermatophyte infections. Drugs have also been implicated and include NSAIDs, sulfonamides, antiepileptics, and antibiotics.

For the purposes of this chapter, this author suggests that *EM major* is a disease with mucosal involvement and systemic symptoms, while *EM minor* does not have mucosal involvement. EM major is now considered a disorder distinct from SJS with similar mucosal erosions but different lesion morphology and distribution.

The overall incidence of EM is unknown, but there is a preponderance for young adults. Recurrences are very likely to occur in individuals with a history of EM.

Table 8.1-4 outlines the EM and SJS spectrum. The focus of this section will be primarily on EM minor.

TABLE 8.1-4	Spectrum Comparison for EM Minor, EM Major, and SJS		
	EM MINOR	**EM MAJOR**	**SJS**
Morphology	Targetoid Atypical papular targetoid	Targetoid Atypical papular targetoid	Purpuric macules Atypical macular targetoid Bullous lesions
Distribution	Elbows, knees, wrists, hands, face	Extremities and face	Trunk and face
Mucosal involvement	None or mild	Severe	Severe
Precipitating factors	HSV Other infections	HSV *Mycoplasma pneumoniae* Other infections Drugs (rare)	Drugs
Prognosis	Often recurrent Low morbidity	Increased morbidity	High morbidity

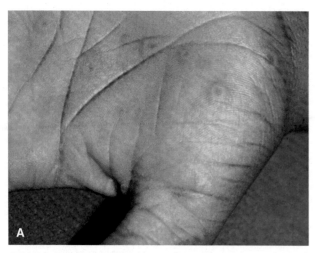 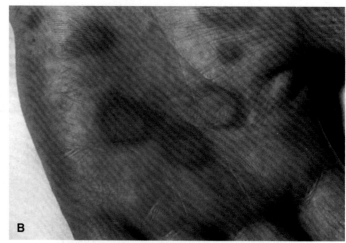

FIG. 8.1-7. **A:** Erythema multiforme minor with small target or iris lesions on the palm. **B:** Larger target papules with central bullae surrounding erythema.

Pathophysiology

EM is a type IV hypersensitivity reaction in response to a stimulus, most often HSV infection. A cell-mediated immune reaction results in destruction of keratinocytes expressing HSV antigen, triggering an inflammatory cascade and causing cell death of HSV-infected keratinocytes and the recruitment of autoreactive T cells. This leads to the epidermal damage and the inflammatory infiltrate that creates classic EM lesions. EM associated with a drug is due to abnormal metabolism resulting in toxic metabolites binding to the surface of keratinocytes and triggering an immune reaction.

Clinical Presentation

The term *multiforme* implies the varied clinical manifestations that can be observed with EM. See Box 8.1-7 regarding clinical distinctions between EM major and minor.

Skin Findings

- The primary and characteristic lesion of EM is a typical *target* or *iris* lesion (Fig. 8.1-7). The typical target size is usually under 3 cm in diameter, round, erythematous, edematous papule that spreads outward, and the center can become cyanotic, purpuric, or vesicular (Fig. 8.1-8). Lesions will evolve during the course of the illness and may develop polycyclic and annular configurations.
- Atypical papular target lesions are round, edematous, and palpable but may have only two zones of color and poorly demarcated edges (Fig. 8.1-9).

Partially formed targets with annular borders, or target lesions on the palms and soles, may resemble urticaria on clinical examination.

- A classic eruption of EM begins symmetrically on extremities, particularly the target lesions favoring the extensor surfaces of the upper extremities and dorsal hands (palms may be involved).
- Lesions then spread centripetally to the trunk, neck, and face.
- Mucosal lesions are usually absent in EM minor and if present are mildly symptomatic and few in number.
- Severe mucosal involvement is characteristic for EM major, with erosions and hemorrhagic crusting on the lips, as well as ulcerations on the buccal mucosa, gingiva, conjunctiva, and genital mucosa.

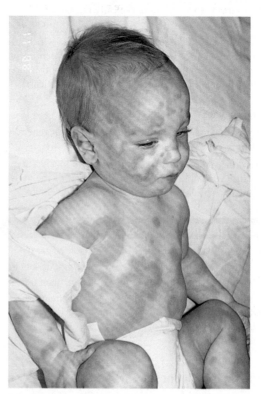

FIG. 8.1-8. Target lesions of EM characterized by a distinct red ring around central clearing (sometimes with a central bull's eye) that can coalesce into large polycyclic plaques. (Photo courtesy of Cathleen Case.)

BOX 8.1-7	Erythema Multiforme Classification	
	Erythema Multiforme Minor	**Erythema Multiforme Major**
Morphology	Targetoid Atypical papular targetoid	Targetoid Atypical papular targetoid
Distribution	Elbows, knees, wrists, hands, face	Extremities and face
Mucosal involvement	None or mild	Severe
Non-skin findings	None	Fever Arthralgias Myalgias

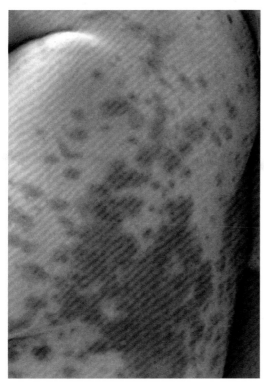

FIG. 8.1-9. Atypical EM secondary to hydroxychloroquine. (Fleisher, G. R., Ludwig, W., & Baskin, M. N. [2004]. *Atlas of pediatric emergency medicine*. Wolters Kluwer Health | Lippincott Williams & Wilkins.)

- The onset of EM lesions is sudden and occurs over about 2 to 3 days. The initial papules and plaques that expand to form targetoid lesions with vesicles are typically monomorphic, fixed, and last at least 7 days.
- These can be differentiated from urticaria, which present as edematous plaques with normal skin in the central portion, a polymorphic eruption, migrate around the body, and last less than 24 hours. (See Section 8.2 for details on urticaria.)

Non-Skin Findings

- Early lesions may burn or be asymptomatic but generally are not pruritic.
- Prodromal symptoms of malaise, fever, and myalgia are not common in EM minor, but occur in about half of the patients with EM major, especially if there is mucosal involvement.

DIFFERENTIAL DIAGNOSIS	Erythema Multiforme
• Stevens–Johnson syndrome	• Pityriasis rosea
• Toxic epidermal necrosis	• Polymorphous light eruption
• Fixed drug eruption	• Urticaria, giant urticaria
• Subacute cutaneous lupus erythematosus	• Viral exanthem
• Bullous pemphigoid	• Urticarial vasculitis

Confirming the Diagnosis

- A complete skin examination is essential since some patients will have target lesions that are not yet typical and only a few completely developed typical target lesions.

- The diagnosis of EM is usually based on clinical presentations with classic morphology of the primary lesion and distribution.
- History of preceding upper respiratory tract infection, HSV, or *M. pneumoniae* illness will further support the diagnosis of EM.
- The presence or absence of mucosal lesions, and signs or symptoms of systemic illness will differentiate EM minor from EM major.
- Skin biopsy may be needed if there is an atypical presentation or severe disease to rule out other skin diseases like vasculitis or lupus erythematosus.
- Additional punch biopsy should be performed for DIF if a blistering disease is suspected.
- Laboratory
  - WBC and ESR may be elevated
  - Viral culture if initial lesion (HSV) is present
- Clinical criteria separate the EM spectrum from the SJS/TEN spectrum, which is usually a severe drug-induced reaction characterized by widespread blisters/epidermal detachment and purpuric macules.

Treatment

The initial treatment of EM is always to identify the precipitating factor and treat appropriate infection or stop the offending medication.

Topical

- In most cases of EM minor, symptomatic treatment is all that is necessary.
- Soothing mouthwashes (e.g., warm saline rinse, or solution of equal parts diphenhydramine, viscous xylocaine, and aluminum/magnesium antacid) may be used. (See Section 13 HFMD Treatment *Magic Mouthwash*.)
- Class II topical corticosteroids for localized skin relief.

Systemic

- Oral antihistamines may reduce swelling, burning, and pruritus of the skin.
- Oral corticosteroid (prednisone 40 to 80 mg/day) can be used for EM major until cleared, then followed by a 1-week taper.
- Acyclovir 400 mg twice daily has been used for suppressive therapy prescribed for patients with more than five attacks a year of herpes-associated EM. Suppressive antiviral therapy can prevent HSV-associated EM, but antiviral therapy started after the EM outbreak has no effect on the course of that outbreak.
- Antiviral suppressive therapy can also be used for idiopathic recurrent EM.
- Valacyclovir and famciclovir are better absorbed and may be used if there is no response to acyclovir.
- In recalcitrant cases, dapsone, azathioprine, and cyclosporine may be considered.

Management and Patient Education

- EM is generally self-limiting and uncomplicated, usually resolving in about 1 month without major sequelae.
- Individual lesions may leave postinflammatory hyper- or hypopigmentation.
- In general, recurrences are common, especially in HSV-associated disease.

- EM major may require hospitalization, and patients with mucosal involvement need specialized care to avoid complications such as infection and sepsis; eye complications, including purulent conjunctivitis with scarring, anterior uveitis, or corneal scarring; pneumoniae; dehydration; gastrointestinal hemorrhage; renal failure.

- Referral to a dermatology specialist is recommended unless the case of EM is mild with no mucosal involvement, and a correlation with HSV is clear.

- Infectious disease specialists may be recommended for intercurrent infections and treatment recommendations.

- Referral to ophthalmology is recommended for topical ophthalmic therapy recommendations.

- Patients should be educated about appropriate symptomatic treatment, and reassurance that EM minor is self-limited. It is also important for patients to be made aware of the risk of recurrent EM, and reminded to avoid any specific etiologic agent.

- Follow-up will depend on individual response to treatment.

- A patient with recurrent HSV-associated EM should be followed up long term by a dermatology specialist.

CLINICAL PEARL

- EM is uncommon in children. When it occurs, it can mimic polymorphous light eruption.

DRUG-INDUCED LUPUS

DIL is an ACDR associated with several drugs capable of triggering a lupus-like illness in patients who have not been previously diagnosed with lupus erythematosus. Recent studies have shown that the proton pump inhibitors (PPIs) are common, and previously underreported triggers of DIL (He & Sawalha, 2018). Older patients are more likely to suffer from DIL than from idiopathic SLE, with a 4:1 ratio of female to males affected. One exception to this trend is the category of young women developing DIL from the use of *minocycline* but this is rare, with only 15 cases of DIL out of 100,000 prescriptions written for this drug (Dalle Vedove et al., 2012). It is estimated that there are about 20,000 cases of DIL each year; however, it is a condition which is often under recognized and therefore underreported. The highest risk of DIL in dermatology patients is associated with minocycline and somewhat less with quinidine. The reaction is dose-related.

Pathophysiology

The etiology of DIL is uncertain but may be related to inhibition of DNA methylation, genetic predisposition (HLA and C_4 alleles), hormonal influences (estrogen), TNF-α inhibition, and reactive drug metabolites.

Clinical Presentation

The onset of DIL can occur weeks to years after the initiation of the drug therapy.

DIL can mimic the signs and symptoms of SLE but typically has a much milder clinical presentation.

Skin Findings

- Erythematous scaly papules and plaques (papulosquamous).

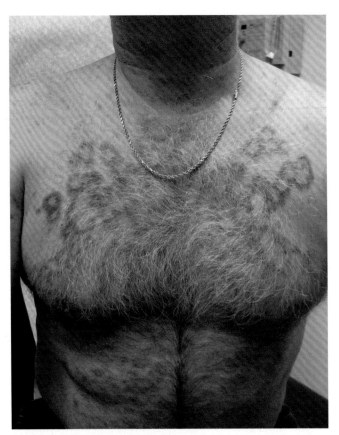

FIG. 8.1-10. Drug-induced cutaneous lupus.

- Annular/Arcuate erythematous papules and plaques.
- Predominantly occurring on photo-exposed areas (Fig. 8.1-10).
- The skin findings may be clinically indistinguishable from subacute cutaneous lupus erythematosus (see Section 9.2).

Non-Skin Findings

- This is a syndrome characterized by fever, arthritis, myalgia, and myositis—all of which can be present in SLE.

DIFFERENTIAL DIAGNOSIS   Drug-Induced Lupus

- Discoid lupus erythematosus
- Subacute cutaneous lupus erythematosus
- Systemic lupus erythematosus
- Psoriasis

Confirming the Diagnosis

- History should determine any signs, symptoms, or diagnosis of SLE or other autoimmune conditions prior to the skin eruption. At least one clinical symptom of SLE should be present after the initiation of drug therapy.
- Serology
  - ANA is usually positive with a homogenous pattern.
  - Anti-histone antibodies are seen in 95% of cases.
  - Anti-SSA/Ro, is positive especially if the causative agent is a thiazide diuretic.

- Anti-dsDNA is usually negative and anti-ssDNA is positive in DIL.
- Histopathology
  - Histology and DIF offer very little diagnostic value in terms of distinguishing DIL from SLE.
- Symptom resolution after discontinuance of the suspected causative drug.

Treatment

Discontinuation of the offending medication is the primary goal.

Topicals

- Topical steroid creams/ointments as needed for pruritus.

Systemic

- NSAIDs for myalgia, joint pain.
- A short course of prednisone will reduce the associated inflammation, thus reducing pain and myalgia. Example: A 2-week taper of prednisone 40 mg daily for 7 days, then 20 mg daily for 7 days. The usual precautions apply, including relative contraindications such as peptic ulcer disease, poorly controlled diabetes, active CHF, concomitant infection, and early dementia (see Section 1.5).

Management and Patient Education

- Clinical symptoms usually resolve within 4 to 6 weeks after the drug is discontinued. Repeat antibody titers may be slow to return to normal. Most patients do not have any further problems or development of SLE.
- Rechallenge can be performed at a later date if there is a question about the causative agent.
- Patients should follow-up in about 2 weeks after the drug has been discontinued to ensure the rash and systemic symptoms have resolved.
- Repeat ANA usually returns to normal but can remain elevated. Patients should be vigilant in avoiding ingestion of the drug (or drug class) in the future.
- The risk of minocycline-induced DIL is relatively low (8.8 cases/100,000 person-years) but the risk does go up with duration of therapy.

See Box 8.1-8.

BOX 8.1-8 Medications Associated with Drug-Induced Lupus

Common medications associated with DIL
- Hydralazine
- Procainamide

Less common medications associated with DIL
- Anti-TNF alphas
- Carbamazepine
- Griseofulvin
- Isoniazid
- Minocycline
- Penicillamine
- Phenytoin
- Sulfasalazine
- Terbinafine

CLINICAL PEARLS

There are some subtle variations in the clinical findings that may help differentiate SLE and DIL.

- DIL uncommonly presents with cutaneous manifestations of SLE.
- Arthralgia and/or myalgia are the predominating symptoms of DIL, making it more difficult to diagnose compared to SLE and its characteristic skin findings.
- Once the diagnosis of DIL is considered, the causative drug usually becomes obvious and once it is discontinued, the disease abates quickly; this is in sharp contrast to SLE.
- When necessary, a rechallenge with the presumed triggering drug will restart the symptoms.
- ANA is usually positive with DIL, in homogenous pattern.
- Antihistone antibodies are positive in most cases of DIL, but less often with minocycline.

URTICARIA AND ANGIOEDEMA

Urticarial drug eruptions are the second most common pattern of ACDRs. Angioedema can also be triggered by medication in addition to other causes. (See Section 8.2 for detailed information about urticaria and angioedema.)

PHOTOSENSITIVITY DRUG REACTIONS

See Section 1.5 for a discussion of photosensitive reactions.

ERYTHRODERMA

Potential triggers for erythroderma include drugs and a number of serious, even life-threatening conditions which must be recognized and managed in a timely fashion.

See Section 4 in this text for a full explanation and description.

RED MAN SYNDROME

Red man syndrome (RMS) is a specific hypersensitivity reaction associated with the administration of intravenous vancomycin. The reaction occurs between 5% and 10% of the time, especially if the infusion is administered in less than a 60-minute period. Patients at greater risk for RMS are individuals 40 years and older or 2 years old and younger. Concurrent use of vancomycin and other antibiotics, opioid analgesics, muscle relaxants, or contrast dyes, increases the risk of RMS attributed to their potential histamine-releasing effects.

N.B. *Erythroderma and "Red man syndrome" are totally different pathologic entities.*

Pathophysiology

RMS is not a true allergic reaction and does not involve drug-specific antibodies. This anaphylactoid reaction is the result of mast cell degranulation and the release of histamine relative to the amount and rate of vancomycin infused.

Clinical Presentation

- Signs of RMS can appear within minutes of initiating a vancomycin infusion or after completion of the treatment but it usually occurs with the first dose.
- In some cases, the reaction may be delayed and appear only after several doses.

Skin Findings

- Flushing or an erythematous rash may involve the face, posterior neck, upper body, and arms.

Non-Skin Findings

- Patients complain of diffuse burning and itching, with a rapid onset of dizziness and agitation.
- Muscle spasms in the back or neck, fever, chills, nausea, vomiting, dyspnea, and hypotension may occur.
- In some patients, there is very subtle pruritus at the completion of the treatment and the reaction may go unnoticed.

Treatment

- As RMS appears, the vancomycin infusion is stopped and diphenhydramine 50 mg is given intravenously.

Management and Patient Education

- The patient should be assessed for developing signs of anaphylaxis, but most cases are mild and result in immediate resolution of symptoms.
- Once symptoms have subsided, consideration can be given to reattempt the infusion of vancomycin. RMS does not prohibit subsequent doses; however, infusion of smaller doses over a longer period (at least 60 minutes) is recommended. Pretreatment with hydroxyzine is recommended for patients with known RMS in the past.

CORTICOSTEROID-INDUCED ACNE

Pustular eruptions resembling acne can occur acutely on the face and upper trunk 1 to 3 weeks after initiation of systemic corticosteroids. True acne is characterized by the presence of *comedones* (plugged follicular units); however, the lesions associated with drug-related acne are monomorphous and not comedonal in nature (see Section 3). Although ideal treatment is the discontinuation of the causative agent, this may not always be possible. Use of topical acne medications such as benzoyl peroxide wash and topical retinoids can be effective until clearance is achieved. Anabolic steroid use can also trigger a form of acne.

DRUG-INDUCED DYSPIGMENTATION

There are multiple medications that are associated with pigmentary changes of the skin including: amiodarone, minocycline, bleomycin, NSAIDs, heavy metals, antimalarials, and psychotropic drugs.

Pathophysiology

There are several mechanisms that can be responsible for drug-induced pigment abnormalities. Pathogenesis includes:

- An accumulation of melanin caused by the drug itself, especially with sun exposure.
- Postinflammatory changes secondary to drug therapy (hemosiderin staining).
- Deposits of the drug or drug metabolites along the basement membrane.

Clinical Presentation

Skin Finding

There is a variable range of color, patterns, and locations of drug-induced pigmentation that is often specific to the offending agent.

Amiodarone dyspigmentation is characterized by a violaceous coloration on sun-exposed skin surfaces, especially the face.

- Cutaneous changes usually develop with long-term, continuous therapy.
- The discoloration may fade after discontinuation of the drug but sometimes remains as a permanent dyspigmentation.

Minocycline can induce a blue-black coloration that affects the skin, nails, sclerae, oral mucosa, and teeth (Fig. 8.1-11A). Scar tissue, such as acne scars, and anterior shins are commonly affected and often confused with bruising. Three patterns of minocycline hyperpigmentation have been described:

- *Type I*: blue-black color that appears in sites of previous inflammation or scarring, typically within facial acne scars. Histology shows iron deposition in the dermis.

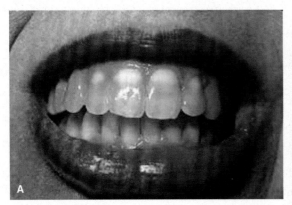

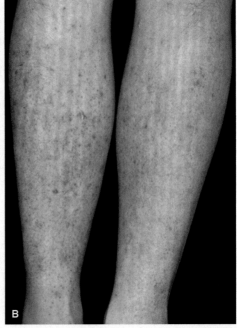

FIG. 8.1-11. Minocycline hyperpigmentation. **A:** Oral mucosa and teeth. **B:** Bluish-black minocycline pigmentation is often on the legs, related to trauma.

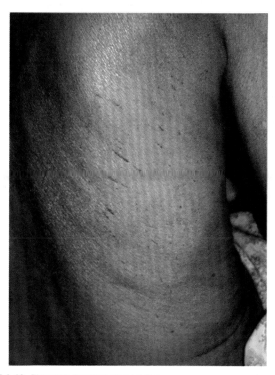

FIG. 8.1-12. Bleomycin flagellate pigmentation.

- *Type II*: blue-gray discoloration that affects otherwise normal skin, often on lower extremities. Histologic analysis exhibits melanin and iron deposits in the deeper dermis and fat (Fig. 8.1-11B).
- *Type III*: muddy brown discoloration accentuated in sun-exposed areas. Histology shows superficial melanin deposition in epidermis or dermis.
- *Type IV*: same etiology as *type III* but is characterized by occurring in preexisting scars on any surface.
- *Bleomycin* causes changes in pigmentation that are characterized as "flagellate pigmentation" (Fig. 8.1-12):
  - Appears as a brown-gray linear hyperpigmentation.
  - The lesions can be diffuse, often developing on the chest, back, and extremities, and can be photo-exacerbated.
  - It develops anywhere from 1 day to 9 weeks after systemic treatment with bleomycin.
  - The discoloration will fade about 3 to 4 months after the bleomycin has been discontinued.
  - Mild pruritus can be managed with low- to mid-potency topical corticosteroids or oral antihistamines.

Treatment

The goal of therapy is avoidance of the medication. Treatment choices include:

- Laser, other photodynamic modalities, used with care to avoid further disruption of pigment, an especially common issue in those with skin of color.
- Photoprotection with complete sunblock should be stressed.

Management and Patient Education

- The pigmentation often fades, albeit quite slowly, becoming a source of serious concern to the patient.

- In general, hyperpigmentation in those with darker skin tends to persist far longer.
- This should be discussed prior to initiation of treatment with such patients, who should be monitored regularly to limit the extent and persistence of darkening.

CLINICAL PEARLS

- Permanent darkening due to medications is rare, but does occur in patients on relatively high doses for longer periods.
- In the practice of dermatology, minocycline is the main offender, and should be watched for at every visit.
- Watch the teeth, gums, and scars for the first signs of hyperpigmentation and stop the minocycline immediately.

VASCULITIS

- Cutaneous small vessel vasculitis has been associated with drugs from almost every drug class.
- Vasculitis typically occurs within 1 to 3 weeks of drug administration.
- Medications associated with drug-induced vasculitis include penicillins, NSAIDs, sulfonamides, and cephalosporins among others.

See Section 9.3 for additional information on vasculitis.

TOXIC ERYTHEMA OF CHEMOTHERAPY

Several chemotherapeutic agents are known to trigger characteristic overlapping skin eruptions now termed toxic erythema of chemotherapy (TEC). TEC may develop as soon as 2 days up to 3 weeks after the initiation of these following medications: cytarabine, anthracycline, 5-fluorouracil, capecitabine, taxanes, and methotrexate.

Pathophysiology

While the pathophysiology of TEC is poorly understood, the reaction represents more of a toxic reaction to medications and not a true hypersensitivity reaction.

Clinical Presentation

Skin Findings

- Erythematous to violaceous scaly painful edematous patches and plaques (Fig. 8.1-13).
- Uncommonly, patients may develop bulla.
- As the process resolves, patients may have desquamation of the skin and postinflammatory hyperpigmentation.
- TEC typically occurs on the hands, feet, and intertriginous areas, and less often the knees, elbows, and ears are also affected (Fig. 8.1-14).

DIFFERENTIAL DIAGNOSIS   Toxic Erythema Chemotherapy

- Graft-versus-host disease
- Contact dermatitis
- Vasculitis
- Cellulitis
- Exanthematous drug eruption
- Viral exanthem

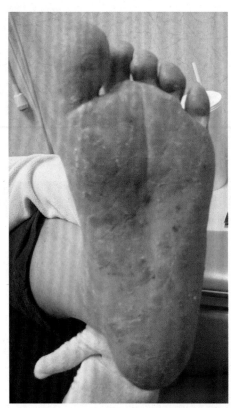

FIG. 8.1-13. Toxic erythema of chemotherapy. Scaly papules and plaques. (Used with permission from Wound, Ostomy and Continence Nurses Society®; Doughty, D. B., & McNichol, L. L. [2015]. *Wound, ostomy and continence nurses society® core curriculum: Wound management.* Wolters Kluwer Health.)

Confirming the Diagnosis

- Accurate diagnosis is critical, since failure to recognize TEC can lead to severe pain, extensive erosions, and increased risk of infection.
- While TEC is typically diagnosed clinically, a skin biopsy is essential for ruling out the other items in the differential.

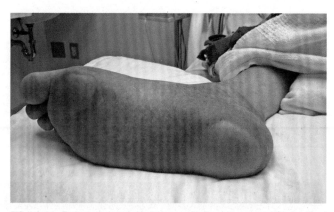

FIG. 8.1-14. Toxic erythema of chemotherapy. Erythematous skin with bulla. (Used with permission from Wound, Ostomy and Continence Nurses Society®; Doughty, D. B., & McNichol, L. L. [2015]. *Wound, ostomy and continence nurses society® core curriculum: Wound management.* Wolters Kluwer Health.)

Treatment

Topical

- Class 1 topical corticosteroids twice daily to affected areas and reevaluate in 1 week.
- Topical analgesics (e.g., lidocaine) prn for pain/dysesthesias

Management and Patient Education

- The condition spontaneously resolves within 2 to 3 weeks of therapy adjustment, and management is primarily supportive.
- The patient's oncologist should be notified immediately upon suspicion of TEC. As the reaction is not a hypersensitivity reaction, the medication does not necessarily have to be stopped. The medication frequency and/or dosage may be adjusted or stopped.
- Cool compresses, ice packs, and emollients can be soothing to the affected areas and local wound care for erosions/ulcerations (see Section 14.1).
- Avoidance of TEC may be assisted by counseling the patient to avoid bathing in hot water, vigorous exercise, and wearing tight clothing (Shi et al., 2016).

Hives and Angioedema

Bethany Grubb

Urticaria and angioedema represent a pathologic inflammatory response to an antigen, either self or foreign, and is referred to as a hypersensitivity reaction. Urticaria and angioedema represent a type 1 reaction which means there is an immediate response involving IgE and histamine. This reaction affects about 9% of the population at some point in their lifetime while 30% to 40% report having both conditions (Antia et al., 2018). Urticaria and angioedema can occur at any age, including children. Those individuals with a history of atopy (i.e., atopic dermatitis or eczema) are slightly more affected. Urticaria is a common presenting complaint in a primary care practice. It may be accompanied by angioedema or both conditions may present separately and the primary care provider (PCP) must understand the significance of each.

URTICARIA

Urticaria is a common vascular reaction of the skin characterized by rapidly fluctuating, transient skin, and/or mucosal edema due to plasma leakage. Wheals (also known as hives) result from edema in the superficial dermis compared to angioedema which occurs in the deep dermis and subcutaneous tissue. Urticaria presents with wheals, and may or may not be accompanied by angioedema. There are three types of urticaria discussed in this section, acute, chronic, and chronic-inducible urticaria.

Acute Urticaria

Acute spontaneous urticaria (ASU) is a mast-cell–mediated inflammatory response of the skin that is characterized by a rapid onset of wheals (30 minutes to <24 hours) that may cause itching/burning but no scarring. ASU is defined as the development of urticaria regularly <6 weeks that resolve spontaneously. ASU accounts for 15% to 25% of urticaria and approximately 80% of cases will resolve in less than 6 weeks (Zuberbier et al., 2018).

Pathophysiology

- The mast cell is the primary effector cell in urticarial reactions. When mast cells are stimulated and subsequently degranulate, histamine and other inflammatory mediators are released. Subsequently, immune cells (e.g., neutrophils, eosinophils) are activated and postcapillary venules dilate causing vascular fluid leakage through vessel walls resulting in localized erythema, tissue edema, and consequently wheal formation.
- There are several types of stimuli that can cause urticaria (Table 8.2-1), which include:
  - Immunologic (rheumatoid arthritis, SLE, Sjögren's)
  - Nonimmunologic (bacterial or viral infections)
  - Physical (cold, heat, pressure)
  - Chemical etiologies (antibiotics, opiates, narcotics)
- When looking at the frequency of urticaria etiology:
  - ~50% of cases are idiopathic
  - 35% are associated with infection (i.e., URI, diarrhea, dental caries, cystitis)
  - 6% are associated with medications
  - 2.5% with insect bite reactions
  - 1% associated with foods

Clinical Presentation

Skin Findings

- Pink or pale raised, well-circumscribed, edematous papules or plaques that change in size and shape (regression or peripheral extension in 24 hours) (Fig. 8.2-1).
- Range in size from a few millimeters to more than 5 cm in size and can coalesce and form annular or polycyclic plaques (Figs. 8.2-2 to 8.2-4).
- Pruritus, sometimes burning.
- Subcutaneous or submucosal edema (angioedema) may be present.

Non-Skin Findings

- Recurrent, unexplained fever, joint or bone pain, or malaise can occur with autoimmune disease.
- Hepatomegaly may occur with viral hepatitis.
- Lymphadenopathy may occur with viral, fungal, or bacterial infection.
- Thyromegaly may occur with concomitant thyroid disease.

TABLE 8.2-1	Causes of Urticaria
CAUSE	**AGENT**
Idiopathic (50%)	No identifiable cause
Infection (40%)	Bacterial (sinus, dental, pulmonary, urinary tract) Viral (preicteric phase of hepatitis B or C, mono- nucleosis, coxsackie) Fungal infections Protozoan and helminthic (intestinal worms, malaria)
IgE mediated (10%)	Medications (penicillin, sulfonamides, aspirin) Insects (stinging or biting) Latex Foods (children: milk, egg, peanuts, tree nuts, wheat, seafood; adults: seafood, tree nuts, peanuts) Food additives (benzoates, salicylates, sulfites) Contact allergens (chemicals, textiles, wood, saliva, cosmetics, perfumes, bacitracin)
Direct mast cell activation	Narcotics/Opiates Muscle relaxants (succinylcholine, curare) Radiocontrast medium Stinging nettle plant
Physical stimuli	Pressure urticarias Exercise-induced anaphylactic syndrome
Internal disease	Serum sickness Systemic lupus erythematosus Rheumatoid arthritis Sjögren syndrome Autoimmune thyroid disease Hyperthyroidism Carcinomas, lymphomas Rheumatic fever Juvenile rheumatoid arthritis Polycythemia vera
Hormones	Pregnancy Premenstrual flare (progesterone)

Adapted from Habif, T. P. (2016). *Clinical dermatology: A color guide to diagnosis and therapy* (5th ed.). Mosby.

- Progression to anaphylaxis is uncommon in urticaria but must be considered in patient history and physical examination.

DIFFERENTIAL DIAGNOSIS Urticaria (Acute and Chronic)

Acute
- Drug eruption
- Acute facial contact dermatitis
- Urticarial phase of bullous pemphigoid
- Dermatitis herpetiformis
- Insect bite reactions
- Other types of urticaria
- Erythema marginatum
- Erythema multiforme
- Urticaria pigmentosa

Chronic: all of the above plus
- Systemic lupus erythematosis
- Sweet syndrome
- Fixed drug eruption

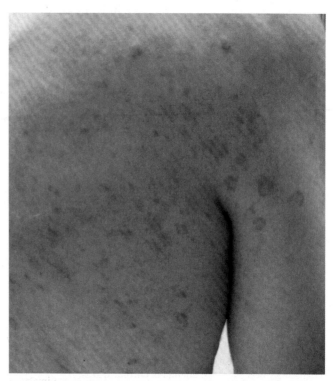

FIG. 8.2-1. Urticaria on a back and arm. Note the pale wheal and erythematous ring. (Photo courtesy of Cathleen Case.)

CONFIRMING THE DIAGNOSIS

History

A detailed history (Box 8.2-1) is essential for the evaluation and diagnosis of urticaria. Determining the duration of urticaria is essential as the diagnostic workup is different.

Laboratory

For ASU, diagnostic workup is warranted if patients fail to respond to initial treatment or an underlying condition is suspected based

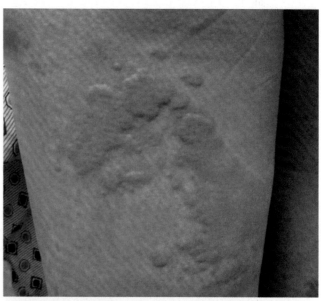

FIG. 8.2-2. Large urticarial plaques with dermal vasodilation and coalescing into polycyclic plaques. (Photo courtesy of M. Bobonich.)

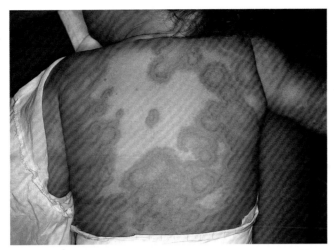

FIG. 8.2-3. Dramatic urticaria on infant with distinct morphologic features: wheal, flare, and central clearing of larger plaques. (Fleisher, G. R., Ludwig, W., & Baskin, M. N. [2004]. *Atlas of pediatric emergency medicine.* Wolters Kluwer Health | Lippincott Williams & Wilkins.)

upon the detailed history. Laboratory diagnostics for acute urticaria may include:

- CBC with differential white count (screening for any infection that may be a trigger or anemia of chronic disease)
- CMP to include liver and renal profile (electrolyte or liver abnormalities)
- Urinalysis to rule out asymptomatic UTI
- ESR or CRP
  - If positive, consider rheumatoid factor, antinuclear antibody panel, C3, C4, and CH50.
- TSH, T3, T4 (30% of patients have thyroid abnormalities)
- Histopathology
  - Skin punch biopsy of the skin is indicated when urticarial lesions are painful or last for more than 24 hours, to rule out urticarial vasculitis

Treatment

See Figure 8.2-5 for algorithm for pharmacologic treatment of urticaria.

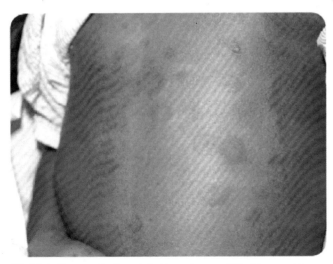

FIG. 8.2-4. Hives or urticaria on dark skin can be more difficult to appreciate.

- In addition to the adjunctive treatments included in the algorithm, patients may benefit from first-generation H_1 antihistamines to assist with sleep at night. Approach adding first-generation antihistamines with caution in older adults or patients with other medications with anticholinergic effects.
- EpiPen should be prescribed for patients with severe reactions or anaphylaxis. Patients should be instructed to proceed to the nearest emergency department following administration of a EpiPen as the effects may be ineffective or only last a few minutes.

Management and Patient Education

- Identifying and avoiding triggers (i.e., NSAIDs) can help prevent recurrence of symptoms. Often, even if the trigger source is not identified, there can be spontaneous remission.
- Rarely, severe anaphylaxis or severe respiratory tract angioedema can develop, and these patients are seen and treated in emergency departments.
- Patients should be counseled to call emergency services (i.e., 911) for symptoms suggestive of anaphylaxis, such as difficulty

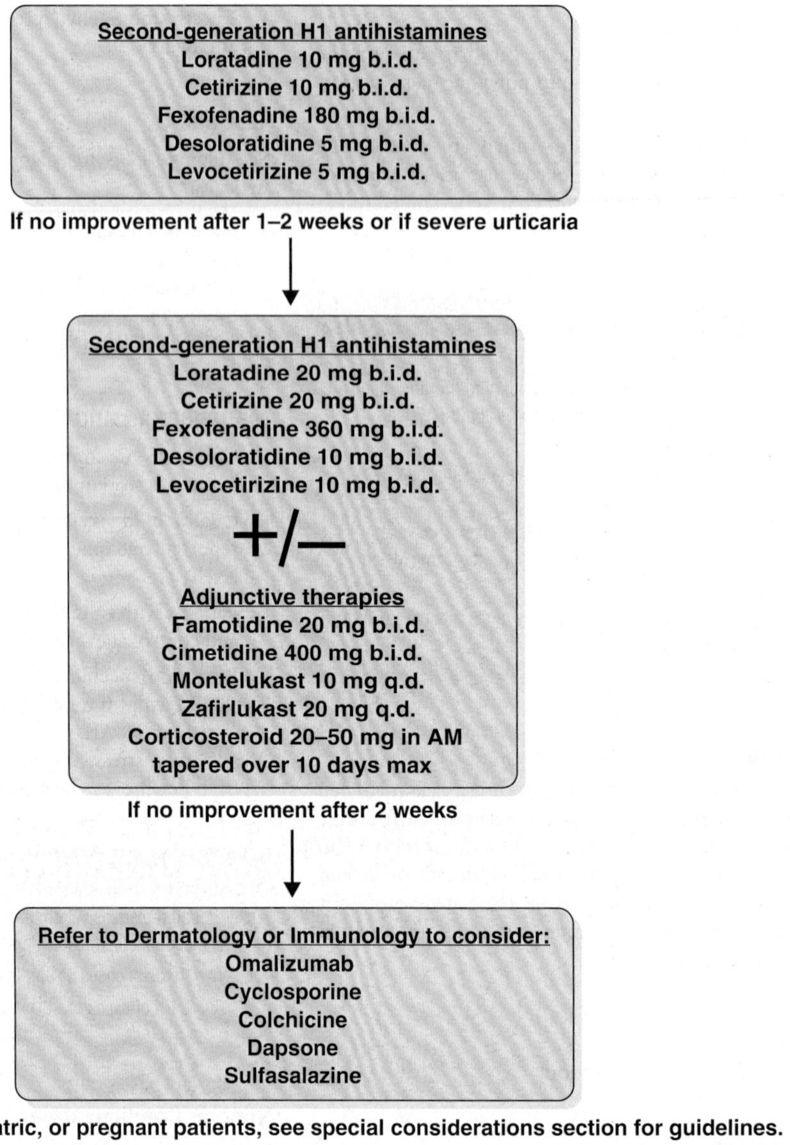

Second-generation H1 antihistamines
Loratadine 10 mg b.i.d.
Cetirizine 10 mg b.i.d.
Fexofenadine 180 mg b.i.d.
Desoloratidine 5 mg b.i.d.
Levocetirizine 5 mg b.i.d.

If no improvement after 1–2 weeks or if severe urticaria

Second-generation H1 antihistamines
Loratadine 20 mg b.i.d.
Cetirizine 20 mg b.i.d.
Fexofenadine 360 mg b.i.d.
Desoloratidine 10 mg b.i.d.
Levocetirizine 10 mg b.i.d.

+/−

Adjunctive therapies
Famotidine 20 mg b.i.d.
Cimetidine 400 mg b.i.d.
Montelukast 10 mg q.d.
Zafirlukast 20 mg q.d.
Corticosteroid 20–50 mg in AM
tapered over 10 days max

If no improvement after 2 weeks

Refer to Dermatology or Immunology to consider:
Omalizumab
Cyclosporine
Colchicine
Dapsone
Sulfasalazine

For pediatric, geriatric, or pregnant patients, see special considerations section for guidelines.

FIG. 8.2-5. Urticaria treatment algorithm. (Adapted from Zuberbier, T., Aberer, W., Asero, R., Abdul Latiff, A. H., Baker, D., Ballmer-Weber, B., Bernstein, J. A., Bindslev-Jensen, C., Brzoza, Z., Buense Bedrikow, R., Canonica, G. W., Church, M. K., Craig, T., Danilycheva, I. V., Dressler, C., Ensina, L. F., Giménez-Arnau, A., Godse, K., Gonçalo, M., … Maurer, M. (2018). The EAACI/GA²LEN/EDF/WAO guideline for the definition, classification, diagnosis and management of urticaria. *Allergy, 73*(7), 1393–1414.)

breathing, tightness in their chest or throat, nausea, vomiting, fainting, and swelling of their eyes, mouth, or tongue.

Special Considerations
Pregnancy

- Treatment of urticaria in pregnant or lactating women is largely the same as nonpregnant adults. However, H_1 antihistamines should be avoided during the 1st trimester.

- First-generation antihistamine chlorpheniramine is preferred during the first trimester when necessary, since it has a long safety record, although it is not approved for this indication. Diphenhydramine is also safe to use during pregnancy, but must be avoided during the 1st trimester due to an association with cleft palate development.

- Second-generation H_1 antihistamines (sgAH) (i.e., loratadine, cetirizine) are preferred and should be used at the lowest possible dose for the shortest period of time possible (Gonzalez-Estrada

& Geraci, 2016). Once the urticaria is controlled with antihistamines, gradually lower dose to the minimum dose required to control the disease.

Pediatrics

- Treatment of urticaria in children is largely the same as adults with a similar increased dose (two to four times) based on weight and age as needed.

- sgAH should be used and first-generation antihistamines (fgAH) should be avoided in infants and children as recommended by the European Academy of Allergy and Clinical Immunology (EAACI), Global Allergy and Asthma European Network (GA²LEN), the European Dermatology Forum (EDF), and the World Allergy Organization (WAO) (EAACI/GA²LEN/EDF/WAO guidelines) (Zuberbier et al., 2018).

- Children are often triggered by a viral or bacterial infection or are experiencing a food-related allergy specifically to milk.

Geriatrics

- The most important consideration for the geriatric patient is the sedative effects of antihistamines due to polypharmacy, comorbidities, and organ insufficiency.
- The second-generation antihistamines which are nonsedating should be used sparingly and may need close monitoring for those with renal or hepatic impairment. First-generation antihistamines should be avoided.

CLINICAL PEARLS

- Most cases of ASU resolve spontaneously.
- Urticaria significantly impacts quality of life secondary to pruritus, sleep disturbance, drug-related side effects, and concerns about physical appearance.
- Shortness of breath or stridor indicates a medical emergency and 911 should be called.
- Lesions lasting longer than 24 hours may indicate an urticarial vasculitis and may require biopsy (i.e., important to confirm the same lesion because urticaria is rapidly fluctuating)
- Patients can monitor specific lesions by drawing a circle around a spot to see if it still present in 24 hours.

Chronic Spontaneous Urticaria

Chronic spontaneous urticaria (CSU) is also a mast-cell–mediated inflammatory response of the skin. CSU is defined as urticaria occurring regularly or intermittently for >6 weeks. It accounts for 0.5% to 5% of cases, is most common during the 3rd to 5th decade of life and is often idiopathic. CSU is more likely to be associated with autoimmune conditions including Hashimoto thyroiditis, rheumatoid arthritis, or pernicious anemia.

Pathophysiology

See acute urticaria pathophysiology section.

Clinical Presentation

Please see acute urticaria clinical presentation section for details as the clinical presentation of CSU is indistinguishable.

DIFFERENTIAL DIAGNOSIS   Acute and Chronic Urticaria

See Urticaria DDx.

Confirming the Diagnosis

A more thorough workup is recommended in the setting of chronic urticaria to rule out any underlying conditions that may require treatment. In addition to the diagnostic workup discussed in ASU, the following labs should be considered in patients with chronic urticaria:

- Cryoglobulin levels
- Hepatitis B and C serologies (only check if clear features on clinical evaluation)
- Stool studies (Ova & Parasites)
- *Helicobacter pylori*

- Chest radiography (screening for autoimmune changes of lungs and heart)

Treatment

See Figure 8.2-5 for algorithm for pharmacologic treatment of urticaria.

- Patients who fail to improve following urticarial treatment algorithm should be referred to dermatology or immunology for the consideration of omalizumab, which is an anti–IgE-humanized monoclonal antibody for the treatment of chronic inducible urticaria (CIU).

Management and Patient Education

- CSU can be considered a diagnosis of exclusion and often requires a workup from a dermatologist or immunologist.
- Quality of life is strongly impacted in CSU and multiple patient-reported outcome tools have been developed to determine the levels.
- Patients with CSU should be assessed for disease activity, impact, and control at every follow-up visit.
- When no specific cause has been identified for CSU, patients should avoid the following: tight clothing, especially straps and waistline, NSAIDs, aspirin, alcohol, opiates, spicy foods, food additives, stress, upper respiratory tract infections, poor sleep, heat, hot showers, and humidity.

CLINICAL PEARLS

- Urticarial plaques >5 cm are at a higher risk to also have associated angioedema (see following section).
- Two thirds of cases of CSU in children remit spontaneously within 5 years.
- One third of cases of CSU in adults remit spontaneously within 5 years.

Special Considerations

Urticarial Vasculitis

- Urticaria must be differentiated from urticarial vasculitis, also known as hypocomplementemic urticarial vasculitis (HUV) or anti-C1q vasculitis, which is a rare immune complex small vessel vasculitis.
- Although most cases are idiopathic, it has been associated with:
  - Connective tissue diseases
  - Infections
  - Medications
  - Malignancies
  - Serum sickness
- In addition to the *painful* urticarial plaques, systemic involvement often may include glomerulonephritis, pulmonary disease, arthritis, and ocular inflammation (see Section 9.3).

Chronic Inducible Urticaria

CIUs are physical urticarias and are listed separately since their presence depends on eliciting a response to a physical factor. Lesions occur with regularity when a specific trigger (e.g., water, cold) is encountered. This type tends to be more severe, longer lasting, and more

difficult to treat. CIUs tend to be diagnosed in childhood and are more severe, longer lasting, and more difficult to treat. Angioedema can be seen with any of the physical urticarias except with symptomatic dermatographism.

Pathophysiology

CIU is a nonimmunologic event, classified by the predominant stimulus (e.g., pressure, cold), and provocative testing can usually confirm the diagnosis. Common causes of CIU include cold, delayed pressure, and an immediate response to stroking the skin (dermatographia). Uncommon causes of CIU include water, vibration, sun, heat, and contact (Hogan et al., 2014).

Subtype CIU

Dermatographism occurs in response to moderate stroking of the skin and is considered an exaggerated physiologic response. Delayed dermatographism will appear 30 to 60 minutes after the stroking stimulus. There is no association with systemic disease, atopy, food allergy, or autoimmunity. The general course is unpredictable, but the tendency is to remain dermatographic for years. A linear wheal develops within several minutes after stroking skin with a tongue blade (Fig. 8.2-6) and occurs in areas of the body associated with friction, such as from clothing. Pruritus may be present before the wheals.

Delayed pressure urticaria presents several hours after physical stimulus and may last for 72 hours or more. Urticarial lesions are induced by prolonged pressure such as standing, walking, manual use of hands, prolonged sitting, tight garments, and sexual intercourse. Systemic symptoms may include malaise, fatigue, fever, headache, or arthralgias. The mean duration for the condition is 6 to 9 years, and many patients have moderate-to-severe disease that is disabling. Pressure urticaria, chronic urticaria, and angioedema will often occur in the same patient with 60% of patients having chronic idiopathic urticaria and 30% having angioedema (Dover et al., 1988).

Cholinergic urticaria starts with itching, burning, tingling, warmth, or irritation of the skin precipitated by overheating the body particularly with exercise, hot shower/bath (Fig. 8.2-7). Up to 20% of young adults are affected by cholinergic urticaria, which typically presents as pinpoint-sized wheals. Concurrent systemic symptoms

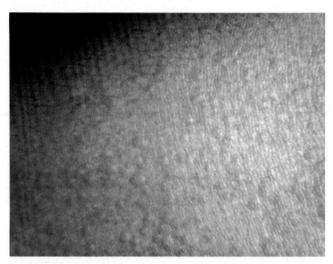

FIG. 8.2-7. Cholinergic urticaria.

are rare but may include angioedema, hypotension, wheezing, and abdominal pain. An episode may last for an hour, and the condition may last for years.

Acquired cold urticaria (ACU) syndromes (Fig. 8.2-8) are a group of conditions in which urticaria, angioedema, or anaphylaxis can occur within minutes of cold exposure, and can reoccur within minutes of rewarming. Within the CIU, the frequency ranges from 5.2% to 33.8% (higher incidence in regions with lower temperatures). A study done on children, found approximately 20% experienced anaphylaxis (grade 3 reaction) and of those almost 80% were triggered by swimming and the remaining by ingestion of cold food, beverage or exposure to cold air (Yee et al., 2019).

Adrenergic urticaria is a distinguishable form of CIU by the presence of blanched vasoconstricted skin surrounding pink wheals that is provoked by sudden stress.

Exercise-induced anaphylaxis (EIA) presents with pruritus, urticaria, respiratory distress, and hypotension after exercise. Attacks of food- and exercise-induced angioedema and anaphylaxis occur when the patient exercises within 30 minutes of ingesting the food (wheat, celery, shellfish, fruit, and fish). EIA is elicited by exercise and not by an increase in core body temperature, differentiating EIA from cholinergic urticaria.

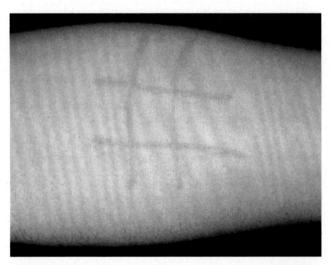

FIG. 8.2-6. Dermatographism or skin writing is an exaggerated response to pressure.

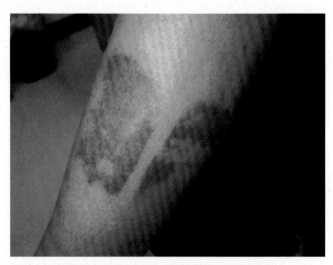

FIG. 8.2-8. Cold urticaria on a lower leg after the use of an ice pack.

Solar urticaria occurs within minutes of sun exposure on sun-exposed areas. The wheals of solar urticaria disappear in less than an hour. Severe reactions can include headache and syncope. Solar urticaria can be caused by natural or artificial UVA and rarely UVB. Patients should be reminded that solar radiation can penetrate light clothing.

Aquagenic urticaria develops after contact with water of any temperature and the eruption will resemble a mild cholinergic urticarial eruption.

Localized heat urticaria is very rare. Itching and whealing occur at the site of contact with heat within minutes of contact. Sources can include warm water, radiant heat, or warm sunlight.

Contact urticaria is triggered by a biologic or chemical agent characterized by the development of wheal and flare at the site of contact with skin or mucosa, or a generalized urticarial attack. The wheal and flare response typically take 30 to 60 minutes to appear.

Allergic contact urticaria is associated with atopic disease, when these young patients become sensitized to environmental allergens like grass, animals, foods, and in some cases latex.

The nonimmunologic type of contact urticaria is most common and most benign. This does not require prior sensitization, is due to the effects of urticants on blood vessels, and may take 30 to 50 minutes to appear. Exposure to histamine-releasing substances such as plants (nettles), animals (caterpillars, jellyfish), medications (dimethyl sulfoxide [DMSO]), bacitracin, cobalt chloride, cinnamic aldehyde, benzoic acid, and sorbic acid are common causes.

DIFFERENTIAL DIAGNOSIS   CIU

- Delayed pressure urticaria
- Cholinergic urticaria
- Adrenergic urticaria
- Exercise-induced anaphylaxis
- Cold urticaria
- Solar urticaria
- Aquagenic urticaria
- Localized heat urticaria
- Contact urticaria
- Allergic contact urticaria

Confirming the Diagnosis

- When the particular CIU is uncertain, patients can be referred to immunology for diagnostics to help with confirming the diagnosis.
- For secondary ACU, consider evaluation for concomitant cryoglobulins, cryofibrinogens, or cold agglutinin.

Treatment

See Figure 8.2-5 for algorithm for pharmacologic treatment of urticaria.

- Patients who fail to improve following urticarial treatment algorithm should be referred to dermatology or immunology for the consideration of omalizumab, which is an anti-IgE humanized monoclonal antibody for the treatment of CIU.

Management and Patient Education

- When the specific trigger is identified, strict avoidance is recommended.
- Clear, written instructions on appropriate avoidance strategies are key.

- Patients should be advised that exposure can lead to not only urticaria but also anaphylaxis.

CLINICAL PEARLS

- Primary acquired/essential cold urticaria most frequently occurs in young adults, and may follow a recent respiratory infection, arthropod bite or sting, drug therapy, or stress.
- Over 50% of children with cold urticaria will have anaphylaxis due to cold exposure (Yee et al., 2019).
- ACU can occur with a sudden drop in air temperature or with exposure to cold water; swimming in cold water can cause a severe reaction with hypotension, shock, and possibly death.

ANGIOEDEMA

Angioedema (angioneurotic edema) is a hive-like swelling in the subcutaneous tissue of skin, mucosa, and submucosal layers of the respiratory and GI tracts. The reaction is similar to that of hives which occurs in the upper dermis. Angioedema without the presence of urticaria is far more uncommon and signals several potentially life-threatening conditions which will be discussed here in detail: allergic angioedema, acquired angioedema (AAE), angiotensin-converting enzyme (ACE) inhibitor-associated angioedema, and hereditary angioedema (HAE).

Allergic Angioedema

Angioedema and hives often occur simultaneously and may have the same histamine driven etiology (see ASU Section).

Pathophysiology

- Mast-cell degranulation (allergic angioedema), as a result of numerous stimuli (Box 8.2-2), results in the release of histamine and numerous other inflammatory mediators that cause increased dilation and permeability of the vasculature.

Clinical Presentation

- Swelling associated with itch and/or urticaria is more suggestive of allergic angioedema (Fig. 8.2-9).

BOX 8.2-2   Common Triggers for Angioedema

- **Foods.** Shellfish, fish, peanuts, tree nuts, soy, wheat, eggs, and milk are frequent offenders.
- **Medication.** Common culprits include penicillin, aspirin, ibuprofen (Advil, Motrin IB, others), and naproxen sodium (Aleve).
- **Airborne allergens.** Pollen and other allergens that you breathe in can trigger hives, sometimes accompanied by upper and lower respiratory tract symptoms.
- **Environmental factors.** Sunlight, vibration such as from using a lawn mower, hot showers or baths, pressure on the skin such as from tight clothing or scratching, emotional stress, insect bites, and exercise.
- **Medical treatments or underlying conditions.** Hives and angioedema also occasionally occur in response to blood transfusions and infections with bacteria or viruses such as hepatitis and HIV.

Adapted from https://www.mayoclinic.org/diseases-conditions/hives-and-angioedema/symptoms-causes/syc-20354908

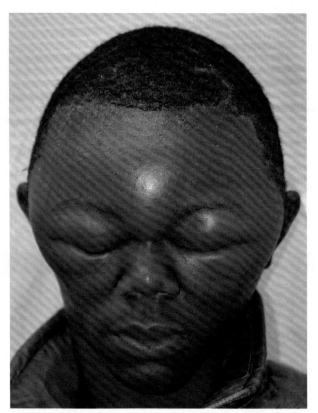

FIG. 8.2-9. Periorbital angioedema from contact allergy to a shampoo. (Photo courtesy of M. Bobonich.)

DIFFERENTIAL DIAGNOSIS Angioedema	
• Contact dermatitis	• Drug eruption
• Erysipelas	• Serum sickness
• Cellulitis	• Delayed pressure urticaria
• Cheilitis granulomatosa	• Eosinophilic cellulitis (Wells syndrome)
• Hereditary angioedema (HAE)	• Insect Bite Reaction

Confirming the Diagnosis

- Performing a comprehensive history, including detailed review of systems, and physical examination to identify potential etiologies of angioedema is essential.
- See acute urticaria section for guidelines.

Treatment

- In addition to antihistamines (see Fig. 8.2-5), patients with severe angioedema benefit from short-term course of oral corticosteroids 40 mg daily in AM tapered over 5 to 7 days.
- Patients with associated anaphylaxis may require intramuscular epinephrine (e.g., EpiPen) and immediately transferred to emergency room for additional management.

Management and Patient Education

- A management plan should be created with the help of dermatology or immunology.

Acquired Angioedema

AAE is an autoimmune response resulting from the formation of acquired anti–C1-INH autoantibodies from a secondary cause. AAE is clinically characterized by recurrent episodes of angioedema, without urticaria or pruritus, involving skin and mucosa of GI tract and upper respiratory tract. Laryngeal involvement can lead to fatal asphyxiation if left untreated. Typically, patients present in later adulthood (fourth decade of life) without a family history. AAE may be associated with: lymphoproliferative diseases (i.e., B-cell lymphoma), neoplastic syndromes (i.e., monoclonal gammopathy (MGUS), and autoimmune diseases (i.e., SLE).

Pathophysiology

- AAE occurs when C1 esterase inhibitor (C1-INH) is lacking, nonfunctional, or have autoantibodies against it; therefore, unrestrained C1 complement activity results in an inflammatory cascade with the downstream effect being increased bradykinin secretion.
- This may occur as a result of lymphoproliferative disorders or other malignancies.
- Additionally, the overproduction or impaired breakdown of bradykinin, a potent stimulator of vasodilation/vascular permeability, can occur as a result of numerous stimuli, but most commonly is associated with angiotensin converting enzyme inhibitors and other blood pressure medications or alterations in C1-INH.

Clinical Presentation

Skin Findings

- Swelling associated with burning and pain is more suggestive of increased bradykinin activity.
- Large, thick, and firm plaques may form on any skin surface but typically involve the lips, eyes, larynx, palms, soles, limbs, trunk, mucosa of the gastrointestinal tract, and genitalia (Fig. 8.2-10).

Non-Skin Findings

- Symptoms of gastrointestinal involvement (abdominal pain, vomiting, diarrhea) could indicate AAE or HAE.

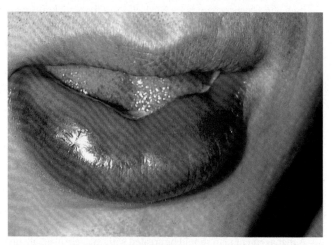

FIG. 8.2-10. Angioedema is a diffuse, nonpitting, tense swelling of the dermis, and subcutaneous tissue that can develop rapidly. Although usually allergic in nature and sometimes associated with hives, angioedema does not itch. (Neville, B. W., Damm, D., White, D., & Waldron, C. [1991]. *Color atlas of clinical oral pathology.* Lea & Febiger.)

- Anaphylaxis may present with dizziness, nausea, vomiting, weak or rapid pulse, wheezing or SOB (due to constriction of airways), or low blood pressure (hypotension), and should not be ignored.

Confirming the Diagnosis

Performing a comprehensive history, detailed review of systems, and physical examination to identify potential etiologies of angioedema is essential.

- Additional diagnostic workup for angioedema is warranted when angioedema is:
  - not associated with urticaria.
  - recurrent episodes of angioedema not associated with exercise, heat, cold, food, medications (ACE inhibitors, NSAIDs), underlying infection, lymphoproliferative disorder, or autoimmune disease process.
- Laboratory
  - Complete blood count with differential to identify potential underlying lymphocytopenia/lymphocytosis.
  - Comprehensive metabolic panel.
  - ESR or CRP.
  - Complement C4 levels and C1-INH antigen.
- If C4 levels or C1-INH levels are low, patients should be referred to immunology for further evaluation for AAE, which may include function of C1-INH and quantitative complement C1q.

DIFFERENTIAL DIAGNOSIS   AAE

- Contact dermatitis
- Erysipelas
- Cellulitis
- Cheilitis granulomatosa
- Hereditary angioedema (HAE)
- Drug eruption
- Serum sickness
- Delayed pressure urticaria
- Eosinophilic cellulitis (Wells syndrome)
- Insect Bite Reaction

Treatment

- AAE should be referred to immunology for treatment. Antihistamines and corticosteroids are NOT effective for bradykinin associated angioedema. For acute attacks (or "on-demand" therapy) icatibant, ecallantide, or berinert may be used to minimize severity of upper airway edema.
  - Prophylaxis with Cinryze, danazol, or lanadelumab is intended to minimize the risk of attacks when avoidance of triggers is not possible, patients experience two or more attacks per month, or those who have recurrent laryngeal attacks.
  - For symptomatic relief, analgesics, antiemetics, and fluids may be used.
  - Tranexamic acid (antifibrinolytic agent) is well tolerated and preferred for pregnant women, children, and patients who do not tolerate androgens.

Management and Patient Education

- A management plan should be created with the help of an allergy expert or an HAE expert (i.e., wallet card with specific treatments) for acute angioedema attacks.
- Due to the rare nature of this condition, it is critical that the patient (and caregivers) become their own advocate (Steiner et al., 2018).

Angiotensin-Converting Enzyme Inhibitor-Induced Angioedema

Angiotensin-converting enzyme inhibitor-induced angioedema (ACE–induced angioedema) is one of the most common causes for emergency treatment for angioedema and occurs in 0.1% to 6% of patients taking ACE inhibitors (Chansakulporn et al., 2014). Most cases occur in the first week of initiation of therapy but up to 33% of cases occur months or years after initiating an ACE inhibitor. ACE inhibitor–induced angioedema has a higher incidence in African Americans, smokers, and females.

Clinical Presentation

- Propensity for the face and tongue.
- The reaction can occur within hours, weeks, months, or years of taking the drug.

DIFFERENTIAL DIAGNOSIS   ACE–Induced Angioedema

- Acquired Angioedema (AAE)
- Drug eruption
- C1 esterase inhibitor (C1-INH) deficiency

Confirming the Diagnosis

- Laboratory
  - C1-INH antigen (usually normal)
  - Function of C1-INH (usually normal)

Treatment

- The primary management of ACE–induced angioedema is stopping the ACE inhibitor.
- ACE–induced angioedema often does not require systemic therapy, and antihistamine and corticosteroids are not effective.
- For acute attacks, icatibant, ecallantide, or berinert may be used to minimize severity of upper airway edema; however, their efficacy have not been proven.

Management and Patient Education

- Episodes of angioedema may occur for up to a month AFTER discontinuing an ACE inhibitor.

CLINICAL PEARL

- Longer-acting ACE inhibitors may present with more severe symptoms than the short-acting form.

Hereditary Angioedema

HAE is characterized by an insufficient production of C1-INH or normal concentrations of C1-INH that are functionally deficient, causing swelling when triggered. HAE has an incidence of 1 in 50,000, is characterized by autosomal dominant inheritance, and affects mostly females. In approximately 30% of HAE patients, clinical symptoms present prior to 5 years old and these patients often have more severe outcomes than those who present later in life (Henao et al., 2016). In contrast, patients with HAE with normal C1-INH often develop symptoms after childhood. Triggers of HAE can lead to a release of vasoactive peptides that produce swelling of the airway and GI tract that can result in death.

Pathophysiology

- There are several types of HAE
  - HAE type 1 (HAE-1)—85% of cases have low C1-INH levels and function.
  - HAE type 2 (HAE-2)—15% of cases have normal C1-INH levels but low function.
  - HAE with normal C1-INH—normal C1-INH level and function.
- One of the main distinctions between the pathophysiology of AAE and HAE is the genetic deficiency of the C1 inhibitor (C1-INH) inherited as an autosomal dominant trait. If C1-INH is lacking, nonfunctional, or autoantibodies against it exist, inhibition of the plasma contact system (e.g., complement, kinin, coagulation cascades) is defective and results in triggering release of vasoactive peptides (e.g., bradykinins) that result in angioedema.
- In patients with HAE with normal C1-INH function, the pathophysiology is not clear but may be due to enhanced bradykinin signaling as a result of genetic mutations in molecules involved in the plasma contact system. For example, patients with mutation in Factor XII have a pronounced response from exogenous estrogen and pregnancy.
- Triggers of HAE include minor trauma, surgery, infection, sudden emotional stress, exogenous estrogen, and fatigue.

Clinical Presentation

Skin Findings

- Most common presentation is nonemergent angioedema including the face, tongue, throat, hands, arms, legs, abdomen, genitalia, or buttocks that lasts 2 to 5 days after onset.
- Edema of the extremities and abdomen is more common in HAE type 1 and 2, whereas facial edema and extremity is more common in HAE with normal C1-INH.
- One third of patients with HAE type 1 and 2 have a prodromal eruption of erythematous annular and polycyclic plaques that spread centrifugally (erythema marginatum). However, HAE with normal C1-INH will not have erythema marginatum.

Non-Skin Findings

- Abdominal pain occurs in up to 93% of HAE patients (Zuberbier et al., 2010).

Confirming the Diagnosis

- If the patient has a positive family history, clinicians should suspect HAE. Patient should be referred to immunology for further evaluation, which will include the following labs:
  - C4 levels
  - C1-INH antigen
  - Function of C1-INH
  - C1q

DIFFERENTIAL DIAGNOSIS   HAE

- Acquired angioedema (AAE)
- Drug eruption
- C1 esterase inhibitor (C1-INH) deficiency

Treatment

The treatment of HAE is similar to C1-INH–induced angioedema. Please see above AAE treatment section for details.

Management and Patient Education

- Patients suspected to have HAE should be referred to immunology for further evaluation and management.
- All family members of patients with HAE type I and II who are one year old or older are recommended to undergo screening for the diagnosis of HAE.
- It is important to have a management plan for acute angioedema attacks that has been created with the help of an allergy expert or an HAE expert.
- Due to the rare nature of this condition, it is critical that the patient (and caregivers) become their own advocate. Early diagnosis and preparation for attacks is imperative to reduce the risk of death (Zuraw et al., 2013).
- US Hereditary Angioedema Association member card can be obtained to identify someone with HAE (https://www.haea.org/).
- Patient advocacy groups are available including the US Hereditary Angioedema Association (US HAEA) (https://www.haea.org/).

CLINICAL PEARLS

- Approximately 50% of HAE patients will experience at least one laryngeal episode within their lifetime (Kanani et al., 2011).
- Laryngeal edema (occurring over several hours) is understood to be the most significant cause of death and must be treated immediately due to the risk of asphyxiation.
- Any patient who experiences recurrent angioedema or abdominal pain in the absence of urticaria should be evaluated for HAE.
- Anaphylaxis may present with dizziness, nausea, vomiting, weak or rapid pulse, wheezing or SOB (due to constriction of airways), or low blood pressure (hypotension), and should not be ignored.

ACKNOWLEDGMENT

We would like to thank the previous authors, Glen Blair, Victoria Griffin, Margaret A. Bobonich, Mary E. Nolen, and Cathleen Case. Many of the figures, tables, and photographs have been reused from the previous edition.

READINGS AND REFERENCES

Adler, N. R., Aung, A. K., Ergen, E. N., Trubiano, J., Goh, M. S. Y., & Phillips, E. J. (2017). Recent advances in the understanding of severe cutaneous adverse reactions. *The British Journal of Dermatology*, *177*(5), 1234–1247. https://doi.org/10.1111/bjd.15423

Antia, C., Baquerizo, K., Korman, A., Alikhan, A., & Bernstein, J. A. (2018). Urticaria: A comprehensive review: Treatment of chronic urticaria, special populations, and disease outcomes. *Journal of the American Academy of Dermatology*, *79*(4), 617–633.

Chansakulporn, S., Pongpreuksa, S., Sangacharoenkit, P., Pacharn, P., Visitsunthorn, N., Vichyanond, P., & Jirapongsananuruk, O. (2014). The natural history of chronic urticaria in childhood: A prospective study. *Journal of the American Academy of Dermatology*, *71*(4), 663–668.

Dover, J. S., Black, A. K., Ward, A. M., & Greaves, M. W. (1988). Delayed pressure urticaria. Clinical features, laboratory investigations, and response to therapy of 44 patients. *Journal of the American Academy of Dermatology*, *18*(6), 1289–1298.

Fan, W.-L., Shiao, M.-S., Hui, R. C.-Y., Su, S.-C., Wang, C.-W., Chang, Y.-C., & Chung, W.-H. (2017). HLA Association with drug-induced adverse reactions. *Journal of Immunology Research*, *2017*, 3186328. https://doi.org/10.1155/2017/3186328

Fedorowicz, Z., van Zuuren, E. J., & Hu, N. (2012). Histamine H2-receptor antagonists for urticaria. *Cochrane Database of Systematic Reviews*, *2012*(3), CD008596.

Gonzalez-Estrada, A., & Geraci, S. A. (2016). Allergy medications during pregnancy. *The American Journal of the Medical Sciences, 352*(3), 326–331.

Habif, T. P. (2015). *Clinical dermatology: A color guide to diagnosis and therapy* (6th ed.). Mosby Elsevier.

Harr, T., & French, L. E. (2010). Toxic epidermal necrolysis and Stevens-Johnson syndrome. *Orphanet Journal of Rare Diseases, 5*(1), 39. https://doi.org/10.1186/1750-1172-5-39

He, Y., & Sawalha, A. H. (2018). Drug-induced lupus erythematosus: An update on drugs and mechanisms. *Current Opinion in Rheumatology, 30*(5), 490–497. https://doi.org/10.1097/BOR.0000000000000522

Henao, M. P., Kraschnewski, J. L., Kelbel, T., & Craig, T. J. (2016). Diagnosis and screening of patients with hereditary angioedema in primary care. *Therapeutics and Clinical Risk Management, 12*, 701–711.

Hogan, S. R., Mandrell, J., & Eilers, D. (2014). Adrenergic urticaria: Review of the literature and proposed mechanism. *Journal of the American Academy of Dermatology, 70*(4), 763–766.

Kanani, A., Schellenberg, R., & Warrington, R. (2011). Urticaria and angioedema. *Allergy, Asthma, and Clinical Immunology, 7*(Suppl 1), S9.

Lavan, A. H., & Gallagher, P. (2016). Predicting risk of adverse drug reactions in older adults. *Therapeutic Advances in Drug Safety, 7*(1), 11–22. https://doi.org/10.1177/2042098615615472

Lazarou, J., Pomeranz, B. H., & Corey, P. N. (1998). *Incidence of adverse drug reactions in hospitalized patients: A meta-analysis of prospective studies.* Centre for Reviews and Dissemination (UK). https://www.ncbi.nlm.nih.gov/books/NBK67323

Lee, H. Y., Walsh, S. A., & Creamer, D. (2017). Long-term complications of Stevens–Johnson syndrome/toxic epidermal necrolysis (SJS/TEN): The spectrum of chronic problems in patients who survive an episode of SJS/TEN necessitates multidisciplinary follow-up. *The British Journal of Dermatology, 177*(4), 924–935. https://doi.org/10.1111/bjd.15360

Pite, H., Wedi, B., Bornego, L. M., Kapp, A., & Raap, U. (2013). Management of childhood urticaria: Current knowledge and practical recommendations. *Acta Dermato-Vereneologica, 93*(5), 500–508. http://www.medicaljournals.se/acta/content/?doi=10.2340/00015555-1573&html=1

Rademaker, M. (2001). Do women have more adverse drug reactions? *American Journal of Clinical Dermatology, 2*(6), 349–351. https://doi.org/10.2165/00128071-200102060-00001

Shi, V. J., Levy, L. L., & Choi, J. N. (2016). Cutaneous manifestations of nontargeted and targeted chemotherapies. *Seminars in Oncology, 43*(3), 419–425. https://doi.org/10.1053/j.seminoncol.2016.02.018

Steiner, U. C., Kölliker, L., Weber-Chrysochoou, C., Schmid-Grendelmeier, P., Probst, E., Wuillemin, W. A., & Helbling, A. (2018). Food as a trigger for abdominal angioedema attacks in patients with hereditary angioedema. *Orphanet Journal of Rare Diseases, 13*(1), 90.

Su, J. R., Haber, P., Ng, C. S., Marquez, P. L., Dores, G. M., Perez-Vilar, S., & Cano, M. V. (2020). Erythema multiforme, Stevens Johnson syndrome, and toxic epidermal necrolysis reported after vaccination, 1999–2017. *Vaccine, 38*(7), 1746–1752. https://doi.org/10.1016/j.vaccine.2019.12.028

Tattersall, I., & Reddy, B. Y. (2016). Fixed drug eruption due to achiote dye. *Case Reports in Dermatology, 8*(1), 14–18. https://doi.org/10.1159/000443949

Vedove, C. D., Simon, J. C., & Girolomoni, G. (2012). Drug-induced lupus erythematosus with emphasis on skin manifestations and the role of anti-TNFα agents. *Journal Der Deutschen Dermatologischen Gesellschaft, 10*(12), 889–897. https://doi.org/10.1111/j.1610-0387.2012.08000.x

Yee, C. S., El Khoury, K., Albuhairi, S., Broyles, A., Schneider, L., & Rachid, R. (2019). Acquired cold-induced urticaria in pediatric patients: A 22-year experience in a tertiary care center (1996–2017). *The Journal of Allergy and Clinical Immunology: In Practice, 7*(3), 1024–1031.

Zuberbier, T., Aberer, W., Asero, R., Abdul Latiff, A. H., Baker, D., Ballmer-Weber, B., Bernstein, J. A., Bindslev-Jensen, C., Brzoza, Z., Buense Bedrikow, R., Canonica, G. W., Church, M. K., Craig, T., Danilycheva, I. V., Dressler, C., Ensina, L. F., Giménez-Arnau, A., Godse, K., Gonçalo, M., … Maurer, M. (2018). The EAACI/GA²LEN/EDF/WAO guideline for the definition, classification, diagnosis and management of urticaria. *Allergy, 73*(7), 1393–1414.

Zuberbier, T., Balke, M., Worm, M., Edenharter, G., & Maurer, M. (2010). Epidemiology of urticaria: A representative cross-sectional population survey. *Clinical and Experimental Dermatology, 35*(8), 869–873.

Zuraw, B. L., Banerji, A., Bernstein, J. A., Busse, P. J., Christiansen, S. C., Davis-Lorton, M., Frank, M. M., Li, H. H., Lumry, W. R., & Riedl, M.; US Hereditary Angioedema Association Medical Advisory Board. (2013). US Hereditary Angioedema Association Medical Advisory Board 2013 recommendations for the management of hereditary angioedema due to C1 inhibitor deficiency. *The Journal of Allergy and Clinical Immunology. In Practice, 1*(5), 458–467.

Approach to a Patient with Blisters

Margaret A. Bobonich

In This Chapter

- Fluid-Filled Lesions
- Approach to a Blister
- Pustular Eruptions
- Vesiculobullous Eruptions
- Autoimmune Blistering Diseases
  - Intraepidermal

- Pemphigus
- Subepidermal
  - Bullous Pemphigoid
  - Linear IgA
  - Dermatitis Herpetiformis
  - Epidermal Bullosa Acquisita

FLUID-FILLED LESIONS

Clinicians often evaluate patients who present with complaints of fluid-filled skin lesions which can be characterized by vesicles, bullae, and pustules. The term *blister* is often interchanged with vesicle, bulla, and pustule which are morphologic descriptions of the lesions and critical to differentiate a wide spectrum of skin diseases. Vesiculobullous and pustular eruptions may be caused by trauma, infection, genetic disorders, immune-mediated, and reactive processes. There is a subgroup of patients who may go undiagnosed or mismanaged if the clinician does not consider underlying systemic diseases or disorders like autoimmune blistering diseases (AIBDs). Although not common, some of these dermatoses may be associated with a high mortality and morbidity. Ultimately, the clinician must determine whether a fluid-filled skin eruption requires supportive care, topical or systemic treatment, or more urgent/emergency measures to preserve life or limb.

This section will focus on a diagnostic approach to fluid-filled skin lesions along with prompt recognition, differential diagnosis, therapeutic options, and referral to experienced clinicians to optimize patient outcomes. Associated underlying causes of fluid-filled lesions, like infection or disease states, will be addressed in their respective chapters in this textbook. This section will offer you more detailed guidance about AIBDs including pemphigus, bullous pemphigoid (BP), linear IgA disease (LAD), and dermatitis herpetiformis (DH). There will be a brief overview of a few other variants.

APPROACH TO A BLISTER

The assessment of any eruption characterized by fluid-filled lesions should follow the same organized history and physical required for any skin disease presentation (Section 1). Actually, fluid-filled lesions are easier to diagnose compared to solid lesions that require further differentiation of morphology including color and scale.

History

Care should be taken to collect a detailed history of past and present illness, family history, medication inventory, and social history. A diary of activities may be necessary if there is a suspicion of an underlying allergic etiology. Any previous prescribed or nonprescribed therapeutics should be noted along with the response to therapy. A review of symptoms may provide subtle clues about associated systemic diseases or reactions.

Pathophysiology

Normal keratinocytes in our skin are bound together by adhesion molecules. Blisters arise when there is a disturbance in the structure or function within epidermis or at epidermal–dermal junction. This disruption may be due to infections, mechanical/physical changes, reaction or aberrancy of the immune system, or underlying genetic etiology. Lesion morphology coupled with a detailed history and physical examination can provide vital clues regarding the pathogenesis of the condition.

Clinical Presentation

A patient presenting with a localized vesicular, bullous, or pustular eruption may only require a focused skin examination of the affected area while a generalized eruption would necessitate a full-body skin examination. However:

- Clinicians must exercise caution not to overlook other skin signs and symptoms that signal a more extensive or complex disease state. An individual may not appreciate that ulcerations in their mouth have any relation to blisters on their arms or genitals.
- Good judgment may dictate that a comprehensive skin examination is necessary in order to accurately assess the patient.
- Care must be taken to look for lesions in the mucous membranes, hair, nails, palms/soles, and genitals.

TABLE 9.1-1	Important Characteristics of Fluid-Filled Skin Eruptions
Tense versus flaccid	The fragility of the blister provides important clues regarding the underlying etiology and diagnosis. A *tense* or firm vesicle/bulla which is intact should guide the clinician to consider a subepidermal skin disease. A *flaccid* lesion is easily ruptured and likely due to a more intraepidermal pathogenesis. The challenge is assessing the fragility of pruritic vesicles/bullae that are eroded secondary to scratching.
Blister stage	Fluid-filled lesions may present at varying stages. An intact blister may signify an earlier stage of lesion formation whereas an erosion/denuded skin can indicate a ruptured lesion that is resolving or one that is fragile.
Distribution	A *generalized* versus *localized* pattern along with symmetry can prove clues for the differential diagnoses, especially for vesiculobullous eruptions. Photodistribution, dermatomal pattern, and flexural or extensor involvement can be helpful in increasing diagnostic accuracy.
Location	Carefully note whether the lesions are present on the trunk, extremities, acral surfaces, mucosal membranes (including ears, nose, throat, vagina, or rectum), or genitals.
Arrangement	Identify whether the lesions are solitary or in clusters. A linear arrangement may indicate a contact dermatitis (i.e., classic poison ivy) compared to a circular pattern (i.e., rosettes of linear IgA) seen in immune-mediated or reactive processes.
Nikolsky sign	A Nikolsky sign is present in Stevens–Johnson syndrome/toxic epidermal necrolysis, Staph scalded skin, and pemphigus vulgaris. A positive Nikolsky is a very concerning sign and should prompt immediate referral to the emergency department or dermatology specialist. The Nikolsky sign is positive when gentle pressure applied to normal-appearing skin, adjacent to a vesicle or bulla, results in a shearing away of the epidermis.
Secondary changes	Crusts (i.e., secondary infection like impetigo) or erosions (from scratching or delicate rupture from pressure or friction).
Skin symptoms	Burning, pruritus, sharp pain, or weakness. Changes in hair or nails.

Assessment of a Blister

Characteristics of fluid-filled lesions are critically important for an accurate assessment (Table 9.1-1). The morphology of the lesion should guide your initial approach and enhance your diagnostic accuracy.

Building Your Differential Diagnoses

Skin Findings

First step—Begin by identifying what type of fluid is inside the blister.

Vesicles—clear fluid-filled lesions, less than 1 cm
Bullae—clear fluid-filled lesions, greater than 1 cm
Pustules—any size fluid-filled lesions with an opaque or purulent liquid
Hemorrhagic vesicles/bullae—filled with clear fluid but contain some red blood cells caused by trauma or inflammation at the site. They are not associated with frank bleeding, but patients may fear they will hemorrhage if the blister ruptures. If present, hemorrhagic blisters should be categorized as vesiculobullous lesions

Second step—Consider the differential diagnoses.

Once the type of fluid-filled lesion is established, proceed to the corresponding algorithm; pustular lesion algorithm (Fig. 9.1-1) or vesiculobullous lesions algorithm (Fig. 9.1-2) to build the differential diagnoses.

Third step—Consider additional characteristics.

The distribution, location, and associated symptoms can help to narrow the diagnoses and aid the decision making to order the appropriate diagnostic tests.

Non-Skin Findings

An ill-appearing individual presenting with a fever or constitutional symptoms accompanied by an eruption of fluid-filled lesions should prompt immediate assessment, treatment, and referral when appropriate. A comprehensive physical examination is essential in identifying underlying systemic conditions that may be limb- or life-threatening.

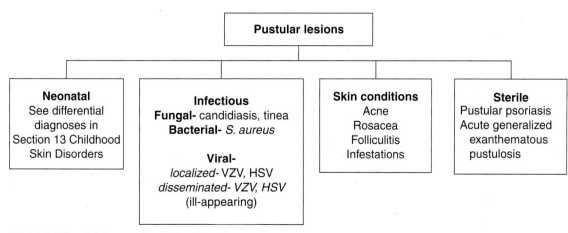

FIG. 9.1-1. Differential diagnoses for pustular skin eruptions.

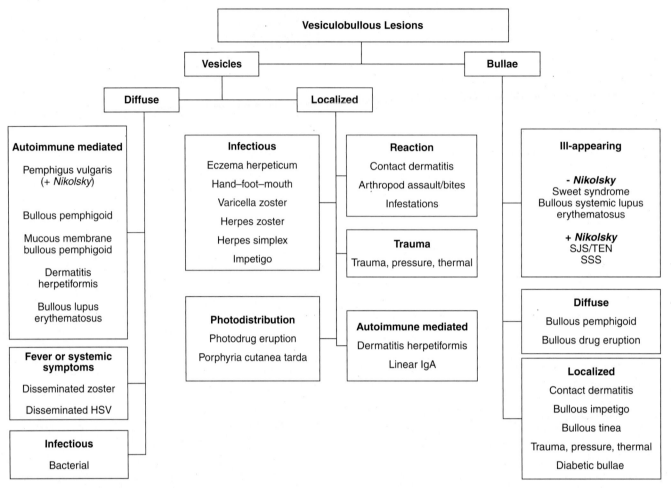

FIG. 9.1-2. Differential diagnoses for vesiculobullous skin eruptions.

PUSTULAR ERUPTIONS

Pustular lesions are often, but not always, caused by an underlying infectious process. The location and distribution of lesions will be one of the most helpful diagnostic clues and will aid the clinician in selecting the appropriate laboratory diagnostics.

- Patients with generalized pustular eruptions, such as disseminated varicella zoster or herpes simplex viruses, are usually ill-appearing and prompt urgent management.
- Localized pustular conditions caused by suspected pathogens can often be managed with topical or systemic antimicrobials. However, topical medications will not be effective if a serum crust covers the lesion. Care of the skin with a gentle cleanser and water will thin the serum crust allowing for better absorption of the topical therapy.

Differential Diagnosis for Pustular Eruptions

See Fig. 9.1-1.

Confirming the Diagnosis

- Appropriate bacterial, fungal, or viral culture and sensitivity
- Viral DNA or RNA detection tests
- Skin scraping for KOH or mineral prep may identify infestations
- Serum IgG may help identify the underlying etiology if there are no skin symptoms
- Skin biopsy is not typically performed for pustular eruptions

Management and Patient Education

- Therapeutic approach to pustular eruptions is based on the underlying cause
- Skin care for pustular lesions includes gentle cleansing and covering with a bandage especially when there is an infectious etiology
- Neonatal eruptions—Section 13
- Infections—Section 6
- Infestations—Section 7
- Other skin conditions—refer to the appropriate content section based on your index of suspicion or diagnostic test results (i.e., infections, eczematous, pediatrics, etc.)

VESICULOBULLOUS ERUPTIONS

Vesicles and bullae may contain clear or blood-tinged (hemorrhagic) fluid from a disruption in the blood vessels. The underlying cause of vesiculobullous eruptions is more expansive compared to pustular eruptions. The size of the lesions and the distribution of the eruption are the key to building the differential diagnosis.

BLISTER FRAGILITY

The fragility of the blister may also provide clues about the pathogenesis of the disease and the level of skin involvement.

Tense vesicles/bullae—usually stay intact and retain fluid. They are not easily ruptured because the underlying etiology is usually lower in the epidermis or epidermal–dermal junction.

Flaccid vesicles/bullae—are fragile and often not intact or fluid-filled when the clinician examines the patient. If they are intact, they are easily ruptured by pressure, friction, or scratching. Flaccid erosions can be an indication that the underlying disease involves the mid to upper epidermis.

Erosions—are often the residual from ruptures or healing fluid-filled lesions. Do not overlook the possibility of any vesiculobullous eruption when a patient presents with numerous erosions (i.e., scratching) or flaccid vesicles/bullae.

Differential Diagnoses for Vesiculobullous Skin Eruptions

See Fig. 9.1-2.

Confirming the Diagnosis

- The appropriate bacterial, fungal, or viral culture and sensitivity.
- Skin scraping for KOH or mineral prep may identify infestations.
- Viral DNA or RNA detection test.
- Serum IgG may help to identify if there are no skin symptoms.
- Punch skin biopsy for tissue culture and sensitivity may be indicated.
- If an autoimmune skin disease is suspected, the patient should be referred to an experienced dermatology provider to perform immunofluorescence and enzyme-linked immunosorbent assay (ELISA) tests.
- Other appropriate tests based on suspicion of underlying causes including culture and sensitivities for infections; patch testing or serologies for allergic reactions; autoimmune serologies associated with AIBDs or connective tissue diseases; and, diagnostics base on the review of symptoms.

Management and Patient Management

A therapeutic approach for patients with vesiculobullous lesions is based on the underlying cause.

- If the eruption is accompanied by a fever or constitutional symptoms, the clinician should elevate their level of concern and refer the patient appropriately.
- Care of the blisters is important to promote healing and prevent infection.
- Gentle cleansing with soap and warm water, then pat dry.
- Try to leave the blister intact to promote healing and prevent infection.
- If the vesicle/bulla is large or tense and causing pain, careful puncture of the blister with a sterile need can relieve the pressure.
- If the blister is punctured, allow the roof of the blister to remain to cover the wound base. This acts like a physiologic bandage.
- Apply white petrolatum and then cover with a protective gauze or dressing.
- See Section 14 for care of wounds.
- Infectious blisters should always be covered to prevent transmission of infection to others as well as reduce the risk of secondary infection.

TABLE 9.1-2	Types of Autoimmune Bullous Diseases and Location of Blisters in the Skin
TYPE OF ADHESION	**LOCATION OF BLISTERS**
Cell-to-cell	Epidermal Pemphigus vulgaris Pemphigus foliaceus Paraneoplastic pemphigus
Cell-to-matrix	Subepidermal Bullous pemphigoid Mucous membrane pemphigoid Linear IgA Epidermolysis bullosa acquisita Bullous systemic lupus erythematosus Dermatitis herpetiformis

AUTOIMMUNE BLISTERING DISEASES

In general, AIBDs are separated into two categories based of the location of the blister in the skin: intraepidermal and subepidermal blistering diseases (Table 9.1-2). Clinicians should always consider an AIBD as a differential diagnosis whenever patients present with blisters or erosions secondary to blisters. The morphology, distribution and location, severity of blisters, and comorbidities are critical for clinical correlation. AIBDs can involve the skin and/or mucous membranes and vary in severity.

Pathophysiology

Individuals with AIBDs develop autoantibodies that target specific adhesion proteins in the epidermis (Fig. 9.1-3).

- *Intraepidermal* blisters are the result of impaired desmosomes and result in characteristically flaccid vesicles/bullae within the epidermis (Fig. 9.1-4A).
- *Subepidermal* blisters involve the hemidesmosomes which are responsible for basal keratinocyte adhesion to the epidermis or cell-to-matrix adhesion in the basement membrane zone (BMZ) (Fig. 9.1-4B). Autoantibodies that target the hemidesmosomes, anchoring fibrils and filaments, and fibrin can result in subepidermal blisters that are tense. The vesicles/bullae are usually tense because the pathology is in the basement membrane of the epidermis.

Confirming the Diagnoses

The diagnosis of an AIBD requires <u>both</u> clinical and immunohistologic correlation usually by a dermatology specialist experienced in AIBDs. Two punch biopsy specimens are recommended: routine hematoxylin and eosin (H&E) and direct immunofluorescence (DIF).

Histopathology

- Routine H&E identifies the location/level of the blister in the skin.
- Punch biopsy should be taken from lesion near the edge of a new blister.
- Placed in formalin for a full-thickness histologic examination.

Direct Immunofluorescence

- A DIF is the gold standard for detecting the presence and location of <u>tissue-bound</u> autoantibodies, complements, and fibrin deposits in skin or mucous membrane.

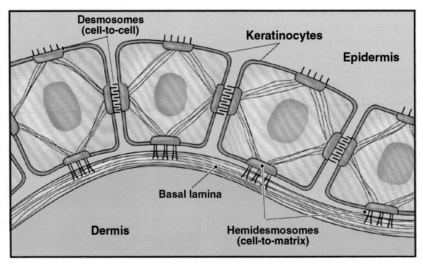

FIG. 9.1-3. Basement membrane zone. Keratinocytes in the epidermis attach to each other (cell-to-cell) with specialized cell junctions called *desmosomes*. Impaired function can result in an intraepidermal blister. *Hemidesmosomes* attach the basal keratinocytes to the dermis (cell-to-matrix) at basal lamina. Disruption of the hemidesmosomes can lead to subepidermal (below the basal keratinocyte) blisters, separating the epidermis from the dermis.

- A DIF identifies the type and location of the autoantibodies. A punch specimen for DIF must be taken from perilesional skin (within 1 cm from the vehicle or blister) and transported in formalin. Do not transport in formaldehyde.

Indirect Immunofluorescence

- Identifies circulating antibodies from the patient's serum and incubated on various substrates to detect the type and location of the autoantigens.
- Indirect immunofluorescence (IIF) provides further differentiation between subepidermal blistering diseases using the salt-split skin technique. Antibodies tagged with immunofluorescence will either bind to the roof (epidermal side) or floor (dermal side) of the BMZ which will help narrow the differential diagnoses.

Enzyme-Linked Immunosorbent Assay

- ELISA detects circulating autoantibodies against the hemidesmosomes (BP 180 and 230 for pemphigoid) and desmosomes (desmogleins 1 and 3 for pemphigus) using the patient's serum.

- These levels can also be used to monitor disease activity and response to therapy.

INTRAEPIDERMAL BLISTERING DISEASE

PEMPHIGUS

Pemphigus is a family of rare skin disorders with immune-mediated, intraepidermal blisters. *Pemphigus vulgaris (PV)*, the most common of the group, has been reported in all ages but is considered a disease of middle age (mean age 40 to 60 years) with increased incidence in Jewish and Mediterranean populations. Subtypes include PV, pemphigus foliaceus (PF) and paraneoplastic pemphigus (PNP). Thymoma and myasthenia gravis have been associated with PV.

Pathophysiology

The blistering that occurs in pemphigus is caused by impaired cell-to-cell adhesion (*acantholysis*) within the epidermis. It is unclear

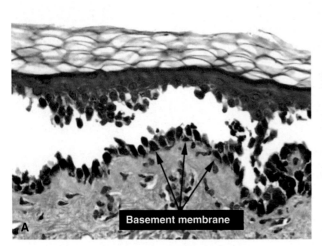

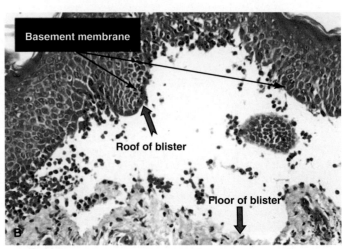

FIG. 9.1-4. **A:** Histopathologic analysis shows intraepidermal separation (blister) that occurs above the basal membrane zone in a patient with PV. **B:** Subepidermal blister below the basal layer (subepidermal) in a patient with pemphigoid.

why IgG autoantibodies target desmogleins 1 and 3, the antigens responsible for keratinocyte adhesion. There is an increasing number of reports that identify thiol drugs (captopril, penicillamine, and gold sodium thiomalate), phenol drugs (aspirin, rifampin, levodopa, and heroin), and nonthiol/nonphenol drugs (NSAIDs, ACE inhibitors, and calcium channel blockers) that may cause pemphigus.

Clinical Presentation

Skin Findings

- Vesicles/bullae can be any size, often coalescing to become generalized erosions. Blisters often favor the head, upper body, and intertriginous areas. They can be localized or generalized.
- Since the defect in pemphigus occurs within the epidermis, vesicles and bullae are *flaccid* and rupture easily.
- There is a positive *Nikolsky sign* where the healthy-appearing skin surrounding the blister shears away when lateral pressure applied.
- The physical examination may only reveal crusted erosions secondary to scratching (Fig. 9.1-5).
- The majority of patients have mucosal involvement which typically precedes the skin eruption. When mucous membranes are involved, erosions and ulcerations are most common on the oral mucosa and gingiva but can also be found on the conjunctiva, nasopharynx, esophagus, urogenital mucosa, and anus (Fig. 9.1-6).
- The pruritus of PV is variable.

Non-Skin Findings

- Mucosal lesions can cause dysphagia, hoarseness, and dehydration due to pain with eating and drinking. Severe burning,

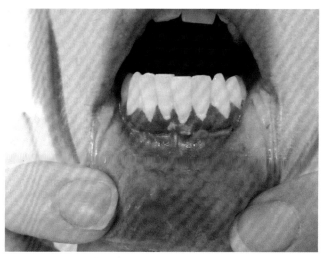

FIG. 9.1-6. Erosions of oral lesions in bullous pemphigoid. (Photo courtesy of M. Bobonich.)

pain, and pruritus are commonly reported. Females with vaginal mucosal involvement may experience dyspareunia, vaginal burning, and burning with urination.

Subtypes

- *Pemphigus vegetans* is considered a variant of PV and has unique mucocutaneous lesions presenting initially as bullae that then develop into hypertrophic granulation or verruciform plaques (Fig. 9.1-7). Lesions are malodorous and favor the extensor surfaces, oral mucosa, and intertriginous areas like the axilla, inguinal folds, and umbilicus.
- *PF* presents as crusted erosions that favor a seborrheic distribution of the scalp, face, upper chest, and back (Fig. 9.1-8). Clinically, PF tends to have more shallow lesions, rarely involves mucous membranes, and has a milder disease course than PV.

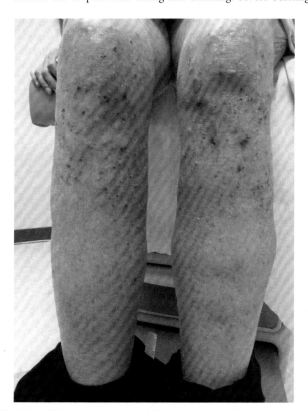

FIG. 9.1-5. Blisters may not be an obvious presentation. Flaccid vesicles and bullae of pemphigus vulgaris often present as crusted erosions. (Photo courtesy of M. Bobonich.)

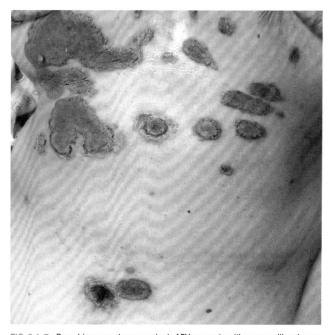

FIG. 9.1-7. Pemphigus vegetans, a variant of PV, presents with verruca-like plaques and pustules favoring intertriginous areas. (Photo courtesy of M. Bobonich.)

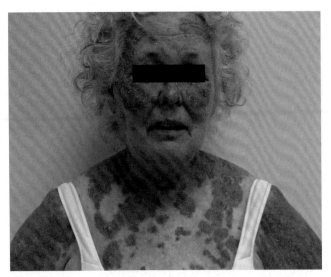

FIG. 9.1-8. Pemphigus foliaceus favors the seborrheic distribution and typically has a milder disease course than PV. (Photo courtesy of M. Bobonich.)

- *PNP* is a rare form of pemphigus characterized by a rapid and extensive stomatitis involving the lips, oral mucosa, throat, and conjunctiva. The oral mucosal lesions of PNP are extremely painful, leading to dehydration and poor nutrition. Dusky targetoid plaques, similar to those in erythema multiforme, may appear on the trunk and extremities. PNP patients have a very ill appearance. Unlike the other pemphigus types, the onset of PNP occurs in patients over 60 years old and is usually associated with an underlying malignancy.

DIFFERENTIAL DIAGNOSIS   Pemphigus Vulgaris

- SJS/TEN (positive Nikolsky sign)
- Other AIBDs
- Erythema multiforme
- Bullous impetigo
- Herpes simplex or zoster
- Drug eruption
- Lupus erythematosus

Confirming the Diagnosis

It is not uncommon for there to be a delay in the diagnosis of pemphigus because erosions, not fluid-filled lesions, are typical on presentation. Thus, AIBDs may not initially be considered in the differential.

- Punch biopsy of lesional skin for H&E shows an intraepidermal blister with acantholysis.
- Punch biopsy of perilesional skin for DIF shows IgG and C3 staining.
- ELISA testing for desmogleins 1 and 3 is highly sensitive for differentiating PV and PF.

Treatment

Corticosteroids

- Systemic corticosteroids have traditionally been the first-line therapy to halt the eruption of vesicles/bullae of pemphigus. The goal is to gain control of the disease with the lowest amount of drug for the shortest period of time. Prednisone is usually initiated at 1 to 2 mg/kg/day but may cautiously be titrated upward until the patient stops getting new lesions.
- Pemphigus has a higher morbidity and mortality than other AIBDs because of the compromised epidermal barrier in a large BSA, increased risk for infections, and fluid/electrolyte imbalance. The use of systemic corticosteroids in pemphigus has significantly reduced the mortality and morbidity of patients, yet the risk of immunosuppression can result in diabetes, hypertension, kidney and liver dysfunction, and hematologic complications.
- Cutaneous complications include secondary infections, hyperpigmentation, scarring, impaired function and psychosocial sequelae.
- Achieving "complete" remission usually takes years for most pemphigus patients.
- Tapering patients with PV off systemic corticosteroids sometimes takes months or years even after the introduction of steroid-sparing agents.
- As with any patient requiring systemic corticosteroids for more than 12 weeks, osteoporosis and peptic ulcer prevention and treatment should be considered along with monitoring for severe side effects (see Section 1.4).

Rituximab

- Rituximab, an anti-CD20 antibody, has become the conventional gold standard for treatment of PV and refractory PF. It was FDA approved in 2018. The goal of therapy is to achieve/maintain remission, allow healing of old lesions, and expedite their taper off systemic corticosteroids.
- Clinical trials of PV patients showed that 90% patients treated with rituximab achieved complete remission and required no systemic steroids by month 24 compared to 28% on placebo (Joly et al., 2017).
- Treatment-related infections associated with patients treated with rituximab were 37% compared to 42% steroids alone.
- The updated 2020 guidelines for PV and PF by the European Academy of Dermatology and Venereology (EADV) recommendations rituximab as first-line therapy for mild and moderate/severe PV (Joly et al., 2020).

Steroid-Sparing Agents

- Systemic agents such as mycophenolate mofetil (CellCept), azathioprine (Imuran), and dapsone are often started at the same time with the goal of tapering off the prednisone as soon as possible. However, the process is done very slowly to avoid flaring of the disease and may take months to years.

Management and Patient Education

- <u>All</u> types of pemphigus require management by a dermatologist experienced in AIBDs due to the high risk for morbidity and mortality from the disease. They should also have the knowledge to utilize high-risk therapies needed to gain control or achieve remission.
- The management approach to PV is dependent on the type, severity of disease, patient age, and comorbidities.
- Monitoring and prevention of steroid-associated side effects and complications are essential (Section 1.4).
- Appropriate specialists should be consulted when there is involvement of mucous membranes.

- Primary care and dermatology should collaborate to screen annually for tuberculosis, as well as age-appropriate health screenings.
- Patients with PV should be educated about recurrence and development of associated diseases (thyroid dysfunction, thymoma, and myasthenia gravis).

Special Considerations

- Women with PV require collaboration between obstetrics and dermatology for management. The autoantibodies of PV can cross the placenta in pregnant women and affect the epidermis of the fetus.
- PV in children is rare but can occur.
- The prognosis for PNP is very poor even with prompt recognition. The treatment approach for PNP differs in that clinicians should immediately perform screening for an underlying malignancy or benign neoplasm. If the initial search does not reveal the underlying etiology, one should maintain a high index of suspicion for an evolving neoplasm. When a malignancy or tumor is identified, treatment or excision must occur without delay.

SUBEPIDERMAL BLISTERING DISEASES

Patients with subepidermal blistering have autoantibodies that target adhesion proteins in the BMZ that are responsible for anchoring keratinocytes to the matrix (cell-to-matrix). The specific type of subepidermal disease is dependent on the specific antigen targeted by autoantibodies.

BULLOUS PEMPHIGOID

BP is the most common AIBD and typically presents in patients 60 years and older with an equal incidence in men and women. It is a chronic disease characterized by exacerbations and remission. There is an increased risk to develop BP in individuals with specific HLA alleles. BP has been associated with a history of neurologic diseases, such as Parkinson, and patients with a history of a cerebral vascular accident. Drug-induced BP has been linked to diuretics, antibiotics, captopril, and neuroleptic agents, contributing to the trigger of an already genetically susceptible individual. The entire gliptin class of antidiabetic agents is known to have a twofold increased risk for BP (Kridin & Ludwig, 2018). More specifically, patients on vildagliptin have an even higher 10-fold increased risk of developing BP.

Pathophysiology

Blister formation occurs in BP when autoantibodies target the hemidesmosomes (BP 180 and 230) triggering complement activation and inflammatory mediators. The result is deposition of IgG and C3 in the BMZ. The recruitment of neutrophils and eosinophils results in the destruction of the BMZ.

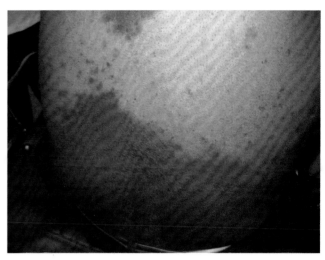

FIG. 9.1-9. The urticarial stage of BP may be present for weeks or months before any fluid-filled lesions erupt. (Photo courtesy of M. Bobonich.)

Clinical Presentation

Skin Findings

- The symptoms of BP are highly variable, often presenting as urticarial plaques (nonbullous phase) that may last from weeks to months then gradually evolve into tense vesicles/bullae (Fig. 9.1-9). This stage may delay the diagnosis since clinicians may not recognize urticaria and pruritus as a key symptom in the early clinical presentation of BP.
- Approximately one third of BP cases are diagnosed before the bullae appear and are referred to as nonbullous pemphigoid (Temel & Murrell, 2019).
- The fluid-filled blisters of BP are located deeper in the skin (compared to pemphigus) and therefore form *tense* bullae that are more difficult to rupture.
- There is a negative *Nikolsky* sign in BP.
- Vesicles/bullae are usually polymorphic and may be filled with either clear or hemorrhagic fluid. Bullae may be solitary lesions but can become very large and extensive, involving the trunk (Fig. 9.1-10).
- Lesions tend to favor the flexural areas on the arms and legs (Fig. 9.1-11).

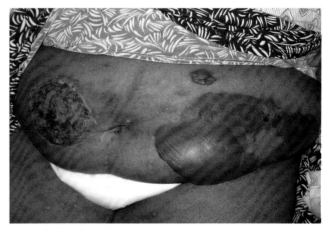

FIG. 9.1-10. Large hemorrhagic bullae in a BP patient who continues to develop new lesions. (Photo courtesy of M. Bobonich.)

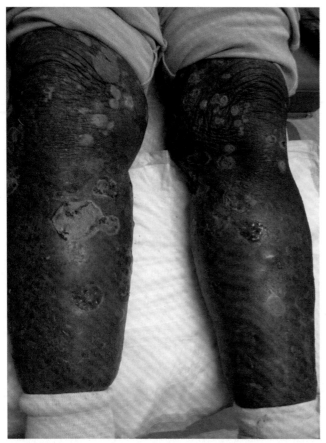

FIG. 9.1-11. BP favoring the lower legs with various stages of blister development and healing. (Photo courtesy of M. Bobonich.)

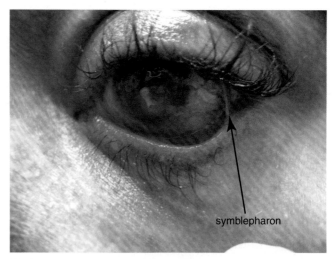

FIG. 9.1-12. Erosions in ocular mucous membrane pemphigoid heal with scarring or symblepharon. (Photo courtesy of M. Bobonich.)

- Once bullae rupture, erosions take days or weeks to heal and may leave abnormal pigmentation.
- Oral lesions may be present in BP but are less common than in pemphigus.

Variants of Bullous Pemphigoid

- *Mucous membrane pemphigoid* (MMP), which has also been referred to as cicatricial (scarring) pemphigoid, is a rare but severe type of localized BP occurring in patients 60 to 80 years old with a higher incidence in women. The most common sites affected in MMP are the oral mucosa and conjunctiva, but may develop in the nasopharynx, esophagus, genitals, and anus. Painful erosions and desquamative gingivitis from the disease can be disabling. Ocular involvement is usually severe and painful, and often progressive from erosions to fibrous conjunctival lesions or symblepharon (Fig. 9.1-12). Patients suffer from corneal opacities and ulcerations, ingrown eyelashes, reduced ability to tear, and ultimately blindness. About one quarter of the patients with MMP also have involvement of the skin usually located on the head, neck, and chest.

- *Pemphigoid gestationis* (PG) is a vesiculobullous eruption that presents during the second and third trimesters of pregnancy and can flare after delivery (Section 12.2). It was previously known as *herpes pemphigoid* which is a misnomer and not related to the herpes virus. PG has been associated with Graves disease. Pruritus, urticarial papules, and plaques erupt on the trunk and the umbilicus is commonly involved (Fig. 9.1-13). Lesions expand and can develop vesicles.

DIFFERENTIAL DIAGNOSIS   Bullous Pemphigoid

- Other AIBDs
- Bullous drug eruption
- Bullous impetigo
- Erythema multiforme
- Contact dermatitis
- SJS/TEN
- Urticaria or urticarial vasculitis
- Pruritic urticarial papules and plaques of pregnancy

Confirming the Diagnosis of Bullous Pemphigoid

- Histopathology of lesional skin in BP will show a subepidermal blister with infiltration of eosinophils and some neutrophils.
- DIF performed on nonlesional skin typically shows a linear deposition of IgG and C3 at the BMZ.
- An IIF on salt-split skin can help differentiate BP with immune deposits on the roof (epidermal side) in comparison to EBA which binds to the floor (dermal side) of the BMZ.

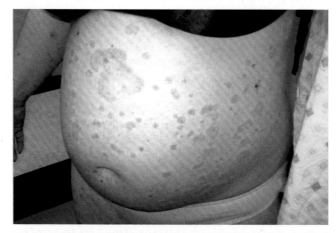

FIG. 9.1-13. Herpes gestationis (gestational pemphigoid) looks similar to PUPPP but is not concentrated in the striae and usually involves the umbilicus. (Photo courtesy of M. Bobonich.)

- ELISA for BP 180 and 230 can be used for diagnostic purposes as well as a prognostic indicator in cessation of therapy and possible relapse.
- Diagnostics for MMP should be ordered and evaluated by an experienced dermatologist. A DIF on salt-split skin may be limited as IgG may bind to both sides but an ELISA for BP 180 and laminin 5 is much more sensitive.

Treatment

Careful consideration must be given to the treatment of patients with BP since it occurs more often in the elderly who are more likely to have comorbid conditions. Additional challenges to managing these patients may be due to their limited resources, ability to monitor for side effects or complications, and adherence to recommendations which can impact outcomes. Treatment approach is based on severity, extent (diffuse vs. localized), and location of the blisters.

Mild and Localized Disease

- BP can be effectively treated with potent topical corticosteroids and immunomodulators.
- Topical corticosteroids are often sufficient to manage AIBDs in children but long-term monitoring for relapse is important.
- Systemic therapies that may be added include nicotinamide, tetracycline class drugs, dapsone, and sulfonamides.

Moderate/Severe Disease

- In severe cases or those involving mucous membranes, dermatologists may initiate systemic corticosteroids starting at low doses.
- Steroid-sparing agents like mycophenolate mofetil, azathioprine, methotrexate, and sulfones, are often started at the same time as prednisone. These agents help control the disease while provider begins to taper the patient off prednisone. Recalcitrant BP or severe oral involvement may require rituximab or IVIG.
- Although considered a more benign disease than PV, BP can result in significant morbidity and death. Close monitoring of the patient cannot be stressed enough as both corticosteroids and steroid-sparing agents can have severe or lethal side effects especially in the elderly.
- Response to therapy can be monitored with serum BP 180 (ELISA) levels to identify disease remission for discontinuation of drug therapy.

Pemphigoid Gestationis

- Women with PG can be treated effectively with mid- to high-potency topical corticosteroids and antihistamines.
- Women with PG require collaboration between obstetrics and dermatology for management.
- Women who develop PG have an increased risk of delivering a low–birth-weight infant, 30% risk of preterm delivery, and less than 5% infants presenting with blisters. Once the infant is delivered, the vesiculobullous lesions resolve. However, there is a risk for flare of PG with subsequent pregnancies, oral contraceptive use, or with menses.

Mucous Membrane Pemphigoid

- The management approach for MMP must be initiated immediately by an experienced dermatology clinician if the patient is to avoid permanent impaired function. Aggressive

immunosuppression often requires more than systemic corticosteroids. A combination of drug therapy and surgical modalities is often necessary.
- The prognosis for MMP is very poor as impaired function of the eyes resulting in blindness is not uncommon. Other mucous membrane involvement of the mouth, nasopharynx, esophagus and trachea, and urogenital tract can also develop scarring and strictures. Patients with BP are at increased risk for adenocarcinoma and solid organ tumors. Additionally, high-risk immunosuppressive agents and long-term therapy increase the risk of complications and secondary infections.
- MMP patients require a multidisciplinary approach dependent of the mucous membrane involved. Ophthalmology, ENT, dentistry, and gastroenterology are commonly consulted.

Management and Patient Education

- Routine and symptomatic follow-up with primary care is vital to any pemphigoid patient. Both patients and providers should have a heightened awareness for signs and symptoms of infection. Age-appropriate and symptomatic cancer screenings are highly advised.
- Patients should understand and monitor for risks and complications of immunosuppressive therapy used to treat their disease.
- UVR protection and avoidance of trauma to the skin can help reduce exacerbations.

LINEAR IgA DISEASE

A rare blistering disease, LAD is a subepidermal disorder presenting in adults over 60 years old. Like many AIBDs, LAD has been associated with patients who have underlying lymphoproliferative or solid organ malignancy, infections, or inflammatory bowel diseases. LAD can be drug-induced by medications such as vancomycin, captopril, lithium, NSAIDs (especially diclofenac), penicillin, furosemide, cephalosporin, and others. There has also been some suggestion of a genetic association with specific HLA alleles.

Pathophysiology

The pathogenesis of LAD is not well understood. IgA autoantibodies target BP 180 antigen along the BMZ which plays a major role in epidermal–dermal adhesion.

Clinical Presentation
Skin Findings

- LAD can have a variable presentation and disease course. In adults, an abrupt onset of vesicles and bullae may develop centrally on an erythematous plaque or as annular lesions.
- LAD is symmetrical and favors the trunk, extensor surfaces of extremities (compared to flexor surfaces of BP), and perineum. Blisters quickly erode due to intense pruritus and scratching.
- The face and perioral mucosa are involved in the majority of adults with LAD.
- The classic lesions of LAD are the small clusters of vesicles or papules that appear on the periphery of erythematous round plaques and are often described as *rosettes, crown of jewels,* or *string of pearls.*
- *Chronic bullous disease of childhood* (CBDC). LAD in children is called CBDC and presents with more generalized symptoms that

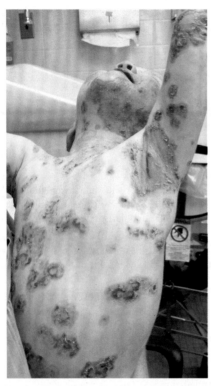

FIG. 9.1-14. Chronic bullous disease of childhood (CBDC). The round "rosettes" of fluid-filled lesions are characteristic of CBDC and LAD. (Photo courtesy of M. Bobonich.)

commonly affect the extremities including hands/feet, genitals, and oral mucosa in about half the cases (Fig. 9.1-14).

DIFFERENTIAL DIAGNOSIS   Linear IgA

- Dermatitis herpetiformis
- Other AIBD
- Bullous impetigo
- Erythema multiforme
- SJS/TEN
- Drug eruption

Confirming the Diagnosis

- A lesional punch biopsy shows a subepidermal blister with an abundance of neutrophils with collections in the dermal papillae.
- DIF reveals linear deposition of IgA along the BMZ (compared to the granular deposition in DH).
- IIF on sera shows circulating IgA bound to the epidermal side (or roof) of salt-split skin.

Treatment

- Patients with LAD that are treated with dapsone usually have a rapid improvement within days of initiating pharmacotherapy.
- Potent topical corticosteroids can be effective for localized lesions on the trunk and extremities.
- Low-potency corticosteroids or calcineurin inhibitors (off-label) are recommended for the face, genitals, or intertriginous regions. If drug-induced LAD is suspected, discontinue the drug immediately.

- First-line therapy for most adults and children with LAD is dapsone. However, the dosing and administration of dapsone should be done by an experienced dermatology clinician. Adverse effects include hemolytic anemia, methemoglobinemia, leukopenia, agranulocytosis, hypersensitivity reaction, and gastrointestinal and hepatic events.
- Patients treated with dapsone should have a laboratory level of their glucose-6-phosphate dehydrogenase (G6PD), an essential enzyme to avoid red blood cell destruction triggered by some medications. Individuals with a G6PD deficiency are vulnerable to hemolytic anemia and therefore should not be used.
- Initially, weekly visits and laboratory monitoring are recommended until the disease is stabilized and risk of complications from drug therapy is lowered. Patients treated with dapsone or other steroid-sparing agents must have regular follow-up and monitoring.
- Severe LAD, disease not responding to dapsone, or patients with a G6PD deficiency may require systemic prednisone or other second-line agents such as sulfapyridine, mycophenolate mofetil, and colchicine.

Clinicians should intermittently attempt to slowly taper off the patient's medications while monitoring for flares.

Management and Patient Education

- The prognosis for CBDC differs from that of adults in that most cases resolve spontaneously within 2 years. Adults with LAD may go into remission for years and then flare again.
- Complications from LAD and CBDC are usually minimal since the lesions do not scar or result in abnormal pigmentation. However, disease involving the mucous membrane can cause scarring and disability.
- Secondary infections as well as conditions inherent with the use of both systemic and topical corticosteroid therapy may occur.
- Patients with LAD or CBDC should be referred immediately to dermatology and consultation with ophthalmology, gynecology, gastroenterology, and otolaryngology depending on the severity and location of the lesions.
- Education regarding side effects and risk of secondary infections is important. Patients are counseled to avoid direct sun and to use sunscreen.

DERMATITIS HERPETIFORMIS

DH is a rare lifelong subepidermal blistering disease associated with gluten sensitivity. Systemic symptoms of gluten-sensitive enteropathy are *celiac disease* (CD) which can range from mild to severe or no intestinal symptoms. DH predominantly affects Caucasians with a higher incidence in individuals with northern European ancestry. It is rarely seen in African Americans and Asians. The onset of DH occurs during the fifth and sixth decades of life with a 2:1 predominance in males to females.

Several autoimmune disorders have been associated with DH, most common are Hashimoto thyroiditis and insulin-dependent diabetes mellitus. Individuals with the immunogenic HLA-DQ2 and HLA-DQ8 genotypes are at higher risk for DH and CD. Patients with DH are at higher risk of developing autoimmune disorders, anemia, and lymphoma (gastrointestinal and nongastrointestinal).

Pathophysiology

There are suggested environmental and genetic influences that play a role in the development of CD and DH. The pathogenesis

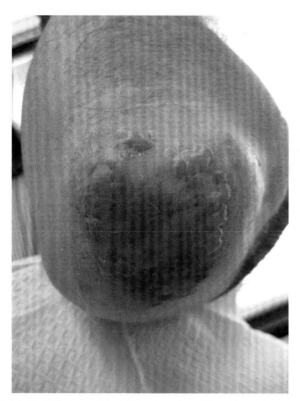

FIG. 9.1-15. Vesicular eruption of DH is extremely pruritic and favors the extensor aspect of the arms and legs. (Photo courtesy of M. Bobonich.)

of DH begins with the ingestion of grains (wheat, barley, and rye) which contain the protein gliadin. Tissue transglutaminase (TG), an enzyme necessary for metabolism, is the target of IgA antiendomysial antibodies (IgA-EmA) resulting in damage to the mucosa in CD. Later, antibodies to epidermal transglutaminase (ET) develop and are more specific to DH. IgA antibodies to ET in the dermis lead to neutrophilic chemotaxis and blister formation in the BMZ at the lamina lucida.

Clinical Presentation

Skin Findings

- DH is symmetrical and favors the extensor aspects of the arms and legs as well as the back and buttocks (Fig. 9.1-15).
- It usually spares the face and genitals but sometimes involves the scalp.
- Erythematous papules, vesicles, and bullae on an urticarial base are clustered in groups (herpetiform arrangement) and can be localized or diffuse, involving the trunk and extremities.
- DH is characterized by severe pruritus associated with the lesions that the clinician often sees only as erosions, ulcers, and crusts secondary to scratching.
- DH is a lifelong skin condition that can go into remission or flares that last weeks to months to years.

Non-Skin Findings

- Most patients with DH also have CD; a gastrointestinal evaluation is vitally important. Almost all patients with DH have evidence of CD on intestinal biopsy; however, they may not have any signs or symptoms of intestinal disease. Subclinical symptoms are easily overlooked by patients and clinicians.

Confirming the Diagnosis

- The histopathology of DH will show a subepidermal blister (at the level of the lamina lucida) with neutrophilic microabscesses in the dermal papillae and perivascular lymphocytic infiltrates.
- DIF from perilesional skin will have *granular* deposition at the BMZ compared to the linear deposition of LAD. Additional diagnostics such as IIF, ELISAs, or serum IgA may be indicated and should be directed by dermatology.
- The initial serum test for screening patients with DH should be IgA transglutaminase 2 (TG2). Antigliadin antibodies lack specificity. The presence of TG2 supports a diagnosis of DH but absence doesn't exclude it. Serum TG2 levels correlate with the small bowel mucosal damage in patients with DH.
- Screening diagnostics for Hashimoto thyroiditis and diabetes are recommended.
- Baseline labs including complete blood count, comprehensive metabolic panel, and G6PD should be ordered in anticipation for treatment with dapsone.
- The pruritic lesions of DH eventually heal but leave hyperpigmentation.
- Secondary infections from erosions and ulcerations are a complication when cutaneous symptoms are not controlled.

Treatment

- *Pharmacologic therapies*
  - Many patients with DH will require pharmacologic therapy in addition to dietary modification.
  - *Dapsone* is considered a first-line drug effective in neutrophilic dermatoses such as DH. Improvement or resolution varies and may occur quickly or take several months. A combination of dietary and drug therapy often allows for a quicker taper off dapsone.
  - Patients on dapsone should be instructed about the risk of side effects and complications, along with the importance of frequent laboratory monitoring.
  - Sulfa-based drugs, such as sulfapyridine and sulfasalazine, do not cause hemolysis and therefore are an option for patients who experience hemolysis with dapsone therapy.
  - Successful treatment with tetracycline and nicotinamide has been reported.
  - Topical corticosteroids can be effective for small, localized outbreaks.
- *Gluten-free* diet (GFD) is the first-line treatment and maintenance of DH which is extremely challenging. Patients must exclude all grains from their diet but are allowed corn, rice, and oat products. Most, but not all, DH patients respond well to the cessation of gluten. Yet it may take months to years to achieve resolution. Patients who knowingly or unknowingly consume

gluten can anticipate and prepare for a flare of their cutaneous symptoms.

Management and Patient Education

- Serum titers of IgA-EmA are indicative of adherence to GFD and will eventually fall to zero if gluten is completely omitted from the diet.
- CD is also a chronic condition and should be addressed with the patient even if they are asymptomatic. Malabsorption can be a chronic problem leading to other systemic disease and illness. Further screening for adults who are at high risk for CD is controversial. If skin biopsies are positive for DH, intestinal biopsies are not warranted but recommend a lifelong gluten-free diet.
- Consultation with a nutritionist can be most valuable in supporting the patient's transition for a gluten-free lifestyle.
- Routine health maintenance screening examinations and symptomatic evaluation are essential. An increased risk for the development of associated diseases (thyroiditis, anemia, diabetes, and lymphoma) should always be at the forefront of the clinician's thoughts. Age-appropriate and symptomatic screening should be current.
- Clinicians should routinely evaluate and reaffirm the importance of lifelong compliance to a gluten-free diet, and avoidance of iodide and NSAIDs.

OTHER AIBDs
Epidermal Bullosa Acquisita

A very rare subepidermal AIBD, epidermal bullosa acquisita (EBA) is an acquired disorder in adults and occasionally in childhood. It should be noted that EBA is different than the inherited blistering disorder, epidermal bullosa (EB). Patients diagnosed with EBA should be screened for a known association with Crohn and systemic lupus erythematosus (Prost & Caux, 2015). EBA has a low mortality rate there but a highly variable prognosis that is difficult to predict.

Pathophysiology

Some case studies have suggested an association between EBA and inflammatory bowel diseases that may predate the blistering disease. IgG autoantibodies targeting type VII collagen in the BMZ, in addition to chronic trauma and friction, are pathogenic for EBA.

Clinical Presentation

- Characteristic blisters erupt on trauma-prone areas like the extensor surfaces of the knees, elbows, dorsal hands, and fingers.
- The chronic inflammation and erosions result in scarring and milia.

Confirming the Diagnosis

- IIF on salt-split skin shows linear deposits of IgG on the floor (dermal side) of the BMZ compared to BP on the roof (epidermal side) of salt-split skin.

DIFFERENTIAL DIAGNOSIS   Epidermal Bullosa Acquisita
- Bullous pemphigoid
- Porphyria cutanea tarda
- Epidermal bullosa

Management and Patient Education

- The primary focus of treatment for EBA is avoidance of trauma or friction. EBA is resistant to treatment and chronic inflammation results in destruction of the hair, skin, nails, and mucous membranes.
- Systemic and topical corticosteroids, colchicine, azathioprine, dapsone, and methotrexate have had reported success but lack data to make recommendations. Complications associated with immunosuppressive therapies (secondary infections, osteoporosis, diabetes, etc.) and malignancies from chronic inflammation should be monitored.
- Patients must be educated about protecting their skin from friction and injury.
- Wound care and healing is paramount to limiting morbidity.
- During flares, patients should be followed monthly. Otherwise, annual follow-up with primary care and age-appropriate cancer screenings.

CLINICAL PEARLS

- All blisters are not AIBDs. Consider infection, injury, hypersensitivity, drugs, and genetic disorders.
- H&E should be performed on an intact vesiculobullous skin eruption if possible.
- Erosions on the skin may have developed secondary to blisters.
- DIF is the gold standard for diagnosing an AIBD. A biopsy for histopathology alone is not sufficient to make the diagnosis.
- Once identified as a blistering condition, it is critical to diagnose the **SPECIFIC AIBD** which guides treatment and prognosis.
- Biopsy for DIF should be performed on perilesional skin and must be transported in Michel's media, NOT formaldehyde.
- Systemic corticosteroids may be necessary for patients with AIBD. However, steroid-sparing agents should be started as soon as possible to allow for the tapering off of corticosteroids.
- Always consider osteoporosis and peptic ulcer prevention for patients treated with systemic corticosteroids for more than 3 months.

READINGS AND REFERENCES

Chen, M., O'Toole, E. A., Sanghavi, J., Mahmud, N., Kelleher, D., Weir, D., & Fairley, J. A. (2002). The epidermolysis bullosa acquisita antigen (type VII collagen) is present in human colon and patients with crohn's disease have autoantibodies to type VII collagen. *Journal of Investigative Dermatology, 118*(6), 1059–1064.

Collin, P., Salmi, T. T., Hervonen, K., Kaukinen, K., & Reunala, T. (2017). Dermatitis herpetiformis: A cutaneous manifestation of coeliac disease. *Annals of Medicine, 49*(1), 23–31. https://doi.org/10.1080/07853890.2016.1222450

Daniel, B. S., & Murrell, D. F. (2019). Review of autoimmune blistering diseases: The pemphigoid diseases. *Journal of the European Academy of Dermatology and Venereology, 33*(9), 1685–1694.

Dinulos, J. (2020). *Habif's clinical dermatology* (7th ed.). Elsevier.

Hertl, M., Jedlickova, H., Karpati, S., Marinovic, B., Uzun, S., Yayli, S., Mimouni, D., Borradori, L., Feliciani, C., Ioannides, D., Joly, P., Kowalewski, C., Zambruno, G., Zillikens, D., & Jonkman, M. F. (2015). Pemphigus. S2 Guideline for diagnosis and treatment–guided by the European Dermatology Forum (EDF) in cooperation with the European Academy of Dermatology and Venereology (EADV). *Journal of the European Academy of Dermatology and Venereology, 29*(3), 405–414. https://doi.org/10.1111/jdv.12772

Joly, P., Horwath, B., Patsatsi, A., Uzun, S., Bech, R., Beissert, S., Bergman, R., Bernard, P., Borradori, L., Caproni, M., Caux, F., Cianchini, G., Daneshpazhooh, M., De, D., Dmochowski, M., Drenovska, K., Ehrchen, J., Feliciani, C., Goebeler, M., ... Schmidt, E. (2020). Updated S2K guidelines on the management of pemphigus vulgaris and foliaceus initiated by the European Academy of Dermatology and Venereology (EADV). *Journal of the European Academy of Dermatology and Venereology, 34*(9), 1900–1913.

Joly, P., Maho-Vaillant, M., Prost-Squarcioni, C., Hebert, V., Houivet, E., Calbo, S., Caillot, F., Golinski, M. L., Labeille, B., Picard-Dahan, C., Paul, C., Richard, M. A., Bouaziz, J. D., Duvert-Lehembre, S., Bernard, P., Caux, F., Alexandre, M., Ingen-Housz-Oro, S., Vabres, P., ... French study group on autoimmune bullous skin diseases. (2017). First-line rituximab combined with short-term prednisone versus prednisone alone for the treatment of pemphigus (Ritux 3): A prospective, multicentre, parallel-group, open-label randomised trial. *Lancet, 389*(10083), 2031–2040. https://doi.org/10.1016/S0140-6736(17)30070-3

Kridin, K. (2018). Emerging treatment options for the management of pemphigus vulgaris. *Therapeutics and Clinical Risk Management, 14*, 757–778. https://doi.org/10.2147/TCRM.S142471

Kridin, K., & Ludwig, R. J. (2018). The growing incidence of bullous pemphigoid: Overview and potential explanations. *Frontiers in Medicine, 5*, 220. https://doi.org/10.3389/fmed.2018.00220

Ljubojevic, S., & Lipozencic, J. (2012). Autoimmune bullous diseases associations. *Clinics in Dermatology, 30*(1), 17–33.

Meijer, J. M., Diercks, G., de Lang, E., Pas, H. H., & Jonkman, M. F. (2019). Assessment of diagnostic strategy for early recognition of bullous and nonbullous variants of pemphigoid. *JAMA Dermatology, 155*(2), 158–165. https://doi.org/10.1001/jamadermatol.2018.4390

Murrell, D. F., Peña, S., Joly, P., Marinovic, B., Hashimoto, T., Diaz, L. A., Sinha, A. A., Payne, A. S., Daneshpazhooh, M., Eming, R., Jonkman, M. F., Mimouni, D.,

Borradori, L., Chan Kim, S., Yamagami, J., Lehman, J. S., Saleh, M. A., Culton, D. A., Czernik, A., ... Werth, V. P. (2018). Diagnosis and management of pemphigus: Recommendations by an international panel of experts. *Journal of the American Academy of Dermatology, 82*(3), 575–585.e1. doi:10.1016/j.jaad.2018.02.012

Salmi, T. T. (2019). Dermatitis herpetiformis. *Clinical and Experimental Dermatology, 44*(7), 728–731. https://doi.org/10.1111/ced.13992

Salmi, T., & Hervonen, K. (2020). Current concepts of dermatitis herpetiformis. *Acta Dermato-Venereologica, 100*(5), 115–121. https://doi.org/10.2340/00015555-3401

Sontheimer, R. D. (2004). Skin manifestations of systemic autoimmune connective tissue disease: Diagnostics and therapeutics. *Best Pract Res Clin Rheumatol, 18*(3), 429–462.

Tan, E. M., Cohen, A. S., Fries, J. F., Masi, A. T., McShane, D. J., Rothfield, N. F., Schaller, J. G., Talal, N., & Winchester, R. J. (1982). The 1982 revised criteria for the classification of systemic lupus erythematosus. *Arthritis Rheum, 25*(11), 1271–1277.

Temel, A. B., & Murrell, D. F. (2019). Diagnostic criteria and phenotypes of pemphigoid and the association with gliptins. *JAMA Dermatol, 155*(2), 147–148. doi:10.1001/jamadermatol.2018.4847

Updating the American College of Rheumatology revised criteria for the classification of systemic lupus erythematosus. American College of Rheumatology website. http://www.rheumatology.org/publications/classification/SLE/1982SLEupdate.asp?aud=mem

Immune-Mediated Connective Tissue Diseases

Margaret A. Bobonich

CUTANEOUS MANIFESTATIONS OF CONNECTIVE TISSUE DISEASE

Connective tissue diseases (CTDs) are autoimmune diseases that cause chronic inflammation leading to the injury and destruction of tissue. Autoantibodies target collagen and elastin that are found in skin and muscles which are essential for structural support and function. These proteins are also present in almost every organ of the body and may cause serious complications in organs like the lungs, heart, and kidneys. Patients with interstitial lung disease associated with CTD have significant risk of high morbidity and mortality (Vij & Strek, 2013). Therefore, it is crucial that clinicians recognize cutaneous signs of a CTD and prompt an early diagnosis for optimal patient outcomes.

LUPUS ERYTHEMATOSUS

Lupus erythematosus (LE) is a multisystem autoimmune disease where most patients manifest mucocutaneous symptoms. The American College of Rheumatology criteria require 4 of 11 symptoms for the diagnosis of systemic lupus erythematosus (SLE)—which could be met in patients who present with four cutaneous symptoms (Tan et al., 1982). The strongest risk factor for SLE is gender with women almost 10-fold higher than men and African Americans at greater risk than Caucasians. Caution should be taken to appreciate that individuals may develop cutaneous lupus erythematosus (CLE) associated with or independent of SLE. The incidence of CLE is also similar to SLE. Discussion of systemic lupus however is beyond the scope of this dermatology text.

CUTANEOUS LUPUS ERYTHEMATOSUS

There are several subtypes of CLE that vary in their pathophysiology, clinical presentation, treatment, and prognoses. Genetic susceptibility, environmental and hormonal factors such as ultraviolet radiation exposure, smoking, family history, medications, infection, and specific HLA phenotypes, play a role in the pathogenesis of CLE. The age of onset disease is variable among the subtypes and is relative to any association with a coexisting SLE.

There is a low risk of patients with CLE progressing to SLE but it is greater in women than men. In studies, approximately 12% to 17% of CLE patients went on to develop SLE with the mean time to diagnosis around 8 years (Durosaro et al., 2009; Wieczorek et al., 2014). Some limited data suggest that antimalarials and prednisone may slow the progression (James et al., 2007). Risk factors identified as predictors of progression of CLE to systemic involvement include clinical symptoms of discoid lesions below the head/neck, periungual telangiectasias, and arthritis (Callen, 1985; Chong et al., 2012).

CLE can be classified into three groups: acute cutaneous lupus erythematosus (ACLE), subacute lupus erythematosus (SCLE), and chronic cutaneous lupus erythematosus (CCLE). Each disease is based on a continuum of systemic and cutaneous involvement (Fig. 9.2-1).

Pathophysiology

In a normal immune system, antibodies identify foreign proteins or organisms that trigger a cascade of inflammatory responses attacking the potential danger. Conversely, CTD can be characterized as a disease where the body's immune system does not recognize "self" and attacks itself. Serum autoantibodies (antibodies directed at one of the body's own cellular components or target antigens) are directed at the body's normal tissue. Autoantibodies that develop are unique for each CTD entity. Autoimmune diseases with systemic

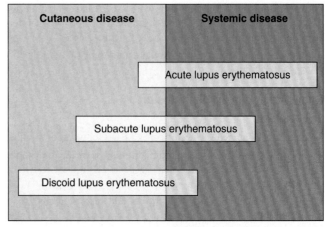

FIG. 9.2-1. The spectrum of systemic and cutaneous involvement related to the three subtypes of chronic cutaneous lupus erythematosus.

BOX 9.2-1 Cutaneous Symptoms of Lupus Erythematosus

- Oral or mucosal ulcers
- Periungual telangiectasias
- Malar "butterfly" rash
- Nonscarring alopecia
- "Lupus hairs"
- Discoid lesions
- Nail fold capillary abnormalities
- Urticaria
- Livedo reticularis
- Photosensitivity
- Raynaud phenomenon

---

involvement are suspected when autoantibodies target nuclear antigens (antinuclear antibodies or ANAs).

Clinical Presentation

Acute Cutaneous Lupus Erythematosus

Skin Findings

- Transient skin eruption lasting for days or weeks.
- Approximately 90% of patients with ACLE have an underlying diagnosis of SLE with multisystem involvement and often accompany the flares (Watanabe & Tsuchida, 1995).
- ACLE can present as localized violaceous plaques or diffuse patches, papules, or plaques often exacerbated by sun exposure on the face, neck, chest, back, and arms.
- There is a wide range of cutaneous symptoms that should alert the clinician to a possible underlying diagnosis of SLE (Box 9.2-1).
- The central face, in particular, often develops erythematous plaques and induration involving the malar prominences and commonly referred to as the *butterfly rash* (Fig. 9.2-2).
- The facial erythema from SLE can be confused with rosacea and seborrheic dermatitis except that it does not involve the nasal labial fold or have acneiform features.
- Cutaneous findings of ACLE may include palmar telangiectasias; edema and erythema of the dorsal fingers (between interphalangeal [IP] joints) (Fig. 9.2-3); periungual erythema and abnormal capillary loops of the nail folds (Fig. 9.2-4A,B); alopecia; and, urticaria.

Non-Skin Findings

- Approximately 90% of patients with ACLE have an underlying diagnosis of SLE with multisystem involvement that often accompanies the flares (Watanabe & Tsuchida, 1995).
- Patients commonly report arthralgia, photosensitivity, fever, and oral ulcerations.

Subacute Lupus Erythematosus

Skin Findings

- In contrast, cutaneous eruptions of SCLE last for weeks or months.
- Involved areas are often photodistributed favoring the upper trunk, extensor arms, and lateral aspects of the face and neck (sparing the central area).
- SCLE is usually more psoriasiform and less indurated than ACLE, sometimes resembling psoriasis or eczema.
- Patches and plaques can be annular or coalescing polycyclic plaques (Fig. 9.2-5A,B).

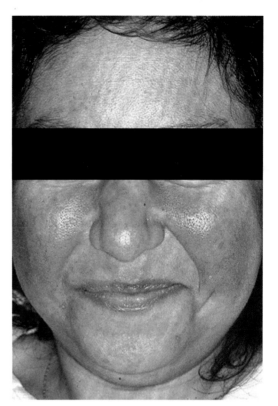

FIG. 9.2-2. The "butterfly" rash of SLE is erythema over the malar prominences and nose but spares the nasolabial folds. It can be very subtle and only about half of the patients with systemic lupus present with this feature.

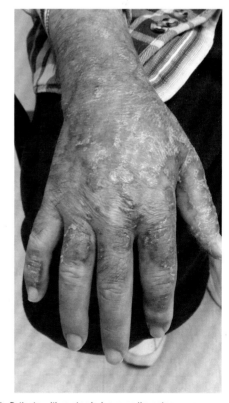

FIG. 9.2-3. Patients with systemic lupus erythematosus may present with erythema on the dorsum of the hands and fingers distributed *between* the interphalangeal (IP) joints. In contrast, patients with dermatomyositis have erythema or Gottron papules *over* the IP joints. (Used with permission from Hall, J. C., & Hall, B. J. [2017]. *Sauer's manual of skin diseases* [11th ed.]. Wolters Kluwer.)

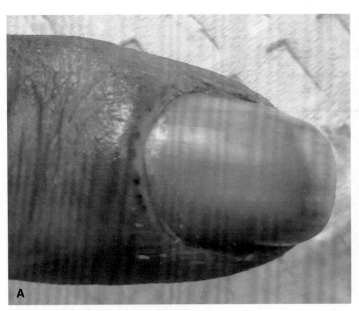
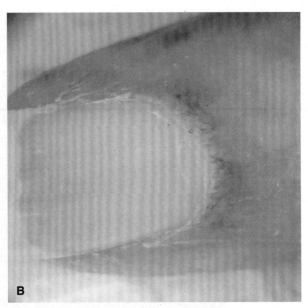

FIG. 9.2-4. A: Periungual erythema, observed by the naked eye, may be an indicator of possible underlying connective tissue disease. **B:** Dermoscopic examination may reveal dilated or tortuous capillary loops in the proximal nail folds. (Photos courtesy of M. Bobonich.)

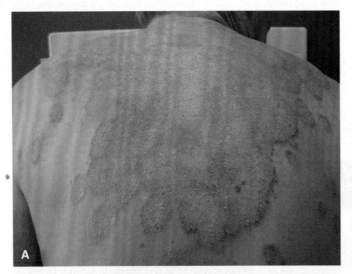
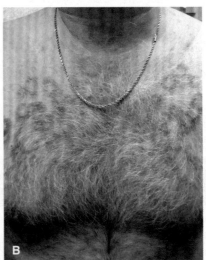
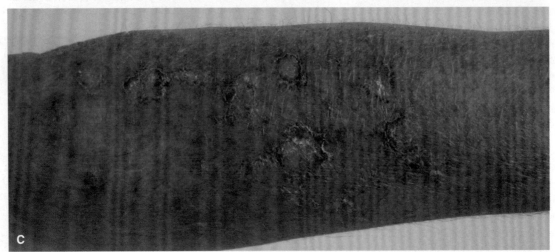

FIG. 9.2-5. A, B: Psoriasiform lesions of subacute lupus erythematous are often annular and can coalesce into polycyclic plaques. **C:** UVR can exacerbate the cutaneous symptoms and result in photodistributed papulosquamous eruptions. (Photos courtesy of M. Bobonich.)

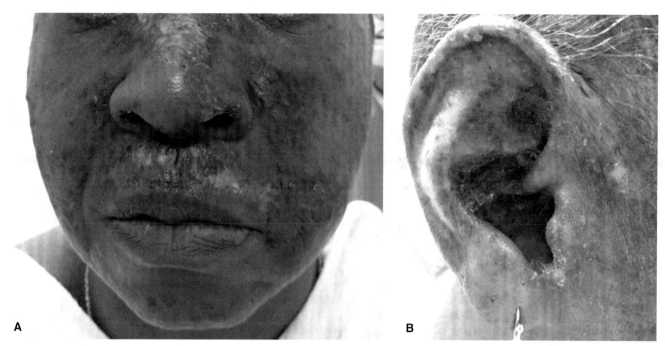

A   **B**

FIG. 9.2-6. **A:** Discoid lupus erythematosus is highest in African-American young women. It can cause significant disfigurement. **B:** The conchal bowl is often involved and should alert the clinician to a possible diagnosis of DLE. (Photos courtesy of M. Bobonich.)

- As lesions resolve, hypopigmentation and telangiectasias may be permanent but scarring is not typical. The course of SCLE is chronic and recurrent.

Non-Skin Findings

- Around 50% of patients with SCLE have underlying SLE (Sontheimer, 2005).

DIFFERENTIAL DIAGNOSIS	Acute Cutaneous and Subacute Cutaneous Lupus Erythematosus
- Sarcoidosis - Psoriasis - Lichen planus - Dermatomyositis - Syphilis drug eruption - Photodermatitis - Seborrheic dermatitis - Tinea corporis - Mycosis fungoides	

Chronic Cutaneous Lupus Erythematosus

There are several types of CCLEs which are not typically associated with underlying SLE. Patients with SLE may however develop CCLE lesions.

Discoid lupus erythematosus (DLE) is present in about one quarter of patients with SLE and may be the only presenting symptom of systemic involvement.

- Lesions are usually distributed above the shoulders and favor the scalp, face, and conchal bowls of the ears (Fig. 9.2-6A,B).

- Because lesions develop deeper in the papillary and reticular dermis (compared to ACLE and SCLE), the result is erythematous, scaly, thick, atrophic, and hyperpigmented plaques that leave scarring and abnormal pigmentation (Fig. 9.2-7).

- Adherent scale near hair follicles causes follicular plugging that can be seen on the underside of the scale ("carpet tack" effect) but progression of the disease can result in severe hair loss (Fig. 9.2-8A,B).

- While most DLE patients have a negative ANA, it is estimated that about 5% to 10% will go on to develop SLE.

Lupus profundus (LP) is also referred to as lupus panniculitis.

- LP is painful, erythematous, nodules caused by subcuticular inflammation and destruction.

- Lesions can occur anywhere but often distributed on the face, breasts, buttocks, arms, and thighs.

- The tender plaques and nodules may ulcerate and then heal with a black hemorrhagic crust, leaving "dents" or atrophic scars (Fig. 9.2-9).

Drug-induced lupus erythematosus (DILE). Drugs can be responsible for inducing a DILE which can mimic SLE (see Section 12.1).

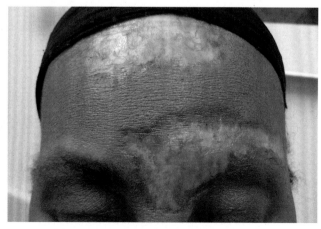

FIG. 9.2-7. Discoid lupus erythematosus can cause both disfiguring hyperpigmentation and depigmentation. (Photo courtesy of M. Bobonich.)

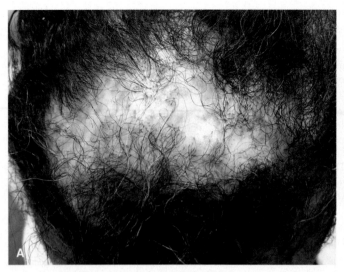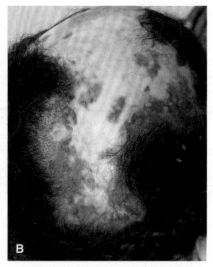

FIG. 9.2-8. **A:** Alopecia is often a complaint in patients with an unknown diagnosis of DLE. **B:** Progression to severe scarring alopecia can result if DLE is not treated. (Photos courtesy of M. Bobonich.)

Neonatal lupus erythematosus (NLE). Neonatal lupus is caused by vertical transmission of maternal autoantibodies (IgG anti-Ro, anti-La, or anti-RNP) to the fetus resulting in cutaneous and systemic manifestations (see Section 13).

Chilblain lupus (perniosis).

- Chilblain presents as small, erythematous (reddish-blue) macules and papules that can be painful or itchy.
- They favor acral sites like the ears, nose, fingers, and toes (Fig. 9.2-10).

- Lesions are a localized form of vasculitis induced by cold exposure and may ulcerate, swell, or bleed.
- One quarter of patients with Chilblain meet the classification ACR criteria for SLE.

DIFFERENTIAL DIAGNOSIS   Discoid Lupus Erythematosus

- Granuloma faciale
- Granulomatous rosacea
- Tinea faciei
- Sarcoidosis
- Tuberculoid leprosy
- ACLE and SCLE

Confirming the Diagnosis

Patients with suspected CLE should be evaluated for possible underlying systemic disease or SLE.

FIG. 9.2-9. Lupus profundus or lupus panniculitis are firm painful nodules often presenting with a necrotic appearance. (Photo courtesy of M. Bobonich.)

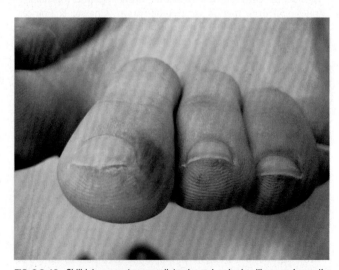

FIG. 9.2-10. Chilblain presents as small, tender, red, or bruise-like macules on the tips of acral skin like fingers, toes, ears, and nose. (Photo courtesy of M. Bobonich.)

Skin Biopsy

A lesional biopsy for histology should be performed initially along with screening laboratories.

- *Histopathology.* Routine histology for an H&E from a punch biopsy and clinical correlation is the preferred diagnostic test to establish a diagnosis of CLE.

- *Immunofluorescence.* A direct immunofluorescence (DIF) performed for suspected diagnosis of CLE should be collected from *lesional* skin which differs from the technique from autoimmune blistering diseases (AIBDs). A positive DIF with deposition of IgG and/or IgM supports the diagnosis, while a negative DIF cannot exclude CLE. A DIF can also be performed on *normal* skin for evidence of strong, continuous antibody deposition (referred to as a "lupus band") at the BMZ.

- To diagnose LP, an excisional biopsy (or deep punch) should be done to ensure subcutaneous fat in the specimen. LP may occur concomitantly with DLE.

Laboratories

- Serologies should include a complete blood count and urinalysis

- An *ANA* titer is the initial screening examination for a patient suspected of any CTD. Autoimmune diseases with systemic involvement are suspected when the ANA is greater than 1:160.

- A negative result makes a CTD unlikely whereas a false-positive finding can be caused by medications, disease, infections, and sometimes healthy individuals. Thus, a positive test does not infer disease but should prompt the clinician to make a clinicopathologic correlation.

- When the ANA is positive, the clinician should order additional autoantibodies, extractable nuclear antigen antibodies (ENA), to identify the antigens relative to the specific type of CTD. Further tests would include ENA panel, anti-dsDNA antibody, ESR/CRP, and C3 and C4 complements. These specific tests may be ordered by the primary care provider or deferred to rheumatology and dermatology for more extensive testing.

Treatment

Treatment for CLE can be complex requiring systemic, topical, and intralesional drug therapy or a combination (Chasset & Francès, 2019). The goals are to promote healthy skin, prevent new skin lesions, and minimize scarring and hair loss.

Mild or Localized CLE

Pharmacologic

- Topical corticosteroids (TCSs) are first-line therapy.

- Treatment of DLE includes potent TCSs, such as fluocinonide 0.05% cream or clobetasol propionate 0.05%, which can be used effectively but should be intermittent and limited to a few weeks due to the side effects. Scalp lesions may be the exception and require longer therapy with potent TCS.

- Topical calcineurin inhibitors can also be used off-label.

- Treatment with intralesional corticosteroids every 4 to 6 weeks has been used in DLE that is not responsive to TCS. It may be especially helpful for scalp lesions with alopecia.

- To diagnose LP, an excisional biopsy (or deep punch) should be done to ensure subcutaneous fat in the specimen. LP may occur concomitantly with DLE.

Chilblain

- Treatment should be focused on the avoidance of cold exposure including gloves, socks, and shoes.

- Topical and oral corticosteroids, calcium channel blockers, and smoking cessation can be efficacious.

Severe or Recalcitrant CLE

Most medications and clinical trials target treatment of SLE with cutaneous symptoms as reported as secondary outcomes. Therefore, systemic therapies for CLE should be referred to rheumatology or dermatology to utilize their expertise in the management and monitoring of these off-label and often high-risk drugs.

- Antimalarials, systemic corticosteroids, methotrexate, retinoids, dapsone, thalidomide and lenalidomide, mycophenolate mofetil, azathioprine, intravenous immunoglobulin

- Biologic therapies currently under investigation for possible treatment of CLE include rituximab, belimumab, sifalimumab, anifrolumab, baricitinib, anti-BDCA2, ustekinumab

Management and Patient Education

- Smoking cessation should be addressed and monitored since smokers have higher CLE disease activity and higher risk of developing SLE. Smokers may be refractory to treatment with hydroxychloroquine and quinacrine.

- Photoprotection is important for the prevention of flares since UV radiation plays a role in the pathogenesis of CLE.

- The importance of referral to dermatology or rheumatology for evaluation and management of CLE cannot be overstated. Dermatology may be involved for the management of cutaneous disease. Regardless of the type of LE diagnosis, the goals of care are control of the disease; early recognition of systemic involvement; and, minimizing morbidity and mortality. This section will focus on the recognition of CLE and not the diagnosis and management of SLE.

- Lifelong management and monitoring are paramount.

Special Populations

- Estrogen has been linked to SLE activity.

- Pregnancy prevention and contraception should be addressed with all women with SLE or CLE who are of childbearing potential.

- Women with SLE and CLE are associated with higher maternal and infant mortality and morbidity including neonatal lupus.

- Regular monitoring and pharmacologic management are key to managing SLE and SLE in high-risk pregnancies.

CLINICAL PEARLS

- The ACR criteria provide guidelines for the diagnosis of SLE but must be individualized for each patient.
- Always consider drug-induced etiology in patient with SCLE. Discontinuation can usually resolve the cutaneous symptoms.

DERMATOMYOSITIS AND POLYMYOSITIS

Dermatomyositis (DM) is a rare autoimmune disease involving idiopathic inflammation of the skin, muscles, joints, and other organs. It has been suggested that there may be a genetic predisposition for

some individuals with HLA phenotypes. DM has a bimodal incidence with peak onset in children between 5 and 10 years old, and adults after the age of 40 years. Women are twice as likely to be affected as men and without racial predilection. There are significant disease associations with DM including interstitial lung disease, cardiac arrhythmias, and inflammatory arthritides. Patients diagnosed with DM are high risk for underlying malignancies.

There is a wide variation of presentation and severity of both cutaneous and systemic manifestations. About 10% of cases are *amyopathic dermatomyositides* ("sine myositis") that do not have any muscle symptoms. An even less common variant is *polymyositis* (PM) which presents with muscle symptoms but lacks cutaneous symptoms.

Pathophysiology

DM is idiopathic and it is difficult to predict the course of the disease or the severity of symptoms. The complex pathogenesis includes both immune and nonimmune mechanisms responsible for the inflammation of muscles and capillaries, leading to muscle weakness and atrophy.

Clinical Presentation

Cutaneous symptoms are usually the first sign of DM but often go unrecognized. Musculoskeletal symptoms may also be overlooked as their onset is insidious.

Skin Findings

- Pathognomonic skin changes of DM include:

  Heliotrope sign—erythema of the upper eyelids (Fig. 9.2-11).

  Shawl sign—appears in photo-exposed areas that develop pigmentary (poikiloderma), eczematous, and erythematous changes on the shoulders, "V" sign on the chest, or lateral upper arms (Fig. 9.2-12A,B).

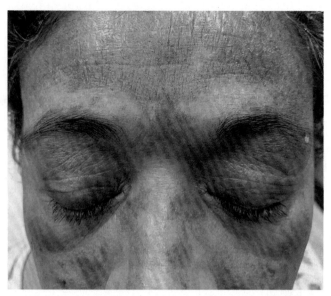

FIG. 9.2-11. Dermatomyositis is characterized by facial erythema. A "heliotrope" eruption is a characteristic violaceous erythema and edema of the upper eyelids. (Photo courtesy of Dr. Ben Farthing.)

  Gottron papules—flat, erythematous papules and plaques over the dorsal IP joints. They are less commonly found on the extensor aspects of the elbows or knees. They have a callus-type appearance and lack pinpoint blood vessels like that of warts (Fig. 9.2-13).

  Periungual telangiectasias—seen on the proximal nail folds. They can appear as generalized erythema with the naked eye. However, evaluation with a dermatoscope can reveal dilated or tortuous capillary loops (Fig. 9.2-4).

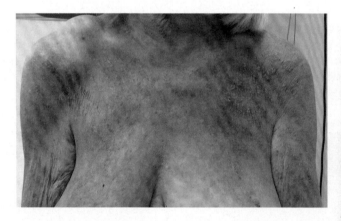

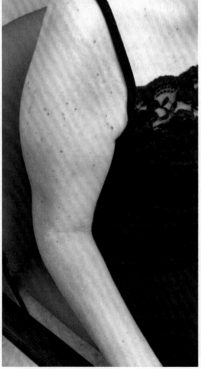

FIG. 9.2-12. **A:** The eczematous lesions of dermatomyositis (DM) often erupt on the shoulders and chest. **B:** Poikiloderma of DM can present as hyperpigmentation or telangiectasias in the photodistributed area of the trunk and extremities. (Photos courtesy of M. Bobonich.)

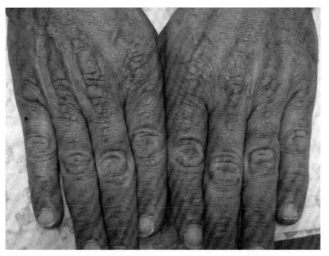

FIG. 9.2-13. *Gottron papules* erupt over the metacarpophalangeal and interphalangeal joints of the extensor surfaces of the hands and fingers. (Photo courtesy of M. Bobonich.)

- Photosensitive poikiloderma (skin changes including reddish-brown hyperpigmentation, dilated blood vessels, and atrophy usually on the neck and chest).

- Scaly or psoriasiform plaques commonly occur on the forehead and scalp.

- Extremely pruritic!!!!

- Erythematous patches/plaques that erupt on the body may have some fine scale but are usually diffuse and can become violaceous.

- Cutaneous symptoms of DM can appear very similar to many other skin diseases and mandates an experienced rheumatology and/or dermatology specialist to provide further evaluation and diagnosis (Table 9.2-1).

Non-Skin Findings

- Myopathies associated with DM can be significant and usually develop as proximal muscle weakness that slowly progresses. Initially, patients may have difficulty raising their hand to brush their hair or lifting their legs to walk and climb steps.

- Esophageal involvement may result in dysphagia.

- Cardiac symptoms including conduction abnormalities may occur.

- Interstitial lung disease has been reported in up to 10% cases of DM (Vij & Strek, 2013).

DIFFERENTIAL DIAGNOSIS   Dermatomyositis

- Contact dermatitis
- Atopic dermatitis
- Seborrheic dermatitis
- Drug eruptions
- Psoriasis
- Polymorphic light eruption
- Acute cutaneous lupus erythematosus
- Subacute cutaneous lupus erythematosus
- Cutaneous T-cell lymphoma
- Tinea corporis
- Lichen planus

Confirming the Diagnosis

For diagnosis of DM, consider the following criteria: proximal muscle weakness (symmetrical); elevated serum muscle enzymes; characteristic skin biopsy findings; electromyography changes; and, classic skin findings (above).

TABLE 9.2-1	Differential Diagnosis for Dermatomyositis. A punch skin biopsy is important to accurately diagnose dermatomyositis which looks like many other dermatoses. A: Cutaneous T-cell lymphoma mycosis fungoides type; B: Dermatomyositis; C: Tinea corporis (Courtesy of M. Bobonich.)

CUTANEOUS T-CELL LYMPHOMA MYCOSIS FUNGOIDES TYPE	DERMATOMYOSITIS	TINEA CORPORIS
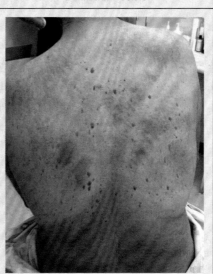		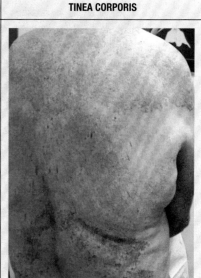

Skin Biopsy

- A punch biopsy of lesional skin for histology and nonlesional skin for DIF are helpful in supporting a suspected diagnosis of DM while eliminating other differential diagnoses.
- Patients with findings suggestive of DM should be referred to rheumatology for further evaluation and diagnostics such as radiographs, electromyography, and MRI-guided muscle biopsy.

Laboratory

- Serologies for suspected DM should include an ANA, anti-Jo, anti-La, and anti-RNP to differentiate it from other CTDs.
- Serum for levels of creatine kinase, glutamic oxaloacetic transaminase (SGOT), alanine aminotransferase (ALT), lactic dehydrogenase (LDH), aldolase, and AST may be elevated.
- A 24-hour urine for creatine is more sensitive than serum markers for DM.

Special Populations

- *Juvenile dermatomyositis* (JDM) can present with symptoms similar to adults (Fig. 9.2-14). There are varied phenotypes of JDM that are associated with presence/absence of autoantibodies that can aid in the diagnosis and therapeutic approach (Li & Tansley, 2019).
- Calcinosis cutis is more commonly reported in childhood DM and the association for underlying malignancy is much lower in JDM.
- Pediatric rheumatologists should be consulted for children suspected with JDM.

Treatment

- TCSs, calcineurin inhibitors, and antipruritics may provide some modest relief from the intense itch.
- Initial systemic agents include hydroxychloroquine or methotrexate.
- Severe or recalcitrant disease may require treatment with systemic corticosteroids, mycophenolate mofetil, or IVIG.
- If symptoms are limited to the skin, patients may achieve complete resolution in a few years.

Management and Patient Education

- Patients with the presumed diagnosis of DM should be referred to rheumatology or dermatology for evaluation of systemic

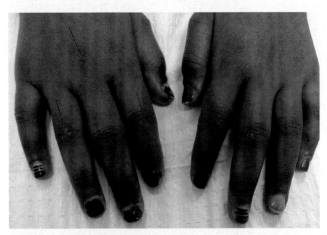

FIG. 9.2-14. Pediatric DM. Very subtle Gottron papules (*arrows*) starting in a 6-year-old African-American girl diagnosed with dermatomyositis. Her initial complaint was swelling in her hands and fingers and hard papules on her elbows (calcinosis cutis). (Photo courtesy of M. Bobonich.)

> **BOX 9.2-2   Risk for Malignancy and Screening Patients with Dermatomyositis**
>
> - Malignancy rates are highest during the first year of diagnosis of and decrease to twofold risk by year 5.
> - The onset of malignancy may precede, occur simultaneously, or follow the diagnosis of DM.
> - Cancer risks are associated with the elevation of specific serum biomarkers:
>   **Anti-TIF1γ**   27-fold increased risk in cancer[1]
>   **Anti-NXP2**   3.68-fold increased risk in cancer[2]
> - There are no official guidelines or consensus for cancer screenings.
> - Annual age-appropriate screening along with those associated with a higher prevalence for the patient's population is paramount.
> - Evidence that supports blind screening for internal malignancy in patients with dermatomyositis.[3]
> - Mammography and gynecologic ultrasound is recommended for women.
> - Whole-body MRI and PET/CT scan are useful. An analysis of two U.S. cohorts with 400 patients showed that 58% patients were diagnosed with asymptomatic cancer–associated dermatomyositis on CT findings.[3] This is important during the first 5 years.
>
> [1]Selva-O'Callaghan et al. (2018); [2]Albayda et al. (2017); [3]Leatham et al. (2018).

involvement and collaborative care in the management and monitoring of their disease.

- Photoprotection is essential as flares can occur especially with UVR exposure.
- Patients should be followed closely for disease control, drug therapy, and side effects.
- Once in remission, patients will not need as frequent office visits but should be monitored as medication is tapered.
- Patients with DM should be carefully evaluated during the first 5 years after the onset for disease when the risk for malignancy is highest.
- Routine cancer screenings and other diagnostics should be performed as indicated (Box 9.2-2).
- Patients must understand the importance of reporting the onset of any new symptoms.

Systemic Scleroderma

Scleroderma is a rare autoimmune disease affecting connective tissue, skin, and internal organs. The disease can be categorized into systemic sclerosis (SSc) and localized scleroderma. The incidence of SSc varies depending on the type but there is an overall female predominance and usually diagnosed between the ages of 30 and 50 years old. It affects African Americans more than Caucasians or those from European descent. There may be some genetic predisposition for SSc but it is not inheritable. Studies suggest that it may be triggered by environmental exposures, infections, and hormonal influences—which are not pathogenic.

Pathophysiology

- SSc is a disruption in the immune system that results in complex extracellular changes in the matrix, including collagen deposition that leads to fibrotic changes or hardening of the skin and organs.
- Patients with SSc have internal organ involvement which will not be addressed here.
- Small blood vessels, like capillaries in the fingers, narrow or develop vasospasms especially with exposure to cold.

BOX 9.2-3 **Cutaneous Symptoms of Systemic Scleroderma**

- Raynaud phenomenon
- Sclerodactyly
- Pitting edema of the fingers/toes
- Changes in skin texture
- Calcinosis (tips of digits and near joints)
- Matted telangiectasias (face, lips, palms)
- Nail folds—tortuous capillaries, dilation or dropout
- Atrophic or thickened patches of skin
- Abnormal pigmentation
- Leukoderma ("salt-and-pepper skin")
- Pitted scars on fingertips
- Ischemic digital ulcerations or contractures of the fingers/toes

---

- Large vessels, such as the renal or pulmonary arteries, vasoconstrict and harden causing disease (i.e., pulmonary hypertension).

Clinical Presentation

Skin Findings

- Patients with SSc have organ involvement are categorized into two subtypes that are differentiated based on their cutaneous involvement.
  - *Limited SSc* has cutaneous manifestations involving the distal extremities and face, whereas
  - *Diffuse SSc* also includes the proximal extremities and trunk. Box 9.2-3 highlights skin findings that are commonly seen in SSc.
- The classic cutaneous manifestations are skin thickening and hardening.
- Pruritus.
- Edema and erythema of the hands/fingers and feet/toes.
- Hands/feet: edema (early stages); erythema; ischemic digits with pits or ulcerations; tightening (later stages) of the skin and autoamputation; and, capillary changes in the proximal nail folds (Fig. 9.2-15).
- Telangiectasias.
- Calcinosis cutis.
- "Salt-and-pepper" abnormal pigmentation.

Raynaud phenomenon is a syndrome that occurs in almost all patients with SSc, often preceding the diagnosis, and in association with other autoimmune diseases. In contrast, Raynaud *disease* is the presence of the syndrome without an underlying disease process. Raynaud phenomenon can be triggered by exposure to cold temperatures or from stress, causing vasoconstriction and/or vasospasms in the arteries and arterioles in the fingers. Patients complain of painful, cold, and numb fingers and toes (Fig. 9.2-16). Their digits become white, cyanotic or bluish, and then red after reactive vasodilation. A close examination of the proximal nail folds may reveal changes in the capillaries (dropout) which would favor Raynaud *phenomenon* and indication for further evaluation for systemic disease.

CREST is the acronym for a syndrome of limited SSC with specific disease characteristics.

Calcinosis cutis which erupts as firm nodules on the fingertips and pads may harden, rupture, and persist as chronic ulcerations
Raynaud phenomenon
Esophageal involvement (usually Barrett's esophagus)
Sclerodactyly
Telangiectasia is a syndrome of limited SSC with specific disease characteristics

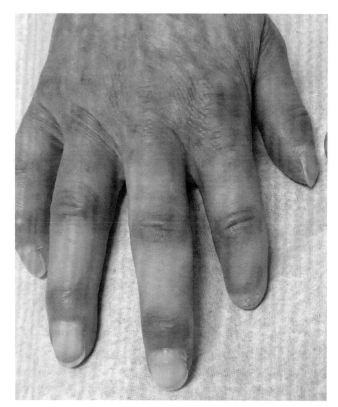

FIG. 9.2-15. Skin tightening, cyanosis, and erythema along with autoamputation of the hands and fingers with SSc. (Photo courtesy of M. Bobonich.)

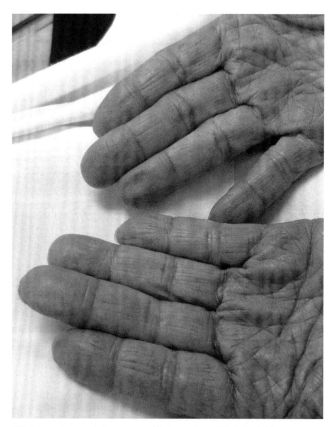

FIG. 9.2-16. Raynaud phenomenon. (Photo courtesy of M. Bobonich.)

Non-Skin Findings

- Myalgia, arthralgia, and fatigue are among the earliest signs and symptoms of SSc.
- The majority of patients have pulmonary involvement presenting with shortness of breath.
- They have an increased risk for lung cancer and thromboembolic event.
- The gastrointestinal system is almost always involved but there may not be symptoms. Patients with SSc complain of dysphagia, hoarseness, choking, cough, bloating, early satiety, constipation, and diarrhea.
- The renal and neurologic systems can be involved.

Confirming Diagnosis

- Patients suspected of SSc should be referred to rheumatology and other specialists for a diagnostic workup.
- Skin biopsy does not diagnose SSc but is helpful in excluding other differential diagnosis.
- Physical examination, laboratory testing, and organ-specific studies are critical in differentiating SSc.
- The presence of these clinical features (Red Flags) should raise clinical suspicion for a patient with a *very early* diagnosis of SSC (Avouac et al., 2011):
  - Raynaud phenomenon
  - Puffy swollen fingers/toes
  - Positive ANA

Treatment

- SSc can have a high mortality and morbidity relative to the type and severity of organ involvement.
- Pain relief using nonsteroidal anti-inflammatories.
- Systemic immunosuppressants are used to slow or halt the progression of cutaneous manifestations and internal organ damage.

Management and Patient Education

- The psychosocial impact of SSc can be devastating for patients and their families and should not be overlooked. Cutaneous lesions can be disfiguring, especially on the face, and should be considered when caring for these patients.
- Dry skin care education.
- Patients diagnosed with SSc require chronic disease management by a multidisciplinary team led by rheumatology.

LOCALIZED SCLERODERMA/MORPHEA

Localized scleroderma, more commonly called *morphea,* affects a younger population with an onset occurring between 20 and 40 years of age but can occur in children. There is a higher incidence of localized scleroderma in individuals of European decent and Caucasians rather than in African Americans. Morphea is NOT associated with SSc or an underlying autoimmune disease.

Pathophysiology

- Inflammation and collagen deposition in the dermis and subcutaneous layer causes a hardening of the skin, leaving atrophic plaques.

- It was once suspected that *Borrelia burgdorferi,* the same spirochete that causes Lyme disease, played a role in the etiology of morphea. However, studies do not support the theory.
- The pathogenesis of morphea is unknown but immune, traumatic, and iatrogenic variables are suspected triggers.

Clinical Presentation

Skin Findings

- *Active* lesions of morphea are papules and plaques of morphea can be solitary or multiple and initially present with erythema and induration. There is no scale.
- As plaques age, they expand centrifugally with the active periphery maintaining a bluish-purple appearance.
- Lesions that maintain an active erythematous border are an indication for treatment.
- Sclerotic plaques have "burned out" and leave atrophic, white, shiny, scar-like (sclerosed) appearance without hair follicles.
- There is variable itch and tenderness associated with the lesions.
- Many patients are unaware of the skin changes until others notice the cosmetic change.
- Additional skin findings vary based on the subtype:
  - *Plaque* or *circumscribed* morphea is the most common type and develops on the trunk. Patients are often unaware of these asymptomatic lesions (Fig. 9.2-17).
  - *Linear* morphea initially presents as a plaque on the arms and legs that begins to extend longitudinally (Fig. 9.2-18). This can be a problem as the thickened, scar-like skin extending

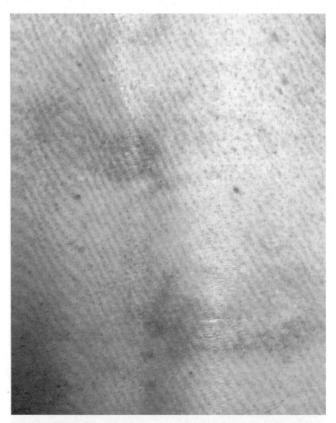

FIG. 9.2-17. Plaque-type morphea showing atrophic plaque with a shiny surface. (Photo courtesy of M. Bobonich.)

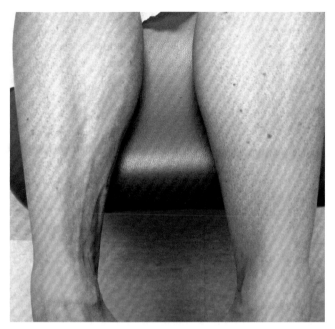

FIG. 9.2-18. Linear morphea in the lower leg of a woman with a notable loss of fat and muscle. This patient does not have a loss of function or mobility that can occur with linear morphea, especially near the joints. (Photo courtesy of M. Bobonich.)

over joints can lead to limited mobility, cause weakness, and shorten limb development.

- *En coup de sabre* is linear morphea involving the face, often the forehead. *Parry–Romberg* syndrome is the loss of subcutaneous tissue that can lead to mild or significant hemifacial atrophy and abnormal development of the underlying facial nerves and vessels (Fig. 9.2-19).
- *Generalized* morphea are large plaques involving large body surface areas of the trunk and extremities including the hands and feet.
- *Eosinophilic fasciitis* is considered by most to be the severe form of morphea. Unlike morphea, the initial lesions begin as pitting edema and erythema, then replaced by a deeper sclerotic plaque. The extracutaneous symptoms may include weight loss, fatigue, myalgia, and weakness.

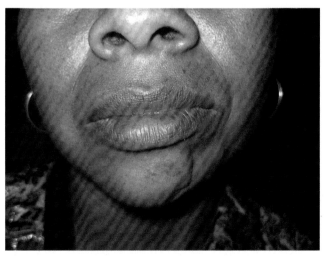

FIG. 9.2-19. Early *Parry–Romberg* syndrome. (Photo courtesy of M. Bobonich.)

Non-Skin Findings

- Patients with morphea do not present with signs or symptoms of Raynaud phenomenon or CREST.

DIFFERENTIAL DIAGNOSIS   Morphea

- Lipodystrophy (medications like injectable corticosteroids)
- Lichen sclerosus
- Graft-versus-host disease
- Eosinophilic folliculitis
- Erythema migrans (early stage of morphea)
- Hamartomas

Confirming the Diagnosis

- Morphea is usually a clinical diagnosis and does not require a skin biopsy.
- If the diagnosis is in question, perform a punch biopsy of the lesion. It is important to communicate the skin features of the biopsy site (erythematous or sclerotic area) to the dermatopathologist for clinicopathologic correlation.
- If the disease is extensive and eosinophilic folliculitis is a concern, a full-thickness skin biopsy containing fascia and muscle is required.
- There are no laboratory studies specifically for morphea.
- Pediatric patients, with morphea diagnosed on the face or head, should have an MRI to evaluate the depth of the lesions.

Treatment

Morphea is usually characterized with mild symptoms, no systemic complications, and can resolve spontaneously. When treatment is indicated for cutaneous disease, therapy is guided by the depth of the lesions, extent or severity of the disease, and evidence of disease activity.

Topical (Mild or Small Lesions)

- Topical and intralesional corticosteroids
- Topical calcineurin inhibitors
- Topical calcipotriol ointment

Systemic (Moderate to Severe Lesions)

For disease that is diffuse or extensive, causing disfigurement (*en coup de sabre*), or limiting function or mobility (linear morphea over joints), systemic therapy is indicated to halt the disease progression.

- Phototherapy (UVA1 wavelength 340 to 400 mm has deeper penetration than NUVB)
- Systemic corticosteroids
- Methotrexate
- Mycophenolate mofetil
- Biologics (off-label) like rituximab and abatacept

Management and Patient Education

- Complications may include hyperpigmentation and "hard" skin which is more cosmetically distressing or disabling.

- Patients with morphea should be referred to dermatology and may require collaboration with rheumatology when there is severe disease or impaired muscle function.

- Ongoing monitoring of morphea is important to ensure that it does not progress.

- Patients with morphea limiting their range of motion or function may benefit from physical therapy.

CLINICAL PEARLS

- Morphea is often misdiagnosed as lichen sclerosus.
- Education of our patients should emphasize that morphea is not the same as systemic scleroderma.
- Close monitoring of active or extensive lesions is important to reduce the progress of disease that can impair function and disfigure.

READINGS AND REFERENCES

Albayda, J., Pinal-Fernandez, I., Huang, W., Parks, C., Paik, J., Casciola-Rosen, L., Danoff, S. K., Johnson, C., Christopher-Stine, L., & Mammen, A. L. (2017). Antinuclear matrix protein 2 autoantibodies and edema, muscle disease, and malignancy risk in dermatomyositis patients. *Arthritis Care & Research, 69*(11), 1771–1776. https://doi.org/10.1002/acr.23188

Avouac, J., Fransen, J., Walker, U. A., Riccieri, V., Smith, V., Muller, C., Miniati, I., Tarner, I. H., Randone, S. B., Cutolo, M., Allanore, Y., Distler, O., Valentini, G., Czirjak, L., Müller-Ladner, U., Furst, D. E., Tyndall, A., Matucci-Cerinic, M., & EUSTAR Group. (2011). Preliminary criteria for the very early diagnosis of systemic sclerosis: results of a Delphi Consensus Study from EULAR Scleroderma Trials and Research Group. *Annals of the Rheumatic Diseases, 70*(3), 476–481. https://doi.org/10.1136/ard.2010.136929

Bogdanov, I., Kazandjieva, J., Darlenski, R., & Tsankov, N. (2018). Dermatomyositis: Current concepts. *Clinics in Dermatology, 36*(4), 450–458. https://doi.org/10.1016/j.clindermatol.2018.04.003

Callen, J. P. (1985). Systemic lupus erythematosus in patients with chronic cutaneous (discoid) lupus erythematosus. Clinical and laboratory findings in seventeen patients. *Journal of the American Academy of Dermatology, 12*(2 Pt 1), 278–288. https://doi.org/10.1016/s0190-9622(85)80036-0

Chasset, F., & Francès, C. (2019). Current concepts and future approaches in the treatment of cutaneous lupus erythematosus: A comprehensive review. *Drugs, 79*(11), 1199–1215. https://doi.org/10.1007/s40265-019-01151-8

Chong, B. F., Song, J., & Olsen, N. J. (2012). Determining risk factors for developing systemic lupus erythematosus in patients with discoid lupus erythematosus. *The British Journal of Dermatology, 166*(1), 29–35. https://doi.org/10.1111/j.1365-2133.2011.10610.x

Durosaro, O., Davis, M. D., Reed, K. B., & Rohlinger, A. L. (2009). Incidence of cutaneous lupus erythematosus, 1965–2005: A population-based study. *Archives of Dermatology, 145*(3), 249–253. https://doi.org/10.1001/archdermatol.2009.21

Eastham, A. B, & Vleugels, R. A. (2013). Cutaneous lupus erythematosus. *JAMA Dermatology, 150*(3), 344.

Florez-Pollack, S., Kunzler, E., & Jacobe, H. T. (2018). Morphea: Current concepts. *Clinics in Dermatology, 36*(4), 475–486. https://doi.org/10.1016/j.clindermatol.2018.04.005

Gilliam, J. N., & Sontheimer, R. D. (1981). Distinctive cutaneous subsets in the spectrum of lupus erythematosus. *Journal of the American Academy of Dermatology, 4*(4), 471–475. https://doi.org/10.1016/s0190-9622(81)80261-7

Guettrot-Imbert, G., Morel, N., Le Guern, V., Plu-Bureau, G., Frances, C., & Costedoat-Chalumeau, N. (2016). Pregnancy and contraception in systemic and cutaneous lupus erythematosus. *Annales de Dermatologie et de Venereologie, 143*(10), 590–600.

James, J. A., Kim-Howard, X. R., Bruner, B. F., Jonsson, M. K., McClain, M. T., Arbuckle, M. R., Walker, C., Dennis, G. J., Merrill, J. T., & Harley, J. B. (2007). Hydroxychloroquine sulfate treatment is associated with later onset of systemic lupus erythematosus. *Lupus, 16*(6), 401–409. https://doi.org/10.1177/0961203307078579

Leatham, H., Schadt, C., Chisolm, S., Fretwell, D., Chung, L., Callen, J. P., & Fiorentino, D. (2018). Evidence supports blind screening for internal malignancy in dermatomyositis: Data from 2 large US dermatology cohorts. *Medicine (Baltimore), 97*(2), e9693. doi:10.1097/MD.0000000000009639

Li, D., & Tansley, S. L. (2019). Juvenile dermatomyositis-Clinical phenotypes. *Current Rheumatology Reports, 21*(12), 74. https://doi.org/10.1007/s11926-019-0871-4

Mertens, J. S., Seyger, M., Thurlings, R. M., Radstake, T., & de Jong, E. (2017). Morphea and eosinophilic fasciitis: An update. *American Journal of Clinical Dermatology, 18*(4), 491–512. https://doi.org/10.1007/s40257-017-0269-x

O'Brien, J. C., & Chong, B. F. (2017). Not just skin deep: Systemic disease involvement in patients with cutaneous lupus. *The Journal of Investigative Dermatology Symposium Proceedings, 18*(2), S69–S74. https://doi.org/10.1016/j.jisp.2016.09.001

Schmidt, E., della Torre, R., & Borradori, L. (2011). Clinical features and practical diagnosis of bullous pemphigoid. *Dermatologic Clinics, 29*(3), 427–438, viii–ix. https://doi.org/10.1016/j.det.2011.03.010

Selva-O'Callaghan, A., Martinez-Gomez, X., Trallero-Araguas, E., & Pinal-Fernandez, I. (2018). The diagnostic work-up of cancer-associated myositis. *Current Opinion Rheumatology, 30*(6), 630–636.

Sontheimer, R. D. (2004). Skin manifestations of systemic autoimmune connective tissue disease: Diagnostics and therapeutics. *Best Practice Research Clinical Rheumatology, 18*(3), 429–462.

Sontheimer, R. D. (2005). Subacute cutaneous lupus erythematosus: 25-year evolution of a prototypic subset (subphenotype) of lupus erythematosus defined by characteristic cutaneous, pathological, immunological, and genetic findings. *Autoimmunity Reviews, 4*(5), 253–263. https://doi.org/10.1016/j.autrev.2004.10.003

Tan, E. M., Cohen, A. S., Fries, J. F., Masi, A. T., McShane, D. J., Rothfield, N. F., Schaller, J. G., Talal, N., & Winchester, R. J. (1982). The 1982 revised criteria for the classification of systemic lupus erythematosus. *Arthritis and Rheumatism, 25*(11), 1271–1277.

Updating the American College of Rheumatology revised criteria for the classification of systemic lupus erythematosus. American College of Rheumatology website. http://www.rheumatology.org/publications/classification/SLE/1982SLEupdate.asp?aud=mem.

Vij, R., & Strek, M. E. (2013). Diagnosis and treatment of connective tissue disease-associated interstitial lung disease. *Chest, 143*(3), 814–824. https://doi.org/10.1378/chest.12-0741

Watanabe, T., & Tsuchida, T. (1995). Classification of lupus erythematosus based upon cutaneous manifestations. Dermatological, systemic and laboratory findings in 191 patients. *Dermatology (Basel, Switzerland), 190*(4), 277–283. https://doi.org/10.1159/000246716

Wieczorek, I. T., Propert, K. J., Okawa, J., & Werth, V. P. (2014). Systemic symptoms in the progression of cutaneous to systemic lupus erythematosus. *JAMA Dermatology, 150*(3), 291–296. https://doi.org/10.1001/jamadermatol.2013.9026

Wolveron, S. E, & Wu, J. J. (2020). *Comprehensive dermatologic drug therapy* (4th ed.). Saunders.

Vasculitis and Purpura

Jeremy Honaker

PURPURA AND VASCULITIS

Purpura is a type of common skin lesion that may represent a simple benign condition (i.e., trauma) or a more ominous condition (i.e., vasculitis, bleeding disorder) associated with high morbidity and mortality. The simplest definition of purpura is hemorrhage or leakage of blood into the skin or mucus membrane. Although commonly purple, purpura may also present as maroon, dark red, blue, or black lesions. The differential diagnosis of purpura is broad and may be associated with inflammatory or noninflammatory etiologies that are inherited or acquired (see Table 9.3-1). Distinguishing between benign and more ominous purpuric lesions for the primary care provider can be difficult. In this chapter, we have created a morphology driven approach that will guide you through your assessment of purpuric lesions and assist you in developing differential diagnoses. Additionally, we provide guidance on selection of diagnostic studies to assist you at arriving at the correct diagnosis, review management of purpura, and know when to refer. Following a review of the morphologic approach to diagnosing purpuric lesions, we will provide an overview of select common and uncommon purpuric conditions.

HOW TO APPROACH A PATIENT WITH PURPURA

The first step in building a differential diagnosis for purpuric lesions (Table 9.3-1) is to assess the lesion:

Lesion Assessment

- Color
  - Purpura presents as purple, maroon, dark red, blue, or black lesions.
  - Red discoloration (i.e., erythema) surrounding the majority of the purpuric lesion suggests an underlying inflammatory condition.
- Blanching
  - Temporary disappearance of the lesion with pressure but reappears once the pressure is removed.
  - *Diascopy* is the use of a glass slide that is applied with firm pressure over a lesion. The glass slide allows the clinician to see whether the lesion disappears (blanching) or is unchanged (nonblanching) in response to the pressure.
  - *Blanching* lesions represent blood vessel dilatation in the dermis. Pressure causes the shifting of blood to the peripheral vessels resulting in the disappearance of the lesion.
  - *Nonblanching* lesions represent the leakage of red blood cells into the dermis/subcutaneous tissue or occlusion of blood vessels. As a result, the application of pressure is unable to cause a shifting of blood to peripheral vessels and the lesion does not disappear.
- Morphology
  - Nonpalpable (flat) purpuric lesions (macules, patches) are typically caused by a noninflammatory process such as an alteration in platelet number, platelet function, coagulation, or due to a compromise in vascular integrity (Fig. 9.3-1A,B).
  - Palpable (raised) purpuric lesions (papules, plaques) are typically caused by an inflammatory process such as inflammation-induced vessel injury with hemorrhage or microvascular occlusion (Fig. 9.3-2).
  - Livedo reticularis lesions are mottled or dusky netlike blue, maroon, or purple patches that occur due to partial or intermittent impaired blood flow (Fig. 9.3-3A).
  - Retiform purpuric lesions are maroon, purple, or black patches or plaques that are angulated or branched that occur due to complete occlusion of the vasculature. These lesions frequently have necrosis (Fig. 9.3-3B).
  - Additional morphologies that may be noted in conjunction with inflammatory purpuric lesions are:
    - Urticaria
    - Nodules
    - Necrotic ulcerations
- Location and distribution of lesions
  - Flat purpura
    - Senile purpura or trauma favors distal extremities.
    - Generalized, truncal, or facial distribution should increase suspicion for underlying bleeding disorder or physical abuse.

TABLE 9.3-1	Using Morphology to Evaluate Purpura

MORPHOLOGY		DIFFERENTIAL DIAGNOSES	
Nonpalpable purpura	Petechiae: <4 mm pinpoint macules Purpura (flat): 4–10-mm macules	Thrombocytopenia	• Medication • Idiopathic • Disseminated intravascular coagulation
		Altered platelet function	• Congenital platelet function defects • Thrombocytosis secondary to myeloproliferative disorder • Medication induced (e.g., NSAIDs) • Chronic kidney disease • Monoclonal gammopathy
		Miscellaneous	• Increased intravascular venous pressure (e.g., Valsalva) • Trauma • Pigmented purpuric dermatoses
	Ecchymoses: >1 cm blue-purple patches	Procoagulant defects	• Disseminated intravascular coagulation • Hemophilia • Hepatic insufficiency • Medications • Vitamin K deficiency
		Altered dermal support of blood vessels	• Actinic purpura • Medications (corticosteroids) • Vitamin C deficiency • Ehlers–Danlos syndrome
		Altered platelet function	• von Willebrand • Thrombocytopenias
	Livedo reticularis: netlike patch of dusky red, maroon, or purple skin	Miscellaneous	• Erythema infectiosum • Erythema ab igne • Cutis marmorata • Vasculitis • Emboli • Medications
Palpable purpura	Purpura (raised): 4–10-mm red-to-purple papules that may coalesce into plaques	Inflammation of blood vessels with hemorrhage	• Infection-induced vasculitis • Medication-induced vasculitis • Autoimmune connective tissue disease vasculitis • Idiopathic vasculitis • Urticarial vasculitis • ANCA vasculitis
		Other small vessel injury	• Erythema multiforme • Pityriasis lichenoides chronica et varioliformis • Arthropod assault • Pigmented purpuric dermatoses
	Retiform purpura: netlike, angulated or branched purpuric patches or plaques	Microvascular platelet plugs Infection-induced vessel occlusion	• Heparin necrosis • Bacterial • Mycobacterial • Fungal
		Hypercoagulopathy	• Coumadin necrosis • Livedoid vasculopathy • Antiphospholipid antibody
		Red blood cell occlusion	• Sickle cell disease
		Miscellaneous	• Calciphylaxis • Brown recluse spider bite
		Miscellaneous—inflammatory	• Vasculitis • ANCA vasculitis • Polyarteritis nodosa • Pyoderma gangrenosum • Chilblains (pernio)

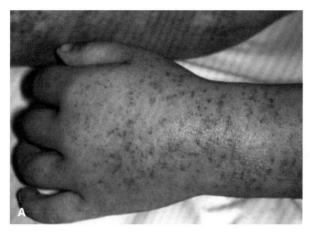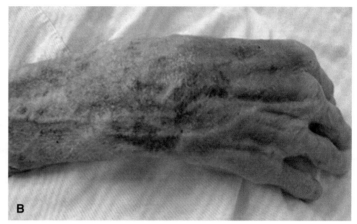

FIG. 9.3-1. **A:** Tiny skin hemorrhages (petechiae) in a child with thrombocytopenia. **B:** Flat purpura in a patient with scurvy. (Photo B used with permission from Wound, Ostomy and Continence Nurses Society®; Doughty, D. B., & McNichol, L. L. [2015]. *Wound, ostomy and continence nurses society® core curriculum: Wound management.* Wolters Kluwer.)

- Raised purpura
  - Favors lower extremities in ambulatory patients.
  - Favors back, buttocks, and posterior thighs in bedbound patients.

History and Comprehensive Physical Examination

Performing a comprehensive history, including detailed review of systems, and physical (see Section 1.2) examination to identify potential etiologies of purpura is essential.

- For flat purpura, an underlying inherited or acquired (see Tables 9.3-2 and 9.3-3) bleeding disorder must be ruled out.

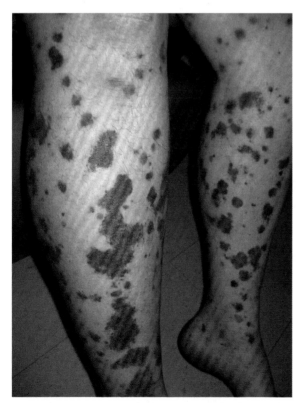

FIG. 9.3-2. Purpura in a patient with small-vessel vasculitis on the lower legs.

- For raised purpura, evaluate for causes and precipitating agents (see Table 9.3-4) and systemic involvement.

Differential Diagnosis

See Table 9.3-1 for morphology-based differential diagnoses.

Confirming the Diagnosis

Flat Purpura

- Laboratory work up if:
  - ≥5 ecchymoses or generalized purpura.
  - Personal or family history of excessive or prolonged bleeding with surgical or dental procedures.
  - Abnormal bruising not associated with an underlying cause (see Table 9.3-3).
- Laboratory evaluation should include:
  - Complete blood count (CBC) with peripheral blood smear
  - Prothrombin (PT)
  - Partial thromboplastin time (PTT)
  - Comprehensive metabolic panel (CMP)

Raised Purpura

- Skin biopsy for histopathology and direct immunofluorescence (DIF)
  - Obtain a full thickness specimen with subcutaneous tissue via punch or excisional biopsy from the center of the lesion.

TABLE 9.3-2	Flat Purpura: Bleeding History

- Age of onset
- Spontaneous development or association with trauma
- Personal or family history of prolonged or excessive bleeding spontaneously or associated with surgical or dental procedure
- Medication history
- Menstrual history
- Nutritional history, including gastrointestinal disorders associated with malabsorption (e.g., Crohn disease, gastric bypass)
- Risk factors for liver disease (e.g., alcohol/drug abuse, viral hepatitis)

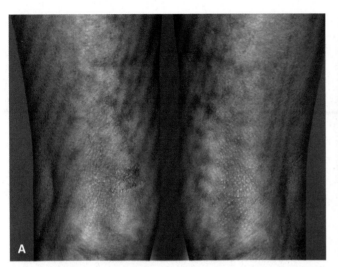 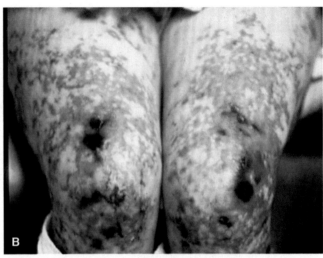

FIG. 9.3-3. A: Livedo reticularis. Net or lace-like erythematous to violaceous patches. **B:** Retiform purpura. Confluent angulated black to purple patches and plaques. (Photo A is used with permission from Lugo-Somolinos, A., McKinley-Grant, L., Goldsmith, L. A., Papier, A., Adigun, C. G., Culton, D., Davey, M., Diamantis, S., Fredeking, A., & Lee, I. [2011]. *VisualDx: Essential dermatology in pigmented skin.* Wolters Kluwer. Photo B is used with permission from Baranoski, B., & Ayello, E. A. [2020]. *Wound care essentials* (5th ed.). Wolters Kluwer.)

TABLE 9.3-3	Flat Purpura: Causes and Precipitating Agents
Inherited	von Willebrand disease Hemophilia A or B Ehlers–Danlos syndrome Marfan syndrome
Disease states	Systemic lupus erythematosus Chronic liver disease Chronic kidney disease Hemolytic uremic syndrome Infection Hypothyroidism
Medications	**Anticoagulants** Factor Xa inhibitors (Apixaban) Thrombin inhibitors (Dabigatran) Heparin Warfarin Vitamin E **Antiplatelets** NSAIDs/Aspirin Thienopyridines (Clopidogrel) Fish oil Selective serotonin reuptake inhibitors **Collagen degradation** Corticosteroids **Thrombocytopenia** Antibiotics (Penicillins, Sulfa) Alcohol Thiazide diuretics Antiseizure (Depakote)
Neoplasm	Leukemia Myeloproliferative disorders
Other	Pregnancy Scurvy Trauma/falls Physical abuse Photodamage (senile purpura)

Adapted from Neutze, D., & Roque, J. (2016). Clinical evaluation of bleeding and bruising in primary care. *American Family Physician, 93*(4), 279–286.

- For histopathology, select a lesion that is 18 to 24 hours old as lesions >48 hours show a nonspecific inflammatory reaction.
- For DIF (preserved in Michel medium), select a lesion that is 8 to 24 hours old as immune complexes may dissipate within 48 hours of onset.
- DIF results will assist in showing the type of immunoglobulins present (e.g., IgA) for patients with vasculitides.
- Laboratory
  - CBC
    - Patients with a primary vasculitis rarely have leukocytosis or thrombocytopenia, which, if present, should prompt further evaluation for an underlying disease, malignancy, or infection.
    - Anemia could signify underlying lupus erythematosus or malignancy.
  - CMP
    - Blood urea nitrogen, creatinine, and electrolyte abnormalities may reflect kidney involvement.
    - Abnormal liver function tests may be associated with underlying liver disease or malignancy.
  - Urinalysis
    - Urinalysis with microscopy that is positive for red blood cell casts is suggestive of glomerulonephritis, while proteinuria is common in lupus nephritis.
  - Estimated sedimentation rate (ESR) or C-reactive protein (CRP)
    - CRP and ESR are usually positive but are nonspecific markers of systemic inflammation.
  - Additional diagnostics to be considered based on past medical history, review of systems, and initial laboratory evaluation:
    - HBV/HCV serologies
    - Streptococcal antibodies
    - HIV
    - Antinuclear antibody

TABLE 9.3-4	Raised Purpura: Causes and Precipitating Agents
Infection	**Bacterial** β-hemolytic *Streptococcus* group A *Staphylococcus aureus* *Mycoplasma pneumoniae* *Mycobacterium tuberculosis* *Neisseria meningococcemia* *Pseudomonas* *Klebsiella* *Escherichia coli* **Viral** Hepatitis A, B, C HSV HIV
Disease state	Systemic lupus erythematosus Rheumatoid arthritis Inflammatory bowel disease
Medications	Anti-TNF agents ACE inhibitors Allopurinol Aspirin/NSAIDs Atypical antipsychotics β-Blockers Cocaine/levamisole contaminated Furosemide Gabapentin Leukotriene inhibitors Selective serotonin-reuptake inhibitors Metformin Phenytoin Retinoids Statins Macrolide antibiotics Minocycline Penicillins Quinolones Sulfonylureas Thiazides Trimethoprim–sulfamethoxazole Vancomycin
Malignancy	Lymphoproliferative disorders Myeloproliferative disorders Solid organ tumors
Other	Chemicals Insecticides Gluten Food allergy

HSV, herpes simplex virus; COX, cyclooxygenase; NSAIDs, nonsteroidal anti-inflammatory drugs; TNF, tumor necrosis factor.

- Rheumatoid factor
- Complement levels (C3, C4, total)
- Serum protein electrophoresis
- ANCA
- Chest radiograph
  - A chest x-ray may be recommended if the patient's review of symptoms or clinical presentation suggests pulmonary involvement and may reveal pulmonary infiltrates, nodules, patchy consolidation, pleural effusion, or cardiomegaly.

- Stool guaiac
  - A stool guaiac will help assess for vasculitis of the bowel in patients with abdominal pain.

Mixed Flat/Raised Purpura
- Follow palpable purpura confirming the diagnosis guidelines.

Retiform Purpura
- Follow palpable purpura confirming the diagnosis guidelines.

Management and Patient Education
- Flat purpura
  - Trauma is a common cause of flat purpura. Patients without a personal or family history of prolonged or excessive bleeding are unlikely to have an underlying bleeding disorder.
  - Spontaneous bleeding should raise suspicion for underlying bleeding disorder.
  - Medications are another common cause for abnormalities in platelets or coagulation, a thorough evaluation of supplements, herbals, over the counter, and prescription medications should be reviewed. If the medication can be stopped, improvement in flat purpura will be noted in 2 to 4 weeks.
  - Patients with distal extremity distribution of flat purpura, negative personal or family history of prolonged bleeding, and no other symptoms of bleeding should be reassured with a follow-up in 3 months for reevaluation.
  - Flat purpura should be referred to Hematology for further evaluation if a patient has:
    - Thrombocytopenia or abnormal coagulation studies not associated with underlying medication.
    - Nonthrombocytopenic purpura with normal coagulation studies and a personal or family bleeding history. These patients need to be evaluated for von Willebrand disease, factor VIII deficiency, or abnormal platelet function.
    - A concern for underlying bleeding disorder with an upcoming planned surgery or pregnancy.
    - Purpura in conjunction with:
      - telangiectasias to the oral mucosa, face, ears, chest, hands, or feet
      - weight loss
      - pallor
      - lymphadenopathy
      - joint swelling
      - fever
- Strategies to assist with preventing ecchymoses include wearing double layer of clothing, minimizing trauma, and keeping skin soft and supple with routine application of moisturizing creams or ointment.
- Patients with suspected bleeding disorder should avoid contact sports and if bleeding does occur to rest, elevate the area above the head if possible, and apply pressure with or without ice to support clotting or wrap the area with compression dressing (e.g., coban).
- Patients with bleeding disorder should have a medic alert bracelet or card.

- Raised purpura
  - The initial presentation and evaluation of raised purpura may begin in the primary care office, and patients with localized or early vasculitis can be managed with supportive care as most cases resolve over 3 to 4 weeks once the causative agent is removed or treated.
  - Ultimately, the best indicator of prognosis in any vasculitis with systemic involvement depends on the size of the vessel and organ involved. Long-term implications include the possibility of multiple episodes with recurrent crops of vasculitic lesions appearing for months or years.
  - Close follow-up of patients with history of systemic vasculitis is essential to halt disease progression, evaluate response to therapy, and the prevention of complications.
  - Patients with raised purpura should be referred to rheumatology or dermatology if there is:
    - extensive cutaneous involvement.
    - systemic involvement.
    - concomitant retiform purpura, nodules, or necrotic ulcerations.
    - relapse or disease progression despite treatment.

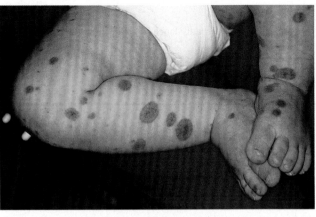

FIG. 9.3-4. Henoch–Schonlein purpura. Lesions are macular and papular, purpuric, varying shades of purple and blue, and necrotizing centers are noted. (Fleisher, G. R., Ludwig, W., & Baskin, M. N. [2004]. *Atlas of pediatric emergency medicine.* Wolters Kluwer Health | Lippincott Williams & Wilkins.)

CLINICAL PEARLS

- Lesions distributed on the arms and legs are more likely caused by trauma.
- Lesions that occur spontaneously or are distributed primarily on the trunk suggest an underlying bleeding disorder.
- Normal platelet counts and coagulation studies do not rule out an underlying bleeding disorder.
- Consider platelet disorder if there is a history of mucocutaneous bleeding (e.g., epistaxis, hematuria).
- Consider physical abuse if:
  - there are unexplained ecchymoses.
  - pattern does not match history.
  - ecchymoses are the shape of an object.
  - ecchymoses occur in unusual locations (e.g., buttock).
- For raised purpura
  - Rule out systemic involvement.
  - Palpable purpura above the waist may be suggestive of concomitant renal involvement.
  - For raised purpura lesions with painful nodules, pustules, necrotic ulcers, livedo, or retiform purpura, consider medium or large vessel vasculitis.

VASCULITIDES

Vasculitides are considered a subcategory of vasculopathy, which is an umbrella term used to describe inflammatory and noninflammatory conditions that develop within and around blood vessels. Vasculitides most commonly present as raised purpura and are defined as conditions that cause inflammation of the blood vessel walls resulting in tissue necrosis.

Occlusive vasculopathies are another subcategory of vasculopathy that present as retiform purpura (Fig. 9.3-4). Occlusive vasculopathies are conditions that cause partial or complete blockage of single or numerous blood vessels that occurs as a result of:

- Concomitant small-to-medium vessel vasculitis
- Emboli

- Microorganism invasion of blood vessels
- Thrombosis due to an underlying coagulopathy

A review of the evaluation and management of occlusive vasculopathies is beyond the scope of this textbook. The following sections will focus on the classification of vasculitides, pathophysiology, and evaluation and management of select small, medium, and large vessel vasculitides.

Vasculitides Classification

In an attempt to classify the vasculitides, several schemes have been proposed with the International Chapel Hill Consensus Conference on the Nomenclature of Systemic Vasculitides (CHCC) being the most widely used nomenclature (i.e., names, definitions) for vasculitis. Based upon the 2018 CHCC nomenclature, cutaneous vasculitides are categorized by:

- ***Vessel type and size.*** All categories of vessels can be affected, including small-, medium-, and large-sized vessels of the arterial and/or venous systems.
  - *Small vessels* include arterioles, capillaries, and postcapillary venules that are found in the dermis of the skin.
  - Medium-sized vessels refer to the main visceral arteries and veins, and the small arteries and veins within the deep dermis or subcutaneous tissue.
  - *Large vessels* are the aorta, its major branches and corresponding veins, and other named arteries such as pulmonary or temporal artery.
- ***Organ distribution***
  - *Single-organ vasculitis* (involves one organ system)
    - Patients with skin-only-involvement may or may not involve other organ systems.
  - *Systemic vasculitis* (involving one or more organs in addition to the skin)
    - Patients with a systemic vasculitis (immunoglobulin A vasculitis) may present with only skin organ involvement initially.
- ***Etiology***
  - Vasculitides should be classified by their cause, whether associated with systemic disease, medications, or infection.
  - For example, if a vasculitis is caused by direct invasion of pathogens, such as *Treponema pallidum,* then the vasculitis should be specified as *syphilitic* vasculitis rather than "infectious vasculitis."

Pathophysiology

- Vasculitis can be broadly labeled as infectious or noninfectious (Table 9.3-4).
- Vasculitis primarily presents as a type III hypersensitivity reaction that is an exaggerated immune system response to a self- or foreign antigen.
- Immune complexes (IgG, M, or A) form with an antigen and deposit in the vessel walls causing activation of the complement system, neutrophil-driven necrosis of blood vessel walls, leakage of red blood cells into the dermal and subcutaneous tissue, and increased clotting.
- The combination of dermal and/or subcutaneous inflammation and leakage of red blood cells produces raised purpura.

SMALL VESSEL VASCULITIS

Small vessel vasculitis is a collection of vasculitides that involves predominantly small arteries, arterioles, capillaries, and venules. The preferred umbrella term for vasculitis that occurs only in the skin (single-organ vasculitis of the skin) is cutaneous small vessel vasculitis (CSVV), with further classification of the cutaneous vasculitis based on diagnostic evaluation (direct immunofluorescence) and etiology (systemic disease or infection). Occasionally, small vessel vasculitides will have concomitant involvement of medium size arteries and veins. When medium vessels are involved, patients will present with livedo reticularis, retiform purpura, or necrotic ulcers. The two major categories of CSVV are immune complex vasculitides and antinuclear cytoplasmic antibody (ANCA)-associated vasculitis.

IMMUNE COMPLEX VASCULITIDES

IgA Vasculitis (Henoch–Schönlein Purpura)

IgA vasculitis (IgAV), formerly known as Henoch–Schönlein purpura, is a multiorgan system small vessel vasculitis that primarily affects children 3 to 12 years old during the fall and winter months. IgAV is less commonly seen in adults with an annual incidence of 0.8 to 1.8 per 100,000 persons (Oni & Sampath, 2019).

Pathophysiology

The pathogenesis for IgAV is not clear, but following observations have been noted:

- Infectious etiology originating from ear, nose, and throat area due to onset in the fall and winter months. Potential organisms include: *Streptococcus, Mycoplasma pneumoniae,* respiratory syncytial virus, influenza, and cytomegalovirus (Piram & Mahr, 2013).
- Vaccinations are not associated with IgAV (Piram et al., 2018).
- Drugs have not been implicated in children. However, several case studies have implicated medications (i.e., nonsteroidal anti-inflammatory, antibiotics, chemotherapy) inducing IgAV in adults (Da Dalt et al., 2016).
- Solid organ malignancies have been associated with IgAV in adults, with lung, prostate, and kidney being the most common (Podjasek et al., 2012).

Clinical Presentation

Skin Findings

- Lesions favor the extensor aspect of the lower extremities and buttocks, but can include arms, face, and ears. Lesions uncommonly present on the trunk (Fig. 9.3-4).
- Early lesions: red to purple macules and occasionally urticarial papules/plaques.
- Later lesions: papular purpura with occasional hemorrhagic blisters/bulla and necrosis.

Non-Skin Findings

- Gastrointestinal
  - Abdominal pain, nausea, vomiting, diarrhea, hematemesis, GI bleeding, and/or melena
  - While rare, intussusception and bowel perforation can be a major complication
- Musculoskeletal
  - Arthralgias (four or fewer) involving ankles, knees, and/or dorsal hands/feet
  - Children will refuse to walk
- Renal
  - Hematuria, proteinuria, nephrotic syndrome, or renal failure can develop
- Male patients may present with scrotal pain, tenderness, or swelling (Fig. 9.3-5)

Confirming the Diagnosis

- Diagnosis can be made on clinical presentation (Table 9.3-5).

The following diagnostics should be considered:

- Blood pressure.
- CBC with differential.
- Complete metabolic panel.
- Early morning urinalysis with microscopy preferred.
- Stool guaiac.
- PTT and PT time (if concerns for coagulopathy).
- Biopsy for histopathology and DIF is not usually necessary unless required to rule out other diagnoses or if skin eruption does not fit typical purpuric eruption involving the buttocks and lower legs.

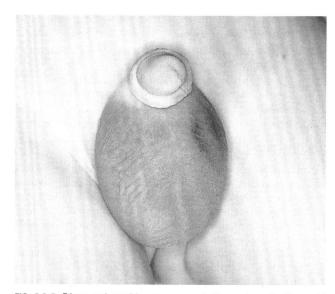

FIG. 9.3-5. Edema and possible purpura seen in the scrotum of a 6-year-old patient referred for possible torsion. (Fleisher, G. R., Ludwig, W., & Baskin, M. N. [2004]. *Atlas of pediatric emergency medicine.* Wolters Kluwer Health I Lippincott Williams & Wilkins.)

TABLE 9.3-5 | **IgAV Diagnostic Criteria**

Mandatory: Purpura or petechiae with lower limb predominance
One of the four criteria must be present:

1. Acute onset diffuse abdominal colicky pain (may include intussusception and gastrointestinal bleeding)
2. Histology showing leukocytoclastic vasculitis or proliferative glomerulonephritis with predominant IgA deposition
3. Acute onset arthralgia or arthritis
4. Either proteinuria or hematuria

Adapted from Ozen, S., Marks, S. D., Brogan, P., Groot, N., de Graeff, N., Avcin, T., Bader-Meunier, B., Dolezalova, P., Feldman, B. M., Kone-Paut, I., Lahdenne, P., McCann, L., Pilkington, C., Ravelli, A., van Royen, A., Uziel, Y., Vastert, B., Wulffraat, N., Kamphuis, S., & Beresford, M. W. (2019). European consensus-based recommendations for diagnosis and treatment of immunoglobulin A vasculitis-the SHARE initiative. *Rheumatology, 58*(9), 1607–1616.

DIFFERENTIAL DIAGNOSIS   IgAV

- Capillaritis
- Erythema multiforme
- Meningococcemia
- Sweet syndrome
- Amyloidosis
- Arthropod assault
- Thrombocytopenia purpura
- Pityriasis lichenoides et varioliformis acuta
- Leukocytoclastic vasculitis
- ANCA-associated vasculitis
- Cryoglobulinemic vasculitis

- Abdominal ultrasonography for patients with severe abdominal symptoms to rule out intussusception.

Treatment

Systemic

- Systemic corticosteroids (1 mg/kg/day × 4 weeks) for severe arthralgias, for mild to moderate abdominal pain, and severe or rapidly progressive renal disease.
- Acetaminophen or NSAIDs if appropriate for milder symptoms (arthralgia, abdominal pain).
- Colchicine can be considered for chronic purpuric lesions. Corticosteroids have not been shown to have any benefit for purpuric lesions.
- Angiotensin converting enzyme inhibitors for mild to moderate proteinuria.
- Mycophenolate mofetil, cyclophosphamide, and rituximab may also be considered as adjunctive therapy in moderate to severe cases.

Management and Patient Education

- Patients with IgAV often require multidisciplinary management (e.g., rheumatology, dermatology, gastroenterology) and may require admission to a tertiary care setting for management.
- Treatment is primarily supportive as IgAV is usually self-limiting and resolves spontaneously in 94% of children within 4 weeks without sequelae (Oni & Sampath, 2019). Recurrent IgAV is uncommon and typically follows a milder severity and shorter duration.

- Nephritis is most likely to occur in the first 2 months after IgAV onset. Early morning urinalysis with microscopy and blood pressure should be checked weekly for the first 2 months after onset, then switch to monthly for 6 to 12 months. Patients with IgAV should have annual urinalysis and blood pressure checks at well child visits (Jauhola et al., 2010).
- Pregnant female patients with history of IgAV or females considering pregnancy should be referred to high-risk obstetrics (Ronkainen et al., 2002).

Special Considerations

- In comparison to children, adults with IgAV typically (Audemard-Verger et al., 2015; Hong et al., 2016):
  - Have lower frequency of abdominal pain and fever.
  - Higher frequency renal disease and arthralgias.
  - More severe disease course requiring immunosuppressive therapy.
  - 20% experience recurrent disease.

CLINICAL PEARL

- For adults with persistent IgAV or failure to respond appropriately to immunosuppressive therapy, rule out underlying solid tumor malignancy.

Cutaneous IgG/IgM Vasculitis (Cutaneous Leukocytoclastic Vasculitis)

Cutaneous IgG/IgM vasculitis affects both genders equally with 15 to 45 cases per 1 million adults per year (Arora et al., 2014). Cutaneous IgG/IgM vasculitis has been associated with (Goeser et al., 2014):

- Idiopathic (45% to 55%)
- Infection (15% to 20%)
- Autoimmune connective tissue disease (15% to 20%)
- Hypersensitivity drug reaction (10% to 15%)
- Malignancy or lymphoproliferative disorder (5% to 10%)

The majority of patients with CSVV experience only one episode. Recurrent CSVV has been reported in up to 30% of the population, and may be associated with:

- Infection
- Autoimmune connective tissue disease
- Idiopathic causes

CSVV reactions range in severity from mild to life-threatening with overall survival rates of 79% at 5 years (Arora et al., 2014). Predictors of survival or mortality have not been identified.

Clinical Presentation

Skin Findings

- Palpable purpura is the classic presentation of CSVV, crops of 3- to 10-mm papules coalesce into purpuric plaques (Fig. 9.3-2).
- Distribution of lesions can occur anywhere on the body, but often favor (Fig. 9.3-6):
  - Areas of dependency (e.g., back, buttocks, lower extremities)
  - Areas associated with tight fitting clothing
  - Areas affected by trauma

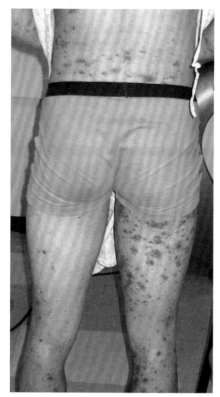

FIG. 9.3-6. Nonpalpable purpura of leukocytoclastic vasculitis, also called single-organ vasculitis, on man with an allergy to shellfish. (Photo courtesy of M. Bobonich.)

- Levamisole vasculitic lesions associated with the intravenous or intranasal use of cocaine contaminated with levamisole presents as purpura and/or necrosis of the ears (Fig. 9.3-7), nose, cheeks, and various other locations including the trunk.
- Lesions evolve within 7 to 10 days of a causative exposure and last approximately 1 to 4 weeks.
- Additional morphologies noted include nonpalpable petechiae/purpura (early stage).
- Urticaria, targetoid lesions, pustules, vesicles, ulcerations, and eschar (Fig. 9.3-8A–C).

Lesions may have associated itch, burning, or pain.

- Edema may develop if nephritis is present.

Non-Skin Findings

While uncommon to have associated extracutaneous involvement, clinicians must evaluate for systemic involvement, which may present as:

- Constitutional: fever, weight loss, or fatigue
- Cardiopulmonary: cough, shortness of breath, hypertension, or hemoptysis
- Gastrointestinal: abdominal pain, melena, weight loss, nausea/vomiting, or diarrhea
- Musculoskeletal: myalgia or arthralgia
- Neurologic: headache, weakness, paresthesias, or visual disturbances
- Renal: proteinuria or hematuria

Differential Diagnosis CSVV

See Table 9.3-1.

Treatment

The initial treatment approach is conservative with a focus on symptomatic management in patients with mild skin disease (no ulcerations, necrosis) and lack of systemic involvement.

Topical Therapy

- Moderately potent topical corticosteroids.
- Best rest, leg elevation, compression stockings if applicable.

Systemic Therapy

- Nonsteroidal anti-inflammatory (NSAIDs) medications for pain if no renal or gastrointestinal involvement.
- Oral antihistamines to attenuate pruritus.
- Prednisone
  - Short course of prednisone 1 mg/kg/day followed by a taper over 4 to 6 weeks for those with widespread disease, severe pruritus/pain/burning, or ulcerative necrotic skin disease.

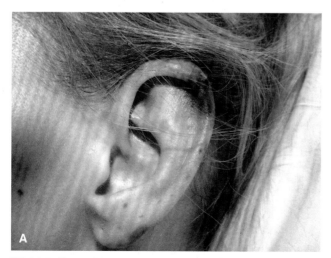
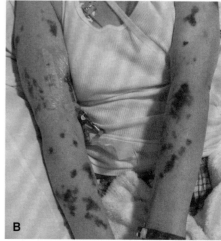

FIG. 9.3-7. Characteristic purpura associated with levamisole (common contaminate in cocaine) induced small-vessel vasculitis on the ear (**A**) and arms (**B**). (Photos courtesy of Lauren Alberta-Wzolek.)

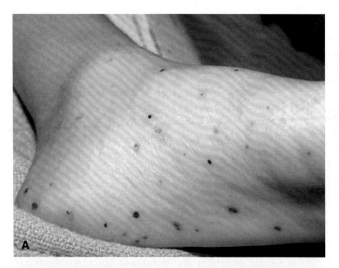

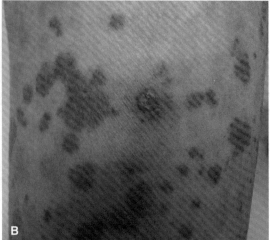

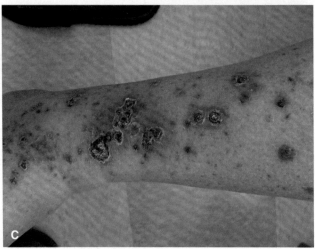

FIG. 9.3-8. A: Petechiae on the foot and sole of a child with HSP with palpable purpura. (Courtesy of M. Bobonich.) **B:** Purpura with a bulla on the lower leg. (Courtesy of M. Bobonich.) **C:** Vasculitis with necrosis. (© Cathleen Case.)

- Higher doses of prednisone may be needed for chronic forms of CSVV, or those with more severe cutaneous disease. Patients requiring long-term corticosteroids should be transitioned to a steroid-sparing agent (i.e., colchicine, dapsone).
- Dapsone
  - Patients on dapsone need G6PD testing prior to initiating therapy and careful monitoring for hemolytic anemia during therapy.
- Other systemic therapies include pentoxifylline, azathioprine, methotrexate, cyclophosphamide, intravenous immunoglobulin, mycophenolate mofetil, rituximab, or plasmapheresis.

Management and Patient Education

- See Management and Patient education subsection of "How to approach a patient with purpura" for common guidelines shared among raised purpura lesions.
- *Management of patients on prednisone*
  - Short-term prednisone taper (<3 months) should be counseled regarding adverse effects including hypertension, glucose intolerance, sleep disturbance, hirsutism, weight gain, and avascular necrosis of the hip.

- Baseline bone mineral density testing should be considered for long-term prednisone (>3 months) use.
- To assist with decreasing bone demineralization patients should be counseled regarding:
  - Weight-bearing exercise
  - Smoking cessation
  - Alcohol cessation
  - Fall prevention
  - Elemental calcium 800 to 1,200 mg cumulative dose daily
  - Vitamin D 800 international units daily
- Blood pressure monitoring at each follow up visit.
- Baseline fasting glucose or hemoglobin A1c to identify potential hyperglycemia.

CLINICAL PEARLS

- Patients with suspected small vessel vasculitis must be screened for systemic organ involvement.
- Drug-induced vasculitis often develops 7 to 10 days after medication exposure.
- Systemic disease–induced vasculitis often develops 6 months after onset.

ANCA-Associated Vasculitides

ANCA-associated vasculitides (AAV) are a group of small-to-medium vessel vasculitides that are uncommon with an estimated incidence of 13 to 20 cases per 1 million people. AAV primarily affects those of European, American, and Asian descent. AAV includes: granulomatosis with polyangiitis (GPA), microscopic polyangiitis (MPA), and eosinophilic granulomatosis with polyangiitis (EGPA).

Pathophysiology

- AAV occurs in those who develop antibodies against specific proteins (i.e., myeloperoxidase [MPO], proteinase 3 [PR3]) found in neutrophils.
- After neutrophils become activated from inflammatory signals (e.g., cytokines, complement) or exposure to bacterial endotoxins, proteins are expressed on the surface of the cell. Antibodies bind to these proteins and cause the activation of surrounding neutrophils and other immune cells causing vessel destruction and tissue necrosis.
- The development of antibodies against MPO and PR3 may develop due to *Staphylococcus* infection, genetics, exposures to hydrocarbons/silica dust, and medications (minocycline, adalimumab).

Clinical Presentation

The clinical presentation of AAV varies and the disease onset can be acute or may have an indolent onset with slow progression over months. Additionally, AAV can present as a single-organ vasculitis or can involve multiple organ systems.

Skin Findings

- Palpable purpura predominantly to the lower extremities but may also affect the trunk, face, and scalp (Fig. 9.3-9). Additional morphologies noted include ulcerated papules, urticarial plaques, vesicles/blisters, necrotic ulcerations, livedo reticularis, or erythematous targetoid macules/papules (EGPA).

Non-Skin Findings

- Constitutional symptoms include fatigue, myalgias, fever, weight loss.

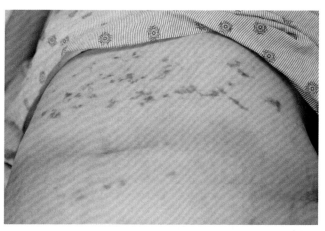

FIG. 9.3-9. GPA with palpable purpura on the abdomen. (Used with permission from Gru, A. A., & Wick, M. [2018]. *Pediatric dermatopathology and dermatology.* Wolters Kluwer.)

- Ear, nose, and throat symptoms are more common in EGPA and GPA and include bloody/purulent nasal drainage, oral/nasal ulcers, otitis media, persistent rhinorrhea, conductive/sensorineural hearing loss. Saddle nose deformity is a common finding in GPA and presents as a sunken depression on the bridge of the nose.
- Pulmonary symptoms are more common in EGPA and GPA and include: cough, dyspnea, hoarseness, hemoptysis, stridor, wheezing.
- Renal symptoms are more common in MPA and include hematuria.
- Neurologic symptoms are more common in MPA and EGPA and include asymmetrical peripheral neuropathy that presents with sharp, burning, aching, tingling pain, cold/heat insensitivity, paresthesias, and weakness.
- Gastrointestinal symptoms are less common but may include nausea, vomiting, abdominal pain, and melena.
- Ocular symptoms are uncommon but may include eye pain, diplopia, foreign-body sensation, visual disturbance, proptosis, erythema of eye structures (conjunctiva, sclera).

DIFFERENTIAL DIAGNOSIS   ANCA Associated Vasculitis

- CSVV
- Systemic lupus erythematosus
- Deep fungal infections (e.g., mucormycosis, coccidioidomycosis)
- Levamisole toxicity
- Pyoderma gangrenosum
- Polyarteritis nodosa
- Systemic lupus erythematosus
- Goodpasture syndrome
- Granulomatosis with polyangiitis
- Eosinophilic granulomatosis with polyangiitis
- Microscopic polyangiitis
- Hypereosinophilic syndrome (EPA only)
- Eosinophilic pneumonia (EPA only)

Confirming the Diagnosis

AAV should be considered in any patients who present with raised purpura with systemic symptoms. The following diagnostics should be performed:

- Skin biopsy
  - See confirming the diagnosis section in "How to approach a patient with purpura" regarding biopsy guidelines for raised purpura.
  - While skin biopsies provide useful information, biopsies from the nasal cavity, lung, or kidneys can also be used to identify AAV.
  - DIF typically shows little to no immunoglobulins or complement for GPA, EGPA, or MPA.
- Antineutrophil cytoplasmic antibody (ANCA) testing
  - ANCA disease associations
    - GPA is associated with a positive PR3/cytoplasmic pattern (cANCA).
    - MPA and EGPA are associated with MPO/perinuclear pattern (pANCA).

- If both pANCA and cANCA are positive, suspect medications.
- While positive ANCA is associated with AAV, positive titers may be seen in the following conditions: inflammatory bowel disease, malignancy, chronic infections (e.g., hepatitis C, human immunodeficiency virus).
- CBC findings may include thrombocytosis, leukocytosis, anemia, and eosinophilia (EGPA only).
- Complete metabolic panel findings may include elevated creatinine/blood urea nitrogen, decreased glomerular filtration rate, and elevated liver enzymes.
- ESR/CRP
- Urinalysis with microscopy findings may include symptomatic hematuria, proteinuria, and casts.
- Chest radiograph and computed tomography scan for all patients with pulmonary symptoms.

While AAV may have overlapping clinical features, the American College of Rheumatology diagnostic criteria are:

GPA (Wegener Granulomatosis)

The presence of two or more of the following criteria:

- Oral or nasal inflammation with ulcers or purulent/bloody drainage
- Abnormal chest radiograph showing cavities, infiltrates, or nodules
- Urinalysis with microscopic hematuria
- Granulomatous inflammation on biopsy from skin, kidney, or lungs

EGPA (Churg–Strauss)

The presence of four or more of the following criteria:

- Asthma
- Peripheral blood eosinophilia >10%
- Neuropathy
- Migratory pulmonary infiltrates
- Paranasal sinus abnormalities
- Biopsy demonstrating tissue eosinophil infiltrate

MPA

Diagnostic criteria for MPA have not been developed. Guidelines for the diagnosis include:

- Biopsy demonstrating necrotizing vasculitis without granulomatous inflammation
- Positive (pANCA)

Treatment

Systemic Therapy

The goals of treatment are to:

- Rapidly suppress the inflammatory process through the use of immunosuppressive medications (induction phase 3 to 6 months)
- Prevent disease relapse (maintenance phase 24 to 48 months)

For the induction phase, a combination of systemic corticosteroids with either cyclophosphamide or rituximab is used. Followed by a gradual taper of systemic corticosteroids over 3 to 5 months. For the maintenance phase, patients are transitioned to corticosteroid sparing agents such as methotrexate, azathioprine, mycophenolate mofetil, or rituximab.

Management and Patient Education

- Patients with AAV require multidisciplinary (e.g., nephrology, rheumatology, immunology, dermatology) management in a tertiary care setting (i.e., hospital).
- AAV is associated with significant morbidity and mortality due to irreversible end-organ damage and complications secondary to chronic immunosuppressive therapy. Early diagnosis and intervention is necessary to preserve organ function and avoid disease progression.
- A 7-year follow-up study of AAV patients showed 91% of patients had permanent end-organ damage as a result of vasculitis and 34% had at least five signs of permanent morbidity. The most common complications from vasculitis and immunosuppressive therapy were hypertension (41.5%), peripheral neuropathy (19%), end-stage renal disease (14%), osteoporosis (14%), malignancy (13%), impaired pulmonary function (12%), and diabetes (10%) (Robson et al., 2015).
- Relapse occurs in 30% to 50% of patients within 5 years of onset, and most commonly 12 to 18 months after stopping maintenance therapy. Risk factors for relapse include GPA phenotype, lower cumulative cyclophosphamide induction dose, and stopping glucocorticoids (Geetha & Jefferson, 2020).
- Venous thromboembolism prophylaxis is necessary as those with AAV have an 8% incidence of venous thrombosis.
- Avoid live vaccines in patients receiving immunosuppressive therapy. However, patients should be up to date on age-appropriate inactivated vaccinations.
- Patients need to be counseled to monitor and notify their health care provider at the onset of skin and non-skin findings so that early identification of relapse can occur. Patients may consider use of urine dipstick at home to monitor for hematuria.

CLINICAL PEARL

- For patients with poorly controlled asthma, consider evaluation for EGPA

Other Small Vessel Vasculitides

For patients who do not match either clinical presentations of IgA vasculitis, cutaneous IgG/IgM vasculitis, or AAV, consider the following more uncommon to rare small vessel vasculitides:

Urticarial Vasculitis

- Urticarial vasculitis can present as a single-organ vasculitis (normocomplementemic) or a systemic vasculitis (hypocomplementemic) and has been associated with medications, infection, malignancy, autoimmune connective tissue diseases, and complement disorders.
- Skin findings include itchy or painful urticarial papules or plaques that last >24 hours (Fig. 9.3-10). In contrast, urticaria lesions resolve <24 hours.

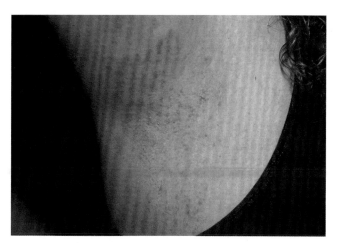

FIG. 9.3-10. Urticarial vasculitis. Urticarial thin papules coalescing into plaques with burning sensation rather than itch. (Used with permission with Hall, J. C., & Hall, B. J. [2017]. *Sauer's manual of skin diseases* [11th ed.]. Wolters Kluwer.)

- Non-skin findings are found in hypocomplementemic urticarial vasculitis and include abdominal pain, nausea, vomiting, arthritis, arthralgias, dyspnea, and conjunctivitis.
- Diagnostic workup prior to referral to dermatology or rheumatology may include skin biopsy for histopathology and DIF, CBC, CMP, UA, complement panel, hepatitis panel, ESR/CRP, and ANA panel.

Cryoglobulinemic Vasculitis

- Cryoglobulinemic vasculitis that is caused by circulating immunoglobulins that when exposed to cold undergo a reversible precipitation (cryoglobulins) and deposition in small vessels causing vasculitis to the cutaneous, glomerular, or peripheral nerves. Associated conditions include hepatitis B/C, autoimmune connective tissue disease, and lymphoproliferative disorders.
- Skin findings that develop following cold exposure include palpable purpura (Fig. 9.3-11), retiform purpura, livedo reticularis, Raynaud phenomenon, ulcerated nodules, and gangrene.
- Non-skin findings include arthralgias, arthritis, peripheral neuropathy, hematuria, dyspnea, and hepatomegaly.
- Diagnostic workup prior to referral to dermatology or rheumatology may include skin biopsy, Hepatitis panel, CBC, CMP, UA, and ANA panel. Contact your laboratory to determine ability to perform cryoglobulin test.

Nodular Vasculitis

- Nodular vasculitis, formerly known as erythema induratum, is a form of small to medium vasculitis that presents as a panniculitis and has been associated with tuberculosis, hepatitis B/C, autoimmune connective tissue disease, bacterial infections, and hematologic disorders.
- Skin findings include tender erythematous to purple nodules predominantly to the calf area that may ulcerate. There are no non-skin findings.
- Diagnostic workup prior to referral to dermatology or rheumatology may include skin biopsy and laboratory workup based on risk factors/history.

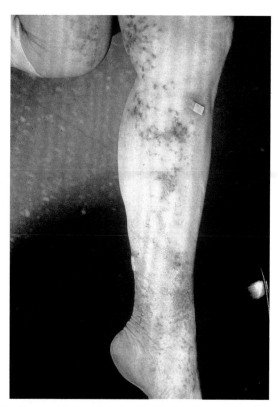

FIG. 9.3-11. Cryoglobulinemia. Erythematous to violaceous papules and plaques. (Used with permission with Hall, J. C., & Hall, B. J. [2017]. *Sauer's manual of skin diseases* [11th ed.]. Wolters Kluwer.)

Erythema Elevatum Diutinum

- Erythema elevatum diutinum is considered a neutrophilic dermatosis with small vessel vasculitis and has been associated with human immunodeficiency virus, monoclonal gammopathies, celiac disease, and inflammatory bowel disease
- Skin findings involving predominantly over the extensor surfaces of joints with painful erythematous to purple plaques or nodules. Non-skin findings occasionally include panuveitis, fever, and fatigue.
- Diagnostic workup prior to referral to dermatology or rheumatology may include skin biopsy and laboratory workup based on risk factors/history.

MEDIUM VESSEL VASCULITIS

Medium vessel vasculitis occurs predominately in medium-sized and small arteries (i.e., visceral arteries and branches) and includes polyarteritis nodosa (PAN) and Kawasaki disease (KD).

Polyarteritis Nodosa

- PAN is a systemic vasculitis that predominantly affects older adults and has been associated with infections, predominantly hepatitis B. There is also a cutaneous PAN subvariant that is more common in children.
- Skin findings include painful subcutaneous nodules, bullae, livedo reticularis, retiform purpura, and necrotic ulcerations.
- Non-skin findings include arthralgias, fatigue, fever, weight loss, testicular pain, peripheral neuropathy, and abdominal pain.
- Patients suspected to have PAN should be referred for further evaluation and management.

Kawasaki Disease

KD, also called mucocutaneous lymph node syndrome, is a self-limiting febrile medium-to-small vessel vasculitis that occurs during the winter and early spring in the United States. KD predominantly affects males more than females (1.5:1) with an incidence of 210–265 and 4–25 cases per 100,000 children <5 years of age in those from Japan and United States, respectively (McCrindle et al., 2017; Vervoort, Donné, & Van Gysel, 2018).

While uncommon, KD is the leading cause of acquired coronary artery disease in children in developed countries with an incidence of 9% to 30%. Approximately 25% of untreated patients with KD develop cardiac abnormalities, while ~5% of children with KD will develop persistent coronary artery aneurysms. Untreated KD can result in KD shock syndrome, arrhythmias, ruptured coronary artery/aortic aneurysm or coronary artery thrombosis resulting in myocardial infarction or sudden death. The vasculitis primarily affects the aorta and main coronary arteries and can rarely lead to death (~0.1%) (McCrindle et al., 2017).

Pathogenesis

- The etiology is unclear, the current hypothesis suggests that a bacterial, viral, or other unidentified antigen elicits an immune response in genetically susceptible individuals (i.e., Japanese, Asian Americans) with subsequent necrotizing vasculitis of the aorta, coronary, or other medium-to-small arteries.

- The infectious hypothesis is further supported by the self-limited and rarely reoccurring nature of the disease process.

Clinical Presentation

The clinical diagnosis of KD is challenging as the clinical features (see Table 9.3-6) often are not all present at one-time point and may develop and abate across the course of the disease process. A thorough history and physical examination is warranted to determine resolution of clinical features of KD (Table 9.3-7).

- The disease course follows three phases:
  - Acute (0 to 14 days)
  - Subacute (2 to 4 weeks)
  - Convalescent (4 to 8 weeks)

TABLE 9.3-6 Clinical Criteria for the Diagnosis of Kawasaki Disease

Persistent fever ≥5 days and the presence of at least four of the following features[a]:
- Bilateral injection of the bulbar conjunctiva (nonexudative)
- Mucositis or changes in oral mucosal membranes and lips (strawberry tongue, hyperemic and fissured lips, injected pharynx)
- Polymorphous eruption
- Cervical lymphadenopathy >1.5 cm (usually obvious)
- Peripheral changes in extremities (erythema of soles, palms, and feet); periungual desquamation of the fingers and toes (usually after 2 wk)

[a]Experienced clinicians can make the diagnoses before 5 days or before day 4 if all five clinical features are present. See also Differential Diagnosis: Kawasaki Disease.
Adapted from McCrindle, B. W., Rowley, A. H., Newburger, J. W., Burns, J. C., Bolger, A. F., Gewitz, M., Baker, A. L., Jackson, M. A., Takahashi, M., Shah, P. B., Kobayashi, T., Wu, M. H., Saji, T. T., & Pahl, E.; American Heart Association Rheumatic Fever, Endocarditis, and Kawasaki Disease Committee of the Council on Cardiovascular Disease in the Young; Council on Cardiovascular and Stroke Nursing; Council on Cardiovascular Surgery and Anesthesia; and Council on Epidemiology and Prevention. (2017). Diagnosis, treatment, and long-term management of Kawasaki disease: A scientific statement for health professionals from the American Heart Association. *Circulation, 135*(17), e927–e999.

TABLE 9.3-7 Clinical Criteria for the Diagnosis of Incomplete Kawasaki Disease

Children with persistent fever ≥5 days *and* the presence of at least two of three of the clinical features or in infants when fever of unknown origin lasts ≥7 days without other explanation in addition to the following:
C-reactive protein ≥3 mg/dL or estimated sedimentation rate ≥40 mm/hr
Suggestive echocardiographic features (e.g., coronary aneurysm)

Or

Three or more of the following laboratory findings
- Anemia for age
- Platelets >450,000 after the 7th day of fever
- Albumin ≤3.0 g/dL
- Elevated ALT
- WBC ≥15,000/uL
- Urine ≥10 WBC/high-power field

Adapted from McCrindle, B. W., Rowley, A. H., Newburger, J. W., Burns, J. C., Bolger, A. F., Gewitz, M., Baker, A. L., Jackson, M. A., Takahashi, M., Shah, P. B., Kobayashi, T., Wu, M. H., Saji, T. T., & Pahl, E.; American Heart Association Rheumatic Fever, Endocarditis, and Kawasaki Disease Committee of the Council on Cardiovascular Disease in the Young; Council on Cardiovascular and Stroke Nursing; Council on Cardiovascular Surgery and Anesthesia; and Council on Epidemiology and Prevention. (2017). Diagnosis, treatment, and long-term management of Kawasaki disease: A scientific statement for health professionals from the American Heart Association. *Circulation, 135*(17), e927–e999.

Skin Findings

- Changes in the oral cavity and lips include erythematous tongue with accentuation of fungiform papillae (Strawberry tongue) (Fig. 9.3-12A); bleeding, cracking, erythema, peeling, and fissuring of lips; diffuse erythema of oropharyngeal mucosa.

- Palms and soles are erythematous and edematous during the acute phase. During the subacute phase, patients will have periungual finger and toe desquamation (Fig. 9.3-13).

- The rash favors the trunk and extremities with accentuation of the perineal area (Fig. 9.3-12C).

- The morphology noted includes erythematous macules/papules, sand paper–like erythematous papules on an erythematous base (scarlatiniform), erythematous targetoid (three zones of color) macules or papules (erythema multiforme like), urticarial, micropustular, and scaly erythematous papules/plaques.

- Nail changes include white discoloration of nail presenting as transverse lines, punctate spots, or involving half the nail often during the acute phase (Leukonychia), deep transverse grooves during the convalescent stage (Beau lines), and separation of nail from proximal nail fold during the convalescent stage (onychomadesis).

Non-Skin Findings

- Prodromal symptoms may include abdominal pain, nausea, vomiting, diarrhea, inconsolable irritability, cough, rhinorrhea, and arthralgias.

- Children often appear very ill (toxic) with fevers (>39°C) lasting on ~1 to 3 weeks and is unresponsive to antipyretics. Resolution of fever after 7 days does not exclude KD.

- Bilateral nonexudative bulbar conjunctivitis shortly after fever onset (80% to 90%)

- Unilateral lymphadenopathy typically involving multiple >1.5-cm lymph nodes in the anterior cervical chain (50% to 60%) (Fig. 9.3-12B).

- Cardiac flow murmurs and gallop rhythm.

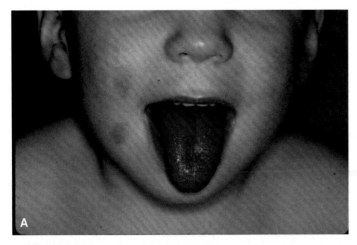

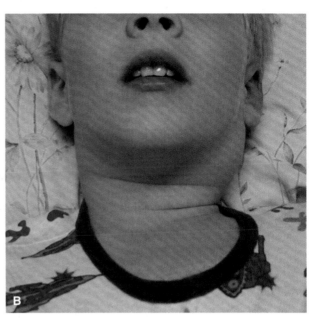

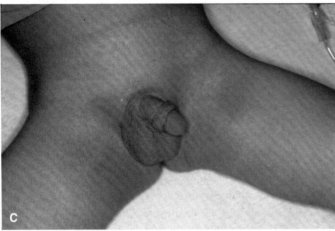

FIG. 9.3-12. Kawasaki disease. **A:** Strawberry tongue. **B:** Unilateral lymphade-nopathy. **C:** Skin eruption favoring perineal area. (Used with permission from Gru, A. A., & Wick, M. [2018]. *Pediatric dermatopathology and dermatology.* Wolters Kluwer.)

- Infants <6 months old with KD may only present with prolonged fever and irritability.
- Ten percent of children who develop coronary artery aneurysms do not meet the outlined criteria for KD.

Confirming the Diagnosis

The diagnosis can be very easy to miss. Laboratory studies are not diagnostic of KD but are important in supporting the diagnosis.

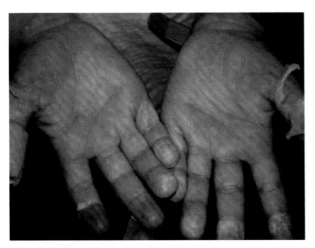

FIG. 9.3-13. Periungual desquamation during the convalescent phase of Kawasaki disease. (Fleisher, G. R., Ludwig, W., & Baskin, M. N. [2004]. *Atlas of pediatric emergency medicine.* Wolters Kluwer Health I Lippincott Williams & Wilkins.)

Please see Tables 9.3-6 and 9.3-7 for American Heart Association guidelines on the diagnosis of Kawasaki and incomplete Kawasaki disease.

The following labs should be ordered when considering the diagnosis of KD:

- CBC with differential
- Complete metabolic panel
- ESR and/or CRP
- Urinalysis with microscopy
- Echocardiography. Coronary artery dilation per echocardiography is not usually identified >1 week

DIFFERENTIAL DIAGNOSIS   Kawasaki Disease

- Viral exanthems (measles, adenovirus, etc.)
- Exudative conjunctivitis or pharyngitis
- Scarlet fever
- Staph scalded skin syndrome
- Toxic shock syndrome
- Rocky Mountain spotted fever
- Stephens–Johnson syndrome
- Serum sickness
- Mercury hypersensitivity
- Juvenile arthritis

Treatment

The initial goal of therapy is to decrease systemic inflammation, reduce/abate arterial damage, and prevent arterial thrombosis. The current American Heart Association KD guidelines recommend:

- Treatment within 10 days of onset of fever *or*
- >10 days after onset of fever in the presence of persistent fever and/or elevated CRP or ESR.

Systemic

- Moderate- to high-dose aspirin.
- Single dose of intravenous immunoglobulins (IVIG).
- Other therapies include high-dose pulse methylprednisolone, corticosteroid taper, infliximab, or cyclophosphamide.

Management and Patient Education

- Patients with KD often require multidisciplinary (e.g., cardiology, rheumatology, dermatology) management in a tertiary care setting (i.e., hospital).
- Although KD is rare and self-limiting, recognition of the clinical presentation is important to avoid cardiac sequelae. Patients should be referred promptly for treatment.
- Reoccurrence of KD is rare with an estimated incidence of 1.7%, but may be associated with increased risk of coronary artery disease.
- Late diagnosis may be accompanied by cardiac abnormalities (pericardial effusion, tachycardia, murmur, arrhythmias, etc.), CNS involvement, lethargy, gastrointestinal symptoms (including hepatic involvement), and long-term cardiac sequelae.
- Patients may be on thromboprophylaxis for 4 to 6 weeks post-acute episode and may be on long-term thromboprophylaxis if coronary dilation is persistent.
- To support continued normal physical and psychosocial development of children and adolescents, exercise guidelines for patients with congenital heart disease can be adapted for KD in the context of arrhythmia, risk of myocardial ischemia, and bleeding associated with thrombocytopenia. Collaborate with pediatric cardiology in establishing an appropriate exercise regimen.
- Patients with history of KD with coronary artery disease of childbearing potential should be referred for reproductive counseling regarding appropriate contraception and pregnancy risk. When contraception is required, the selection of low estrogen or progesterone would be preferred. When in doubt, consultation with OB/GYN is necessary. For those contemplating pregnancy should be referred to high-risk obstetrics for counseling and management.
- Counsel parents that KD has not been shown to have detrimental effects on cognitive or academic performance.
- Immunization guidelines post-IVIG are as follows:
  - Avoid Measles, Mumps, and Rubella vaccinations for up to 11 months after receiving high-dose IVIG infusion.
  - Alternatively, if the child is at high risk for exposure, a Measles, Mumps, and Rubella vaccination should be given and then the child should be revaccinated at 11 months after IVIG administration.

LARGE VESSEL VASCULITIS

Large vessel vasculitis involving the aorta and large arteries means that affected patients have systemic involvement and appear much sicker. Ulcerations and sometimes gangrenous digits are seen with large vessel involvement.

Giant Cell Arteritis (GCA)

- GCA is a large and medium vessel vasculitis that predominantly occurs in those >50 years old and primarily affects the aorta, temporal artery, or cranial arteries. GCA is frequently associated with polymyalgia rheumatic.
- Skin findings may include palpable purpura, painful subcutaneous nodules, retiform purpura, erythema nodosum, and necrosis.
- Non-skin findings include temporal artery tenderness and enlargement, frequently absent temporal pulse, visual loss, headache, and jaw claudication.
- Patients suspected to have GCA should be referred emergently to a tertiary care center for multidisciplinary management.

Takayasu Arteritis

- Takayasu arteritis is a large and medium vessel vasculitis that predominantly affects young adult females with Asian ancestry.
- Skin findings include palpable ulcerated purpuric papules or plaques, painful subcutaneous nodules, targetoid papules or plaques, and Raynaud phenomenon.
- Non-skin findings include blood pressure >10 mm Hg between arms, extremity claudication, decreased brachial pulse, subclavian/aorta bruit, hypertension, headache.
- Patients should be referred to rheumatology for further evaluation and management.

VARIABLE VESSEL VASCULITIS

The final category of vasculitis is variable vessel vasculitis and is characterized by effecting vessels of all sizes including the aorta, aortic/mitral valves, arteries, arterioles, capillaries, postcapillary venules, and veins. The two conditions associated with variable vessel vasculitis are Behçet disease and Cogan syndrome, and are considered rare.

PIGMENTED PURPURIC DERMATOSIS

Pigmented purpuric dermatoses (PPD), also known as capillaritis, are a collection of chronic benign skin conditions. Schamberg disease is the most common PPD and tends to occur in middle–older aged adults with no gender predilection.

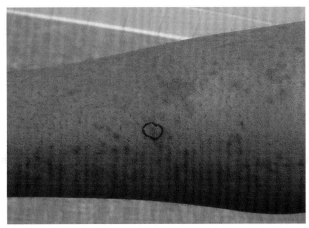

FIG. 9.3-14. Schamberg purpura; cayenne pepper spots on lower leg. (Photo courtesy of M. Bobonich.)

Pathophysiology

- The etiology of PPD is unclear. Current evidence suggests that there is dilation and fragility of capillaries secondary to a combination of increased orthostatic pressure, humoral, and lymphocyte-driven inflammation (Coulombe et al., 2015).
- Numerous cofactors have been reported including infections, medications, gravitational dependency, venous hypertension, and exercise (Kim et al., 2015).
- Potential medications implicated in PPD include acetaminophen, nonsteroidal anti-inflammatory medications, thiazide diuretics, statins, beta blockers, glipizide, interferon-alpha, and injection medroxyprogesterone.

Clinical Presentation

While there are six subvariants of PPD, Schamberg disease is the most common presentation.

Skin Findings

- Nonblanchable red-brown pinpoint "cayenne pepper" macules and patches that coalesce into pink-yellow, brown-yellow, or orange-brown patches (Fig. 9.3-14).
- Commonly occurs below the knees but could occur anywhere on the body.

Non-Skin Finding

- Lower extremity edema

DIFFERENTIAL DIAGNOSIS	Pigmented Purpuric Dermatoses

- Postinflammatory hyperpigmentation
- Venous stasis dermatitis (hemosiderin staining)
- Thrombocytopenic purpura
- Drug-induced purpura
- Hypergammaglobulinemic purpura
- Fixed drug eruption
- Lichen planus
- Contact dermatitis
- Nummular eczema
- Leukocytoclastic vasculitis

Confirming the Diagnosis

Clinical presentation is usually diagnostic, but further diagnostic tests should be considered if:

- The clinical presentation does not match traditional clinical presentation.
- The review of systems is suggestive of an underlying condition (e.g., connective tissues disease).
- There is suspicion regarding an underlying thrombocytopenia/coagulation defect.

Additional diagnostic tests to consider include:

- Skin biopsy for histopathology
- CBC with differential
- PTT/PT
- Antinuclear antibody
- Rheumatoid factor

Treatment

There are no topical or systemic agents that have demonstrated clinical superiority in the management of PPD.

Topical

- Daily application of 20 to 30 compression therapy stockings in patients with concomitant venous insufficiency. For patients without palpable pulses, an ankle brachial index diagnostic should be performed. For ankle brachial index <0.9, refer to vascular specialist for management.
- Midpotency topical (e.g., triamcinolone, mometasone) corticosteroids therapy trial with taper over 4 weeks for pruritus and extensive erythema. If no improvement by 4 weeks, discontinue therapy.
- Topical calcineurin inhibitors (tacrolimus) b.i.d.
- For narrowband ultraviolet B therapy, refer to dermatology.

Systemic

- Pentoxifylline 400 mg three times daily for 2 to 3 weeks.
- Griseofulvin 500 to 750 mg daily.
- Oral rutoside 50 mg twice daily and vitamin C 1,000 mg once daily.

Management and Patient Education

PPD follows a benign chronic course that may resolve over a period of months to years. While the erythema may resolve, the hyperpigmentation often persists.

Special Considerations

- Pediatric PPD
  - Pediatric PPD follows an indolent course with spontaneous resolution from 6 months to 9 years.
  - PPD is an idiopathic phenomenon in children with a lack of evidence showing a connection with disease conditions, infections, or medications.
  - Topical corticosteroids and narrowband ultraviolet B have both shown modest efficacy for pediatric PPD.

ACKNOWLEDGMENT

Jeremy Honaker would like to thank the previous author Cathleen Case. Many of the figures, tables, and photographs have been edited or reused from the previous edition.

READINGS AND REFERENCES

Arora, A., Wetter, D. A., Gonzalez-Santiago, T. M., Davis, M. D. P., & Lohse, C. M. (2014). Incidence of leukocytoclastic vasculitis, 1996 to 2010: A population-based study in Olmsted County, Minnesota. *Mayo Clinic Proceedings*, *89*(11), 1515–1524. https://doi.org/10.1016/j.mayocp.2014.04.015

Audemard-Verger, A., Pillebout, E., Guillevin, L., Thervet, E., & Terrier, B. (2015). IgA vasculitis (Henoch-Shönlein purpura) in adults: Diagnostic and therapeutic aspects. *Autoimmunity Reviews*, *14*(7), 579–585. https://doi.org/10.1016/j.autrev.2015.02.003

Corral-Gudino, L., González-Vázquez, E., Calero-Paniagua, I., Pérez-Garrido, L., Cusacovich, I., Rivas-Lamazares, A., Quesada-Moreno, A., González-Fernández, A., Mora-Peña, D., Lerma-Márquez, J. L., & Del-Pino-Montes, J. (2020). The complexity of classifying ANCA-associated small-vessel vasculitis in actual clinical practice: Data from a multicenter retrospective survey. *Rheumatology International*, *40*(2), 303–311. https://doi.org/10.1007/s00296-019-04406-5

Coulombe, J., Jean, S. E., Hatami, A., Powell, J., Marcoux, D., Kokta, V., & McCuaig, C. (2015). Pigmented purpuric dermatosis: Clinicopathologic characterization in a pediatric series. *Pediatric Dermatology*, *32*(3), 358–362. https://doi.org/10.1111/pde.12519

Da Dalt, L., Zerbinati, C., Strafella, M. S., Renna, S., Riceputi, L., Di Pietro, P., Barabino, P., Scanferla, S., Raucci, U., Mores, N., Compagnone, A., Da Cas, R., Menniti-Ippolito, F., & Italian Multicenter Study Group for Drug and Vaccine Safety in Children. (2016). Henoch-Schönlein purpura and drug and vaccine use in childhood: A case-control study. *Italian Journal of Pediatrics*, *42*(1), 60. https://doi.org/10.1186/s13052-016-0267-2

Geetha, D., & Jefferson, J. A. (2020). ANCA-Associated Vasculitis: Core Curriculum 2020. *American Journal of Kidney Diseases*, *75*(1), 124–137. https://doi.org/10.1053/j.ajkd.2019.04.031

Georgesen, C., Fox, L. P., & Harp, J. (2020a). Retiform purpura: A diagnostic approach. *Journal of the American Academy of Dermatology*, *82*(4), 783–796. https://doi.org/10.1016/j.jaad.2019.07.112

Georgesen, C., Fox, L. P., & Harp, J. (2020b). Retiform purpura: Workup and therapeutic considerations in select conditions. *Journal of the American Academy of Dermatology*, *82*(4), 799–816. https://doi.org/10.1016/j.jaad.2019.07.113

Goeser, M. R., Laniosz, V., & Wetter, D. A. (2014). A practical approach to the diagnosis, evaluation, and management of cutaneous small-vessel vasculitis. *American Journal of Clinical Dermatology*, *15*(4), 299–306. https://doi.org/10.1007/s40257-014-0076-6

Grau, R. G. (2015). Drug-induced vasculitis: New insights and a changing lineup of suspects. *Current Rheumatology Reports*, *17*(12), 71. https://doi.org/10.1007/s11926-015-0545-9

Hamad, A., Jithpratuck, W., & Krishnaswamy, G. (2017). Urticarial vasculitis and associated disorders. *Annals of Allergy, Asthma & Immunology*, *118*(4), 394–398. https://doi.org/10.1016/j.anai.2017.01.017

Harrison, L. B., Nash, M. J., Fitzmaurice, D., & Thachil, J. (2017). Investigating easy bruising in an adult. *BMJ*, *356*, j251. https://doi.org/10.1136/bmj.j251

Jauhola, O., Ronkainen, J., Koskimies, O., Ala-Houhala, M., Arikoski, P., Holtta, T., Jahnukainen, T., Rajantie, J., Ormala, T., Turtinen, J., & Nuutinen, M. (2010). Renal manifestations of Henoch-Schonlein purpura in a 6-month prospective study of 223 children. *Archives of Disease in Childhood*, *95*(11), 877–882. https://doi.org/10.1136/adc.2009.182394

Jennette, J. C., Falk, R. J., Bacon, P. A., Basu, N., Cid, M. C., Ferrario, F., Flores-Suarez, L. F., Gross, W. L., Guillevin, L., Hagen, E. C., Hoffman, G. S., Jayne, D. R., Kallenberg, C. G. M., Lamprecht, P., Langford, C. A., Luqmani, R. A., Mahr, A. D., Matteson, E. L., Merkel, P. A., … Watts, R. A. (2013). 2012 revised International Chapel Hill Consensus Conference Nomenclature of Vasculitides. *Arthritis and Rheumatism*, *65*(1), 1–11. https://doi.org/10.1002/art.37715

Kim, D. H., Seo, S. H., Ahn, H. H., Kye, Y. C., & Choi, J. E. (2015). Characteristics and clinical manifestations of pigmented purpuric dermatosis. *Annals of Dermatology*, *27*(4), 404–410. https://doi.org/10.5021/ad.2015.27.4.404

Marzano, A. V., Raimondo, M. G., Berti, E., Meroni, P. L., & Ingegnoli, F. (2017). Cutaneous manifestations of ANCA-associated small vessels vasculitis. *Clinical Reviews in Allergy & Immunology*, *53*(3), 428–438. https://doi.org/10.1007/s12016-017-8616-5

McCrindle, B. W., Rowley, A. H., Newburger, J. W., Burns, J. C., Bolger, A. F., Gewitz, M., Baker, A. L., Jackson, M. A., Takahashi, M., Shah, P. B., Kobayashi, T., Wu, M. H., Saji, T. T., Pahl, E., & American Heart Association Rheumatic Fever, Endocarditis, and Kawasaki Disease Committee of the Council on Cardiovascular Disease in the Young; Council on Cardiovascular and Stroke Nursing; Council on Cardiovascular Surgery and Anesthesia; and Council on Epidemiology and Prevention. (2017). Diagnosis, treatment, and long-term management of Kawasaki Disease: A scientific statement for health professionals from the American Heart Association. *Circulation*, *135*(17), e927–e999. https://doi.org/10.1161/CIR.0000000000000484

Micheletti, R. G., & Werth, V. P. (2015). Small vessel vasculitis of the skin. *Rheumatic Diseases Clinics of North America*, *41*(1), 21–32, vii. https://doi.org/10.1016/j.rdc.2014.09.006

Momen, S. E., Jorizzo, J., & Al-Niaimi, F. (2014). Erythema elevatum diutinum: a review of presentation and treatment. *Journal of the European Academy of Dermatology and Venereology*, *28*(12), 1594–1602. https://doi.org/10.1111/jdv.12566

Nagata, S. (2019). Causes of Kawasaki Disease-from past to present. *Frontiers in Pediatrics*, *7*, 18. https://doi.org/10.3389/fped.2019.00018

Neutze, D., & Roque, J. (2016). Clinical evaluation of bleeding and bruising in primary Care. *American Family Physician*, *93*(4), 279–286.

Oni, L., & Sampath, S. (2019). Childhood IgA vasculitis (Henoch Schonlein Purpura)-advances and knowledge gaps. *Frontiers in Pediatrics*, *7*, 257. https://doi.org/10.3389/fped.2019.00257

Ozen, S. (2017). The changing face of polyarteritis nodosa and necrotizing vasculitis. *Nature Reviews Rheumatology*, *13*(6), 381–386. https://doi.org/10.1038/nrrheum.2017.68

Ozen, S., Marks, S. D., Brogan, P., Groot, N., de Graeff, N., Avcin, T., Bader-Meunier, B., Dolezalova, P., Feldman, B. M., Kone-Paut, I., Lahdenne, P., McCann, L., Pilkington, C., Ravelli, A., van Royen, A., Uziel, Y., Vastert, B., Wulffraat, N., Kamphuis, S., & Beresford, M. W. (2019). European consensus-based recommendations for diagnosis and treatment of immunoglobulin A vasculitis-the SHARE initiative. *Rheumatology* , *58*(9), 1607–1616. https://doi.org/10.1093/rheumatology/kez041

Piette, W. W. (1994). The differential diagnosis of purpura from a morphologic perspective. *Advances in Dermatology*, *9*, 3–23; discussion 24.

Piram, M., & Mahr, A. (2013). Epidemiology of immunoglobulin A vasculitis (Henoch-Schönlein): Current state of knowledge. *Current Opinion in Rheumatology*, *25*(2), 171–178. https://doi.org/10.1097/BOR.0b013e32835d8e2a

Piram, M., Gonzalez Chiappe, S., Madhi, F., Ulinski, T., & Mahr, A. (2018). Vaccination and risk of childhood IgA vasculitis. *Pediatrics*, *142*(5), e20180841. https://doi.org/10.1542/peds.2018-0841

Podjasek, J. O., Wetter, D. A., Pittelkow, M. R., & Wada, D. A. (2012). Cutaneous small-vessel vasculitis associated with solid organ malignancies: The Mayo Clinic experience, 1996 to 2009. *Journal of the American Academy of Dermatology*, *66*(2), e55–65. https://doi.org/10.1016/j.jaad.2010.09.732

Robson, J., Doll, H., Suppiah, R., Flossmann, O., Harper, L., Höglund, P., Jayne, D., Mahr, A., Westman, K., & Luqmani, R. (2015). Damage in the anca-associated vasculitides: Long-term data from the European Vasculitis Study group (EUVAS) therapeutic trials. *Annals of the Rheumatic Diseases*, *74*(1), 177–184. https://doi.org/10.1136/annrheumdis-2013-203927

Ronkainen, J., Nuutinen, M., & Koskimies, O. (2002). The adult kidney 24 years after childhood Henoch-Schönlein purpura: A retrospective cohort study. *Lancet*, *360*(9334), 666–670. https://doi.org/10.1016/S0140-6736(02)09835-5

Silva, F., Pinto, C., Barbosa, A., Borges, T., Dias, C., & Almeida, J. (2019). New insights in cryoglobulinemic vasculitis. *Journal of Autoimmunity*, *105*, 102313. https://doi.org/10.1016/j.jaut.2019.102313

Sunderkötter, C. H., Zelger, B., Chen, K.-R., Requena, L., Piette, W., Carlson, J. A., Dutz, J., Lamprecht, P., Mahr, A., Aberer, E., Werth, V. P., Wetter, D. A., Kawana, S., Luqmani, R., Frances, C., Jorizzo, J., Watts, J. R., Metze, D., Caproni, M., … Jennette, J. C. (2018). Nomenclature of cutaneous vasculitis: Dermatologic addendum to the 2012 revised international chapel hill consensus conference nomenclature of vasculitides. *Arthritis & Rheumatology*, *70*(2), 171–184. https://doi.org/10.1002/art.40375

ten Holder, S. M., Joy, M. S., & Falk, R. J. (2002). Cutaneous and systemic manifestations of drug-induced vasculitis. *The Annals of Pharmacotherapy*, *36*(1), 130–147. https://doi.org/10.1345/aph.1A124

Vervoort, D., Donné, M., & Van Gysel, D. (2018). Pitfalls in the diagnosis and management of Kawasaki disease: An update for the pediatric dermatologist. *Pediatric Dermatology*, *35*(6), 743–747.

White Lesions

Katie B. O'Brien

In This Chapter

- Biology of Pigmentation
- Disorders of Pigment Loss
- Pityriasis Alba
- Idiopathic Guttate Hypomelanosis

- Progressive Macular Hypomelanosis
- Tinea Versicolor
- Vitiligo
- Lichen Sclerosis

The presence of color plays a significant role throughout our lives as we learn to recognize objects and conditions. In childhood we learn that blood is red and the sky is blue. So it is also true that in dermatology, color can be a very helpful clue to diagnosis. This section is designed to help one consider certain disorders when specific colors are manifest and assist in ruling in or ruling out a diagnosis. Clinicians must also appreciate that the presence or the absence of color does not always reflect the presence or absence of pigment. In this section, we will present common dermatoses and neoplasms grouped according to color and we will begin with a discussion of pigmentation.

The presence of pigmentation in the skin is largely determined by genetic makeup. Skin type is related to the amount of melanin that is produced by an individual. A general understanding of the process of melanin synthesis is essential to understanding the conditions of dyspigmentation. Disturbances in the process of pigment production can yield significant alterations in one's appearance. Cosmetic and physiologic changes may occur as a result of genetic, environmental, and even pharmacologic influences. The sun alone can play a major role, not only in the overproduction of pigmentation which is seen in normal tanning, but as a predisposing factor in the development of skin cancer. We will review the biology and function of melanocytes, the role of melanosomes in the production of the melanin, and the common types of dyspigmentation which can result when this normal process is interrupted.

BIOLOGY OF PIGMENTATION

Melanocytes are derived from the neural crest and migrate to the epidermis, hair follicles, uveal tract of the eye (choroid, ciliary body, and iris), the leptomeninges, and the inner ear (cochlea). They contain the melanin-producing cells called melanosomes, where, under genetic influence, and with the aid of the enzyme tyrosinase, melanin is synthesized. There are two types of melanin: eumelanin (brown/black) and pheomelanin (yellow-red). The melanocyte resides in the basal layer of the epidermis and via its dendritic processes attaches to the keratinocytes and deposits the melanin-containing melanosome. A person's skin color is determined by the size and number of these melanosomes, the amount of melanin they produce, and their distribution within the epidermis.

DISORDERS OF PIGMENT LOSS

Hypopigmentation and depigmentation can occur if there is a loss of melanocytes, an inability of melanocytes to produce melanin, or an inability to transport melanin correctly. The term hypopigmentation refers to a partial loss of melanocytes, while depigmentation refers to a total loss of melanocytes. Patients with large body surface areas (BSAs) of pigment abnormality may be challenging for the clinician to identify their normal skin color.

Pityriasis Alba

Pityriasis alba is a common dermatosis in which patients present with ill-defined patches of hypopigmentation. It is most commonly seen in children and adolescents who have a history of atopy. Males and females are affected equally. It is more cosmetically distressing for those with darkly pigmented skin.

Pathophysiology

- The exact etiology of pityriasis alba is unknown but the cause of this hypopigmentation has been classified as postinflammatory and often seems to appear after a flare of eczema or atopic dermatitis.
- The hypopigmentation resolves spontaneously, usually before young adulthood.
- Histopathology reveals a reduction in the number of melanocytes.

Clinical Presentation

- This condition is asymptomatic.
- Small slightly elevated hypopigmented, ill-defined patches are most commonly distributed on the cheeks but may also appear on the proximal upper and lower extremities.
- In early stages, lesions may be mildly erythematous, then become hypopigmented and scaly.
- The lesions are more apparent on skin that has become tanned, creating an even greater contrast next to the hypopigmented patches (Fig. 10.1-1A,B).

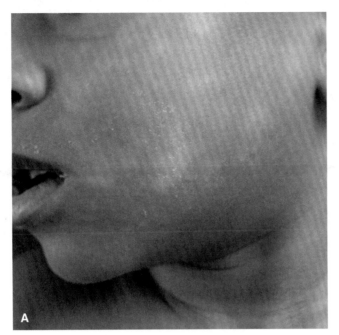
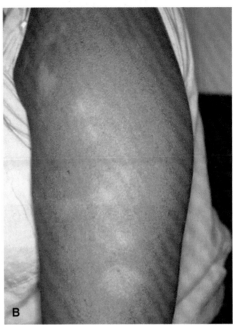

FIG. 10.1-1. A: Pityriasis alba on the face. Pityriasis alba. Hypopigmented patches with fine overlying scale and minimal erythema. (Used with permission from Gru, A. A. [2018]. *Pediatric dermatopathology and dermatology.* Wolters Kluwer Health.) **B:** Pityriasis alba on arm. (Photo courtesy of M. Bobonich.)

DIFFERENTIAL DIAGNOSIS   Pityriasis Alba

- Vitiligo
- Chemical leukoderma
- Tinea versicolor
- Eczematous dermatitis

Confirming the Diagnosis

- A negative KOH prep can differentiate pityriasis alba from tinea versicolor or other fungal infections.
- Wood light examination does not demonstrate or accentuate the white spots as it would in vitiligo.

Treatment

- Mild topical corticosteroids or topical immunomodulators may be helpful, as they can reduce subtle inflammation allowing repigmentation to occur.
- Phototherapy has not shown an improvement in pigmentation.
- Emollients should be encouraged one to two times a day.

Management and Patient Education

- Refer to dermatology if the pityriasis alba fails to resolve spontaneously, spreads despite treatment, or if the patient's atopic dermatitis is poorly controlled.
- It is important to listen to the patients' concerns, be empathetic, and reassure them that the hypopigmentation will resolve.
- Sun protection should be encouraged, as tanning may make hypopigmentation more noticeable.
- If they are being treated with topical corticosteroids, the side effects and risks should be discussed, and the duration of use limited.

Idiopathic Guttate Hypomelanosis

Idiopathic guttate hypomelanosis (IGH) is a common dermatosis of unknown etiology. It consists of photodistributed, hypopigmented macules on the upper and lower extremities. It affects 50% to 70% of people over the age of 50 and 80% of patients over the age of 70. It seems to be more common in females, perhaps because females seek medical attention for this more frequently than men.

Pathophysiology

- IGH is thought to be a result of actinic damage, as patients exhibit signs of photoaging in the same locations.
- Others propose that it is simply a degenerative sign of aging.
- Histopathology shows a loss of melanocytes in the skin, but not a complete absence. Some melanocytes function normally, while others do not.

Clinical Presentation

- Patients usually present with IGH out of cosmetic concern.
- There are well-demarcated 2- to 5-mm, hypopigmented macules distributed on the sun-exposed (extensor) surfaces of the upper and lower extremities.
- Lentigines (light brown macules) and xeroses are usually present.
- Once these hypopigmented macules present, they do not usually become larger and are permanent (Fig. 10.1-2).

DIFFERENTIAL DIAGNOSIS   Idiopathic Guttate Hypomelanosis

- Pityriasis alba
- Vitiligo
- Tinea versicolor
- Flat warts

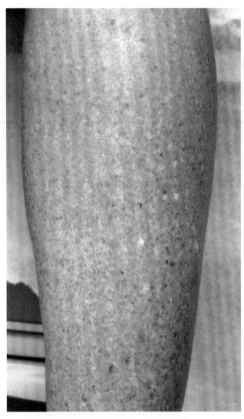

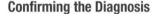

FIG. 10.1-2. Idiopathic guttate hypomelanosis.

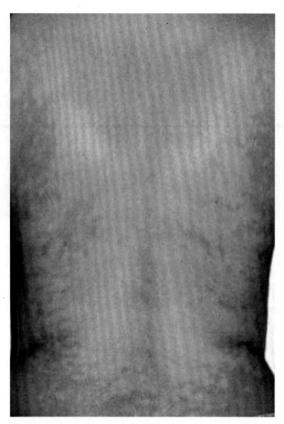

FIG. 10.1-3. Progressive macular hypomelanosis. (Photo courtesy of M. Bobonich.)

Confirming the Diagnosis

- IGH is usually a clinical diagnosis.

- A biopsy is not usually needed, but may confirm incomplete loss of melanocytes and melanin.

- A KOH prep may be done if tinea versicolor is suspected but will be negative in IGH.

Management and Patient Education

- Patients should be aware of the risk of leukoderma or postinflammatory hyperpigmentation (PIH) after treatment with cryotherapy.

- Tinted makeup, such as Dermablend or Covermark, can be used to cover hypopigmented macules.

- Self-tanners are not helpful as the macules do not absorb the topical product.

- Patients should be reassured that treatment is not medically necessary as it is a benign condition.

- Patients should be counseled on sun protection.

- Regular skin cancer screening should be performed on these patients.

Progressive Macular Hypomelanosis

Progressive macular hypomelanosis (PMH) is a common disorder of pigmentation resulting in areas of hypopigmentation. It is a benign and asymptomatic eruption which occurs primarily in women ages 13 to 38 and typically lasts for years. It does not seem to be preceded by infection, inflammation, or trauma but is more common in darker skin types.

Pathophysiology

It is suggested that the dyspigmentation is caused by the bacteria that people associate with acne namely *Cutibacterium acnes* (formerly known as *Propionibacterium acnes*). It is thought that the bacteria produce a substance which interferes with melanogenesis.

Clinical Presentation

- Macules and coalescing patches of hypopigmentation (Fig. 10.1-3).

- Lesions are ill defined, symmetric, and without scale.

- Primarily affects the trunk, lumbar, and abdominal areas.

- Rarely affects proximal upper extremities and neck.

DIFFERENTIAL DIAGNOSIS	Progressive Macular Hypomelanosis
• Tinea versicolor	• IGH
• Postinflammatory hypopigmentation	• Vitiligo
• Pityriasis alba	• Sarcoidosis

Confirming the Diagnosis

- Wood light examination reveals a classic follicular red fluorescence.

- Negative KOH.

- Absence of pruritus or inflammation.

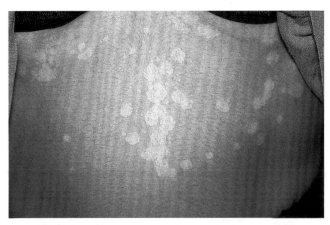

FIG. 10.1-4. Tinea versicolor. This patient has hypopigmented lesions. Note the similarity to vitiligo. (Used with permission from Goodheart, H., & Gonzalez, M. [2015]. *Goodheart's photoguide to common pediatric and adult skin disorders* [4th ed.]. Wolters Kluwer Health.)

Treatment

- Topical antibacterial wash daily, such as benzoyl peroxide.
- Topical clindamycin can also be used in combination.
- Narrowband ultraviolet B (NBUVB) phototherapy two to three times per week × 1 month.
- Isotretinoin orally has been used with mixed results (Damevska et al., 2017; Kim et al., 2012).

Management and Patient Education

- Patients can be reassured the condition is not contagious and often resolves spontaneously in 3 to 5 years.
- Even with treatment, this eruption may recur.
- Treatments are strictly cosmetic.

Tinea Versicolor

This is a superficial fungal infection which usually occurs on the trunk and presents as both hypopigmentation and hyperpigmentation (Fig. 10.1-4). You will likely see pink to light brown patches with powdery scale in discrete patches or coalescing macules.

See Section 6.1 for details.

Vitiligo

Vitiligo is an unpredictable disease of depigmentation. It affects males and females equally, and is present in all ethnicies. The prevalence of vitiligo is estimated to be 0.5% to 2% of the world's population, with 50% of all cases occurring before the age of 20 years. Thirty percent of patients with vitiligo have other family members with the disease. Some people attribute the initial onset to emotional stress, illness, or skin trauma such as sunburn.

Pathophysiology

- The mechanism of depigmentation in vitiligo is not well understood. It is thought that there is an absence of functional melanocytes caused by both genetic and nongenetic factors.
- In addition to the belief that vitiligo is hereditary, it is theorized that specific autoantibodies are directed against tyrosinase, the enzyme that converts tyrosine into melanin, resulting in pigment loss.

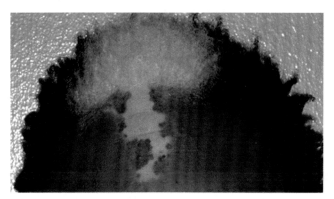

FIG. 10.1-5. Poliosis. A localized loss of pigment in the hair and skin on a 17-year-old male with a white forelock and leukoderma of the forehead. (Used with permission from Gru, A. A. [2018]. *Pediatric dermatopathology and dermatology.* Wolters Kluwer Health.)

- Others suggest that vitiligo is caused by an intrinsic defect in the structure and function of melanocytes or that there is a defective free-radical defense, which results in the destruction of melanocytes, leading to depigmentation.

Clinical Presentation

- Patients present with well-demarcated, depigmented macules or patches surrounded by normal skin.
- The onset of lesions is insidious which expand centrifugally into irregularly shaped patches that rarely have inflamed borders.
- Hair follicles present in the depigmented patch are usually white.
- When scalp area is involved, it usually presents as a solitary patch called *poliosis* or *white forelock* (Fig. 10.1-5). The eyebrows and eyelashes may also be affected.
- There may also be focal blue-gray hyperpigmented macules on the skin representing melanin incontinence.
- Clinically, vitiligo can be classified into two different types: generalized and localized.

  Generalized vitiligo is the most common type, accounting for 90% of all cases. It is usually symmetrically distributed on the face, upper chest, dorsal hands, axillae, and groin (Fig. 10.1-6A). It has a predilection for orifices, including the eyes, nostrils, mouth, nipples, umbilicus, and anogenital areas. Sites of trauma are commonly affected. *Areas of vitiligo may present with various shades of pigmentation* (Fig. 10.1-7). This classification also includes *Universal* vitiligo where the entire skin surface is depigmented, *Mixed* type which combines segmental and generalized, and *Acrofacial vitiligo* which affects facial orifices and/or distal fingers and toes (think "lips and tips"). *Localized* vitiligo may affect one nondermatomal site, or asymmetrically affect one region (e.g., an extremity). Examples of localized vitiligo are *segmental vitiligo* (Fig. 10.1-8A,B) which is often dermatomally distributed, seen more often in younger patients, and is less likely to be related to autoimmune disease and *mucosal vitiligo,* as its name clearly states, which affects the mucous membranes alone, and is commonly seen on the lips, genital, and perianal areas (Fig. 10.1-9).

- *Inflammatory vitiligo* is uncommon and presents with "raised inflammatory borders" (Fig. 10.1-10). It can be present in any type (Bolognia et al., 2017).

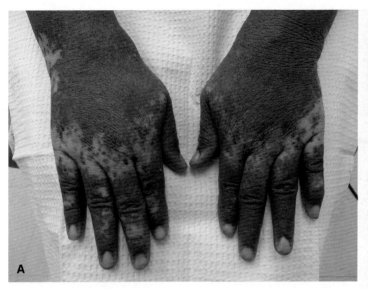

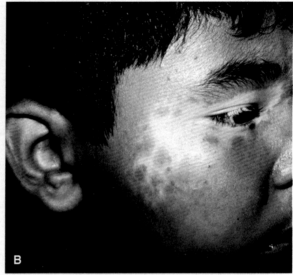

FIG. 10.1-6. **A, B:** Vitiligo hands. Well-demarcated, depigmented, coalescing symmetric patches on the hands. (**A:** Photo courtesy of M. Bobonich; **B:** Used with permission from Goodheart, H. P. [2003]. *Goodheart's photoguide of common skin disorders* [2nd ed.]. Lippincott Williams & Wilkins.)

DIFFERENTIAL DIAGNOSIS   Vitiligo

- Chemical leukoderma
- Leukoderma associated with melanoma
- Postinflammatory depigmentation
- Tinea versicolor
- Morphea
- Lichen sclerosus
- Pityriasis alba

Confirming the Diagnosis

- The diagnosis of vitiligo is usually made based on clinical findings.
- Laboratory studies should include CBC, TSH, T_3, T_4, glycosylated hemoglobin, thyroid antibodies (antithyroglobulin and antithyroid peroxidase antibodies), and antinuclear antibody (ANA) screening to rule out systemic disease associated with pigment loss.
- A skin biopsy will show an absence of melanocytes and some inflammation.
- Vitiligo macules/patches may not be obvious upon a general examination, especially around the eyes, nose, axilla, hands/fingers, and groin.
- Wood light examination is a low-cost and convenient diagnostic tool that can help differentiate depigmented lesions from hypopigmented lesions. Vitiligo lesions become markedly enhanced on Wood light examination and help to define specific areas of depigmentation (Fig. 10.1-11A,B).

See Section 15 Common Dermatology Procedures for Wood light examination.

Treatment

Topical Treatment

- *Topical corticosteroids* (TCSs) are the treatment of choice for vitiligo when small areas of skin are involved and for children. High-potency TCSs should be initiated with these patients and continued for 2 months. If there is no response, then the treatment should be discontinued. If the lesions are regaining their color, a slow taper to lower potency TCSs should be initiated with these patients and continued for 4 to 6 months. An exception to this general approach is lesions located around the eyes due to concern for increased intraocular pressure. Clinicians should regularly monitor patients for side effects and response to treatment. Pulse dosing can be used to minimize these side effects by alternating days of application with several days off. A common example is to apply Monday to Friday and omit the weekend.
- *Topical calcineurin inhibitors* (TCIs). Off-label use of pimecrolimus (Elidel) and tacrolimus 0.3% to 0.1% (Protopic) are alternatives to TCS and have been effective in treating facial vitiligo. Some studies have shown that these drugs are more efficacious when used in combination with narrowband ultraviolet light (NBUVB) phototherapy (Bolognia et al., 2017). However, TCIs should not be on the skin while the patient is receiving phototherapy treatment.

FIG. 10.1-7. Trichrome vitiligo. At times, vitiligo can appear with different stages of depigmentation, called trichrome vitiligo. (Used with permission from Edwards, L., & Lynch, P. [2017]. *Genital dermatology atlas and manual* [3rd ed.]. Wolters Kluwer Health.)

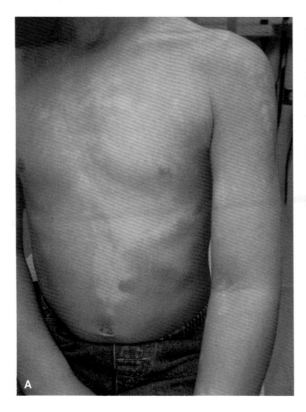

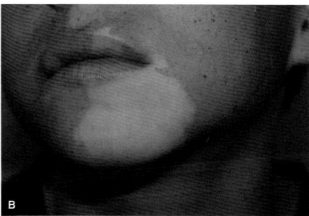

FIG. 10.1-8. A, B: Segmental vitiligo. (**A:** Image provided by Stedman's; **B:** Used with permission from Chung, E. K., Atkinson-McEvoy, L. R., Lai, N. L., & Terry, M. [2014]. *Visual diagnosis and treatment in pediatrics* [3rd ed.]. Wolters Kluwer Health.)

- *Calcipotriol.* Topical calcipotriol has also proven to be effective in producing repigmentation of vitiligo when used in combination with topical corticosteroid treatments or as a monotherapy. In general, Cochrane review (2015) states that most of the trials assessed combination therapies using phototherapy to enhance repigmentation.

- *Chemical depigmentation.* Depigmentation is usually reserved for vitiligo patients with a 40% or greater BSA involvement.

The treatment approach considers that it is easier to remove the remaining normal pigment to match the large depigmented areas. This is permanent and requires lifelong sun protection. A 20% cream of monobenzylether of hydroquinone may be applied b.i.d. for 6 to 18 months. Referral to dermatology is needed.

Systemic Treatment

- *Systemic corticosteroids* and immunosuppressants are not commonly used in the treatment of vitiligo. They should only be used to arrest rapidly spreading disease. Referral to dermatology is needed.

- *Phototherapy.* Narrowband UVB (NBUVB) and psoralen with UVA (PUVA) have been shown to be effective treatments for

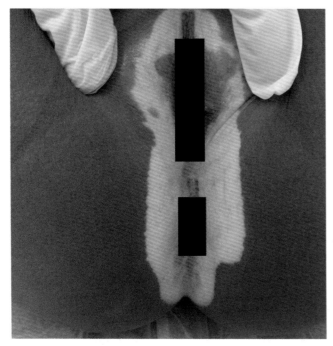

FIG. 10.1-9. Vitiligo at the anogenital area. (Photo courtesy of M. Bobonich.)

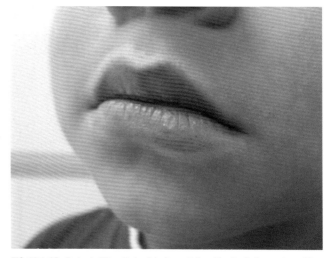

FIG. 10.1-10. Perioral vitiligo. Perioral depigmentation. Marginal inflammatory vitiligo with an erythematous, raised border. (Used with permission from Gru, A. A. [2018]. *Pediatric dermatopathology and dermatology.* Wolters Kluwer Health.)

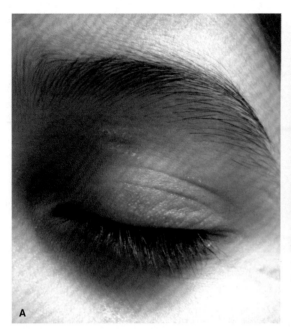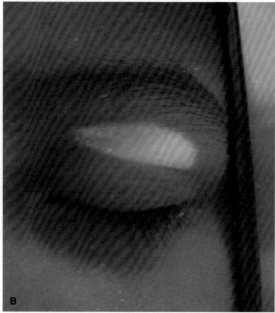

FIG. 10.1-11. **A, B:** Vitiligo. Vitiligo can have a subtle presentation that is difficult to discern especially in fair skin. Wood light examination can be used to accentuate areas of pigment loss and aid in diagnosis. (Photos courtesy of M. Bobonich.)

vitiligo; however, their exact mechanism of action is unknown. The primary objective is to stimulate the few remaining melanocytes which reside in the hair follicle. Ultraviolet light (UVL) activates the melanocytes, which migrate up the hair follicle and then spread to the surrounding area. Initially, repigmentation occurs at the hair follicle and presents as small hyperpigmented dots within the area of depigmentation. Phototherapy can be inconvenient for the patient, as it is an in-office therapy to whole body and usually recommended two to three times per week. Treatment considerations must also include increased risk for skin cancer if the treatment is prolonged.

- *Excimer laser* is a more focused beam of UVL and can be employed to target smaller areas such as the face and hands but requires twice weekly treatments for 24 to 48 sessions.

- *Janus kinase (JAK) inhibitors* target interferon gamma–inhibiting JAK1/2 but are not currently FDA approved for this purpose.

Surgical Treatment

- *Micropigmentation.* Medical tattooing or micropigmentation may be useful for sites that have a poor response to treatment, such as the lips and distal fingers, and are cosmetically concerning.

- *Punch grafting* may be successful for carefully chosen individuals who fail to respond to other therapies. Small punch grafts (1 to 2 mm) are taken from uninvolved skin and implanted 5 to 8 mm apart into the depigmented areas. Criteria for punch grafting include stable vitiligo for at least 6 months, no Koebner phenomenon, no tendency to develop keloid scars, a positive mini-grafting test, and at least 12 years of age (Bolognia et al., 2017).

Special Considerations

Pediatrics

- Pigment loss in children is either congenital or acquired; therefore, the onset of the disease can provide important diagnostic clues.

- Congenital depigmentation is an uncommon occurrence that presents at birth or during infancy and is usually associated with a genetic disorder.

- A white forelock on an infant would be concerning for autosomal dominant piebaldism in comparison to patients with vitiligo that may develop a forelock later in life. Children have a higher propensity for autoimmune disease than adults.

Pregnancy

- Corticosteroids, pimecrolimus, tacrolimus, calcipotriol, monobenzone, and psoralens have all been classified historically as pregnancy category C. It is best to postpone topical vitiligo treatment until after pregnancy.

- NBUVB treatment is safe during pregnancy.

Ocular Disease

- An uncommon ophthalmologic condition called *Vogt–Koyanagi–Harada (VKH) syndrome* is characterized by uveitis and facial vitiligo, therefore vitiligo patients should be advised to have an ophthalmologic examination if they have eye problems as well. Typically, however, the cutaneous symptoms occur later in the disease process (Bolognia et al., 2018).

Management and Patient Education

- In patients with fair skin, no treatment may be an option as the disfigurement from vitiligo may not be severe. Patients should be counseled on their increased risk for skin cancer and the importance of UVR protection. A broad-spectrum sunscreen containing zinc oxide or titanium dioxide should be used and sun-protective clothing encouraged.

- Camouflage makeup can be used as well. Some brand-name products available for dyspigmentation are Dermablend, Dermacolor, Keromask, Veil Cover, Perfect Cover and, Covermark.

- Aestheticians can be helpful in assisting patients with applying cosmetics and matching their skin tone.

- Manage patient expectations appropriately. Lesions may not resolve, may take a while to improve, or can recur. Facial lesions achieve greater than 90% improvement in pigmentation with

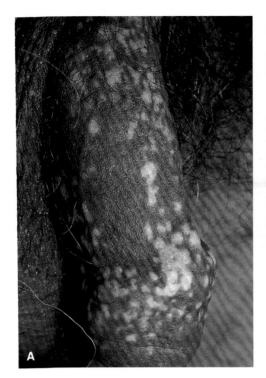

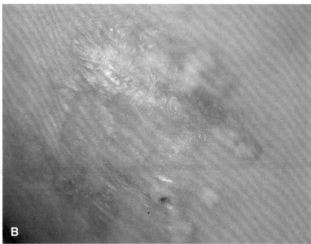

FIG. 10.1-12. **A, B:** Genital lichen sclerosus. Although at first glance, these very light papules mimic vitiligo, the crinkled texture change is pathognomonic for lichen sclerosus rather than vitiligo. (Used with permission from Edwards, L., & Lynch, P. J. [2017]. *Genital dermatology atlas* [3rd ed.]. Wolters Kluwer Health; **B:** From Edward, S., & Yung, A. [2011]. *Essential dermatopathology.* Wolters Kluwer Health.)

TCS, whereas lesions located on the trunk only achieve a 40% response to treatment.

- Darker skin tones are more responsive to TCS than lighter skin.

- Repigmentation of facial lesions occurs diffusely, but it occurs perifollicularly in lesions on the trunk. Cochrane review (2015) also states that none of the studies reported long-term benefit, that is, sustained repigmentation for at least 2 years.

- Refer to dermatology if vitiligo fails to respond to topical treatment or expands to involve large BSA as the patient may require advanced therapies.

- Newborns and infants with depigmented skin should be referred immediately to a pediatric dermatologist if available.

The following section refers to a disorder which presents with white color change but does not represent a disorder of pigmentation.

Lichen Sclerosus (Extragenital)

Lichen sclerosus is a chronic skin disease that most often affects the genital area, but can affect extragenital areas as well. Genital lichen sclerosus is discussed in Section 11.4. It is most common in females over the age of 50 and is often seen in conjunction with another autoimmune disease, for example, thyroid disease. In Figure 10.1-12A you can see how it mimics vitiligo at first glance.

Pathophysiology

- The etiology of extragenital lichen sclerosus is unclear, but it is thought to be influenced by genetics, hormones, infection, and sometimes occurs in sites of irritation or trauma.

Clinical Presentation

- Dry white plaques with cigarette paper texture and epidermal atrophy. Most commonly affects the buttocks, inner thighs, upper back, breasts, and inframammary areas (Fig. 10.1-12B).

- Lesions may also affect the periorbital areas and other areas on the face. Oral lesions are rare.

- Erythema, depigmentation, hyperpigmentation, telangiectasia and follicular plugs may be present.

- Most patients who have extragenital lichen sclerosus also have genital involvement.

- Pruritus may be present in extragenital lesions but is more profound in genital lesions.

DIFFERENTIAL DIAGNOSIS Lichen Sclerosus

- Lichen planus
- Vitiligo
- Morphea
- Trauma/scar
- Postinflammatory hypopigmentation
- Atopic dermatitis
- Discoid lupus erythematosus

Confirming the Diagnosis

- The diagnosis can be made clinically and confirmed with biopsy.

Treatment

- High potency topical steroid ointment may seem paradoxical but is the most commonly used first-line therapy. Apply b.i.d. × 3 months.

- Tacrolimus or pimecrolimus one to two times a day have been tried but must be continued for 3 to 6 months.

- If no response, intralesional steroids, oral retinoids, methotrexate, or cyclosporine can be used and the patient should be referred to dermatology.

Brown Lesions

Katie B. O'Brien

In This Chapter

- Erythema ab Igne
- Confluent and Reticulated Papillomatosis of Gougerot and Carteaud
- Melasma
- Post Inflammatory Hyperpigmentation

- Café au Lait Macules
- Lentigo
- Fixed Drug Eruption
- Phytophotodermatitis

The first two conditions present with a reticulated (lacy) pattern of hyperpigmentation.

Disorders of Pigment Excess

Erythema Ab Igne

Erythema ab igne (EAI), also known as *toasted skin syndrome* or *fire stains,* describes a local area of erythema and *reticulated* hyperpigmentation. The incidence of this condition had dramatically declined with the invention of central heating; however, the introduction of the laptop computer has brought a resurgence in the condition especially on the anterior thighs.

Pathophysiology

- EAI is caused by chronic exposure of the skin to heat sources such as heating pads, or open fire. Other heat sources include hot water bottles, electric heaters, radiators, car heaters, heated reclining chairs, and electric blankets.

- EAI develops from long-term exposure to heat below 113°F. The exposure is not hot enough to cause a thermal burn but does cause injury to the epidermis and superficial vasculature. The exact pathogenesis is unknown.

- Patients will usually have a history of chronic local heat exposure. There may be a history of chronic back pain where the patient often uses a heating pad. If the heat source is not obvious, the provider should inquire about occupation and hobbies. Children and adults in underdeveloped countries may have EAI from lying close to a fire for warmth.

Clinical Presentation

- Early EAI presents with reticular, net-like erythema that blanches easily, followed by reticulated hyperpigmentation.

- It is most commonly seen in the lumbosacral region, abdomen, and anterior legs (Fig. 10.2-1).

- Over time, the erythema evolves into hyperpigmentation and does not blanch.

- Lesions are typically asymptomatic.

DIFFERENTIAL DIAGNOSIS   Erythema Ab Igne

- Livedo reticularis
- Cutis marmorata telangiectatica congenita
- Poikiloderma
- Vasculitis

Confirming the Diagnosis

- EAI is usually a clinical diagnosis when the source of heat exposure has been identified.

- A punch biopsy may be done if diagnosis is uncertain.

Treatment

- Discontinuing the offending heat source is most important.

- If caught early, EAI may be responsive to topical therapies such as off-label use of tretinoin, corticosteroids, and combination products of both such as Tri-Luma.

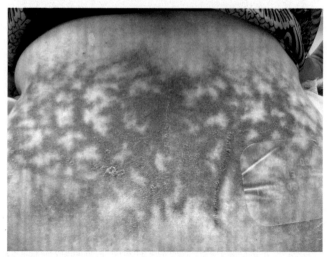

FIG. 10.2-1. Erythema ab igne. (Photo courtesy of M. Bobonich.)

- Chronic changes of EAI are very stubborn and not usually responsive to treatment.

Management and Patient Education

- EAI is more likely to resolve if it is found early and the heat source is removed.
- Epithelial atypia can develop from the chronic inflammation and potentially lead to squamous cell carcinoma (SCC) and Bowen disease.
- Skin cancer education should be provided. Patients should be advised to follow up for any changes in the skin.
- If the patient is applying heat chronically, the source of pain and discomfort must be identified.

Confluent and Reticulated Papillomatosis of Gougerot and Carteaud

Confluent and reticulated papillomatosis of Gougerot and Carteaud (CARP) is a disorder of reticulated or net-like hyperpigmentation that typically occurs on the chest and upper back. Young adult females are affected more often than males, and individuals with dark skin are affected more often than those with light skin. There have been some familial cases reported.

Pathophysiology

- The exact etiology of CARP is unknown. A genetic defect in keratinization, overproduction of yeast (*Malassezia* or *Pityrosporum*) and bacteria, endocrine abnormalities, and response to UVR exposure are among the suspected causes.

Clinical Presentation

- Scaly hyperpigmented macules and papules begin on the midsternal chest or midline of the back.
- Lesions coalesce to form larger plaques with reticular or net-like borders (Fig. 10.2-2A,B).

- Lesions may be itchy or asymptomatic.
- Sometimes lesions appear to be hypopigmented with fine white scale and are often mistaken for tinea versicolor.

DIFFERENTIAL DIAGNOSIS   **Confluent and Reticulated Papillomatosis of Gougerot and Carteaud**

- Tinea versicolor
- Postinflammatory hyperpigmentation
- Acanthosis nigricans
- Terra firma-forme

Confirming the Diagnosis

- KOH preparation should eliminate the diagnosis of tinea versicolor.
- A biopsy should be sent however, if KOH prep is equivocal, for periodic acid–Schiff (PAS) fungal staining to help detect the presence of a fungal organism.
- CARP associated with metabolic and hormonal disturbances should include patient screening for diabetes, thyroid disease, and polycystic ovary syndrome.

Management and Patient Education

- While the cause of CARP is unclear, several therapies have been effective in treating it.
- Minocycline 100 mg b.i.d. for 6 weeks is effective in most cases.
- Amoxicillin, azithromycin, and topical mupirocin have also been successful.
- Topical tretinoin and/or oral retinoids (isotretinoin or acitretin) have been used successfully, as they reduce abnormal cell turnover and reduce the hyperkeratotic surface of the papules/plaques.
- CARP has responded to oral contraceptives when occurring along with polycystic ovary syndrome.

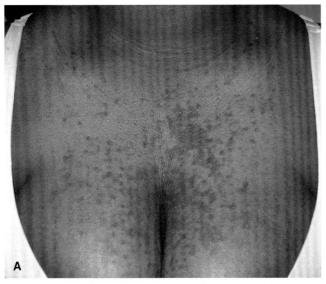

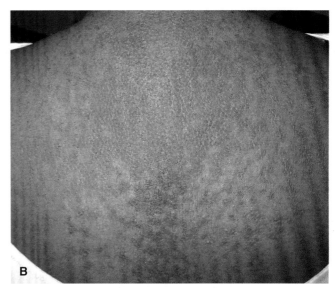

FIG. 10.2-2. A, B: CARP. The chest and back are the most commonly affected areas. Note the raised, hyperkeratotic coalesced papules on upper back that are sometimes misdiagnosed as acanthosis nigricans.

- Systemic or topical antifungal agents have also been effective if fungal elements are present.
- Patients should have the expectation that this is a chronic condition with exacerbations and remissions and there is no cure.

Melasma

Melasma is a common disorder of hyperpigmentation. It is also known as chloasma when associated with pregnancy. Melasma is more common in females of childbearing age, and those with darker skin phenotypes.

Pathophysiology

- The exact cause of melasma is unknown. It is theorized that the melanocytes in the affected skin produce greater amounts of melanin than they do in the uninvolved skin.
- This increased functioning of the melanocytes is thought to be triggered by UV exposure, hormonal or other systemic conditions such as thyroid disease.
- These stimuli can cause increased levels of nitric oxide which stimulates tyrosinase activity causing increased localized melanin production.
- Genetics is suspected to play a role in melasma in Asian and Hispanic ethnicities.
- Sun exposure is the greatest risk factor for the development of melasma.
- Hormones have also been implicated. Therefore, pregnant women and those taking oral contraceptives or hormone replacement therapy are at higher risk.

Clinical Presentation

- Tan to dark brown irregularly bordered, symmetric patches are most commonly distributed on the face and sometimes forearms (Fig. 10.2-3A,B).

- Three patterns of hypermelanosis are observed and are described as centrofacial, malar, and mandibular. The central facial pattern is the most common affecting the forehead, cheeks, nose, upper lip, and chin. The malar and mandibular patterns exclusively affect the cheeks, nose and, the mandible.

DIFFERENTIAL DIAGNOSIS   Melasma

- Drug-induced hyperpigmentation
- Postinflammatory hyperpigmentation
- Solar lentigines
- Nevus of Ota
- Discoid lupus

Confirming the Diagnosis

- It is important to determine if the patient has epidermal or dermal type of melasma, as dermal lesions do not respond well to bleaching agents.
- In the epidermal type, Wood light examination reveals an enhanced color contrast between normal skin and affected skin.
- In dermal type, there is no enhancement of color contrast seen under the Wood light.
- Keep in mind that in very darkly skinned patients, melasma lesions will not be visible under the Wood light.
- A biopsy may be required to determine if the lesions are epidermal or dermal.

Treatment

Topical Treatment

- Treatment of melasma is generally managed with topical lightening agents such as hydroquinone either alone or in combination

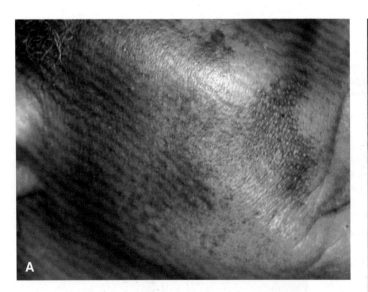
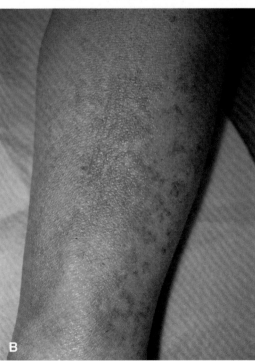

FIG. 10.2-3. **A:** Melasma frequently occurs in heavily pigmented skin. **B:** Melasma forearms. (Photos courtesy of M. Bobonich.)

with a topical retinoid (tretinoin or adapalene) and at times a mild TCS to counteract the irritation from the retinoid.

- Hydroquinone blocks the production of tyrosinase and selectively damages melanosomes and melanocytes. Hydroquinone 2% to 4% cream may be applied twice daily to affected areas. Hydroquinone 2% can still be purchased without prescription.

- Tretinoin cream 0.025%, 0.05%, and 0.1% is effective as monotherapy but has greater efficacy if used in combination with the hydroquinone. Caution should be used with higher strengths of topical retinoids (tretinoin 0.1%) as they can often cause significant inflammation.

- Tri-Luma Cream, which is a combination of hydroquinone, tretinoin, and fluocinolone, is often prescribed for efficacy and ease of administration. The hyperpigmentation should be reassessed after 2 months of treatment and is more likely to improve and less likely to recur if patients avoid the sun and any causative agent.

- Azelaic acid is a naturally occurring acid which has antibacterial and anti-inflammatory properties and is often used for the treatment of acne. Many users find improvement with areas of PIH. It is therefore often used off-label to treat conditions such as melasma in conjunction with other products.

- Recently, a number of skin-lightening agents without hydroquinone have become available. They contain numerous agents that claim to be more natural and nontoxic, such as vitamin C. Most cosmetic companies have a skin-lightening product available over the counter.

- Chemical peels are only mildly effective, so are best used in combination with other treatments. Glycolic acid and trichloroacetic acid (TCA) peels are most effective. Peels pose a risk of PIH.

Systemic Treatment

- Tranexamic acid 250 mg PO daily × 8 to 12 weeks is effective, but relapse is common.

- Treatment would likely need to be long term. Potential side effects include nausea, vomiting, and diarrhea (Spierings, 2019). Refer to a cosmetic dermatologist for treatment.

Surgical Treatment

- *Laser therapy.* Laser treatment has not been consistently effective, and the side effects may be greater than the benefits. As this condition exists primarily in patients with darker skin, hypopigmentation from the laser is a definite concern. Low-fluence Q-switched Nd:YAG laser is the most effective.

Management and Patient Education

- Epidermal melasma typically has a better response to treatment than the dermal process. Melasma usually improves or resolves slowly over a few months postpartum or after discontinuing oral contraceptives. Melasma commonly relapses.

- Patients using high-strength hydroquinone for long periods may be at risk for worsening pigmentation which can be a sign of ochronosis, a known side effect of long-term use.

- Therefore, it is advised to have patients follow up 2 months after beginning a hydroquinone-based treatment to evaluate response and transition to a suitable, long-term treatment alternative, such as azelaic acid.

- Strict sun protection with broad-spectrum physical sunblocks, hats, and sun avoidance is imperative for patients with melasma. Patients should be advised that their treatment will fail if they do not adhere to these sun protection practices.

- Patients taking oral contraceptives should decide if discontinuation or changing to a low-estrogen oral contraceptive is necessary.

Special Considerations

Pregnancy

The state of pregnancy is often the cause of melasma; so care must be taken to avoid most of the usual treatments. The risks and benefits of hydroquinone use during pregnancy and lactation should be weighed, as there is a possible risk of fetal harm, though inadequate human data is available. Tretinoin should absolutely be avoided during pregnancy, but may be used during breastfeeding. Azelaic acid was historically rated as category B but package insert information in 2019 states it should be used in pregnancy only if necessary and is not recommended while breastfeeding. Pregnant patients should be reassured that melasma usually fades postpartum.

Postinflammatory Hyperpigmentation

PIH can occur commonly as a result of inflammatory dermatoses and as a complication of many therapeutic interventions and mechanical injuries. PIH is more common in those with darker skin tones but also affects Caucasians. Many patients confuse PIH with scarring.

Pathophysiology

- An increase in pigment deposition in surrounding keratinocytes.

- The inflammation may have an endogenous cause from systemic disease or cutaneous skin conditions such as acne or cystic lesions.

- Exogenous inflammation can be induced by many mechanisms such as friction/scratching or manipulation of acne lesions.

Clinical Presentation

- Patients who have PIH have a history of preceding inflammation or injury to the skin.

- Lesions can range from light brown color occurring in the epidermis to a deeper dermal melanosis appearing dark brown, gray, or bluish.

- PIH will appear differently on various skin types. It will appear darker in those with darker skin tones and pink or light purple in individuals with skin types I to III (Fig. 10.2-4).

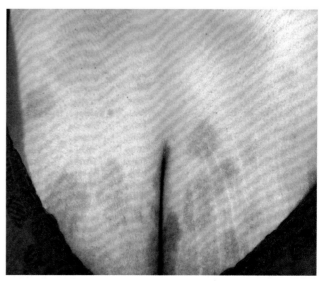

FIG. 10.2-4. Postinflammatory hyperpigmentation. (Photo courtesy of M. Bobonich.)

- PIH commonly results from acne, lichen planus, systemic lupus erythematosus, and chronic eczematous dermatitis.
- Some lesions may fade significantly, while others may be permanently disfiguring.
- PIH can worsen with sun exposure.

DIFFERENTIAL DIAGNOSIS	Post Inflammatory Hyperpigmentation

- Melasma
- Acanthosis nigricans
- Drug-induced hyperpigmentation
- Systemic lupus
- Discoid lupus
- Sarcoidosis

Confirming the Diagnosis

- The diagnosis of PIH is typically made clinically by history and physical examination.
- Epidermal lesions have accentuated borders with Wood light examination, while dermal lesions are not accentuated and are poorly demarcated.
- A skin biopsy may be performed if definitive diagnosis cannot be made.
- Discoid lupus is often accompanied by hyperpigmentation; scarring is also seen.

Management and Patient Education

- Treatment of PIH requires time and patience, as it may take 6 to 12 months.
- Acne should be treated early and efficiently to prevent PIH, especially in darkly pigmented skin.
- Topical preparations, such as tretinoin and azelaic acid, are used to treat acne and may also be effective at minimizing hyperpigmentation.
- Patients should also be advised to wear sunscreen daily to avoid worsening of the symptoms.
- Other topical therapies may be used for PIH such as the ones listed above in Management of Melasma. Response is variable.
- Caution must be used in darkly skinned individuals because of the increased risk of hypopigmentation.
- PIH can be emotionally difficult for adolescents and those with darker skin types. PIH usually fades within 6 to 12 months, but may not resolve completely in severe inflammatory conditions such as lichen planus or cutaneous lupus.
- If PIH is severe and/or refractory to topical treatment, then a referral to a cosmetic dermatology provider who has experience in laser treatment, specifically one who has experience using lasers on darkly pigmented skin may be helpful.
- Patients often think that PIH is the same as scarring and must be informed of the difference.

Café au lait Macules

Café au lait macules (CALMs) are well-demarcated light brown patches, which measure approximately 2 to 5 cm. CALMs are usually noted during early childhood and may persist into adulthood.

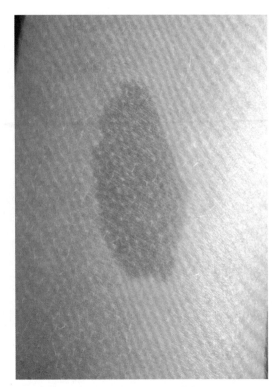

FIG. 10.2-5. Café au lait macule. (Photo courtesy of M. Bobonich.)

The term "café au lait" refers to the lesion's color, which resembles coffee with milk, which can be light tan to brown. Single CALMs are found in 10% to 20% of the population. Multiple lesions (>5) can be an indicator of various genetic syndromes. African Americans are affected more often than Caucasians, but it is reported less.

Pathophysiology

The hyperpigmentation seen in CALMs is due to increased amounts of melanin within the keratinocytes. The underlying cause of this is not known.

Clinical Presentation

- CALMs are typically oval-shaped, completely macular patches, which may be located anywhere on the body, except the mucous membranes (Fig. 10.2-5).
- Their size ranges from 2 to 5 cm, but may sometimes be smaller or larger.
- CALMs tend to grow as the body grows and are not associated with malignancy.
- Rarely, CALMs are associated with an underlying systemic disorder such as neurofibromatosis. (See Section 13 Childhood Disorders for details.)

DIFFERENTIAL DIAGNOSIS	Café au lait Macules

- Linear nevoid hyperpigmentation
- Early nevus spilus (before nevi appear within the tan patch)
- Postinflammatory hyperpigmentation (PIH)
- Phytophotodermatitis
- Neurofibromatosis (if number and size of lesions match NF criteria)

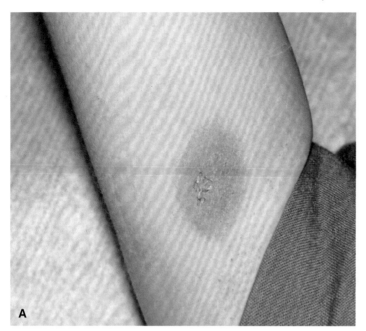
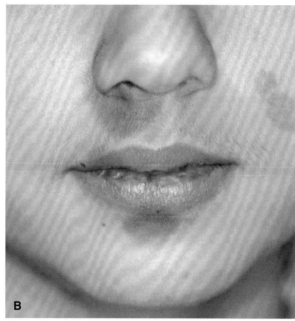

FIG. 10.2-6. **A:** Fixed drug eruption. In the early phase, the oval lesion occurred at the identical site where it had occurred previously. In both episodes, the rash emerged after this patient ingested a sulfonamide antibiotic. Note the eroded blister in the center of the lesion. (Used with permission from Goodheart, H., & Gonzalez, M. [2015]. *Goodheart's photoguide to common pediatric and adult skin disorders* [4th ed.]. Wolters Kluwer Health.) **B:** Over time, the lesions become more hyperpigmented as seen here. (Used with permission from Gru, A. A. [2018]. *Pediatric dermatopathology and dermatology.* Wolters Kluwer Health.)

Treatment

- Treatment is not medically necessary as malignant transformation has not been reported.
- Hydroquinone is not effective, and laser treatment has had variable results.
- The risks of laser surgery include scarring, dyspigmentation, incomplete clearance, and recurrence.

Management and Patient Education

- If there is clinical suspicion for any associated syndromes with CALMs, referral to the appropriate specialists for evaluation and management should be done promptly. Genetic counseling and testing may be indicated. If neurofibromatosis is suspected, multidisciplinary evaluation and management are essential.
- Patients and their parents should be reassured that CALMs are typically benign lesions.
- Patients should notify their provider if any change develops within the lesion(s).
- A full skin examination should be performed on patients with CALMs to look for other signs of associated syndromes.

Lentigo

A lentigo is a small pigmented macule. A single lesion or multiple lesions (lentigines) may be present at birth or more commonly first develop in early childhood. Lentigo simplex is not induced by sun exposure, and it is not associated with any medical diseases or condition.

See Section 2.1 for complete discussion.

Fixed Drug Eruption

A fixed drug eruption is a cutaneous adverse drug reaction that typically presents with a hyperpigmented patch that recurs in the same site whenever the offending drug is taken.

See Section 8.1 for further details.

Clinical Presentation

- Fixed drug eruption usually starts as an erythematous round or oval patch, sometimes with a blister. It fades to a purple-brown color. There can be multiple patches.
- Commonly occurs on hands, feet, legs, chest, or genitals (Fig. 10.2-6).
- Lesions occur within hours to days of starting the offending drug and recur when the drug is reintroduced.

Management and Patient Education

- Stop offending medication.
- Drugs that can cause fixed drug eruption include ASA, NSAIDs, sulfonamides, aminopenicillins, tetracyclines, TMP/SMX, phenolphthalein, barbiturates.

Phytophotodermatitis

Phytophotodermatitis (PPD) is a phototoxic reaction that occurs when the skin is exposed to plants or fruits which contain chemical compounds called furocoumarins. In the presence of UVL, these chemicals produce an inflammatory reaction which can range from erythema to blisters and always results in hyperpigmentation when inflammation subsides and is usually how the patient presents.

See Section 12.3 for complete description.

Blue-Gray Pigmentation

Katie B. O'Brien

In This Chapter

- Blue Nevus
- Nevus Ito/Ota
- Drug Induced Hyperpigmentation

Blue Nevus

A blue nevus is a melanocytic nevus in which the melanocytes are deeper than the ones in brown nevi. These lesions appear blue because of the way the light is scattered by these deep melanocytes. This is called the Tyndall effect (Fig. 10.3-1).

See Section 2.1 for details.

Nevus of Ito/Ota

Nevus of Ito/Ota are examples of oculodermal melanocytosis. They are similar in pathophysiology but different in clinical location. There is an increased prevalence in women and Asian, African-American, and Indian races.

Pathophysiology

It is thought to be due to the failure of the melanocytes to migrate from the dermis up to the epidermis during embryonic development.

Clinical Presentation

- Nevus Ota presents with a dark blue hyperpigmented patch, usually with a unilateral distribution along the trigeminal nerve (V1 and V2 branches) on the forehead and face and around the eye area. Hyperpigmentation of parts of the eye may occur (sclera, cornea, iris, retina) (Fig. 10.3-2).

- The underlying mucosa, conjunctiva, and tympanic membranes may also be pigmented and may darken with age.

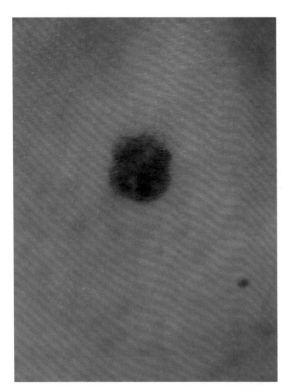

FIG. 10.3-1. Blue nevus. The dark color represents the depth of the pigment. (Photo courtesy of M. Bobonich.)

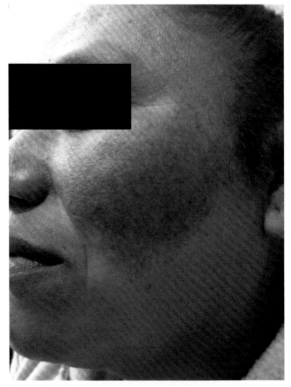

FIG. 10.3-2. Nevus Ota. (Photo courtesy of M. Bobonich.)

377

- Nevus of Ota has been associated with glaucoma.
- Nevus of Ito presents also with blue-gray pigmentation but is present on the shoulder scapular or deltoid regions (shoulder girdle) and is usually unilateral (Fig. 10.3-3).

DIFFERENTIAL DIAGNOSIS   Nevus Ito/Ota

- Ota/ecchymosis or venous malformation
- Ito/extrasacral Mongolian spot

Confirming Diagnosis

- Diagnosis is clinical.
- Biopsy will confirm dermal hypermelanosis.

Management and Patient Education

- Although usually benign, these often can have a psychological impact on the patient's body image.
- Camouflage makeup is often used, but topicals have no effect.
- Q-switched laser, requiring repeated treatments, provides the most promising cosmetic results.

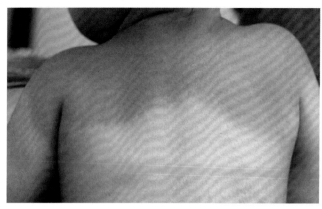

FIG. 10.3-3. Nevus Ito. Nevus of Ito showing blue-gray pigmentation on scapular area and shoulder. (Photo courtesy of M. Bobonich.)

Drug-Induced Hyperpigmentation

Multiple drugs including amiodarone, minocycline, bleomycin, NSAIDs, heavy metals, antimalarials, and psychotropic drugs can induce a blue-black coloration that affects the skin, nails, sclerae, oral mucosa, and teeth. This typically is related to high doses over a longer period of time. For greater details involving minocycline, amiodarone, and bleomycin, please see Section 8.2 for details.

Yellow Lesions

Katie B. O'Brien

In This Chapter

- Xanthelasma/Xanthomas
- Eruptive Xanthoma
- Juvenile Xanthogranuloma

- Necrobiosis Lipoidica
- Sebaceous Hyperplasia

Xanthelasma/Xanthomas

Xanthomas are lipid deposits in the skin. They typically occur after age 50 and can be associated with hyperlipidemia. Xanthelasma is a common condition of flat, yellowish, well-demarcated papules and plaques usually occurring on the eyelids (Fig. 10.4-1).

See Section 2.3 for complete discussion.

Eruptive Xanthoma

These papules appear as a result of increased lipid levels.

Pathophysiology

- This may be the result of familial lipoproteinemia, lipoprotein lipase deficiencies, or secondary causes such as excessive alcohol intake, hypothyroidism, nephrotic syndrome, or DM.
- Skin lesions caused by accumulation of fat in macrophages within the skin.
- Often seen with hypertriglyceridemia. Triglyceride levels often are 3,000 to 4,000 mg/dL.

Clinical Presentation

- Small red-yellow papules on the buttocks, shoulders, arms, and legs (Fig. 10.4-2) which appear abruptly.

- Rarely affects the face.
- Usually itchy or tender.

DIFFERENTIAL DIAGNOSIS   Eruptive Xanthoma

- Sarcoidosis
- NLD
- Xanthogranuloma
- Granuloma annulare

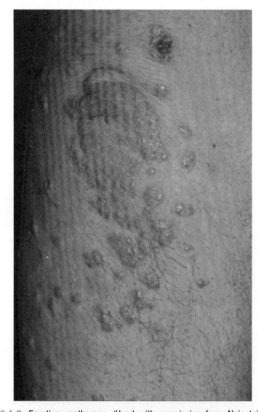

FIG. 10.4-2. Eruptive xanthomas. (Used with permission from Neinstein, L. S., Katzman, D. K., Callahan, T., Gordon, C. M., Joffe, A., & Rickert, V. [2016]. *Neinstein's adolescent and young adult health care* [6th ed.]. Wolters Kluwer Health.)

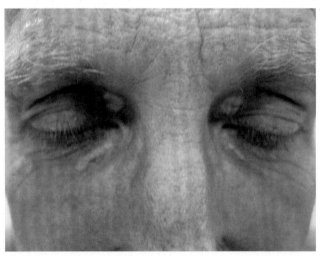

FIG. 10.4-1. Xanthelasma. (Image provided by Stedman's.)

379

Confirming the Diagnosis

- Skin biopsy should be performed to confirm the diagnosis which will show foamy histiocytes.
- Serum triglyceride levels will be marked elevated.

Treatment

- Treat triglycerides if elevated. Fibrates and Niacin work best to lower triglycerides.
- Healthy lifestyle modification and pharmacologic treatment are important.
- Discontinue medications that may be increasing triglycerides. Systemic retinoids, estrogens, protease inhibitors, cyclosporine, and prednisone have all been known to increase triglycerides.

Management and Patient Education

- Usually lesions resolve within 6 months after lipid levels normalize.
- If persistent, surgery, laser, or cryosurgery may be utilized.

Juvenile Xanthogranuloma

Juvenile xanthogranulomas (JXGs) are skin lesions seen predominantly in infants and young children, more often in males, and present at birth in 20% of cases. About 10% of cases are seen in adults. It is more common in Caucasians than in those of Asian origin.

Pathophysiology

- The cause is unknown.
- It represents a type of non-Langerhans cell histiocytosis.

Clinical Presentation

- Initially they appear as smooth pink bumps that later become yellow in color (Fig. 10.4-3).
- Most are under 0.5 cm but giant variant can occur up to 2.0 cm.

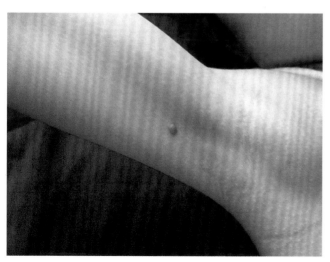

FIG. 10.4-3. Juvenile xanthogranuloma. (Littlekidsdoc, CC BY-SA 4.0 https://creativecommons.org/licenses/by-sa/4.0, via Wikimedia Commons.)

- Most frequently they appear on the trunk and upper extremities. Occasionally they also appear in the eye or internal organs.

DIFFERENTIAL DIAGNOSIS   Juvenile Xanthogranuloma

- Benign cephalic histiocytosis
- General eruptive histiocytosis
- Papular xanthogranuloma

Confirming the Diagnosis

- JXG has a characteristic appearance on dermoscopy known as "setting sun," in which there is a central yellow area surrounded by reddish periphery.
- Biopsy shows collections of histiocytes, older lesions show "foamy" histiocytes and enlarged histiocytes (giant cells).

Treatment

- Since JXGs are benign, treatment is not necessary unless symptomatic.

Management and Patient Education

- Reassure parents and/or patients that these lesions usually regress within 3 to 6 years.
- JXG rarely occurs extracutaneously. The most common extracutaneous site, occurring in less than 0.05% of patients with cutaneous lesions, is the eye. This usually occurs before the age of 2, so early referral to an ophthalmologist is recommended.
- Despite the presence of fat-filled histiocytes in the skin, the levels of lipids in the blood are quite normal and JXG and related disorders are not usually associated with any serious abnormality.
- 20% of patients with JXG also have CALMs therefore, careful physical examination is recommended to identify the number and size of CALM and referral to dermatology may be prudent.

Necrobiosis Lipoidica

Necrobiosis lipoidica is a disorder of collagen degeneration with a granulomatous response. 15% to 65% of patients with NLD have or will develop DM. It most commonly affects females in their 30s and 40s.

Pathophysiology

- Etiology is unclear.
- Immune-mediated vascular disease has been suggested as a cause.
- Small vessel changes present in diabetics may lead to breakdown of collagen and development of inflammation.

Clinical Presentation

- Lesions are most often seen on the shins and are multiple and bilateral.
- They may begin as firm brown papules and then enlarge into violaceous, shiny, well-demarcated patches or thin plaques with palpable peripheral rims and yellow-brown atrophic centers with telangiectasias (Fig. 10.4-4).

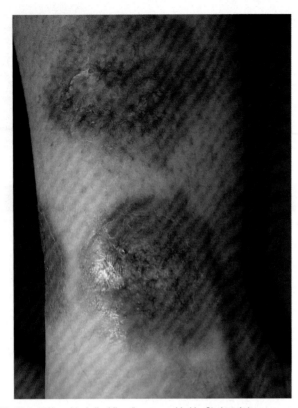

FIG. 10.4-4. Necrobiosis lipoidica. (Image provided by Stedman's.)

- Lesions are often tender or itchy, but may be asymptomatic.
- Minor trauma can result in ulceration.

DIFFERENTIAL DIAGNOSIS	Necrobiosis Lipoidica
• Granuloma annulare	• Lichen sclerosus
• Early erythema nodosum	• Pretibial myxedema
• Cutaneous sarcoidosis	• Xanthomas
• Nonmelanoma skin cancer	• Stasis dermatitis
• Morphea	

Confirming the Diagnosis

- Diagnosis is often clinical.
- Skin biopsy would reveal palisading granulomatous dermatitis that involves the deep dermis and extends to the septae of fat with layers of inflammation surrounding the destroyed collagen.

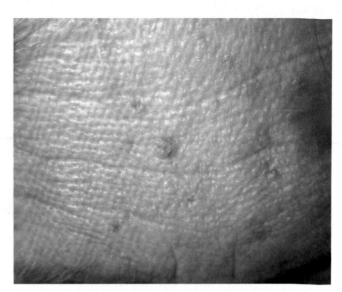

FIG. 10.4-5. Sebaceous hyperplasia. (Photo courtesy of M. Bobonich.)

Treatment

- Topical, intralesional, or systemic corticosteroids may slow the progression.
- Sometimes they resolve spontaneously.

Management and Patient Education

- It is important to minimize trauma to the area, as it can lead to nonhealing ulcers.
- Side effects of topical, oral, and intralesional steroids should be discussed.
- Patients with active lesions should be monitored every couple of weeks until stable.
- If indicated, screen for diabetes and refer to endocrinology.

Sebaceous Hyperplasia

- Sebaceous hyperplasia is a disorder of enlarged sebaceous glands. It affects both females and males equally. There is an increased incidence in the elderly, in transplant patients, and in pregnancy.
- They present as soft yellowish 1- to 3-mm papules, either solitary or scattered on the forehead and central face.
- Lesions have central umbilication and telangiectasias along the outer rim (Fig. 10.4-5).
- Primary differential diagnosis is BCC.

See Section 2.3 for more details.

Red-Purple Lesions

Katie B. O'Brien

In This Chapter

- Angiomas
- Pyogenic Granuloma
- Angiokeratoma

- Purpura
- Petechiae

Angiomas

- Cherry angiomas are bright red, dome-shaped papules typically appearing on the trunk and proximal extremities (Fig. 10.5-1A).
- They typically start appearing during one's third decade and can increase in number during pregnancy.
- There is a characteristic appearance on dermoscopy (Fig. 10.5-1B).
- Unless there are cosmetic concerns, no treatment is necessary.
- Cherry angiomas are commonly treated with electrodessication, laser, or excision.

See Section 2.3 for more details and Section 13 for childhood angiomas.

Pyogenic Granuloma

- Pyogenic granulomas are solitary, friable red papules or polyps that erupt rapidly (Fig. 10.5-2).
- These lesions often occur at sites of trauma.
- They can occur on the skin or mucosal surface.

- Pyogenic granulomas are usually treated with shave removal and electrodessication of the base.
- Patients should be aware that they commonly recur after treatment.

See Section 2.3 and Section 13 for more details.

Angiokeratoma

Angiokeratomas are benign, dermal vascular papules. There is often epidermal change as well. Several types of angiokeratoma exist.

Pathophysiology

Pathophysiology is unknown but may be related to increased venous pressure.

Clinical Presentation

- There are several subtypes, however the most common presentation is single or multiple 2- to 3-mm, smooth, red, or violaceous papules seen on the scrotum or vulva (Fig. 10.5-3).

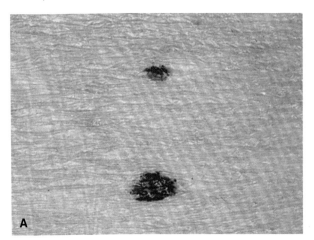

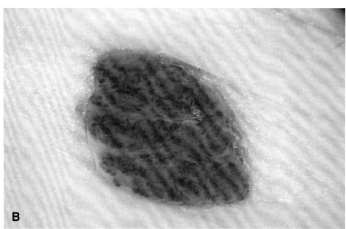

FIG. 10.5-1. **A:** Infantile hemangioma. Angiomas are characterized by well-demarcated red to blue-red or blue-black to maroon, round or oval structures (lacunae). (**A:** Used with permission from Bickley, L. S., & Szilagyi, P. [2003]. *Bates' guide to physical examination and history taking* [8th ed.]. Lippincott Williams & Wilkins.) **B:** These clinically flat or slightly elevated lesions are red, with vascular red lacunae on dermoscopy. These structures are collections of blood vessels. When thrombosed, they appear as a homogeneous, confluent dark bluish-black pigment. (**B:** Used with permission from Markowitz, O. [2017]. *A practical guide to dermoscopy*. Wolters Kluwer Health.)

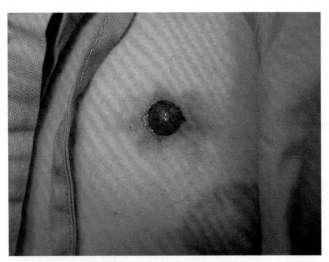

FIG. 10.5-2. Pyogenic granuloma. (Image provided by Stedman's.)

DIFFERENTIAL DIAGNOSIS   Angiokeratoma

- Hemangioma
- Blue rubber bleb nevus
- Melanocytic nevus
- Melanoma
- Pigmented BCC
- Condyloma acuminata
- Kaposi sarcoma

Confirming the Diagnosis

- Dermoscopy reveals a lacuna pattern of round to oval areas with red-blue to black coloration. There may be some keratotic areas as well which strongly suggest angiokeratoma.
- Biopsy will show large dilated blood vessels in the superficial dermis with overlying hyperkeratosis.

Treatment

- These lesions are benign and require no treatment unless there is cosmetic concern.

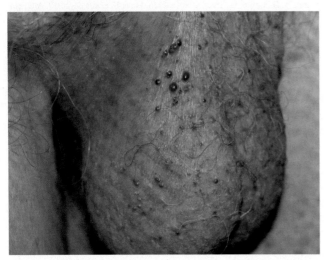

FIG. 10.5-3. Angiokeratoma. (Used with permission from Edwards, L., & Lynch, P. J. [2017]. *Genital dermatology atlas* [3rd ed.]. Wolters Kluwer Health.)

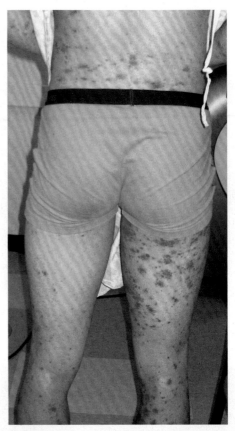

FIG. 10.5-4. Purpura.

- They can be treated with electrocautery if lesions are irritated or bleeding.
- Simple excision or laser can be used if lesions are large.

Management and Patient Education

- Reassurance

Purpura

- The term purpura is used to define a visible hemorrhage on the skin (Fig. 10.5-4).
- Ecchymoses are nonpalpable purpura >1 cm in diameter and may occur from minor trauma, anticoagulant use, liver disease, vitamin K deficiency, overuse of topical steroids, sun damage (actinic purpura), and thrombocytopenia.
- Palpable purpura are purpura that can be felt on palpation. This can be a sign of vasculitis and a biopsy should be done to confirm the diagnosis (Fig. 10.5-5A,B).
- Purpura appear purple, then fade to orange, brown, then blue or green.

See Section 9.3 for complete discussion.

Petechiae

- Petechiae are small (<4-mm-diameter) purpuric macules (Fig. 10.5-6).
- Can occur from thrombocytopenia, or disseminated intravascular coagulation.

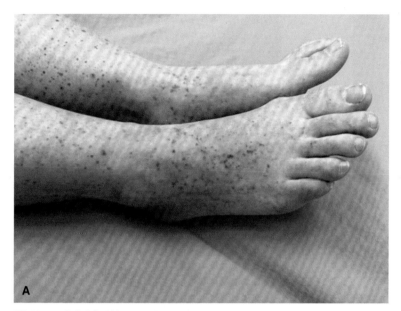

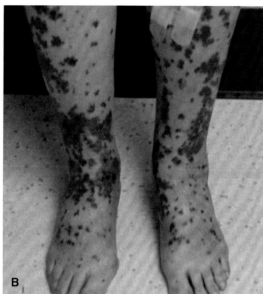

FIG. 10.5-5. **A, B:** Palpable purpura. Leukocytoclastic vasculitis is characterized by palpable purpura. (Used with permission from Gru, A. A. [2018]. *Pediatric dermatopathology and dermatology.* Wolters Kluwer Health.)

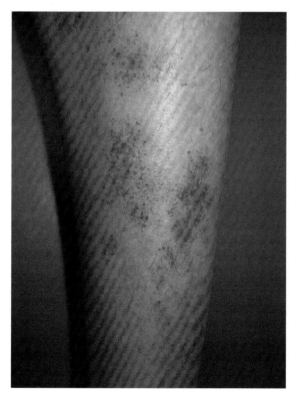

FIG. 10.5-6. Petechiae. Schamberg disease (progressive pigmented purpura) is groups of small purpuric macules that give a cayenne pepper appearance. (Image provided by Stedman's.)

- They can also occur from trauma, venous stasis, repetitive vomiting, childbirth, severe coughing, or seizures.

- Perifollicular petechiae are seen with scurvy, most commonly found on shins.

See Section 9.3 for details of petechiae.

READINGS AND REFERENCES

Alikha, A., Felsten, L., Daly, M., & Petronic-Rosic, V. (2011). Vitiligo: A comprehensive overview Part I. Introduction, epidemiology, quality of life, diagnosis, differential diagnosis, associations, histopathology, etiology, and work-up. *Journal of the American Academy of Dermatology*, 65(3), 473–491. https://doi.org/10.1016/j.jaad.2010.11.061

Bolognia, J. L., Schaffer, J., & Cerroni, L. (2017). *Dermatology* (4th ed.). Elsevier.

Bolognia, J. L., Schaffer, J., & Cerroni, L. (2018). *Dermatology* (4th ed.). Elsevier.

Damevska, K., Pollozhani, N., Neloska, L., & Duma, S. (2017). Unsuccessful treatment of progressive macular hypomelanosis with oral isotretinoin. *Dermatologic Therapy*, 30(5). doi:10.1111/dth.12514

Habif, T. P. (2004). Clinical dermatology. *A color guide to diagnosis and therapy* (6th ed.). Elsevier.

James, W. D., Elston, D., Treat, J., Rosenbach, M., & Neuhaus, I. (2019). Andrews' diseases of the skin. *Clinical dermatology* (13th ed.). Elsevier.

Kim, Y., Lee, D., Lee, J., & Yoon, T. (2012). Progressive macular hypomelanosis showing excellent response to oral isotretinoin. *Journal of Dermatology*, 39(11), 937–938. doi:10.1111/j.1346-8138.2012.01605.x

Rothstein, B., Joshipura, D., Saraiya, A., Abdat, R., Ashkar, H., Turkowski, Y., Sheth, V., Huang, V., Au, S. C., Kachuk, C., Dumont, N., Gottlieb, A. B., & Rosmarin, D. (2017). Treatment of vitiligo with the topical Janus kinase inhibitor ruxolitinib. *Journal of the American Academy of Dermatology*, 76(6), 1054–1060.e1.

Spierings, N. M. K. (2019). Melasma: A critical analysis of clinical trials investigating treatment modalities published in the past 10 years. *Journal of Cosmetic Dermatology*, 19(6), 1284–1289.

Whitton, M., Pinart, M., Batchelor, J., Leonardi-Bee, J., González, U., Jiyad, Z., Eleftheriadou, V., & Ezzedine, K. (2015). Interventions for vitiligo. *Cochrane Database of Systematic Reviews*, 24(2), CD003263. doi:10.1002/14651858.CD003263.pub5

Hair Disorders

Martha Sikes

In This Chapter

Hair is an important appendage of the skin that serves for both protection and self-esteem. Changes that involve these structures can provide valuable clues to both localized and systemic diseases. Disorders involving hair loss or excess have significant social and psychological implications for men and women. Hairstyles and hair care can communicate much about a person, and diseases of the hair can have a significant impact on one's self-esteem. Knowledge of the anatomy and growth cycle of hair is fundamental to understanding the causes of hair growth abnormalities. In this section, we will discuss how to recognize disorders involving both hair loss and hair excess.

TYPES AND STRUCTURE OF HAIR

Hair follicles differentiate and produce three different types of hair:

- *Lanugo*—short, soft, and nonpigmented hair that develops over all over the body of an embryo, starting in the 12th week of gestation. This immature hair is shed about 1 month before birth and is replaced with vellus and terminal hairs.
- *Vellus*—relatively nonpigmented hair that is not associated with a sebaceous gland.
- *Terminal*—hairs associated with sebaceous glands which cover the head and often arms, legs, and other parts of the body.

Hair has two separate structures that work together, the follicle and the hair shaft.

- The inferior portion of the follicle includes the hair bulb and the dermal papillae from which the hair shaft is formed and is rooted in the subcutaneous fat.

- The emerging hair shaft consists of an outer cuticle which is tightly compacted to support the cortex, and the interior of the follicle with rapidly dividing and growing cells.
- Melanocytes in the hair bulb give the cortex its color. Each hair shaft has a tapered tip, and the hair is lubricated by the sebum produced by the sebaceous gland (Fig. 11.1-1).

HAIR GROWTH CYCLE

The cycle of hair growth has three phases: anagen, catagen, and telogen.

- *Anagen phase*—this is the growth phase, which occurs when the cells in the bulb and the dermal papilla are actively dividing and forming a new hair shaft. Normally, 90% to 95% of hairs are in the anagen phase, which can last 2 to 6 years and enables some to achieve hair of extraordinary lengths. The anagen phase, which is genetically determined, is the longest on the scalp and much shorter on other areas such as eyelashes and brows.
- *Catagen phase*—a short transitional phase lasting a few days to weeks, with only a few hairs (<1%) at any given time. During this phase, the hair bulb goes through an involution and the outer sheath shrinks and detaches from the follicle but attaches to the hair shaft to develop a tighter club hair. The inferior portion of the hair shaft detaches from the dermal papilla, comes to rest at the level of the arrector pili muscle, and is eventually pushed out. The dermal papilla rests under the hair follicle bulge before it starts to reform a new hair shaft.
- *Telogen phase*—known as the resting phase and lasts 2 to 3 months, accounting for the average loss of 50 to 100 hairs

385

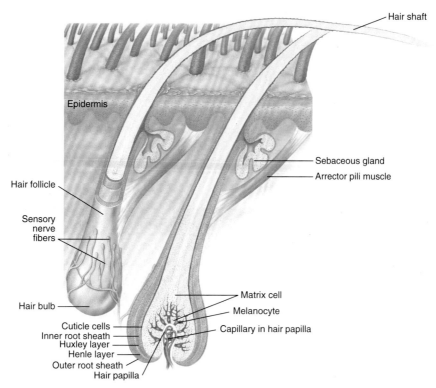

FIG. 11.1-1. Anatomy of hair. (Courtesy of Anatomical Chart Co.)

daily. In many animals, telogen and shedding are seasonal but in humans it is random (Fig. 11.1-2).

HAIR LOSS

As with most medical problems, a good assessment of a patient with the complaint of alopecia, or hair loss, begins with a complete history and physical examination. History alone is sometimes sufficient to determine the diagnosis, especially in nonscarring alopecia. A physical examination should begin by assessing the entire scalp surface and the hair shaft. Other hair-bearing areas, such as eyebrows, eyelashes, beard and moustache, axillae, genitals, and extremities, should be inspected if indicated. Specific characteristics of the

alopecia can guide the clinician to develop differential diagnoses and appropriate diagnostics (Box 11.1-1).

Alopecia, or hair loss, can be divided into two main categories: nonscarring (noncicatricial) and scarring (cicatricial).

- *Nonscarring (noncicatricial) alopecia* is seen more commonly and comprises patchy hair loss, thinning, or shedding without any scarring features.

- *Scarring (cicatricial) alopecia* is less common and associated with an inflammatory or infectious etiology. It is characterized by an area of complete destruction of the follicles with resulting scar formation. The hair loss is most often permanent and irreversible.

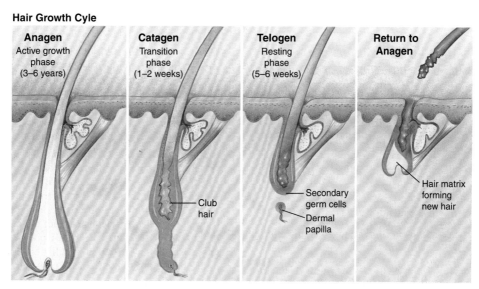

FIG. 11.1-2. Hair growth cycle. (Courtesy of Anatomical Chart Co.)

BOX 11.1-1 Important Findings in Patients with Hair Loss

Physical Examination
- Location and pattern of hair loss
- Diffuse or localized
- Complete loss or thinning
- Hair texture, length, and color
- Presence of scarring
- Presence of erythema, pustules, scale, or abnormal pigmentation
- Nail findings
- Acne or hirsutism
- Patient affect and behaviors (i.e., anxiety)

Diagnostics (If Indicated)

Part Width Test
Performed with the patient's head tipped forward, begin by parting the hair on the frontal scalp with a comb (if available) or the wooden end of a cotton-tipped applicator. Observe the width of the part and then compare the part width of the crown with many parallel parts on the temporal areas and occipital areas. Check to see if the part width is consistent in all sections.

Hair Pull Test
Grasp 50 to 60 or so hairs on the crown. Pull gently but with enough pressure to tent the scalp and slide the fingers along the hair shafts distally to pull some hairs out. Examine the bulbs of the extracted hairs with a magnifier. Telogen hairs will appear as white bulbs at the end of the shaft. Fewer than six bulbs is considered normal

(5% to 10%). This may need to be repeated on two to three additional areas.

Punch Biopsy
Aids in the diagnosis of scarring alopecias. Indicated if the diagnosis is uncertain, the patient has multiple characteristics, or fails to respond to treatment. A 4-mm (not any smaller) punch biopsy should be performed on the scalp area affected and close to the active edge of the scalp area. Be sure to get a sample of hair follicles and punch deep enough to get subcutaneous tissue where the bulb of anagen hairs will be located. Many clinicians will send two specimens, one indicated for vertical and one for horizontal sectioning, allowing for a good examination of the hair bulb. The specimen should be labeled for hair evaluation. Avoid specimens from the bitemporal area, which normally have some miniaturized hairs.

Laboratory Diagnostics
- Not often necessary but are guided by specific differential diagnoses.
- KOH and/or fungal cultures can help to confirm tinea.
- Serologies help identify underlying disease causing alopecia: complete blood count and ferritin (iron-deficiency anemia); RPR (syphilis); antinuclear antibodies (autoimmune diseases); and TSH, T4, and thyroid antibodies (hypothyroidism).
- In women, serum testosterone (free and total), dehydroepiandrosterone sulfate (DHEAS), and prolactin levels (if galactorrhea is present).
- Additional hormonal studies should be done in the presence of menstrual irregularities or hormonal abnormalities.

Each of these categories can be further divided into diffuse or localized (patchy) hair loss. These four characteristics of alopecia are important clues for an accurate assessment and differential diagnoses (Table 11.1-1).

Nonscarring Hair Loss Diffuse

Male Pattern Hair Loss

Patterned hair loss in men (MPHL), also known as androgenic alopecia, is the most common cause of progressive hair loss in men. It is estimated that 30% of Caucasian men present with MPHL by age 30 and up to 80% by the age of 70 years, but is seen slightly less in Japanese, Chinese, or African American men (Lolli et al., 2017). While it is viewed by some as inevitable and tolerable, others find it unacceptable. Health risks associated with MPHL include increased penetration of ultraviolet radiation on the scalp and increased incidence of benign prostatic hypertrophy and myocardial infarction.

Pathophysiology

MPHL is caused by a genetically predetermined influence of androgens on hair follicles. Normally, 5α-reductase converts testosterone to the more potent dihydrotestosterone (DHT) and increases scalp and beard growth in the male adolescent. Later in life, however, the DHT binds to the androgen receptor in the follicle, causing a shortening of the anagen cycle and miniaturization of hair follicles. The result is finer, shorter, and fewer hairs that can ultimately lead to baldness. Inheritance patterns of MPHL is generally viewed as being multifactorial with a significant increase risk for development in men with a bald father and/or a positive maternal family history of balding (Lolli et al., 2017) (Table 11.1-2).

Clinical Presentation

- Partial or complete hair loss at temples and crown ("M" distribution) (Fig. 11.1-3).
- Usually spares the sides and back ("horseshoe" pattern).
- Hamilton–Norwood classification is used to document and monitor the extent of hair loss (Fig. 11.1-4).
- Seborrheic dermatitis is also commonly seen.

TABLE 11.1-1	Characteristics of Alopecia for Differential Diagnosis	
TYPE	**DIFFUSE**	**PATCHY/FOCAL**
Nonscarring	Androgenic alopecia (thinning) Telogen effluvium (shedding) Anagen effluvium	Alopecia areata Trichotillomania Tinea capitis or infection[a]
Scarring	Lichen planopilaris Chronic cutaneous lupus erythematosus Dissecting cellulitis	Discoid lupus Central centrifugal cicatricial alopecia Acne keloidalis Traction alopecia

[a]If not treated early, can result in scarring alopecia.

DIFFERENTIAL DIAGNOSIS   Male Pattern Hair Loss

- Alopecia areata (diffuse)—acute onset

  Telogen effluvium—acute onset; associated with underlying condition

  Anagen effluvium—sudden loss of hair usually associated with chemotherapy treatment
- Thyroid disease—expand review of systems (ROS) and physical examination
- Iron-deficiency anemia—expand ROS and physical examination

TABLE 11.1-2 | Evaluation of Hair Loss: History

PERSONAL HISTORY	MEDICAL HISTORY	FAMILY HISTORY
Ask the patient: • When did you first notice hair loss? • When did your hair last seem normal? • Was it sudden or gradual? • Is hair falling out (and seen in the drain or brush) or do you notice thinning (not as thick)? • Is the hair loss diffuse or patchy? • Is it only on the scalp or in other areas? • Any recent trauma, physical, or emotional? If yes, when did this occur? • What treatments have you tried? • Detailed inquiry about hair care, products, styling, use of tools (hot combs), relaxers or dyes, heat, use of extensions or weaves, and styling that pulls or binds (corn rows, ponytails, etc.)	• List medications, especially new medications • Consider undeclared use of anabolic corticosteroids • Corticosteroids use of prescription or over-the-counter herbs or supplements • Recent illness, surgeries, anesthesia, weight loss (diets) • Thyroid disease • Ob/gyn issues: menstrual irregularities, infertility • Skin conditions: acne, hirsutism, etc.	Balding male or female family members Thyroid disease

Confirming the Diagnosis

- Clinical presentation is typically sufficient.
- Thyroid-stimulating hormone (TSH) if thyroid dysfunction suspected.
- Hair pull test, skin biopsy, and/or serum iron levels if telogen effluvium (TE) suspected.

Treatment

Topical

- Minoxidil
    - Increases the anagen cycle and decreases miniaturization ultimately increasing diameter of existing hairs rather than dramatically increasing hair count (Lolli et al., 2017).
    - 2% or 5% Solution; 5% Foam—FDA approved for MPHL.
    - Applied twice a day to dry scalp and should remain on for at least 1 hour.

    - Treatment response should be assessed at the end of 6 months and continued indefinitely to maintain results.
    - Most efficacious in young males with new onset of hair loss on the vertex. Less effective in bitemporal loss.
    - Adverse effects include telogen shedding within the first 8 weeks, contact dermatitis, and increased facial hair if product comes in contact with the face (i.e., transfer from pillowcase at night or touching face while sleeping). Treatment continued indefinitely to maintain results.
- Latanoprost or dutasteride
    - Topical use is not FDA approved but has also been reported to have some success.
- Low-level laser light therapy (LLL)—Over-the-counter red-light hairbrush device with 510K FDA approval for safety only (not efficacy), may improve hair regrowth.
- Surgical treatments—hair transplantation and scalp reduction. Refer to dermatology surgeons or plastic surgeons skilled in these procedures.
- Camouflage—hair weaves, powder scalp dye, or wigs

Systemic

- Minoxidil
    - Originally used as an antihypertensive drug for vasodilatory effects, later discovered to increase the anagen cycle and decrease miniaturization. Literature reports successes at doses ranging from 0.25 to 2.5 q.d., but its use is limited by systemic adverse effects.
- Finasteride 1-mg tablets
    - While originally approved for treatment of benign prostatic hyperplasia, it is now FDA approved for MPHL in males aged 18 years and older.

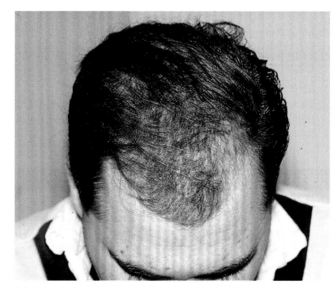

FIG. 11.1-3. Male pattern hair loss. Note the M pattern on frontal hairline. (Used with permission from Arndt, K. A., Hsu, J. T., Alam, M., Bhatia, A. C., & Chilukuri, S. [2014]. *Manual of dermatologic therapeutics* [8th ed.]. Wolters Kluwer.)

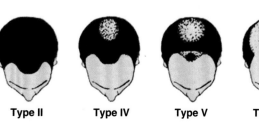

Type II   **Type IV**   **Type V**   **Type VII**

FIG. 11.1-4. Hamilton–Norwood classification of male pattern baldness.

- Inhibits 5α-reductase type I and II by blocking conversion of testosterone to DHT, slowing the binding to androgen receptors and therefore slowing miniaturization of hair.
- Lowers DHT in serum, prostate, and scalp by 60% to 70% (Lolli et al., 2017).
- Dosed once daily with treatment response assessed at the end of 6 months but may take up to 12 months in some men.
- Adverse effects are uncommon, but may include gynecomastia, reduced libido, erectile dysfunction, and ejaculatory disorders (Lolli et al., 2017). These typically resolve with continued use and usually reverse when discontinued.
- Most effective in preventing progression of hair loss.
- Treatment continued indefinitely to maintain results.
- Other—combination use of minoxidil and finasteride, although there is no supporting evidence of improved efficacy.

Management and Patient Education

- MPHL is a cosmetic concern where both medical and surgical treatments are available. Determining how aggressive your patient wants to be is important when suggesting therapies.
- Medical therapies do not cure, but instead slow the progression and promote a thicker hair shaft. They also cannot grow hair on bald areas void of hair follicle.
- Realistic patient expectations should be emphasized at each visit as the process to "see" a change is slow. Serial photographs can be a helpful tool in gauging treatment success.
- Remember, it is important to treat any concomitant scalp conditions like seborrheic dermatitis or TE, and patients should be reminded at each visit to avoid any harsh treatments on the hair or scalp.
- Referral to providers who specialize in hair transplantation or cosmetic camouflage may be necessary.

CLINICAL PEARLS

- Serial photography will help document treatment success.
- Minoxidil and finasteride are the only two FDA-approved treatment options; and if these medical treatments are successful, they will need to be continued indefinitely.
- Surgical options include autologous hair transplantation.

Female Pattern Hair Loss

Female pattern hair loss (FPHL), the preferred term for androgenic alopecia in women, is the most common disorder of hair loss in women (Fabbrocini et al., 2018). Approximately 12% of women initially present with FPHL by age 30 years, and more than 50% by age 80 years (Fabbrocini et al., 2018). Just as with MPHL, FPHL is more commonly seen in Caucasian females and less in Asian women. These differences may depend on genetic and biochemical factors that regulate hair growth as hirsutism is also less commonly present in Asian women (Carmina et al., 2019). As with men, the hair loss is diffuse and nonscarring with a typical presenting complaint of "I can see my scalp" or "I am getting a sunburn on my scalp."

The most common comorbidities associated with FPHL are endocrine in nature—polycystic ovarian syndrome, metabolic syndrome, which can lead to an increased risk of coronary artery diseases. The association between low ferritin levels and FPHL is controversial.

Pathophysiology

- FPHL results from progressive miniaturization of the hair follicle with subsequent conversion of terminal follicles into vellus-like follicle; however, unlike MPHL, the miniaturization is not uniform and there are no complete areas of baldness in most cases (Fabbrocini et al., 2018).
- Although FPHL and MPHL share a final common pathway that results in follicular regression, hair loss in women may occur even in the absence of elevated androgen levels.
- Estrogen protects against hair loss and therefore FPHL is seen to some degree in all women who are postmenopausal. It is believed that currently unidentified genetic, nonandrogenic factors along with environmental influence may play a role in the development of FPHL.

Clinical Presentation

- The presenting hair loss is usually thinning noticed on the central hairline with frontal accentuation. Rarely will they present with the vertex/male pattern (Carmina et al., 2019).
- Excess shedding is not a symptom.
- The part width is increased when compared to the temporal and occipital areas and is often described as a Christmas tree pattern (Fig. 11.1-5).
- There can be significant miniaturization and thinning of the crown, but the frontal border of hair is always preserved (Fig. 11.1-6). The presence of follicular ostia (opening) is a sign that regrowth is possible. Loss of these ostia implies a scarring process as there is loss of the follicular unit and sebaceous gland (Carmina et al., 2019).

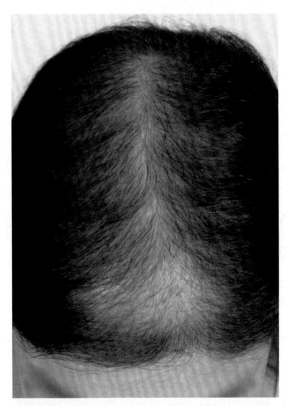

FIG. 11.1-5. Female pattern hair loss begins with widening central part and diffuse thinning. Hair is thinning over the crown and vertex with sparing of the frontal hairline. (Used with permission from Hall, J. C., & Hall, B. J. [2017]. *Sauer's manual of skin diseases* [11th ed.]. Wolters Kluwer.)

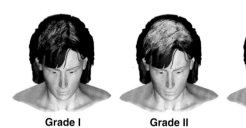

Grade I	Grade II	Grade III

FIG. 11.1-6. Ludwig classification of female pattern hair loss. Note the retention of the frontal hairline despite the increasing severity of hair loss. (LifeART image copyright © 2014 Wolters Kluwer Health | Lippincott Williams & Wilkins. All rights reserved.)

- Small areas with no hair on the central scalp are seen in 44% of women and more common in late-onset FPHL (Carmina et al., 2019).

DIFFERENTIAL DIAGNOSIS   Female Pattern Hair Loss

- Telogen effluvium (acute and chronic)—generalized, persistent shedding; + hair pull test; underlying conditions/medications
- Postpartum hair loss—occurs 2 to 3 months post delivery
- Alopecia areata—acute onset
- Central centrifugal cicatricial alopecia—loss of follicular openings; associated with burning, itching, tenderness
- Frontal fibrosing alopecia—symmetrical hair and eyebrow loss; postmenopausal

---

Confirming the Diagnosis

- Hair pull test—used to evaluate the number of hairs shed after slight traction of about 50 to 60 hairs between the thumb and index finger. More than six (10%) grasped hairs shed indicates a positive test. Fewer than six hairs is considered normal shedding (Fabbrocini et al., 2018).
- Modified wash test—helps to distinguish between FPHL and TE. Patients refrain from hair washing for 5 days, then after shampooing, the number of shed hairs are counted and divided into groups by length (<3 cm or >5 cm). Approximately 10 to 100 hairs ≥5 cm indicates FPHL (Rebora, 2019).
- Scalp biopsy—4-mm punch biopsy.
- Dermoscopy—can help determine if follicular ostia are present.
- Laboratory evaluation for total and free testosterone.
- Additional laboratory evaluation including iron indices, vitamin D, zinc, TSH, and prolactin if history and physical examination warrant.

Treatment

Topical

- Minoxidil
  - 2% or 5% Solution; 5% foam—FDA approved and considered first-line treatment.
  - The 2% solution twice daily is considered equivalent to 5% foam applied once daily (Fabbrocini et al., 2018).
  - Same treatment course, adverse effects, and follow-up evaluation as MPHL.
- LLL, platelet-rich plasma (PRP), and microneedling may be used as adjuvant therapy (Fabbrocini et al., 2018).

- Hair transplant, combination therapy of the above treatments, and camouflage methods are similar to MPHL.
- Ketoconazole 2% shampoo—may be beneficial in FPHL with hyperandrogenism due to its antiandrogen effects at follicular androgen receptors (Fabbrocini et al., 2018). While not considered a monotherapy, it can be used in combination with the above treatments.

Systemic

- Finasteride
  - Off-label use in FPHL with several studies conducted in postmenopausal women with some data supporting cautious use in premenopausal women with androgen excess and hair loss.
  - Usually dosed at 2.5 mg once daily.
  - Contraindicated in pregnancy and lactation due to risk of feminization of male fetus (Carmina et al., 2019).
- Spironolactone
  - Potassium-sparing diuretic used for its antiandrogen activity.
  - Dosed 100 to 200 mg daily, its off-label use in FPHL has shown to stabilize hair loss and promote hair regrowth in 44% to 74% of patients (Carmina et al., 2019).
  - Best results noted in patients with FPHL and hirsutism or acne (Carmina et al., 2019).
  - Adverse effects include postural hypotension, electrolyte disturbances, menstrual irregularities, breast tenderness, and fatigue (Fabbrocini et al., 2018).
- Cyproterone acetate (CPA)—CPA is used as a progestin and antiandrogen in hormonal birth control formulations and has been used in the treatment of androgen-dependent conditions with mixed results; it is not available in the United States.

Management and Patient Education

- Management of FPHL is the same as MPHL. If androgen levels are elevated and/or abnormal, a referral to an endocrinologist may be necessary.
- Patient counseling should emphasize that FPHL is a lifelong problem with no cure, and most treatments will need to be continued indefinitely.

Telogen Effluvium

Telogen effluvium (TE) is a nonscarring, noninflammatory diffuse hair loss with a sudden onset that affects both sexes and all age groups. TE can be classified as acute or chronic (lasting >6 months). The chronic form tends to occur more often in women aged 30 to 60 years. TE is considered to be a common form of hair loss, but the exact incidence is unknown. Many patients initially report, "I am noticing a lot of hair in the shower drain." This can cause significant psychological stress and require empathy and time on the part of the clinician to appropriately treat these patients.

Pathophysiology

- A physiologic or emotional stressor leads to an alteration of the hair cycle, which results in 70% of hairs entering the telogen phase. These hairs shed 3 to 5 months later.
- Triggers implicated in the development of TE include chronic illnesses, pregnancy and childbirth, surgery, high fever, nutritional deficiencies, endocrine disorders, emotional events, and

medications (i.e., warfarin, isotretinoin, β-blockers, ACE inhibitors, oral contraceptives, antithyroid medications) to name a few (Phillips et al., 2017).

- Hair loss in TE is actually a sign of hair regrowth as the resting hair is pushed out by new hairs.

Clinical Presentation

- Uniform hair shedding with no erythema, scaling, or changes in hair distribution, hair shaft caliber, length, or fragility (Phillips et al., 2017).
- No noticeable scalp abnormalities.
- Usually asymptomatic, but some will complain of itching, discomfort, or a feeling like a needle prick on the scalp (Rebora, 2019).
- Nails (as they grow under the same influence as hair) may show Beau lines that will help determine when the inciting event occurred.
- All other hair-bearing areas will be normal.

DIFFERENTIAL DIAGNOSIS   Telogen Effluvium

- Female pattern hair loss—not acute; progressive hair loss
- Male pattern hair loss—not acute; progressive hair loss
- Diffuse alopecia areata—will show lymphocytic perifollicular infiltrate on biopsy
- Diffuse anagen effluvium—more severe hair loss

Confirming the Diagnosis

- Diagnosis is usually based on clinical presentation and history. It takes approximately 100 days for hairs to shed; therefore, the diagnosis of TE depends on the chronology of past events and symptoms.
- The precipitating event is usually identified and precedes the hair loss by approximately 3 to 4 months. The shedding continues for about 1 to 2 months but may last 4 to 6 months before it subsides.
- Hair pull test—as described above, will be positive. A negative test may indicate FPHL or MPHL. A test with more than 70% to 80% telogens should prompt the clinician to investigate an underlying metabolic or drug-associated etiology.
- Modified wash test—as described above with more than 100 hairs (median ~300 hairs) >5 cm (Rebora, 2019).
- Scalp biopsy—rarely needed. Would show normal ratio of vellus to terminal hairs, increased number of telogen hairs, and no inflammation.

Treatment

- Usually self-limited and no specific treatment is required except assurance, patience, and time.
- On occasion, patients can be quite anxious and request some form of treatment. For these individuals, clobetasol 0.05% solution or foam for 3 months (Rebora, 2019). The effectiveness is difficult to ascertain as the very nature of the condition will improve despite treatment.
- The use of minoxidil 2% or 5% solution can cause synchronization of the hair cycles and is not recommended.
- Recognition and treatment of triggering events is very important.

Management and Patient Education

- Continue to counsel patients that TE is self-limited, will not result in permanent baldness, and will resolve spontaneously. It can recur and become chronic in some individuals.
- New hairs may not have the thickness or texture of the original hair.
- Lack of regrowth in a timely manner should prompt the clinician to exclude other diseases like iron-deficiency anemia or endocrinopathies, with referral as needed.
- Reassurance and psychological support is vital. Patients should be advised that although they feel that they have less hair, they have the same number of hair follicles and hair shafts as before.
- Patient follow-up is necessary if there is no resolution in the anticipated time frame discussed above.

CLINICAL PEARLS

- Patients report increased shedding even if the density of the hair appears normal to the examiner.
- Patients may begin to shampoo less often in hopes of preserving hair. They fail to realize that the average number of hairs lost daily is more evident on days they shampoo.

Anagen Effluvium

Anagen effluvium is the sudden loss of hair, either partial or complete. The most common cause is chemotherapy, radiation, and, rarely, severe emotional or physical trauma. Chemotherapy-induced anagen effluvium occurs in approximately 65% of patients (Phillips et al., 2017). Other causes include severe protein malnutrition, alopecia areata (AA), systemic disease (systemic lupus erythematosus [SLE], secondary syphilis), exposure to mercury, and rarely medications (i.e., levodopa, bismuth, allopurinol, colchicine, and cyclosporine) (Kanwar & Narang, 2013).

Pathophysiology

- In this process, the rapidly dividing cells of the matrix are affected, leaving hair shafts that are narrowed, weakened, and easily broken.
- Additionally, hair follicles do not convert (or progress) into a growth phase (Kanwar & Narang, 2013). The hairs are then shed in unison, about 1 to 3 weeks after the insult.
- The hair loss is usually reversible within a few weeks following cessation of chemotherapy and regrowth is visible within 1 to 3 months (Kanwar & Narang, 2013).
- Occasionally, hair texture and color are different than pretreatment.
- Radiation-induced anagen effluvium may not be completely reversible (Kanwar & Narang, 2013) (Fig. 11.1-7).

Clinical Presentation

As with TE, the examination of the scalp shows no erythema, scaling, pigmentation or scarring, and follicular ostia are intact (Kanwar & Narang, 2013).

- The amount of hair loss in anagen effluvium can be profound (80% to 90%), as the majority of the hairs are in the anagen phase of growth.
- Other hair-bearing areas (i.e., eyebrows, eyelashes, and body hair) may also be affected.

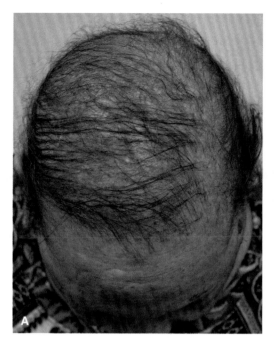

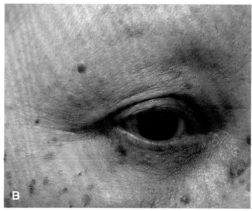

FIG. 11.1-7. A: Anagen effluvium is the sudden and complete loss of hair, usually occurring 2 to 3 weeks after chemotherapy. **B:** The scalp, eyebrows, or eyelashes can be affected. Regrowth occurs after therapy is discontinued, but the texture and color may be different. (Photos courtesy of M. Bobonich.)

DIFFERENTIAL DIAGNOSIS   Anagen Effluvium

- Telogen effluvium—shedding onset is 2 to 4 months after insult; less profound hair loss; normal hair shaft
- Female pattern hair loss
- Male pattern hair loss
- Trichotillomania—localized patch of alopecia with irregular hair lengths; eyebrows may be affected

Confirming the Diagnosis

The diagnosis of anagen effluvium is mainly clinical and based on the history and physical examination.

- Hair pull test—will show tapered fracture of hair shafts
- Biopsy—4-mm punch biopsy rarely needed. Will show <15% of hair follicles in the telogen phase (normal) and no inflammation (Kanwar & Narang, 2013).
- Laboratory workup as dictated by cause (i.e., systemic disease, nutritional deficiency, etc.)

Treatment

Topical

- A scalp tourniquet or scalp hypothermia have been utilized; however, these methods are typically only effective with chemotherapy agents with a short half-life (Kanwar & Narang, 2013).
- Topical minoxidil can shorten the time of baldness by an average of 50 days, aiding in faster regrowth of hair once chemotherapy has been discontinued.
- Anagen effluvium is typically reversible without special treatment.

Management and Patient Education

- Patient management should focus on addressing the psychological aspects of the disorder.

- Reassure patients that the hair loss is usually temporary and will regrow normally within a few weeks (complete regrowth takes 3 to 6 months) after completion of chemotherapy, but color and hair texture may change.
- General hair care recommendations include avoiding physical or chemical trauma to the hair, using a satin pillowcase (less likely to pull on fragile hair), and gentle brushing and shampooing.
- Cutting the hair short may give a fuller appearance to the hair and shedding may be less noticeable (Kanwar & Narang, 2013).
- Camouflage techniques may also be useful.

NONSCARRING ALOPECIA—LOCALIZED

Alopecia Areata

Alopecia areata (AA) is a total loss of hair at a specific site. While it affects only approximately 2% of the population, men and women are affected equally. The age of onset can vary but the first occurrence is before the age of 20 years in 60% of cases. AA can occur as a single episode or have a remission/recurrence pattern, especially in patients with early onset, extensive involvement, or rapid progression. AA is associated with higher than expected rates of thyroid disease, atopy, vitiligo, and lupus erythematosus, and can have a significant psychological impact on patients' lives (Renert-Yuval & Guttman-Yassky, 2017).

Pathophysiology

- The exact cause of AA is unknown but is believed to have a genetic predisposition with an environmental trigger.
- This results in T-cell accumulation with release of cytokines and chemokines at the hair bulb.
- In the area of hair loss, the follicles have entered the telogen phase. As a result, the hair shaft is poorly formed and breaks at the scalp. However, the follicle remains intact.

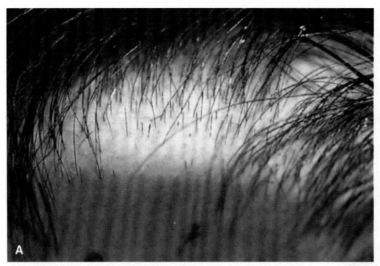

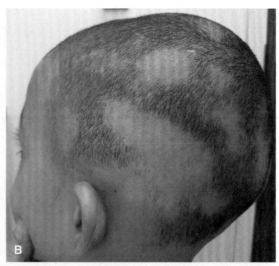

FIG. 11.1-8. Alopecia areata. **A:** "Exclamation" hairs (tapering at the proximal end with "!" appearance) are noted at the periphery of a well-circumscribed patch of alopecia. Typically, this condition responds to intralesional corticosteroids. **B:** AA in children can appear similar to tinea capitis (noninflammatory), which should be considered in the differential diagnosis. (Photos courtesy of M. Bobonich.)

Clinical Presentation

- Patients complain of a sudden "bald spot." The area may be preceded by a feeling of itching or burning. *Areata* means circumscribed areas with distinct borders, which in AA begins as round 1- to 4-cm areas of spot loss.

- The involved skin is normal in color and smooth, without scarring, scale, or erythema. Hairs on the periphery of the area break at the surface and resemble an "exclamation point" because of a narrow proximal end, widening into the thicker distal shaft (Fig. 11.1-8A,B).

- AA is most common on the scalp but sometimes affects the beard, eyelashes, eyebrows—places that should also entertain a possible diagnosis of trichotillomania.

- A pattern of hair loss surrounding the head like a band is referred to as an *ophiasis* pattern (Fig. 11.1-9). Complete loss of hair on the scalp is termed *alopecia totalis* (Fig. 11.1-10), while the loss of hair on the entire body, including eyelashes and eyebrows, is referred to as *alopecia universalis*.

- Be sure to check the nails, as nail changes are present in about 20% of AA patients. Proximal nail shedding, longitudinal ridging, and pitting have been observed (see Section 11.2 for Nail Disorders).

DIFFERENTIAL DIAGNOSIS   Alopecia Areata

- Tinea capitis—will see scale, crust
- Trichotillomania—hair of varying length; unusual shape of hair loss
- MPHL—slow onset; progressive loss
- Syphilis—patchy, "moth-eaten" appearance
- Telogen effluvium—diffuse hair loss; no balding

Confirming the Diagnosis

- AA is often a clinical diagnosis supported by the presence of exclamation-point hairs. Further diagnostic testing is usually not

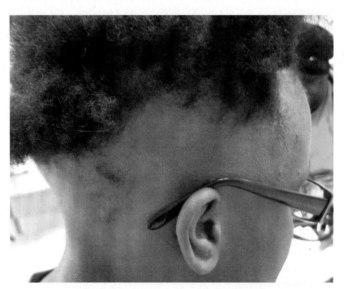

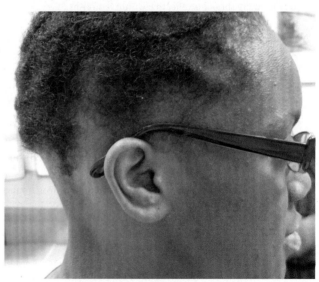

FIG. 11.1-9. Ophiasis pattern AA, a band-like distribution around the scalp. It usually has a poor prognosis for hair growth. (Photo courtesy of M. Bobonich.)

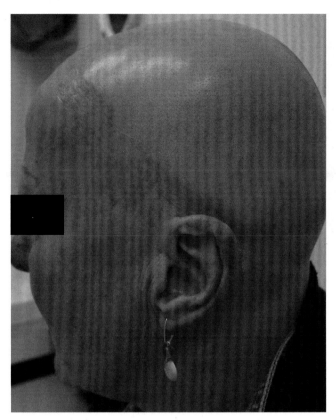

FIG. 11.1-10. Alopecia totalis. (Image provided by Stedman's.)

indicated. However, clinicians should have a high index of suspicion if the history and physical examination indicate a possible associated autoimmune disease. In those cases, a punch biopsy can be helpful.

- Fungal culture and lymphatic examination can rule out tinea.
- RPR or VDRL testing if secondary syphilis is suspected.

Treatment

Topical

- Topical mid- to high-potency topical corticosteroids (TCS) once to twice daily should be effective within 3 months.
- Topical minoxidil 2% to 5% can be used as monotherapy or in combination with the TCS. Warn patients of the risk of increased hair shedding with initial therapy.
- Topical therapy with anthralin (a tar derivative), diphenylcyclopropenone (DCHP), or squaric acid (which are not widely available) has been used effectively by experienced dermatology providers.

Systemic

- Psoralen plus UVA and excimer laser have reported good results.
- Intralesional triamcinolone 10 mg/mL diluted 1:1 with lidocaine or normal saline can be effective for limited areas to stimulate new hair growth (Fig. 11.1-8). Injections can be repeated every 4 to 6 weeks for 3 months. If the AA is in the beard area, the concentration of triamcinolone should be reduced to 2.5% per mL. Clinicians performing these injections should be experienced and the patient advised of the risks and side effects of atrophy, telangiectasias, and abnormal pigmentation.
- Systemic corticosteroids should be avoided.

- Referral to dermatology for systemic therapies which could include finasteride, spironolactone, and/or novel Janus kinase (JAK) inhibitor drugs.

Management and Patient Education

- Treatment depends on age, location, extent of hair loss, and the length of time the alopecia has persisted. Small areas will regrow, and treatment may not be necessary. The goal of treatment is to stimulate regrowth in affected areas.
- Hair regrowth can be spontaneous, but timing is unpredictable. Regrowth commonly occurs within 1 to 3 months, and total hair regrowth is seen most of the time.
- Treatment does not affect the course of the disease nor does it prevent new areas of loss.
- The hairs may be the original color or they may be fine and white initially, but their presence on a follow-up examination can be encouraging for the patient. Alopecia totalis, universalis, and ophiasis patterns have a poor prognosis for regrowth.
- If a topical or intralesional corticosteroid has been used over a 2- to 3-month period without improvement, or if the hair loss involves large areas, referral to a dermatology provider is essential to confirm the diagnosis and consider other treatment options.
- Consultation with a reputable wig maker and/or psychological counseling may be helpful to patients in dealing with this skin disease.
- The National Alopecia Areata Foundation provides information and support for both patients and providers.

CLINICAL PEARLS

- Failure to grow back may warrant consideration of trichotillomania.
- Associated autoimmune disorders may be discovered as a result of the patient's presentation of AA.

Trichotillomania

Trichotillomania is classified by the Diagnostic and Statistical Manual of Mental Disorders (DSM-5) as an obsessive-compulsive or related disorder where the person repeatedly pulls or twists their hair until it is extracted, creating noticeable hair loss (Henkel et al., 2019). The age of onset is between 10 and 13 years old, is more common in females in late adolescence, and has a lifetime prevalence of 1% to 3% (Henkel et al., 2019). The most commonly affected sites are the scalp, eyebrows, eyelashes, and pubic area. Often a parent or teacher will report the behavior; however, the behavior may not be seen if the child does it only in private or at bedtime. Trichotillomania can have significant psychosocial sequelae.

Pathophysiology

- This is a self-induced impulse control disorder. Trauma from twisting or rubbing results in hair loss by extraction. This continued trauma to the hair follicle can potentially lead to skin infections and permanent scarring.
- Trichotillomania is associated with depressive or anxiety conditions or may be a habit or tic. The act of pulling hair provides a sense of relief, satisfaction, or pleasure to the patient.

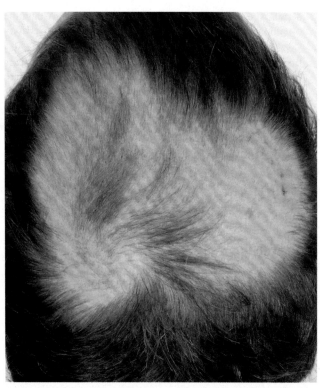

FIG. 11.1-11. Trichotillomania is characterized by irregular-shaped patches of hair loss along with varied lengths of remaining hairs. Note the excoriations on the right. (Used with permission from Hall, J. C., & Hall, B. J. [2017]. *Sauer's manual of skin diseases* [11th ed.]. Wolters Kluwer.)

- Trichophagia (ingestion of pulled hair), a rare subset of pica, can occur concomitantly and result in formation of trichobezoars (hair balls in the stomach), which can lead to significant gastro-intestinal complications (Henkel et al., 2019).

Clinical Presentation

- Hallmark sign of trichotillomania is an area of hair loss with irregular borders and hairs of various lengths present at the same time.
- Commonly seen in the easily reached frontoparietal region of the scalp and should always be suspected when there is hair loss of the eyebrows or eyelashes.
- No inflammation or scarring present (Fig. 11.1-11).

DIFFERENTIAL DIAGNOSIS   Trichotillomania

- Tinea capitis—scaling, erythema, crusting
- Alopecia areata—complete, smooth loss of hair at the site
- Pressure alopecia—due to helmet
- Traction alopecia—associated with hair styles/care

Confirming the Diagnosis

- Direct examination of hairs under a microscope or with a derma-toscope will usually reveal a normal tapered end.
- Hair pull test—negative.
- Wood lamp—negative for fungal infection.

- Punch biopsy—majority of the hairs are in anagen phase and not in telogen, differentiating it from TE.

Therapeutics and Management

- No optimal therapy for trichotillomania exists. Current treatments ideally include a combination of cognitive behavioral therapy, electronic devices that monitor habits, hypnotherapy, support groups, N-acetylcysteine, and tricyclic antidepressants or selective serotonin inhibitors (especially in the setting of comorbid anxiety and/or depression) (Henkel et al., 2019).
- Identification and awareness of hair pulling behavior is crucial to improving the disorder.
- Referral for psychological evaluation and behavioral modification is key to the treatment of trichotillomania.

Traction Alopecia

Traction alopecia (TA) is hair loss caused by prolonged stress or pulling on an area of the scalp usually by hairstyles such as braids, ponytails, cornrows, weaves, dreadlocks, hot combs, hair straighteners, or rollers. The risk of TA is higher when aforementioned hairstyles are done on hair that has been chemically relaxed (Billero & Miteva, 2018). Development of TA is highest in women and children of African descent due in large part to the characteristic curved African hair follicle and cultural hairstyling practices. (Billero & Miteva, 2018).

Pathophysiology

Usually caused by hairstyles such as braids, ponytails, cornrows, weaves, dreadlocks, hot combs, hair straighteners, or rollers. If prolonged, can result in scarring.

Clinical Presentation

- Alopecia is usually seen on the periphery, most commonly the frontal and temporal scalp, although any area can be affected depending on the hairstyle (Billero & Miteva, 2018).
- Scalp usually normal early on, but some evidence of inflammation, papules or pustules, and broken hairs may be present. Over time, follicular loss and scarring occur (Fig. 11.1-12).

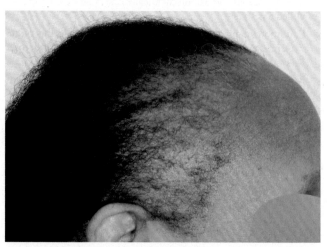

FIG. 11.1-12. Traction alopecia caused by the pulling or traction associated with hair styles like corn rows. (Used with permission from Hall, J. C., & Hall, B. J. [2017]. *Sauer's manual of skin diseases* [11th ed.]. Wolters Kluwer.)

- Trichotillomania—history of self-induced hair pulling
- Alopecia areata—acute onset
- Frontal fibrosing alopecia—lichen planopilaris variant; typically seen only on frontal hairline
- Central centrifugal cicatricial alopecia—begins on scalp vertex and spreads

Confirming the Diagnosis

- In most cases, the diagnosis is made clinically and further testing is not necessary.
- Trichoscopy (dermoscopic imaging of scalp and hair)—decreased hair density with absence of follicular ostia or absence of hairs with preserved ostia. Hair casts (yellowish-white cylinders around traumatized hair shaft) may be present.
- Punch biopsy—similar findings to trichotillomania; preservation of sebaceous gland and no perifollicular inflammatory infiltrate.

Treatment

- Early awareness of the causative action usually results in a change in style or hair care regime. Avoidance of any traction or chemical stress on hair is advised.
- Topical or intralesional corticosteroids are useful in early disease to combat inflammatory changes (Billero & Miteva, 2018).
- Topical or systemic antibiotics to treat infection and for their anti-inflammatory properties.
- Topical minoxidil 2% or 5% may also offer some benefit. Adverse effects and clinical course similar to use in patterned hair loss.
- Hair transplantation for advanced stages of TA as scarring and follicular atrophy is not responsive to medical management.

Management and Patient Education

- The hair loss is usually temporary unless the traction is continued after the initial symptoms and then permanent scarring changes may occur.
- Patients should be encouraged to engage in gentle hair care practices and avoid the use of chemical relaxers along with tightly pulled hairstyles.
- Education of high-risk populations should include the motto "Tolerate pain from a hairstyle and risk hair loss" (Billero & Miteva, 2018).
- Referral to a dermatology provider or specialist in hair transplantation may be necessary if initial therapy is unsuccessful.

CLINICAL PEARLS

- The early terminal hairs present on the back of the infant's head are shed at 3 to 4 months of age. This is often thought to be related to rubbing while sleeping, but is in fact a natural and expected occurrence.

SCARRING ALOPECIA—LOCALIZED

- *Primary* scarring (cicatricial) alopecias represent a series of conditions that usually involve a significant inflammatory process that targets and destroys hair follicles, creates scarring in the reticular dermis, and subsequent permanent hair loss. Categorizing these conditions is often confusing, and there is considerable overlap.
- *Secondary* scarring alopecias are the result of a disease process unrelated to the follicle but which ultimately results in follicular destruction and hair loss. Examples of secondary scarring alopecia are chronic infections, deep burns, and radiation dermatitis. In this section, however, we will only discuss the primary scarring alopecias.

Discoid Lupus Erythematosus

Discoid lupus erythematosus (DLE), the most common form of chronic cutaneous lupus erythematosus, is an autoimmune, inflammatory process which results in scarring of the affected areas. It affects females more than males, is slightly more common in African American women, and occurs between the ages of 20 and 45, with peak occurrence in the fourth decade. DLE is usually limited to the skin. The incidence of developing SLE has been estimated to be 5% to 10%, with some newer evidence that this occurs in approximately 16% of cases. The most significant complication of DLE is the depigmentation, scarring, and alopecia, which are permanent. Repigmentation can occur after treatment, but is less likely when there is scarring or destruction of hair follicles.

Pathophysiology

- While there is more known about SLE as an autoimmune disorder, DLE is less well understood.
- It is thought to occur in genetically predisposed individuals; however, the genetic connection is unclear.
- Environmental factors, such as ultraviolet light exposure or trauma, are thought to be precipitating factors.
- A heat-shock protein is then induced within keratinocytes, leading to T-cell–mediated destruction of the epidermal cells.

Clinical Presentation

- Early lesions are erythematous papules evolving into well-demarcated plaques with adherent scale; usually localized but can produce generalized lesions. It is commonly seen on the face, scalp, ears, and upper trunk.
- The scale penetrates the follicles and if lifted, reveals the characteristic spines on the undersurface, which is said to resemble a *carpet tack*, the hallmark sign of DLE.
- Plugging of the follicles is a characteristic finding as the lesions progress, and is often seen in the conchal bowl of the ear.
- Areas of involvement may also exhibit telangiectasia and central hypopigmentation with peripheral hyperpigmentation (Fig. 11.1-13A,B).
- Scarring alopecia can be widespread and disfiguring with progressive and advanced disease.

DIFFERENTIAL DIAGNOSIS Discoid Lupus Erythematous

- Granuloma annulare—no scaling; rarely occurs on the face or scalp, no scarring
- Subacute cutaneous lupus erythematosus—slight scale; on sun exposed areas
- Plaque psoriasis—thicker, scaling lesions; location on elbows, knees
- Lichen planus—commonly seen on flexural areas of limbs
- Lichen planopilaris

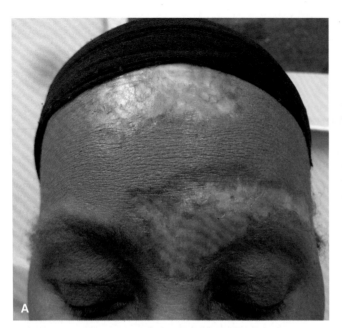
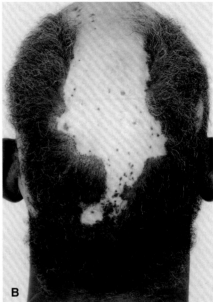

FIG. 11.1-13. Discoid lupus erythematosus. **A:** Scarring (permanent) alopecia and red scaly atrophic plaques are seen on the crown of the scalp. (Photo courtesy of M. Bobonich.) **B:** Depigmented atrophic plaques with hyperpigmented borders are typical of "burnt out" inactive discoid lupus; these changes are permanent. (Used with permission from Hall, J. C., & Hall, B. J. [2017]. *Sauer's manual of skin diseases* [11th ed.]. Wolters Kluwer.)

Confirming the Diagnosis

- Antinuclear antibody (ANA) testing—to rule out SLE, but is negative most of the time.

- Punch biopsy—from lesional skin, usually confirmatory and demonstrates hyperkeratosis, follicular plugging, and a lymphocytic infiltrate.

- Direct immunofluorescence biopsy—lesional and/or nonlesional, will be positive the majority of the time.

Treatment

Topical

- Initial treatment of DLE consists of complete UV light protection and use of broad-spectrum sunscreens at all times.

- High-potency TCS, such as clobetasol ointment 0.05%, should be used in early lesions to minimize inflammation and scarring. Patients should be cautioned about risk of atrophy, telangiectasia, striae, purpura, and hypertrichosis with long-term use.

- Intralesional injections of triamcinolone at concentrations of 3 to 5 mg/mL can be used on the scalp. If newer lesions continue to occur or existing ones continue to be active, systemic treatment may be needed.

- Topical calcineurin inhibitors (TCI), such as pimecrolimus 1% or tacrolimus 0.3% or 0.1%, alone or in combination with TCS or antimalarials, have been shown to improve DLE. Most common adverse effects include burning and stinging, which usually resolves with continued use (Company-Quiroga et al., 2019).

Systemic

- Hydroxychloroquine is considered first-line oral treatment, and can be used alone or in combination with other treatment modalities. Adverse effects include skin rashes (including hyperpigmentation, urticaria, morbilliform rash), gastrointestinal symptoms, and ophthalmic effects. The American Academy of Ophthalmology recommends a baseline examination within the first year of hydroxychloroquine use and again in 5 years in a low-risk individual. Individuals at high risk for developing maculopathy should continue to have screening every 6 months. CBC, LFTs, and G6PD are performed before initiating hydroxychloroquine use and annually thereafter.

- Other treatments include methotrexate, azathioprine, systemic retinoids, thalidomide, dapsone, and biologic agents (Company-Quiroga et al., 2019).

Management and Patient Education

- Patient education should focus on lifestyle modifications, photoprotection, and smoking cessation.

- Studies confirm that smoking is associated with worsening of DLE, worse quality of life, and potentially decreased efficacy of antimalarial agents.

- High-potency TCS should be started early in the disease.

- If cutaneous lesions of DLE remain active, follow-up visits at 4- to 6-week intervals are recommended.

- Patients should be advised to return if they develop any systemic symptoms. Routine follow-up depends on the drug therapy.

- Referral to a rheumatologist is recommended if patients present with symptoms of SLE or if the clinician has any suspicion of systemic disease.

Central Centrifugal Scarring Alopecia

Central centrifugal scarring alopecia (CCCA) is a progressive, scarring alopecia that can occur in all races and both sexes, but is generally seen in African American women. It typically presents in the third decade and affects approximately 3% to 6% of the population (Dlova et al., 2017). CCCA has been referred to as "hot comb alopecia," "follicular degeneration syndrome," "pseudopelade," "folliculitis

decalvans," and "tufted folliculitis." There is a suspected association between CCCA and development of diabetes mellitus but there is no evidence to support it at this time.

Pathophysiology

The cause of CCCA is multifactorial. Genetic inheritance combined with certain hair care practices, heat (hot combs, flat irons, or hair relaxers), chemical treatments, and hairstylings that use traction, are considered to increase the risk for development of CCCA (Dlova et al., 2017).

Clinical Presentation

- Hair breakage is often an initial sign and is commonly seen with the use of chemical hair products.
- Hair loss initially presents at the crown and remains most severe on the crown or vertex of the scalp, gradually expanding in a centrifugal fashion (Fig. 11.1-14).
- Affected scalp may appear smooth and shiny with loss of follicular ostia, and in some areas, a few short, brittle hairs remain within the scarred expanse.
- Pustules and crusting may be found, and folliculitis decalvans may overlap.
- Patients may complain of mild pruritus or tenderness in the affected areas.
- The condition progresses slowly, but long-standing or severe disease can result in scarring of the entire crown.

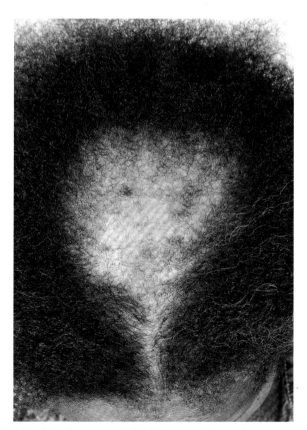

FIG. 11.1-14. Central centrifugal cicatricial alopecia. This condition occurs most commonly in African Americans and affects the crown and vertex scalp. Hair loss is permanent. (Used with permission from Hall, J. C., & Hall, B. J. [2017]. *Sauer's manual of skin diseases* [11th ed.]. Wolters Kluwer.)

Confirming the Diagnosis

- Punch biopsy of the scalp—required for definitive diagnosis. Demonstrates specific findings of hyalinization of dermal collagen and broad tree trunk–like fibrous tracts.
- Dermoscopy—shows perihilar white/gray halos around follicles (Dlova et al., 2017).

Treatment

Topical

- Cessation of all heat treatments and relaxers as well as avoiding hairstyles that require traction must be initiated.
- Similar to treatment of DLE on the scalp, high-potency TCS, intralesional corticosteroids TCI have been used with some success.
- Minoxidil 2% to 5% solution may be used to regrow hair in patients with viable follicles.
- Hair transplantation in patients with stable disease for 9 to 12 months, with absence of inflammation, can be considered (Dlova et al., 2017).

Systemic

- Oral antibiotics such as doxycycline or minocycline, may be used in addition to TCS if pustules are present on examination.
- Hydroxychloroquine has been used with some success.

Management and Patient Education

- Early intervention may minimize the scarring process.
- Patient education should focus on a thorough understanding of the etiology of CCCA and discontinuation of hair care practices that contribute to the development of this scarring alopecia.
- Cicatricial Alopecia Research Foundation (CARF) has abundant literature and resources for these patients, and certain communities, especially near large teaching hospitals, have chapters of CARF that hold regular educational meetings.
- Patients should be referred to a dermatology provider as soon as possible as early treatment may minimize additional scarring.
- Due to existing scarring, transplanted hairs may not survive.

Lichen Planopilaris

Lichen planopilaris (LPP) is a cicatricial alopecia that is referred to by some authors as a follicular form of lichen planus, but only 30% present with characteristic lesions of lichen planus on the skin of the extremities and mucous membranes.

- LPP has two clinical variants, frontal fibrosing alopecia and Graham-Little-Piccardi-Lasseur syndrome.
- LPP is more commonly seen in women and Caucasians, with a peak incidence in the third to sixth decade of life (Errichetti et al., 2018).

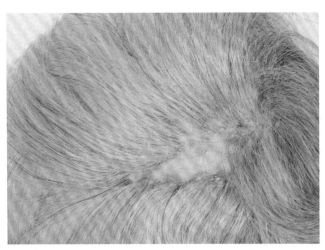

FIG. 11.1-15. Lichen planopilaris. LPP has a characteristic perifollicular erythema and scale. (Used with permission from Hall, J. C., & Hall, B. J. [2017]. *Sauer's manual of skin diseases* [11th ed.]. Wolters Kluwer.)

Pathophysiology

- LPP pathogenesis is largely unknown, but is thought to be a hair-specific, inflammatory, autoimmune disorder involving T-lymphocytes that attack the hair follicle stem cells.
- Recent evidence suggests decreased PPAR-γ expression may play a role in the destruction of the pilosebaceous unit seen in LPP (Errichetti et al., 2018).

Clinical Presentation

- Classic presentation is a centrifugal pattern on the frontal and vertex scalp. There are hyperkeratotic follicular papules with characteristic perifollicular scale and perifollicular erythema (Fig. 11.1-15).
- May also see smooth, atrophic patches of alopecia.
- Lesions tend to spread outward, leaving the scarred areas in the center.
- Patients may also complain of pruritus, pain, and/or burning sensation in lesional areas.
- In frontal fibrosing alopecia, postmenopausal women present with bitemporal and frontal recession accompanied by eyebrow loss and erythema.

> **DIFFERENTIAL DIAGNOSIS Lichen Planopilaris**
> - Discoid lupus erythematosus—can occur also on face, ears, extremities
> - Alopecia areata—acute onset; lack of scale and inflammation
> - Central centrifugal cicatricial alopecia—associated hairstyling practices; hair breakage; pustules
> - Folliculitis decalvans—presents with erythema, swelling, and pustules around hair follicle

Confirming the Diagnosis

- Punch biopsy—shows a lichenoid dermatitis at the dermal–epidermal junction. There may be fibrosis around the hair follicles in advanced disease.
- Direct immunofluorescence is positive 50% of the time.

- Dermoscopy—"collar" of perifollicular scaling on proximal hair shaft, fibrotic white dots, loss of follicular ostia, hair tufts, and scattered hyperpigmentation (Errichetti et al., 2018).

Treatment

LPP is very difficult to treat and no studies have shown truly effective treatment. Disease improvement may be due to the normal fluctuation in disease rather than treatment success.

Topical

- High-potency TCS are often first line of treatment.
- Intralesional triamcinolone 5 to 10 mg/mL can also be tried if the areas are small. Widespread and worsening disease may require systemic agents.

Systemic

- Hydroxychloroquine—generally considered a first-line systemic agent. See DLE for adverse effects and monitoring.
- Methotrexate, cyclosporine, mycophenolate mofetil, and pioglitazone (for its immunomodulatory effects on PPAR-γ) are proposed second- and third-line agents for LPP (Errichetti et al., 2018).
- Doxycycline or minocycline 100 mg b.i.d. for their anti-inflammatory effects have been used with some success.
- Trials with biologic agents are also being attempted.

Management and Patient Education

- Treatment of LPP is difficult and is best treated by a dermatology specialist. Early intervention may be helpful to minimize scarring.
- Camouflage with styling or hair pieces can help patients feel more confident in social settings.
- Hair transplantation may be used in advanced disease with varying results due to scarring.

Dissecting Cellulitis

Dissecting cellulitis (DC) is an uncommon scarring alopecia which occurs most frequently in African American men between 20 and 40 years of age, but can occur in any age, race, or sex. DC is known to occur concomitantly with hidradenitis suppurativa, acne conglobata, and pilonidal cysts. The long-term prognosis is poor (Scheinfeld, 2014).

Pathophysiology

The etiology is unknown, but thought to be the result of an inflammatory reaction to hair follicle components, particularly microorganisms.

Clinical Presentation

- Large, inflammatory nodules which evolve into fluctuant boggy, oval, and linear ridges that progress to form extensive interconnected sinus tracts; usually at the crown, vertex, or occiput.
- Fibrosis and permanent hair loss ensue.
- Painful draining nodules may be present and scarring can be extensive (Fig. 11.1-16).

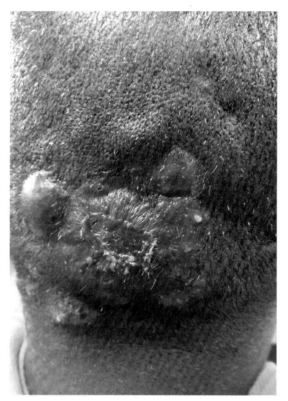

FIG. 11.1-16. Dissecting cellulitis. (Used with permission from Hall, J. C., & Hall, B. J. [2017]. *Sauer's manual of skin diseases* [11th ed.]. Wolters Kluwer.)

DIFFERENTIAL DIAGNOSIS	Dissecting Cellulitis

- Folliculitis decalvans—tufts of hair seen
- Folliculitis keloidalis (acne keloidalis)—small, firm inflammatory papules/pustules at hairline on occiput of scalp
- Fungal kerion
- Ruptured pilar cysts
- Furunculosis

Confirming the Diagnosis

- Physical examination by an experienced dermatology practitioner will generally result in a diagnosis.
- Punch biopsy may be helpful to confirm the diagnosis.
- Bacterial culture

Treatment

Topical

- Intralesional triamcinolone 5 mg/mL to a few affected areas.
- Surgical intervention to drain any large, painful nodules.
- Laser hair removal with resulting patches of alopecia has been successful in some cases.
- Camouflage with the use of wigs and hair pieces may be a last resort.

Systemic

- Antibiotics are used extensively to minimize the inflammatory process and must be continued for the long term with immediate referral to a dermatology specialist.

- Drugs of choice are minocycline 100 mg b.i.d., doxycycline 100 mg b.i.d., and erythromycin 500 mg b.i.d.
- Other antibiotics such as clindamycin and rifampin may be initiated by a specialist.
- A course of systemic antibiotics should be initiated by the primary care clinician, with immediate referral to a dermatology specialist.
- Oral corticosteroids may be used for a short time to decrease inflammation.
- Retinoids such as isotretinoin or acitretin have been used to decrease the follicular keratinization as is seen in cystic acne.
- Dapsone and biologic agents which inhibit TNF-α may be considered for long-term use.

Management and Patient Education

- Patients must understand that the prognosis for this condition is poor and that treatment of new lesions should be done promptly.
- A good skin care regimen with antibacterial cleansers may help discourage secondary infection.
- Loss of weight has been shown to be helpful if the patient is overweight.
- This condition should be managed by dermatology specialists until condition is stable.

HAIR EXCESS

Hirsutism

Hirsutism in females is defined as the presence of male-pattern dark, coarse terminal hairs on the face, chest, lower abdomen, and areola (postpubertal growth areas). Longer, thicker hair may also occur on limbs and trunk. It typically manifests in late teens and progresses with age.

- Hirsutism may be seen with or without virilization (development of male sex characteristics).
- Hirsutism without virilization may simply be the result of genetic, racial, or familial differences. Although, it may represent endocrine dysfunction such as hypothyroidism or be related to drug use, particularly glucocorticoids, minoxidil, oral contraceptives, and phenytoin.
- When hirsutism is associated with virilization, high androgen levels may be caused by polycystic ovary syndrome (PCOS), Cushing syndrome, adrenal hyperplasia, or androgen-secreting tumors. Idiopathic hirsutism can be seen in women with normal ovarian function and normal circulating androgen levels.

Pathophysiology

Hirsutism is usually the result of hyperandrogenism or an increased sensitivity of the hair follicle to androgens. These high androgen levels convert the normal vellus hairs on the body to terminal hairs.

Clinical Presentation

- Hirsutism by definition is excessive hair growth in nine specific areas: face, chest, lower back, upper back, buttocks, inner thighs, external genitalia, linea alba, and areola (Fig. 11.1-17).
- Virilization may be manifested as acne, deepening of the voice, reduction in breast size, clitoral hypertrophy, frontal–temporal balding, increased muscle mass, infrequent or absent menses, heightened libido, and malodorous perspiration.

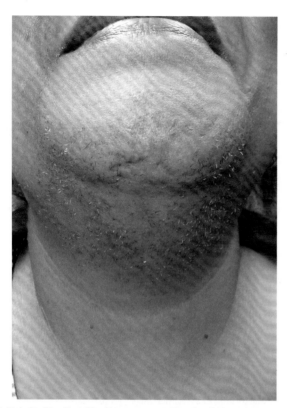

FIG. 11.1-17. Hirsutism. Hirsutism: a woman with extensive terminal hair growth of the beard area. (Used with permission from Hall, J. C., & Hall, B. J. [2017]. *Sauer's manual of skin diseases* [11th ed.]. Wolters Kluwer.)

DIFFERENTIAL DIAGNOSIS Hirsutism

- Idiopathic hirsutism
- Polycystic ovary syndrome
- Congenital adrenal hyperplasia
- Androgen-secreting tumors (adrenal and ovarian)
- Exogenous androgens

Confirming the Diagnosis

- Detailed history should include a timeline of hair growth, presence or absence of other signs of virilization, family history of hirsutism, and medication use (including anabolic corticosteroids).
- Physical examination should include presence or absence of skin changes such as acne, androgenic alopecia, and acanthosis nigricans.
- Laboratory studies include 17-hydroxysteroid, TSH, and prolactin if menses are irregular or absent, total testosterone, and dehydroepiandrosterone sulfate.
- If PCOS is suspected, a complete workup is required, including ultrasound, fasting glucose tolerance test (GTT), and lipid panel.

Treatment

- Oral contraceptives and antiandrogens such as spironolactone or finasteride. Patients are usually followed by an endocrinologist or gynecologist for treatment.
- Eflornithine (Vaniqa) applied b.i.d. alone or in combination with laser hair removal can slow the rate of regrowth.

Management and Patient Education

- Treatment and long-term management depend upon the cause of hirsutism.
- If PCOS or other androgen-related disorders are suspected, referral to an endocrinologist is required.
- Laser therapy may be used in combination with other hair removal methods

---

CLINICAL PEARLS

- Hirsutism in children may occur as a result of familial or ethnic traits and usually begins during puberty.
- Hirsutism that occurs before puberty (precocious puberty) may be a sign of an underlying disease such as congenital adrenal hyperplasia (CAH) and usually occurs in early childhood.
- Late-onset CAH may occur with hirsutism after puberty.

Hypertrichosis

Hypertrichosis is the overgrowth of hair on the scalp and body. Unlike hirsutism, hypertrichosis affects both men and women and in a nonsexual pattern. The cause is often heredity, and may be congenital or acquired.

Pathophysiology

- *Medications have* been implicated in the development of hypertrichosis, and include oral corticosteroids, bimatoprost, minoxidil, phenytoin, and cyclosporine (Fig. 11.1-18).

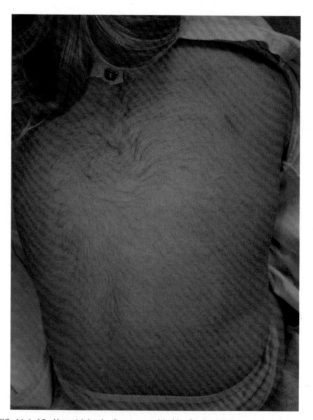

FIG. 11.1-18. Hypertrichosis. (Image provided by Stedman's.)

- Porphyria cutanea tarda (inherited disorder in which an enzymatic defect causes disruption in the body's production of heme), malnutrition, and malignancy are also associated with hypertrichosis.
- Etiology is unknown, but the congenital form may result from inherited genetic disorder or due to spontaneous mutation.

Clinical Presentation

- Congenital form presents with excessive hair growth at birth with lanugo (rather than vellus) hair covering most of the body. This continues throughout life.
- Acquired forms may be generalized or cover most of the body.

Confirming the Diagnosis

- Clinical presentation
- Thorough medical and medication history
- Laboratory workup or imaging if malnutrition or malignancy is suspected

Treatment

- Hair removal via shaving, waxing, electrolysis, or laser.
- Discontinuation of medications (listed above) that are reported to cause hypertrichosis.

Management and Patient Education

- Patient education should not focus on the need for regular, repeated removal of hair because it will typically grow back.
- Laser hair removal may offer a more long-lasting result.

READINGS AND REFERENCES

Billero, V., & Miteva, M. (2018). Traction alopecia: The root of the problem. *Clinical, Cosmetic and Investigational Dermatology, 11*, 149–159.

Blattner, C., Polley, D. C., Feritto, F., & Elston, D. M. (2013). Central centrifugal cicatricial alopecia. *Indian Dermatology Online Journal, 4*(1), 50–51.

Bolognia, J. L., Jorizzo, J. L., & Rapini, R. P. (2008). *Dermatology* (2nd ed., pp. 965–1035). Mosby Elsevier.

Carmina, E., Azziz, R., Bergfeld, W., Escobar-Morreale, H. F., Futterweit, W., Huddleston, H., Lobo, R., & Olsen, E. (2019). Female pattern hair loss and androgen excess: A report from the multidisciplinary androgen excess and PCOS Committee. *Journal of Clinical Endocrinology and Metabolism, 104*(7), 2875–2891.

Company-Quiroga, J., Alique-García, S., & Romero-Maté, A. (2019). Current insights into the management of discoid lupus erythematosus. *Clinical, Cosmetic and Investigational Dermatology, 12*, 721–732.

Dinulos, J. (2021). *Habif's clinical dermatology: A color guide to diagnosis and therapy* (7th ed.). Elsevier.

Dlova, N. C., Salkey, K. S., Callender, V. D., & McMichael, A. J. (2017). Central centrifugal cicatricial alopecia: New insights and a call for action. *Journal of Investigative Dermatology Symposium Proceedings, 18*(2), S54–S56.

Errichetti, E., Figini, M., Croatto, M., & Stinco, G. (2018). Therapeutic management of classic lichen planopilaris: A systematic review. *Clinical, Cosmetic and Investigational Dermatology, 11*, 91–102.

Fabbrocini, G., Cantelli, M., Masarà A., Annunziata, M. C., Marasca, C., & Cacciapuoti, S. (2018). Female pattern hair loss: A clinical, pathophysiologic, and therapeutic review. *International Journal of Women's Dermatology, 4*(4), 203–211.

Freedberg, I. M., Eisen, A. Z., Wolff, K., Austen, K. F., Goldsmith, L. A., & Katz, S. I. (Eds.). (2003). *Fitzpatrick's dermatology in general medicine* (6th ed., pp. 148–163, 633–671). McGraw Hill.

Henkel, E. D., Jaquez, S. D., & Diaz, L. Z. (2019). Pediatric trichotillomania: Review of management. *Pediatric Dermatology, 36*(6), 803–807.

Kanwar, A. J., & Narang, T. (2013). Anagen effluvium. *Indian Journal of Dermatology, Venereology, and Leprology, 79*(5), 604–612.

Linton, C. P. (2012). Describing the hair and related abnormalities. *Journal of the Dermatology Nurses' Association, 4*(3), 207–208.

Lolli, F., Pallotti, F., Rossi, A., Fortuna, M. C., Caro, G, Lenzi, A., Sansone, A., & Lombardo, F. (2017). Androgenetic alopecia: A review. *Endocrine, 57*(1), 9–17.

Phillips, T. G., Slomiany, W. P., & Allison, R. (2017). Hair loss: Common causes and treatment. *American Family Physician, 96*(6), 371–378.

Rebora, A. (2019). Telogen effluvium: A comprehensive review. *Clinical, Cosmetic and Investigational Dermatology, 12*, 583–590.

Renert-Yuval, Y., & Guttman-Yassky, E. (2017). The changing landscape of alopecia areata: The therapeutic paradigm. *Advances in Therapy, 34*(7), 1594–1609.

Nail Disorders

Martha Sikes

NAIL DISORDERS

Although the primary function of the nail is protection and the enhancement of tactile sensation, changes in the nails can also be useful as a diagnostic sign. Nail changes occur normally as a process of aging or may accompany cutaneous disease, but can also provide clues to the diagnosis of certain systemic diseases. Understanding the structure and function of the nail will allow you to identify and explain abnormalities.

NAIL ANATOMY

The nail unit consists of the following structures (Cashman & Sloan, 2010) (Fig. 11.2-1):

- Nail bed—contains vascular capillaries, begins where lunula ends and extends to hyponychium, and is where the nail plate adheres. Its function is to support the nail plate.

- Nail plate—made of hard and soft keratin, provides protection for nail unit, and is generally what is referred to as the "fingernail" or "toenail." Pinkish color is due to the vascular layer in nail bed.

- Nail matrix—thick portion of nail bed where nail is developed.

- Lunula—white, half-moon shaped area located at the most distal portion of the nail matrix and determines the shape of the nail plate.

- Eponychium—also known as the "cuticle," is part of proximal nail fold that seals the nail plate. It provides protection against microorganisms that can infect the nail.

- Hyponychium—epidermis located between distal portion of nail plate free edge and nail bed. It provides protection to the nail matrix.

- Nail folds (proximal and lateral)—provide support and growth direction for nail plate.

The normal growth of the nail plate is very slow, with fingernails taking approximately 5 to 6 months to completely regenerate from the matrix to the hyponychium, and toenails 12 to 18 months. The rate of growth is slowest at birth, increases through childhood, peaks in the teens and 20s, and sharply decreases after the age of 50. Understanding the nail growth process can provide clinicians with information concerning response rates to nail treatments, disorders

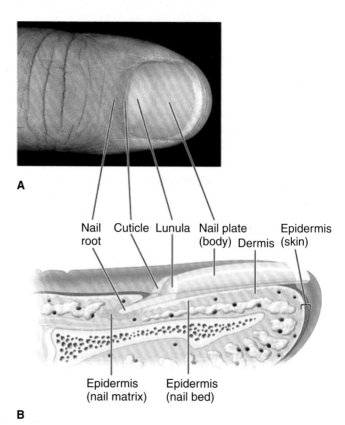

A

Nail root | Cuticle | Lunula | Nail plate (body) | Dermis | Epidermis (skin)

Epidermis (nail matrix) | Epidermis (nail bed)

B

FIG. 11.2-1. Fingernail. **A:** External view. **B:** Anatomy of a nail.

that affect the nail itself, and/or systemic conditions that occurred months prior. Nails can also store information such as toxicology exposure and DNA.

EVALUATION OF NAILS

- Perform a detailed history
  - Duration present
  - Which nails were affected first and which nails are now affected
  - Any previous trauma (this one can be difficult for patients—may help to give them a time frame based on where findings are in the nail)
  - Occupation—noting repeated exposure to water, chemicals, trauma
    Hobbies—noting repeated exposure to water, chemicals, trauma
  - Nail habits (i.e., picking, biting, etc.)
  - Nail care routine (i.e., use of polish, artificial nails, manicures)
  - Other skin conditions (i.e., psoriasis, atopic dermatitis, lichen planus [LP], tinea cruris)
  - Other medical history (including medications taken in the last year, surgeries, etc.)
  - Family history of nail problems
  - Diet (nutritional deficiencies can influence nail growth and appearance)
- Physical examination
  - Inspect *all* 20 nails (the entire nail unit)
  - Note any findings (pitting, peeling, thickening, onycholysis, etc.). Photograph nails if possible, for future comparisons

COMMON NAIL CHANGES

Variations seen in the nail apparatus can be the result of normal aging or can be related to infection, trauma, cutaneous disorders, or may reflect systemic disease such as liver dysfunction, pulmonary disorders, iron and other nutritional deficiencies, malabsorptive and inflammatory gastrointestinal diseases, among others (Box 11.2-1). See Tables 11.2-1 and 11.2-2.

Nail Changes Caused by Infection

Onychomycosis

The most common cause of a nail infection is fungus and is caused by dermatophytes, yeast, or nondermatophyte molds. See Section 6.1

BOX 11.2-1   Nail Assessment: What to Look for

- Textural changes: any abnormalities in nail plate surface (smooth, crumbled, ridges)?
- Discoloration of the nail plate or surrounding skin (black, brown, red)?
- Abnormalities in cuticle or nail fold (is nail fold present, missing, ragged)?
- Abnormalities in the shape of the nail (spoon shaped or overly curved)?
- Is the nail plate present or partially or completely destroyed by pathology?
- Growths or lesions around the nail (warts, pyogenic granuloma, digital fibroma)?

---

for a detailed discussion of fungal nail infections and treatment (Fig. 11.2-2).

Acute Paronychia

An infection in the nail fold which is often caused by *Staphylococcus aureus,* but other organisms such as *Candida, Pseudomonas,* or dermatophytes can be involved. Trauma and/or chronic exposure to moisture predispose patients to developing paronychia.

Clinical Presentation

- Erythema, pain, and swelling of the nail fold. See Table 11.2-1.
- Purulent material may be trapped behind the cuticle and should be relieved by gently separating the cuticle from the nail plate to release the purulent drainage.

Treatment

- Releasing purulent drainage is usually adequate treatment.
- If the patient does not improve, oral antibiotics or anticandida/fungal treatments with incision and drainage of the lesion may be indicated.

Management and Patient Education

- Be sure to ask patients how the paronychia occurred—compulsive manipulation of the cuticle or nail folds is a common finding.
- Note that 30% of paronychia patients are continuous carriers of *S. aureus,* which may increase risk of developing skin infections (Kang et al., 2019).

Chronic Paronychia

Evolves slowly over time and is not a result of acute paronychia but is caused by repeated contact or irritant exposure.

Pseudomonas (Chloronychia or Green Nail Syndrome)

Infection of the nail bed with *Pseudomonas aeruginosa,* a gram-negative bacterium, is typically caused by repeated exposure to water and that result in softening of the hyponychium thus allowing the microorganism to enter beneath the nail plate. This infection can be seen in women who wear artificial nails, where moisture becomes trapped under the cosmetic aid. It is more common in the elderly.

Clinical Presentation

- Appears as a green/black discoloration of the nail bed, known as "green nail syndrome." Often mistaken for hemorrhage from trauma, the greenish-black coloration is the result of the pigments secreted by the bacteria. See Table 11.2-1.
- Often presents as a proximal nontender chronic paronychia and distolateral onycholysis.

Confirming the Diagnosis

- Clinical appearance of a greenish-yellow, greenish-brown, or greenish-black nail is usually enough for diagnosis but it can be easily confused with onychomycosis; therefore nails clippings can be sent for bacterial or fungal culture.
- This infection lacks a history of injury thus ruling out subungual hemorrhage.

TABLE 11.2-1 | Nail Abnormalities Associated with Localized Disease

Onychoschizia
Age, dehydration, trauma

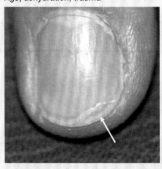

Onycholysis
Separation of nail plate from nail bed; many causes

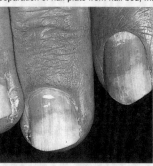

Onycholysis and Nail Dystrophy
Psoriasis, infection, many causes

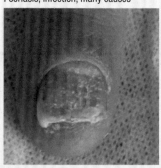

Nail Dystrophy
Lichen planus

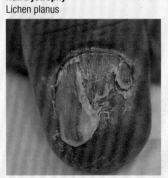

Median Nail Dystrophy
Habit tic

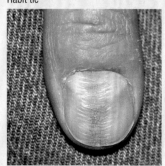

Chronic Paronychia

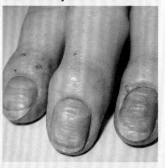

Acute Paronychia
Bacterial or candida infection

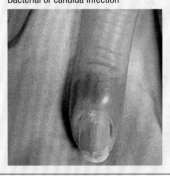

Pseudomonas Infection
Green nail syndrome

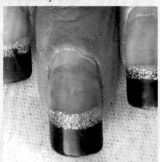

Nail Pitting
Psoriasis, lichen planus, alopecia areata

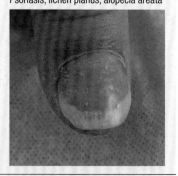

Longitudinal Melanonychia

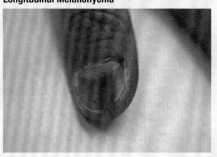

Onychomycosis

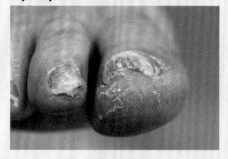

Subungual Hematoma

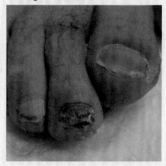

TABLE 11.2-2	Nail Abnormalities Associated with Systemic Disease

Lindsay's Nails (Half & Half)
Kidney disease

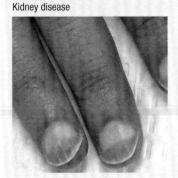

Beau Lines
Horizontal ridges: infection, trauma, systemic disease

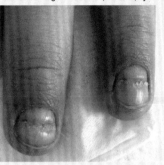

Pincer Nail
Inherited, Kawasaki disease, β-blockers, genodermatoses

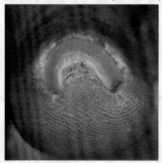

Terry Nails (80/20 Nails)
Liver disease

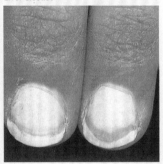

Chemotherapy

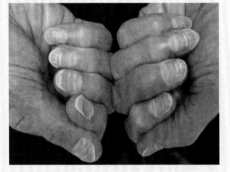

Yellow Nail Syndrome

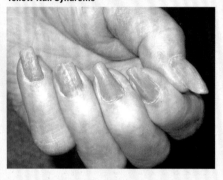

(Figure: "Nail Changes Due to Chemotherapy"—Image provided by Stedman's.)

Treatment

- *Pseudomonas* can be treated with a white vinegar or bleach solution of 1:4 parts water. Distal fingers are submerged to soak where the separation has occurred.
- Trimming the nail or removing the artificial nail helps to remove the reservoir of moisture and hasten resolution of the infection.
- Oral quinolones or topical fluoroquinolone solutions (ofloxacin otic solution; one drop under nail twice a day; off-label) may be necessary.

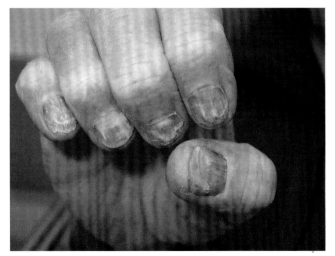

FIG. 11.2-2. Onychomycosis. (Image provided by Stedman's.)

Nail Abnormalities Associated with Localized Skin Disorders

Nail Psoriasis

Nail changes are a common manifestation in patients diagnosed with psoriasis, and are rarely the only symptom of psoriasis. Approximately half to three quarters of patients with skin psoriasis, and as much as 80% of patients with psoriatic arthritis, present with nail psoriasis (Bardazzi et al., 2019). This nail disease can greatly impact patients' functionally and socially if not treated. The number of nails affected may range from a few toenails or fingernails to all 20 nails (Bardazzi et al., 2019).

Pathophysiology

Nail psoriasis, just as with plaque psoriasis, is the result of environmental, genetic, and immune-mediated factors. The extent of nail changes largely depends on the affected site of the nail. The nail bed, nail matrix, nail folds, and/or the hyponychium may be involved. Focal defects in the keratinization process of the proximal matrix are the mechanism that creates nail pitting (Bardazzi et al., 2019). Nail crumbling is the result of severe involvement in the nail matrix (Bardazzi et al., 2019).

Clinical Presentation

Clinical findings depend on where psoriatic disease affects the nail matrix and/or nail bed.

- Common changes are pitting, oil-staining, lunulae red spots, nail plate crumbling, subungual hyperkeratosis, and nail dystrophy (see Psoriasis, Section 4.4). See Table 11.2-1.

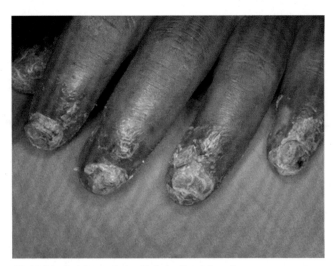

FIG. 11.2-3. Pustular psoriasis with destruction of the nail.

- Nail bed alterations can lead to onycholysis of the nail(s).
- A border of erythema that surrounds the area of onycholysis is diagnostic of nail bed psoriasis. (Bardazzi et al., 2019).
- A severe form of pustular psoriasis may occur, producing significant destruction of the nails and periungual skin (Fig. 11.2-3).
- Be sure to look at the scalp, arms, legs, joints, and potentially even the anogenital region to look for other possible signs and symptoms of psoriasis and/or psoriatic arthritis.

DIFFERENTIAL DIAGNOSIS   Nail Psoriasis

- Alopecia areata
- Eczema
- Lichen planus
- Onychomycosis

Confirming the Diagnosis

- Clinical presentation is usually sufficient. Dermoscopy can help differentiate nail psoriasis from onychomycosis. Look for other clues of psoriasis: plaques in scalp, around umbilicus, in skin folds, or on scalp.
- Punch biopsy of the nail matrix or nail bed is recommended if the diagnosis is not clinically apparent. Use of ultrasound to aid in diagnosis is being investigated.

Treatment

- Topical therapies include high-potency TCS or vitamin D analogs (i.e., calcipotriol) alone, or combination therapy with topical calcineurin inhibitors, tazarotene, or 5-fluorouracil (Bardazzi et al., 2019).
- Systemic therapy includes traditional agents used in plaque psoriasis (i.e., methotrexate, cyclosporine, acitretin, phototherapy), biologic agents (i.e., TNF-α antagonists, IL-17 inhibitors), and small molecule inhibitors such as apremilast.

See Section 4.4 for treatment details.

Management and Patient Education

- Diagnosis and treatment of nail psoriasis is best done by dermatology providers familiar with the treatment of psoriasis.

Alopecia Areata

Nail changes occur in approximately 30% of patients with alopecia areata (AA). These changes are often overlooked on physical examination, and can occur at any point during the course of AA. Nail involvement is more prevalent in patients with severe alopecia areata (AA universalis and AA totalis). It usually presents in the fingernails and can involve a few nails to all 20 nails. While many patients are asymptomatic, extensive nail involvement can cause discomfort, significantly impact quality of life, and may indicate a risk of progress to more severe forms of AA. Nail changes in AA are poorly understood and thought to occur from genetic and immunologic factors that affect the nail matrix (Chelidze & Lipner, 2018).

Clinical Presentation

- Pitting is the most predominant feature, but is more geometric and appears shallower than the pitting of psoriasis. In AA, the pits are generally arranged in longitudinal rows. In psoriasis, they are more haphazard (Table 11.2-1).
- Trachyonychia and red lunula are also usually seen.
- Nail changes occur at increased frequency in children and women, while trachyonychia occurs more often in men (Chelidze & Lipner, 2018).

DIFFERENTIAL DIAGNOSIS   Alopecia Areata Nail

- Nail psoriasis
- Lichen planus
- Onychomycosis
- Eczema

Confirming the Diagnosis

- Clinical examination of hair-bearing areas is usually significant and will be positive for findings of hair loss associated with AA (see Hair Disorders, Section 11.1).
- Nail fungal culture may be necessary to rule out onychomycosis.
- Punch biopsy of nail matrix is rarely necessary.

Treatment

- High-potency TCS, intralesional corticosteroids, topical tazarotene, and systemic corticosteroids have been used with some success, but recurrence of nail changes is common.

Management and Patient Education

- Prompt referral to a dermatology provider is essential as nail changes are considered an independent risk factor associated with treatment-resistant AA, and are often present in patients with more severe forms of AA (Chelidze & Lipner, 2018).

Lichen Planus

LP is a chronic, inflammatory disorder that can affect skin, hair, nails, and mucous membranes in children and adults, most often

perimenopausal women, and has a peak incidence in the third to sixth decades of life. The nail changes of LP are seen in about 10% of patients, and are usually associated with disseminated disease.

Pathophysiology

The exact etiology is poorly understood but thought to be autoimmune (T-cell mediated) in nature. It is known to coincide with other autoimmune conditions such as vitiligo and AA. Development of LP has been associated with hepatitis C virus infection. Nail changes are the result of inflammatory effects on the nail matrix and if severe enough, can cause a nail pterygium due to permanent destruction of the nail matrix (Usatine & Tinitigan, 2011).

DIFFERENTIAL DIAGNOSIS Lichen Planus of Nail

- Nail psoriasis
- Eczema
- Onychomycosis
- Alopecia areata
- Twenty-nail dystrophy of childhood

Clinical Presentation

- The most common changes are longitudinal grooves, ridging, and hyperpigmentation. Onycholysis may also occur (Fig. 11.2-4).

- In more extensive disease, a nail pterygium may occur when the proximal nail fold adheres to the matrix, resulting in destruction of the cuticle and a permanent scar (Fig. 11.2-5). This is also known as "angel wing deformity" for its characteristic shape.

- Be sure to look for other cutaneous signs and symptoms as LP can affect the skin (typically extensor surfaces), scalp, oral mucosa, and genitalia. See Section 4.5 for details.

- Pay close attention to the oral mucosa as LP in this area is associated with the development of oral cancer.

Treatment

- High-potency topical corticosteroids, intralesional corticosteroids by an experienced clinician, or systemic corticosteroids if extensive involvement of other cutaneous areas.

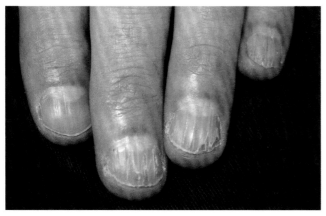

FIG. 11.2-4. Lichen planus. (Image provided by Stedman's.)

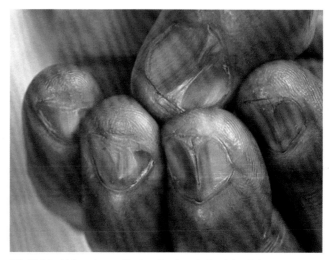

FIG. 11.2-5. Lichen planus with pterygium (angel wing deformity).

Management and Patient Education

- Patients should be tested for presence of hepatitis C virus as 10% to 20% of patients may be infected.

- Reassurance that the condition is typically self-limited.

Benign Tumors of the Nail

Digital Mucous Cysts

These benign ganglion cysts arise on the dorsum or lateral aspect of the distal digit adjacent to the DIP joint or in the proximal nail fold. Digital mucous cysts (DMCs) usually occur in patients aged 50 to 70 years; females are affected more than males. The exact mechanism responsible for development of the cyst is not known, but is believed to be caused by the degeneration of connective tissue and is thought to coexist with osteoarthritis. Trauma has also been cited as a cause.

Clinical Presentation

- DMCs appear as solitary or multiple translucent bluish cysts, located just off midline of digits, and may be tender when pressure is applied (Fig. 11.2-6).

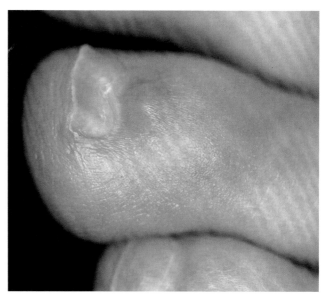

FIG. 11.2-6. Digital mucous cyst. Note the linear depression distal to the cyst.

- Grooving or depression of nail plate may occur if DMC involves the proximal nail fold.

DIFFERENTIAL DIAGNOSIS   Digital Mucous Cyst

- Heberden node
- Xanthoma epidermoid cyst
- Squamous cell carcinoma

Confirming the Diagnosis

- Clinical presentation with or without transillumination with a penlight may be sufficient to make the diagnosis.
- As a result of pressure on the nail matrix at the site of the cyst, a vertical depression will appear in the nail and may be present even if the cyst is not visible.
- Aspiration of the cyst will produce a clear gelatinous substance, helping to confirm diagnosis.
- Plain radiographs are nondiagnostic. CT images may be useful if lesions are to be surgically excised.

Treatment

- Digital compression, intralesional corticosteroids, and/or repeated incision and drainage (most effective) are all viable treatments.
- Aspiration—the area should be prepped with alcohol and a no. 11 surgical blade or a medium-gauge needle (25G) is used to pierce the cyst approximately 1 to 2 mm. The cyst is then drained by manual pressure. The cysts tend to recur but may become smaller or asymptomatic with repeated drainage.
- Osteophyte excision and debridement by a hand surgeon may be needed for recalcitrant lesions.

Management and Patient Education

- Patients should be reassured these lesions are not associated with malignancy.
- Referral to a hand surgeon may be necessary.

Pyogenic Granulomas

Pyogenic granuloma (PG) is a common, benign, acquired vascular tumor that can occur on the skin and mucous membranes. These lesions, also known as lobular capillary hemangiomas, occur most often on children and young adults and are associated with medications (i.e., oral retinoids, oral contraceptives, BRAF inhibitors, rituximab, epidermal growth factor receptor inhibitors), viral infections, trauma, and pregnancy. The exact mechanism for the development of PG is unknown, but overexpression of certain growth factors (i.e., vascular endothelial growth factor) may lead to inappropriate activation of proangiogenic pathways (Mashiah et al., 2019).

Clinical Presentation

- Painless, solitary, friable (easy to bleed), red papule or nodule commonly found on the fingers (usually the lateral nail fold), but can occur on the head, gingiva, or upper extremities (Fig. 11.2-7).
- PG lesions grow quickly, bleed with trauma, and carry risk of ulceration (Mashiah et al., 2019).

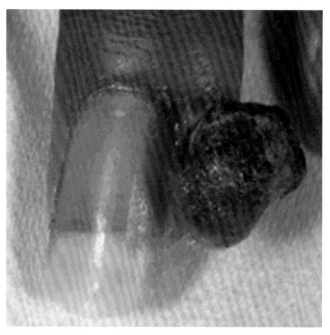

FIG. 11.2-7. Pyogenic granuloma. Friable papule on lateral nail fold.

DIFFERENTIAL DIAGNOSIS   Pyogenic Granuloma

- Hemangioma
- Foreign body reaction
- Angiosarcoma
- Basal cell carcinoma
- Amelanotic melanoma

Confirming the Diagnosis

- Clinical presentation and history are usually sufficient.
- Shave biopsy if concern for other benign or malignant tumor.

Treatment

- Although some lesions may spontaneously resolve, treatment is usually required and recurrence is common.
- Excision, curettage, electrodessication, cryosurgery, laser therapy, imiquimod 5%, and intralesional injection with corticosteroids or bleomycin have all been utilized with some success.
- Multiple treatment options exist due to reported lack of efficacy with any one therapy.
- Use of topical beta blockers (i.e., propranolol) has been successful in recent case reports (Goetze et al., 2019).

Management and Patient Education

- Reassure patients that PG lesions are benign, but have a high recurrence rate.
- If removal of PG is performed, the entire lesion should be removed to prevent reoccurrence, and sent for histologic examination by the dermatopathologist, as these tumors may mimic an amelanotic melanoma.

TABLE 11.2-3	Acral Lentiginous Melanoma of Nail Unit

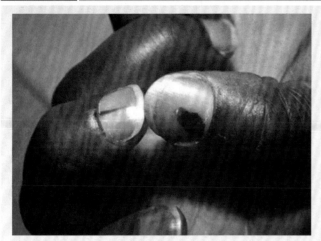

Melanoma. Note nail bed pigmented lesions of the thumb and middle finger. (Centers for Disease Control and Prevention. PHIL#13433)

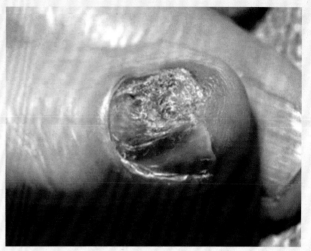

Melanoma. Nail bed pigmentation and deformation due to a neoplastic condition. (Centers for Disease Control and Prevention. PHIL# 13434)

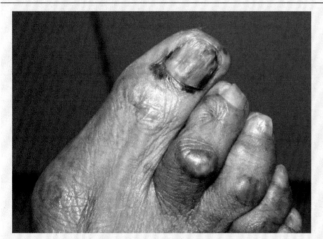

Melanoma. Note the location of these lesions, and the irregularly demarcated margins, as well as the Hutchinson sign represented by staining of the proximal nail fold. (Centers for Disease Control and Prevention. PHIL# 13432)

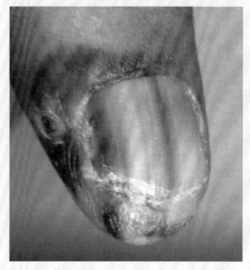

Melanoma. Note the pigmented proximal and lateral nail folds, known as "Hutchinson sign."

MALIGNANT TUMORS OF THE NAIL

Melanoma

Melanomas of the nails are classified as acral lentiginous melanomas (Table 11.2-3). They grow slowly and painlessly and are often diagnosed too late (see Section 2.1 for melanoma details).

As clinicians, when we examine nail changes that may possibly be malignant, there are some important signs that are suspicious for melanoma which we must recognize (Box 11.2-2).

Squamous Cell Carcinoma

Squamous cell carcinoma (SCC) of the nail bed is rare (see Section 2.2) but can masquerade as a wart or even benign tumor such as a pyogenic granuloma or a mucoid digital cyst (Figs. 11.2-8 and 11.2-9).

BOX 11.2-2	Suspicious Signs of Nail Melanoma

A Age (peak fifth to seventh decades)
Abnormal nail plate surface or texture
African Americans, Asians, Native Americans
B Black or brown streaks >3 mm
Borders variegated
C Change: recent or rapid increase in size of nail band
D Digits involved most often thumb, great toe
E Extension of pigmentation onto the skin of proximal nail fold (Hutchinson sign)
F Family or personal history

Adapted from Levit, E. K., Kagen, M. H., Scher, R. K., Grossman, M., & Altman, E. (2000). The ABC rule for clinical detection of subungual melanoma. *Journal of the American Academy of Dermatology, 42*(2 Pt 1), 269–274.

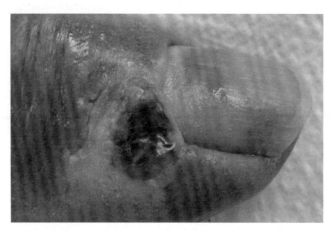

FIG. 11.2-8. Squamous cell carcinoma. (Photo courtesy of M. Bobonich.)

Periungual warts are a common complaint in dermatology practice but lesions that resist treatment or frequently recur should be evaluated for possible carcinoma.

READINGS AND REFERENCES

Bardazzi, F., Starace, M., Bruni, F., Magnano, M., Piraccini, B. M., & Alessandrini, A. (2019). Nail psoriasis: An updated review and expert opinion on available treatments, including biologics. *Acta Dermato-Venereologica*, *99*(6), 516–523.

Cashman, M., & Sloan, S. (2010). Nutrition and nail disease. *Clinics in Dermatology*, *28*(4), 420–425.

Chelidze, K., & Lipner, S. R. (2018). Nail changes in alopecia areata: An update and review. *International Journal of Dermatology*, *57*(7), 776–783.

Goetze, A. C., Sasaya, E. M. K., Cerci, F. B., Talkachjov, S. N., & Werner, B. (2019). Pyogenic granuloma of the lip with complete resolution after topical propranolol. *Journal of Drugs in Dermatology*, *18*(10), 1061–1062.

Habif, T. P. (2004). *Clinical dermatology: A color guide to diagnosis and therapy* (4th ed., pp. 834–891). Mosby.

Kang, S., Amagai, M., Bruckner, A. L., Enk, A., Margolis, D. J., McMichael, A. J., & Orringer, J. S. (2019). *Fitzpatrick's dermatology*. New York: McGraw Hill Education.

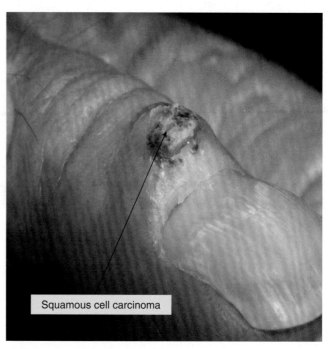

Squamous cell carcinoma

FIG. 11.2-9. Squamous cell carcinoma.

Linton, C. P. (2012). Describing nail abnormalities. *Journal of the Dermatology Nurses' Association*, *4*(2), 149–150.

Linton, C. P. (2012). Describing the hair and related abnormalities. *Journal of the Dermatology Nurses' Association*, *4*(3), 207–208.

Mashiah, J., Hadj-Rabia, S., Slodownik, D., Harel, A., Sprecher, E., & Kutz, A. (2019). Effectiveness of topical propranolol 4% gel in the treatment of pyogenic granuloma in children. *Journal of Dermatology*, *46*(3), 245–248.

Omori, M. S. (2012). Herpetic whitlow. http://emedicine.medscape.com/article/788056-overview

Tosti, A. (2013). Onychomycosis. http://emedicine.medscape.com/article/1105828-overview

Usatine, R. P., & Tinitigan, M. (2011). Diagnosis and treatment of lichen planus. *American Family Physician*, *84*(1), 53–60.

Oral Cavity, Lips, Gums, and Tongue

Travis M. Hayden, Joleen M. Volz, and Jennifer Winter

In This Chapter

- Lips
  - Angular Cheilitis
  - Actinic Cheilitis
- Gingiva/Buccal Mucosa
  - Gingivitis
  - Mucocele
  - Irritation Fibroma
- Tongue
  - Fissured Tongue
  - Hairy Tongue
  - Migratory Glossitis
- Oral Cavity
  - Aphthous Ulcers
  - Torus Palatinus
  - Leukoplakia
  - Lichen Planus

Clinicians are often called upon to evaluate dermatoses and/or lesions involving the oral cavity, lips, gums, and tongue. Pathology in any of these areas may represent either local disease or can be the early sign of a systemic disease. Making the initial assessment is very important as is the appropriate referral to either a dental professional or an otolaryngologist who understands the anatomy of the oral cavity region and is comfortable in further diagnosing and treating these disorders. This chapter is divided into sections that will cover common disorders a provider may encounter that involve the oral cavity, lips, gums, and tongue.

LIPS

Angular Cheilitis

Angular cheilitis, also known as perlèche, is an acute or chronic inflammation of the skin at the lateral commissures of the mouth (either unilateral or most often bilateral). It is associated with an increase in moisture causing maceration of the skin at the commissures (most often from salivation, particularly at sleep), which can then become secondarily infected (most commonly with *Candida albicans,* or less commonly with *Staphylococcus aureus*). Angular cheilitis can occur at any age without sex predilection. It is common among patients who wear dental apparatus and/or dentures.

Pathogenesis

- Common predisposing factors include drooling/thumb-sucking/ or lip licking (among children), wearing of orthodontic appliances, or ill-fitting dentures, xerostomia (dry mouth due to either an underlying disease [e.g., type 2 diabetes, Sjögren syndrome, immunodeficiency], infection [e.g., fungal] and/or medications [e.g., systemic retinoids]), poor oral hygiene, irritant or allergic dermatitis reactions to either oral hygiene products or denture materials, and age-related anatomical changes of the mouth (either due to loss of dentition and/or a sagging face causing more prominent marionette lines at the lateral commissures).

- Less common causes include nutritional deficiencies, such as B9 (folic acid), zinc (B6, pyridoxine), B2 (riboflavin), or B3 (niacin) (Park et al., 2011).

Clinical Presentation

- Erythema, scale, and/or maceration found in the oral commissures (Fig. 11.3-1)
- Fissuring common with chronic cases
- Pain, soreness, or irritation when opening mouth wide, yawning

DIFFERENTIAL DIAGNOSIS Angular Cheilitis

- Trauma
- Herpes simplex infection
- Contact dermatitis (irritant or allergic)

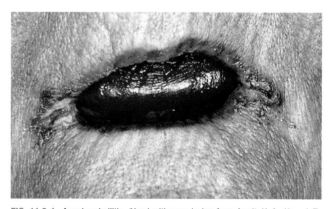

FIG. 11.3-1. Angular cheilitis. (Used with permission from Arndt, K. A., Hsu, J. T., Alam, M., Bhatia, A. C., & Chilukuri, S. [2014]. *Manual of dermatologic therapeutics* [8th ed.]. Wolters Kluwer.)

Confirming the Diagnosis

- Diagnosis is based on history and clinical findings and can be confirmed with laboratory studies (clinical diagnosis is made most often of angular cheilitis).
- Potassium hydroxide (KOH) preparation—confirms or rules out *Candida* infection.
- Bacterial and fungal swabs for cultures are recommended for recalcitrant angular cheilitis.

Treatment

Treatment is directed at identifying and controlling or eliminating the underlying predisposing factors:

- *Candida* infections are best managed with a topical azole antifungal (e.g., miconazole, clotrimazole) ointment applied two to three times per day for 1 to 3 weeks.
- *Staphylococcal* infections are best managed with topical mupirocin ointment applied two times per day for 1 to 2 weeks.
- Severe or recalcitrant cases may require systemic yeast or antibiotic therapy.
- Barrier products (zinc oxide or petrolatum-based products).

Management and Patient Education

General measures to reduce skin maceration occurring from saliva collecting at the lateral commissures of the mouth:

- Encourage optimal oral hygiene.
- Improve orthodontic/denture fit and encourage proper cleaning.
- Treatment of xerostomia symptoms.
- Use of a barrier product to the lateral commissures of mouth frequently throughout the day and at bedtime (zinc oxide or petrolatum-based products).

CLINICAL PEARLS

- Very common presentation seen among elderly patients wearing dentures.
- Recurrence of angular cheilitis is common due to the difficulty in fully controlling or eliminating the underlying predisposing factors.

Actinic Cheilitis

Actinic cheilitis is a precancerous condition resulting from chronic sun exposure. It predominantly affects adults with fair skin and chronic sun damage. It has a male–female preference as high as 10:1 (Lee et al., 2008). It is the equivalent to an actinic keratosis that presents on the lips and vermilion border. The lesions develop slowly making it difficult for patients to notice the change. Early diagnosis and treatment is recommended to decrease the risk of progression into an invasive lip squamous cell carcinoma (SCC), a malignant disease with poor prognosis.

Clinical Presentation

- Atrophy of lower lip or vermilion border; or smooth-surfaced, blotchy pale areas.

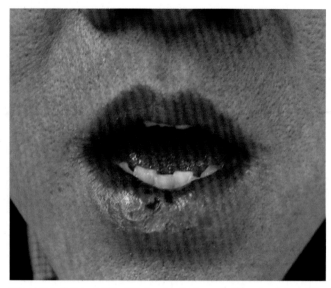

FIG. 11.3-2. Actinic cheilitis. Note the chronically cracked hyperkeratotic patches on the lower lip.

- Blurring of margin between vermilion and cutaneous lip.
- Hyperkeratotic patches, chronic dry sensation, cracked lips, focal erosions that are more common on the lower lip, usually spares commissures (Fig. 11.3-2).
- Hyperkeratotic patches return a few days after they are scraped off.
- Usually painless.

DIFFERENTIAL DIAGNOSIS   Actinic Cheilitis

• Herpes simplex virus	• Exfoliative cheilitis
• Lichen planus	• Factitious cheilitis
• Lupus erythematosus	• Glandular cheilitis
• Radiation damage	• Granulomatous cheilitis
• Allergic, contact, or photosensitive cheilitis	• Plasma cell cheilitis
• Angular cheilitis or perlèche	

Confirming the Diagnosis

- Clinical diagnosis; the lip may have a texture similar to rubbing across sandpaper.
- Shave biopsy if cancer or other inflammatory etiology suspected.
- Pathology demonstrates variable hypertrophy or atrophy, solar elastosis, partial-thickness epidermal hyperplasia, and dermal inflammation.

Treatment

- Topical: retinoids, 5-fluorouracil, imiquimod, chemical peel (TCA).
- Photodynamic therapy.
- Physical therapies: cryotherapy, electrocautery, laser ablation, vermilionectomy.

Management and Patient Education

- Encourage smoking cessation.
- Discuss daily sun protection; limit midday sun exposure, recommend a hat with wide brim, frequent application of lip balm with SPF30+.
- Long-term follow-up for skin cancer screening.

CLINICAL PEARL

Actinic cheilitis is more common in smokers as well as those with immunosuppression, alcohol abuse, and oncogenic factors such as human papillomavirus (wart).

Venous Lake

A venous lake is a benign, slow-growing vascular lesion first described in the literature in 1956 by Bean and Walsh. They most often occur on sun-exposed skin in adults older than 50 years of age, and are distributed on areas of the lips, ears, face, and neck. The worldwide incidence of venous lakes is unknown, but they are believed to be common. No racial predilection has been identified and men have been reported to have venous lakes more often than women.

Pathophysiology

Venous lake lesions have an unknown etiology, and are cutaneous vascular malformations resulting from a collection of dilated venules. Typical pathology demonstrates a single large dilated space (or several interconnecting dilated spaces) observed in the superficial dermis. The dilated space is lined by a single layer of endothelium and is supported by a thin wall of fibrous connective tissue. Solar elastosis and other evidence of actinic damage are typically seen in the adjacent dermis (Jay & Borek, 1998).

Clinical Presentation

- Asymptomatic, but may bleed easily and become tender after minor trauma.
- Color ranges from blue to violaceous (Fig. 11.3-3).

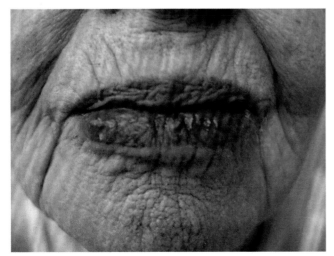

FIG. 11.3-3. Venous lake. (Image provided by Stedman's.)

- Soft, well-demarcated macule or papule with a smooth surface.
- Compressible with a slow venous refill to its original size and shape.

DIFFERENTIAL DIAGNOSIS   Venous Lake

- Blue nevus
- Cherry angioma
- Angiokeratoma circumscriptum
- Pyogenic granuloma
- Basal cell carcinoma
- Lentigo
- Melanocytic nevus
- Melanoma

Confirming the Diagnosis

- The diagnosis is generally made clinically.
- Diascopy is positive for blanchability (i.e., applying pressure with a finger or glass slide induces blanching). In this case, the color changes as the blood content is emptied from the space.
- Dermoscopy is also useful to differentiate vascular lesions from melanocytic neoplasms (a venous lake under dermoscopy will lack pigment network structures and will have a homogenous reddish-blue to reddish-black color).
- Biopsy may be indicated if malignancy or other inflammatory etiology is suspected.

Treatment

- Cryotherapy
- Electrocautery
- Sclerotherapy
- Vascular laser ablation (Wall et al., 2007)
- Surgical excision

Management and Patient Education

- Reassurance.
- Venous lakes are benign and typically require no treatment unless they bleed repeatedly from minor trauma or are cosmetically unacceptable to the patient. In such cases, the previously listed treatments can be utilized to remove venous lakes, but patients should be warned that while rare, hyper- or hypopigmentation and/or scarring can result at the site(s) of treatment.
- Venous lakes most often occur on sun-damaged skin; it is therefore important to counsel patients on the importance of daily sun protection and to recommend regular skin cancer screening.

Oral Melanotic Macule

Oral melanotic macules are the most common mucosal pigmented lesions. They are benign, slow growing, and occur on the lips and/or oral mucosa of adults. Oral melanotic macules are more commonly seen in individuals with darker skin types and typically present as a solitary lesion. If multiple lesions are present, one should consider

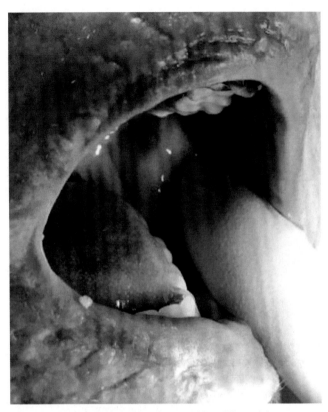

FIG. 11.3-4. Oral melanocytic lesion. (Courtesy of Doug DiRuggerio.)

a systemic or genetic etiology for the oral pigmentation. The most common location is the lower lip, with a higher prevalence reported in females.

Clinical Presentation

- Lesions are asymptomatic.
- Color varies from tan, brown, to darkly pigmented (Fig. 11.3-4).
- They are well demarcated and symmetrical.

DIFFERENTIAL DIAGNOSIS   Oral Melanotic Macule

- Oral melanocytic nevus
- Oral melanoma
- Oral melanoacanthoma
- Smoker's melanosis
- Drug-induced pigmentation
- Amalgam tattoos
- Peutz–Jeghers syndrome
- Laugier–Hunziker syndrome

Confirming the Diagnosis

- Clinical diagnosis. History may be helpful.
- Diascopy to rule out a vascular lesion.
- Biopsy if suspicious for malignancy, other melanocytic etiology, or nonmelanocytic pigmentation is suspected. Don't miss a melanoma!

Treatment

- Shave or complete excision for removal and confirmation of pathology.

Management and Patient Education

- Reassurance. Oral melanotic macules are benign and typically require no treatment unless they are perceived to be cosmetically unacceptable to the patient. In such cases, surgical or shave excision can be utilized, but patient should be warned that scarring may result at the site.
- If cosmetic, insurance may not cover removal.
- Oral melanotic macules tend to be solitary in nature. If multiple macules are present, a thorough workup is needed to rule out an acquired hyperpigmentation disorder: Peutz-Jeghers syndrome (CBC, fecal blood, iron studies, upper GI endoscopy); Laugier-Hunziker syndrome (a diagnosis of exclusion); primary adrenal failure (corticotropin level); connective tissue diseases (ANA panel); or hemochromatosis (iron studies).

GINGIVA/BUCCAL MUCOSA
Gingivitis

Gingivitis is a common condition characterized by inflammation of the gums. It often favors women over the age of 40. Most commonly caused by plaque buildup but can also be associated with substance use, smoking, hormones, infections, immunocompromised and nutritional deficiencies. If not well controlled, gingivitis progresses to a more advanced disease called periodontitis. Periodontitis is classified as gingival inflammation (gingivitis) as well as the loss of supportive connective tissues, periodontal ligament, and alveolar bone. As the disease progresses, the consequence is accelerated tooth mobility that may lead to eventual tooth loss. The disease can begin in early childhood and incidence and severity increase with age.

Pathophysiology

Most commonly, gingivitis is caused by plaque buildup but can also be associated with substance use, smoking, hormones, infections, immunocompromised and nutritional deficiencies.

Clinical Presentation

- Edematous, erythematous, swollen, tender gums that bleed easy especially when brushing or flossing (Fig. 11.3-5).

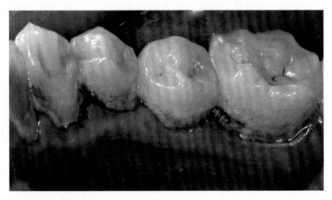

FIG. 11.3-5. Gingivitis.

- Varying degrees of sloughing and erosion.
- Halitosis.

DIFFERENTIAL DIAGNOSIS   Gingivitis

- Oral lichen planus
- Cicatricial pemphigoid
- Pemphigus vulgaris
- Bullous pemphigoid
- Chronic ulcerative stomatitis
- Lupus erythematosus
- Linear immunoglobulin A disease
- Dermatitis herpetiformis
- Chronic viral, bacterial, or fungal infection
- Reaction to medication or other substance in contact with gums
- Squamous cell carcinoma

Confirming the Diagnosis

- Thorough examination of mouth including teeth, cheeks, gums, and tongue.
- Probes to examine gingival pockets.
- X-rays to evaluate underlying damage.

Treatment

- Referral to dentist or periodontist for teeth cleaning and descaling, to remove plaque and tartar.
- Oral antibiotics if infection present.
- NSAIDs to reduce inflammation.
- Chlorhexidine (0.12%) oral rinse.

Management and Patient Education

- Good oral hygiene, brushing at least twice daily with soft-bristled brush, mouthwash, and flossing as directed by dentist.
- Smoking cessation.
- Regular dental evaluation.
- Treat any underlying condition.

Mucocele

Mucocele (or mucous cyst) is a pseudocyst that does not have an epithelial lining. It is most often found on the lower mucosal surface of the lip, but can also occur on the floor of the mouth, gingiva, buccal mucosa, or tongue. Ranula is the term for the variant that affects the ducts on the floor of the mouth where it originates from the sublingual or submandibular gland.

Pathophysiology

Trauma is often the causative factor for this common benign self-limiting condition. Disruption of the minor salivary ducts results, causing mucus or saliva to escape into the surrounding tissue which creates a smooth gelatinous fluid-filled nodule.

Clinical Presentation

- A compressible translucent to bluish papule or nodule on the lower mucosal surface of the lip (Fig. 11.3-6).
- It is painless and appears suddenly.

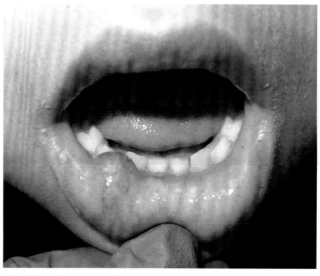

FIG. 11.3-6. Mucocele. A painless, translucent compressible papule usually found on the mucosal lip. (Used with permission from Gru, A. A., & Wick, M. [2018]. *Pediatric dermatopathology and dermatology.* Wolters Kluwer.)

DIFFERENTIAL DIAGNOSIS   Mucocele

- Soft tissue abscess
- Fibroepithelial polyp
- Venous lake
- Pyogenic granuloma
- Gingival cyst
- Soft irritation fibroma
- Gingival cysts
- Hemangioma
- Herpes simplex
- Neurofibroma
- Lipoma
- Salivary gland tumor
- Oral lymphangioma

Confirming the Diagnosis

- Biopsy to rule out other mucocutaneous lesions. Presence of salivary gland tissue and sialomucin is diagnostic (More et al., 2014).

Treatment

- Lesions often rupture and resolve spontaneously.
- If persistent, excision or other destructive procedure such as cautery, cryotherapy, laser ablation, or micromarsupialization.
- Intralesional corticosteroid.

Management and Patient Education

- Avoidance of local trauma to help prevent occurrence.
- Recurrent mucocele may result in a permanent lump to the area.

Irritation Fibroma

Irritation fibromas are common, benign slow-growing tumors composed of fibrous or connective tissue. They develop over weeks to months and can be greater than 1 cm in diameter. They affect 1% to 2% of adults but can occur at any age.

Pathophysiology

They result from chronic local trauma forming a scarlike reaction. They can develop from biting, dentures, or a rough tooth.

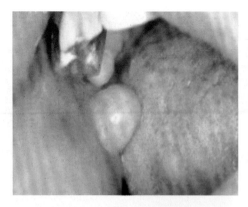

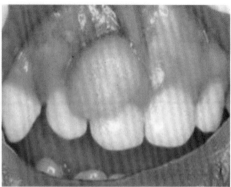

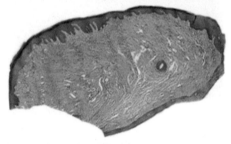

FIG. 11.3-7. Irritation fibroma. (Courtesy of SlideShare.)

Clinical Presentation

- Asymptomatic other than the awareness of lesion.
- Firm, smooth, dome-shaped pale pink papule in the mouth (tongue, lip, palate, or buccal mucosa or other oral mucosal surface (Fig. 11.3-7).
- Usually less than 1 cm, solitary lesion with a pedunculated base.
- If multiple lesions present, then consider tuberous sclerosis, Cowden syndrome, familial fibromatosis, and fibrotic papillary hyperplasia of the palate.

DIFFERENTIAL DIAGNOSIS   Irritation Fibroma

- Squamous papilloma
- Giant cell fibroma
- Neurofibroma
- Mucocele
- Benign and malignant salivary gland tumors
- Peripheral giant cell granuloma

Confirming the Diagnosis

- Clinical suspicion.
- Biopsy to exclude other conditions and to remove lesion if bothersome. Biopsy shows a typical dense, avascular fibrous stroma with few lymphocytes, no capsule, often atrophic epithelium.

Treatment

- Surgical excision with narrow margins if warranted.

Management and Patient Education

- May recur despite excision if irritation continues
- Remove potential irritant

TONGUE
Fissured Tongue

Fissured tongue is a common variation of a "normal"-appearing tongue. Its incidence increases with age, affecting approximately 2% to 5% of the U.S. population and up to 30.5% worldwide (Yarom et al., 2004). It is synonymous with scrotal tongue, hamburger tongue, grooved tongue, furrowed tongue, lingua fissurata, and lingua plicata. It can be associated with the following disorders: Melkersson–Rosenthal syndrome, Down syndrome, Sjögren syndrome, psoriasis, acromegaly, benign migratory glossitis (geographic tongue).

Pathophysiology

It is a permanent benign condition of unknown etiology. Fissured tongue may have a hereditary predisposition.

Clinical Presentation

- Multiple furrows and deep grooves with anterior–posterior orientation on the dorsal and lateral aspects of the tongue (Fig. 11.3-8)
- Asymptomatic unless debris within the grooves or if associated with geographic tongue
- May lead to halitosis

DIFFERENTIAL DIAGNOSIS   Fissured Tongue

- Cheilitis granulomatosa
- Geographic tongue

Confirming the Diagnosis

- Diagnosis based on clinical appearance.
- Biopsy is rarely required, but usually demonstrates hypertrophic lamina propria, loss of filiform papillae of the surface mucosa,

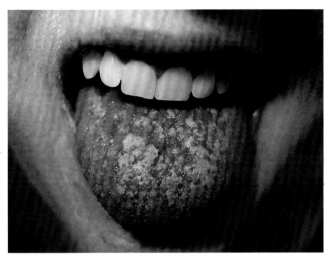

FIG. 11.3-8. Fissured tongue. (Image provided by Stedman's.)

hyperplasia of the rete pegs, neutrophilic microabscesses within the epithelium, and a mixed inflammatory infiltrate in the lamina propria (Rogers, 1996).

Treatment

- No treatment required

Management and Patient Education

- If symptomatic, encourage brushing the tongue or using an oral irrigator to eliminate debris
- Appropriate referral for Melkersson–Rosenthal syndrome, especially if cranial nerve VII (facial nerve) is affected

Hairy Tongue

Hairy tongue, also known as lingua villosa (nigra), is commonly referred to as black or white hairy tongue despite the variance of color presentation. The condition is benign and generally asymptomatic. Incidence varies geographically between 0.6% and 11.3% (Gurvits & Tan, 2014). Contributing factors to hairy tongue are numerous and include tobacco use, alcohol, coffee or tea consumption, poor oral hygiene, mouth breathing, *C. albicans,* trigeminal neuralgia, general debilitation, xerostomia, dehydration, and certain medications.

Pathophysiology

It is characterized by hypertrophy and elongation of the filiform papillae due to defective desquamation and retention of keratin. This results in hairlike projections on the dorsal surface of the tongue.

Clinical Presentation

- It can present as black, brown, white, green, pink, or other coloration on tongue depending on the etiology.
- Asymptomatic hairlike lesions or furry plaques on the dorsum of the tongue (Fig. 11.3-9).
- Patients may report gagging sensation, altered taste, halitosis, cosmetic imperfection.

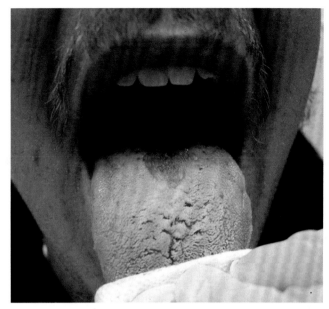

FIG. 11.3-9. Black hairy tongue. (Image provided by Stedman's.)

DIFFERENTIAL DIAGNOSIS   Hairy Tongue
• Pseudo hairy tongue
• Acanthosis nigricans
• Oral hairy leukoplakia
• Pigmented fungiform papillae of the tongue
• Congenital melanocytic/melanotic nevi/macules
• Drug-induced hyperpigmentation

Confirming the Diagnosis

- Visual intraoral examination with detailed history and evaluation.
- Distinguish from oral candidiasis (thrush)—lesions of thrush can be scraped away.
- Consider KOH or culture.
- Biopsy rarely required, but would show elongated filiform papillae on the dorsal aspect of the tongue greater than 3 mm in length; microbial colonies between the filiform papillae.

Treatment

- Remove the predisposing factors (smoking, alcohol, etc.).
- Routine brushing of tongue's surface.
- If *C. albicans* present, treat with antifungal agents as you would treat thrush.

Management and Patient Education

- Reassurance

Migratory Glossitis

Migratory glossitis, often referred to as geographic tongue, is a benign condition that occurs in up to 3% of the general population. It is more common in adults and there is a 2:1 preference for females. It may wax and wane over years.

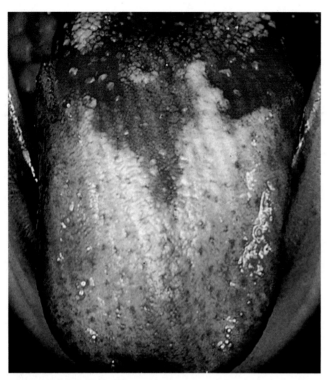

FIG. 11.3-10. Migratory glossitis.

Pathophysiology

The etiology is unknown, however there may be increased incidence in patients with psoriasis, especially the pustular psoriasis, as well as atopic dermatitis and Reiter syndrome. Loss of the filiform papillae of the tongue causes depapillated, erythematous circumferential areas with a white border on the dorsal aspect of the tongue in a maplike appearance. It may wax and wane over years.

Clinical Presentation

- Irregular shaped, erythematous maplike smooth or swollen areas surrounded by a well-demarcated white border on surface of tongue (Fig. 11.3-10).
- Lesions of migratory glossitis can change in location (migratory), size, and shape rapidly.
- Usually asymptomatic, however burning and irritation may occur.
- Can occur suddenly and persist for months or longer, and may often recur.

DIFFERENTIAL DIAGNOSIS	Migratory Glossitis
• Oral candidiasis	• Oral cancer
• Lichen planus	• Fissured tongue
• Leukoplakia	• Chemical burns
• Systemic lupus erythematosus	• Fissured tongue
• Herpes simplex virus	• Contact stomatitis
• Drug reaction	• Manifestation of psoriasis

Confirming the Diagnosis

- Diagnosis is usually made by clinical presentation
- Biopsy if questionable; histology comparable to pustular psoriasis (Assimakopoulos et al., 2002)

Treatment

- No treatment usually required
- Symptomatic treatment if needed, topical and systemic antihistamines, topical corticosteroids, topical retinoids, topical tacrolimus (Ishibashi et al., 2011)
- Cyclosporine for more severe/chronic presentation if oral involvement of psoriasis is a strong consideration (Abe et al., 2007)

Management and Patient Education

- Reassurance
- Most cases resolve without treatment

ORAL CAVITY

Aphthous Ulcers

Aphthous ulcers, also known as canker sores, are most commonly caused by recurrent aphthous stomatitis (RAS). These painful ulcerations occur on the oral mucous membranes. RAS occurs in up to 66% of the population, most commonly in adolescents and young adults (rare in adults over 40), and in those in higher socioeconomic classes. A familial predilection has been noted with a slight female predominance. With no known cure, management is based on symptom control.

Pathophysiology

Despite research to determine etiology, the cause of RAS remains unknown. In those with an underlying cause, pathophysiology is specific to that condition. In addition to RAS, known triggers of aphthous ulcers include trauma, recurrent intraoral herpes simplex virus (HSV) stomatitis, cyclic neutropenia, certain foods, psychological stress, medications, and hormonal fluctuations. Associated systemic disorders are more likely to be seen with complex aphthosis and can include anemia, hematinic or mineral deficiencies, inflammatory bowel disease, and gluten-sensitive enteropathy.

Pertinent History

It is important to know if the lesions are few or many, if they recur infrequently or are frequent/continuous, how rapidly the lesions heal, the level of associated pain and disability, and whether there are lesions on other mucous membrane sites.

Clinical Presentation

- *Minor aphthae* generally present with a few, small (<5-mm) ulcers on the nonmasticatory, soft oral mucosal surfaces of the cheeks, lips, and tongue.
- Ulcers can be round to ovoid, and shallow with yellowish-white to gray (Fig. 11.3-11) pseudomembranous base, well-defined border, and prominent erythematous rim.
- Outbreaks occur three to six times per year and last up to 14 days.
- *Major aphthae*—by contrast, are over 1 cm and usually deeper, lasting up to 6 weeks.
- They may occur on keratinized mucosa such as the dorsal tongue and hard palate and may scar. Herpetiform (grouped) aphthae are numerous small aphthae that develop simultaneously and may coalesce. They favor nonkeratinized mucosa unlike recurrent oral HSV lesions which favor keratinized mucosa.
- *Complex aphthae*—are less common, but are more painful, leading to greater disability. They may be episodic or continuous and

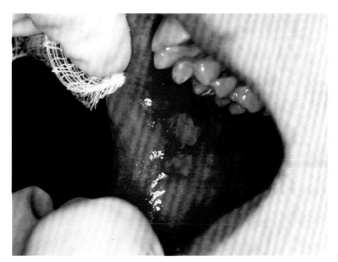

FIG. 11.3-11. Aphthous ulcers. (Used with permission from Arndt, K. A., Hsu, J. T., Alam, M., Bhatia, A. C., & Chilukuri, S. [2014]. *Manual of dermatologic therapeutics* [8th ed.]. Wolters Kluwer.)

are slower to heal with usually more ulcers per outbreak. There may be genital involvement.

- Pain is frequently associated with aphthous ulcers of all types.

DIFFERENTIAL DIAGNOSIS	Aphthous Ulcers
• HSV • Herpes zoster • HIV infection • Erosive lichen planus • Hand–foot–mouth disease • Mucous membrane pemphigoid • Oral candidiasis • SCC	• Chemotherapy-induced mucositis • Behçet disease—especially if genital and ocular involvement • Gluten-sensitive enteropathy—if bowel symptoms • Inflammatory bowel disease—if bowel symptoms

Confirming the Diagnosis

- Diagnosis is clinical and the lesions must be distinguished from ulcers occurring from an underlying cause.
- Biopsy is rarely necessary.
- Findings consistent with complex aphthae should prompt a possible workup to rule out systemic disease initially: CBC, iron studies with ferritin, B12 levels, serum antiendomysium antibodies, and transglutaminase assay.
- GI consult with recurrent ulcers and persistent bowel symptoms.

Treatment
Topical

- Avoid any known triggers such as spicy, acidic, and hard-edged foods such as toast or chips. Minimize trauma by brushing with a soft rounded toothbrush.
- Manage pain with topical agents: A mixture of equal parts Benadryl and Maalox can be held in the mouth for 2 to 5 minutes before meals to reduce pain; viscous lidocaine 2% can be added to the mixture. A coating substance such as sucralfate can be applied to individual lesions.

- Topical steroids can suppress immunologic mechanisms. The use of a topical fluorinated corticosteroid such as 0.05% fluocinonide in orabase, applied every 1 to 2 hours while awake, may prevent full-blown development of lesions of RAS.
- Conversion of the painful ulcer to a painless wound using escharotics or laser can speed healing.

Systemic

- Systemic therapy should be specific to the underlying condition, such as treating inflammatory bowel disease or replenishing a deficiency.
- Nonspecific systemic therapy should be used if there is sufficient severity or duration of symptoms. These treatments could include steroids, dapsone, colchicine, tetracycline, thalidomide, biologic agents, and levamisole. These treatments should be used by those familiar with their use and risks (Saikaly et al., 2018).

Management and Patient Education

- Fortunately, most patients with aphthae have RAS, which is characterized by simple aphthae, few lesions per episode, few episodes per year, mild symptoms, and the expectation of eventual remission.
- Avoidance of triggers or treatment to manage symptoms is all that is required.
- For those with more severe disease or complex aphthae, further workup will likely reveal an underlying cause and therefore identify available treatments.
- For those with no underlying cause identified and not managed adequately by local topical therapy, consider referral for nonspecific immunomodulating agents.
- Most treatments do not prevent recurrence of outbreaks.

CLINICAL PEARLS

- First identify whether it is simple or complex aphthae and proceed accordingly with management of simple or workup of complex symptoms. Most patients will fall into the simple category and do well.
- Reserve workup for those likely to have an identifiable underlying cause and then treat accordingly.
- Be sure to reassure RAS patients that spontaneous remission is likely in time.

Torus Palatinus

Torus palatinus is a benign bony tumor of the maxilla that affects 20% to 30% of people in the United States.

Pathophysiology

Etiology is unknown though genetic factors, superficial injuries, and palate stress from mastication are thought to play a role (Aron et al., 2017).

Clinical Presentation

- Asymptomatic, usually located along the longitudinal ridge of the hard palate
- Shape can be flat, nodular, fusiform, unilobular, multilobulated, or pedunculated (Fig. 11.3-12)
- Usually flat and symmetrical with a smooth appearance

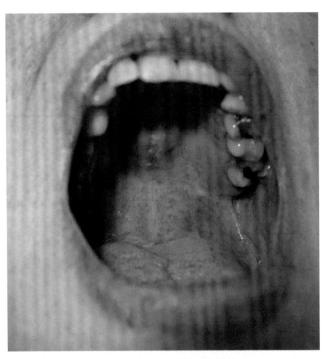

FIG. 11.3-12. Torus palatinus. (Image provided by Stedman's.)

- Covered by thin mucosa with sensitivity during trauma (Bouchet et al., 2019)

DIFFERENTIAL DIAGNOSIS   Torus Palatinus

- Benign or malignant tumor

Confirming the Diagnosis

- Clinical diagnosis when classic presentation
- Radiographs may be used for confirmation

Treatment

- No treatment usually required
- Surgical removal is indicated if the torus is large enough to interfere with surgical airway management, subject to trauma or causes trapping of food

Management and Patient Education

- Benign and asymptomatic
- Reassurance and management only if problems arise

Leukoplakia

Leukoplakia is a relatively common, oral, potentially malignant disorder that presents as white patches of the oral mucosa. Although leukoplakia itself is a benign and asymptomatic condition, the potential for malignancy requires that the lesions have appropriate monitoring and biopsy when indicated with treatment based on histologic results.

Leukoplakia is found in between 1.5% and 4.3% of the general population (Mello et al., 2018) with greater risk in those over 40. Risk factors are similar to those for SCC and include use of tobacco

and alcohol, as well as infection with human papillomavirus (HPV). It should be noted the oral hairy leukoplakia is commonly triggered by the Epstein–Barr virus and is most often seen in immunocompromised individuals, especially those with HIV.

Pathophysiology

Leukoplakia usually demonstrates benign features, with simple hyperkeratosis seen most frequently. Epithelial dysplasia, if present, ranges from mild to severe, although carcinoma in situ or even invasive SCC may be encountered.

Clinical Presentation

- White plaques or patches adherent to the underlying mucosa, such that it cannot be easily removed with gauze—and an attempt to remove it forcibly may induce bleeding.
- May be homogeneous with a uniformly white, thin, thick, or verrucous plaque with well-defined margins; or nonhomogeneous with mixed red and white lesions that can be nodular, speckled, or granular (van der Waal, 2019) (Fig. 11.3-13).
- Increased risk of progression to SCC is found in those lesions that are nonhomogeneous, large, localized to the lateral border of the tongue and the floor of the mouth, and demonstrate dysplasia on histologic examination.

DIFFERENTIAL DIAGNOSIS   Leukoplakia

- Frictional keratosis
- Lichen planus
- Discoid lupus erythematosus
- Candidiasis
- Oral hairy leukoplakia
- SCC
- Oral HPV

Confirming the Diagnosis

- If lesion is persistent after elimination of possible causative factors (such as trauma or candida), a biopsy is warranted.
- Referral to oral surgeon, dermatology surgeon, or otolaryngologist for biopsy of several foci of a large lesion is recommended.

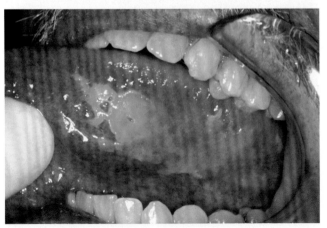

FIG. 11.3-13. Leukoplakia. (Used with permission from DeLong, L., & Burkhart, N. [2012]. *General and oral pathology for the dental hygienist* [2nd ed.]. Wolters Kluwer.)

- If histology suggests a benign process (such as lichen planus [LP], or trauma), then treatment is based on those findings.
- If pathology reveals moderate to severe dysplasia, or the lesion is in a high-risk area as above, then prompt referral and more aggressive management is warranted.

Treatment

- Treatment decisions should be made based on clinical experience, patient preference, lesion size and location, and the presence of histologic dysplasia.
- Surgical management is recommended for small lesions with moderate to severe dysplasia, in high-risk locations, or that are clinically nonhomogeneous.
- Many nonsurgical destructive options exist such as laser ablation, cryosurgery, and medical therapy. These options do not have the advantage of histologic evaluation of the entire lesion which may show changes not present in biopsy samples.

Management and Patient Education

- For all patients, regardless of treatment or observation status, cessation of high-risk habits (tobacco and alcohol use) should be encouraged and reinforced at each visit.
- Any lesion showing clinical evidence of recurrence or change suggestive of cancer should be biopsied.
- Clinical and histologic surveillance should be ongoing. Recommend lifelong follow-up at intervals of 3 to 18 months depending on patient-specific characteristics.

Lichen Planus

LP is a mucocutaneous inflammatory condition that can present as pruritic violaceous, slightly shiny papules and plaques on the body, or as lesions on the conjunctiva, genitalia, anus, mucosal membranes, tonsils, or larynx. Oral LP has many forms, may occur separately or concurrently, and can be severe and erosive. The reticular form is most common and appears as white plaques with a lacelike pattern, called "Wickham striae," affecting the buccal mucosa or lateral tongue (Fig. 11.3-14). It most commonly affects middle-aged adults, with a slightly higher prevalence in females. Studies report a high incidence of hepatitis C virus (HCV), chronic hepatitis, and

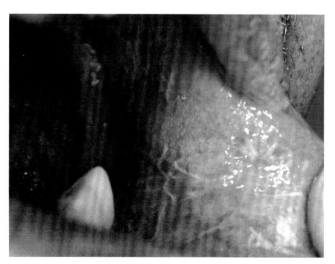

FIG. 11.3-14. Lichen planus.

primary biliary cirrhosis in patients with LP. Refer all patients with erosive LP to a specialist.

Please refer to Section 4.5 (LP, PR, and other Scaly Stuff) for detailed diagnostic, treatment, and management information. LP in the genital area is discussed in Section 11.4.

KOPLIK SPOTS—MEASLES

This highly contagious respiratory virus (*Measles morbillivirus*), which is known to present with high fever, purple to red macular and papular rash, and the three "Cs" (coryza, cough, and conjunctivitis).

Clinical Presentation

- An oral presentation of erythematous mucous membranes with gray-white to red papules on the buccal mucosa (Koplik spots) is pathognomonic for measles.

Treatment and Management

Please refer to Section 13.2 (Common Childhood Infections) for detailed information.

READINGS AND REFERENCES

Abe, M., Sogabe, Y., Syuto, T., Ishibuchi, H., Yokoyama, Y., & Ishikawa, O. (2007). Successful treatment with cyclosporin administration for persistent benign migratory glossitis. *Journal of Dermatology*, 34(5), 340–343. https://doi.org/10.1111/j.1346-8138.2007.00284.x

Aron, J., Raithel, S. J., & Mannes, A. J. (2017). Images in anesthesiology: Torus palatinus and airway management. *Anesthesiology*, 127(1), 164. https://doi.org/10.1097/ALN.0000000000001566

Assimakopoulos, D., Patrikakos, G., Fotika, C., & Elisaf, M. (2002). Benign migratory glossitis or geographic tongue: An enigmatic oral lesion. *American Journal of Medicine*, 113(9), 751–755. https://doi.org/10.1016/s0002-9343(02)01379-7

Bean, W. B., & Walsh, J. R. (1956). Venous lakes. *American Medical Association Archives of Dermatology*, 74(5), 459–463.

Bouchet, J., Hervé, G., Lescaille, G., Descroix, V., & Guyonet, A. (2019). Palatal torus: Etiology, clinical aspect, and therapeutic strategy. *Journal of Oral Medicine and Oral Surgery*, 25(2), 18. https://doi.org/10.1051/mbcb/2018040

Gurvits, G. E., & Tan, A.˙ (2014). Black hairy tongue syndrome. *World Journal of Gastroenterology*, 20(31), 10845–10850. https://doi.org/10.3748/wjg.v20.i31.10845

Ishibashi, M., Tojo, G., Watanabe, M., Tamabuchi, T., Masu, T., & Aiba, S. (2011). Geographic tongue treated with topical tacrolimus. *Journal of Dermatological Case Reports*, 4(4), 57–59. https://doi.org/10.3315/jdcr.2010.1058

Jay, H., & Borek, C. (1998). Treatment of a venous-lake angioma with intense pulsed light. *Lancet*, 351(9096), 112.

Lee, C., Neville, B. W., Damm, D. D., Allen, C., & Bouquot, J. (2008). *Oral and maxillofacial pathology*. Elsevier Health Sciences.

Mello, F. W., Miguel, A., Dutra, K., Porporatti, A., Warnakulasuriya, S., Guerra, E., & Rivero, E. (2018). Prevalence of oral potentially malignant disorders: A systematic review and meta-analysis. *Journal of Oral Pathology & Medicine*, 47(7), 633–640.

More, C. B., Bhavsar, K., Varma, S., & Tailor, M. (2014). Oral mucocele: A clinical and histopathological study. *Journal of Oral and Maxillofacial Pathology*, 18(Suppl 1), S72–S77. https://doi.org/10.4103/0973-029x.141370

Park, K. K., Brodell, R. T., & Helms, S. E. (2011). Angular cheilitis, part 2: Nutritional, systemic, and drug-related causes and treatment. *Cutis; Cutaneous Medicine for the Practitioner*, 88(1), 27–32.

Rogers, R. S. (1996). Melkersson-Rosenthal syndrome and orofacial granulomatosis. *Dermatologic Clinics*, 14(2), 371–379. https://doi.org/10.1016/s0733-8635(05)70363-6

Saikaly, S. K., Saikaly, T. S., & Saikaly, L. E. (2018). Recurrent aphthous ulceration: A review of potential causes and novel treatments. The *Journal of Dermatological Treatment*, 29(6), 542–552. https://doi.org/10.1080/09546634.2017.1422079

van der Waal, I. (2019). Oral leukoplakia; a proposal for simplification and consistency of the clinical classification and terminology. *Medicina Oral, Patologia Oral y Cirugia Bucal*, 24(6), e799–e803.

Wall, T., Grassi, A., & Avram, M. (2007). Clearance of multiple venous lakes with an 800-nm diode laser: A novel approach. *Dermatologic Surgery*, 33(1), 100–103.

Warnakulasuriya, S., Johnson, N., & van der Waal, I. (2007). Nomenclature and classification of potentially malignant disorders of the oral mucosa. *Journal Oral Pathology & Medicine*, 36(10), 575–580.

Yarom, N., Cantony, U., & Gorsky, M. (2004). Prevalence of fissured tongue, geographic tongue and median rhomboid glossitis among Israeli adults of different ethnic origins. *Dermatology*, 209(2), 88–94. https://doi.org/10.1159/000079590

Genital Disorders

Elizabeth Drumm and Jeffrey Viveiros

In This Chapter

- Benign Genital Skin Lesions
- Genital Anatomy
- Diagnostic Approach
  - History
  - Genital Examination
- Genital Pruritus
  - Atopic Dermatitis
  - Allergic Contact Dermatitis
  - Irritant Contact Dermatitis
- Inflammatory Conditions
  - Lichen Planus
  - Lichen Sclerosis
  - Zoon Balanitis
- Infections
  - Genital Herpes Virus
  - Genital Human Papillomavirus
  - Candidiasis
- Premalignant and Malignant
  - Intraepithelial Neoplasia
  - Extramammary Paget Disease

Numerous skin conditions can affect the genitalia of men and women and can be common manifestations of disorders involving other areas of the body. Often, genital dermatoses go untreated because of embarrassment, shame, and physical or emotional discomfort in treating these problems. Genital disorders may be painful, affect sexual function and relationships, impact self-esteem, and alter the quality of life. They may be related to infection, inflammation, and sometimes skin cancer. Variants of normal and common benign growths can also be concerning for patients until they have been reassured. It behooves all providers to be aware of and be able to recognize them to avoid any unnecessary biopsy or treatment. See Table 11.4-1.

GENITAL ANATOMY

Skin in the genital area is a combination of keratinized, modified mucous membrane and membranous skin which makes the clinical

TABLE 11.4-1	Benign Genital Skin Lesions	
CONDITION	**DESCRIPTION**	**PRESENTATION**
Angiokeratoma (Fig. 11.4-1)	Small (2–5 mm), red, blue, or purple papules that can occur as solitary or multiple lesions on scrotum, penile shaft, glans penis, labia minora, or labia majora. No treatment required	FIG. 11.4-1. Angiokeratoma. (Used with permission from Edwards, L., & Lynch, P. [2018]. *Genital dermatology atlas and manual* [3rd ed.]. Wolters Kluwer.)

(continued)

TABLE 11.4-1	Benign Genital Skin Lesions (*Continued*)	
CONDITION	**DESCRIPTION**	**PRESENTATION**
Fordyce Spots (sebaceous glands) (Fig. 11.4-2)	Asymptomatic, small (2–3 mm) papules of varying color from white to red on scrotal sac and penile shaft labia minora, majora. No treatment required	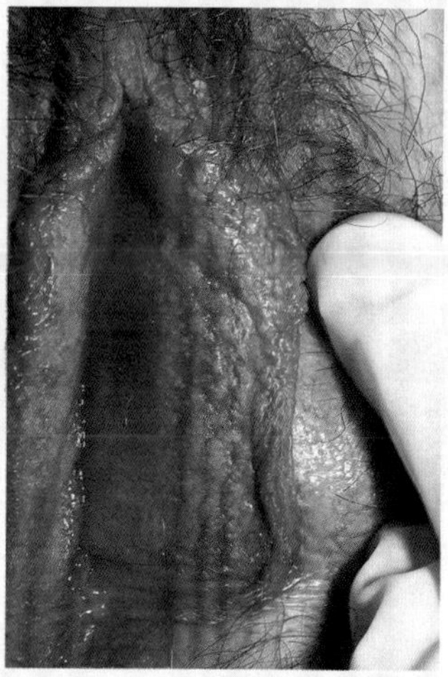 FIG. 11.4-2. Fordyce spots. (Used with permission from Edwards, L., & Lynch, P. [2018]. *Genital dermatology atlas and manual* [3rd ed.]. Wolters Kluwer.)
Pearly Penile Papules (Fig. 11.4-3)	Present in two or three rows of uniform skin colored, smooth, rounded papules (1–2 mm) around the coronal margin or sulcus and rarely involves the glans penis. No treatment required	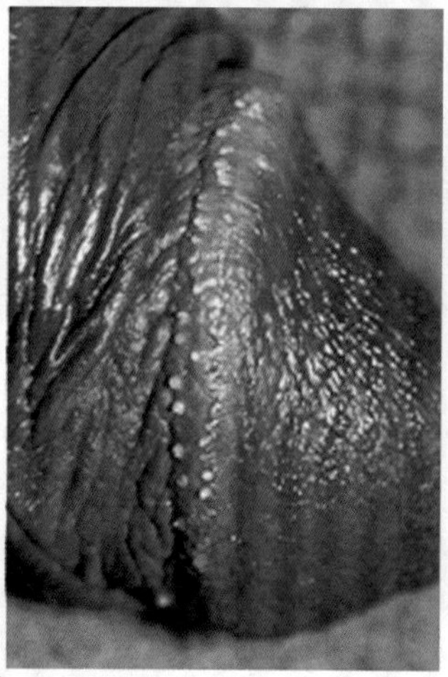 FIG. 11.4-3. Pearly penile papules.
Epidermal Cysts (Fig. 11.4-4)	2-1-mm white or yellow cystic papules commonly see in men and women	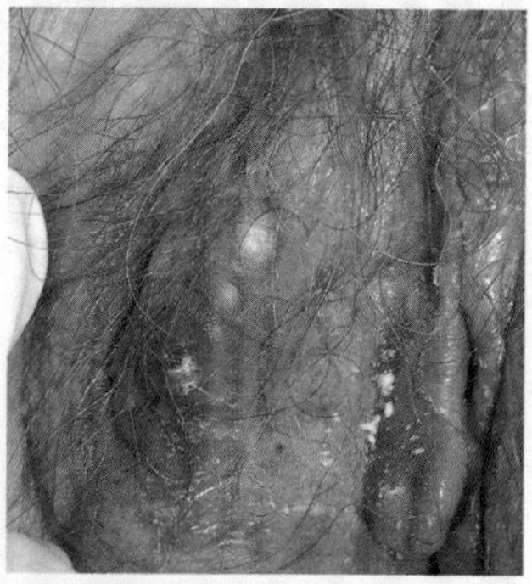 FIG. 11.4-4. Epidermal cysts. (Used with permission from Edwards, L., & Lynch, P. [2018]. *Genital dermatology atlas and manual* [3rd ed.]. Wolters Kluwer.)

CONDITION	DESCRIPTION	PRESENTATION
Lichen Nitidus (Fig. 11.4-5)	Discrete and uniform, flat topped, itchy 1–2-mm micropapules; pruritus may be an associated feature; usually seen in young school-aged children. Seen in anogenital area, shaft, and glans of penis It rarely affects the genitals of adult men	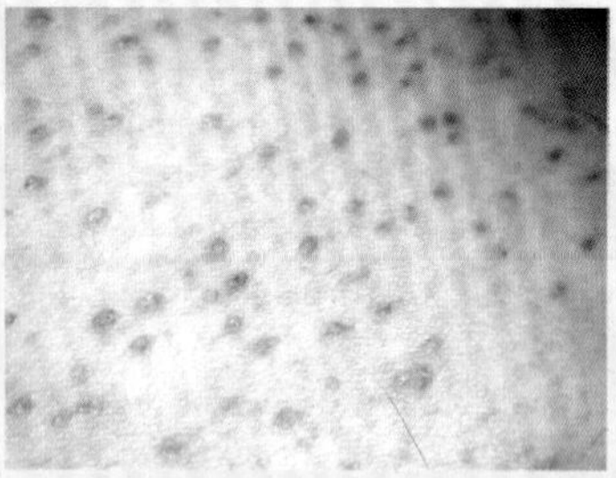 FIG. 11.4-5. Lichen nitidus.
Vestibular Papillae (Fig. 11.4-6)	It can be confused with viral warts and Bowenoid papulosis Labia minora, labia majora, penis	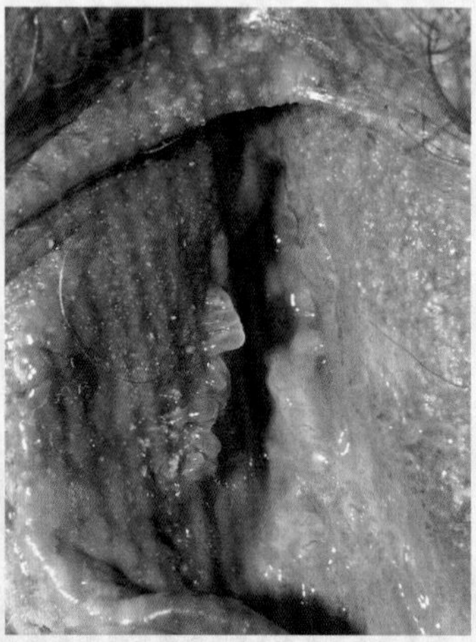 FIG. 11.4-6. Vestibular papillae. These benign papillae are often misdiagnosed as warts. (Used with permission from Edwards, L., & Lynch, P. [2018]. *Genital dermatology atlas and manual* [3rd ed.]. Wolters Kluwer.)
Normal Labial Rugae (Fig. 11.4-7)	Vestibule Mistaken warts Labia majora	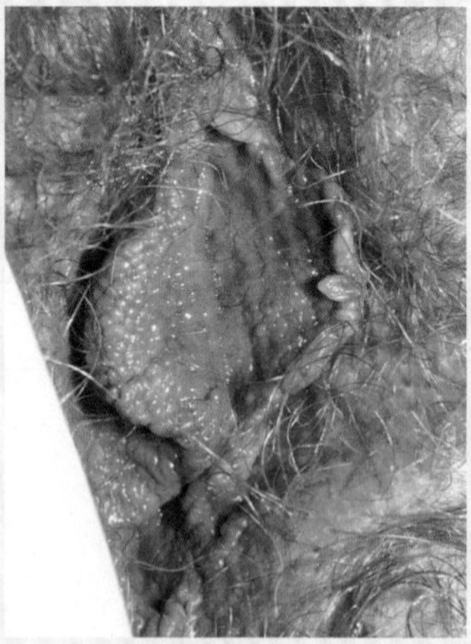 FIG. 11.4-7. Normal labial rugae. (Used with permission from Edwards, L., & Lynch, P. [2018]. *Genital dermatology atlas and manual* [3rd ed.]. Wolters Kluwer.)

presentation unique and challenging to diagnose disease. Knowledge of the normal male and female genital anatomy is paramount to correctly identifying abnormal signs and symptoms.

- Inflammatory dermatoses on the genitalia may be difficult to appreciate and appear hyperpigmented instead of red. Typical scaly plaques of a papulosquamous disease on the trunk may lack the defined borders, erythema, and scale when it involves the genitalia.

- The normal rugae of the labia majora and the scrotum may mask lichenification.

- Normal papillae on the vulva or pearly papules on the corona of the glans penis may be mistaken for verrucous papules.

- The secretory glands on the glans penis and the vulva, as well as cervical and vaginal mucous secretions, can alter the appearance of the genitalia, especially when inflammation is present.

FEMALE

- The skin on the mons pubis which extends to the lateral aspect of the labia majora is dry, keratinized, and usually hair bearing.
- Medial aspects of the labia majora, including the labia minora, are partially keratinized and partially modified mucous membrane which is generally moist and hair bearing (Fig. 11.4-8A).

MALE

- The pubis and part of the shaft of the penis and scrotum have dry, keratinized skin that may be hair bearing.
- The penile shaft is modified mucosa, as well as the glans of the penis and the border of the glans or corona, and most often these areas contain no hair.

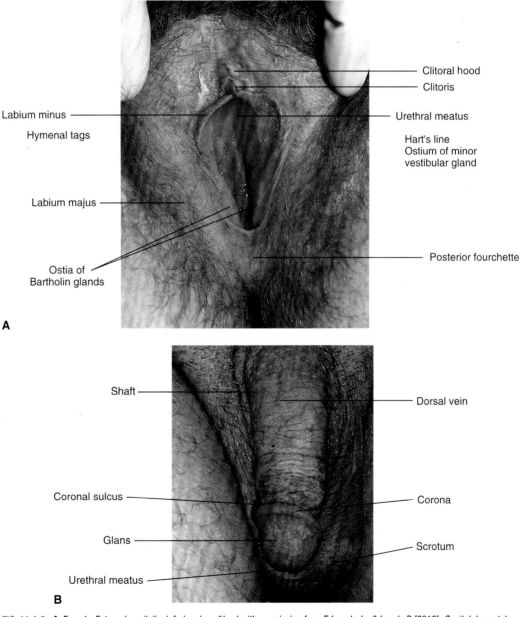

FIG. 11.4-8. **A:** Female. External genitalia, inferior view. (Used with permission from Edwards, L., & Lynch, P. [2018]. *Genital dermatology atlas and manual* [3rd ed.]. Wolters Kluwer.) **B:** Male. External genitalia, inferior view. (Used with permission from Edwards, L., & Lynch, P. [2018]. *Genital dermatology atlas and manual* [3rd ed.]. Wolters Kluwer.)

- The urethra at the tip of the glans is composed of mucous membrane.

- In uncircumcised males, the glans and corona are covered by the prepuce (foreskin).

- Careful examination of this otherwise obstructed area is important because of the increased incidence of psoriasis, lichen planus (LP), lichen sclerosus (LS), balanitis, and squamous cell carcinoma (Fig. 11.4-8B).

HYGIENE

With the variation of skin of the genitalia in mind, we must also consider personal hygiene practices and how they can affect the skin barrier and clinical presentation. Many people wash frequently or apply multiple products to the genitals in an effort to "clean" the area. Over cleansing may contribute to a compromised skin barrier and irritant or allergic dermatitis, making it more susceptible to infectious organisms and inflammation. Likewise, urine and feces left on the skin can result in chronic irritation. Adult incontinence products are widely utilized and may be tight or occlusive resulting in friction and increased moisture, all of which may affect the skin barrier of the genitalia.

DIAGNOSTIC APPROACH

Males and females may present with similar complaints but may have vastly different diagnoses.

The chief complaint is often pruritus or discomfort. A thorough history will begin to refine the differential and help focus the physical examination (Box 11.4-1).

Genital Skin Examination

- First, examine extragenital areas which may reveal the presence of inflammatory dermatoses such as psoriasis, offering clues to the genital problem.

- Retracting the foreskin (if possible) is important to observe the glans and perhaps clues to urinary incontinence and possible irritants.

- Women who present with vulva pain should have a Q-tip test to locate the exact area of discomfort.

- Observe for discharge from urinary meatus or vagina.

- Observe for papules, pustules, vesicles, excoriations, rash, or lichenification.

- Examine the genital, perineal, and perianal areas for lesions, erythema, lichenification, or areas of hyper or hypopigmentation.

GENITAL PRURITUS

Anogenital pruritus is a very common complaint of patients in dermatology departments.

BOX 11.4-1 Important Aspects of History

Symptom onset, duration, location, aggravating and alleviating factors
Sexual dysfunction/dyspareunia
Urinary dysfunction/incontinence
Circumcision
Drug history
Contraception measures
Personal/family history/atopy
Sexual history/risk factors
Menstrual cycle/pregnancy

The very nature of the location causes embarrassment and often reluctance to seek advice.

It is experienced by men and women and can reflect a myriad of problems both local and systemic. Section 5 discusses the pathophysiology of pruritus, along with the careful evaluation, diagnosis, and management of symptoms.

In this section, however, we will focus our discussion on common dermatoses associated with this most annoying symptom in the genital area. A broad range of conditions can present with itching including infection such as human papillomavirus (HPV) or HSV, dermatoses such as atopic dermatitis (AD), inflammatory conditions such as LP, and some dermatoses which may have some potential for cancerous transformation such as lichen sclerosis. A careful history and physical examination as discussed above should be completed at the outset. It is important to provide an environment of comfort and acceptance in your professional approach to these patients with genital concerns.

Eczematous Disorders

Eczema is a common inflammatory skin condition and a common cause of chronic pruritus in the genital area. Eczematous disorder encompasses *AD, seborrheic dermatitis, irritant contact dermatitis (ICD), and allergic contact dermatitis (ACD).* These dermatoses may affect areas of the body outside of the genital area, and they are discussed in detail in Section 4.

Atopic Dermatitis

AD is an inflammatory disorder usually associated with atopy, which includes a possible family or personal history of seasonal allergies, medication allergies, skin allergies, and/or asthma.

- It is the itch that induces scratching, resulting in the changes seen on the skin, and can include the genital area. People with AD usually have a sensation of itch in response to irritation of the skin, rather than soreness.

- For these patients, scratching can offer a sense of temporary relief, but in turn may keep the itch/scratch cycle active and eventually produces a secondary rash.

See Section 4.1 for Pathophysiology AD.

Clinical Presentation

Skin Findings

- Erythematous scaling, intensely itchy plaques or patches, often affecting flexural surfaces of the skin.

- Adults may have a flare involving the genitalia and sparing other regions of the body, which can appear different than AD on the arms and legs.

- Often what is seen on the genitalia is thickening of the tissue with accentuated skin lines, known as *lichen simplex chronicus* (Fig. 11.4-9), which occurs after prolonged pruritus and scratching.

- The erythema and scaling may also affect the thighs and perianal area but spare other extensor surfaces.

- There is hyperkeratosis of the stratum corneum and thickening of the epidermis analogous to a callus.

- In men, AD usually involves the scrotum, where skin lines may blend with the normal rugae or the skin may appear somewhat shiny (Fig. 11.4-10). The shaft of the penis can also be involved.

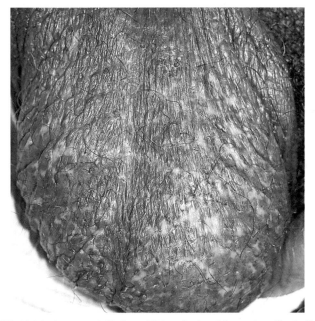

FIG. 11.4-9. Accentuated skin lines of lichen simplex of the scrotum. (Used with permission from Edwards, L., & Lynch, P. [2018]. *Genital dermatology atlas and manual* [3rd ed.]. Wolters Kluwer.)

- In women, AD usually involves the labia majora, which may appear smooth with a wrinkled appearance, hyperpigmented, excoriated, and lichenified (Fig. 11.4-11).
- Fissuring in these areas may occur, and candida may be found in the fissures.
- If there is crusting, pustules, or moist scale, there may be a bacterial infection.

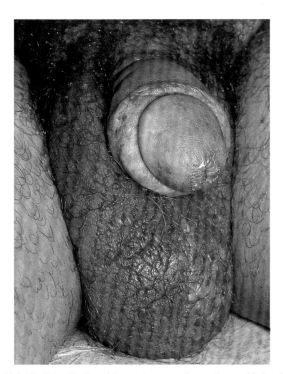

FIG. 11.4-10. Lichenification of the scrotum as well as erythema, dried vesicles, and scale in a patient with a history of atopic dermatitis. (Used with permission from Edwards, L., & Lynch, P. [2018]. *Genital dermatology atlas and manual* [3rd ed.]. Wolters Kluwer.)

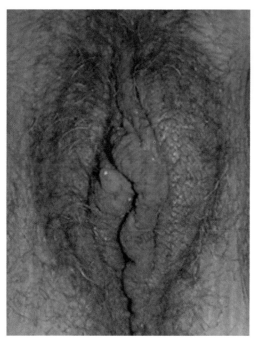

FIG. 11.4-11. Atopic dermatitis female. Even patients who are not naturally dark sometimes exhibit hyperpigmentation that obscures the inflammation of lichen simplex chronicus, as seen on this left labium majus.

DIFFERENTIAL DIAGNOSIS   Atopic Dermatitis

- Psoriasis
- Irritant contact dermatitis (ICD)
- Allergic contact dermatitis
- Scabies
- Pediculosis
- Candida
- Dermatophyte infection (e.g., tinea cruris)
- Seborrheic dermatitis
- Pityriasis rosea
- Secondary syphilis
- Mycosis fungoides

Confirming the Diagnosis

- The diagnosis may be made by clinical appearance and personal history.
- Patients are prone to bacterial, fungal, or viral superinfections, which can further exacerbate dermatitis flares.
- Culture if secondary infection suspected.
- KOH test may be helpful to rule out candida or dermatophyte as a source of the itch.
- Careful history of the patient's hygiene practices and use of cleansing products will be helpful to rule out irritant or allergic dermatitis.
- A biopsy is rarely needed unless the patient does not respond to standard treatment.

Treatment

Treatment for AD in genital area follows the same principles as AD anywhere.

BOX 11.4-2   Common Allergens in Genital Dermatitis (Men and Women)

Topical treatments—corticosteroids, antimicrobials
Bacitracin, triple antibiotic
Latex (found in condoms or contraceptive devices)
Personal lubricants (K-Y jelly contains propylene glycol), spermicides, preservatives
Perfumed hygiene sprays (fluorinated hydrocarbons)
Lipstick (octyl gallate) transferred to genitals
Nail polish from the hand
Fragrances (Balsam of Peru)

Panty liners: adhesive (acetyl acetonate or cull-acetylacetonate) fragrance or blue dye
Resin in the wax for string instruments (colophony) transferred to genitals
Medicated wipes contain methylisothiazolinone and methylchloroisothiazolinone found in Huggies and Cottonelle brands
Benzocaine or other topical anesthetics
Para-aminobenzoic acid
Hemorrhoidal medication

See Section 4 for treatment and management options.

- The treatment goal is to eliminate the itch and subsequent rash by identifying and removing any triggers or treating infections that are present.
- Daily use of emollients and barrier treatments (e.g., petrolatum or zinc oxide) should be used to restore the skin barrier.
- Consider referral to dermatology with extensive involvement, any disease that is not responding to a reasonable course to topical treatment, or if there is an uncertainty of the diagnosis.

Allergic Contact Dermatitis

ACD occurs more frequently from exposures to products applied or transferred to the genitalia, and less commonly from personal hygiene pads or undergarments.

Topical medications, including local anesthetics (such as benzocaine or lidocaine) and corticosteroids, are the most common genital allergens for men and women (Box 11.4-2). Other typical allergens include fragrances, preservatives, adhesives, dyes, and rubber products (Yale et al., 2018).

Pathophysiology

ACD of the genitalia is a T-cell–mediated, or type IV delayed hypersensitivity reaction to exogenous agents. This means that it can take hours, months, or years for the skin to react. Section 4.2 discusses the pathophysiology of ACD in detail.

Clinical Presentation

- The clinical presentation of ACD in the genitalia is usually localized and with the distribution providing very important clues for diagnosis.
- Allergens may be introduced or transferred to the genitalia from touching or rubbing.
- Chemicals on the patient's, caregiver's, or patient's partner's hand or mouth (e.g., latex condom) may be the offending agent.

Skin Findings

- Erythema, swelling, weeping, crusting, vesicles, and bullae can be seen in acute ACD (Fig. 11.4-12).
- Scaling, lichenification, fissures, and cracks can be seen in chronic ACD.
- Secondary lesions can occur from scratching.
- Geometric shapes with well demarcated borders may be seen.

Non-Skin Finding

- Pruritus and burning are usually present.

DIFFERENTIAL DIAGNOSIS   Allergic Contact Dermatitis

- Irritant contact dermatitis
- Atopic dermatitis
- Candidiasis
- Balanitis
- Seborrheic dermatitis
- Atrophic vaginitis
- Tinea cruris
- Lichen simplex chronicus
- Psoriasis
- Drug eruption
- Secondary syphilis
- Scabies
- Herpes simplex virus infection
- Bacterial vaginosis
- Impetigo
- Bowen disease

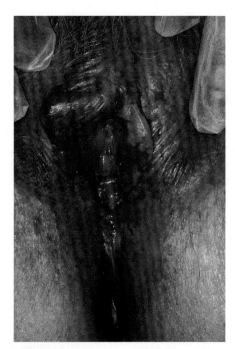

FIG. 11.4-12. Allergic contact dermatitis. Allergic contact dermatitis from an over-the-counter anti-itch medication characterized by blisters that have resulted in small round erosions. (Used with permission from Edwards, L., & Lynch, P. [2018]. *Genital dermatology atlas and manual* [3rd ed.]. Wolters Kluwer.)

Confirming the Diagnosis

- ACD of the genitalia can be difficult to diagnose, but a good history and timeline may be helpful in identifying possible allergen(s).

- Appropriate cultures and serologies may be indicated to rule out other causes of genital dermatitis, including sexually transmitted infections (STIs).

- KOH to rule out candidiasis or dermatophyte infection.

- Consider biopsy for diagnostic confirmation if there is no improvement in 2 to 3 weeks.

- Patch testing by dermatology, or other specialist (e.g., allergist or immunologist) can be helpful if the allergen is not identified through a thorough history and physical examination.

- Collaboration between the primary care provider, gynecologist, and dermatologist may be necessary for complete resolution.

Treatment

Topical

- In the absence of infection, a short course of topical corticosteroids (TCS) may be prescribed.

- Topical nonsteroidal agents (Tacrolimus ointment or Pimecrolimus cream) can also be used.

See Section 4 Treatment Atopic Dermatitis.

Systemic

- For severe ACD, oral prednisone 40 to 60 mg/day × 7 to 10 days may be required (longer courses may be required if the reaction persists but referral to dermatology is recommended).

- If there is any suspicion of HSV, concurrent use of a systemic antiviral agent is recommended.

- Consider treatment with oral antimicrobials for possible bacterial, yeast, or viral infections, if indicated.

- Oral antihistamines may be added as needed for symptomatic relief of itch.

Management and Patient Education

- The treatment goals are relief of symptoms, identification and removal of the allergen, and restoration of the skin barrier.

- Complete resolution of ACD may take several weeks even when the allergen is identified and eliminated.

- Supportive care, sitz baths, or cool soaks followed by petrolatum can calm and protect the genitalia.

- Avoidance of personal products with known common allergen. Consider any wet wipes being used to cleanse as culprit (many with preservatives).

- Fragrance-free and dye-free detergents should be used exclusively.

- Avoid tight, occlusive clothing or those that are newly purchased.

- Refer to dermatology for patch testing if avoidance and treatment does not control the outbreak after 4 weeks.

Irritant Dermatitis

ICD is an inflammatory skin condition that results from direct physical or chemical injury to the epidermis; it may be acute or chronic.

> **BOX 11.4-3 Common Irritants to Genital Area**
>
> Frequent cleansing with soap/water
> Perfumed products
> Douches
> Fragrances
> Sprays
> Nylon underwear
> Feminine hygiene pads (brands can vary)
> Tampon strings
> Alcohols
> Spermicides
> Prescribed vaginal medications
> Personal lubricants

Unlike ACD, it is not immunologically mediated. Patients with a history of eczema or AD may be at greater risk for ICD. Diaper dermatitis is discussed in detail in Section 13.

Pathophysiology

- The etiology of ICD is related to direct or indirect irritation of the skin of the genitalia.

- The offending agent can be water, moisture, and humidity, or chemicals from soaps, detergents, and personal hygiene products.

See Box 11.4-3.

- Moisture and humidity in the genital area can lead to a change in the pH and increase microbial growth.

- Irritation can also occur from exposure to a strong irritant, or repeated exposures to weaker agents.

- Exposure over time to any irritant may increase the severity of the dermatitis.

- ICD may be exacerbated by continuous cleansing, which breaks down the skin barrier, causing an increase in the inflammation and irritation.

Clinical Presentation

Skin Findings

- The genitalia may be erythematous, shiny, edematous, and with secondary erosions from scratching (Fig. 11.4-13).

- In the acute stages, vesicles may be present, but easily ruptured and go unnoticed; because the skin is thin and not well keratinized on the glans, vulva, and inner prepuce, erosions may be left in their place (Fig. 11.4-14).

- When the irritation is chronic, hypo or hyperpigmentation with lichenification may be present.

- Patients who wear incontinence garments (both infants and adults) may already have alterations in the epidermal barrier from continuous moisture, ammonia from urine, and friction from undergarments or pads.

Non-Skin Findings

- Patients with genital ICD may complain of soreness, burning, stinging, and a feeling of being "raw" or tender but the initial symptoms may be mild and go unnoticed.

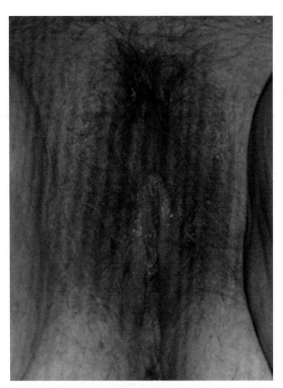

FIG. 11.4-13. Irritant contact dermatitis.

DIFFERENTIAL DIAGNOSIS   Irritant Dermatitis

- Atopic dermatitis
- Lichen simplex chronicus
- Psoriasis
- Candidiasis
- Intertrigo
- Tinea cruris
- Seborrheic dermatitis
- Scabies
- Herpes simplex virus infection

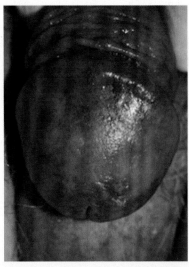

FIG. 11.4-14. This acute ICD produced by a reaction to OTC medication exhibits erythema and edema sufficient to produce some crust on glans penis.

BOX 11.4-4   Indications for Genital Biopsy

- To confirm diagnosis
- To confirm or rule out the possibility of a malignancy or precancerous dermatosis
- To identify premalignant or malignant transformation in area of erosive, hyperkeratotic, or verrucous change in lichen sclerosus and lichen planus
- To identify an abnormal melanocytic proliferation in pigmented areas, especially for those with a history of lichen sclerosus

Adapted from Shim, T. N., Ali, I., Muneer, A., & Bunker, C. B. (2016). Benign male genital dermatoses. *British Medical Journal, 354*, i4337. doi: 10.1136/bmj.i4337.

Confirming the Diagnosis

- The diagnosis of ICD can be made based on history, symptoms, clinical presentation, and exclusion of other conditions.
- ICD in the genitalia is usually localized to the area of contact, which may spare the intertriginous areas.
- ACD, in contrast may include the folds of the skin and multifocal areas.
- A KOH scraping can identify or rule out candidiasis or dermatophyte infection.
- Biopsy is not generally indicated, but histology would show spongiosis, dermal inflammatory infiltrate, and possible vesicles.

See Box 11.4-4.

Treatment
Topical

- TCS may be prescribed, as mentioned previously in Section 4 Treatment for AD.
- Topical calcineurin inhibitors (TCIs) (Tacrolimus ointment or Pimecrolimus cream) also as described in Section 4.1.

INFLAMMATORY GENITAL DERMATOSES
Lichen Planus

- LP is a chronic, inflammatory dermatosis which affects the skin, mucous membranes, hair follicles, and nails. There are several variants of LP, including the *classic cutaneous form* (skin only*), erosive LP (ELP)* involving mucous membranes (oral, anogenital bladder, conjunctiva, and esophagus), and a variant with both types. Other subtypes exist but are beyond the scope of this text. Mucosal LP is a more chronic condition with exacerbations and remissions. The cutaneous variant often resolves spontaneously after a few years. While LP in extragenital areas poses no risk for cancer transformation, genital LP has been recognized as an associated condition in penile SCCs that are HPV-negative. The association of vulvar LP and SCC has not been as well established (Regauer et al., 2014).

Section 4.5 provides a general overview of the *epidemiology* and *pathophysiology* of LP. This section will only focus on the disease as it affects the genitalia.

Clinical Presentation
Skin Findings

- In genital LP, the clinical findings will depend on location. The classic lesions of the purple, planar, polygonal, pruritic, papule, and plaques will likely not be seen.

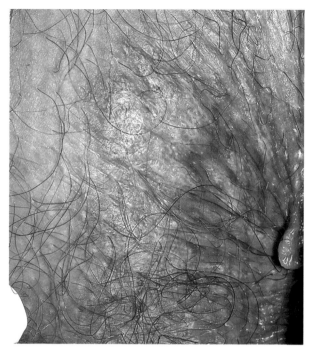

FIG. 11.4-15. Lichen planus. (Used with permission from Edwards, L., & Lynch, P. [2018]. *Genital dermatology atlas and manual* [3rd ed.]. Wolters Kluwer.)

- The hair-bearing skin of mons pubis and labia majora and minora, clitoris and perineum will have individual white or skin-colored papules or plaques (Fig. 11.4-15).

- The erosive type of LP will present with the more typical adherent scales that form fine, grayish-white streaks (Wickham striae) on the mucosa (Fig. 11.4-16).

- In patients with darker skin, lesions are often dark violet or slate-blue color with prominent postinflammatory hyperpigmentation.

- Koebner phenomenon may occur, with lesion formation in areas of trauma or friction.

- In males, LP involves the genitalia in 25% of cases, with the glans penis the most common location. Nonerosive, annular plaques are often located near the coronal rim.

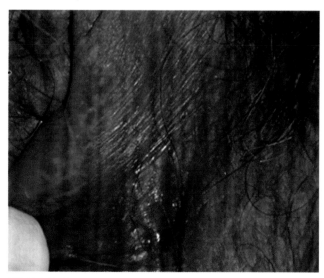

FIG. 11.4-16. Erosive LP female. This erosion is pathognomonic for LP because of the surrounding white, reticular papules.

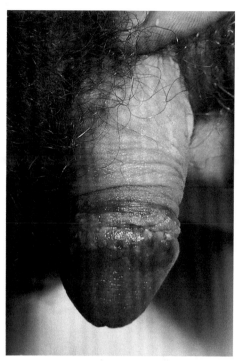

FIG. 11.4-17. Erosive LP male. The uncircumcised male with erosions. (Used with permission from Edwards, L., & Lynch, P. [2018]. *Genital dermatology atlas and manual* [3rd ed.]. Wolters Kluwer.)

- ELP occurs less frequently and results in erosions and white reticular striae (Fig. 11.4-17).

- Approximately 50% of females diagnosed with oral LP also have genital lesions, often a combination of nonerosive and ELP types.

- The mucosa may become very thin and shiny, similar to LS. These lesions frequently itch, burn, and cause dyspareunia (Fig. 11.4-18).

- ELP on the genitalia may be extremely painful and debilitating, and can cause vaginal discharge or urethral stenosis.

Non-Skin Findings

- Sequelae of ELP are more profound than those of non-ELP and can lead to phimosis, urethral strictures, scarring, alopecia, pigmentary alterations, vulvar and vaginal adhesions, and fissures.

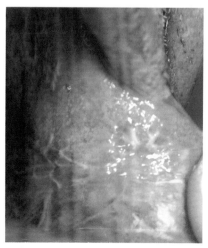

FIG. 11.4-18. Wickham striae.

- Patients with genital LP can experience dysuria, dyspareunia, depression and anxiety, loss of function, and overall altered quality of life

---

DIFFERENTIAL DIAGNOSIS Genital Lichen Planus

- Drug eruption
- Lichen sclerosus
- Contact dermatitis
- Herpes simplex virus
- Psoriasis
- Secondary syphilis
- Stevens–Johnson syndrome
- Autoimmune blistering diseases
- Squamous cell carcinoma
- Seborrheic dermatitis

Confirming the Diagnosis

- Diagnosis of LP can often be made clinically.
- Biopsy when clinically indicated will confirm the diagnosis.
- Bacterial and viral cultures may be indicated to exclude an infectious etiology or identify a secondary infection.

Treatment

Topical

- TCS are the treatment of choice.
  - Fluocinonide 0.05% ointment b.i.d. × 1 to 2 weeks
  - Clobetasol 0.05% ointment b.i.d. × 1 to 2 weeks
- Vulvovaginal LP can also be treated using intravaginal hydrocortisone 25-mg suppositories (1 to 1½) b.i.d. × several months.
  - Taper dose to twice a week for maintenance (Anderson et al., 2002).
- Topical Calcineurin Inhibitors (TCIs) may be used as well.
  - Tacrolimus ointment (0.03%, 0.1%) b.i.d.
  - Pimecrolimus cream (1%) b.i.d.

See Section 4.5 for further suggestions.

Management and Patient Education

- LP has been described in association with hepatitis C, predominantly in certain geographical areas (Japan and Mediterranean regions). Consider obtaining serologic tests for hepatitis B and C as well as a liver function panel.
- Any patients with genital erosions who do not respond to antimicrobial therapies (viral, bacterial, mycologic) or topical steroids, should be referred appropriately to gynecology, dermatology, or urology for further evaluation and management.
- Often, oral LP occurs concomitantly and requires dental care with an experienced provider.
- Classic lesions of LP in the genital area are not commonly associated with scarring, however, architectural features of the labia and perineum disappear over time.
- Adhesions at the vaginal introitus may require surgical removal or use of graduated dilators. Ultrapotent TCS may also be useful for their side effect of atrophy (thinning).
- Uncircumcised males often see improvement after circumcision.

CLINICAL PEARLS

- Wickham striae, a hallmark lesion of LP may be present: lacey (reticular), white papules on the vulva and vaginal mucosa with surrounding erythema (Fig. 11.4-18).
- Koebner phenomenon may occur, where lesions develop in areas of trauma or friction.
- The risk for SCC may be increased in sites of lesions, particularly in males.
- Erosive lesions on penis or vulva should be treated in conjunction with gynecology and dermatology.

Lichen Sclerosus

LS is a chronic inflammatory skin disorder that can occur on any cutaneous site, but tends to have a predilection for the genital area. It occurs in children and then in adults in fourth decade of life. In this condition, scarring and atrophy occurs on the skin shortly after an inflammatory phase, therefore early detection is important. Dyspareunia may be the most prominent symptom.

Additionally, if genital lesions are left untreated, there is a risk of development of squamous cell carcinoma at the site. It does have a strong association with other autoimmune disorders such as other thyroid disorders.

Pathophysiology

The etiology and pathogenesis of LS are not completely understood. In women, a heritable risk is considered due to cases within families, as well as associations with certain HLA and other haplotypes (Bolognia et al., 2018). Additionally, there are known associations to other autoimmune disorders, such as thyroid disease, supporting the genetic risk. While less common in males, one study of 56 males with genital lichen sclerosis found a history of urinary micro-incontinence or dribbling in 95% of participants (Bunker et al., 2013). Other triggers such as viruses (EBV), trauma, and hormones have been postulated.

Clinical Presentation

Skin Findings

- Fixed, atrophic plaques (*sclerotic*) with telangiectasia, purpura, erythema, and erosions.
- Hypopigmentation to white (porcelain) in color with a smooth or waxy appearance (Fig. 11.4-19).
- Inguinal and gluteal fold involvement may be present.
- Follicular plugging may be present from follicular destruction.
- Young women and children with LS may initially report an eruption of small pink or white coalescing papules.
- Older lesions may take on a different appearance and become thickened and hyperkeratotic, some of which may occur as a result of rubbing or scratching.

Women

- Characteristic finding: "figure eight" (or key hole) distribution. The affected area surrounds the vulvar and perianal region (Fig. 11.4-20).
- There is a risk of fusion of labia minora and/or midline fusion with subsequent burying of the clitoris. If left untreated, architectural changes may result with total loss of labia minora and a narrowed vaginal opening (Fig. 11.4-21).

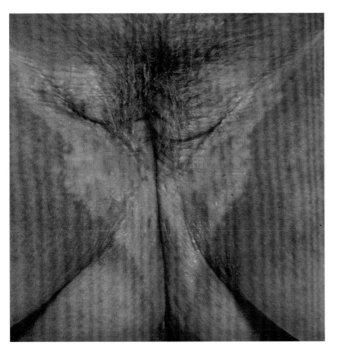

FIG. 11.4-19. Lichen sclerosis. Although hypopigmentation is the most striking abnormality in LS, the texture change is the key to diagnosis including the crinkled or tissue-paper-like appearance.

- This creates great discomfort and dyspareunia for a sexually active woman.
- Postmenopausal women may have further atrophy due to the thinning effects from diminished estrogen.

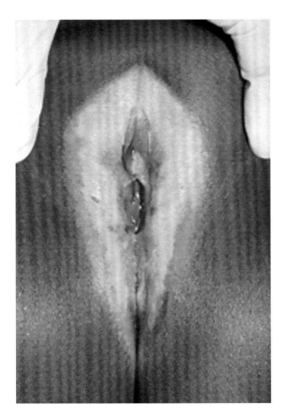

FIG. 11.4-20. Lichen sclerosus in keyhole distribution.

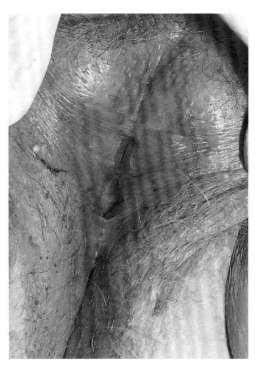

FIG. 11.4-21. Lichen sclerosis female. Note the significant atrophy and complete loss of architectural features of labia. (Used with permission from Edwards, L., & Lynch, P. [2018]. *Genital dermatology atlas and manual* [3rd ed.]. Wolters Kluwer.)

Men

- LS affects glans penis and foreskin typically, without perianal involvement.
- When it occurs on glans and foreskin, it is termed balanitis xerotica obliterans (BXO). It can occur, though less commonly, on the shaft or scrotum.
- Uncircumcised men make up majority of cases.
- Often misdiagnosed as phimosis (foreskin cannot be retracted) or balanitis. Retracting the foreskin may become impossible, and stenosis of the meatus may be noted.
- Sclerotic plaques around the glans may be friable and bleed easily with intercourse, or result in urethral strictures (Fig. 11.4-22).

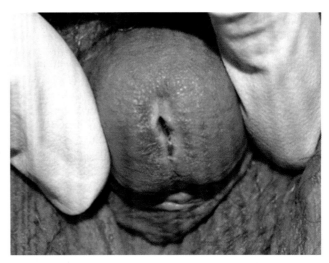

FIG. 11.4-22. Lichen sclerosis male. Lichen sclerosus often affects the urethral meatus and can cause strictures.

Non-Skin Findings

- Pruritus, soreness, dyspareunia
- Children may have GI/GU symptoms, recurrent balanitis, poor urinary stream, and constipation.

DIFFERENTIAL DIAGNOSIS   Lichen Sclerosis

- Lichen planus
- Lichen simplex chronicus
- Sexual abuse
- Erythroplasia of Queyrat
- Balanitis
- Postmenopausal atrophy

Confirming the Diagnosis

- Scarring and architectural changes from genital LS may be a clue to diagnosis and are not reversible, emphasizing the importance of prompt diagnosis and treatment.
- KOH to rule out yeast or fungal infection could be done.
- Urine culture to rule out urinary tract infection if symptomatic.
- Clinical diagnosis can be confirmed with a skin biopsy which should be taken from thin, tissue-paper-like skin. Multiple biopsies may be required to obtain diagnosis and therefore patients should be referred to dermatology, gynecology, or urology.
- Additional biopsies should be taken if there is change or growth, due to risk for SCC.

Treatment

- TCS (class II) and ultrapotent (class I) are the gold standard treatment for genital LS.
- Clobetasol 0.05% or Halobetasol 0.05% ointment is recommended as initial therapy 1–2×/day for 3 months or until clinical signs (texture and color) have improved.
- TCIs, such as Tacrolimus 0.1% b.i.d., have been used with good results and can provide a safer, long-term, nonsteroidal alternative for treatment and maintenance of the disease.
- Circumcision followed by topical Tacrolimus 0.1% postoperatively for 3 weeks may be beneficial. However, men treated with high-potency TCS for about 8 weeks may be able to avoid circumcision.
- Testosterone creams are no longer recommended due to risk for virilization and a similar response rate to petrolatum.

Maintenance and Patient Education

- The goal of treatment is to alleviate the symptoms and prevent progression quickly without side effects.
- Given the side effects of these TCS, the patient should be reevaluated in 4 to 6 weeks and referred to dermatology if no improvement.
- After initial control, the topical steroid should be tapered over 2 weeks and a maintenance regimen, such as twice weekly is recommended.
- Due to the chronicity of the disease, clinicians must be sure to monitor the use of TCS by monitoring for adverse effects, and tapering appropriately when indicated.
- Good skin hygiene is fundamental for any genital dermatosis for the promotion of healing and prevention of infection.
- Treatment of genital LS often requires a multidisciplinary approach with primary care, dermatology, gynecology, and urology (as appropriate).

- For males, urethral obstruction from LS can interfere with urination and lesions can also cause pain with erection. Consider recommending counseling regarding sexual dysfunction or dyspareunia.
- In women, the most common site of SCC is near the clitoris or on the labia. The length of time from diagnosis to the possible development of SCC is unknown.
- Self-examination should be taught and encouraged so that patients can report early recognition of new or changing lesions.

CLINICAL PEARLS

- In adult females, lichen sclerosus (LS) is the most common reason for chronic vulvar symptoms, especially itching.
- LS in women has the characteristic finding of "figure eight" (or key hole) distribution.
- Although it seems contradictory due to the atrophic appearance of skin, ultra-potent to potent steroids are used to treat this condition.

Zoon Balanitis/Vulvitis

Zoon plasma cell balanitis is a condition which appears in uncircumcised males. It may also be present in postmenopausal women but clinically is difficult to distinguish from erosive LP. It is thought to be related to poor hygiene and chronic irritation.

It is usually seen between the ages of 40 and 80. It may present with pruritus but typically, patients notice a red patch that is resistant to topical home remedies such as antifungal or hydrocortisone cream.

Pathophysiology

Chronic irritation and poor hygiene result in an inflammatory plasma cell infiltrate in the upper dermis. In women lack of hormones may play a role.

Clinical Manifestation

Skin Findings

- On the glans penis is a red or orange-red flat, shiny patch or plaque.
- There is a cayenne pepper speckled appearance.
- Because it is covered by foreskin, there is no scale or crust and usually no swelling.
- There may be some erosion.
- Lesions occur on opposing surfaces of the glans and overlying foreskin (Fig. 11.4-23).

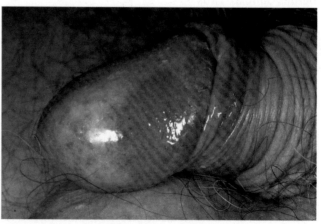

FIG. 11.4-23. Zoon balanitis male. (Courtesy T. Habif.)

- In women, there are erythematous plaques with superficial erosions present anywhere on vulva.
- Lesions may be asymptomatic or be associated with dyspareunia, dysuria, itching, or pain.

DIFFERENTIAL DIAGNOSIS   Zoon Balanitis/Vulvitis

- Psoriasis
- Candidiasis
- Irritant dermatitis
- Allergic contact dermatitis
- Bowen disease
- SCCIS
- Erythroplasia of Queyrat
- Extramammary Paget disease
- Erosive lichen planus
- Fixed drug eruption
- HSV
- Pemphigus vulgaris

Confirming the Diagnosis

- A therapeutic trial of low- to medium-potency steroid cream b.i.d. for 2 weeks will often result in complete resolution.
- If no improvement or frequent recurrences, a biopsy may be needed to confirm the diagnosis.

Treatment

- Hydrocortisone cream 1% to 2.5% b.i.d. × 2 weeks
- Desonide cream or ointment 0.05% b.i.d.
- Alclometasone cream or ointment 0.05% b.i.d.
- Mometasone cream or ointment 0.01% b.i.d.
- TCIs may be helpful
- Vaginal estrogen cream may be helpful for women
- If diagnosis confirmed in men, circumcision is usually curative

Management and Patient Education

- Reassurance and improved hygiene is encouraged.

GENITAL INFECTIONS

Herpes Simplex Virus

- Herpes simplex virus type 1 (HSV-1) and herpes simplex virus type 2 (HSV-2) are common infections worldwide and both can cause genital herpes.
- The Centers for Disease Control and Prevention (CDC) estimates that, annually, 776,000 people in the United States get new genital herpes infections.
- Risk factors include low socioeconomic status, early age of first intercourse, a high number of sexual partners, and a history of sexually transmitted disease (STD).

Pathophysiology

- Most cases of genital herpes are caused by HSV-2 (Habif, 2016, p. 429). However, HSV-1 has been associated with an increasing proportion of cases of genital herpes infection (Bernstein et al., 2013). A *primary infection* occurs after exposure to the virus in an

---

DIFFERENTIAL DIAGNOSIS   Genital Herpes Simplex Virus

- Cellulitis/Infected traumatic erosions
- Contact dermatitis
- Intertrigo
- Fixed drug eruption
- Chancroid usually presents as a deep solitary and nonpainful ulcer compared to the multiple shallow and painful ulcers of HSV (see Section 6.4)
- Lymphogranuloma venereum
- Candidiasis
- Bullous impetigo
- Herpes zoster
- Syphilis
- Erosive lichen planus
- Fournier or gas gangrene
- Behçet syndrome
- Pyoderma gangrenosum
- Ecthyma gangrenosum
- Granuloma inguinale
- Cytomegalovirus (CMV)

---

individual who has no antibodies to HSV-1 or HSV-2, whereas a *recurrent infection* occurs when there is a reactivation of the virus after a period of latency.

- A *nonprimary infection* occurs in an individual with antibodies to one HSV type, who then acquires a new infection to the other HSV type. Each of these types can be either symptomatic or asymptomatic.
- Immunosuppressive therapy, organ transplant recipients, and immunologic disorders are at greater risk for a severe HSV outbreak.

Transmission

- Infections are transmitted through direct contact with HSV in active herpetic lesions, mucosal surfaces, genital secretions, or oral secretions, and may occur during periods of subclinical viral shedding. HSV can also be acquired by autoinoculation.
- Transmission commonly occurs from contact with an infected partner who does not have visible lesions and who may not know that he or she is infected. According to the CDC, in persons with asymptomatic HSV-2 infections, genital HSV shedding occurs on 10.2% of days, compared to 20.1% of days among those with symptomatic infections.
- Asymptomatic infection can occur in the cervix, prostate, or urethra, as a result of antibody acquisition to HSV without a history of "active" disease.
- This may cause a "silent" first outbreak that later in life emerges as a symptomatic outbreak; resulting from a change in the person's immune function.

Clinical Presentation

Primary Infection

- Average incubation period after exposure is 4 days (ranges from 2 to 12 days).
- In women, the HSV lesions are found primarily on the labia, fourchette, cervix, buttocks, thighs, and occasionally the nipples (Fig. 11.4-24).

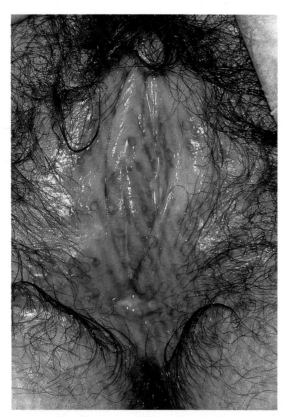

FIG. 11.4-24. HSV-2. Note the punched-out quality to the erosions. (Used with permission from Edwards, L., & Lynch, P. [2018]. *Genital dermatology atlas and manual* [3rd ed.]. Wolters Kluwer.)

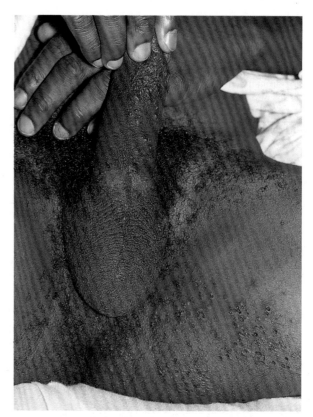

FIG. 11.4-25. HSV-2 presenting as vesicles and pustules on the shaft and discrete punched-out erosions on upper thigh. (Used with permission from Edwards, L., & Lynch, P. [2018]. *Genital dermatology atlas and manual* [3rd ed.]. Wolters Kluwer.)

- In men, the HSV lesions can be found on the penis, buttocks, or thighs (Fig. 11.4-25), and erosive balanitis can occur (especially in immunosuppressed patients).

- Symptoms tend to be more severe in women than in men.

Skin Findings

- Erythematous papules or vesicles that become umbilicated (depressed in the center) and then coalesce into eroded, "punched out," irregularly bordered ulcerations.

- Erosions on the mucous membranes or intertriginous areas may appear macerated or as linear fissures due to the moist environment.

- Cutaneous lesions usually resolve in 1 to 3 weeks (with a mean of 19 days), and can leave behind scarring if the inflammation was intense (Habif, 2019, p. 431).

Non-Skin Findings

- First-episode infections are more extensive and have more constitutional symptoms, including fever, nausea and vomiting, myalgias, headache, malaise, and lymphadenopathy.

- There may be itching, tingling, or an intense burning pain at the site of the outbreak, as well as dysuria.

- Acute urinary retention with loss of sacral sensation can occur due to lumbosacral radiculomyelitis secondary to severe primary HSV infection.

- Primary genital herpes is commonly associated with viremia, or disseminated herpes, which can lead to organ failure and death.

First Non-Primary Infection

- The first non-primary infection is associated with fewer lesions and less systemic symptoms than primary infection.

- This is attributed to the antibodies that the patient already has to one type of HSV.

- Cutaneous symptoms may be similar to those in primary HSV infection, except the ulceration number and severity is milder.

- Lesions usually heal faster and have fewer recurrences.

Recurrent Infection

- Cutaneous symptoms tend to be more localized and milder than those in primary HSV infection, and often resolve sooner.

- Recurrences may occur four to seven times per year and are thought to be triggered by illness, stress, tight clothing, abrasion, or friction from the lack of lubrication with sexual contact.

- The frequency of recurrence depends on the severity and duration of the initial episode, the infecting serotype (HSV-2), and the host.

- Recurrent infection is more common with HSV-2 than HSV-1.

- It is estimated that 80% to 90% of persons with a symptomatic primary HSV-2 infection will have a recurrent episode within the following year, compared with 50% to 60% of persons with a symptomatic primary HSV-1 infection (Habif, 2016, p. 436).

Skin Findings

- Erythematous papules or vesicles that become umbilicated and then coalesce into eroded, "punched out," irregularly bordered

ulcerations. HSV is classically defined as "grouped vesicles on an erythematous base."

Non-Skin Findings

- Prodromal symptoms (e.g., tingling, itching or pain) may precede cutaneous symptoms, and may last hours to 3 days.
- May be accompanied by lymphadenopathy, but usually no vaginal discharge or urinary symptoms.

Confirming the Diagnosis

Viral culture

- Perform within 7 days of the first episode and within 2 days of a recurrence
- 50% to 75% rate of sensitivity with higher yield in the early stages of disease (vesicular lesions).
- Sensitivity declines rapidly as the lesions begin to heal. Higher sensitivity with primary infection, rather than recurrent infection.
- Viral culture can distinguish between HSV-1 and HSV-2.
- To obtain the optimal specimen, unroof a vesicle and sample the exudate at the base by rolling the culturette across the wound base.
- If the first culture is negative, repeat the culture during a recurrence.

Polymerase chain reaction (PCR)

- PCR assays are rapid, highly sensitive tests for both HSV-1 and HSV-2 detection.
- PCR is especially advantageous during asymptomatic shedding, cerebrospinal fluid (CSF) infection, neonates, and for monitory antiviral suppression therapy.
- Specimens are collected from serum, CSF, vesicle fluid, tissue, or endocervical sampling (thin prep).
- The use of PCR can be limited due to cost and availability.

Serologic testing

- In the absence of a lesion, serologic testing for HSV antibodies can also be performed if no lesions are present and will detect evidence of past or recent infection (IgG and IgM) of HSV-1 and HSV-2
- Patient with true primary infections have seronegative test results, as they have never been infected with any type of herpes virus in the past (Habif, 2016, p. 431)

Tzanck prep

- Tzanck prep can be done to identify multinucleate giant cells.
- It is necessary to scrape the contents of a freshly opened vesicle, place on a slide and fix with methanol and Wright or Giemsa stain.
- If available in office, it will provide an immediate result.

Biopsy

- When diagnosis is unclear or presentation is atypical, a biopsy can be helpful.

Treatment

Systemic Therapy

Antiviral therapy can shorten the duration and reduce the severity of an outbreak. Initiate as early as possible, ideally 72 hours after lesions erupt. Oral Therapy for HSV infection (Table 6.3-2), discusses systemic antivirals and dosing based on the type of infection: primary versus recurrence, episodic or suppressive, and the immune status of the patient.

Supportive Care

- Encourage good personal hygiene to help keep the area free of irritants and reduce the risk for secondary infection.
- Recommend tepid baths to soothe the perineal area and alleviate dysuria, and therefore prevent secondary urinary retention.
- Avoid tight or occlusive clothing in an effort to reduce irritation and promote healing.
- Advise patients to abstain from sexual contact to reduce transmission of HSV and to reduce friction that can be painful.
- Recommend an emollient, like white petrolatum, to provide a soothing barrier and reduce painful friction.
- Recommend cool packs or compresses to reduce pain and itching.

Special Considerations

Pregnancy

- Transmission to a fetus can occur during pregnancy, delivery, or postpartum.
- The greatest risk for neonatal infection occurs when the mother develops a primary HSV-2 infection within the last 3 months of pregnancy.
- Women who have had a previous infection develop IgG antibodies that cross the placenta and may offer protection to the fetus.
- Neonatal infection is rare but can be serious and possibly fatal to the newborn.
- Prevention is the primary goal, especially in the last weeks of pregnancy.
- Consult obstetrics if the patient is pregnant.

Immunosuppression

- May include extensive mucocutaneous involvement, variable appearance of genital lesions, and the development of chronic and recurrent ulcers.
- Recurrences are often more frequent, more extensive, and of longer duration than in immunocompetent.
- Immunosuppressed patients may have prolonged viral shedding.
- Patients with systemic symptoms, severe mucocutaneous disease, and at-risk or immunosuppressed individuals (e.g., human immunodeficiency virus [HIV]-infected patients and other immunodeficiency states with T-cell defects) may warrant hospitalization for evaluation for viremia, IV antiviral therapy, and supportive care.

HSV-2 and Risk of HIV Transmission

- HSV-2 genital ulcer disease has been linked to an increased risk for acquisition of HIV infection (Looker et al., 2017).
- HIV incidence in general populations was found to be roughly tripled by exposure to prevalent HSV-2 infection.
- Newly acquired HSV-2 infection is associated with an increased frequency and severity of genital ulceration, viral shedding, and inflammation in the genital tract.
- These biologic mechanisms of HSV-2 infection are thought to increase the risk of HIV acquisition.

- Symptomatic HSV-2 genital ulcers frequently cause local inflammation and mucosal disruption in the genital tract, which can facilitate HIV entry during exposure to HIV-infected genital fluids.
- Genital HSV-2 ulcers selectively increase local recruitment of CD4 positive cells, which may serve as targets for HIV attachment in mucosal tissue (Rebbapragada et al., 2007).
- Replication competent virus has been isolated in HSV-2 lesions.

Management and Patient Education

- The diagnosis of genital herpes and the knowledge that it can recur during one's lifetime can be devastating. Patients and their partners may struggle with a new diagnosis and all of the important patient education.
- STD education and testing should be offered including the use of latex condoms with sexual contact.
- Encourage lubricants to reduce friction that may cause pain or trigger a recurrence.
- Avoid direct contact when an active lesion appears, emphasize good hand washing, and discourage the use of shared personal items.

CLINICAL PEARLS

- First-episode infections are more extensive and have more constitutional symptoms, including fever, nausea and vomiting, myalgias, headache, malaise, and lymphadenopathy.
- Transmission to a fetus can occur during pregnancy, delivery, or postpartum.
- Suppressive antiviral therapy for frequent recurrences is detailed in Section 6.3.

Genital Human Papilloma Virus

Genital warts are the most common sexually transmitted infection, with an estimated lifetime risk for infection in sexually active adults as high as 80%. The CDC estimates that about 1% of the sexually active adolescent and adult population in the United States have clinically apparent genital warts.

- In the United States, anogenital HPV infection is the most common genital wart infection, with an estimated 79 million infected persons.
- Additionally, there are an estimated 14 million new HPV infections diagnosed annually.
- Condyloma acuminatum (or genital warts), squamous cell carcinoma in situ (SCCIS), Bowenoid papulosis, erythroplasia of Queyrat (or SCCIS of glans penis), cervical dysplasia, and cervical cancers are all associated with HPV infections.
- Although, HPV types 6 and 11 are low risk and nononcogenic, more than 90% of anogenital wart cases are associated with 6 and 11. Additionally, they may cause benign or low-grade cervical dysplasia and laryngeal papillomas.
- According to the CDC, in 2019, in addition to cervical cancer, HPV is believed to be responsible for 90% of anal cancers, 71% of vulvar, vaginal, or penile cancers, and 72% of oropharyngeal cancers. The oncogenic potential in HPV differs by type. HPV type 16, 18, 31, 33, 45, 52, and 58 are seen in approximately 90% of cervical cancers (Bolognia et al., 2018). HPV 16 alone is detected in about 50% of cervical cancers and high-grade cervical intraepithelial neoplasia (CIN).

Nongenital HPV is discussed in Section 6.3.

Pathophysiology

- HPV are small, double-stranded, circular DNA viruses. The virus infects the squamous cells and creates characteristic koilocytes within the cell.
- They initially enter the skin or mucous membrane through tiny tears or abrasions that may be created through trauma or friction during sexual contact. The virus enters the basaloid epithelium and is able to evade immune surveillance.
- Most HPV DNA becomes undetectable spontaneously over time with only 9% persistence detected after 2 years (Bolognia et al., 2018, p. 1384).
- Some viral types can cause the p53 protein and RB proteins to be inactivated and therefore, a normal cell becomes a cancerous one. It takes days, months, or years to develop the condyloma, if it will at all. Often the body is able to clear the virus in time through cell-mediated immunity and antibodies induced by the viral infection itself.

Transmission

- The most common path of transmission is through sexual contact or direct skin-to-skin contact. It takes only one sexual contact with a partner who does (or does not) know that he or she has HPV to transmit the virus.
- Sexual contact with a new partner who has a different strain of HPV can trigger an outbreak of warts. Nongenital warts can also be spread to the genital area (Fig. 11.4-26).
- Condoms are often limited in preventing transmission because they cover only the shaft of the penis. Risk for infection includes a high number of sexual partners or a partner who had multiple contacts previously.
- The frequency of sexual intercourse also increases risk.

Clinical Presentation

Skin Findings
Genital warts (condyloma acuminata)

- Small, discrete, flat, smooth red, brown, or flesh colored papules (Fig. 11.4-27A).
- May be filiform, pedunculated like a skin tag or verrucous coalescing papules.
- May resemble pearly, penile papules that are a normal variant (Fig. 11.4-27B).

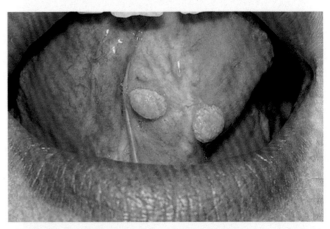

FIG. 11.4-26. HPV. It can be transmitted through orogenital contact, increasing risk for oropharyngeal SCC.

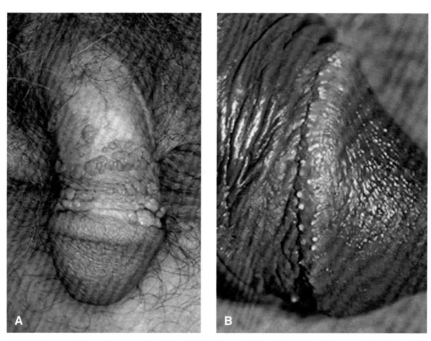

FIG. 11.4-27. A: Penile warts; verrucal papules of HPV on the penis. These skin-colored, brown, and slightly hypopigmented lobular papules on the penis are a very common morphology of genital warts. **B:** Pearly penile papules (*arrow*) can be differentiated from genital warts by the monomorphous, symmetric appearance and by the finding that each is discrete. These papules are most often located on the corona in circumferential, parallel rows.

- White and keratotic on moist mucosal surfaces.
- In males, they may involve pubis, shaft of the penis, scrotum, foreskin, meatus, urethra, or perianal area (Fig. 11.4-28).
- In females, they may involve the pubis, vulva, vagina, urethra, or anal area.

- Cervical warts (*condylomata plana*) are flat and require the aid of colposcopy to visualize.
- Giant condyloma (Buschke-Lowenstein) is a rare, slow growing warty plaque that is easily misdiagnosed as genital wart but considered to be a type of squamous cell carcinoma (Fig. 11.4-29).

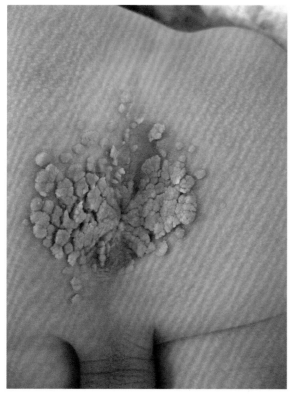

FIG. 11.4-28. Perianal warts. (Photo courtesy of M. Bobonich.)

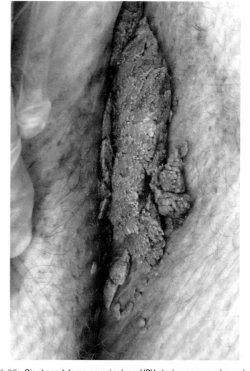

FIG. 11.4-29. Giant condyloma acuminatum. HPV starts as verrucal papules before coalescing into plaque. Giant condyloma acuminatum (Buschke and Löwenstein) is at risk for transformation into a malignancy. (Photo courtesy of M. Bobonich.)

Non-Skin Finding

- Genital HPV may bleed easily and cause dyspareunia.

DIFFERENTIAL DIAGNOSIS	HPV Infections	
Genital Warts	*Bowenoid Papulosis*	*Erythroplasia Queyrat*
• Condyloma lata	• Lichen Planus	• Erosive balanitis
• Molluscum contagiosum	• Condyloma	• Psoriasis
• Pearly penile papules (Fig. 11.4-3)	• Psoriasis	• Lichen planus
• Vestibular papillae (Fig. 11.4-6)	• Fordyce spots	• Fixed drug eruption
• Vulvar papillomatosis	• Lichen nitidus	• Pemphigus or pemphigoid
• Fox–Fordyce	• Molluscum	• Herpes simplex virus
• Lichen nitidus	• Lichen simplex chronicus	• Candidiasis
• Bowenoid papulosis	• Scabies	

Confirming the Diagnosis

- Diagnosis is based on clinical presentation and symptoms.

- Any persistent and unresponsive lesion should be biopsied.

- Histopathology that reveals koilocytosis can help the clinician eliminate many of the differential diagnoses.

- Condyloma lata, sometimes confused with condyloma, are associated with secondary syphilis; therefore, serologic screening, including rapid plasma reagin (RPR), may be necessary.

- Curettage of a lesion and KOH prep revealing Henderson–Patterson bodies can differentiate molluscum contagiosum from HPV (see Section 15 for KOH procedure).

- Acetic acid whitening test may help identify genital warts. However, not specific to HPV-induced lesions and may also be positive in other inflammatory or infectious conditions.

Treatment

See Boxes 11.4-5 to 11.4-7.

Management and Patient Education

- No treatment offers a 100% cure rate; prevention is the best approach.

BOX 11.4-5 Physical Destruction Treatment Genital Warts

Cryotherapy (liquid nitrogen)
- Often first-line in-office therapy is inexpensive, effective, and safe during pregnancy

See Section 15 for application details.
- Blisters and small erosions begin to develop in 1 to 3 days and heal completely in 1 to 2 weeks
- Side effects include discomfort, blistering, dyspigmentation, and scarring with a very small risk for infection and paresthesias

Electrosurgery
- Destruction of the lesions by electrocautery should only be performed by a dermatologist or gynecologist and may require local anesthesia
- Loop electrosurgical excision procedure (LEEP) uses a high-frequency current to cut and cauterize tissue and is generally used for cervical treatment and performed by urology and gynecologic specialists

Laser vaporization
- YAG or CO_2 laser can be used to treat a group of lesions
- This should be done by someone experienced in laser surgery, usually a dermatologist
- Special care must be taken to control the plume from laser treatment, which can aerosolize the virus and pose a potential hazard for patients and staff

Surgery
- Scissor snip, shave excision, or excisional surgery is reserved for large lesions as a debulking process and may require general anesthesia
- Postoperative pain may be significant and warts can recur after removal

---

- Treatment is aimed at eliminating the visible condyloma and any associated discomfort.

- Treating visible lesions may reduce the chance of transmission of the virus, however, subclinical infection does exist in the surrounding tissue.

- Selection of treatment should consider cost to the patient, potential discomfort and scarring, recurrence rate, and effectiveness.

- Scarring and hypo- or hyperpigmentation can occur with any of the physical destruction methods and should be discussed with the patient beforehand.

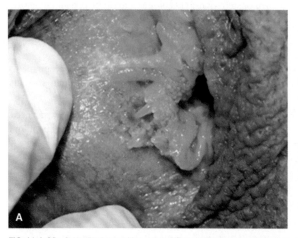
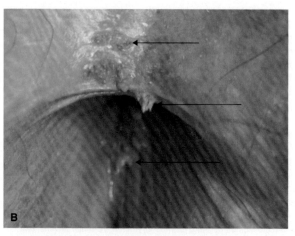

FIG. 11.4-30. A: Vestibular papillae mimic HPV infection, but the tips are rounded, and individual papillae are discrete to the base. **B:** Some genital warts are spiky, or acuminate, leading to the term *condylomata acuminata*. There are small lobular warts just above these acuminate lesions.

BOX 11.4-6   Chemical Destruction Treatment Genital Warts

Trichloroacetic acid (TCA) and Bichloracetic acid (BCA)
- Strong topical keratolytics that result in chemical cauterization (similar to cryotherapy or electrodessication) of the skin and destruction of local tissue
- In-office application
- Vaseline should be applied to the surrounding skin as protection
- TCA and BCA are applied with the wooden end of the cotton-tipped applicator

Apply a small amount to the wart and allow time to dry. When dry, the lesion develops a white frost
- It may be used in pregnancy on external lesion
- Treatment requires weekly applications for 4 to 6 weeks and has a high recurrence rate
- Side effects include burning at the application site

Podophyllotoxin
- This is the most active constituent of podophyllin which is no longer recommended, due to low efficacy and potential toxicity
- Contraindicated in pregnancy
- Regimen: self-application of podophyllotoxin 0.5% solution twice daily × 3 days and repeat weekly (Condylox)
- If the lesion is located on the perianal area, the application is once daily for 3 days a week, repeated for 4 weeks
- Allow to dry completely, therefore not recommended on moist surfaces
- Surrounding skin should be protected with petrolatum before application
- Side effects include irritation, erythema, and erosions

- For suspected *atypical* lesions or carcinomas of the external genitalia, refer appropriately to a dermatology specialist, obstetrician/gynecologist, or urologist for evaluation and treatment.
- A gastroenterologist or colorectal surgeon should be consulted for the evaluation of anal warts or suspected anal carcinomas.
- Educate patients about the risk factors for contracting the infection, risk for cancer, and preventative behaviors.
- Advise patients to notify their sexual contacts to be evaluated for HPV and other STDs.

BOX 11.4-7   Immune-Based Treatment Genital Warts

Imiquimod
- Topical immune enhancer which induces cell-mediated activity against HPV
- Approved by FDA for treatment of condyloma acuminata
- Higher response rate occurs in warts treated on mucosal sites
- Patient-applied imiquimod, in addition to in-office destructive modalities, is preferred to monotherapy using one treatment alone
- Regimen: apply three times per week at night for 16 weeks
- Similar recurrence rate to cryotherapy
- Side effects include application-site reactions

Sinecatechins 15%
- FDA-approved topical treatment for external genital warts
- Produced from green tea leaves and thought to have an immunostimulatory effect. Apply 0.5 cm (maximum amount per treatment) ointment to the warts, t.i.d. for up to 16 weeks
- Do not use on the genital mucosa (urethra, vagina, or rectum) or open wounds
- Caution the patient that use may decrease the effectiveness of condoms and diaphragms, recommend backup contraceptive method
- Side effects include burning, pruritus, erythema, vesicular lesions, and discomfort at the treatment site

---

- Advise condoms, however, note that there is still a risk for viral spreading without active lesions.
- Patients undergoing treatment for HPV genital warts should be followed every 2 to 4 weeks until there is no clinical evidence of infection.
- If no evidence of condyloma after 6 months, annual visits are indicated.
- STD tests should be completed based on sexual history. HPV can occur in presence of other disorders related to sexual activity.

Prevention HPV Vaccine

- The CDC Advisory Committee on Immunization Practices (ACIP) recommends the 9-valent HPV vaccine (Gardisal 9) to be given routinely to males and females between the ages of 11 and 26 years.
- HPV vaccine is not routinely recommended in adults aged 27 to 45 years due to decreasing exposure with age, however, it is recommended that there be shared patient-provider clinical decision making to vaccinate those in this age group with a high risk for exposure (Meites et al., 2019).
- HPV vaccine is not indicated in those aged >45 years.
- The current vaccine contains HPV types 6, 11, 16, 18, 31, 33, 45, 52, and 58.
- Vaccination is also recommended to those who have not already been vaccinated and fall into below categories:
  - Females aged 13 to 26 years
  - Males aged 13 to 21 years
  - Men who have sex with men (up to age 26 years)
  - Immunocompromised (including HIV)
- It is not recommended in pregnancy, but if a pregnancy occurs after a dose is given, the remaining doses would be postponed until after delivery.

Special Considerations

Pregnancy

- Warts tend to grow during pregnancy because of the hormonal changes and immune suppression.
- Visible warts should be treated after the first trimester. Liquid nitrogen is the treatment of choice for genital warts.
- An obstetrician/gynecologist should be consulted before treating the patient.
- Interferon, 5-fluorouracil, podophyllin, and TCA are contraindicated in pregnancy.
- Animal data on use of imiquimod during pregnancy suggests a low risk, however, data is limited in human subjects (CDC, 2015b).
- In pregnancy, transmission of HPV to the newborn can occur during vaginal delivery and can cause laryngeal papillomatosis.

High-Risk Populations

- Men having sex with men and anal sexual contact may increase the risk of developing anal cancers from HPV.

Children

- Autoinoculation resulting in genital warts in children is not uncommon, however, 50% of cases occur as a result of sexual abuse.

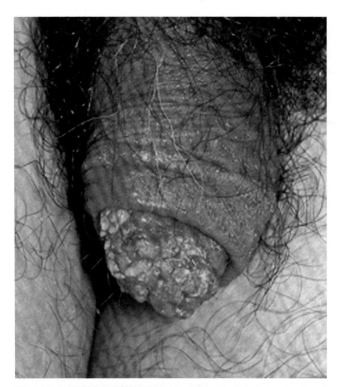

FIG. 11.4-31. SCC. This SCC is the color of the patient's skin, verrucous, and precipitated by HPV.

Immunosuppression

- Genital warts tend to resist common treatments in immunosuppressed patients and have a greater risk for transformation into carcinoma, such as SCC (Fig. 11.4-31).
- Patients who have extensive or atypical infections, or are recalcitrant to treatment, should be screened for HIV and immunosuppression.

CLINICAL PEARLS

- HPV infection on genitalia can cause genital warts and squamous cell carcinoma, depending on the HPV type.
- A gastroenterologist or colorectal surgeon should be consulted for the evaluation of anal warts or suspected anal carcinomas.
- The Gardisil 9 HPV vaccine is recommended to be given routinely to males and females between the ages of 11 and 26 years.
- It is recommended that there be shared patient–provider clinical decision making to vaccinate those aged 27 to 45 with a high risk for exposure.

Candidiasis

Candidiasis is included in genital dermatoses as it is often a concomitant infection that occurs with other genital dermatoses. It can be a primary or secondary infection involving the vaginal and vulva areas of women and the glans penis in men.

Seventy-five percent of women will have one symptomatic yeast infection in their lifetime, and 5% have recurrent infections.

According to the CDC, it is estimated that 20% of women have asymptomatic active vulvovaginal candida infections. There are an estimated 1.4 million clinic visits annually for vaginal candidiasis; as it is the second most common vaginal infection.

Pathophysiology

- The causative agents in the majority of yeast infections in the genitalia are *Candida albicans* and *Candida tropicalis*.
- *C. albicans* is part of the normal flora in the vagina and gastrointestinal tract. However, sweating, interruption of the skin barrier (i.e., chronic moisture from urinary incontinence), oral antibiotic therapy, obesity, diabetes, use of oral contraceptives, pregnancy, and immunosuppression can result in an overgrowth of the yeast.
- Vaginal intercourse with an infected partner may cause candida balanitis in men, especially uncircumcised males. It may also be transmitted to the neonate through an infected vaginal tract.

Clinical Presentation

Skin Findings

- Erythematous and moist plaques that may be macerated, favoring intertriginous areas such as the inframammary, inguinal, and abdominal areas.
- Acute infections may have violaceous papules or pustules that extend just beyond the border of the plaque known as "satellite" papules, pustules, or collarettes (Fig. 11.4-32A).
- Scale may not always be evident (Fig. 11.4-32B).
- Males typically have ill-defined erythema with itching and burning. Erythematous pustules or erosions may extend to the glans and/or shaft of the penis.
- Uncircumcised men can have white plaques or erosions under the prepuce (Fig. 11.4-33).
- On the female genitalia, there may be swelling and shiny erythema as well as a clumpy white, adherent discharge in the vagina or spreading onto the vulva.

Non-Skin Finding

- Burning, pruritus, dyspareunia, dysuria, vaginal discharge

DIFFERENTIAL DIAGNOSIS	Candidiasis
Male	*Female*
• Zoon balanitis	• Lichen sclerosus
• Lichen planus	• Lichen simplex chronicus
• Lichen sclerosus	• Contact dermatitis
• Contact dermatitis	• Psoriasis
• Erythroplasia of Queyrat	• Paget disease

Confirming the Diagnosis

- Most commonly a clinical diagnosis.
- KOH prep is an easy and inexpensive in-office test that can confirm the presence of hyphae, pseudohyphae, and spores. See Section 15 for instructions on KOH prep procedure. A negative KOH and wet prep may occur in truly positive candida infections.
- A biopsy and/or culture with sensitivity may be helpful if symptoms are severe, recurrent, and/or not responsive to anti-yeast medications.

Treatment

See Section 6, Table 6.3 for complete listing.

- External genital candida infections respond well to topical "azole" therapy, such as Miconazole cream applied b.i.d. × 10 days or Clotrimazole cream applied b.i.d. × 10 days.

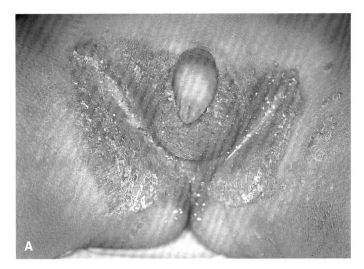

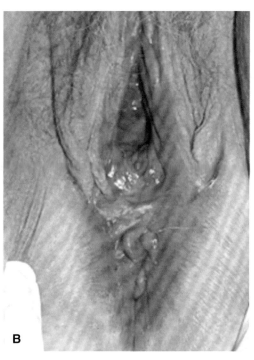

FIG. 11.4-32. **A:** In acute candidiasis infections, papules and pustules may extend beyond the border of the violaceous plaque. **B:** Vaginal candidiasis frequently infects the vulva with characteristic redness, fissuring, and shiny skin, but it may lack scale. (Used with permission from Edwards, L., & Lynch, P. [2018]. *Genital dermatology atlas and manual* [3rd ed.]. Wolters Kluwer.)

- Intravaginal agents are used for vulvovaginal candidiasis.
- Oral therapy may be used, in addition to topical therapy, for quicker resolution and relief.

Management and Patient Education

- If the patient has more than four candida infections per year, consider a non-albicans species and treat with an alternate medication based on culture result.
- Recurrent candida infections should also prompt screening for diabetes, HIV, or immunosuppression, and may require longer therapy or maintenance regimens.
- In recurrence, consider reinfection with an infected partner. Examine and treat partner.

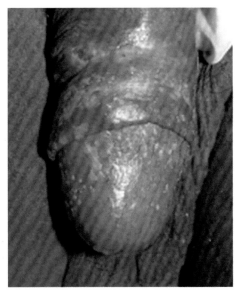

FIG. 11.4-33. Candidiasis. This uncircumcised man with candidiasis also exhibits white papules and erosions.

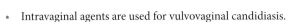

CLINICAL PEARL

- Satellite papules, pustules, or collarettes are a hallmark sign of candidiasis.

Genital Ulcerations

- Superficial erosions and ulcerations on the genital area are hallmark signs of infection. See Box 11.4-8 for differential diagnosis of genital ulcers.

PREMALIGNANT AND MALIGNANT

Intraepithelial Neoplasia Vulvar/Penile

Intraepithelial neoplasia is a term used to describe premalignant changes on anogenital epithelium. Depending on location, the more descriptive terminology includes vulvar intraepithelial neoplasia (VIN), penile intraepithelial neoplasia (PIN), and anal intraepithelial neoplasia (AIN). VIN is further described as *usual type VIN* (or *high-grade squamous intraepithelial lesion [HSIL]*), both terms referring to VIN as a result of HPV infection or *differentiated type VIN*, which arises in LS or LP (Bolognia et al., 2018).

Pathophysiology

In many cases, these premalignant lesions are a consequence of infection with the oncogenic HPV. Immunosuppression, including HIV, smoking, and LS and LP have all also been associated with disease.

Clinical Manifestation

Bowenoid Papulosis-Like Lesions

- Clinically resemble genital warts; however, on pathology review, they represent high-grade lesions or SCCIS.
- Lesions are often brown in color, but may also be whitish, pink, red-brown to dark brown, violaceous, and black.

BOX 11.4-8   DDx Genital Ulcers

Disease	Clinical Lesion	Organism
Genital herpes	Eroded, "punched out," irregularly bordered ulcers; painful	Herpes simplex virus type 1 (HSV-1) and herpes simplex virus type 2 (HSV-2)
Primary syphilis	Painless, firm ulcer; usually single; nonpurulent	*Treponema pallidum*
Lymphogranuloma venereum	Painless ulcer; heals within days to 1 week	*Chlamydia trachomatis* serovars L1, L2, and L3
Grauloma inguinale	Superficial ulcer; raised, rolled margin with granulation tissue–like base raised above the skin surface; beefy red	*Klebsiella granulomatis* (formerly known as Calymmatobacterium granulomatis)
Chancroid	Painful, well demarcated, purulent ulcer with undermined borders; often multiple ulcers	*Haemophilus ducreyi*

- Often present on the penile shaft, with multiple red-brown papules to confluent plaques (Fig. 11.4-34). The glans penis, foreskin, and scrotum may be involved.
- On the vulva, lesions may resemble leukoplakia with white to grayish hyperkeratotic patches.

Erythroplasia of Queyrat (or SCCIS of Glans or Vulva)

- Appears on glans penis or vulva and/or adjacent mucosal surfaces.
- Solitary or multiple, well-demarcated red papules and plaques (Fig. 11.4-35).
- Lesions may be smooth, verrucous, or velvety.

DIFFERENTIAL DIAGNOSIS   Intraepithelial Neoplasia

- Lichen sclerosus
- Condyloma acuminatum
- Zoon balanitis/vulvitis
- Invasive SCC

Confirming Diagnosis

- The definitive diagnosis is established with a skin biopsy.
- It is vital to biopsy any genital erythema or lesion that is persistent despite attempted therapies.

Treatment

- The treatment decision should take into consideration the patient's age, along with the site and extent of their disease.
- Excision of localized disease is preferred. Although, if possible, a mutilating surgery should be avoided. Differentiated VIN, which is associated with LP and LS, has a higher risk for invasion and must be excised.
- Cryosurgery and laser surgery have high recurrence rates.
- Topical imiquimod and fluorouracil can require prolonged regimens with low tolerability, though these may be helpful in certain cases.
- In select cases, where risks of treatment outweigh benefits, it is reasonable to opt for observation with a plan for the necessary surgical excision in the event of any progression.
- Circumcision is recommended in uncircumcised men to reduce the risk of invasion.

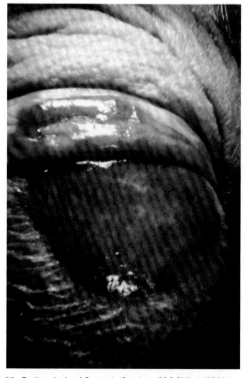

FIG. 11.4-35. Erythroplasia of Queyrat. (Courtesy CDC PHIL #17536.)

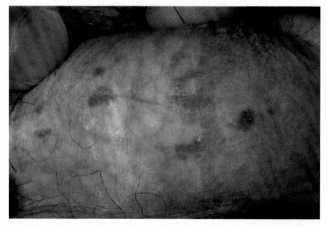

FIG. 11.4-34. Bowenoid papulosis. Clinical appearance is very similar to warts. (Courtesy T. Habif.)

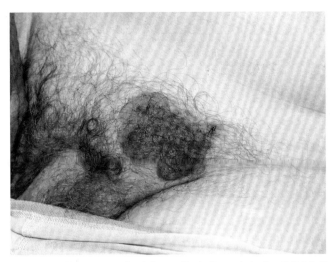

FIG. 11.4-36. Extramammary Paget disease. (Used with permission from Hall, J. C., & Hall, B. J. [2017]. *Sauer's manual of skin diseases* [11th ed.]. Wolters Kluwer Health.)

Extramammary Paget Disease

Extramammary Paget Disease (EMPD) is a rare neoplasm which can be primary, arise as a cutaneous adenocarcinoma, or secondary, due to extension of an underlying adenocarcinoma (Fig. 11.4-36). About 10% to 25% of patients have a contiguous malignancy at the time of diagnosis, but 10% of patients with a new diagnosis of EMPD are diagnosed with a noncontiguous malignancy within 12 months of diagnosis. In women, the most common area involved is the vulva. In men, the most common area is the scrotum followed by perianal disease, penis, and groin. These may spread to the labia, mons pubis, vagina, and thighs. Perianal lesions may extend up into the anal canal.

In men, the most common area is the scrotum followed by peri-anal disease, penis, and groin. The location of EMPD is useful in predicting the risk of associated cancer. The most commonly associated malignancies are cancers of the prostate, urinary tract, and breast. Associated carcinomas of the cervix, vagina, endometrium, bladder, and Bartholin glands have also been described. EMPD around the anal region is associated with an underlying colorectal cancer 25% to 35% of the time. EMPD is thought to invade and metastasize via lymphatics (Wagner & Sachse, 2011).

Clinical Manifestation

Skin Findings
- Present as red, sharply demarcated plaque with erosions and white scale, leading to the appearance of "strawberries and cream."
- Lesions expand slowly, and are similar in appearance to eczematous dermatoses, often leading to delays in diagnosis.
- Usually a single plaque is present.
- Lesions most commonly appear on the vulva in women and in the perianal area in men.

Non-Skin Finding
- May be asymptomatic but early symptoms are often itching and burning of persistent plaques.

Confirming the Diagnosis
- The diagnosis is confirmed by skin biopsy.

DIFFERENTIAL DIAGNOSIS   Extramammary Paget Disease
- Eczematous dermatitis
- Lichen simplex chronicus
- Psoriasis
- Erosive lichen planus
- Pemphigus vegetans
- Candidiasis
- Tinea cruris
- Intertrigo

Treatment
- Surgical treatment by wide local excision or Mohs micrographic surgery (MMS) is often first-line therapy.
- Refer to medical oncology and radiation oncology if patients are not surgical candidates or have extensive disease.

Management and Patient Education
- All age-appropriate malignancy screening should be performed
- Refer to gastroenterology for a colonoscopy
- Refer female patients to gynecology for mammography and Pap Smear
- Male patients should have a PSA blood test checked
- Lesions recur about 20% to 30% of the time, therefore patients will require frequent follow-up

READINGS AND REFERENCES

Anderson, M., Kutzner, S., & Kaufman, R. H. (2002). Treatment of vulvovaginal lichen planus with vaginal hydrocortisone suppositories. *Obstetrics and Gynecology, 100*(2), 359–362.

Bernstein, D. I., Bellamy, A. R., Hook, E. W. 3rd, Levin, M. J., Wald, A., Ewell, M. G., Wolff, P. A., Deal, C. D., Heineman, T. C., Dubin, G., & Belshe, R. B. (2013). Epidemiology, clinical presentation, and antibody response to primary infection with herpes simplex virus type 1 and type 2 in young women. *Clinical Infectious Diseases, 56*(3), 344–351.

Bolognia, J., Cerroni, L., & Schaffer, J. V. (2018). *Dermatology.* Elsevier.

Brenninkmeijer, E. E., Schram, M. E., Leeflang, M. M., Bos, J. D., & Spuls, P. I. (2008). Diagnostic criteria for atopic dermatitis: A systematic review. *British Journal of Dermatology, 158*(4), 754–765.

Bunker, C. B., Patel, N., & Shim, T. N. (2013). Urinary voiding symptomatology (micro-incontinence) in male genital lichen sclerosus. *Acta Dermato-Venereologica, 93*(2), 246–248.

Centers for Disease Control and Prevention. (2015a). *Anogenital warts—2015 STD treatment guidelines.* https://www.cdc.gov/std/tg2015/warts.htm.

Centers for Disease Control and Prevention. (2015b). *Human papillomavirus (HPV) infection—2015 STD treatment guidelines.* https://www.cdc.gov/std/tg2015/hpv.htm.

Centers for Disease Control and Prevention. (2019). *HPV.* https://www.cdc.gov/hpv/hcp/index.html.

Centers for Disease Control and Prevention. (2019). *Vaginal candidiasis.* https://www.cdc.gov/fungal/diseases/candidiasis/genital/index.html.

Chi, C. C., Kirtschig, G., Baldo, M., Lewis, F., Wang, S. H., & Wojnarowska, F. (2012). Systematic review and meta-analysis of randomized controlled trials on topical interventions for genital lichen sclerosus. *Journal of the American Academy of Dermatology, 67*(2), 305–312.

Fistarol, S. K., & Itin, P. H. (2013). Diagnosis and treatment of lichen sclerosus: An update. *American Journal of Clinical Dermatology, 14*(1), 27–47.

Habif, T. (2016). *Clinical dermatology: A color guide to diagnosis and therapy* (6th ed.). Mosby, Elsevier.

Hendi, A., Brodland, D. G., & Zitelli, J. A. (2004). Extramammary Paget's disease: Surgical treatment with Mohs micrographic surgery. *Journal of the American Academy of Dermatology, 51*(5), 767–673.

Ito, T., Kaku-Ito, Y., & Furue, M. (2018). The diagnosis and management of extramammary Paget's disease. *Expert Review of Anticancer Therapy, 18*(6), 543–553.

James, W., Berger, T., & Elston, D. (2016). Diseases resulting from fungi and yeasts. *Andrews' Diseases of the Skin: Clinical Dermatology* (12th ed; pp. 291–323). Philadelphia, PA: Saunders Elsevier.

Kang, Z., Zhang, Q., Zhang Q., Li, X., Hu, T., Xu, X., Wu, Z., Zhang, X., Wang, H., Xu, J., Xu, F., & Guan, M. (2015). Clinical and pathological characteristics of extramammary Paget's disease: Report of 246 Chinese male patients. *International Journal of Clinical and Experimental Pathology, 8*(10), 13233–13240.

Karam, A., & Dorigo, O. (2014). Increased risk and pattern of secondary malignancies in patients with invasive extramammary Paget disease. *British Journal of Dermatology, 170*(3), 661–671.

Kirtschig, G., Becker, K., Günthert A., Jasaitiene, D., Cooper, S., Chi, C-C., Kreuter, A., Rall, K. K., Aberer, W., Riechardt, S., Casabona, F., Powell, J., Brackenbury, F., Erdmann, R., Lazzeri, M., Barbagli, G., & Wojnarowska, F. (2015). Evidence-based (S3) Guideline on (anogenital) Lichen sclerosus. *The Journal of the European Academy of Dermatology and Venereology 29*(10), e1–e43.

Kundu, R. V., & Garg, A. (2012). Yeast infections: Candidiasis, tinea (pityriasis) versicolor, and Malassezia (Pityrosporum) folliculitis. In: Goldsmith, L. A., Katz, S. I., Gilchrest, B. A., Paller, A. S., Leffell, D. J., Wolff, K., eds. *Fitzpatrick's Dermatology in General Medicine.* 8th ed. New York, NY: McGraw-Hill; 2298–2307.

Kyle, A. A., & Dahl, M. V. (2004). Topical therapy for fungal infections. *American Journal of Clinical Dermatology, 5*(6), 443–451.

Lewis, F. M., Tatnall, F. M., Velangi, S. S., Bunker, C. B., Kumar, A., Brackenbury, F., Mohd Mustapa, M. F., & Exton, L. S. (2018). British Association of Dermatologists guidelines for the management of lichen sclerosus, 2018. *British Journal of Dermatology, 178*(4), 839–853.

Looker, K. J., Elmes, J. A. R., Gottlieb, S. L., Schiffer, J. T., Vickerman, P., Turner, K. M. E., & Boily, M. C. (2017). Effect of HSV-2 infection on subsequent HIV acquisition: An updated systematic review and meta-analysis. *The Lancet, Infectious Diseases, 17*(12), 1303–1316

Meites, E., Szilagyi, P. G., Chesson, H. W., Unger, E. R., Romero, J. R., & Markowitz, L. E. (2019). Human papillomavirus vaccination for adults: Updated recommendations of the advisory committee on immunization practices. *MMWR Morbidity and Mortality Weekly Report, 68*(32), 698–702. doi:10.15585/mmwr.mm6832a3

Nyirjesy, P. (2008). Vulvovaginal candidiasis and bacterial vaginosis. *Infectious Disease Clinics of North America, 22*(4), 637–652.

Pappas, P. G., Kauffman, C. A., Andes, D., Benjamin, D. K. Jr., Calandra, T. F., Edwards, J. E. Jr., Filler, S. G., Fisher, J. F., Kullberg, B-J., Zeichner, L. O., Annette, C., Reboli, A. C., Rex, J. H., Walsh, T. J., & Sobe, J. D. (2009). Clinical practice guidelines for the management of candidiasis: 2009 update by the Infectious Diseases Society of America. *Clinical Infectious Diseases, 48*(5), 503–535.

Rebbapragada, A., Wachihi, C., Pettengell, C., Sunderji, S., Huibner, S., Jaoko, W., Ball, B., Fowke, K., Mazzulli, T., Plummer, F. A., & Kaul, R. (2007). Negative mucosal synergy between herpes simplex type 2 and HIV in the female genital tract. *AIDS, 21*(5), 589–598.

Regauer, S., Reich, O., & Eberz, B. (2014). Vulvar cancers in women with vulvar the risk of human immunodeficiency virus type 1 acquisition in India. *Journal of Infectious Diseases, 187*(10), 1513–1521.

Schacker, T., Ryncarz, A. J., Goddard, J., Diem, K., Shaughnessy, M., & Corey, L. (1998). Frequent recovery of HIV-1 from genital herpes simplex virus lesions in HIV-1-infected men. *Journal of the American Medical Association, 280*(1), 61–66.

Sobel, J. D. (2007). Vulvovaginal candidosis. *Lancet, 369*(9577), 1961–1971.

Tong, L. X., Sun, G. S., & Teng, J. M. (2015). Pediatric lichen sclerosus: A review of the epidemiology and treatment options. *Pediatric Dermatology, 32*(5), 593–599.

Wagner, G., & Sachse, M. M. (2011). Extramammary Paget disease—Clinical appearance, PATHOGENESIS, management. *Journal Der Deutschen Dermatologischen Gesellschaft, 9*(6), 448–454.

Wald, A., & Link, K. (2002). Risk of human immunodeficiency virus infection in herpes simplex virus type 2-seropositive persons: A meta-analysis. *Journal of Infectious Diseases, 185*(1), 45–52.

Yale, K., Awosika, O., Rengifo-Pardo, M., & Ehrlich, A. (2018). Genital allergic contact dermatitis. *Dermatitis, 29*(3), 112–119.

Williams, H. C. (2005). Clinical practice. Atopic dermatitis. *New England Journal of Medicine, 352*(22), 2314–2324.

The Sweaty Patient

CHAPTER
11.5

Wayne Emineth

In This Chapter

- Hyperhidrosis
- Dyshidrosis
- Miliaria
- Hidradenitis Suppurativa

- Erythrasma
- Pitted Keratolysis
- Chromhidrosis
- Bromhidrosis

HYPERHIDROSIS

Hyperhidrosis is the production of increased amounts of sweat beyond what is necessary for thermoregulation. Known to have a genetic predisposition, this condition affects 1% to 3% of the population (males more than females) and can have a significant social and emotional impact. It has an increased occurrence at puberty and a tendency to improve after the age of 25. When hyperhidrosis is limited to certain areas of the body it is referred to as focal hyperhidrosis, which most commonly affects the palms, soles, axilla, and face. When the sweating is generalized, it suggests a secondary cause. Secondary causes include increased hypothalamic activity, acetylcholine, or alpha/beta-adrenergic hyperfunction, hypersensitive sweat gland receptors, anxiety, increased body temperature, and certain medications such as opioids, cholinesterase inhibitors, selective serotonin reuptake inhibitors, and tricyclic antidepressants (see complete list below) (Fig. 11.5-1).

Pathophysiology

Hyperhidrosis is usually a primary, idiopathic condition, but it can be secondary to other medical conditions or medications. Sweat glands are either eccrine or apocrine (Fig. 11.5-2).

Eccrine Sweat Glands

- Primarily responsible for creating sweat when the body needs to regulate temperature via evaporation. There are up to 2,000 per square inch on the palms and soles and as few as 300 per square inch on the elbows and knees.

- While essential for thermoregulation, they also excrete heavy metals, toxins, and some drugs. Eccrine sweat production is largely dependent on increased skin temperature and hypothalamic/sympathetic/acetylcholine signaling.

- Anxiety or febrile conditions can increase sensitivity of these pathways causing an increased propensity for hyperactivity years beyond the precipitating event. In short, with primary hyperhidrosis, the eccrine glands appear histologically and

FIG. 11.5-1. Hyperhidrosis. Note the shiny moist skin on the plantar foot. (Photo used with permission from Altchek, D. W. [2012]. *Foot and ankle sports medicine.* Wolters Kluwer.)

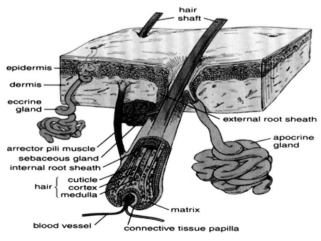

FIG. 11.5-2. Eccrine and apocrine glands. (Courtesy of SlideShare.)

448

functionally normal, but are receiving abnormal sympathetic stimuli.

Apocrine Sweat Glands

- These are part of the hair follicle unit and are primarily involved in pheromone production. Commonly referred to as "scent glands," they are largely responsible for body odor.
- Apocrine sweat is high in protein, which bacteria break down with odiferous consequences.
- Abnormal or offensive body odor is called bromhidrosis. As a result of genetic factors, 1% to 2% of people do not produce detectable armpit body odor when they perspire and thus do not need deodorant.
- Apocrine sweat glands are located in the axillae, inguinal/gluteal creases, and other body fold areas.
- They are a rare site of pathology but are believed to be the nidus for the autoimmune condition called hidradenitis suppurativa (Fig. 11.5-6).

Clinical Presentation

Primary Focal Hyperhidrosis

- Symptoms develop in childhood or adolescence and usually persist into the 20s, but sometimes throughout life.
- Typically bilateral and symmetrical, may be episodic or continuous.
- Rarely associated with bromhidrosis, but commonly associated with emotional stress.

Generalized Secondary Hyperhidrosis

- Usually presents in adults and is said to be present during sleep as well as waking hours.

DIFFERENTIAL DIAGNOSIS   Generalized Hyperhidrosis

- Hyperthyroidism, hyperpituitarism, hypoglycemia
- Carcinoid tumors, lymphoma, pheochromocytoma
- Cystic fibrosis, Parkinson disease, polycythemia vera
- Reflex hyperhidrosis due to spinal injury and spinal lesions
- Infections (TB, malaria, brucellosis, any febrile infection)
- Medications (methylphenidate, amphetamines, fluoxetine and many other antidepressants, oseltamivir (flu), tramadol, cholinesterase inhibitors/stigmine class of drugs, anabolic steroid use/abuse)
- Organophosphate poisoning (nerve agents and insecticides)
- Obesity
- Menopause

Confirming the Diagnosis

- Diagnostic criteria for primary hyperhidrosis:
  - Focal, visible excessive sweating for at least 6 months, with no apparent cause.
  - At least two of the following: bilateral and relatively symmetrical sweating; impairment of daily activities; at least one episode per week; age of onset less than 25; positive family history; lack of sweating during sleep.

- A brief medical examination, but thorough medical history and medication review, can help identify possible secondary causes of hyperhidrosis, which can include hyperthyroidism, infections, kidney dysfunction, diabetes, neurologic disorders, malignancy, connective tissue disorders, or a medication side effect. Appropriate subsequent lab tests can include CBC, CMP, thyroid panel, ANA, chest x-ray, hemoglobin A1c, and sedimentation rate (Brackenrich & Fagg, 2020).

Treatment

Topicals

Antiperspirants

- Over-the-counter (OTC) antiperspirants are usually a 3% to 6% solution of aluminum chloride (or other aluminum chlorohydrate variants) and may be useful for mild sweating. OTC "Clinical Strength" products containing 15% to 20% aluminum chloride are more successful, including: Certain Dri 20% aluminum chloride roll on and soft solid; Sweat Block towelettes allow for application to hands, axillae, and other areas; Vanicream hypoallergenic 20% aluminum zirconium chlorohydrex which can be less irritating for sensitive skin.
- Patients should apply nightly until the sweating has ceased and then as often as needed to maintain control. Application of antiperspirants at night, when sweat glands are less active, allows more time for absorption and subsequent reduction of perspiration.
- Showering in the morning does not wash away the benefits of nighttime application and can help minimize potential skin irritation from prolonged use.
- In vitro studies using human skin indicate that insignificant amounts of aluminum chloride are absorbed into the body to cause concern or harm (Pineau et al., 2012).
- Prescription antiperspirants include Drysol/Hypercare 20% aluminum chloride. Best applied before bed when not sweating to avoid prickly needle sensation. Glycopyrronium pad and roll on block acetylcholine at the site of application and may be used in combination with prescription and OTC antiperspirants.
- Topical glycopyrronium (Qbrexza): A prescription wipe FDA indicated for axillary use but also safely used off-label for palmar sweating. If the individual packages are carefully opened and reused, patients may get two to three uses out of one pad. A roll-on version may be approved soon. Patients should be instructed to wash hands thoroughly after handling the pads and to avoid rubbing their eyes, as prolonged pupillary dilation could result.
- Deodorants are not the same as antiperspirants. True deodorants only reduce bacteria and thus odor, but do not reduce perspiration. Being less irritating, true deodorants are helpful for patients prone to irritant axillary dermatitis. Gentle deodorants include deodorant stones (actual salt stones) and Tussy deodorant.

Systemics

Anticholinergics

- Both topical and oral acetylcholine antagonists can be effective in controlling hyperhidrosis.
- Oral glycopyrrolate (Robinul, Robinul Forte) is used off-label for hyperhidrosis. It is available in 1- and 2-mg tablets and is best

dosed QAM and titrated to the lowest dose that achieves the desired reduction of sweating. Tablets can be cut in half to further titrate the dose.

- Oral glycopyrrolate and topical glycopyrronium do not cross the blood–brain barrier and thus have minimal, if any, CNS effects.

- Mild side effects include reduced secretion and excretion of saliva, tears, GI fluids, stomach acid, respiratory mucus, and perspiration.

- While it has a 3- to 4-hour half-life, its anticholinergic (hyperhidrosis-reducing) effects tend to last 6 to 9 hours. Morning dosing allows the drug to clear during the night, thus reducing potential side effects.

- Typically, a steady state level of drug (dosed t.i.d.) is **not** required unless the hyperhidrosis is very severe. The desired side effect of anhidrosis can cause overheating during exercise, therefore these activities should take place either prior to, or 8 hours after, the morning dose.

- Other anticholinergic side effects include dry mouth, dry eyes, dry mucous membranes, reduced gastric acid production, blurred vision, exacerbation of glaucoma, urinary retention, temporarily reduced GI motility, constipation, HTN, arrhythmias, and CHF.

- *It should not be taken with antacids or H-blockers. Be cautious prescribing with patients over 40 years old, or with those on multiple medications, as side effects and interactions can be compounded.*

Iontophoresis

- A nonsurgical and drug-free treatment that uses direct current electricity from a small battery and tap water to suppress sweat production. The mechanism by which it works is not fully known but this treatment can be very effective.

- These medical devices are cleared by the FDA for treatment of axillary, palmar, and plantar hyperhidrosis. Utilize three times a week for 4 weeks, then reduce frequency based on the desired clinical response. Drionic, Iontoderma, and other manufacturers offer compact and easy-to-use home units (Fig. 11.5-3).

Botulinum Toxin

- Used for more severe cases. Affected areas are mapped out with a 1-cm grid and the toxin is methodically injected intradermally with a 30-G needle. The injections are expensive and can be painful (especially in the palms), but significant sweat reductions can last for 6 to 12 months.

- Temporary weakness in thenar eminence muscles has been reported with palmar injections.

- Refer patients to experienced dermatology providers for botulinum toxin injections.

Energy Devices and Perspiration Reduction

- Microwave energy device, Miradry, is an in-office, noninvasive treatment proven effective for axillary hyperhidrosis. Multiple treatments are required and patients can encounter significant out-of-pocket expense. While not approved as a hair destruction device, axillary hair reduction has been reported by patients.

Surgical Sympathectomy

- Sympathetic nerve fibers in the shoulder area between second, third, and fourth thoracic nerve ganglia are treated with cryoablation, radiofrequency ablation, or are surgically severed. This procedure blocks sympathetic nerve stimulation of sweat glands in the axilla, arm, and hand.

- Referral to an experienced neurosurgeon is required but is only considered for only the most severe and recalcitrant hyperhidrosis cases.

Management and Patient Education

- First-line treatment with topical medications includes glycopyrronium (Qbrexza) QAM or Drysol/Hypercare 20% aluminum chloride applied QPM.

- Second-line treatments include oral glycopyrrolate and/or battery-powered iontophoresis.

- Third-line treatments include Miradry, botulinum toxin, and as a last resort, surgical sympathectomy.

- Patients should be advised of all side-effects to anticholinergics.

Sweat Gland–Associated Conditions
Dyshidrotic Eczema/Pompholyx

- Dyshidrotic hand/foot eczema is associated both with higher dietary nickel intake as well as with hyperhidrosis (Fig. 11.5-4).

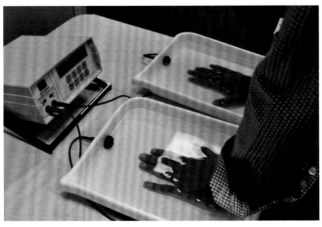

FIG. 11.5-3. Iontophoresis device. (Reprinted with permission, © International Hyperhidrosis Society, www.sweathelp.org)

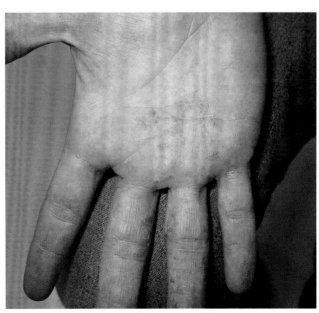

FIG. 11.5-4. Dyshidrotic eczema. (Image provided by Stedman's.)

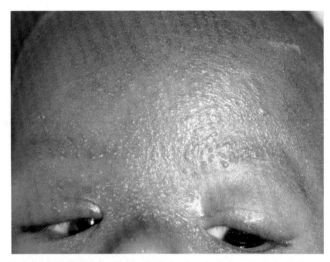

FIG. 11.5-5. Miliaria. (Used with permission from Lugo-Somolinos, A., McKinley-Grant, L., Goldsmith, L.A., Papier, A., Adigun, C. G., Culton, D., Davey, M., Diamantis, S., Fredeking, A., & Lee, I. [2011]. *VisualDx: Essential dermatology in pigmented skin.* Wolters Kluwer.)

- Treatment includes trial of a nickel-free diet (no nuts, beans/legumes, seeds, peanut, chocolate, coconut), superpotent topical steroids, and occasional systemic steroids for severe flares.
- Atopic dermatitis (eczema) patients have been found to sometimes have IgE autoantibodies against antigens in their own sweat and/or to excreted metals like nickel and mercury.

Miliaria/Prickly Heat

- Miliaria is due to occlusion of the sweat ducts (leading to maceration of the skin), thick lotion/sunblock, and/or skipping a baths. Sweat duct occlusion causes hypertonic sweat and salt crystals to leak within the epidermis causing prickles/pain/stinging (Fig. 11.5-5).
- Treatment: utilize cool water compresses, a cool shower, or relocate to an air-conditioned environment. May apply camphor and menthol lotion like Sarna. Alpha hydroxy acid lotion like Am Lactin 12% can break down plugging.

Hidradenitis Suppurativa

- An autoimmune inflammatory disorder of the apocrine sweat glands which causes inflammatory localized abscesses in body fold areas, namely the axillae, gluteal cleft, and inguinal creases.
- For evaluation and treatment (see Section 3.2) (Fig. 11.5-6).

Erythrasma

- Superficial overgrowth of *Corynebacterium minutissimum* with a similar appearance to tinea cruris (jock itch) (Fig. 11.5-7).
- Diagnostic feature is a pink fluorescence on Wood lamp examination.
- Treatment is 1% clindamycin solution and OTC benzoyl peroxide cleansers.
- If co-infection is suspected, naftifine 2% gel may treat both conditions as it has both antifungal and antibacterial benefits.

Pitted Keratolysis

- An overgrowth of sweat-dependent *Corynebacterium minutissimum* that causes a strong and foul odor of the feet.

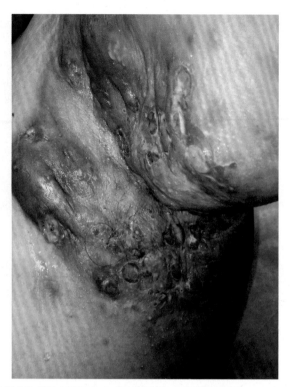

FIG. 11.5-6. Hidradenitis suppurativa. (Courtesy of D. DiRuggiero.)

- Presents with tiny pits sometimes with subtle retained black material within the pits (Fig. 11.5-8).
- Treatment: clindamycin or erythromycin solution with the addition of a benzoyl peroxide wash for flares and unscented antiperspirant sprays for prevention.

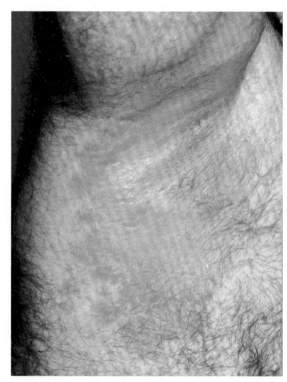

FIG. 11.5-7. Erythrasma. (Used with permission from Berg, D., & Worzala, K. [2006]. *Atlas of adult physical diagnosis.* Lippincott Williams & Wilkins.)

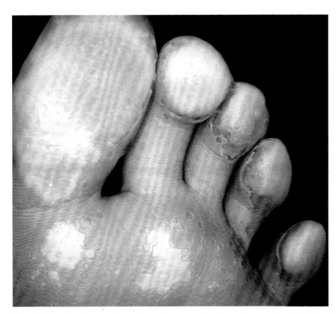

FIG. 11.5-8. Pitted keratolysis. Note the maceration from the sweaty foot. (Used with permission from Gru, A. A., & Wick, M. [2018]. *Pediatric dermatopathology and dermatology.* Wolters Kluwer.)

- Patients should alternate pairs of shoes daily to allow more time for them to dry. Merino wool socks have antibacterial properties and therefore may be a better choice than socks made of plastics like nylon, rayon, polyester, acrylic, dacron, etc.

- If co-infection of pitted keratolysis and tinea pedis is suspected, topical naftifine 2% gel is a good choice as it has antifungal and antibacterial benefits.

Chromhidrosis

- A rare condition where the apocrine glands, usually face and axilla, secrete a colored sweat. It is thought to be secondary to lipids and proteins (lipofuscin) being excreted from sweat glands. Other theories suggest that chromogenic pigments produced by bacteria (*Corynebacterium*) are excreted.

- While concerning for patients, chromhidrosis does not indicate or result in any disease or disorder.

- Treatment options are limited but reports include use of capsaicin cream and botulinum toxin injections in the affected areas.

Bromhidrosis

- An undesirable odor produced by the secretions of the sweat glands and the actions of bacteria on these secretions. Foods containing volatile sulfur compounds like onions, garlic, cruciferous vegetables, and fermented foods can be significant contributors.

- Antiperspirants, deodorants, antibacterial cleansers, and dietary changes.

READINGS AND REFERENCES

Brackenrich, J., & Fagg, C. (2020). *Hyperhidrosis.* In *StatPearls [Internet].* StatPearls Publishing. https://www.ncbi.nlm.nih.gov/books/NBK459227

Genius, S. J., Birkholz, D., Rodushkin, I., & Beesoon, S. (2011). Blood, urine, and sweat (BUS) study: Monitoring and elimination of bioaccumulated toxic elements. *Archives of Environmental Contamination and Toxicology, 61*(2), 344–357.

Hussain, J. N., Mantri, N., & Cohen, M. M. (2017). Working up a good sweat—the challenges of standardising sweat collection for metabolomics analysis. *Clinical Biochemistry Reviews, 38*(1), 13–34.

Pineau, A., Guillard, O., Favreau, F., Marrauld, A., & Fauconneau, B. (2012). In vitro study of percutaneous absorption of aluminum from antiperspirants through human skin in the Franz™ diffusion cell. *Journal of Inorganic Biochemistry, 110,* 21–26.

Thornhill, R., Gangestad, S. W., Miller, R., Scheyd, G., McCollough, J. K., & Franklin, M. (2003). Major histocompatibility complex genes, symmetry, and body scent attractiveness in men and women. *Behavioral Ecology, 14*(5), 668–678. https://doi.org/10.1093/beheco/arg043

Skin Findings in Systemic Disease

Susan T. Voss

CHAPTER 12.1

In This Chapter

Of all the organs of the human body, the skin is the largest. There are many conditions of the skin which affect the skin only. However, there are several conditions of the skin that may signal to the clinician an internal issue. The patient will often seek the advice of their primary care provider (PCP) when these skin conditions arise. The ability to identify these cutaneous manifestations of internal or systemic conditions and malignancy is important.

ENDOCRINE SYSTEM DISORDERS

The endocrine system is one of the most complex systems of the human body. The glands and hormones of the endocrine system regulate every cell in the body, impacting growth and metabolism. This section will focus on the cutaneous manifestations related to diabetes mellitus (DM), type I and II, and thyroid dysfunction.

With the current obesity epidemic in the United States, the incidence of DM is escalating. Individuals are being diagnosed in greater numbers and at a younger age. Early diagnosis of DM and initiation of treatment can decrease the long-term sequelae of the disease. DM impacts all systems of the body and there are distinct cutaneous features that indicate the potential for DM.

ACANTHOSIS NIGRICANS

Acanthosis nigricans (AN) is a skin condition that often presents in primary care. It can be very distressing for the patient and their family. It can impact them physically, mentally, and socially. AN impacts males and females equally and can occur at any age. It is more common in dark skin tone races, including Native Americans, Hispanics, and African Americans (Lause et al., 2017). AN can be benign but can also represent a red flag for an existing or developing medical condition such as: Type II DM, hypothyroidism, Addison disease, polycystic ovarian syndrome, acromegaly, pituitary or adrenal adenomas, Cushing syndrome, lymphoma, or GU/GI malignancies.

Pathophysiology

- The cause of AN is not fully known. AN may be caused by stimulation of insulin-like binding growth factor receptors on keratinocytes and dermal fibroblasts resulting in hyperproliferation.
- The darkened skin appearance and thickening of the epidermis is therefore caused by increased keratinocyte and fibroblast proliferation and not excessive melanin.
- The roughened appearance is the result of the multiple small, flesh colored papules or finger like growths called papillomatosis.
- AN may also be genetically inherited.

Clinical Presentation

Skin Findings

- The onset is insidious as the lesions start out as flat patches that thicken and darken over time (Fig. 12.1-1A,B).
- The typical presentation of AN involves hyperpigmentation and hyperkeratinization that results in velvety thickening of the skin folds (Fig. 12.1-2) and areas of friction (Fig. 12.1-3).
- The most common site is around the neck. Initially, patients may attempt to wash or exfoliate it off but have no success.
- The axillae, groin, umbilicus, areolae, submammary regions, and hands can develop these characteristic lesions.

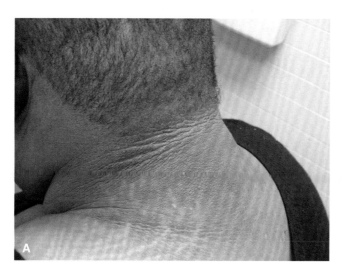

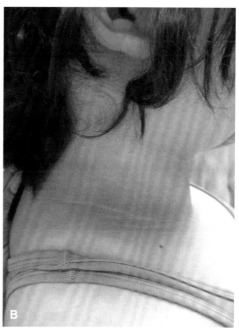

FIG. 12.1-1. A: Woman with classic ANs with a thick, hyperpigmented, velvety plaque. **B:** A 10-year-old girl with early ANs and the "dirty" appearance of an early plaque forming around her neck.

Non-Skin Findings

- The affected skin may be pruritic and have a foul odor. Children and adolescents with AN often experience ridicule and are called "dirty" (Fig. 12.1-1B).

DIFFERENTIAL DIAGNOSIS   Acanthosis Nigricans
• Addison disease
• Hemochromatosis
• Pellagra
• Erythema dyschromicum perstans
• Terra firma-forme dermatosis
• Confluent and reticulated papillomatosis
• Becker nevus

Confirming the Diagnosis

A basic workup for underlying malignancy in a patient with AN should be considered with the following presentations (Higgins et al., 2008):

- Older adult
- Rapid onset of extensive AN accompanied by unintentional weight loss
- Atypical locations such as mucosal involvement (Fig. 12.1-2), velvety plaques (Fig. 12.1-3) on the palms (tripe palms) or soles
- Accompanied by sign of Leser–Trélat (rapid onset of multiple seborrheic keratosis)

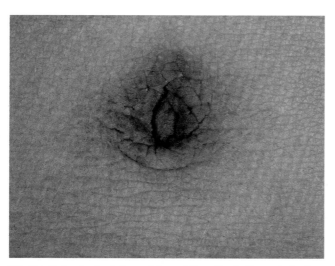

FIG. 12.1-2. Acanthosis nigricans of the umbilicus. (Used with permission from Lugo-Somolinos, A., McKinley-Grant, L., Goldsmith, L. A., Papier, A., Adigun, C. G., Culton, D., Davey, M., Diamantis, S., Fredeking, A., & Lee, I. [2011]. *VisualDx: Essential dermatology in pigmented skin.* Wolters Kluwer.)

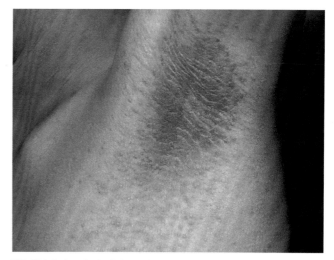

FIG. 12.1-3. Acanthosis nigricans of the axilla. (Used with permission from Lugo-Somolinos, A., McKinley-Grant, L., Goldsmith, L. A., Papier, A., Adigun, C. G., Culton, D., Davey, M., Diamantis, S., Fredeking, A., & Lee, I. [2011]. *VisualDx: Essential dermatology in pigmented skin.* Wolters Kluwer.)

Laboratory

Serologic testing based on a thorough history and physical examination may identify potential underlying disease. Specific monitoring is suggested for:

- Polycystic ovarian syndrome
  - Follicle-stimulating hormone (FSH)
  - Luteinizing hormone (LH)
  - Testosterone
  - Estrogens
  - Sex hormone binding globulin (SBGH)
- Addison disease
  - AM serum cortisol level
  - AM ACTH stimulation test
  - Serum aldosterone level
- Cushing disease
  - 24-hour urine sample for free cortisol and creatinine
- Acromegaly
  - Serum insulin-like growth factor (IGF)—1 level
- Terra firma-forme dermatosis
  - Cleansing area with a 70% isopropyl alcohol-soaked pad will remove entire lesion (regular soap and water will not)
- Insulin resistance
  - Glycosylated hemoglobin (hemoglobin A1c) and fasting blood sugar, although a normal level does not rule out insulin resistance
  - Plasma insulin level to rule out hyperinsulinemia
- Biopsy
  - AN is easily identified by the experienced practitioner and rarely requires biopsy. If, however, a biopsy is performed, it should be a punch biopsy for H&E within the area of affected skin

Treatment

- When obesity is a factor, weight loss can eliminate or improve the lesions. Low-carbohydrate diets and exercise can help to moderate the insulin resistance.

Topical

Cosmetic improvement may be achieved with application of topical treatments (Higgins et al., 2009).

- Topical retinoids, tretinoin 0.1% daily
- Calcipotriene 0.005% cream daily to affected area
- Preparations with salicylic acid (CeraVe SA lotion or cream)
- 12% ammonium lactate lotion or cream (Lac-Hydrin)
- 20% urea cream
- Laser and dermabrasion

Systemic

- Oral retinoids
- Fish oil
- Metformin 500 mg b.i.d.

Management and Patient Education

- Benign AN can usually be managed in the primary care setting and has few physical complications.
- AN associated with underlying disease carries a prognosis directly related to the disease and treatment.
- The psychologic complications from AN can have an impact on the patient's self-esteem, especially children and young adults.
- Patients should be empowered with the knowledge that control of AN (benign) is within their ability.
- Utilizing the topical therapies and following the lifestyle changes and medication when appropriate can greatly reduce, if not eliminate the condition.
- Topical remedies are rarely covered by insurance since considered cosmetic.
- Follow-up should be done to evaluate the efficacy of therapy and to monitor the insulin resistance. Periodic screening for DM is advised.
- Referral to dermatology is only needed if the diagnosis is not obvious, the patient is not responding to treatment, or if they desire cosmetic treatment.
- Endocrinology may be consulted as needed to assist in the diagnosis and management of a possible metabolic disorder.
- Patients with AN likely have multiple diabetes risk factors (Kong et al., 2010).

CLINICAL PEARL

- Patients need reassurance that AN is not related to hygiene.

NECROBIOSIS LIPOIDICA

Necrobiosis lipoidica (NL) is a chronic granulomatous dermatitis. There is an association between NL and type I DM and, to a lesser extent, type II DM. Few patients with DM develop NL. In contrast, 75% of patients with NL have or will develop DM. However, since not all patients with NL have diabetes, there is decreased use of the previous term, NL diabeticorum. NL is three times more common in females (Lima et al., 2017), and the average age of onset is 30 to 40 years of age.

Pathophysiology

The actual etiology and cause of NL continues to be elusive. Most experts agree that microangiopathy plays a significant role. Histologic analysis shows a degeneration of collagen and granulomatous inflammation (Reid et al., 2013).

Clinical Presentation

Skin Findings

- Most commonly presents on the pretibial region of the lower leg.
- Less often may present on face, scalp, trunk, and upper extremities.
- Begins as 1- to 3-mm shiny erythematous papules or sharply defined violaceous patches (Fig. 12.1-4).
- Slowly evolves and coalesces into larger plaques with central waxy yellow and brown appearance with telangiectasias (Fig. 12.1-5).
- At risk for development of ulceration occurring in 33%.
- Lesions may develop in areas of minor injury (Koebnerization).

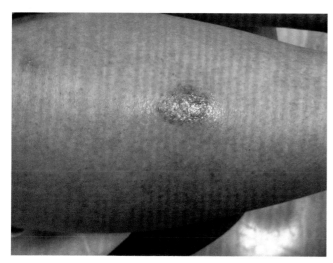

FIG. 12.1-4. Necrobiosis lipoidica. Early necrobiosis lipoidica can begin as a violaceous plaque, often found on the anterior lower legs. (Photo courtesy of M. Bobonich.)

Non-Skin Findings

- Asymptomatic or may experience tenderness, pruritus, or paresthesia.

DIFFERENTIAL DIAGNOSIS Necrobiosis Lipoidica
• Granuloma annulare
• Majocchi granuloma
• Diabetic dermopathy
• Pyoderma gangrenosum
• Sarcoidosis
• Xanthomas
• Chronic venous insufficiency
• Morphea

Confirming the Diagnosis

- Usually a clinical diagnosis.
- If necessary to confirm the diagnosis, a punch biopsy for histopathology may be done at the leading edge of a lesion. This should be avoided if possible since NL is already at risk for developing ulcers and a biopsy can increase the risk and cause a nonhealing area. Performing the biopsy centrally should be avoided.
- Appropriate glucose monitoring (e.g., fasting blood glucose, Hgb A1c).

Treatment

Topical

- No one treatment has proven effective.
- Focus of treatment is preventing and healing ulcers.
- Cautious use of class I-III topical corticosteroids b.i.d. for 2 to 4 weeks for active lesions remains the mainstay of treatment. For thicker lesions, application of class I-III topical corticosteroids under occlusion may improve efficacy.
- Tacrolimus ointment 0.1% twice daily to affected lesions can be used.
- Topical tretinoin daily in varying strengths based on thickness of lesions, 0.025%, 0.05%, and 0.1% cream or gel. Reevaluate in 4 to 6 weeks after initiating therapy.

Systemic

- Patients requiring systemic therapy should be referred to dermatology for the consideration of the following therapies:
  - Intralesional steroids for the raised borders (triamcinolone acetonide 2.5 mg/cc). Avoid the central aspect (Lause et al., 2017)
  - Three to five-week course of oral steroids to arrest active extensive cases, keeping in mind the impact on glycemic control

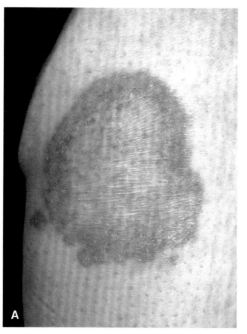
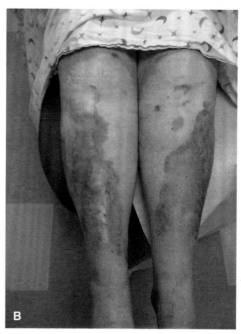

FIG. 12.1-5. **A:** Necrobiosis lipoidica can expand with waxy, yellow centers and erythematous borders. **B:** Larger lesions may become shiny and atrophic with telangiectasias. (Photos courtesy of M. Bobonich.)

- Pentoxifylline 400 mg t.i.d.
- Aspirin 325 mg daily
- Dipyridamole 2 to 3 mg/kg per day
- Narrow-band UVB and PUVA
- Tumor necrosis factor (TNF) inhibitors
- Other disease-modifying antirheumatic drugs

Surgical

- Skin grafting for very extensive cases.

Management and Patient Education

- No treatment has shown efficacy for prevention of NL and lesions can be resistant to treatment.
- Tight glycemic control does not modify lesions.
- Patients should be monitored closely for development of ulcers.
- Risk and benefits of specific treatments must be considered.

CLINICAL PEARLS

- In a small number of cases, NL has evolved to squamous cell carcinoma (SCC). Referral to dermatology is advised for nonhealing ulcers and suspected SCC (Reid et al., 2013).
- Close surveillance is advised to prevent and address ulcers early.

GRANULOMA ANNULARE

Granuloma annulare (GA) is a relatively common, self-limited, idiopathic dermatosis of the dermis and subcutaneous tissue. The frequency of GA is unknown but is two times more common in women. Localized GA is more common in those under the age of 30 while disseminated GA is more common in those 30 to 60 years of age. The PCP should be alert for signs and symptoms and screen the patient appropriately for association with other conditions. GA has been associated with type I DM, and less often with type II DM and thyroid dysfunction. The association between disseminated GA and DM has been established while an association between localized GA and DM has not (Ferringer & Miller, 2003). It has also been suggested but not proven to be associated with a myriad of other conditions such as thyroiditis, trauma, sun exposure, insect bites, viral infections (HIV, hepatitis, herpes zoster, Epstein–Barr).

Pathophysiology

The exact cause of GA is not known. A delayed hypersensitivity and cell-mediated immune response to an antigen or component of the dermis is suggested by the presence of T-helper cells with histiocytes in the inflammatory infiltrate in GA lesions.

Clinical Presentation

Localized

Skin Findings

- Most common on distal extremities.
- Flesh-colored to erythematous papule that undergoes central involution.

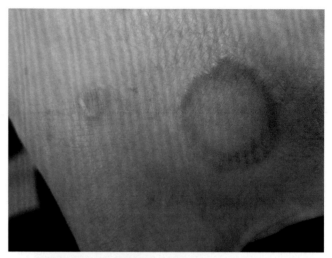

FIG. 12.1-6. Localized GA on the dorsal hand with the classic plaques with a raised border and central clearing. (Photo courtesy of M. Bobonich.)

- Over months, a ring of papules slowly increases in diameter from 0.5 to 5 cm with a raised palpable border (Fig. 12.1-6).

Non-Skin Findings

- Asymptomatic
- Variable duration
- May undergo spontaneous evolution or last for years. Duration of the disease is highly variable. Many lesions undergo spontaneous involution without scarring, whereas others last for years.

Generalized

Skin Findings

- Presents as few to thousands of scattered 1- to 2-mm papules (disseminated type) arranged in groups 10 cm in diameter favoring the skin folds. Large coalescing annular plaques (3 to 6 cm) may enlarge centrifugally over weeks to months or nodules ranging from flesh-colored to erythematous may occur (Fig. 12.1-7).

Non-Skin Findings

- Asymptomatic

DIFFERENTIAL DIAGNOSIS   Granuloma Annulare

- Tinea corporis
- Majocchi granuloma
- Pityriasis rosea
- Necrobiosis lipoidica
- Nummular eczema
- Psoriasis
- Lichen planus
- Sarcoidosis
- Erythema migrans (Lyme disease)
- Subacute cutaneous lupus erythematosus
- Erythema annulare centrifugum

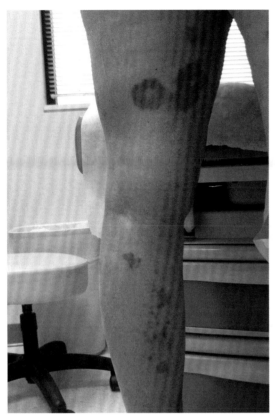

FIG. 12.1-7. The generalized form of GA presents as chronic lesions, as on legs of this 62-year-old woman with diabetes. (Photo courtesy of M. Bobonich.)

Confirming the Diagnosis

- Diagnosis is usually made based on the presentation and history of the lesions.
- Punch biopsy at the leading border of a lesion for histopathology can confirm the diagnosis.
- A biopsy for direct immunofluorescence (DIF) is usually not needed but can be helpful to rule out other causes.

Treatment

Treatment success varies greatly and no treatment may be needed if lesions spontaneously involute.

Topical

- High potency corticosteroids with or without occlusion.
- Intralesional steroid injections with triamcinolone acetonide with strength varied by the severity/thickness of the lesion.
- Cryotherapy
- Topical calcineurin inhibitors, tacrolimus 0.1% ointment or pimecrolimus 1% cream twice daily to lesions.

Systemic

If patients fail topical therapy, refer to dermatology where multiple systemic therapies can be tried such as narrow-band ultraviolet B radiation phototherapy, pentoxifylline, allopurinol, antibiotic cocktail (rifampin, ofloxacin, minocycline), dapsone, systemic steroids, DMARDs, and certain biologic medications.

Management and Patient Education

- If the diagnosis is not clear or if GA fails to respond to topical therapy, refer to dermatology. Many of the systemic treatment options have potential adverse effects and should only be administered by a clinician with experience with the treatment.
- Patients with GA should be given reassurance that it is typically a benign condition. There is conflicting data regarding generalized GA representing a paraneoplastic condition. Older adults with generalized GA with symptoms suggestive of malignancy (e.g., weight loss, fatigue) should have age-appropriate cancer screenings completed.
- Patients and their family should be educated that GA is not contagious.
- Some struggle with the cosmetic aspect of the lesions, especially when generalized.
- They should be informed that new lesions may form independent of whether or not they treat current lesions.

> **CLINICAL PEARLS**
>
> - Often, patients will present to primary care after attempting to treat with OTC antifungals since localized GA looks similar to "ringworm." GA tends to be smooth whereas fungal infections tend to be scaly. The clinician should consider GA when treatment for "ringworm" fails.

DIABETIC DERMOPATHY

Diabetic dermopathy (DD) is commonly known as "shin spots" or "pigmented pretibial papules." It is the most common cutaneous manifestation of DM. DD predominantly affects men over the age of 50 and impacts 70% of adult persons with DM (Lause et al., 2017).

Pathophysiology

- The etiology of DD is unclear though trauma seems to be a modifying factor.
- It is speculated that microangiopathic changes associated with DM play a role in the development of DD.
- Research has failed to demonstrate a correlation between glucose control and DD.

Clinical Presentation

Skin Findings

- Multiple, bilateral, asymmetrical, annular, or irregular, red papules or plaques on the anterior aspect of the lower legs.
- Lesions gradually evolve into atrophic hyperpigmented finely scaled macules (Fig. 12.1-8).
- While it is most common on the "shins," DD can present on the lateral malleoli, thighs, or forearms.

> **DIFFERENTIAL DIAGNOSIS   Diabetic Dermopathy**
>
> - Necrobiosis lipoidica
> - Stasis dermatitis
> - Pigmented purpura
> - Posttraumatic scarring
> - Postinflammatory hyperpigmentation
> - Lymphedema

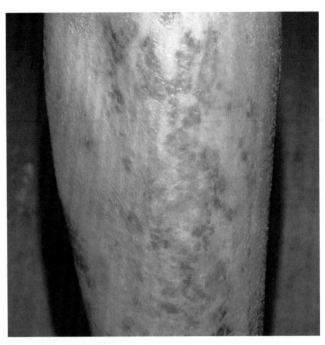

FIG. 12.1-8. Diabetic dermopathy.

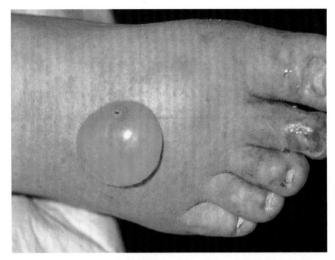

FIG. 12.1-9. Large clear bulla on the foot or lower leg is characteristic of diabetic bullae.

Confirming the Diagnosis

- DD is a clinical diagnosis and skin biopsy is usually not necessary.
- If considered, the benefit of biopsy must be weighed against the risk of slow healing, infection, and ulceration on the lower extremities of a diabetic patient.

Management and Patient Education

- DD is largely asymptomatic and rarely progresses to ulceration.
- The lesions should be monitored, but there is no effective treatment.
- It is largely a cosmetic issue.
- DD is a common problem managed by PCPs and rarely requiring referral to dermatology unless the diagnosis is uncertain.
- Patients should be educated on importance of good glycemic control and proper skin care avoidance of trauma to the affected areas.

DIABETIC BULLAE

Diabetic bullae or bullosis diabeticorum develop in approximately 0.5% of individuals with DM. It has been reported only in adults and is most common in men. Diabetic bullae are prevalent in those 17 to 84 years old. It is more common in long-term diabetics who suffer from neuropathy (Ferringer & Miller, 2003).

Pathophysiology

- The pathogenesis of diabetic bullae is poorly understood and is likely multifactorial.
- Evidence suggests an abnormality of anchoring fibrils that are essential for the integrity of the dermo-epidermal junction.
- The prominence of bullae on acral surfaces is suggestive of trauma. The threshold for suction-related blister formation is lower for diabetics than nondiabetics.
- Ultraviolet radiation (UVR) also seems to play a role. Recurrence is not uncommon.

Clinical Presentation

Skin Findings

- Bullae appear suddenly and favor acral skin areas, especially the dorsal and lateral aspects of the lower legs and feet.
- Diabetic bullae are painless with clear fluid lesions ranging in size from a few millimeters to several centimeters (Fig. 12.1-9).
- After rupture, the bullae heal in 2 to 5 weeks without treatment.

DIFFERENTIAL DIAGNOSIS   Diabetic Bullae
- Bullous pemphigoid
- Autoimmune blistering diseases
- Porphyria cutanea tarda
- Bullous impetigo
- Erythema multiforme
- Bullous tinea
- Arthropod assault

Confirming the Diagnosis

- A tissue punch biopsy for histology and DIF is indicated to exclude other blistering disorders of the skin.
- This will be best accomplished by dermatology since it would require a lesional biopsy for histology and a perilesional specimen for direct immunofluorescence (requires Michel's solution, no formaldehyde).
- If porphyria cutanea tarda is in the differential (especially if bullae are located on the dorsal hands), porphyrin levels should be evaluated.
- Bacterial and fungal cultures may be necessary if an infection is suspected.

Treatment

- Since the bullae heal spontaneously, treatment is focused on the avoidance and treatment of secondary infections.
- If there is discomfort, bullae can be aspirated with a sterile small-bore needle.

- Appropriate antibiotics should be utilized for secondary bacterial infections.

Management and Patient Education

- Refer diabetic bullae patients to dermatology for appropriate biopsy if needed to rule out other blistering skin disorders.
- Good skin care and diabetic foot care should be taught and stressed. Patients should continue with appropriate diabetic care and monitoring.
- Since the bullae are prone to recur, the patient should be evaluated with each episode.
- Patients with diabetic bullae should be monitored closely until the bullae have healed and resolved. Should the blister become unroofed, aggressive wound healing measures should be taken (see Section 14.1). If wounds from unroofed blisters are resistant to healing, refer to dermatology as soon as possible to avoid ulceration and necrosis. Once necrosis occurs, the patient may require referral to a surgeon for debridement and skin grafting.

THYROID DISEASE

Thyroid hormones are primarily responsible for regulation of metabolism and can affect any organ in the body. There are a wide variety of skin changes and disorders that are associated or caused by dysregulation of the thyroid gland. Skin changes may be the patient's chief complaint and should prompt the clinician to consider evaluation of thyroid function. Correcting the thyroid hormone levels can lead to resolution of the skin conditions.

Hypothyroidism

Low levels of circulating thyroid hormone or cell resistance to thyroid hormone action can result in hypothyroidism. The most common cause for hypothyroidism is the autoimmune disease Hashimoto thyroiditis, which results in glandular failure. Hypothyroidism can also occur as a result of genetics, treatment to correct hyperthyroidism, drug induced (e.g., lithium), pregnancy, and iron deficiency.

Hyperthyroidism

Hyperthyroidism results when there are excessive levels of circulating thyroid hormones usually due to an autoimmune disease called Graves disease. Hyperthyroidism can also develop due to thyroid adenomas, inflammation of the thyroid, excess iron intake, postpartum period, and can be drug induced by amiodarone and some IV contrasts.

Pathophysiology

- Thyroid hormones appear to play a pivotal role in cellular metabolism, including the growth and formation of hair, nails, skin, and sebum production. The skin responds when there are inadequate or excessive amounts of circulating thyroid hormone.
- There can be a direct or indirect effect on the skin as thyroid dysfunction affects all organs and body systems, thus resulting in cutaneous system effects.
- In a hyperthyroid state, many cutaneous manifestations are due to increased cutaneous blood flow and peripheral vasodilatation.
- In a hypothyroid state, symptoms may be associated with a reduced core body temperature and reflex cutaneous vasoconstriction (Doshi et al., 2008).

Clinical Presentation

In addition to the skin changes noted in Table 12.1-1, other cutaneous manifestations may be present from disease or conditions associated with thyroid disease. For example, dyslipidemia resulting from hypothyroidism may manifest symptoms of AN.

TABLE 12.1-1	Cutaneous Symptoms of Thyroid Dysfunction	
	HYPERTHYROID (GRAVES OR THYROTOXICOSIS)	**HYPOTHYROID (MYXEDEMA)**
Skin	Vasodilatation Thin Warm Moist Smooth Excessive sweating Pruritus	Vasoconstriction Weight gain Cool Dry/Xerosis Pale Decreased sweating Thickening of palms and soles Impaired wound healing
Hair	Soft and fine Diffuse, nonscarring alopecia	Dry, coarse, and brittle Diffuse or partial alopecia Loss of lateral ⅓ eyebrow "Queen Anne" sign (Fig. 12.1-10)
Nails	"Plummer's nail" or separation from the nail bed Swelling and tenderness Soft, friable	"Plummer's nail" or separation from the nail bed Brittle nails
Pigmentation	Hyperpigmentation (palms and soles, gingival and buccal mucosa) Vitiligo	Yellowish hue on the skin (palms, soles, and nasolabial folds)
Myxedema changes	Scleromyxedema: firm, white, yellow, or pink papules scattered on the face, trunk, axillae, and extremities	Myxedema, facial and/or generalized: thickened, nonpitting edematous changes to the soft tissues

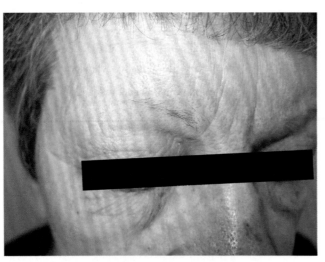

FIG. 12.1-10. Queen Anne sign of hypothyroidism; lateral third of the eyebrow is missing.

Confirming the Diagnosis

Laboratory

Serologic Screening for Thyroid Disease

- Thyrotropin or thyroid-stimulating hormone
- A free or total T4

May be affected by pregnancy, disease states such as end-stage renal disease and major cardiac surgery, or genetic predisposition.

- Free T3 levels are important when hyperthyroidism is suspected
- If considering autoimmune thyroid disease:
  - Anti-thyroid peroxidase (anti-TPO)
  - Anti-thyroglobulin (anti-Tg)
    - May be elevated with infertility

Radiologic Screening

- Thyroid scans
- Ultrasound of the neck
- Scintigraphy

Treatment

- The goal of therapy is to normalize thyroid hormone levels. After the initiation of thyroid hormone replacement, and thyroid hormone levels stabilize, the majority of the symptoms resolve.
- In hyperthyroidism, ablation with radioactive therapy or surgical thyroidectomy is the most common treatment.

Management and Patient Education

- Prognosis is good for individuals with thyroid dysfunction.
- Once corrected, symptoms usually resolve but may be dependent on the severity, chronicity, comorbidities, and treatment.
- Hyperthyroid patients undergoing thyroid ablation should be monitored for hypothyroidism.
- Half of the patients with Graves disease have ocular symptoms, with about 5% having severe ophthalmopathy. Graves disease requires management by an endocrinologist and often an ophthalmologist (Doshi et al., 2008).

- Thyroid disease is often managed by a PCP but may necessitate referral to an endocrinologist for complex cases. Dermatology may be consulted for specific cutaneous manifestations and OB/GYN for women with fertility problems.
- It is not uncommon for resolution of symptoms of hypo- and hyperthyroidism to lag behind normalization of thyroid levels. Patients can become frustrated when their thyroid level is normal but symptoms have not resolved.
- Educating patients on palliative treatment of the symptoms while the evaluation and treatment is ongoing can be helpful. Patients should know the signs and symptoms of abnormal thyroid function and report them immediately.
- Regular monitoring of serum levels should occur, more often when there is a change in dose or for changes in symptoms.
- Since thyroid regulation occurs in a slow negative feedback loop, it can take several weeks for the thyroid levels to normalize once appropriate therapy has been instituted.
- TSH levels should be checked every 2 to 3 months until it normalizes and after any changes in dosage.

CLINICAL PEARLS

- Patients experiencing issues with hair loss may be taking over-the-counter biotin supplements, commonly marketed as "Hair and Nail" supplements.
- These high-dose biotin supplements can lead to inaccurate thyroid function test. Patients should be advised to hold their supplement for at least 1 week prior to any thyroid testing.

HEPATIC SYSTEM DISORDERS

Several diseases of the hepatic system can result in dermatologic conditions or manifestations. Porphyria cutanea tarda (PCT) is associated with viral hepatitis C. Lichen planus, a pruritic rash, can be associated with hepatitis C, chronic hepatitis, and primary biliary cirrhosis. Some patients in the early phase of hepatitis B can suffer from a serum sickness-like illness. Polyarteritis nodosum, a vasculitis, may also be associated with chronic hepatitis B. Cirrhosis of the liver may also have cutaneous manifestations.

PORPHYRIA

Porphyria refers to a group of diseases caused by enzymatic defects in the heme biosynthetic pathway (Balwani & Desnick, 2012). Porphyrias may be classified by the primary site of enzymatic defect or clinically as acute and nonacute types (Fig. 12.1-11). Of the nonacute types, PCT is the most common and will be the focus of this section.

Porphyria Cutanea Tarda

PCT is the most common and most readily treated type of porphyria (Balwani & Desnick, 2012).

It is estimated that PCT rates are one case per 10 to 25,000 individuals. Both genders and all races are affected. The majority of PCT is acquired (80%) with a few familial cases (20%). The onset of PCT is usually in the third or fourth decade. In contrast, other nonacute porphyrias begin during infancy or early childhood. It is associated with individuals who have hepatic iron overload and liver disease. There is a strong association between PCT and HCV and with mutations of the hemochromatosis gene (Garcovich et al., 2015).

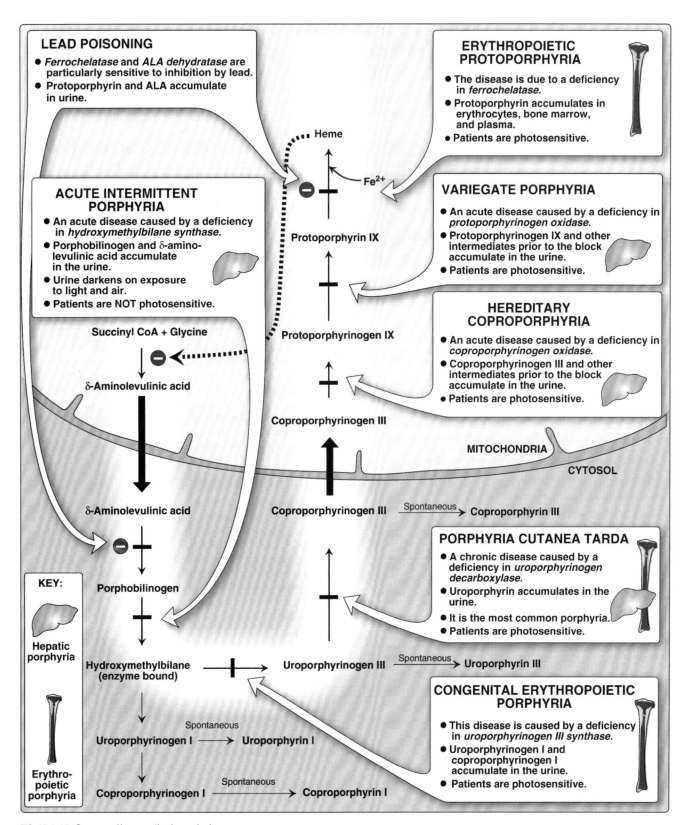

LEAD POISONING
- *Ferrochelatase* and *ALA dehydratase* are particularly sensitive to inhibition by lead.
- Protoporphyrin and ALA accumulate in urine.

ERYTHROPOIETIC PROTOPORPHYRIA
- The disease is due to a deficiency in *ferrochelatase*.
- Protoporphyrin accumulates in erythrocytes, bone marrow, and plasma.
- Patients are photosensitive.

ACUTE INTERMITTENT PORPHYRIA
- An acute disease caused by a deficiency in *hydroxymethylbilane synthase*.
- Porphobilinogen and δ-aminolevulinic acid accumulate in the urine.
- Urine darkens on exposure to light and air.
- Patients are NOT photosensitive.

VARIEGATE PORPHYRIA
- An acute disease caused by a deficiency in *protoporphyrinogen oxidase*.
- Protoporphyrinogen IX and other intermediates prior to the block accumulate in the urine.
- Patients are photosensitive.

HEREDITARY COPROPORPHYRIA
- An acute disease caused by a deficiency in *coproporphyrinogen oxidase*.
- Coproporphyrinogen III and other intermediates prior to the block accumulate in the urine.
- Patients are photosensitive.

PORPHYRIA CUTANEA TARDA
- A chronic disease caused by a deficiency in *uroporphyrinogen decarboxylase*.
- Uroporphyrin accumulates in the urine.
- It is the most common porphyria.
- Patients are photosensitive.

CONGENITAL ERYTHROPOIETIC PORPHYRIA
- This disease is caused by a deficiency in *uroporphyrinogen III synthase*.
- Uroporphyrinogen I and coproporphyrinogen I accumulate in the urine.
- Patients are photosensitive.

Heme

Fe^{2+}

Protoporphyrin IX

Protoporphyrinogen IX

Succinyl CoA + Glycine

δ-Aminolevulinic acid

Coproporphyrinogen III

MITOCHONDRIA

CYTOSOL

δ-Aminolevulinic acid

Coproporphyrinogen III → Spontaneous → Coproporphyrin III

KEY:

Hepatic porphyria

Porphobilinogen

Hydroxymethylbilane (enzyme bound)

Uroporphyrinogen III → Spontaneous → Uroporphyrin III

Erythropoietic porphyria

Uroporphyrinogen I → Spontaneous → Uroporphyrin I

Coproporphyrinogen I → Spontaneous → Coproporphyrin I

FIG. 12.1-11. Summary. Heme synthesis porphyria.

BOX 12.1-1	Porphyria Cutanea Tarda Skin Signs and Common Triggers	

Clinical Signs	Common Triggers
Photosensitivity(most common)	Ultraviolet light
Primarily affects the neck, preauricular area, chest, and back	Exogenous estrogen (OCP)
Vesicles, bulla, erosions (sun-exposed areas)	Alcohol
Mila, atrophic scarring	HCV
Hyper/Hypopigmentation	HIV
Skin fragility	Iron supplements
Facial hypertrichosis temples, lateral cheeks	Multiple blood transfusions
Red to violaceous coloration face, neck, upper chest	
Indurated and waxy plaques	

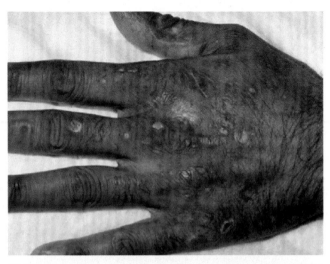

FIG. 12.1-13. Healing lesions of PCT with milia, scars, and abnormal pigmentation.

Pathophysiology

- In PCT, the activity of the heme synthetic enzyme uroporphyrinogen decarboxylase is deficient, thus leading to increased uroporphyrin.

- UVR triggers the photoactivation of porphyrins, which causes oxidative damage to biomolecular targets and activation of the complement system. The result is the release (or activation) of dermal mast cells, leading to skin fragility, vesicles, and bullae.

- The development of PCT can be influenced by both genetic and environmental factors (see Box 12.1-1).

Clinical Presentation

Skin Findings

- Features present on sun-exposed areas include: vesicles, bullae, erosions, burning, and edema (Fig. 12.1-12).

- The dorsum of the hands is a common site and may reveal scars, milia, and hyper- or hypopigmentation from previous lesions (Fig. 12.1-13).

- Increased skin fragility and scleroderma-like plaques (indurated and waxy) may be present on the neck, preauricular area, chest, and back.

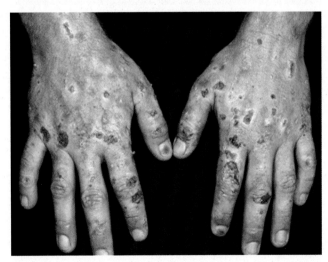

FIG. 12.1-12. Erosions, vesicles, and skin fragility on the dorsum of a hand suggest the need to test for PCT.

- Patients may report similar changes on their face and scalp in addition to violaceous coloration of the periorbital and malar areas.

- Facial hypertrichosis is a hallmark characteristic that occurs on the zygoma and malar prominences. This can be cosmetically distressing in females and may be the impetus for their visit to a PCP or dermatologist. Males may complain about an increased growth in beard. It has been suggested that the hypertrichosis of PCT led to the myth of werewolves.

DIFFERENTIAL DIAGNOSIS   Porphyria Cutanea Tarda

- Epidermolysis bullosa (children)
- Epidermolysis bullosa acquisita (adults)
- Erythropoietic porphyria
- Pemphigus vulgaris
- Hydroa vacciniforme
- Bullous lupus erythematosus
- Pseudoporphyria

Confirming the Diagnosis

Laboratory

- **Serology**
  - Plasma is obtained for red blood cell porphyrins.
  - Complete blood count to assess for elevated hemoglobin.
  - Serum ferritin levels, which may be elevated in patients with PCT.
  - Chemistry panel with special attention to liver function studies is important to evaluate the patient for liver disease.
  - HCV
  - HIV
- **Urine**
  - A 24-hour urine sample will have elevated levels of uro- and coproporphyrins, which confirms the diagnosis of PCT (Balwani & Desnick, 2012).
  - If PCT is suspected, the clinician can perform a simple screening test and collect a random urine sample in the office. Using the Wood light in a dark room, the urine specimen will fluoresce a bright red-pink (Fig. 12.1-14). However, the absence of fluorescence does not exclude the diagnosis of PCT.

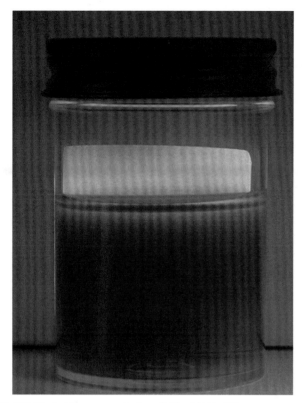

FIG. 12.1-14. Red fluorescence of urine with Wood light in PCT.

- *Stool*
  - Stool samples may only have trace amounts of uroporphyrinogen, coproporphyrinogen, and protoporphyrinogen.
- *Skin biopsy*
  - While not essential for the diagnosis of PCT, a biopsy for histopathology may show:
    - subepidermal blister
    - extension of rigid dermal papillae into subepidermal blister (festooning)
    - Minimal to no inflammatory infiltrate
  - Perilesional biopsy (5 cm away from active eruption) for direct immunofluorescence can help differentiate PCT from an immunobullous disease.

Treatment

The goal of therapy is to identify and avoid triggers such as sun exposure, alcohol, and estrogen therapy. Removal of the offending agents can result in improving symptoms.

Topical

- High-potency topical corticosteroids applied to affected areas may provide some relief.
- Sunscreens with zinc or titanium oxide (physical blockers).

Systemic

- Phlebotomy is the most common treatment used to reduce the iron overload and performed regularly until ferritin levels normalize.

- Low-dose antimalarials, iron chelators, and cholestyramine have been effective (Balwani & Desnick, 2012).
- Equally important, any associated HCV or HIV must be managed.

Management and Patient Education

- Given appropriate treatment, prognosis for PCT is very good.
- Fragility, blistering, and associated pain make performing certain jobs difficult, if not impossible.
- Mila, scarring, and pigment abnormalities are usually permanent.
- Secondary skin infections are common and should be treated appropriately.
- There may be an association between PCT and the development of hepatocellular carcinoma.
- Since PCT is a hepatic form of porphyria, consultation with a gastroenterologist or hepatologist is essential.
- Consultation with a dermatology provider for skin evaluation and biopsy may be considered.
- Phlebotomy and iron chelation therapies may best be managed by a referral to a hematologist.
- Females with PCT should be evaluated and counseled regarding birth control methods other than estrogen containing therapies.
- Patients with PCT, who have alcohol dependency, should be referred to counseling and support for avoidance.
- Patients should be educated on the importance of following the prescribed treatment plan and follow-up.
- Physical sunscreens like titanium dioxide and zinc oxide, which reflect UVR, are the best type of sunscreens for these patients. However, sun avoidance and UV-protective clothing including gloves, are the most important recommendation to help the patient achieve remission and avoid exacerbations.
- PCT patients must be monitored closely for response to therapy. Hemoglobin, serum ferritin, and serum or plasma porphyrin levels must be monitored at least quarterly. Regular health maintenance and monitoring for complications including hepatic tumors should be emphasized.

CLINICAL PEARL

- Referral to the proper provider for help with alcoholism is necessary but may not be welcomed by the patient. Developing a trusting relationship with the patient is important.

Pseudoporphyria

- Pseudoporphyria is a bullous photosensitivity disorder that mimics PCT both clinically and histologically, but without porphyrin abnormalities in blood, urine, or stool. Many think that it is not uncommon and is underreported in the literature. Pseudoporphyria affects males and females equally. No specific race is impacted. It has a higher incidence in children (fair-skinned) compared to adults, and women more than men. Reported cases have ranged from 2 to 81 years of age.

Pathophysiology

- It is attributed often to medications but not fully understood. Naproxen is the most frequent offending agent in drug-induced

pseudoporphyria. Other causative medications include antibiotics (tetracyclines and quinolones), furosemide, hydrochlorothiazide, amiodarone, dapsone, voriconazole, nabumetone, metformin, oral contraceptives, and oxaprozin.

- UVA radiation from tanning beds or UVA plus psoralen therapy and chronic renal failure with hemodialysis have been implicated.
- It has a higher incidence in children (fair-skinned) compared to adults, and women more than men.

Clinical Presentation

- Similar to PCT, patients with pseudoporphyria develop vesicles or bullae on the hands, arm, face, and less often to the legs/feet.
- Skin fragility, scars, and milia may be present.
- Pseudoporphyria patients do not have hypertrichosis, hyperpigmentation, or sclerodermoid changes—important diagnostic clues distinguishing the condition from PCT.

DIFFERENTIAL DIAGNOSIS   Pseudoporphyria

- Bullous pemphigoid
- Bullous lupus erythematosus
- Epidermolysis bullosa (children)
- Epidermolysis bullosa acquisita (adults)
- Erythropoietic porphyria
- Porphyria cutanea tarda

Confirming the Diagnosis

- True porphyria must be ruled out in patients suspected of having pseudoporphyria.
- Unlike PCT, pseudoporphyria will have normal porphyrin levels in the urine, blood, and stools.
- Biopsy for histopathology will not differentiate pseudoporphyria from PCT.

Management and Patient Education

- Elimination of the offending drug is usually adequate for cure. However, it can take several months for remission and skin lesions to heal.
- If pseudoporphyria was drug induced, it is important for the patient to avoid that drug and all others in the drug classification.
- The patient should be instructed to avoid excessive sun exposure and tanning beds.
- Periodic follow-up is helpful to make sure that the patient is following the recommended plan of avoidance therapy.

LICHEN PLANUS

Lichen planus (LP) is a self-limiting pruritic inflammatory, mucocutaneous condition of unknown etiology. It can occur at any age but two thirds of all cases occur between the ages of 30 and 60 years. LP occurs in 1% of the population. Men and women are equally affected. The association of LP with HCV is controversial as the data has not identified a clear causal relationship. The cutaneous manifestation of LP may be the chief complaint of a patient who is unaware of their HCV infection. Therefore, patients with LP in the United States or from the Mediterranean basin should be evaluated to rule

out underlying HCV. LP has been associated with other immune-mediated conditions including ulcerative colitis, morphea, vitiligo, alopecia areata, lichen sclerosis, dermatomyositis, and myasthenia gravis. See Section 4.5 for additional LP details.

Serum Sickness-Like Reaction (SSLR)

It is estimated that 10% to 30% of patients in the pre-icterus acute phase of hepatitis B virus (HBV) will experience SSLR. The duration of the SSLR often relates to the level of viremia (Akhter & Said, 2015).

Pathophysiology

- The syndrome is believed to be due to circulating immune complexes causing reactions in the skin, joints, muscles, and kidneys. These complexes are composed of hepatitis B surface antigen (HBsAg) with subsequent depletion of normal complement.

Clinical Presentation

Skin Findings

Rashes of varied presentation (Fig. 12.1-15)

- Discrete or diffuse
- Urticaria
- Petechial, nodular, or palpable purpura.
- Erythema multiforme
- Lichenoid dermatitis
- Rash may or may not be tender.

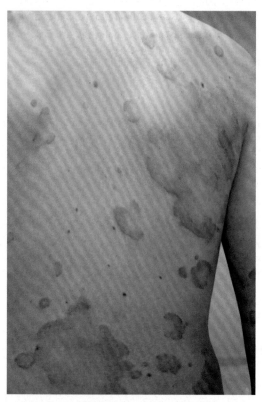

FIG. 12.1-15. Serum sickness. Erythematous urticarial and morbilliform eruption on the upper back. (Used with permission from Gru, A. A., & Wick, M. [2018]. *Pediatric dermatopathology and dermatology.* Wolters Kluwer.)

Non-Skin Findings

- Diffuse polyarthralgias of the spine and neck.
- Glomerulonephritis
- Vasculitis

Confirming the Diagnosis

Laboratory
- HBV DNA
- HBsAg
- HBeAg

Management and Patient Education

- Patients should have appropriate testing done for HBV.
- Those diagnosed with HBV should be referred to the appropriate specialist such as gastroenterology or infectious disease.

POLYARTERITIS NODOSA

- Polyarteritis nodosa (PAN), also referred to as generalized necrotizing vasculitis, is one of the more serious syndromes associated with chronic hepatitis B virus infection.
- It involves the small, medium, and large vessels. It is estimated that 7% to 8% of chronic HBV patients will experience PAN.

Skin Findings

- Cutaneous manifestations include palpable purpura, nodules, and erythematous rashes in 10% to 15% of patients with PAN.
- Painful subcutaneous nodules along the arteries of the lower legs, livedo reticularis, and ulcerations represent the triad of PAN cutaneous manifestations (Akhter & Said, 2015).

CIRRHOSIS

- Cirrhosis is a diffuse hepatic process characterized by fibrosis and conversion of the normal liver architecture into structurally abnormal nodules.
- The progression of liver injury to cirrhosis may occur over weeks to years.

Skin Findings

- Cutaneous manifestations of cirrhosis include vascular alterations/lesions, coagulation defects (petechiae, purpura, delayed clotting time), jaundice and pigmentary changes, and hair and nail changes.
- Pruritus, which is also present, is discussed in Section 5.

Cardiovascular Disease

Several conditions of the cardiovascular system will demonstrate specific cutaneous findings (Table 12.1-2). Clubbing, or the distal curvature of the nails, may be observed with congenital heart disease or endocarditis. The diagonal earlobe crease is considered by some as an independent marker for coronary artery disease (Uliasz & Lebwohl, 2008).

TABLE 12.1-2	Skin Manifestations of Cardiovascular Disease
DISEASE	**SKIN FINDINGS**

Infective endocarditis	• Petechiae
	  • Conjunctival
	  • Palatal
	• Subungual splinter hemorrhages
	• Osler nodules
	  • Painful erythematous nodules
	  • Flesh of fingertips and toes
	• Janeway nodules
	  • Nontender, red or hemorrhagic macules
	  • Palms and soles

Acute rheumatic fever	• Erythema marginatum
	  • Nonpruritic, blanching, erythematous with raised serpiginous margin
	  • Trunk and proximal extremities
	  • Facial sparing
	  • May disappear and reappear within hours
	• Subcutaneous nodules
	  • After first week
	  • Present up to 1 mo
	  • Millimeters to 2-cm size
	  • Small, firm, painless
	  • Tendons, bony surfaces, especially elbows

Lipid disorders	• Xanthomas
	  • Yellow-orange superficial papules, plaques, nodules
	• Xanthelasma
	  • Soft yellow macules or plaques
	  • Eyes, neck, palms, chest
	  • Millimeters to several cm in size
	  • May coalesce
	• Eruptive xanthomas
	  • Sudden onset
	  • Crops of papules or nodules on erythematous base
	  • Buttocks, extensor surfaces of extremities

Cardiac amyloidosis	• Smooth, waxy papules or nodules
	  • Face, chest, periumbilical region, perineum, and intertriginous regions
	• Periorbital purpura
	  • "Pinch purpura"
	  • After emesis, Valsalva maneuver, or proctoscopy

Kawasaki disease (see Section 9.3 for details)	• Nonspecific rash
	  • Diffuse, macular, papular, erythematous
	  • Five days after onset of fever
	  • Scarlatiniform or erythema multiforme-like with target lesions
	  • Perineal region first, followed by extremities
	• Extremities
	  • Edema, hands, and feet
	  • Erythema of palms and soles progressing to sheet-like desquamation
	  • Beau lines 1–2 mo after onset
	  • Traverse linear nail crease

RENAL DISEASE

CALCIPHYLAXIS

Calciphylaxis is a rare syndrome involving vascular calcification, intensely painful lesions, and skin necrosis. It is associated mainly with individuals with chronic renal disease, especially those with end-stage renal disease (ESRD). Sometimes referred to as calcific uremic arteriolopathy. This term is less accurate since there are cases of calciphylaxis with normal kidney function. Majority of patients are Caucasians 50 to 70 years old with a female to male ratio 3:1. Calciphylaxis impacts 1% to 4% of those with ESRD. Higher incidence in those with peritoneal dialysis versus hemodialysis (Nigwekar et al., 2018).

Pathophysiology

- The pathogenesis of calciphylaxis is poorly understood.
- Accumulation of calcium deposits in the tunica media of the walls of small- and medium-sized vessels results in occlusion, endothelial injury, microthrombosis, and ultimately tissue necrosis from infarction.
- It has been suggested that it may be due to a uremic-induced defect, chronic inflammation, or other processes that impact bone metabolism and calcification.

Clinical Presentation

Skin Findings

- Early presentation of calciphylaxis resembles livedo reticularis with the mottled pattern of cyanosis.
- Rapid progression into the subcutaneous tissue, as purple nodules expand into large, stellate, and necrotic ulcers (Fig. 12.1-16).
- May be one or several lesions that are commonly located on the lower legs, thighs, buttocks, and lower abdomen.
- Secondary infections are common.

Non-Skin Findings

- Intense cutaneous pain with no skin changes may be present with sudden onset.
- Excruciating and unremitting pain persists.

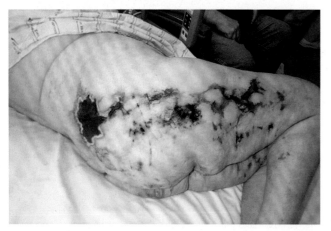

FIG. 12.1-16. Retiform purpura and frank necrosis in a patient with calciphylaxis. (Used with permission from Baranoski, S., & Ayello, E. A. [2020]. *Wound care essentials* [5th ed.]. Wolters Kluwer.)

DIFFERENTIAL DIAGNOSIS   Calciphylaxis

- Brown recluse spider bite
- Bullous pemphigoid
- Cellulitis
- Erythema nodosum
- Hypersensitivity vasculitis (leukocytoclastic vasculitis)
- Lupus erythematosus, bullous
- Necrotizing fasciitis
- Pyoderma gangrenosum
- Venous ulcer
- Vibrio vulnificus infection
- Wegener granulomatosis

Confirming the Diagnosis

- Patients suspected of having calciphylaxis should be referred to dermatology immediately for proper diagnosis.
- Biopsy with a deep excisional specimen is required to ensure that subcutaneous tissue is submitted for histologic analysis and accurate diagnosis.
- Need to weigh benefit versus risk of causing new, nonhealing ulcer or infection.
- If the patient has a history of ESRD and has the traditional clinical presentation, a biopsy can be deferred.
- If early, atypical presentation in patient without ESRD may justify biopsy.
- Contraindicated for acral and penile lesions or if infection suspected.
  - Double-punch method may be utilized
  - Patients should be screened for diabetes and hypercoagulability conditions. Serum calcium, phosphorus, parathyroid hormone, aluminum, urea nitrogen, creatinine, and albumin are critical.
- Imaging may be ordered to identify calcium deposits.

Treatment

- A treatment plan for the calciphylaxis patient should begin with ongoing assessment and treatment of renal failure by nephrology.
- Correction of hypercalcemia and hyperphosphatemia is important.
- Hemodialysis may require increased length and frequency.

Management and Patient Education

- Calciphylaxis, especially when it has progressed to ulcerations, has a high mortality rate of 60% to 80% (Nigwekar et al., 2018).
- The most common cause of death is secondary sepsis (Cordova et al., 2009).
- Patients presenting with lesions suspicious for calciphylaxis are typically diagnosed and managed by dermatology or wound care specialist in consultation with a PCP and nephrologist.
- Patients with calciphylaxis should be referred to wound care or surgical specialists for wound management and consideration of debridement.
- Patients should be referred to pain management as calciphylaxis is often associated with severe pain that is difficult to manage.

Counseling can be important in helping patients and their families deal with this physically and psychologically devastating disease.

PULMONARY DISEASE

Sarcoidosis

Sarcoidosis is a chronic inflammatory disease that can impact multiple organs of the body. The skin, lungs, and intrathoracic lymph nodes are the primary locations. Approximately 25% to 30% of cases will experience skin involvement (Yanardag et al., 2013). The Male to female ratio is 1:2 and the peak age is 24 to 35 years with a second peak for women at 45 to 65 years. The incidence of sarcoidosis is 34 per 100,000 for African Americans and 11 per 100,000 for Caucasians (Wanat & Rosenbach, 2014).

Pathophysiology

- Sarcoidosis is characterized by noncaseating epithelioid granulomas on biopsy.
- The exact etiology for sarcoidosis is unknown and probably multifactorial, with numerous genetic, immunologic, and environmental interactions.
- T cells likely cause an overactive cellular immune response to a trigger (Yanardag et al., 2013).

Clinical Presentation

Skin Findings

- Violaceous to erythematous to brown papules, macules, and plaques frequently appearing on head, face, and neck (Fig. 12.1-17).

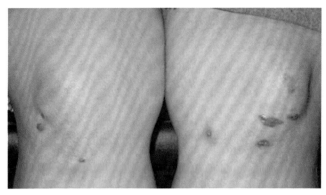

FIG. 12.1-18. Persistent nodules on the legs of a patient with systemic sarcoidosis. (Photo courtesy of M. Bobonich.)

- Subcutaneous nodules present in the Darier–Roussy type of sarcoidosis (Fig. 12.1-18).
- Violaceous nodules and plaques over the nose, cheeks, and ears (lupus pernio) are common locations (Fig. 12.1-19).
- Lesions can occur as infiltration or thickening of old scars which is highly suggestive of sarcoidosis.

Associated Skin Findings

- Erythema nodosum
- Erythema multiforme
- Calcinosis cutis
- Pruritus

Non-Skin Findings

- Weight loss
- Loss of appetite
- Fatigue
- Fever
- Chills and night sweats.
- Cough

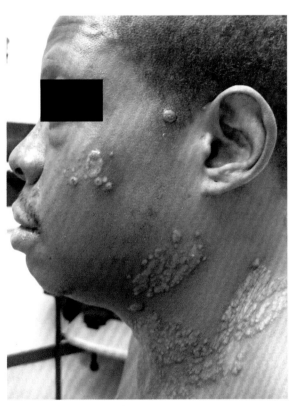

FIG. 12.1-17. Reddish-brown plaques and nodules of cutaneous sarcoidosis frequently occur on the head, face, and neck. (Photo courtesy of M. Bobonich.)

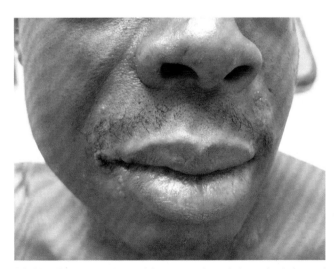

FIG. 12.1-19. Lupus pernio are violaceous papules and plaques located around the nose, mouth, and cheeks. They are associated with systemic sarcoidosis and a higher prevalence of lung and respiratory tract involvement. (Photo courtesy of M. Bobonich.)

DIFFERENTIAL DIAGNOSIS   Sarcoidosis

- Granuloma annulare
- Necrobiosis lipoidica
- Rheumatoid nodules
- Erythema nodosum
- Xanthogranulomas
- Granulomatous vasculitis
- Cutaneous tuberculosis
- Leprosy
- Drug eruptions
- Granuloma faciale
- Lamellar ichthyosis
- Lichen planus
- Discoid lupus erythematosus
- Subacute cutaneous lupus erythematosus
- Lymphocytoma cutis
- Plaque psoriasis
- Syphilis
- Tinea corporis

Confirming the Diagnosis

- Some lesions have a distinctive yellow-brown color that looks like "apple jelly" on diascopy. Diascopy refers to the practice of applying pressure to a lesion with a clear microscope slide which will reveal the unique "apple jelly sign." This is considered a diagnostic clue for granulomatous disease, especially sarcoidosis (Fig. 12.1-20).
- Skin biopsy can confirm cutaneous sarcoidosis.
- Tissue culture can rule out fungal or atypical mycobacterial infection.
- Evaluation of other organ involvement can determine the extent of the disease.
  - Chest x-ray
  - Liver and kidney function tests
  - Angiotensin-converting enzyme
  - Pulmonary function testing

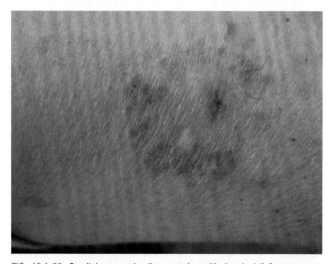

FIG. 12.1-20. Small brown-red-yellow papules with "apple jelly" appearance characteristic of cutaneous sarcoidosis. This patient does not have systemic involvement. (Photo courtesy of M. Bobonich.)

- TB screening
- Ophthalmology screening
- ECG

Treatment

Topical

- Watchful waiting may be the best approach for possible spontaneous resolution for the majority of mild cutaneous cases. For plaques that are symptomatic:
  - TCS with strength dependent on location.
  - Topical tacrolimus ointment 0.1% b.i.d.
  - Topical retinoids 0.025% at bedtime in cases with scaling and dyspigmentation (Wanat & Rosenbach, 2014).
  - Intralesional corticosteroids, triamcinolone acetonide with strength based on body location.

Systemic

- Cutaneous sarcoidosis which affects the cosmetic areas or the ulcerative type should be referred to dermatology for systemic therapy with the following agents:
  - Antimalarials (chloroquine, hydroxychloroquine)
  - Minocycline 100 mg b.i.d. or Doxycycline 100 mg b.i.d.
  - Numerous immunosuppressant drugs have been used and include methotrexate, oral/systemic steroids, azathioprine, mycophenolate mofetil, TNF inhibitors, isotretinoin, thalidomide, or pentoxifylline.

Management and Patient Education

- PCPs may want to refer patients with cutaneous sarcoidosis to dermatology for confirmation of the diagnosis.
- Many of the systemic treatment options have potential adverse effects and should only be administered by a clinician with experience with the treatment.
- Patients with pulmonary symptoms should be referred to pulmonary for management. Patients with other organ involvement should be referred to the proper specialty.
- Duration of the disease may vary from a shorter self-limited course to a chronic long-term disease. Therefore, follow-up monitoring should occur frequently and long term.
- Facial lesions in sarcoidosis can be very troubling for patients and can impact their daily and social life.

ERYTHEMA NODOSUM

Erythema nodosum (EN) is an inflammation of the subcutaneous fat known as panniculitis, and EN is the most common form. The majority of EN is idiopathic in nature and occurs in approximately 1 to 5 per 100,000 individuals. Children and older adults may experience EN, but the peak age is in young adults 18 to 34 years. Women experience EN more than men at a 4:1 ratio (Chowaniec et al., 2016). EN frequently occurs in association with granulomatous disease, including sarcoidosis (discussed previously), tuberculosis, and granulomatous colitis.

Pathophysiology

- Experts believe that EN probably is a delayed hypersensitivity reaction to a wide variety of antigens and disorders that manifests in the subcutaneous fat (Table 12.1-3).

TABLE 12.1-3	Causes of Erythema Nodosum	
COMMON		
Infections (28–48%)	Streptococcus (URI) Other: Yersinia Mycoplasma Chlamydia Histoplasmosis Coccidioidomycosis Mycobacteria	
Sarcoidosis (11–25%)	Lofgren syndrome	
Drugs (3–10%)	Sulfonamides Penicillin Oral contraceptives	
Pregnancy (2–5%)	1st trimester	
Enteropathy (1–4%)	Crohn disease Chronic ulcerative colitis	
Idiopathic (≤55%)	Unknown	
UNCOMMON (<1%)		
Viral infections	Herpes simplex virus, Epstein–Barr virus Hepatitis B virus Hepatitis C virus Human immunodeficiency virus	
Bacterial infections	Campylobacter Rickettsia Salmonella Bartonella Syphilis	
Parasitic infections	Amoebiasis Giardiasis	
Paraneoplastic	Lymphoma Leukemia	

Adapted from Schwartz, R. A., & Nervi, S. J., (2007). Erythema nodosum: A sign of systemic disease. *American Family Physician, 75*(5), 695–700; Chowaniec, M., Starba, A., & Wiland, P. (2016). Erythema nodosum—review of the literature. *Reumatologia, 54*(2), 79–82.

- Subcutaneous fat is a homogeneous tissue that responds to insult in a limited number of ways, and thus histologically, there is an overlap of different forms of panniculitis. EN is considered the prototypic septal panniculitis; the biopsy specimens show inflammatory infiltrate involving the connective tissue septa between fat lobules.

- It has been proposed that EN is a circulating immune complex–mediated process. The potential pathogenic role of circulating immune complexes is not clear since they are not found in idiopathic and uncomplicated cases.

Clinical Presentation

Skin Findings

- Erythematous subcutaneous nodules symmetrically involving the pretibial aspect of the lower legs.

- Tender to touch.

- Initial lesions are 2 to 6 cm, with poorly defined borders (Fig. 12.1-21).

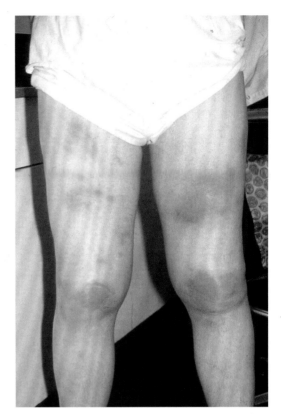

FIG. 12.1-21. Initially, EN can present as tender, bruise-like nodules on the legs. (Used with permission from Hall, J. C., & Hall, B. J. [2017]. *Sauer's manual of skin diseases* [11th ed.]. Wolters Kluwer.)

- Over 1 to 2 weeks, lesions progress from being tense, hard, and painful to fluctuant. Color evolves to bluish or dark bluish gray. Eventually, color resembles that of a bruise (Fig. 12.1-22).

- EN does not become suppurative and uncommonly ulcerates.

- New lesions may continue for up to 6 weeks.

Non-Skin Findings

- Lesions are usually preceded by acute onset of fever, generalized aching, and arthralgias.

- Leg discomfort and swelling may persist.

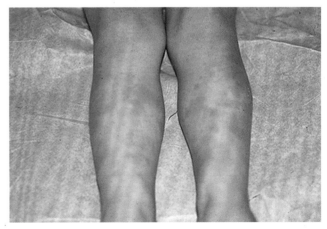

FIG. 12.1-22. Bilateral and tender nodules of EN on the pretibial aspects of lower legs. (Photo courtesy of George A. Datto III.)

Confirming the Diagnosis

- Diagnosis is usually made clinically.

Laboratory

- Throat culture to exclude group A streptococcus.
- Erythrocyte sedimentation rate or C reactive protein.
- Antistreptolysin titer (ASLO) to determine previous Streptococcal infection.
- Stool culture, based on GI complaints.
- TB screening if suspected.

Biopsy

- If unable to confirm, referral to dermatology for biopsy for histopathology is suggested.
    - A punch biopsy may not be adequate. May require a deep incisional skin biopsy since subcutaneous tissue must be included (Gupta et al., 2016).
    - Tissue culture and PCR can be done to rule out infectious panniculitis.

Imaging

- Chest x-ray to exclude sarcoidosis and TB and to confirm or disprove hilar adenopathy.

Treatment

Topical

- EN is a self-limited disease in most cases and requires only symptomatic supportive care.
- Elevation of the legs and bed rest in the acute phase.
- Cool wet compresses.

Systemic

- Nonsteroidal anti-inflammatory drugs (NSAIDs) such as aspirin, naproxen, indomethacin, and colchicine.
- Systemic steroids if needed and contraindications have been ruled out.
- Oral potassium iodide prepared as a supersaturated solution in a dosage of 400 to 900 mg daily for 1 month. Long term use may lead to thyroid dysfunction.

Management and Patient Education

- Reassure the patient that EN is usually benign and prognosis is good.
- Resuming activities too soon is discouraged since it may lead to return of symptoms.

- Usually resolves in 3 to 6 weeks.
- EN is usually cared for by PCPs. Identification of the cause is important to prevent relapses and prolongation of what is usually a short-term condition.
- Infections must be diagnosed and treated appropriately.
- Offending drugs must be identified and eliminated.
- Identification and management of the underlying cause may require consultation with dermatology and/or internal medicine.

COVID-19

Coronavirus 2019 (COVID-19) is a highly contagious new novel coronavirus that can result in asymptomatic disease to mild disease to severe acute respiratory syndrome. The new COVID-19 virus resulted in a global pandemic involving 188 countries and millions of people worldwide. COVID-19 is a single-stranded RNA virus that infects host cells via the angiotensin-converting enzyme 2 receptor (ACE2R). Following viral infiltration of ACE2R rich cells, tissue damage is proposed to occur as a result of viral mediated cell damage, alteration in renin angiotensin aldosterone system, dysregulated immune response, and endothelial damage/thrombo-inflammation. While there is a high concentration of ACE2R in the pulmonary system, other organ systems (i.e., skin, gastrointestinal, cardiovascular) are also rich in ACE2R and may experience tissue damage that accounts for the numerous extrapulmonary symptoms reported.

Clinical Presentation

Skin Findings

- Erythematous to violaceous papules or plaques in an acral (fingers, toes) distribution (pernio-like skin eruption) that develops in the absence of cold exposure (Fig. 12.1-23).

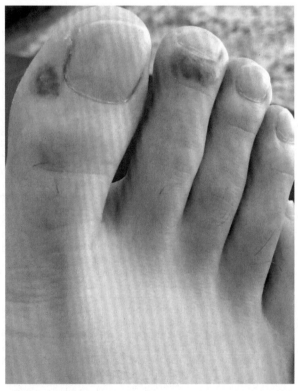

FIG. 12.1-23. Pseudo-chilblains. Erythematous to violaceous papules or plaques involving the toes.

TABLE 12.1-4 Paraneoplastic Conditions

DISEASE	BACKGROUND	CLINICAL PRESENTATION	DIAGNOSTICS	MANAGEMENT
Carcinoid syndrome	Neuroendocrine tumors that secrete biologic compounds (e.g., serotonin, histamine) and are often found in the small intestine, respiratory, or colorectal areas.	Episodes of flushing without sweating (face, neck, chest). May be associated with dyspnea, diarrhea, palpitations, tachycardia, or fatigue.	24 hour urinary 5-HIAA Plasma chromogranin A levels CT scan of abdomen and pelvis	Refer medical/surgical oncology. Flushing may be triggered by **food** (eggs, avocado, banana, coffee), **medications** (opioids, anesthesia, catecholamines), **alcohol**, **stress**, and **exercise**. Carcinoid crisis medic alert bracelet.
Erythroderma (see Section 4.5)	Extensive erythema and scaling **involving 90% of the body surface** that may be associated with the following malignancies: solid tumors, mycosis fungoides, or Sézary syndrome.	Erythema and scaling, progressing into a dull scarlet color with extensive exfoliation of the skin. Palmar–plantar keratoderma Severe pruritus Fatigue or shivering	Punch biopsy for histopathology CBC with diff. CMP +/– skin/blood cultures	May require emergency management if associated hypothermia, hypotension, or electrolyte imbalances. Immediate referral to dermatology for subacute patients. Erythrodermic patients are high risk for secondary skin infections.
Paraneoplastic pemphigus (see Section 9.2)	Vesiculobullous condition associated with non-Hodgkin lymphoma, chronic lymphocytic leukemia, thymoma, Castleman disease, and Waldenström macroglobulinemia.	Painful erosive ulcerative stomatitis Polymorphic cutaneous eruption including erythema, papules, bullae, or erosions Dyspnea Melena, hematochezia, or hematemesis due to gastrointestinal bleeding.	Punch biopsy for histopathology and DIF IIF ELISA desmoglein 1 and 3 CBC with diff. S-PEP Chest x-ray CT scan chest, abdomen, and pelvis	Refer to dermatology. 90% mortality rate due to gastrointestinal bleeding, sepsis, or bronchiolitis obliterans. Patients should be evaluated for lung involvement (e.g., bronchiolitis obliterans).
Sign of Leser–Trélat (Fig. 12.1-24)	Sudden appearance of numerous seborrheic keratoses may be associated with the following malignancies: gastric, colorectal, breast, lung, or lymphoma.	Skin colored, tan, brown, or black "warty" stuck on appearing scaly papule or plaque.	Seborrheic keratoses are a clinical diagnosis.	Patients should be up to date on their age appropriate screenings.
Dermatomyositis (see Section 9.2)	Autoimmune connective tissue disease that can be associated with the following malignancies: ovarian, cervical lung, prostate, pancreatic, gastric carcinomas, or non-Hodgkin lymphoma.	Periorbital erythematous to violaceous patch +/– scale (heliotrope). Erythematous to violaceous papules on dorsal hand bony prominences (Gottron papules). Scaly erythematous patches or plaques, especially over the back/shoulders (Shawl sign) Proximal nailfold dilated capillaries. Weakness in distal extremities.	Punch biopsy for histopathology ANA panel Aldolase CPK LDH ESR or CRP CMP Referral for EMG or muscle biopsy	Refer to dermatology and rheumatology for further evaluation and management.
Sister Mary Joseph nodule (Fig. 12.1-25)	Localization of metastatic tumors to the umbilicus that may be associated with the following malignancies: stomach, colon, ovaries, or pancreas.	Scaly erythematous patches or plaques, especially over the back/shoulders (Shawl sign).	Punch biopsy for histopathology.	Usually the primary malignancy has been diagnosed prior to the presentation of the nodule.
Vasculitis (see Section 9.3)	Hypersensitivity reaction characterized by inflammation of small, medium, or large blood vessels and can be associated with solid tumor malignancies, lymphoma, and leukemia.	Petechiae, palpable purpura, subcutaneous nodules, and ulcerations. Large variation of systemic symptoms based upon vessels affected.	Punch biopsy for histopathology CBC with diff. CMP Urinalysis ESR or CRP	Refer to dermatology or rheumatology for further evaluation.

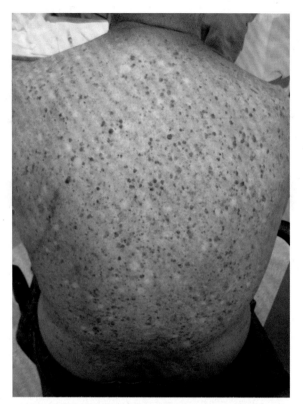

FIG. 12.1-24. Sign of Leser–Trélat, or sudden onset of numerous seborrheic keratoses, may be associated with an underlying malignancy. (Photo courtesy of M. Bobonich.)

- Erythematous maculopapular skin eruption (morbilliform).
- Monomorphic and polymorphic vesicular skin eruption that can be localized or diffuse.
- Erythematous edematous papules or plaques (urticaria).
- Erythematous to violaceous reticulated patches or plaques (livedo reticularis/retiform purpura).
- Erythematous targetoid papules and plaques (erythema multiforme-like eruptions).
- Petechial rash.
- Erythematous scaly papules and plaques (papulosquamous).
- Skin eruptions may be asymptomatic or associated with itch, burning, or pain.

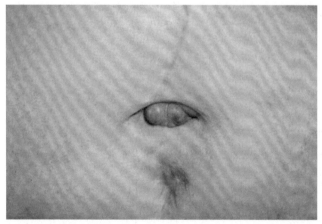

FIG. 12.1-25. Sister Mary Joseph nodule.

Non-Skin Findings

- Constitutional findings include fever.
- Pulmonary findings include dyspnea, cough, sputum production, interstitial pneumonia, and respiratory failure.
- Neurologic findings include stroke, headache, anosmia, ageusia, myalgias, dizziness, and encephalopathy.
- Renal findings include hematuria, proteinuria, and acute kidney injury.
- Hepatic findings include elevated liver transaminases.
- Gastrointestinal findings including abdominal pain, anorexia, diarrhea, nausea, vomiting, and abdominal pain.
- Cardiovascular findings include arrhythmias, cardiomyopathy, cardiogenic shock, cor pulmonale, and myocardial infarction.
- Endocrine findings include hyperglycemia and diabetic ketoacidosis.

Confirming the Diagnosis

- The majority of skin eruptions develop following after the onset of COVID-19 symptoms, but have been reported to develop at the onset of symptoms. Uncommonly, skin eruptions may be noted prior to onset of COVID-19 symptoms.
- The skin eruptions were reported to resolve anywhere from days to up to 4 weeks.
- Acral (pernio-like skin eruptions) are primarily seen in younger patients with milder symptoms and often have a longer duration of up to 4 weeks. Interestingly, patients with acral lesions are predominantly COVID-19 laboratory negative (Daneshgaran et al., 2020; Freeman et al., 2020).
- Patients with purpura, livedo reticularis, or retiform purpura lesions often develop at onset of COVID-19 symptoms and are seen more often in older adults with more severe disease.

Treatment

- There are no evidence-based guidelines for the treatment of COVID-19 skin eruptions at the time of this publication. As the skin eruptions are self-resolving following resolution of viral infection, the treatment focus is supportive only.

Management and Patient Education

- Management of patients with COVID-19 depends upon disease severity. The majority of cases will resolve with only supportive care. However, patients with severe disease may require management in a tertiary care setting (i.e., hospital).
- Patients at risk of severe illness include older adults or those of any age with the following comorbidities: cardiac disease, chronic obstructive pulmonary disease, chronic kidney disease, diabetes, obesity, immunodeficiency, or those receiving immunosuppressive therapy (e.g., solid organ transplant).

Paraneoplastic Conditions

Involvement of the skin by visceral tumors may be either direct or indirect. There are a multitude of syndromes, tumors, and dermatoses that are manifestations of internal malignancy. There are some characteristic cutaneous signs of specific internal malignancies that should be a "red flag" to clinicians (Table 12.1-4). These associations are not always based on evidence but are empiric. A keen awareness of these associations may aid the clinician in earlier recognition and a diagnosis that may improve the patient outcomes or prognosis.

Pregnancy and the Skin

Melissa Davis

In This Chapter

- Physiologic Changes of Pregnancy
- Polymorphic Eruption of Pregnancy
- Atopic Eruption of Pregnancy

- Pemphigoid Gestationis
- Intrahepatic Cholestasis of Pregnancy

Many skin changes can present during pregnancy and the postpartum period. Some of these changes are physiologic, and others are pregnancy-related dermatoses. A few physiologic changes you might see in pregnancy include darkening of melanocytic lesions, linea nigra, striae gravidarum, and melisma (Table 12.2-1). There are four major pregnancy-related dermatoses: polymorphic eruption of pregnancy (PEP), atopic eruption of pregnancy (AEP), pemphigoid gestationis (PG), and intrahepatic cholestasis of pregnancy (IHCP).

Recognizing these conditions, knowing how to treat them within limitations of pregnancy (Table 12.2-2), and when to refer, are vital for the care of your pregnant patient.

Polymorphic Eruption of Pregnancy

PEP, also called pruritic urticarial papules and plaques of pregnancy (PUPPP), is a very common dermatosis affecting pregnant women.

TABLE 12.2-1	Physiologic Changes of Pregnancy		
CONDITION	CLINICAL CHARACTERISTICS	TREATMENT/MANAGEMENT	PATIENT EDUCATION
Melasma ("Mask of Pregnancy") See Section 10.2	Hyperpigmented tan/brown macules and patches. Most common on cheeks, forehead, and upper lip. Occurs in approximately 75% of pregnancies.	Sunscreen during pregnancy	Sun avoidance and/or sun protection are very important to prevent or minimize melasma. Often pregnancy induced melasma resolves within 1 yr postpartum.
Linea nigra	Hyperpigmented line down midline of abdomen. Most common pigmentary change in pregnancy.	None	Darkening typically resolves after pregnancy but can take up to 1 yr.
Pigmented nevi	Patient's current nevi may darken with pregnancy. Patients may also develop new nevi in pregnancy.	Lesions that are suspicious should be biopsied regardless of pregnancy. There should not be a delay in biopsy.	Patients should do monthly skin checks and bring any changing lesions to the attention of their dermatology provider.
Striae gravidarum	Pink/Violaceous atrophic lines, most common on the abdomen, breasts, and thighs that occur in the third trimester.	No proven treatment or prevention and many treatments postpartum are not effective.	Excessive weight gain can lead to striae gravidarum. Genetics often play a role.
Pyogenic granuloma	Violaceous friable papules on face, neck, hands, or oral mucosa.	New suspicious lesions or symptomatic (bleeding) lesions should be biopsied/treated by a dermatology provider.	Many lesions that are benign may regress postpartum. Any questionable lesion should be biopsied.
Postpartum hair loss	Sudden shedding of hair in the 3–6 mo postpartum period.	No treatment. Reassurance that 12–15 mo postpartum it usually resolves. There may be a small amount of' loss that is permanent.	Scalp hair stays in the anagen "growing" phase longer during pregnancy which results in thicker hair. During the postpartum period, many hairs convert to the telogen phase, resulting in a sudden hair loss or telogen effluvium. Reassure patients that this is common.

TABLE 12.2-2	Preferred Therapeutics During Pregnancy
CLASS	**MEDICATIONS**
Analgesics	Acetaminophen
Anesthetics	Lidocaine
Antibacterial	Penicillins, erythromycin
Antifungal	Itraconazole[a], clotrimazole[b], miconazole[b], nystatin[b]
Antiviral	Acyclovir
Antiscabietic/ Antipediculocide	Permethrin
Antihistamines	Chlorpheniramine, cetirizine[a], loratadine[a]
Topical corticosteroids	Class IV–VII topical corticosteroids
Oral corticosteroids	Prednisone[c], prednisolone[c], methylprednisolone[c]
Acne	Azelaic acid, clindamycin, erythromycin

Adapted from Lee, K. B., & Greiling, T. M. (2021). Dermatologic drugs during pregnancy and lactation. In *Comprehensive dermatologic drug therapy* (4th ed., pp. 710–724.e4). Elsevier.
[a]Avoid use during the first trimester.
[b]Avoid use after membrane rupture.
[c]Avoid high doses during first trimester.

It is seen most frequently in primigravidas, and usually begins in the third trimester or very early in the postpartum period. The incidence is estimated to be 1 in 160 pregnancies (Ambros-Rudolph, 2011).

Pathophysiology

- Pathogenesis is unknown. The correlation with the distension of the abdomen and the onset of the symptoms in the striae suggests that it is related to connective tissue damage and subsequent inflammation. Other theories that have not been proven to be the cause are birth weight of the baby, fetal sex, or maternal hormone changes.
- PEP may be associated with rapid and excessive weight gain, multiple gestations, labor induction, and hypertensive disorders.
- With PEP, there is no concern for fetal involvement or risk.

Clinical Presentation

- PEP usually begins within the striae on the abdomen (Fig. 12.2-1A). The lesions present with pink or red papules, surrounded by a narrow pale halo that will coalesce to large urticaria-like plaques.
- The eruption may be broadly erythematous with discrete papules; papulovesicles may develop, but blisters are not seen (Fig. 12.2-1B).
- The distribution includes the abdomen, upper thighs, umbilicus, face, and palms.
- The periumbilical area and soles are usually spared.

DIFFERENTIAL DIAGNOSIS	Polymorphic Eruption of Pregnancy

- Contact dermatitis
- Drug eruption
- Urticaria
- Viral exanthem
- Urticarial pemphigoid gestationis
- Erythema multiforme

Confirming the Diagnosis

- Diagnosis is made on clinical presentation; however, a biopsy may be indicated if there is suspicion for PG.
- Evaluation by dermatology is recommended if unsure of diagnosis.

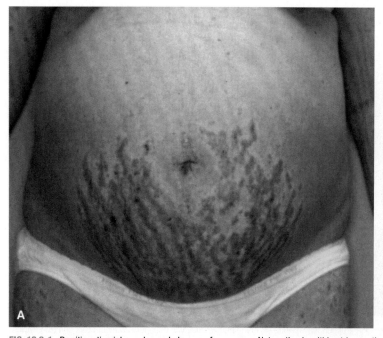

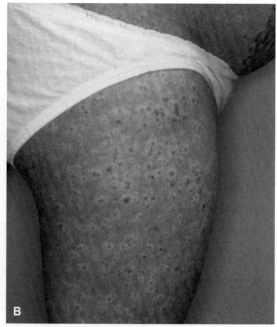

FIG. 12.2-1. Pruritic urticarial papules and plaques of pregnancy. Note urticaria within striae on the abdomen (**A**) and on the thighs (**B**). (Photo courtesy of Callen, J. P.)

Treatment

- Treatment is mainly supportive with cool baths or compresses for relief of pruritus.
- For relief of pruritus, utilize class III-V topical corticosteroids, antipruritic topical lotions with menthol, or second-generation antihistamines as needed.

Management and Patient Education

- This condition is self-limiting.
- Closer follow-up and dermatology referral are warranted if symptoms worsen or aren't able to be controlled with initial therapy.
- If systemic steroids are needed to control symptoms, co-management with patient's OB/GYN would be suggested. The typical duration is 4 to 6 weeks. Provide patient reassurance that lesions typically clear within 1 week of delivery.

> **CLINICAL PEARLS**
>
> ■ PEP typically does not recur with subsequent pregnancies.
> ■ PEP onset occurs during the third trimester or immediately postpartum.
> ■ No cutaneous involvement in the fetus/newborn.

ATOPIC ERUPTION OF PREGNANCY

AEP is the most common dermatosis of pregnancy, and encompasses 50% of all pregnancy-related dermatoses. The occurrence is approximately 1:5 to 1:20 pregnancies (Sävervall, 2015). Patients who develop AEP often have a history of atopy. However, that history isn't necessary for the diagnosis as it is thought that up to 80% of patients with AEP have no history of atopic dermatitis (Ambros-Rudolph, 2011). AEP often recurs in subsequent pregnancies.

Pathophysiology

Pathophysiology is proposed to be a pregnancy-related reduction in Th1 cytokines and an increase in Th2 cytokines, which mediate itch (Ambros-Rudolph, 2011).

Clinical Presentation

- AEP typically presents in the first or second trimester.
- Eczema type AEP (E-type AEP)
  - The eruption is often more widespread.
  - Itchy erythematous scaly patches and papules in the flexural areas. During the acute phase, occasionally blisters and vesicles may be noted (Fig. 12.2-2).
  - This is the same distribution you would typically see in non-pregnant patients with atopic dermatitis.
  - Generalized dry scaly skin is often present.
- Prurigo type AEP (P-type AEP)
  - This is a less common presentation.
  - Itchy excoriated papules over the trunk and extremities.
  - These patients often have prurigo nodules as well.
- Pruritic folliculitis of pregnancy
  - This is a less common variant of AEP.
  - Presents with itchy perifollicular pustules and papules.
- The patient may also have generalized xerosis.

> **DIFFERENTIAL DIAGNOSIS   Atopic Eruption of Pregnancy**
>
> - Polymorphic eruption of pregnancy
> - Allergic contact dermatitis
> - Pemphigoid gestationis
> - Bacterial folliculitis (if pustules present)
> - Pustular psoriasis of pregnancy

Confirming the Diagnosis

- Diagnosis is based on clinical presentation and patient history.
- P-type AEP and pruritic folliculitis of pregnancy can be more difficult to distinguish from other pregnancy dermatoses.
- If unsure, punch biopsy for direct immunofluoresence (DIF) of perilesional (uninvolved skin) **and** a punch biopsy of involved

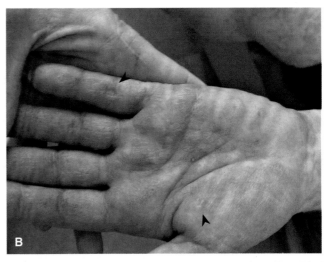

FIG. 12.2-2. AEP E-type. During the acute phase AEP E-type (<2 weeks), skin eruption may include (**A**) erythematous macules or papules without scale and (**B**) vesicles/blisters (see *arrowheads*).

skin to be sent for standard biopsy could be considered to rule out PG, pustular psoriasis or other nonpregnancy-related dermatoses.

- DIF specimens should be sent in Michels medium and can **NOT** be submitted in formaldehyde like a standard hematoxylin and eosin biopsy.

Treatment

- Low- to mid-potency topical steroids are used to control pruritus and inflammation as needed.
- Second-generation antihistamines, such as cetirizine, can be used to control pruritus.

Management and Patient Education

- Atopic skin care routine should be recommended to patients. This consists of the following:
  - Using sensitive skin soap (fragrance free).
  - Bathing with lukewarm water.
  - Moisturizing with emollients (creams or ointments) daily.
  - Using unscented laundry detergent.
- There is no fetal risk if the diagnosis is AEP.
- Refer to dermatology for further evaluation, management, and biopsy if the diagnosis is unclear.

Special Considerations

- Not all experts agree that eczema in pregnancy, prurigo of pregnancy, and pruritic folliculitis of pregnancy should all be lumped together under the AED heading.
- Pustular psoriasis of pregnancy (PPP) is a widespread pustular rash that could put the mother and fetus at risk. The patient with PPP is often very ill with fever. Careful examination of the patient to distinguish pruritic folliculitis of pregnancy and early PPP is very important. Referral to dermatology for evaluation is vital if you are unsure of the diagnosis.

CLINICAL PEARLS

- If pustules are present, recommend culture to rule out bacterial folliculitis and consider biopsy to evaluate for pustular psoriasis or pemphigoid gestations (as discussed above).
- No cutaneous involvement in the fetus/newborn.
- Typically presents in subsequent pregnancies.

PEMPHIGOID GESTATIONIS

PG, previously called herpes gestationis, is a pregnancy-related autoimmune blistering disorder. The incidence is rare, occurring 1:20,000 to 1:50,000 (Sadik et al., 2016).

Pathophysiology

- As in bullous pemphigoid, blister formation occurs when autoantibodies target the hemidesmosomes (BP 180 and BP 230). The function of BP 180 and BP 230 is to attach the basal keratinocytes to the dermis in the basement membrane zone.

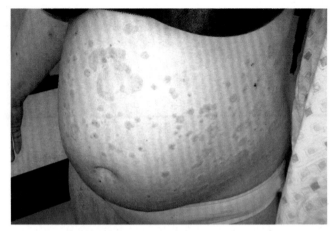

FIG. 12.2-3. Pemphigoid gestationis papules and plaques.

- For PG, autoantibodies attach to BP 180 causing inflammation, which subsequently causes separation of the epidermis and dermis resulting in subepidermal blisters.
- In pregnancy, this autoimmunity is due to maternal antibodies formed from the paternal major histocompatibility complex (MHC) antigens in the placenta.
- These autoantibodies target the amniotic membrane zone as well as the maternal and sometimes fetal basement membrane zones.

Clinical Presentation

- Presents during the second and third trimester of pregnancy and can flare during/after delivery.
- Patients can improve in few weeks prior to delivery but approximately 75% relapse at delivery (Huilaja et al., 2014).

Skin Findings

- Intensely itchy urticarial papules and/or plaques that typically begins around umbilicus and then spreads to involve the trunk, arms, and legs (Fig. 12.2-3).
- Lesions expand and develop tense vesicles/bullae, although they may not be present at the onset of the rash (Fig. 12.2-4).
- The face and mucous membranes are typically spared.

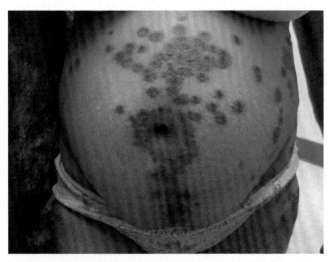

FIG. 12.2-4. Pemphigoid gestationis blisters and bulla adjacent to the umbilicus. (Photo courtesy of M. Bobonich.)

DIFFERENTIAL DIAGNOSIS   Pemphigoid Gestationis

- Polymorphic eruption of pregnancy
- Erythema multiforme
- Intrahepatic cholestasis of pregnancy
- Urticaria
- Allergic contact dermatitis
- Erythema multiforme

Confirming the Diagnosis

- Perilesional punch biopsy for DIF shows linear deposition of complement C3 in the basement membrane zone.
- Occasionally, immunoglobulin G may also be noted on DIF but is not required for diagnosis of PG.
- Lesional punch biopsy will show subepidermal blister.
- ELISA for BP 180 is very sensitive (97%) and specific (100%) for PG. BP 230 is not involved in PG (Al Saif et al., 2017).

Treatment

- Goals of therapy are to improve pruritus, prevent the development of vesicles/bullae, and hasten resolution of vesicles/bullae.
- Topical therapy includes mid- to high-potency topical steroids. Select potency and duration of topical steroid based on potency needed to control symptoms and the risk for systemic absorption. See Section 1.4 for more information on topical and systemic steroids in pregnancy.
- Second-generation oral antihistamines, such as cetirizine, can be used to help control pruritus.
- Phototherapy (UVB) can be utilized for widespread disease.
- After consultation with the patient's obstetrician, if necessary, begin oral prednisolone 0.25 to 0.5 mg/kg/day. If pruritus is not controlled, and blister formation does not cease, increasing the dose may be necessary (Huilaja et al., 2014).
- For patients with numerous erosions, the use of nonadherent dressings such as Vaseline-based gauze can be used in conjunction with gauze wrap or ACE wrap to support wound healing.

Management and Patient Education

- The patient should be managed closely with her obstetrician.
- Patients should be urgently referred to dermatology for evaluation and management with the obstetrician at first suspicion of PG.
- Patients should be counseled that PG will persist from diagnosis through delivery and sometimes flare postpartum. Occasionally, patients will have a slight improvement in symptoms prior to delivery.
- The risk to the fetus in PG is fetal growth restriction and preterm delivery.
- Early onset in the first or second trimester and presence of blisters at time of diagnosis, may result in increased fetal complications, such as low birth weight and premature birth (Chi et al., 2009).
- There is risk for PG in subsequent pregnancies. However, the incidence is not 100%.

Special Considerations

- In the pre-bullous phase of the disease, it is very difficult to differentiate from PEP. Close follow-up to monitor the progression of the lesions is necessary.
- The probability of blisters present in the newborn is approximately 10%. These typically resolve a few weeks following delivery (Sadik, 2016).

CLINICAL PEARLS

- The previous name of herpes gestationis is a misnomer, as PG is not related to the herpes virus.
- Lesions may recur postpartum with hormonal contraception or menstruation.
- Patients with PG have an increased risk for Graves disease.

INTRAHEPATIC CHOLESTASIS OF PREGNANCY

IHCP is the only pregnancy-related dermatosis without a primary skin rash. The main symptom is intense pruritus. Skin changes are secondary due to pruritus and self-induced excoriation. Women over the age of 35 are at increased risk.

Ethnic variability and geography also may play a role in the risk of the patient developing IHCP.

Incidence in middle European descent patients is around 2% while Scandinavian and Chilean patients have the highest incidence of this disease with the highest incidence around 25% (Ambros-Ruolph, 2011). Multiparity increases incidence. Family history of IHCP also increases a patient's risk of developing the disease. Close management with the patient's obstetrician and dermatology is necessary due to fetal risk.

Pathophysiology

- Cholestasis can be caused by genetics, elevated hormone levels, infections (most common Hepatitis C), and environmental factors.
- These triggers lead to an increase in serum transaminases and serum bile acids, which results in intense pruritus.

Clinical Presentation

- The most common onset is in the third trimester, although it could present as early as week 7.

Skin Findings

- Pruritus is mainly on palms and soles but can progress to generalized pruritus.
- Skin changes found on physical examination are secondary.
- These are typically self-induced excoriations or prurigo nodules due to the patient's response to the intense pruritus.

Non-Skin Findings

- Some patients develop jaundice.

DIFFERENTIAL DIAGNOSIS   Intrahepatic Cholestasis of Pregnancy

- Causes of primary pruritus (see Section 5)
- Polymorphic eruption of pregnancy
- Atopic eruption of pregnancy
- Scabies
- Hepatitis

Confirming the Diagnosis

- Lab test showing serum bile acid level elevation confirms the diagnosis. Normal range is 0 to 10 μmol/L.

- Hepatic panel may show elevated transaminases (ALT/AST), alkaline phosphatase (ALP), and bilirubin.

- If vitamin K is abnormal, there is a risk of hemorrhage.

- A biopsy is only necessary if pemphigus gestationis is suspected.

Treatment

- Ursodeoxycholic acid was previously the mainstay of treatment, but recent studies show that it may not improve fetal outcomes. However, it can still be utilized to improve pruritus (Chappell et al., 2019).

- Biophysical profiles (BPPs) are utilized to monitor fetal health two times weekly.

- The patient's obstetrician may choose to induce early labor at 36+0 weeks' gestation to reduce fetal risk. However, they may decide to induce earlier based on the results of the BPP or history of previous fetal complications in a prior pregnancy.

Management and Patient Education

- Patient needs to be closely followed by their obstetrician. If you suspect IHCP, communicate quickly with the obstetrician.

- Fetal risk is associated and correlated with elevated serum bile acids. Risk is significantly increased when levels are above 100 μmol/L (Palmer et al., 2019).

- Complications include premature birth, intrauterine fetal distress and/or death, meconium staining, and stillbirths.

- Pruritus resolves soon after delivery.

- Educate the patient that this can be recurrent with subsequent pregnancies.

- Continue to follow serum bile acid levels postpartum and evaluate mother for ongoing liver disease. Increased risk of future hepatobiliary disease is present for the mother.

CLINICAL PEARLS

- There is a higher incidence in winter months.
- Incidence in subsequent pregnancies is up to 70% (Ambros-Rudolph, 2011).

ACKNOWLEDGMENT

Melissa Davis would like to thank the previous authors of the pregnancy dermatoses material, Margaret Bobonich and Cathleen Case. Many of the figures, tables, and photographs have been reused from the previous edition.

READINGS AND REFERENCES

Akhter, A., & Said, A. (2015). Cutaneous manifestations of viral hepatitis. *Current Infectious Disease Reports, 17*(2), 452.

Al Saif, F., Jouen, F., Hebert, V., Chiavelli, H., Darwish, B., Duvert-Lehembre, S., & Joly, P.; French Study Group on Autoimmune Bullous Skin Diseases. (2017). Sensitivity and specificity of BP180 NC16A enzyme-linked immunosorbent assay for the diagnosis of pemphigoid gestationis. *Journal of the American Academy of Dermatology, 76*(3), 560–562. https://doi.org/10.1016/j.jaad.2016.09.030

Ambros-Rudolph, C. M. (2011). Dermatoses of pregnancy—clues to diagnosis, fetal risk and therapy. *Annals of Dermatology, 23*(3), 265–275. https://doi.org/10.5021/ad.2011.23.3.265

Ambros-Rudolph, C. M., Müllegger, R. R., Vaughan-Jones, S. A., Kerl, H., & Black, M. M. (2006). The specific dermatoses of pregnancy revisited and reclassified: Results of a retrospective two-center study on 505 pregnant patients. *Journal of the American Academy of Dermatology, 54*(3), 395–404. https://doi.org/10.1016/j.jaad.2005.12.012

Artantaş, S., Gül, U., Kiliç, A., & Güler, S. (2008). Skin findings in thyroid diseases. *European Journal of Internal Medicine, 20*(2), 158–161.

Balwani, M., & Desnick, R. J. (2012). The porphyrias: Advances in diagnosis and treatments. *Blood, 120*(23), 4496–4504.

Barnadas, M. A., Rubiales, M. V., González, M. J., Puig, L., García, P., Baselga, E., Pujol, R., Alomar, A., & Gelpí, C. (2008). Enzyme-linked immunosorbent assay (ELISA) and indirect immunofluorescence testing in a bullous pemphigoid and pemphigoid gestationis. *International Journal of Dermatology, 47*(12), 1245–1249. https://doi.org/10.1111/j.1365-4632.2008.03824.x

Bieber, A. K., Martires, K. J., Driscoll, M. S., Grant-Kels, J. M., Pomeranz, M. K., & Stein, J. A. (2016). Nevi and pregnancy. *Journal of the American Academy of Dermatology, 75*(4), 661–666. https://doi.org/10.1016/j.jaad.2016.01.060

Bishnoi, A., Raj, D., Vinay, K., & Dogra, S. (2019). Refractory generalized granuloma annulare treated with oral apremilast. *JAMA Dermatology, 15*(11), 1318–1320.

Bohdanowicz, M., Ghazarian, D., & Rosen, C. F. (2019). Targetoid form of polymorphic eruption of pregnancy: A case report. *SAGE Open Medical Case Reports, 7*, 2050313X19882841. https://doi.org/10.1177/2050313X19882841

Bolognia, J. L., Schaffer, J. V., Duncan, K. O., & Ko, C. J. (2014). Erythroderma. In *Dermatology essentials* (pp. 76–83). Elsevier Saunders.

Chakradeo, K., Narsinghpura, K., & Ekladious, A. (2016). Sign of leser-trélat. *British Medical Journal Case Report, 2016*. https://doi.org/10.1136/bcr-2016-215316

Chappell, L. C., Bell, J. L., Smith, A., Linsell, L., Juszczak, E., Dixon, P. H., Chambers, J., Hunter, R., Dorling, J., Williamson, C., & Thornton, J. G.; PITCHES study group. (2019). Ursodeoxycholic acid versus placebo in women with intrahepatic cholestasis of pregnancy (PITCHES): A randomised controlled trial. *The Lancet, 394*(10201), 849–860. https://doi.org/10.1016/S0140-6736(19)31270-X

Chi, C.-C., Wang, S.-H., Charles-Holmes, R., Ambros-Rudolph, C., Powell, J., Jenkins, R., Black, M., & Wojnarowska, F. (2009). Pemphigoid gestationis: Early onset and blister formation are associated with adverse pregnancy outcomes. *The British Journal of Dermatology, 160*(6), 1222–1228. https://doi.org/10.1111/j.1365-2133.2009.09086.x

Chi, C.-C., Wang, S.-H., & Kirtschig, G. (2016). Safety of topical corticosteroids in pregnancy. *JAMA Dermatology, 152*(8), 934–935. https://doi.org/10.1001/jamadermatol.2016.1009

Chowaniec, M., Starba, A., & Wiland, P. (2016). Erythema nodosum—review of the literature. *Reumatologia, 54*(2), 79–82.

Cordova, K. B., Oberg, T. J., Malik, M., & Robinson-Bostom, L. (2009). Dermatologic conditions seen in end-stage renal disease. *Seminars in Dialysis, 22*(1), 45–55.

Daneshgaran, G., Dubin, D. P., & Gould, D. J. (2020). Cutaneous manifestations of COVID-19: An evidence-based review. *American Journal of Clinical Dermatology, 21*(5), 627–639. https://doi.org/10.1007/s40257-020-00558-4

Dasari, A., Shen, C., Halperin, D., Zhao, B., Zhou, S., Xu, Y., Shih, T., & Yao, J. C. (2017). Trends in the incidence, prevalence, and survival outcomes in patients with neuroendocrine tumors in the United States. *JAMA Oncology, 3*(10), 1335–1342.

Degnan, A. J., Tocchio, S., Kurtom, W., & Tadros, S. S. (2017). Pediatric neuroendocrine carcinoid tumors: Management, pathology, and imaging findings in a pediatric referral center. *Pediatric Blood Cancer, 64*(9).

Doshi, D., Blyumin, M., & Kimball, A. (2008). Cutaneous manifestations of thyroid disease. *Clinics in Dermatology, 26*(3), 283–287.

Driscoll, M. S., & Grant-Kels, J. M. (2007). Hormones, nevi, and melanoma: An approach to the patient. *Journal of the American Academy of Dermatology, 57*(6), 919–931. https://doi.org/10.1016/j.jaad.2007.08.045

Edmund, W., & Kelly, R. (2017). Pentoxifylline: An effective therapy for necrobiosis lipoidica. *Australasian Journal of Dermatology, 58*(1), 65–68.

Ferringer, T., & Miller, F. (2003). Cutaneous manifestations of diabetes mellitus. *Dermatologic Clinics, 20*(3), 483–492.

Floreani, A., & Gervasi, M. T. (2016). New insights on intrahepatic cholestasis of pregnancy. *Clinics in Liver Disease, 20*(1), 177–189. https://doi.org/10.1016/j.cld.2015.08.010

Freeman, E. E., McMahon, D. E., Lipoff, J. B., Rosenbach, M., Kovarik, C., Desai, S. R., Harp, J., Takeshita, J., French, L. E., Lim, H. W., Thiers, B. H., Hruza, G. J., & Fox, L. P. (2020). The spectrum of COVID-19–associated dermatologic manifestations: An international registry of 716 patients from 31 countries. *Journal of the American Academy of Dermatology, 83*(4), 1118–1129. https://doi.org/10.1016/j.jaad.2020.06.1016

Garcovich, S., Garcovich, M., Capizzi, R., Gasbarrini, A., & Zocco, M. (2015). Cutaneous manifestations of hepatitis C in the era of new antiviral agents. *World Journal of Hepatology, 7*(27), 2740–2748.

Geenes, V., & Williamson, C. (2009). Intrahepatic cholestasis of pregnancy. *World Journal of Gastroenterology, 15*(17), 2049–2066. https://doi.org/10.3748/wjg.15.2049

Geraghty, L. N., & Pomeranz, M. K. (2011). Physiologic changes and dermatoses of pregnancy. *International Journal of Dermatology, 50*(7), 771–782. https://doi.org/10.1111/j.1365-4632.2010.04869.x

Ghosn, S. H., & Kibbi, A. (2008). Cutaneous manifestations of liver disease. *Clinics in Dermatology, 26*(3), 274–282.

GISED. (1990). Lichen planus and liver diseases: A multicentre case-control study. Gruppo Italiano Studi Epidemiologici in Dermatologia. *BMJ (Clinical Research Ed.), 300*(6719), 227–230.

Grin, C. M., Rojas, A. I., & Grant-Kels, J. M. (2001). Does pregnancy alter melanocytic nevi? *Journal of Cutaneous Pathology, 28*(8), 389–392. https://doi.org/10.1034/j.1600-0560.2001.028008389.x

Gupta, A., Madhavan, M. V., Sehgal, K., Nair, N., Mahajan, S., Sehrawat, T. S., Bikdeli, B., Ahluwalia, N., Ausiello, J. C., Wan, E. Y., Freedberg, D. E., Kirtane, A. J., Parikh, S. A., Maurer, M. S., Nordvig, A. S., Accili, D., Bathon, J. M., Mohan, S., Bauer, K. A., . . . Landry, D. W. (2020). Extrapulmonary manifestations of COVID-19. *Nature Medicine, 26*(7), 1017–1032. https://doi.org/10.1038/s41591-020-0968-3

Gupta, P., Saikia, U. N., Arora, S., De, D., & Radotra, B. D. (2016). Panniculitis: A dermatopathologist's perspective and approach to diagnosis. *Indian Journal of Dermatopathology and Diagnostic Dermatology, 3*(29), 29–41.

Higgins, S. P., Freemark, M., & Prose, N. S. (2008). Acanthosis nigricans: A practical approach to evaluation and management. *Dermatology Online Journal, 14*(9), 2.

Higgins, S. P., Freemark, M., & Prose, N. S. (2008). Acanthosis nigricans: A practical approach to evaluation and management. *Dermatology Online Journal, 49*(9), 2.

Huilaja, L., Mäkikallio, K., & Tasanen, K. (2014). Gestational pemphigoid. *Orphanet Journal of Rare Diseases, 9*(1), 136. https://doi.org/10.1186/s13023-014-0136-2

Ingelfinger, J. R., Thadhani, R., & Brandenburg, V. (2018). Calciphylaxis. *The New England Journal of Medicine, 378*(18), 1704–1712.

Ito, T., Lee, L., & Jensen, R. T. (2018). Carcinoid-syndrome: Recent advances, current status and controversies. *Current Opinion in Endocrinology, Diabetes and Obesity, 25*(1), 22–35.

Jones, S. V., Ambros-Rudolph, C., & Nelson-Piercy, C. (2014). Skin disease in pregnancy. *BMJ (Clinical Research Ed.), 348*, g3489. https://doi.org/10.1136/bmj.g3489

Kong, A. S., Williams, R. L., Rhyne, R., Urias-Sandova, V., Cardinali, G., Weller, N. F., Skipper, B., Volk, R., Daniels, E., Parnes, B., & McPherson, L.; PRIME Net Clinicians. (2010). Acanthosis Nigricans: High prevalence and association with diabetes in a practice-based research network consortium—a PRImary care Multi-Ethnic network (PRIME Net) study. *Journal of the American Board of Family Medicine, 23*(4), 476–485.

Lause, M., Kambo, A., & Faith, F. F. (2017). Dermatologic manifestations of endocrine disorders. *Translational Pediatrics, 6*(4), 300–312.

Lima, A., Illing, T., Schliemann, S., & Elsner, P. (2017). Cutaneous manifestations of diabetes mellitus: A review. *American Journal of Clinical Dermatology, 18*(4), 541–553.

Massone, C., Cerroni, L., Heidrun, N., Brunasso, A. M. G., Nunzi, E., Gulia, A., & Ambros-Rudolph, C. M. (2014). Histopathological diagnosis of atopic eruption of pregnancy and polymorphic eruption of pregnancy: A study on 41 cases. *The American Journal of Dermatopathology, 36*(10), 812–821. https://doi.org/10.1097/DAD.0000000000000067

Mistry, N., Gupta, A., Alavi, A., & Sibbald, R. G. (2015). A review of the diagnosis and management of erythroderma (generalized red skin). *Advances in Skin and Wound Care, 28*(5), 228–236.

Nigwekar, S., Thadhani, R., & Brandenburg, V. (2018). Calciphylaxis. *The New England Journal of Medicine, 378*(18), 1704–1714.

Ovadia, C., Seed, P. T., Sklavounos, A., Geenes, V., Di Ilio, C., Chambers, J., Kohari, K., Bacq, Y., Bozkurt, N., Brun-Furrer, R., Bull, L., Estiú, M. C., Grymowicz, M.,

Gunaydin, B., Hague, W. M., Haslinger, C., Hu, Y., Kawakita, T., Kebapcilar, A. G., . . . Williamson, C. (2019). Association of adverse perinatal outcomes of intrahepatic cholestasis of pregnancy with biochemical markers: Results of aggregate and individual patient data meta-analyses. *The Lancet, 393*(10174), 899–909. https://doi.org/10.1016/S0140-6736(18)31877-4

Palmer, K. R., Xiaohua, L., & Mol, B. W. (2019). Management of intrahepatic cholestasis in pregnancy. *The Lancet, 393*(10174), 853–854. https://doi.org/10.1016/S0140-6736(18)32323-7

Puljic, A., Kim, E., Page, J., Esakoff, T., Shaffer, B., LaCoursiere, D. Y., & Caughey, A. B. (2015). The risk of infant and fetal death by each additional week of expectant management in intrahepatic cholestasis of pregnancy by gestational age. *American Journal of Obstetrics and Gynecology, 212*(5), 667.e1–667.e5. https://doi.org/10.1016/j.ajog.2015.02.012

Reid, S. D., Ladinzinski, B., Lee, K., Baibergenova, A., & Alvai, A. (2013). Update on necrobiosis lipoidica: A review of etiology, diagnosis, and treatment options. *Journal of the American Academy of Dermatology, 69*(5), 783–791.

Roth, M-M. (2011). Pregnancy dermatoses. *American Journal of Clinical Dermatology, 12*(1), 25–41. https://doi.org/10.2165/11532010-000000000-00000

Rubin de Celis Ferrari, A. C., Glasberg, J., & Riechelmann, R. (2018). Carcinoid syndrome: Update on the pathophysiology and treatment. *Clinics, 73*(1), 1–9.

Rudolph, C. M., Al-Fares, S., Vaughan-Jones, S. A., Müllegger, R. R., Kerl, H., & Black, M. M. (2006). Polymorphic eruption of pregnancy: Clinicopathology and potential trigger factors in 181 patients. *British Journal of Dermatology, 154*(1), 54–60. https://doi.org/10.1111/j.1365-2133.2005.06856.x

Sadik, C. D., Lima, A. L., & Zillikens, D. (2016). Pemphigoid gestationis: Toward a better understanding of the etiopathogenesis. *Clinics in Dermatology, 34*(3), 378–382. https://doi.org/10.1016/j.clindermatol.2016.02.010

Sävervall, C., Sand, F. L., & Thomsen, S. F. (2015). Dermatological diseases associated with pregnancy: Pemphigoid gestationis, polymorphic eruption of pregnancy, intrahepatic cholestasis of pregnancy, and atopic eruption of pregnancy. *Dermatology Research and Practice, 2015*, 979635.

Schwartz, R. A., & Nervi, S. J. (2007). Erythema nodosum: A sign of systemic disease. *American Family Physician, 75*(5), 695–700.

Sethi, K., Shareef, N., & Bloom, S. (2018). The Sister Mary Joseph nodule. *British Journal of Hospital Medicine, 79*(2), C27–C29.

Shengyuan, L., Songpo, Y., Wen, W., Wenjing, T., Haitao, Z., & Binyou, W. Y. (2009). Hepatitis C virus and lichen planus. *JAMA Dermatology, 145*(9), 1040–1047.

Thiers, B. H., Sahn, R. E., & Callen, J. P. (2009). Cutaneous manifestations of internal malignancy. *Cancer Journal for Clinicians, 59*(2), 73–98.

Uliasz, A., & Lebwohl, M. (2008). Cutaneous manifestations of cardiovascular diseases. *Clinics in Dermatology, 26*(3), 243–254.

Vaughan-Jones, S. A., & Black, M. M. (1999). Pregnancy dermatoses. *Journal of the American Academy of Dermatology, 40*(2), 233–241. https://doi.org/10.1016/S0190-9622(99)70194-5

Wanat, K., & Rosenbach, M. (2014). A practical approach to cutaneous sarcoidosis. *American Journal of Clinical Dermatology, 15*(4), 283–297.

Wee, E., & Kelly, R. (2017). Pentoxyflline: An effective therapy for necrobiosis lipoidica. *Australasian Journal of Dermatology, 58*(1), 65–68.

Wee, S., & Possick, P. (2006). Necrobiosis lipoidica. *Dermatology online journal, 10*(3), 18.

Yanardag, H., Tetikkurt, C., Bilir, M., Demirci, S., & Iscimen, A. (2013). Diagnosis of cutaneous sarcoidosis; Clinical and the prognostic significance of skin lesions. *Multidiscipline Respiratory Medicine, 8*(2), 26.

The Neonate

Victoria Garcia-Albea

This chapter is dedicated to common pediatric dermatologic conditions. When faced with a pediatric patient, consider the patient's age, recent exposures, immunization status, immune status, genetic factors, developmental stage, mobility, and environmental factors. The patient may be unable to communicate, so thorough history taking, a high index of suspicion and diagnostic skills are important. Patterns of distribution and the patient's overall appearance, mood, and effect are important clues. Biopsy is often not possible, so a conservative approach to management may be necessary.

Always exercise caution with topical treatments, as higher body surface area to weight ratios increases percutaneous absorption.

Newborn skin is different from adult skin in several ways: it is thinner, has less hair, and the adherence between the epidermis and dermis is weaker. Infants have a body surface area to weight ratio that is up to five times higher than adults. For these reasons, infant skin is at higher risk for skin infection and injury, as well as increased percutaneous absorption. Infants have a higher rate of transepidermal water loss, which can lead to dehydration, electrolyte imbalance, and temperature instability.

Newborn Skin Care

At birth, the skin is covered with vernix caseosa, a grayish-white thick greasy material, which is comprised of water, proteins, lipids, and antimicrobial peptides (Coughlin & Taieb, 2014). Allowing the vernix to be retained provides greater moisture accumulation and hydration in the skin. Wipe the vernix caseosa from the face, but allow the vernix on the body to slough off spontaneously.

Newborns lack the normal skin flora that protects against infection and do not need to be bathed daily. Washing the buttocks and perianal area with warm soapy water at diaper changes will suffice. Once weekly tub bathing should be quick, to prevent thermoregulatory problems. Sponge bathing is more likely to cause changes in body temperature than tub bathing, especially in preterm or extremely preterm infants. After bathing, application of topical emollients helps to prevent transepidermal water loss and improve

barrier function. Safe ingredients for full-term neonates include white petrolatum ointment and lanolin. In preterm and extremely preterm infants, use of petrolatum ointment was associated with higher rates of candida and coagulase-negative *Staphylococcus* infection (Kusari et al., 2019). Parents should look for products that are free of fragrances and dyes.

The Umbilicus

There may be one or two surgical wounds present after birth—the umbilical stump and the circumcision site. To prevent infection, skin care should involve gentle cleansing with nontoxic, nonabrasive material. There is no single standard of care for the umbilical stump. Avoid the use of povidone-iodine, as absorption of iodine can cause transient hypothyroxinemia or hypothyroidism. The cord site can be left dry, without bandages until the crust falls off on its own, usually about 10 days after birth. The site can become irritated, red, and sometimes painful, usually from diapers or clothing rubbing or pulling on the scab.

Infection of the umbilical stump is not common but can occur and may present as periumbilical erythema and induration (*omphalitis*). *Staphylococcus aureus*, introduced through the umbilical stump, is the most common pathogen and necessitates treatment to prevent sepsis. Systemic antibiotics are first line, but prevention should be the primary focus. Daily washing with regular soap and water is usually enough to prevent infection.

Circumcision Site

Care of the circumcision site is similar to that of the umbilical stump. Keep the area clean by washing the area gently with soap and water at least once a day. Apply petrolatum ointment to the tip of the penis at each diaper change to prevent the penis from sticking to the diaper. The penis may initially be red, swollen, and bruised, and can have a yellow crust. Infection is rare; perform a culture if there is pus or drainage. The wound will heal in about 7 to 10 days.

Common Infections

Victoria Garcia-Albea

In This Chapter

- Measles
- Varicella
- Rubella
- Scarlet Fever
- Roseola
- Erythema Infectiosum

- Hand-Foot-Mouth Disease
- Eczema Herpeticum
- Eczema Coxsackium
- Mycoplasma Exanthem
- Staphylococcal Scalded Skin Syndrome

Exanthem

An exanthem is a local or widespread skin eruption usually in response to a viral infection. It can also be in response to bacterial illnesses, toxins produced by pathogens, or drug ingestion. The term *exanthem* actually refers to lesions found on the skin while *enanthem* refers to those on the mucosa. Some causative infectious agents can be potentially harmful to specific patient populations, such as pregnant women or the immunocompromised. Vaccinations are available to prevent and control many infectious diseases, including several childhood exanthems discussed in this chapter. Each year, the CDC's Advisory Committee on Immunization Practices (ACIP) publishes recommended vaccination schedules that guide clinician practice and public health (http://www.cdc.gov/vaccines/schedules/).

The evaluation of a child presenting with an exanthem should include a thorough history, review of systems, and physical examination. Lesion morphology, distribution pattern, prodrome, concurrent symptoms, known exposures, and local epidemiology are key for diagnostic accuracy (Table 13.2-1). Additionally, the primary morphology of the eruption including morbilliform, vesicular, and pustular lesions can guide the clinician in building their differential diagnosis (Table 13.2-2).

MEASLES

Measles, or *rubeola,* is a highly contagious respiratory virus. Since the introduction of the measles vaccine in 1963, the incidence in the United States dropped dramatically. Recent outbreaks have been reported and attributed to people who contracted the virus outside the country (such as while on vacation). In 2019, the CDC reported 1276 confirmed cases in 31 states. More than 75% of those cases were linked to outbreaks in New York City. Most of the cases were among people who were unvaccinated. People who are not vaccinated are at risk of contracting the virus and spreading it to others.

Pathophysiology

- *Measles morbillivirus,* formerly called *measles virus* (MeV), is a single-stranded, negative-sense, enveloped, nonsegmented RNA virus of the genus *Morbillivirus within the family Paramyxoviridae*.

- Humans are the natural hosts of the virus; no animal reservoirs are known to exist.
- The virus is spread via respiratory droplets.

Clinical Presentation

Skin Findings

- Red mucous membranes
- *Koplik spots*, gray-white to red papules on the buccal mucosa, are pathognomonic for measles (Fig. 13.2-1)
- Classic skin lesions are described as *morbilliform* which are 2 to 4 mm erythematous macules that coalesce
- Lesions start on the face or behind the ears and spread cephalo-caudally and will fade in the same order that they appeared

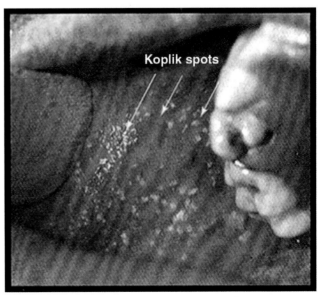

FIG. 13.2-1. Koplik spots measles.

TABLE 13.2-1 Overview of Childhood Exanthems

EXANTHEM	CAUSATIVE AGENT	AGE	PRODROME	SKIN FINDINGS	ASSOCIATED FINDINGS	SEASON	COMMENTS
Roseola	*HHV-6* *HHV-7*	Infant to preschool	High fever 3 days Mild URI symptoms	When fever breaks, rash appears and last 1–2 days • Erythematous macules and papules • Circumoral pallor	Mostly well appearing Complication including febrile seizures	Spring	• Supportive care
Erythema Infectiosum *(Slapped Cheek, Fifth disease)*	*Human parvovirus B19*	Early school age	Low-grade fever, malaise, sore throat	Three stages: 1. "Slapped-cheeks" 2. Erythematous patches on trunk spreading to extremities (spares palms/soles) 3. Lacey/reticulated pattern as it clears 4. Can wax/wane for weeks	Arthritis	Late Winter Early Spring	• Supportive care • Risk of fetal hydrops, anemia, and intrauterine death if congenital infection in 1st or 2nd trimester • Not teratogenic
Hand-Foot-and-Mouth Disease	*Coxsackie A6, A16, and enterovirus 71*	Infant to preschool	Fever, sore throat, URI, GI distress	Rash appears 1–2 days after fever • Vesicles on an erythematous base in oral cavity (herpangina) • Red macules or vesicles on knees, elbows, palms, soles, buttocks	Dysphagia that can result in dehydration, eczema coxsackium	Late Summer Early fall	• Supportive care • Very contagious • Slight increased risk of miscarriage and still birth, greater risk near delivery
Rubeola *(Measles)*	*Measles virus*	Pre- and early- school aged	Moderate fever, malaise, conjunctivitis, coryza, cough	Morbilliform eruption—erythematous macules and papules • Koplik spots (buccal mucosa) • Eruption begins on face or around/behind ears and spreads cephalocaudally • Rash clears after 1 wk in the same sequence	Infectious complications	Winter Spring	• Supportive care • Highly infectious • Increased risk of premature labor and delivery, and fetal loss. • Increased risk of maternal death
Rubella *(German measles)*	*Rubivirus*		Low-grade fever, headache, URI, conjunctivitis, lymphadenopathy	Rash (1–3 days) appears at same time • Rose-pink macules and papules • Petechial macules on palate (Forchheimer spots) • Spreads cephalocaudally	Arthralgias	Late Winter Early Spring	• Supportive care • Vaccination • Congenital Rubella syndrome with increased risk in 1st trimester

(continued)

483

TABLE 13.2-1 Overview of Childhood Exanthems (*Continued*)

EXANTHEM	CAUSATIVE AGENT	AGE	PRODROME	SKIN FINDINGS	ASSOCIATED FINDINGS	SEASON	COMMENTS
Scarlet Fever (*mild form is scarlatina*)	*Streptococcus pyogenes*	Age 5–15 yr Rare <5 yr old	Fever, exudative pharyngitis, malaise, cervical lymphadenopathy	Generalized red-orange sandpaper eruption • Forchheimer spots • Strawberry tongue • Pastia lines • Desquamation after 4–5 days • Starts on head/neck and axillae, then spreads cephalocaudally	• Abdominal pain • Complications: Rheumatic fever Acute glomerular nephritis	Fall Spring	Treatment • Full 10 days of penicillin to prevent rheumatic fever • Isolation until after 24 hr antibiotic
Varicella (*Chickenpox*)	*Varicella virus*		Fever	Eruption starts as same time as fever • Pruritic vesicles on erythematous base, often in crops • Progress to crust over • Mucous membranes involved • Starts on scalp and trunk then rapidly spread centrifugally		Late Winter Early Spring	• Supportive care • Vaccination • Very contagious • Antivirals not routine unless severe
Kawasaki disease	Presumed infectious	Children 1–5 yr old	High fever lasting 5 days	In addition to fever, dx includes four of the following criteria: 1. Erythema, edema hands/feet and desquamation (esp. periungual) 2. Bilateral conjunctival injection 3. Oral mucosal injection and strawberry tongue 4. Cervical lymphadenopathy 5. Truncal morbilliform rash (not vesicular) 6. Perineal erythema with desquamation in 48 hr	Most common cause of acquired heart disease in children • Carditis • Coronary aneurysms • arthritis		Treatment • IVIG • High dose aspirin • Not infectious
Gianotti–Crosti Syndrome (Papular acro-dermatitis of childhood)	Presumed viral Suspected causes: • Hepatitis B • Epstein–Barr virus • Cytomegalovirus • Enteroviruses • Respiratory syncytial virus (RSV)	6 mo to 12 yr	Low-grade fever for 3–4 days Malaise Diarrhea	Mild illness • Pink, skin colored, or dull red-brown papules that can coalesce into plaques beginning on thighs and buttocks and spreading to lateral arms and eventually the face • Lesions are 5–10 mm erythematous to deep red • May develop vesicles • Usually not itchy • Typically spares the chest, abdomen and back	Mild lymphadenopathy in axillae and groin, which can last for months If associated with Hepatitis B, patients may develop enlarged liver but usually do not develop jaundice.	Spring Summer	Supportive care Mild topical steroid ointments for itch Can last up to 8 wk Usually not recurrent It is not necessary to keep children home from daycare, school, or activities

TABLE 13.2-2	Differential Diagnosis for Eruptions Based on Morphology

MORBILLIFORM ERUPTIONS	PAPULAR VESICULAR ERUPTIONS
Rubeola (measles)	Herpes simplex
Roseola erythema	Varicella (chickenpox)
Infectious mononucleosis	Herpes zoster (shingles)
Pityriasis rosea	Coxsackievirus (especially HFM)
Hepatitis	Influenza
Mumps	Echoviruses
Echoviruses	Variola
Adenoviruses	Vaccina (cowpox)
Parvoviruses (fifth disease)	
Echoviruses	
Epstein–Barr virus (EBV)	
Coxsackieviruses	
Respiratory syncytial virus (RSV)	
Cytomegalovirus	
Dengue	
MORBILLIFORM WITH PETECHIAE	**NEONATAL PUSTULAR ERUPTIONS**
Rubella	Infectious
Epstein–Barr virus	Bacterial
Parvovirus B19	Fungal—usually yeast
RSV	Viral
Echoviruses	Noninfections
Hepatitis	Acne neonatorum
Measles (atypical)	Erythema toxicum neonatorum
Dengue	Miliaria pustulosa
Coxsackievirus A9	Benign neonatal cephalic pustulosis
	Transient pustular melanosis
	Infantile acropustulosis
	Pustular psoriasis
	Fever and pustular rash = CAUTION for systemic infection

Modified from Weston, W. L., Lane, A. T., & Morelli, J. G. (2007). *Color textbook of dermatology.* (4th ed.). St Louis, Mosby.

Non-Skin Findings

- Patients with measles appear very ill
- High fever
- The three "C"s: coryza, cough, and conjunctivitis

DIFFERENTIAL DIAGNOSIS	Measles
Common	*Uncommon*
• Drug reaction	• Toxic shock syndrome
• Other viral exanthems	• Systemic lupus erythematosus
	• Serum sickness
	• Syphilis

Confirming the Diagnosis

- Diagnosis is based on history and clinical findings and can be confirmed with laboratory studies.

- The CDC recommends reverse transcriptase-polymerase chain reaction (RT-PCR) and IgM blood testing.
- Ideally, serum should be collected within 3 days of the onset of the rash.
- All suspected or laboratory confirmed cases must be reported to the CDC.

Treatment

- Treatment is supportive
- No specific antiviral therapy is available

Management and Patient Education

- There is no cure for measles.
- Most patients recover without complications in 7 to 10 days.
- Children with measles should be kept out of daycare and school until 4 to 5 days after the rash initially appeared.
- Some parents worry that the vaccine for measles can cause autism. This concern has been proven false by numerous research studies.
- Parents who do not vaccinate their children can contribute to new outbreaks of measles, mumps, and rubella.
- Complications include pneumonia, bronchitis, otitis, gastroenteritis, myocarditis, and encephalitis.

Special Considerations

Pregnancy

- Measles is not teratogenic, but can cause miscarriage and premature labor.

Vaccination

- A measles vaccine is available as a combination with mumps and rubella.

> **CLINICAL PEARLS**
> - Low vitamin A levels are associated with increased measles-related morbidity and mortality
> - The World Health Organization (WHO) recommends treating with vitamin A daily for 2 days after diagnosis is made

VARICELLA

Varicella zoster virus (VZV) is a highly contagious virus and is the causative agent of varicella (*chicken pox*) and herpes zoster (*shingles*, which is discussed in Section 6.3).

Like other herpesviruses, VZV has the capacity to persist in the body after the primary (first) infection as a latent infection. Active disease or vaccination, discussed in Section 6, usually confers lifetime immunity. Recurrence can occur, but is uncommon.

Pathophysiology

- VZV is a DNA virus and is a member of the herpesvirus group.
- Primary infection with VZV causes the cutaneous eruption known commonly as *chicken pox*, which is highly contagious via respiratory droplet spread.

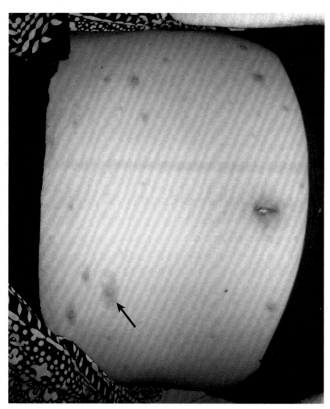

FIG. 13.2-2. Varicella dewdrop on rose petal. Note the clear juicy vesicle on a "rose petal" base. (Used with permission from Gru, A. A., & Wick, M. (2018). *Pediatric dermatopathology and dermatology.* Wolters Kluwer Health.)

- Patients are contagious until at least 5 days after the appearance of the rash, or until all of the lesions are dried and crusted.

Clinical Presentation

Skin Findings

- The skin lesions appear 1 to 2 days after the prodrome begins (see non-skin findings).
- Lesions are initially erythematous macules and papules.
- Macules and papules quickly evolve into pustules and vesicles that appear like "dewdrops on rose petal" (Fig. 13.2-2).
- New lesions develop for several days.
- Lesions become dried and crusted by day 6 or 7.

Non-Skin Finding

- There is a prodrome characterized by malaise, fever, chills, headache, and arthralgia.

DIFFERENTIAL DIAGNOSIS Varicella	
Common	*Uncommon*
• Eczema herpeticum	• Disseminated herpes simplex virus
• Eczema coxsackium	
• Bullous impetigo	• Urticaria
• Arthropod assaults (bites or stings)	• Dermatitis herpetiformis
• Drug reaction	
• Measles	• Smallpox infection
• Other viral exanthem	

Confirming the Diagnosis

- Diagnosis of primary VZV is based on history and physical findings.
- Diagnosis can be confirmed with viral culture of a vesicle for PCR.
- Serum IgG and IgM antibody titers are not recommended for diagnosis because they are less sensitive.

Treatment

Topical Treatment

- Cool compresses and colloidal oatmeal baths for pruritus
- Use of topical antibiotics should be reserved for cases of secondary infection

Systemic Treatment

- No specific antiviral therapy is available.
- Treatment is symptomatic for otherwise healthy patients.
- Oral analgesics for pain (acetaminophen, ibuprofen).
- Oral antihistamines for pruritus (diphenhydramine, loratadine, cetirizine).
- Secondary bacterial infection, usually due to *Staphylococcus aureus* or group A *strep*, is the most common complication and can result in scarring.
- Use of oral antivirals should be reserved for cases of confirmed secondary infection.

Management and Patient Education

- For most immunocompetent patients, VZV infection is a mild and self-limited illness.
- The course of disease usually lasts 5 to 10 days.
- Most children recover without complications.
- VZV is highly contagious until fever resolves and lesions are dried and crusted.
- Patients may return to daycare or school when they are afebrile, and lesions are dried and crusted. Until then, patients should not be in public places.

Special Considerations

- Adults have a greater risk for complications than children.
- Complications such as recurrence, disseminated infection, secondary infections, or pneumonia are more common in patients who are immunocompromised.
- VZV infection during pregnancy can cause congenital varicella syndrome, which will not be discussed in this chapter.
- Patients with disseminated VZV or pneumonia require immediate hospitalization and intravenous antiviral therapy.

Vaccination

- There is a live attenuated vaccine available; refer to http://www.cdc.gov/vaccines/schedules

RUBELLA

Rubella, also known as *German measles* or *three-day measles,* is a viral exanthem spread through droplet contact from infectious nasopharyngeal secretions.

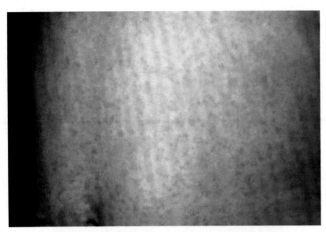

FIG. 13.2-3. Rubella. Rash of rubella on skin of child's back. Distribution is similar to that of measles, but the lesions are less intensely red. (CDC Public Health Image LibraryPHIL_4514_lores Rubella.)

Pathophysiology

- Rubella is caused by an RNA virus in the *Togaviridae* family
- The virus is spread through droplet contact from nasopharyngeal secretions
- Patients are contagious from onset of symptoms until 7 days after the onset of the rash
- The incubation period is 14 to 21 days

Clinical Presentation

Skin Findings

- The exanthem is light, "rose-pink" macules and papules that begin on the head (Fig. 13.2-3)
- The exanthem spreads cephalocaudally.
- Pink macules and papules become confluent.
- Lesions begin to fade in 1 to 3 days, in the same order in which they appeared.
- In severe cases, there may be fine flaky desquamation.
- The enanthem: *Forchheimer spots* are erythematous and petechial macules on the soft palate and are usually seen early in disease. They are not diagnostic for rubella because they may also be noted in scarlet fever and measles.
- Up to 25% of infected patients do not have the exanthem.

Non-Skin Findings

- The prodrome occurs 2 to 5 days before the skin eruption.
- Patients develop a low-grade fever (compared to the high fever associated with measles).
- Patients may experience headache, malaise, eye pain (particularly with eye movement), myalgias, sore throat, rhinorrhea, and cough.
- Up to 50% of cases are asymptomatic.
- Patients can develop generalized lymphadenopathy in suboccipital, postauricular, and cervical areas.
- Arthralgias and arthritis (fingers, wrists, or knees) can occur, especially in adolescent females, and may continue for several months after the infection has resolved.

DIFFERENTIAL DIAGNOSIS	Rubella
Common	*Uncommon*
• Hypersensitivity reaction	• Acute HIV seroconversion
• Contact dermatitis	
• Scarlet fever	
• Other viral exanthems	

Confirming the Diagnosis

- The vague and often mild symptoms of rubella can make diagnosis challenging.
- Nasal secretions can be cultured for the virus.
- Serology for rubella-specific IgM antibody identifies recent infection.
- Rubella titers taken 1 to 2 weeks apart, showing a fourfold or greater increase, indicates acute infection.

Treatment

- NSAIDs are used for arthralgia
- Vaccination is the best prevention and is available in combination with mumps and measles vaccine. http://www.cdc.gov/vaccines/schedules

Management and Patient Education

- Management is symptomatic.
- Disease is self-limiting.
- Infection most often occurs in spring and summer.
- Arthritis may continue for several weeks following the resolution of infection.
- Monitor for adequate fluid intake during illness.
- Once symptoms improve, no special follow-up is needed, unless complications occur.

Special Considerations

Immunosuppression

- Even patients with immunosuppression usually have mild illness

Pregnancy

- Rubella is teratogenic
- *Congenital rubella syndrome* (CRS) results from viral infection during pregnancy and can cause miscarriage, stillbirth, and birth defects, including cataracts, congenital heart disease, hearing impairment, and developmental delay.
- Mothers who are not immune to rubella are at risk for CRS and therefore should avoid all contact or exposure with individuals suspected of being infected.

SCARLET FEVER

Scarlet fever, or *scarlatina*, results from a *group A beta-hemolytic Streptococcus* (GABHS) infection. It is rare in infants and is most common in 1- to 10-year olds.

Pathophysiology

- Scarlet fever is a GABHS or *Streptococcus pyogenes* infection.
- Exotoxins from a GABHS infection cause the characteristic rash of scarlet fever.

- While most cases are associated with GABHS infections of the pharynx and tonsils, it can originate from the skin as well.
- Patients not previously exposed to GABHS have no antibodies to it and therefore develop the exanthem.
- Ordinary "strep throat" can present with a sore throat and a fine macular rash but does not present with the classic eruption of scarlet fever as presented below.
- GABHS is transmitted via respiratory secretions.
- Scarlet fever is contagious from about 4 to 5 days before the onset of the rash, until about 4 to 5 days after it fades, or 24 hours after antibiotics are initiated.

Clinical Presentation

Skin Findings

- On day 1 or 2 of illness, the tongue develops a white coating with red, edematous papillae called "strawberry tongue" (Fig. 13.2-4).
- Forsheimer spots may also be seen on the soft palate (similar to Rubella).
- One to 5 days after the fever starts, a fine, erythematous macular and papular eruption appears on the ears, chest, and axillae.
- The exanthem spreads to the trunk and extremities (Fig. 13.2-5).
- It is accentuated in the flexural areas with petechiae and hyperpigmentation, called *Pastia lines*.
- The face may be flushed with circumoral pallor.
- The skin has a classic "sandpaper" or rough texture.
- In patients with dark skin, the erythema can be difficult to appreciate, but the skin will still have the "sandpaper" texture. The exanthem lasts 4 to 5 days, followed by desquamation (Fig. 13.2-6).

Non-Skin Findings

- Scarlet fever presents with abrupt onset of fever, sore throat, headache, and chills.
- There may be painful anterior cervical adenopathy.
- Rhinorrhea and cough are notably absent in most cases.

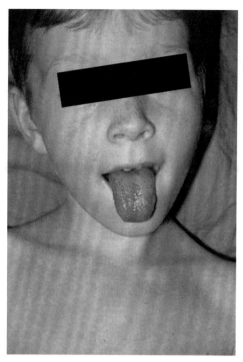

FIG. 13.2-4. Scarlet fever. Strawberry tongue. (Photo courtesy of Hans B. Kersten.)

DIFFERENTIAL DIAGNOSIS	Scarlet Fever
Common	*Uncommon*
• Viral infection	• Kawasaki disease
• Hypersensitivity reaction	• *Chlamydia* infection
• Drug eruption	• Unusual viral infection such as hepatitis
• *Mycoplasma* infection	

Confirming the Diagnosis

- Diagnosis is based on clinical findings and laboratory testing.
- Throat culture will be positive for GABHS.
- Antistreptolysin O (ASO) serologic testing can be useful.

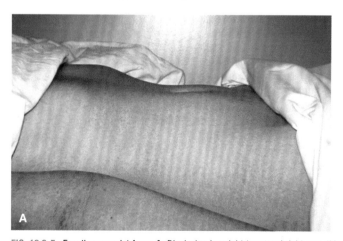

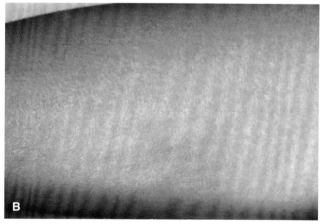

FIG. 13.2-5. Exanthem scarlet fever. **A:** Displaying her right torso and right arm, this female patient who was lying prone in a clinical setting, revealed a patchy mottled skin rash, which was diagnosed as being a case of scarlet fever caused by a bacterium referred to as group A *Streptococcus*, or group A strep (GAS). Scarlet fever is a rash that sometimes occurs in people who have strep throat. People with scarlet fever typically also have a high fever, and a strawberry-like appearance of the tongue. The rash of scarlet fever is usually seen in children under the age of 18. (CDC Public Health Image Library #15772.) **B:** This image depicts a close view of a patient's skin, revealing a scarlet fever rash on the volar surface of the forearm due to group A *Streptococcus* bacteria. (CDC Public Health Image Library #5163.)

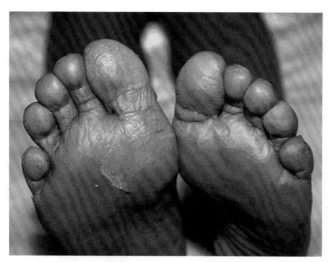

FIG. 13.2-6. Desquamation of exanthem after 5 days.

Treatment

Topical Treatment

- Topical treatment is supportive care but does not negate the need for systemic antibiotics.
- Cool baths help alleviate symptoms.

Systemic Treatment

- The treatment of choice for scarlet fever is penicillin for a complete 10-day period.
- For penicillin allergic patients, first-generation cephalosporin (some risk of cross reaction) and macrolides provide alternatives.
- Intramuscular penicillin G is used when compliance is a concern.
- Antipyretics and increased fluid intake help to alleviate symptoms.

Management and Patient Education

- Most patients can be managed in the outpatient setting with supportive care.
- There is no vaccine available.
- If patients appear toxic or are experiencing decreased fluid intake, referral to the emergency department may be necessary.
- Complications include pneumonia, pericarditis, meningitis, hepatitis, post-streptococcal glomerulonephritis, and rheumatic fever.

- Parents should be educated about the importance of completing the antibiotic therapy to avoid complications like post-strep glomerulonephritis or acute rheumatic fever.
- Reassure parents that previously healthy children tend to fully recover in a matter of days.
- Children can return to school or daycare when they are afebrile and have been on an antibiotic for at least 24 hours.

CLINICAL PEARLS

- The morphology of scarlet fever is referred to as *morbilliform*, which is a term used to describe other rashes with similar characteristics
- Patients over 10 years old have usually been exposed to GABHS and therefore have developed antibodies and do not develop the rash

Erythema Infectiosum

- Erythema infectiosum (EI) is a contagious viral infection also called *fifth disease* or *human parvovirus*. EI usually affects preschoolers and school-aged children.

Pathophysiology

- Caused by *parvovirus* B19.
- EI is spread by respiratory droplets, through blood products, and from mother to fetus.
- Patients are contagious for 5 to 10 days from onset of symptoms, or until the exanthem appears.

Clinical Presentation

Skin Findings
See Table 13.2-1 and Fig. 13.2-7A,B.

Non-Skin Findings

- Prodrome consists of headache, low-grade fever, myalgias and chills, rhinorrhea, and cough.
- Prodrome usually lasts 7 to 10 days before the exanthem appears.
- Arthralgia or arthritis may occur in up to 10% of cases. It is more common in females and favors the fingers, hands, wrists, ankles, and knees.
- Joint involvement is more common in adults with B19 infection.

TABLE 13.2-3	Stages of Erythema Infectiosum	
STAGE I	**STAGE II**	**STAGE III**
Begins 5–10 days after the prodrome begin Classic bright red erythema "slapped-cheek" rash appears suddenly (Fig. 13.2-7) Spares nasal bridge and perioral areas	Begins 1–4 days after the facial rash starts Lesions begin as erythematous macules and papules Lesions progress to a pink to erythematous, lacy, reticulated, macular eruption on the extremities Trunk becomes involved later Spares palms and soles Can be pruritic In adolescents, lesions tend to be petechial and more prominent in acral and periflexural areas Lasts 1–3 wk or occasionally longer	Final 2–3 wk of the exanthem Lesions on trunk and extremities fade completely Lesions can wax and wane during this stage

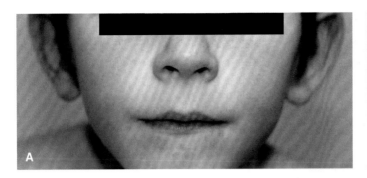

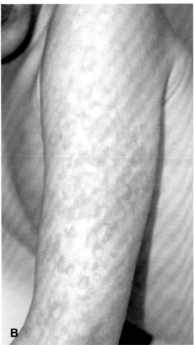

FIG. 13.2-7. Erythema infectiosum (*fifth disease*). **A:** "Slapped cheek" with a symmetric erythema of bilateral cheeks in erythema infectiosum. **B:** Erythematous macules in a "lacy" pattern on the arm, the extremities, and trunk in a reticulated, "lacy" pattern appearing after the "slapped cheeks" in erythema infectiosum. (A and B: Used with permission from Gru, A. A., & Wick, M. [2018]. *Pediatric dermatopathology and dermatology.* Wolters Kluwer Health.)

DIFFERENTIAL DIAGNOSIS	Erythema Infectiosum Fifth Disease
Common	*Uncommon*
• Contact dermatitis	• Systemic lupus erythematosus
• Phototoxic reaction	• Juvenile idiopathic arthritis (Still disease)
• Other viral exanthems	
• Rosacea	
• Drug reaction	

Confirming the Diagnosis

- When needed, serology for anti-B19 IgM antibody is the preferred method for diagnosis.
- Presence of anti-B19 IgM antibody indicates infection within the past 2 to 4 months.
- Serology for anti-B19 IgG antibody can be detected 3 weeks after onset of symptoms, which is approximately when the rash and arthralgias appear, but at this stage patients are no longer contagious.

Treatment

- No specific antiviral therapy is available
- Treatment is supportive care
- NSAIDs for arthropathy
- Antipyretics for fever

Management and Patient Education

- EI is self-limiting.
- Most cases are mild.
- Patients usually make a full recovery without complications.
- Arthritis resolves spontaneously.

- Patients are contagious until the onset of the rash.
- Once the rash appears, they are no longer contagious and can return to daycare or school.

Special Considerations

Pregnancy

- Mothers can be infected without showing any symptoms
- **Pregnant women exposed to Parvovirus B19 should be referred to their obstetrician for monitoring and management**
- The highest risk for fetal compromise is in cases when infection occurs before 20 weeks gestation
- Parvovirus B19 is not teratogenic
- About 30% to 66% of adult females are immune, so their fetuses are not at risk
- In most cases of maternal infection, the fetus is delivered without developmental or neurologic problems
- *Congenital infection* can cause anemia, high-output congestive heart failure, hydrops fetalis, and intrauterine fetal demise
- Most fetal losses occur between 9 and 28 weeks gestation
- Severely affected surviving fetuses can be treated with *in utero* digitalization and blood transfusions
- *Papular-purpuric gloves and socks syndrome* (PPGSS)
- Caused by numerous viruses, including parvovirus B19
- Edema and erythema of hands and feet, especially palms and soles
- Petechiae and purpura
- Spontaneous resolution in 1 to 2 weeks

Transient Aplastic Crisis

- Parvovirus B19 affects red blood cell (RBC) production, causing transient anemia.
- Patients at risk include those with low RBC production, increased RBC destruction or loss, Sickle cell disease, iron deficiency anemia,

thalassemia, and glucose-6-phosphate dehydrogenase (G6PD) deficiency.

- Patients with aplastic crisis may require RBC transfusions.

Roseola

Roseola, *roseola infantum, exanthema subitum,* or *sixth disease,* is a mild and common exanthem that usually occurs in children under 2 years.

Pathophysiology

- Roseola is caused by human herpesvirus types 6 and 7.
- It is thought to spread via saliva.
- Horizontal transmission from mother to child has been well documented.

Clinical Presentation

Skin Findings

- The classic presentation is a cutaneous eruption that presents just AFTER the fever breaks.
- Subtle, light pink, erythematous macules and papules on the face, neck, and extremities, and sometimes chest (Fig. 13.2-8).
- The rash usually resolves in 1 to 3 days.

Non-Skin Findings

- Prodrome includes 3 to 5 days of high fever.
- With or without irritability, diarrhea, bulging fontanelle, cough, cervical lymphadenopathy, and eyelid edema.
- Children are otherwise well-appearing.

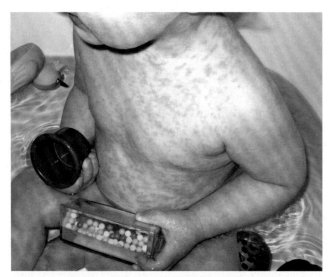

FIG. 13.2-8. Roseola. Erythematous macules and papules over the trunk which then spread to the extremities and face in roseola. (Used with permission from Gru, A. A., & Wick, M. [2018]. *Pediatric dermatopathology and dermatology.* Wolters Kluwer Health.)

Confirming the Diagnosis

- Diagnosis is based on history and physical findings.
- In rare severe cases, diagnosis is based on exclusion of other illnesses and diseases.
- HHV-6 and 7 can be isolated in the saliva and stool of infected patients.

Therapeutics

- No specific antiviral therapy is available
- Treatment of roseola is symptomatic and supportive

Management and Patient Education

- Mild and short-lived infection
- Most children recover without long-term sequelae
- Follow-up is not necessary unless infection is severe or complicated

HAND-FOOT-AND-MOUTH DISEASE

Hand-foot-and-mouth disease (HFMD) is a mild viral exanthem most commonly seen in children 1 to 4 years old but is often seen in adults within the same household. These viruses can spread from person-to-person through direct contact with unwashed hands or contaminated surfaces. A more severe form of HMFD called eczema coxsackium is discussed later in the chapter.

Pathophysiology

- Hand-foot-and-mouth disease is caused by an enterovirus, most commonly coxsackievirus A16 (CV-A16) and human enterovirus 71 (HEV71), but it has been linked to multiple coxsackievirus subtypes.
- HFMD is spread via fecal–oral exposure.
- Incubation period is 3 to 5 days.

Clinical Presentation

Skin Findings

- Starting 1 to 2 days after the fever begins
- Characteristic exanthem of vesicular lesions on the palms, soles, buttocks, and perineum
- Dorsal hands and feet may also be involved
- Classic enanthem of vesicles and erosions on the buccal mucosa, palate, tongue, uvula, gingivae, and anterior tonsillar pillars (Fig. 13.2-9)
- Lesions are painful

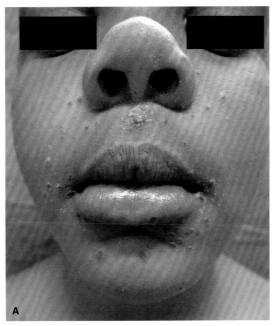
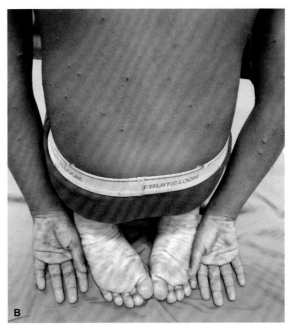

FIG. 13.2-9. A,B: Hand-foot-and-mouth disease. Widespread vesicles around the mouth and scattered over extensor arms and legs and over the trunk along with erythematous macules on palms and soles seen in the more dramatic eruption of "atypical hand-foot-and-mouth disease" associated with coxsackievirus A6. (Used with permission from Gru, A. A., & Wick, M. [2018]. *Pediatric dermatopathology and dermatology.* Wolters Kluwer Health.)

Non-Skin Findings

- Prodrome of fever, malaise, sore throat, decreased oral intake
- Young children may be irritable
- There may be cervical and submandibular lymphadenopathy

DIFFERENTIAL DIAGNOSIS	Hand Foot and Mouth Disease
• Erythema multiforme	• Aphthous ulcers
• Herpes simplex	• Streptococcal throat infection
• Herpangina	• Dyshidrotic eczema

Confirming the Diagnosis

- Diagnosis of HFMD is usually based on clinical findings.
- Viral culture can be collected from an intact vesicle.
- An important clue to diagnosis is local epidemiology
- Outbreaks are common in summer and fall, but sporadic cases occur throughout the year.

Treatment

Topical Treatment

- *"Magic mouthwash"* is a common off-label pain medication used for HFMD in children.
  - A mixture of diphenhydramine solution and Maalox (calcium carbonate) solution, 1:1; with or without viscous lidocaine 2%, 1:1:1.
  - Only add lidocaine if the child is able to spit the solution out because if lidocaine is ingested, there is a risk of arrhythmia.
  - Parents can paint the oral cavity with an oral sponge swab in younger children.
  - Magic mouthwash is administered every 4 to 6 hours for pain from oral vesicles and erosions.

- It should be swished around in the mouth for 30 seconds and then spit out.
- Salt-water mouth rinses using ½ teaspoon of salt in 8 ounces of warm water may be soothing.
- Use petroleum-based ointment for ulcers in the diaper area.
- If erosions and ulcers in the diaper area become infected, treat with mupirocin 2% ointment.

Systemic Treatment

- No specific antiviral therapy is available
- Antipyretics and analgesics for fever and pain

Management and Patient Education

- HFMD is usually a benign, mild, short-lived infection requiring only supportive treatment.
- Illness usually spontaneously resolves after about 7 to 10 days, with low rates of complications.
- It is important to counsel parents on pain management, fever control, and prevention of dehydration.
- Instruct parents to watch for dry mucous membranes, sunken fontanelle, weight loss, or decreased urine output.
- Encourage increased fluid intake of cold water and milk, especially if the patient has a fever.
- Fever is not usually high; febrile seizures are possible but uncommon.
- Acidic juices and sodas can cause burning pain if there are mucosal erosions.
- Monitor infants and toddlers for dehydration related to anorexia from painful oral erosions.
- Encephalitis, aseptic meningitis, acute flaccid paralysis, and myocarditis are uncommon complications (Paller & Mancini, 2015).
- Follow-up is required if the patient becomes lethargic or irritable, or has other signs or symptoms of dehydration.

- Onychomadesis, nail shedding, occurs 1 to 2 months after infection due to temporary nail matrix arrest associated with the viral infection.

ECZEMA COXSACKIUM

Eczema coxsackium is an atypical presentation of HFMD. It was first described in 1968 when a child with severe eczema developed an extensive vesicular eruption caused by CV-A16 (Miller et al., 2017). It was described again in 2011–2012 during an outbreak of the CV-A6-associated North America enterovirus (Ganguly & Kuruvila, 2016). Since then, several case reports and case studies have been published describing this entity. One report described four characteristic morphologies of severe CV-A6 (Miller et al., 2017). See Clinical Presentation below.

Pathophysiology

- Similar to HFMD, eczema coxsackium is caused by a coxsackievirus, usually CV-A6 and less commonly CV-A16.
- Typically, this occurs in patients with atopic dermatitis with altered skin barrier function.
- It has been described in areas of preexisting diaper dermatitis, sunburn, healing lacerations, and tinea pedis.

Clinical Presentation

Skin Findings

- Vesicles, pustules, hemorrhagic bullae, hemorrhagic crusts, and erosions in areas of preexisting dermatitis
- Four characteristic morphologies exist (Fig. 13.2-10)
  - Widespread vesiculobullous
  - Localized vesicles/erosions in areas of atopic dermatitis
  - Gianotti–Crosti-like eruption in acrofacial distribution
  - Petechial/Purpuric papulovesicles on the palms and soles
- *Onychomadesis* (an idiopathic shedding of the nails beginning at the proximal end, possibly caused by the temporary arrest of the function of the nail matrix) is common.

- *Beau lines* (horizontal depressions in nail plate, which can result from any systemic disease process or illness that is severe enough to affect the growth plate of the nail) are common but will not appear for several months after the disease has resolved.
- Desquamation of the palms and soles can occur a few weeks after the rash resolves.

Non-Skin Findings

- Most patients experience brief and mild symptoms such as fever or diarrhea prior to developing the rash.
- Children are at risk for dehydration due to oral lesions.

DIFFERENTIAL DIAGNOSIS	Eczema Coxsackium
Common	*Uncommon*
Bullous impetigo	Eczema herpeticum
Varicella	Primary immunobullous disease
Contact dermatitis	Vasculitis
Bullous drug eruption	Erythema multiforme

Confirming the Diagnosis

- Diagnosis is based on clinical presentation.
- Skin biopsy at the periphery of a lesion will confirm the diagnosis.
- Culture from vesicular fluid, mucosal fluid, or a stool sample should be sent to confirm the diagnosis.
- It is important to rule out eczema herpeticum (EH) and varicella. Enterovirus PCR can sometimes be obtained from a vesicle or bulla, or from a nasopharyngeal swab.
- Serum testing for antibody is available.

Treatment

Topical Treatment

- Low- to mid-potency topical corticosteroids can be used for pruritus.
- *"Magic mouthwash"* is a common off-label pain medication used for HFMD in children (see HFMD section above for details).
- Salt-water mouth rinses using ½ teaspoon of salt in 8 ounces of warm water may be soothing.
- Treat lesions that are secondarily infected with mupirocin 2% ointment.

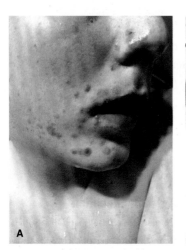 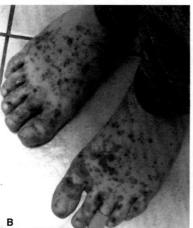 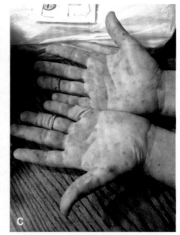

FIG. 13.2-10. A–C: Eczema coxsackium. Localized vesicles/erosions on face and purpuric papulovesicles on the palms and soles. (Photos courtesy of Victoria Garcia-Albea.)

Systemic Treatment

- No specific antiviral therapy is available.
- Pain management is achieved with acetaminophen and ibuprofen.

Management and Patient Education

- Disease is self-limited.
- Care is supportive.
- Encourage patients to eat and drink normally.
- Hospitalization is rarely necessary.
- Isolation is not necessary. Prevent spread of the virus with good hand hygiene.
- Treat secondary bacterial infection appropriately
- Lesions crust over and heal within about 2 weeks.
- Aseptic meningitis has been reported, but is rare.
- Secondary bacterial infection can occur due to scratching.
- There is no vaccine.

CLINICAL PEARLS

- It is important to rule out eczema herpeticum and varicella
- In contrast to eczema herpeticum, patients are usually well-appearing, without fever, decreased appetite, or decreased activity

---

ECZEMA HERPETICUM

EH, or Kaposi varicelliform eruption, is a disseminated infection with herpes simplex virus (HSV) typically seen in patients with atopy, Darier disease, burns, seborrheic dermatitis (SD), autoimmune blistering disorders, or other chronic skin disease where skin barrier is altered.

Pathophysiology

- EH can occur as a primary infection with HSV, or by autoinoculation
- An impaired skin barrier is thought to be the cause of the extensive viral invasion

Clinical Presentation

Skin Findings

- Widespread painful, disseminated, monomorphic, umbilicated vesicles, or pustules on an erythematous base
- Pustules and vesicles become the classic "punched-out" erosions that then coalesce into painful erosions and ulcerations with a scalloped border (Fig. 13.2-11)
- Lesions may appear in multiple crops over several days
- The lesions are most severe in areas of active dermatitis
- Lesions occur most commonly on the head, neck, and trunk

Non-Skin Findings

- Sudden fever
- Malaise
- Lymphadenopathy

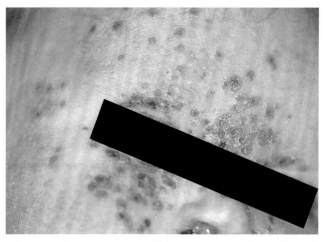

FIG. 13.2-11. Eczema herpeticum. (Fleisher, G. R., Ludwig, W., & Baskin, M. N. [2004]. *Atlas of pediatric emergency medicine.* Wolters Kluwer Health | Lippincott Williams & Wilkins.)

DIFFERENTIAL DIAGNOSIS	Eczema Herpeticum
Common	*Uncommon*
• Varicella	• Disseminated zoster
• Disseminated molluscum	• Eczema coxsackium
• Vesicular viral exanthem	• Erysipelas
• Contact dermatitis	• Acute generalized exanthematous pustulosis
• Bullous impetigo	• Dermatitis herpetiformis

Confirming the Diagnosis

- Tzank preparation taken from the base of a vesicle, looking for multinucleated giant cells
- Direct fluorescent antibody (DFA) testing
- Viral culture
- PCR for HSV DNA
- Bacterial culture to rule out secondary infection

Treatment

Topical Treatment

- Cool compresses help with pruritus
- Bland emollients initially
- Topical glucocorticosteroids
- Anti-inflammatory ointments

Systemic Therapy

- Initiate systemic antiviral therapy as soon as possible
- Supportive care is often required, including hydration and electrolyte balance
- Treatment of secondary bacterial infection
- Oral analgesics for pain control

Management and Patient Education

- Patients with severe disease require hospitalization
- Patients with EH can develop serious complications including keratoconjunctivitis, secondary bacterial superinfection, fluid loss, and viremia

- Patients are considered infectious until all lesions have crusted over
- Proper hand washing is needed to prevent dissemination by autoinoculation
- Perform bacterial culture to rule out secondary infection

Gianotti–Crosti Syndrome

Gianotti–Crosti syndrome or *papular acrodermatitis of childhood* is a common viral exanthem, most common in children between 1 and 6 years of age.

Pathophysiology

- When this entity was first described in the 1950s, it was thought to be due to hepatitis B virus infection.
- Now that hepatitis B vaccination is a standard, many other viruses have been implicated including Epstein–Barr virus (EBV), cytomegalovirus, coxsackievirus, adenovirus, respiratory syncytial virus, parainfluenza virus, parvovirus B19, rotavirus, and HHV-6.
- In the United States, EBV virus is the most common cause.
- It is thought to be immunologically mediated, possibly related to immune complexes or a delayed hypersensitivity reaction.
- Most cases occur in spring and summer.
- Patient under 4 years of age are most often affected.
- It occurs most commonly in patients with atopic dermatitis, family history of atopy, or elevated IgE syndrome.

Clinical Presentation

Skin Findings

- A few days after the prodrome, symmetric, edematous, erythematous, monomorphic papules and vesicles erupt.
- As the name *acrodermatitis* implies, lesions typically occur on the acral surfaces (face, extensor surfaces of extremities, ears) (Fig. 13.2-12).

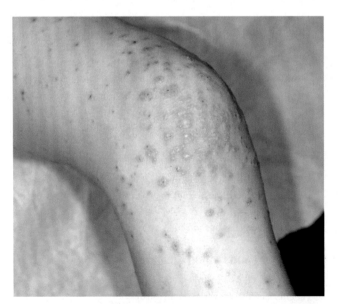

FIG. 13.2-12. Gianotti–Crosti. Juicy, pink papules on extensor surfaces with concentration over elbows in Gianotti–Crosti syndrome. Similar papules occur in high number over knees, buttocks, and cheeks. (Used with permission from Gru, A. A., & Wick, M. [2018]. *Pediatric dermatopathology and dermatology.* Wolters Kluwer Health.)

- The buttocks may be involved, but the trunk is almost always spared.
- There may be larger coalescing erythematous plaques.
- Patient can have localized purpura.

Non-Skin Findings

- There is a common prodrome of upper respiratory symptoms, fever, and lymphadenopathy.
- Mild pruritus.
- Hepatitis, jaundice, or liver function abnormalities can occur.

DIFFERENTIAL DIAGNOSIS	Gianotti–Crosti Syndrome
Common	*Uncommon*
• Other viral illnesses	• Urticaria pigmentosa
• Contact dermatitis	• Langerhans cell histiocytosis
• Arthropod assault	
• Phototoxic dermatitis	
• Drug reaction	
• Urticaria	

Confirming the Diagnosis

- Diagnosis is based on history and physical findings
- Screen patients for any potential risk factors for hepatitis B
- Examine patients for jaundice, hepatosplenomegaly, and lymphadenopathy
- If these symptoms are present, screen for hepatitis B and LFT abnormalities
- In the absence of risk factors or symptoms, serum studies for hepatitis are not indicated
- Viral cultures from nasal secretions or saliva may or may not be helpful
- Skin biopsy helps to confirm the diagnosis by ruling out other diseases

Treatment

Topical Treatment

- Use mild topical corticosteroids like desonide 0.05% ointment twice daily for 1 week on the face and groin.
- Use mid-potency topical corticosteroids like triamcinolone 0.1% ointment twice daily for up to 2 weeks on the extremities.
- If topical corticosteroids are prescribed, counsel patients on the proper usage, risks, and side effects.
- If scratching causes impetigo, treat with mupirocin 2% ointment three times per day until clear.

Systemic Treatment

- If patients develop secondary bacterial infection from scratching, treat appropriately with antibiotics
- Treat pruritus with oral antihistamines

Management and Patient Education

- Most cases of Gianotti–Crosti are benign and self-limited.
- Symptoms usually last 2 to 4 weeks.

- Skin lesions can persist up to 12 weeks and heal without scarring.
- If hepatitis is detected, referral to appropriate specialists is recommended.
- Patients without hepatitis B history usually recover fully.

MYCOPLASMA-INDUCED RASH AND MUCOSITIS

This entity is also referred to as, *Mycoplasma* exanthem, atypical Stevens–Johnson syndrome (SJS), incomplete SJS, Fuchs syndrome, mycoplasma mucositis, or *Mycoplasma pneumoniae*–associated mucositis. It is a rash that occurs in up to 25% of people infected with *M. pneumoniae* (Schalock & Dinulos, 2009). It is a diagnosis that should be considered in a patient with an exanthematous eruption and respiratory symptoms.

Pathophysiology

- *M. pneumoniae* is a common cause of respiratory tract infection and pneumonia in children and adolescents.
- It has a long, 2- to 3-week incubation period and can cause outbreaks among children, those living in military housing, in schools, and in families.
- *M. pneumoniae* is not a *true* bacteria because it lacks cell walls.

Clinical Presentation
Skin Findings

- Lesions can be morbilliform, vesicular, bullous, targetoid, or urticarial (Fig. 13.2-13)
  - Patients may have cutaneous lesions and mucosal lesions, or they may only have mucous membrane involvement (Martinez-Perez et al., 2016)
- Distribution of cutaneous lesions:
  - Acral (46%)
  - Widespread (31%)
  - Truncal (23%)
- Distribution of mucosal lesions:
  - Oral lesions (94%)
  - Bilateral conjunctivitis (82%)
  - Urogenital involvement (63%) (Martinez-Perez et al., 2016)

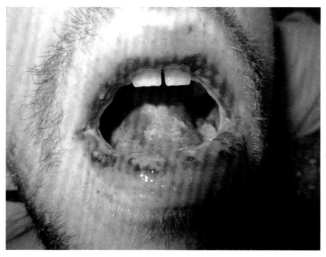

FIG. 13.2-13. MIRM. (Courtesy Anar Mikailov, MD.)

Non-Skin Findings

- The illness presents slowly with sore throat, malaise, cough, and fatigue and gradually worsen
- Headache
- Conjunctivitis
- Photophobia
- Symptoms can persist for 1 to 2 weeks; but illness is generally mild

DIFFERENTIAL DIAGNOSIS	Mycoplasma-Induced Rash and Mucositis
Common	*Uncommon*
• Viral exanthem	• Stevens–Johnson syndrome
• Hypersensitivity reaction	• Erythema multiforme

Confirming the Diagnosis

- PCR from nasopharyngeal secretions early in the disease.
- PCR is highly sensitive and specific.
- Measuring serum IgM antibody titers to *M. pneumoniae* is only useful later in disease, as levels will not be elevated until 7 to 10 days after onset of symptoms.
- IgG antibodies rise approximately 2 weeks after IgM antibodies.
- Both IgG and IgM titers may be negative in early stages of the disease.

Treatment
Topical Treatment

- Topical steroids twice daily can help manage pruritus
- Treat impetigo with mupirocin 2% ointment
- *Magic Mouthwash* for oral skin lesions (as described above for HFMD)
- Topical treatment is supportive
- Bland emollients can be applied judiciously for erosions and crusts on the skin or mucosal surfaces

Systemic Treatment

- Treatment with oral antibiotics for 10 days can hasten recovery
- Infants and children can be treated with azithromycin, clarithromycin, or erythromycin
- Children over 8 years old can be treated with doxycycline or tetracycline
- Most patients are treated with antibiotics (80%)
- Fewer are treated with systemic steroids (35%)
- IVIG and glucocorticosteroids may be effective in treating mucocutaneous disease (Yang & Lee, 2017)
- Plasmapheresis has been used less commonly

Management and Patient Education

- Most cases follow a benign course
- Patients usually recover spontaneously
- Treatment is supportive and symptomatic; maintain hydration and control pain
- It may be necessary to consult with dermatology, infectious diseases, ophthalmology, and urology depending on disease severity

- Patients with mucocutaneous disease should receive a chest x-ray due to the high risk of pulmonary complications
- Four percent of patients required ICU care

Special Considerations

- It is thought that the mortality rate is about 3%.
- Complications are rare and can include hepatitis, meningitis, pericarditis, arthritis, and acute hemolytic anemia.

> **CLINICAL PEARLS**
>
> ■ Some classify it on the spectrum of erythema multiforme and Stevens–Johnson syndrome
> ■ Others consider it a distinct entity

STAPHYLOCOCCAL SCALDED SKIN SYNDROME

- Staphylococcal scalded skin syndrome (SSSS), previously called Ritter disease or pemphigus neonatorum, is a blistering disease caused by certain strains of *S. aureus* that produce epidermolytic toxins (ETs).

Pathogenesis

- SSSS can occur in the setting of any infection with ET-producing *S. aureus*
- These ETs target desmoglein 1, a cell-to-cell adhesion molecule found in the superficial epidermis
- Children are susceptible to SSSS because they lack neutralizing antibodies to *S. aureus* and because they have decreased renal excretion of the ETs
- Neonates and children under 5 years of age are at higher risk for SSSS (Mishra et al., 2016)
- Fifteen to 40% of the population carry *S. aureus* on their skin without any symptoms

Clinical Presentation

Skin Findings

- SSSS usually starts as a localized infection
- In neonates and young children, site of infection is often nasopharynx, umbilicus, conjunctivae, or perineum
- Diffuse erythema develops and is more pronounced in flexural and perioral area
- Characteristic radial fissures extending out from the oral commissures, lateral canthi, and around the nose
- Erythema progresses to large, superficial, flaccid bullae
- Bullae rupture easily and leave behind denuded, erythematous, and tender skin (Fig. 13.2-14)

Non-Skin Findings

- Infection may begin as pneumonia, septic arthritis, endocarditis, or polymyositis.
- Patients will initially experience a sudden fever, irritability, lethargy, malaise, and poor feeding.
- Patients experience skin pain.

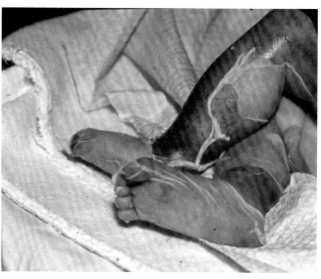

FIG. 13.2-14. SSSS. (Photo courtesy of Samuel Moschella.)

DIFFERENTIAL DIAGNOSIS	Staphylococcal Scalded Skin Syndrome
Common	*Uncommon*
• Scarlet fever	• Toxic epidermal necrolysis
• Other viral exanthem	• Epidermolysis bullosa
• Exanthematous drug eruption	• Graft versus host disease
• Burns	• Bullous ichthyosis
• Bullous impetigo	• Toxic shock syndrome (TSS)
• Nutritional deficiency	• Kawasaki disease
	• Drug-induced eosinophilia with systemic symptoms (DRESS)

Confirming the Diagnosis

- Diagnosis is usually based on clinical findings
- Diagnosis is confirmed by culturing *S. aureus*
- Culture the conjunctiva, nares or nasopharynx, and blood
- The blisters are sterile as they are due to the exotoxins and not the bacteria itself
- Skin biopsy in SSSS shows that the blister occurs in the superficial epidermis at the level of the granular level

Treatment

Topical Treatment

- Topical treatment alone is not sufficient to treat true SSSS
- Topical mupirocin 2% ointment for impetigo
- Bland emollients to promote skin healing

Systemic Treatment

- Treatment with antistaphylococcal antibiotics is required.
- Resistance to penicillin is common.
- SSSS responds to penicillinase-resistant synthetic penicillins, first- or second-generation cephalosporin, and clindamycin.
- Methicillin-resistant *Staphylococcus aureus* (MRSA) infection requires longer antibiotic treatment.
- Vancomycin or linezolid have been used for SSSS due to MRSA.

Management and Patient Education

- The first 2 days of the blistering and desquamation are the most critical.
- Once appropriate antibiotic therapy has been initiated, disease improves rapidly.
- After a few days of intravenous antibiotic therapy, patients may be transitioned to oral treatment.
- Most children improve within 1 to 2 days of starting antibiotics.
- Patients require fluid and electrolyte management, prevention of secondary infection, and pain management.
- Wound care is similar to care of second-degree burns with bland emollients and careful bandaging.
- Skin lesions usually heal within a few days without scars.
- Mild skin desquamation can be seen for up to 7 to 10 days.
- SSSS can be spread to neonates and children by an asymptomatic adult.
- Infection can be mild to severe.
- Patients are expected to make a full recovery.

Special Considerations

- SSSS must be distinguished from toxic epidermal necrolysis (TEN), which is typically drug-induced and has a high mortality rate.
- In neonates and young children, infection can be severe, requiring hospitalization.
- Severe cases may best be handled in an intensive care unit or burn unit.
- In more severe cases, patients are at risk for fluid loss, thermoregulatory disturbance, electrolyte imbalance, secondary infection, and sepsis.
- In older children and adolescents, infection is usually mild and outpatient therapy may be an option.

CLINICAL PEARLS

- This distinguishing feature of SSSS is that mucous membranes are not involved in SSSS as they are involved in TEN
- The *Nikolsky* sign (pressure on the edge of an intact bulla causes the blister to extend) is positive in SSSS

Inflammatory Disorders

Victoria Garcia-Albea

In This Chapter

- Seborrheic Dermatitis
- Diaper Dermatitis
- Slime Dermatitis
- Neonatal Lupus
- Gianotti–Crosti

SEBORRHEIC DERMATITIS

SD, or "cradle cap," is a benign erythematous scaly or crusting dermatosis of the scalp that is common in infants and adolescents.

Pathophysiology

- The exact cause of SD is unknown.
- It occurs in "seborrheic areas," which contain the highest concentration of sebaceous glands such as scalp and face.
- This suggests an association with sebum and sebaceous glands.
- The yeast *Malassezia furfur* has also been implicated.

Clinical Presentation

Skin Findings

- In infants with SD, scalp involvement has variable erythema with thin, white-yellow scale (Fig. 13.3-1).
- In the diaper area, lesions are redder and without scale (Fig. 13.3-2).
- In older children and adolescents, central face and nasolabial folds can have red to salmon-colored patches and plaques with greasy scale and sharply defined borders.
- Pinpoint red papules may be present near the nasal ala.
- Older children and adolescents may complain of dandruff.
- Pruritus is usually minimal.

DIFFERENTIAL DIAGNOSIS	Seborrheic Dermatitis
Common	*Uncommon*
• Atopic dermatitis	• Langerhans cell histiocytosis
• Acneiform dermatoses	
• Contact dermatitis	
• Psoriasis	

Confirming the Diagnosis

- SD is usually diagnosed clinically.
- Its clinical features can resemble many other disorders so it can be difficult to differentiate from other papulosquamous, eczematous, and infectious dermatoses.

- Irritant diaper dermatitis usually spares the skin in contrast to SD which usually involves the skin folds.
- Inverse psoriasis does usually involve the skin folds but lacks scale in the intertriginous areas.
- Figure 13.3-3 shows an algorithm for use in diagnosing scaly scalp.

Treatment

Topical Treatment

- For infants and children, application of mineral or baby oil can be left on the scalp overnight.

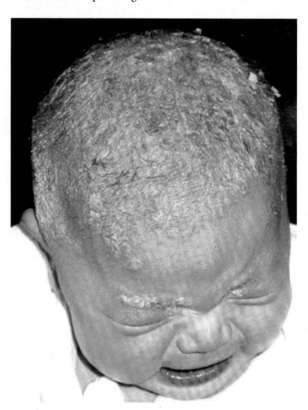

FIG. 13.3-1. Seborrheic dermatitis "cradle cap."

499

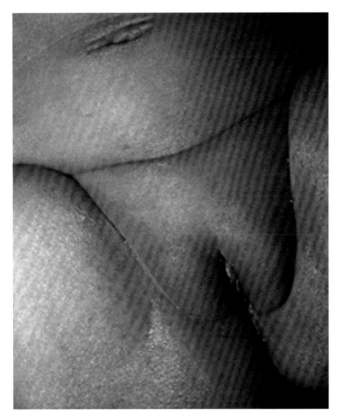

FIG. 13.3-2. Seborrheic dermatitis in diaper area.

- Shampooing in the morning will allow for gentle removal of the scale with a soft hairbrush or toothbrush.
- Over-the-counter keratolytic or antiseborrheic shampoos containing zinc, salicylic acid, or tar are safe to use daily for flares.

- Antifungal shampoos, such as ketoconazole and ciclopirox, are used if *M. furfur* is suspected.
- Ketoconazole 1% shampoo is available over-the-counter whereas 2% shampoo is available by prescription.
- Low-potency topical corticosteroid oils, lotions, or shampoos can be used twice daily for up to 2 weeks.
- Calcineurin inhibitors (pimecrolimus cream or tacrolimus ointment) can reduce inflammation and help control pruritus.
- Diluted bleach baths reduce bacterial colonization.
- Mupirocin 2% ointment can be used for secondary bacterial infection.
- Tea tree oil is a naturopathic alternative used by many, but lacks supporting studies.

Systemic Treatment

- Oral antibiotics may be required for more significant secondary bacterial infection.

Management and Patient Education

- SD is a benign condition with no cure.
- Reassure parents that infantile cradle cap will self-resolve, usually by 8 to 12 months of age.
- In older children and adolescents, SD has a more chronic course and may wax and wane.
- Watchful waiting and reassurance are acceptable treatment choices.
- Children who scratch or pick off waxy plaques from their scalp are also at increased risk for bacterial infection.
- If oozing occurs, a culture should be obtained, and antimicrobials prescribed as needed.
- Daily use of medicated shampoos and antipruritic agents can control symptoms.

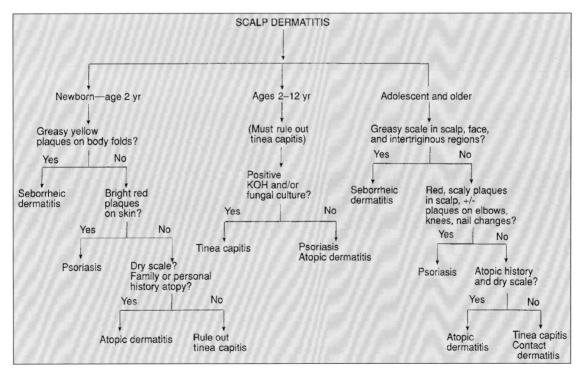

FIG. 13.3-3. Algorithm for diagnosis of scaly scalp.

DIAPER DERMATITIS

Diaper dermatitis, also called *napkin dermatitis* or *diaper rash*, is one of the most common skin conditions of childhood, affecting about 25% of children under 2 years. "Diaper dermatitis" describes a number of different clinical disorders characterized by acute inflammation in the diaper area. Inflammation develops when the integrity of the epidermal barrier is compromised by excessive moisture, heat, or irritation. The warm, moist environment of diapers can exacerbate skin irritation. In this section, chafing dermatitis (the most common), irritant dermatitis, and diaper candidiasis are discussed.

Pathophysiology

- *Chafing dermatitis* is due to friction and rubbing.
- *Irritant contact dermatitis* occurs when irritating substances come in contact with the skin. Most common irritating substances are urine or feces.
- *Candida albicans* lives in the lower intestine of infants and is usually the causative organism in diaper candidiasis.

Clinical Presentation

Skin Findings

- *Chafing dermatitis* occurs in areas with the most friction (thighs, genitalia, buttocks, and abdomen) and presents with mild erythema and fine scale.
- *Irritant contact dermatitis* results from direct skin contact with urine, stool, or chemicals (soap, detergent, creams, etc.) and causes bright red erythema, fine scale, skin breakdown, and superficial erosions on the convex surfaces of the buttocks, vulva, lower abdomen, proximal thighs, and perineum.
- *Diaper candidiasis* appears as bright red plaques with white scaly borders and bright pink-red satellite papules and pustules on the buttocks, lower abdomen, and inner thigh.

Non-Skin Finding

- Extracutaneous findings are uncommon.

DIFFERENTIAL DIAGNOSIS Diaper Dermatitis	
Common	*Uncommon*
• Seborrheic dermatitis	• Nutritional deficiency (e.g., acrodermatitis enteropathica)
• Psoriasis	
• Intertrigo	• Granuloma gluteale infantum
• Folliculitis	• Langerhans cell histiocytosis
• Impetigo	• Epidermolysis bullosa
• Scabies	• Streptococcal perianal cellulitis
• Contact dermatitis	
• Atopic dermatitis	
• Tinea cruris	

Confirming the Diagnosis

- Begin by differentiating between the types of diaper dermatitis
- A thorough history focusing on diaper care helps confirm the diagnosis
- Ask about products used in the bath and during diapering, topical ointments and pastes, cleansing wipes, type of diapers, and frequency of diaper changing
- Perform a KOH or fungal culture to rule out yeast
- If *C. albicans* is present, microscopic KOH examination will show budding yeasts with short hyphae
- If not responsive to antifungals, a bacterial culture and sensitivity can rule out bacterial infection
- See Figure 13.3-4.

Treatment

Topical Treatment

- Treatment depends on the underlying cause of diaper dermatitis.
- For *chafing dermatitis*, reduce the friction by loosening the securing tabs on the diapers, using larger-sized diapers, or using barrier creams, which help reduce friction.
- Primary management of *irritant dermatitis* is to keep the area as clean and dry as possible.
- Skin will improve with more frequent diaper changes, nonirritating, fragrance-free wipes, chemical-free disposable diapers or cloth diapers, exposure to air whenever possible, and liberal use of barrier creams (petrolatum, zinc oxide).
- In the absence of *C. Albicans*, conservative use of low-potency (nonfluorinated) topical corticosteroid ointments (hydrocortisone 2.5% ointment, desonide 0.05% ointment) can be used cautiously for up to 2 weeks, or less if the dermatitis resolves.
- *Diaper candidiasis* can be treated with topical anti-yeast/fungal creams (nystatin, clotrimazole, ketoconazole).
- The authors suggest avoiding combination topical antifungal/corticosteroid products.

Systemic Treatment

- Oral fluconazole is reserved for severe cases.

Management and Patient Education

- Once the cause of diaper dermatitis is determined, treatment and management can be administered, and clearance should be completed within days to weeks.
- Any diaper dermatitis present for more than 3 days is at high risk for developing a secondary candidiasis.
- *Chafing dermatitis* and *diaper candidiasis* are both prone to recurrences.
- Prevention is the focus of patient education for all diaper dermatoses.
- Close follow-up is not needed, as parents should notice improvement after a few days of proper treatment.
- If improvement is not rapid, and in severe or complicated cases, more frequent monitoring may be indicated with phone calls or in-office checkups, especially if oral medications are required.

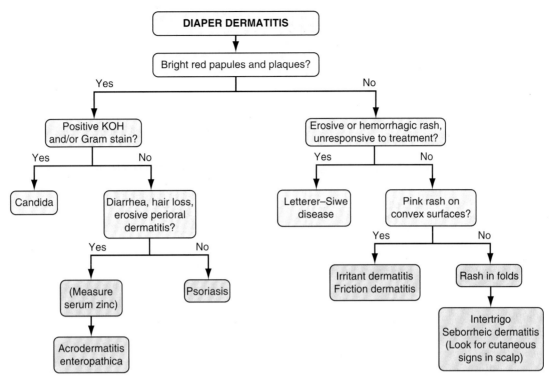

FIG. 13.3-4. Algorithm for diaper dermatitis.

- If treated with topical corticosteroids, the clinician must educate that caregiver about administration, risks, benefits, and side effects of therapy.

Special Considerations

- There are combination antifungal/corticosteroids available.
- These products can lead to overtreatment with topical steroids because the yeast takes longer to resolve than the inflammation.
- Nystatin/Triamcinolone (mid-potency topical corticosteroid) available as Mycolog II and is FDA approved for children >2 years old, but should not be used under occlusion (diapers or plastic pants).
- Clotrimazole/Betamethasone dipropionate, available as Lotrisone, contains a high-potency topical corticosteroid and has been prescribed by some clinicians for diaper dermatitis but is not recommended.
- The manufacturer reports that treatment of diaper dermatitis with clotrimazole/betamethasone in children under 17 years has been reported to cause adrenal suppression in up to 30% of patients.

CLINICAL PEARLS

- In chafing dermatitis, the leg openings and waist are most commonly affected
- If diaper candidiasis is suspected, examine the oral mucosa for oral thrush
- Fungal infection is rare in infants

SLIME DERMATITIS

Slime is a homemade or store-bought material that children enjoy playing with. It is stretchy and gooey, can be made in any color, and resembles Silly Putty. Many varieties exist (glitter slime, glow in the dark slime, uniform slime, etc.). Common ingredients used to make homemade slime include glue, borax, baking soda, shaving cream, and contact lens solution. School glues (common brand Elmer's glue) contains methylchloroisothiazolinone (MCI) and/or methylisothiazolinone (MI), which are a common contact allergens. MCI and MI are commonly found in cosmetics, shampoos, conditioners, shoe glue, wallpaper glue, and many washable glues. Slime dermatitis can be due to irritant contact dermatitis and/or allergic contact dermatitis.

Pathophysiology

- Slime allergic contact dermatitis is most commonly due to an allergic reaction to MCI/MI
- Slime irritant contact dermatitis is due to irritation to any of the other ingredients

Clinical Presentation

Skin Findings

- Acute signs include erythema, edema, scale, papules, and vesicles consistent with allergic contact dermatitis (Fig. 13.3-5).
- If exposure is frequent and repeated, skin findings include lichenification, thicker scale, and fissured plaques consistent with chronic hand dermatitis.

Non-Skin Findings

- Pruritus
- Pain

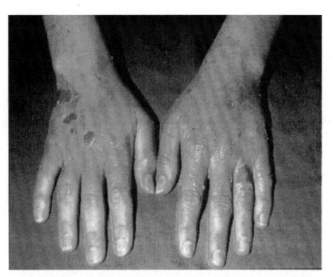

FIG. 13.3-5. Slime dermatitis. (CDC Centers for Disease Control and Prevention. The National Institute for Occupational Safety and Health [NIOSH].)

DIFFERENTIAL DIAGNOSIS   Slime Dermatitis

- Hand eczema
- Dyshidrotic eczema
- Psoriasis
- Tinea manuum

Confirming the Diagnosis

- Thorough history is crucial. Ask about hobbies, interests, art projects, school projects, and class activities at school
- Slime dermatitis will usually spare the dorsal hands as the slime does not come in contact with these areas
- History will confirm that the eruption will come and go, depending on exposure
- Perform KOH to rule out tinea
- Skin biopsy will show allergic contact dermatitis

Treatment

- Removal of offending agent
- Topical steroids. Choose steroid potency depending on the age of the patient and the severity of the dermatitis
- Triamcinolone 0.1% ointment twice daily for up to 1 week is safe and effective in most cases
- If cases are severe, betamethasone 0.05% ointment can be used sparingly
- Apply topical steroids to wet or damp skin to increase treatment response
- Frequent use of emollients to repair skin barrier

Management and Patient Education

- Patch testing to confirm allergies
- If found to be allergic to MCI/MI, patients must avoid exposure to MCI/MI

- Patients who wish to continue to play with slime may do so wearing gloves

---

CLINICAL PEARLS

- The most common allergen identified in slime dermatitis is MCI/MI
- The other ingredients in slime can also cause irritant or allergic contact dermatitis
- Borax has been reported to cause irritant contact dermatitis
- Contact lens solution can contain MCI/MI, propylene glycol, myristamidopropyl dimethylamine, and fragrance, all of which can cause allergic contact dermatitis
- Shaving cream can contain sodium lauryl sulfate, which can cause allergic contact dermatitis

---

NEONATAL LUPUS ERYTHEMATOSUS

Neonatal lupus erythematosus (NLE) is a spectrum of cutaneous, cardiac, and systemic symptoms that occurs in infants whose mothers have antibodies to Ro/SSA and La/SSB, or less commonly U1-ribonucleoprotein (U1-RNP). Some mothers have a known diagnosis of systemic lupus erythematosus (SLE). However, 40% to 60% of mothers are asymptomatic at time of delivery. Many have no known history of connective tissue disease or autoimmune disease. These mothers have a tendency for SLE, rheumatoid arthritis, Sjögren syndrome, or mixed connective tissue disease.

Pathophysiology

- NLE occurs when autoimmune antibodies are passively transferred to the neonate from the mother.
- Antibodies against 52/60-kD Ro/SSA and 48-kD La/SSB ribonucleoproteins are associated with heart block.
- Antibodies against 50-kD La/SSB ribonucleoproteins are associated with cutaneous disease.
- Only about half of mothers who give birth to babies with NLE have a previously diagnosed connective tissue disease.

Clinical Presentation

Skin Findings

- Half of patients display cutaneous symptoms at some point and can be present at birth
- Scaly atrophic erythematous plaques are the most common clinical presentation (Fig. 13.3-6)
- Lesions can be discoid with atrophy and hypopigmentation
- Facial erythema is common, especially around the periorbital areas, termed *raccoon eyes* (Fig. 13.3-7)

Non-Skin Findings

- Almost one quarter of infants with NLE have systemic symptoms at birth
- Cardiac symptoms
  - Congenital heart block, the most common cardiac complication usually develops in utero
  - Heart murmur
  - Bradycardia
- Pancytopenia

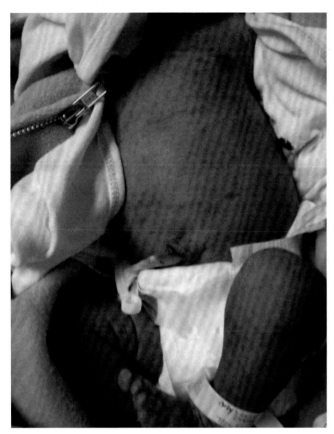

FIG. 13.3-6. Neonatal lupus trunk. (Photo courtesy of Jessica Galvin.)

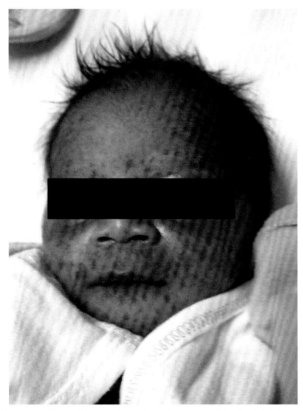

FIG. 13.3-7. Neonatal lupus periorbital. (Photo courtesy of Jessica Galvin.)

- Thrombocytopenia
- Leukopenia
- Elevated transaminases

DIFFERENTIAL DIAGNOSIS	Neonatal Lupus
Common	*Uncommon*
• Seborrheic dermatitis	• Langerhans-cell histiocytosis
• Atopic dermatitis	• Congenital syphilis
• Neonatal acne	• Congenital rubella
• Tinea corporis	• Bloom syndrome
• Granuloma annulare	• Rothmund–Thomson syndrome
• Psoriasis	
• Erythema multiforme	

Confirming the Diagnosis

- Diagnosis requires a thorough history and physical examination.
- Diagnosis is based on cutaneous findings, systemic symptoms, and serology: CBC with platelets, liver function tests, antinuclear antibody (ANA), anti-Ro/SS (present in 90% of cases), anti-La/SSB, U1-RNP, C_3 and C_4, urinalysis.
- Electrocardiography and echocardiography if bradycardia or a heart murmur is detected.
- Mothers should also be screened (regardless of their symptoms) for ANA, anti-Ro, anti-La, anti-U1-RNP, anti–double-stranded DNA.

Treatment
Topical Treatment

- Treatment with low- to mid-potency topical corticosteroids or topical immune modulators can improve erythema, but will not reduce permanent skin changes.

Systemic Treatment

- Patients with bradycardia may require pacemakers.

Management and Patient Education

- Treatment focuses on associated systemic disease and complications.
- If neonatal lupus is suspected, consult with dermatology and cardiology.
- Skin lesions usually fade by age 6 to 12 months, as maternal antibodies wane, but can last longer.
- Lesions heal with telangiectasias.
- One quarter of patients have permanent telangiectasia, hyper- or hypopigmentation, atrophic scars, and/or alopecia.
- Reassure parents that patients do not have a higher risk of developing SLE or other autoimmune disorders.
- NLE patients should have regular well-child visits with a pediatrician and any other specialties needed to manage other complication.

Special Considerations
Pregnancy

- Mothers with one child with NLE have a 22% risk of having another child with NLE.

KAWASAKI DISEASE

Kawasaki disease (KD) or mucocutaneous lymph node syndrome is a multisystem vasculitis that involves small- and medium-sized arteries and has a predilection for coronary vessels. It is the most common vasculitis of childhood (Cohen & Sundel, 2016) and primarily affects infants and children.

Pathophysiology

- The etiology is unknown but clinical and epidemiologic features resemble a viral illness that causes an abnormal immune response in genetically predisposed individuals.
- The disease occurs primarily in children younger than 6 years, and in most cases, it occurs in individuals who live in East Asia or are of Asian ancestry.

Clinical Presentation

Diagnostic criteria: Fever for 5 or more days plus at least four of the five clinical signs:

- Bilateral conjunctival injection without exudate
- Oral mucous membrane changes (injected pharynx, infected or fissured lips, strawberry tongue)
- Peripheral extremity changes (acute: edema and/or erythema; convalescent: periungual desquamation of fingertips)
- Polymorphous skin eruption
- Cervical lymphadenopathy (at least 1.5 cm), usually unilateral

Skin Findings

- Nonexudative bilateral bulbar conjunctival injection
- Dry, red, fissured, crusted lips
- Red, strawberry tongue
- Nonpitting edema of the dorsal hands and feet
- Erythema of the palms and soles
- Polymorphous eruption with nonspecific, diffuse morbilliform or urticarial erythematous eruption, "sandpapery" papules with background erythema, or multiforme-like lesions (Fig. 13.3-8)
- Vesicles, bullae, and purpura are almost never seen
- Skin lesions are accentuated in intertriginous areas, particularly the groin, and on the lower abdomen, perineum, and buttocks
- Periungual desquamation later in the disease, starting on the tips of the fingers and progressing to fingers, toes, palms, and soles

- Beau lines (transverse linear grooves in the nail plates) can be observed months after disease onset

Non-Skin Findings

- Persistent fever for more than 5 days and unresponsive to antipyretics
- Irritability, inconsolability, lethargy
- Gastrointestinal involvement—hepatomegaly, hepatitis, diarrhea, jaundice
- Cardiac sequelae—pericardial effusion, myocarditis, tachycardia, gallop rhythm, congestive heart failure, arrhythmias, mitral valve regurgitation, dilatation, or aneurysms of coronary arteries
- CNS involvement—cerebral infarction, sensorineural hearing loss, cranial nerve palsies, CSF pleocytosis
- Increased ESR

DIFFERENTIAL DIAGNOSIS Kawasaki Disease	
Common	*Uncommon*
• Viral exanthems	• Toxic shock syndrome
• Scarlet fever	• Rocky Mountain spotted fever
• MIRM	• Drug reactions including SJS and TEN
• SSSS	
• Erythema infectiosum	• Connective tissue disorder

Confirming the Diagnosis

- KD is idiopathic, so there are no specific tests used to confirm the diagnosis.
- Lab tests used to support the diagnosis include the following: CBC, ESR, CRP, urine dip for blood and protein, LFTs, serum albumin, EKG, and echocardiogram.
- Lab tests used to rule out other diseases include the following: ASO titer (to rule out strep), nasal swab to check for other viruses, blood culture to rule out sepsis, autoantibody profile to rule out connective tissue disease, serology for tick-borne illnesses, IgM and IgG for *mycoplasma pneumonia*, measles, EBV, enterovirus, parvovirus, and adenovirus.

Treatment

Topical Treatment

- There are no topical treatments for KD other than routine skin care.

Systemic Treatment

- Standard treatment is IV corticosteroids, IVIG, and aspirin.
- Treatment is customized to each individual patient based on symptoms.

Management and Patient Education

- Most patients with KD follow a benign course.
- Twenty to 25% of untreated patients develop a coronary artery aneurysm.
- Patients with lab test abnormalities, early evidence of coronary artery dilatation and those under 6 months of age are at higher risk for complications and should be referred to a KD specialist.

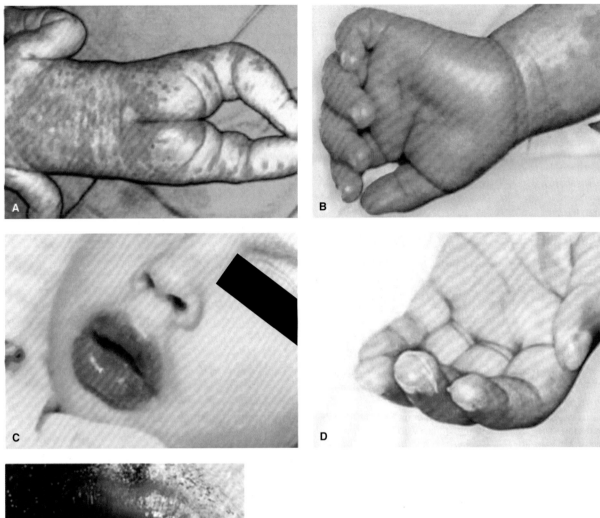

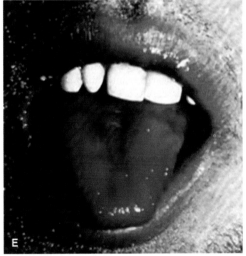

FIG. 13.3-8. Kawasaki disease. **A:** Rash of Kawasaki disease in a 7-month-old child on the fourth day of illness. **B:** Conjunctival injection, lip edema in a 2-year-old boy on the sixth day of illness. **C:** Erythema and edematous hand of a 1.5-year-old girl on the sixth day of illness. **D:** Periungual desquamation in a 3-year-old child on the 12th day of illness. **E:** Strawberry tongue. (A–D: Reprinted with permission from Council on Cardiovascular Disease in Young; Committee on Rheumatic Fever, Endocarditis, and Kawasaki Disease; & American Heart Association. (2001). Diagnostic guidelines for Kawasaki disease. *Circulation, 103*(2), 335–336; E: Reprinted with permission from Goodheart, H. P. [2003]. *Goodheart's photoguide of common skin disorders* [2nd ed.]. Lippincott Williams & Wilkins.)

- These patients should be identified early and treated with corticosteroids and IVIG to improve outcomes.
- There are treatment algorithms for managing "incomplete KD" when patients do not satisfy classic diagnostic criteria.

Special Consideration

Adults

KD in adults is rare, therefore delay in diagnosis is common. Adults present with the same constellation of symptoms.

CLINICAL PEARLS

- KD is a multisystem disease that involves infectious disease, rheumatology, immunology, and cardiology
- Multiple specialties are routinely consulted for suspected and confirmed cases
- KD is the leading cause of acquired heart disease in children
- With appropriate treatment, over 95% of KD cases resolve without sequelae (Cohen & Sundel, 2016)
- Live virus vaccines should not be given for at least 11 months after IVIG

Genetic Disorders

Victoria Garcia-Albea

In This Chapter

- Neurofibromatosis
- Tuberous Sclerosis Complex

NEUROFIBROMATOSIS

Neurofibromatosis (NF) is a genetic disorder with an increased propensity to develop tumors of the nerve sheath. There are two distinct types: NF type 1 (NF1) or von Recklinghausen disease and NF type 2 (NF2) or bilateral acoustic or central NF. This chapter will only discuss NF1 which comprises more than 90% of NF cases.

Neurofibromas are benign tumors that are made up of neuro-mesenchymal tissue. They commonly occur as a single lesion in healthy individuals. When accompanied by other clinical criteria, they can be a marker of *NF*.

Pathophysiology

- NF is an autosomal dominant genetic disorder.
- NF1 and NF2 occur because of an inherited or spontaneous genetic mutation.

Clinical Presentation

Skin Finding
There is great variability in the number and severity of neurofibromas.

Cutaneous Neurofibromas

- Soft, skin-colored papules, 2 mm to 2 cm in diameter (Fig. 13.4-1).
- Occasionally, they can be red, blue, or brown.
- As they enlarge, they may become globular, pear-shaped, or pedunculated.
- Neurofibromas display the "buttonhole" sign defined as easy invagination into the dermis when direct pressure is applied on top of the lesion.

Subcutaneous Neurofibromas

- Firmer lesions that occur deeper in the dermis.
- Less well circumscribed than cutaneous neurofibromas.

Plexiform Neurofibromas

- Tender, firm nodules or masses in the subcutaneous tissue.
- They can occur in the skin, fascia, muscle, and internal structures.

Additional Skin Findings

- Café au lait macules (Fig. 13.4-2)
- Axillary or inguinal freckling (Crowe sign)
- Small juvenile xanthogranulomas may also exist

Non-Skin Findings

- Short stature
- Macrocephaly
- Hypertension
- Hearing loss
- Learning disabilities
- Cardiovascular complications
- Skeletal anomalies
- Ocular manifestations: Lisch nodules and optic gliomas

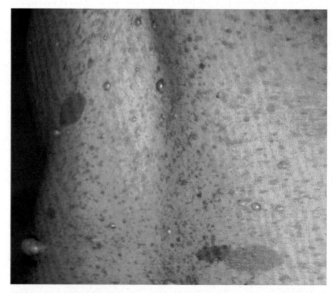

FIG. 13.4-1. Neurofibromatosis multiple neurofibromas. (Photo courtesy of M. Bobonich.)

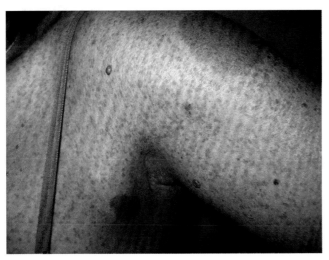

FIG. 13.4-2. Café au lait macules. (Photo courtesy of M. Bobonich.)

Confirming the Diagnosis

- Table 13.4-1 lists diagnostic criteria for NF1 and NF2.
- Genetic testing is available for NF1.

DIFFERENTIAL DIAGNOSIS	Neurofibromatosis
Common	*Uncommon*
• Café au lait macule	• Partial unilateral lentiginosis
• Congenital melanocytic nevi	• McCune–Albright syndrome
• Nevus spilus	

Treatment

- Neurofibromas require no treatment unless they are symptomatic or cosmetically disturbing to the patient.

Management and Patient Education

- If NF1 is suspected, refer patients to a dermatologist, neurologist, or genetic counselor.

TABLE 13.4-1	Diagnostic Criteria for Neurofibromatosis Types 1 and 2
NEUROFIBROMATOSIS TYPE 1	**NEUROFIBROMATOSIS TYPE 2**
Must have at least two of the following: Six café au lait macules at least 0.5 cm in diameter before puberty or at least 1.5 cm in diameter after puberty Axillary freckling A plexiform neurofibroma Two or more derma Neurofibromas Two or more Lisch nodules Optic nerve glioma Pathognomonic skeletal Dysplasia An affected first-degree relative	Bilateral vestibular schwannomas seen on MRI or a first-degree relative with NF2 *and* unilateral vestibular schwannoma or two of the following: Meningioma Glioma Schwannoma Juvenile posterior subcapsular cataract

- Once the diagnosis is established, care may be transferred to a multidisciplinary team specializing in NF.
- Referral should occur as early as possible to optimize patient outcomes.
- Counsel patients about the benign nature of neurofibromas or the association with underlying disease.
- Perform a physical and developmental examination, detailed family history, and examination of family members if indicated.
- Patients with NF1 have a 5% lifetime risk of developing malignancy, including malignant peripheral nerve sheath tumors, nonlymphocytic leukemia, carcinoid, and pheochromocytomas.
- Perform appropriate diagnostic tests if there are positive findings at any time.

CLINICAL PEARLS

- Patients should have annual ophthalmology examinations and complete blood counts
- The presence of neurofibromas alone is not diagnostic for NF, but it should alert the clinician to look for other clinical signs of the disease
- Both sexes and all races are equally affected
- More serious involvement or complications from NF typically present in childhood or adolescence
- If an at-risk patient does not meet diagnostic criteria by age 10 years, they are unlikely to be affected
- The number of cutaneous lesions does not correlate with disease severity

Tuberous Sclerosis Complex

Tuberous sclerosis (TSC) is a genetic disorder characterized by excessive development of hamartomas of the skin, brain, eyes, heart, kidneys, lungs, and bones. Hamartomas are abnormal overgrowths of cells in the skin resulting in benign, tumor-like masses. Nevi are examples of hamartomas. Most patients diagnosed with TSC are between 2 and 6 years of age. TSC affects all races equally and there is no sex predilection. The many cutaneous and systemic features of TSC are reviewed below.

Pathophysiology

- TSC is an autosomal dominant disorder caused by a mutation in one of two genes: *TSC1*, encodes hamartin, and *TSC2* encodes tuberin
- These mutations demonstrate variable expressivity
- Patients with *TSC1* mutation tend to have milder disease

Clinical presentation
Skin Findings

Hypopigmented Macules or Patches

- Lesions range from millimeters to centimeters in diameter
- They do not evolve over time
- They can occur anywhere on the body, but are usually on the trunk

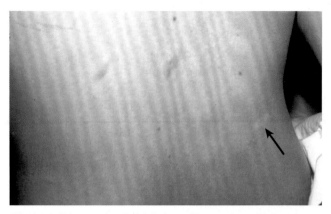

FIG. 13.4-3. Tuberous sclerosis. Ash leaf spot. (Photo courtesy of M. Bobonich.)

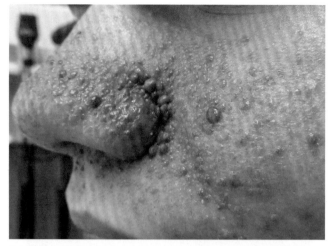

FIG. 13.4-4. Tuberous sclerosis: angiofibromas. (Courtesy S. Moschella, MD.)

- They can take the shape of a "thumbprint," "confetti," or an "ash leaf" (Fig. 13.4-3)

Facial Angiofibromas

- Hamartomas that contain fibrous and vascular tissue
- 1- to 4-mm pink-to-red, smooth, dome-shaped soft papules
- Commonly found on the face, especially around the nose
- Facial angiofibromas can mimic acne in teenagers (Fig. 13.4-4)

Fibrous cephalic (forehead) plaques are histologically similar lesions that can occur unilaterally on the forehead.

Collagenomas

- Connective tissue nevi on the forehead, cheeks, scalp, or trunk
- On the trunk, they are called *shagreen patches* and are more likely to be present at birth (Fig. 13.4-5)
- There may be one or many flesh colored papules in varied sizes that have a leathery texture and follicular openings

Periungual Fibromas

- Benign, small periungual papules (Fig. 13.4-6)
- Common on the toenails and proximal nail folds
- Can be tender
- Can bleed
- Can cause longitudinal droves in the nail

Non-Skin Findings

- Cortical tubers occur in the brain and often precede development of skin lesions by years.
- The more the cortical tubers, the greater the severity of seizures.
- The majority of patients will have epilepsy and a developmental delay.
- Renal lesions include angiomyolipomas, lymphangiomas, benign cysts, renal cell carcinoma.

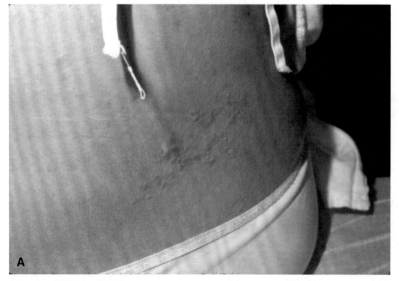
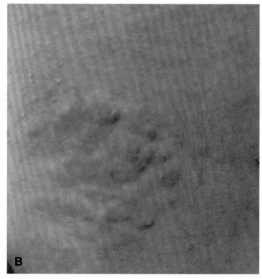

FIG. 13.4-5. **A,B:** Tuberous sclerosis: Shagreen patch. (Courtesy Moschella, MD.)

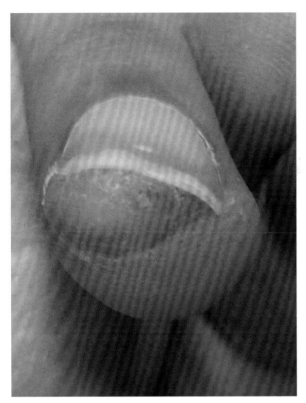

FIG. 13.4-6. Subungual fibroma. (Photo courtesy of M. Bobonich.)

- As angiomyolipomas enlarge, they can cause pain, bleeding, and impaired renal function.
- Cardiac involvement in the form of rhabdomyomas.
- Pulmonary involvement is not common but patients can have lymphangioleiomyomas.
- Dental enamel pits.
- Intraoral fibromas.

TSC-associated neuropsychiatric disorders (TAND)

- Newly described entity
- Behavioral and clinical symptoms
- Aggressive behavior
- Autism spectrum disorder

- Intellectual disability
- Psychiatric disorder
- Neuropsychological deficits
- School and occupational challenges

DIFFERENTIAL DIAGNOSIS	**Tuberous Sclerosius**
Common	*Uncommon*
• Acne	• Nevus depigmentosus
• Vitiligo	• Nevus anemicus
• Multiple endocrine neoplasia type 1 (MEN1)	• Other genetic disorders
• Birt–Hogg–Dube syndrome	
• Nail trauma	

Confirming the Diagnosis

- Diagnosis can be a challenge because the manifestations may initially be very subtle and can involve many organ systems.
- Diagnostic criteria, set forth in the *Recommendations of the 2012 International Tuberous Sclerosis Complex Consensus Conference* (Northrup et al., 2013), identifies the genetic and clinical (major and minor) criteria for a definitive, probable, and possible diagnosis of TSC (Table 13.4-2).
- Blood tests for TSC1 and TSC2 mutations are available.
- Dermatologic and dental manifestations are present in almost 100% of patients so a thorough oral examination is recommended if suspicions are high.
- Thorough skin examination should reveal multiple markers for the disease and should result in a prompt referral for evaluation and diagnosis.
- If TSC is suspected, refer to a dermatologist, neurologist, or genetic counselor.

Treatment

Topical Treatment

- Skin lesions do not require treatment because they are benign.
- Angiofibromas respond to sirolimus 0.2% gel and rapamycin 1% ointment, which are topical mTOR inhibitors.
- Angiofibromas can be treated with laser, cryotherapy, curettage, chemical peels, or excision if they are of cosmetic concern.

TABLE 13.4-2	Cutaneous Manifestations in the Diagnostic Criteria for Tuberous Sclerosus		
CUTANEOUS/DERMATOLOGIC SYMPTOM	**CRITERIA**	**PROPORTION WITH CUTANEOUS MANIFESTATION**	**ONSET OF SYMPTOMS**
Hypomelanotic macules (≥3, at least 5 mm diameter)	Major	90%	Birth or infancy
Angiofibromas (≥3), or	Major	75%	2–5 yr of age
Fibrous cephalic (forehead) plaque	Major	25%	Usually present at birth
Ungual fibromas (≥2)	Major	20% in children; 80% adults	Second decade or later
Shagreen patch	Major	50%	First decade of life
"Confetti" skin lesions	Minor	5–58%	First decade of life

From Northrup, H., & Krueger, D. A.; International Tuberous Sclerosis Complex Consensus Group. (2013). Tuberous sclerosis complex diagnostic criteria update: Recommendations of the 2012 International Tuberous Sclerosis Complex Consensus Conference. *Pediatric Neurology, 49*(4), 243–254.

Systemic Treatment

- Oral sirolimus, a systemic mTOR inhibitor can reduce seizure activity and glioneuronal hamartoma growth.

Management and Patient Education

- Treatment is directed at symptoms.
- Care is multidisciplinary.
- Referral to a specialty center is recommended once diagnosis is made.
- Prognosis depends on disease severity and the extent of neurologic involvement.
- Parents should receive genetic counseling, especially if they are considering having more children.
- Patient follow-up depends on disease severity and system involvement.

CLINICAL PEARLS

- The onset of cutaneous features varies by age, so continued vigilance is important
- Lesions that occur within the first few years of life
  - Hypomelanotic macules
  - Fibrous forehead papule
- Lesions that can occur at any time
  - Facial angiofibromas
- Lesions that occur anytime during childhood
  - Shagreen patch
- Lesions that occur from childhood to adolescence
  - Ungual and periungual fibromas
  - Confetti-like macules
- Cutaneous and dental manifestations are present in nearly all patients with TSC

Birthmarks and Vascular Malformations

Victoria Garcia-Albea

Vascular Disorders of Infancy

Vascular lesions can be classified into two categories: tumors and malformations. Although both can be present at birth, their pathogenesis, clinical presentation, and evolution during the first few months of life are different.

Understanding the progression of various vascular lesions can aid in an accurate diagnosis. Vascular lesions may be associated with or an indication of systemic disease or genetic syndromes.

In this chapter, specific vascular tumors and malformations will be discussed, but tumor and malformation syndromes are beyond the scope of this textbook.

Vascular Tumors

Vascular tumors are benign vascular growths that include infantile hemangiomas (IHs) and pyogenic granulomas (PGs). They also include tufted angioma and kaposiform hemangioendothelioma, which will not be discussed in this chapter.

Infantile Hemangiomas

IHs or hemangiomas of infancy are the most common benign soft tissue tumor of childhood. They occur in 4% to 10% of full-term infants. IHs are more common in girls than in boys (3-5:1) and premature infants. Most are not present at birth, but develop in the first 4 weeks of life, and are often first noticed by the parents.

Pathophysiology

- Angiogenesis and vasculogenesis possibly play a role
- Glucose transporter protein type-1 (GLUT-1) is present only in IHs
- Vascular endothelial growth factor (VEGF) may also play a role as patients with proliferating IHs have higher levels of VEGF compared to involuting IHs and negative controls
- IHs evolve in three phases:
  - The *Proliferation phase* occurs within the first 8 weeks of life, much earlier than previously thought, and is characterized by rapid growth. During proliferation, an imbalance in angiogenic factors and an increase in VEGF are seen
  - *Plateau phase* follows for up to 6 months and usually has no growth of the lesion
  - *Involutional phase* is the final phase, in which there is dramatic color change from bright red to dull red, purple, or gray. During the involution phase, the center of the hemangioma begins to involute or flatten

Clinical Presentation

Skin Findings

- IHs can be categorized as superficial, deep, or mixed, and are described by phases
  - *Superficial* hemangiomas present as bright red, flat or raised papules, plaques, or nodules
  - *Deep* hemangiomas appear as subcutaneous nodules with an overlying blue discoloration and may have telangiectasias or a prominent venous network
  - *Mixed* hemangiomas, the most common type, have both a superficial and deep component causing them to appear bright red with a nodular blue component
- All types tend to be compressible, slightly more solid than a lipoma, but not as firm as a lymph node or cyst
- IHs are most common on the head and neck, but can appear anywhere on the body, including internally (Fig. 13.5-1)

Non-Skin Findings

- More than five cutaneous IHs increases the likelihood of having internal involvement. The liver is the most common internal site affected
- Visceral hemangiomas (such as in the liver) predispose patients to high-output heart failure
- Large segmental facial hemangiomas can indicate PHACE syndrome (posterior fossa malformations, hemangiomas, arterial abnormalities, coarctation of the aorta and cardiac defects, and eye abnormalities)

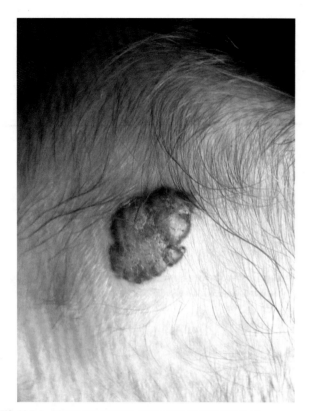

FIG. 13.5-1. Infantile hemangioma. (Photo courtesy of M. Bobonich.)

TABLE 13.5-1	Features of High-Risk Infantile Hemangiomas
LOCATION	**ASSOCIATED RISKS**
Periorbital hemangiomas	Impaired development of normal binocular vision, amblyopia, astigmatism, strabismus, proptosis, and optic atrophy
Nasal tip hemangiomas	Distortion of nasal anatomy and disfigurement
Lip hemangiomas	Increased risk of ulceration, bleeding, scarring Feeding problems
Ear hemangiomas	Possible obstruction of the auditory canal and conductive hearing loss Cosmetically problematic
"Beard area" hemangiomas (neck, lower lip, chin, preauricular, mandibular area)	Increased risk for airway obstruction, feeding difficulties, respiratory stridor, and hoarseness Patients may require immediate laryngoscopy
Genital and perineal hemangiomas	Frequent ulceration and bleeding Increased risk for infection, pain, and scarring
Lumbosacral hemangiomas	Possible occult spinal dysraphism or spinal cord defect (tethered cord most common) Anorectal, urogenital, and renal abnormalities
Segmental hemangiomas	Higher incidence of urogenital anomalies
PHACES syndrome	Genetic disorder with constellation of features: P—posterior fossa abnormality (brain and especially cerebellum) H—hemangiomas (head, face, and/or neck) A—arterial anomalies (brain) C—cardiac anomalies or aortic coarctation E—eye abnormalities S—sternal clefting, supraumbilical abdominal raphe, or thyroid abnormalities
Five or more lesions anywhere on the body	At risk for visceral involvement, further workup is recommended

DIFFERENTIAL DIAGNOSIS	Infantile Hemangiomas
Common	*Uncommon*
• Cyst	• Congenital hemangioma
• Lipoma	• Venous malformation
• Trauma	• Glioma
• Port wine stain	• Nevus anemicus
• Pyogenic granuloma	• Leukemia cutis
	• Plexiform neurofibroma
	• Tufted angioma

Confirming the Diagnosis

- IHs are usually diagnosed clinically with the help of the history of the lesion as provided by parents, photos, or in-office monitoring.

- Hemangiomas can be differentiated from vascular malformations, as the latter are more likely to be present at birth and do not proliferate or involute.

- If the distinction cannot be made based on history and physical examination, it is highly recommended that an experienced dermatology provider or surgical specialist evaluate the patient.

- If the IH has any high-risk features, additional imaging, biopsy, and other studies are indicated to carefully diagnose the extent and severity of the vascular tumor (Table 13.5-1).

Treatment

Topical Treatment

- For IHs that are small, solitary, and do not pose a risk of life or function-threatening or disfigurement, no treatment is necessary.

- The β-blocker, timolol, is effective and is available as a topical gel.

- Children must be monitored closely for side effects including hypoglycemia, hypotension, and bronchospasm.

- Ulcerated IHs require local wound care, antifungal and antibiotic therapy as needed.

Surgical Treatment

- Pulsed dye laser (PDL) can be used to treat and reduce pain of ulcerated hemangiomas.

Systemic Treatment

- Until a few years ago, oral corticosteroids were the gold standard of treatment for large, life-threatening, or function-threatening hemangiomas and oral corticosteroids are still used to hasten involution in some cases.

- Current therapies include the oral β-blocker propranolol, which has been shown to rapidly stop proliferation and induce involution.

- Oral antibiotics if ulcerated IHs become superinfected.

Management and Patient Education

- Over time, IHs become smaller, softer, and less warm.
- Most IHs can be monitored and do not require treatment.
- The management goals are to prevent life-threatening complications, minimize disfigurement, prevent or reverse functional impairment, and reduce psychosocial stress.
- Multidisciplinary teams providing care have protocols for initiation and monitoring of treatment.
- Approximately 10% to 15% of IHs ulcerate, which usually occurs during the proliferation phase.
- IHs in the diaper area are at higher risk for ulceration.
- When the skin breaks down, the IH bleeds, becomes painful, and increases risk for secondary infection and possible scarring.
- Care of ulcerated IHs includes warm compresses, topical antibiotics, and petrolatum-based nonstick gauze dressings.
- A culture should be taken if IHs become deeply ulcerated, have drainage, or exudate.
- Infection requires appropriate use of oral antibiotics.
- Involution is completed by age 10 years in 90% of cases.
- Once the IH has involuted, there are usually residual telangiectasias, atrophy, scarring, or a fibro-fatty mass (like a lipoma).

Special Considerations

- High-risk IHs that are life and function-threatening require prompt referral to a specialist, ideally a multidisciplinary team dedicated to children with vascular anomalies (usually academic centers), for evaluation and treatment.
- Large IHs may be more resistant to treatment and require multidisciplinary approach.
- **Ulceration** approximately 10% to 15% of IHs ulcerate which usually occurs during the proliferation phase.

Pyogenic Granuloma

A pyogenic granuloma (PG) is a common benign lobular capillary hemangioma. The incidence is higher in children and pregnant women.

Pathophysiology

- The etiology is unknown, but they often develop following minor trauma.
- PGs are exophytic papules comprised of blood vessels.

Clinical Presentation

Skin Findings

- Well-circumscribed, small (<1 cm) red papules
- Rapidly growing
- Polypoid red mass
- Can ulcerate and bleed easily
- The most common site is on the face and acral areas, particularly the fingers and toes (Fig. 13.5-2)
- Biopsy shows a lobular vascular proliferation with inflammation

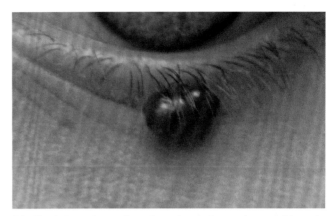

FIG. 13.5-2. Pyogenic granuloma. Pyogenic granuloma on lower eyelid margin. (Used with permission from Gru, A. A., & Wick, M. [2018]. *Pediatric dermatopathology and dermatology.* Wolters Kluwer Health.)

DIFFERENTIAL DIAGNOSIS	Pyogenic Granuloma
Common	*Uncommon*
• Melanocytic nevus	• Glomus tumor
• Hemangioma	• Amelanotic melanoma
• Irritated nevus	
• Verruca vulgaris	
• Spitz nevus	

Confirming the Diagnosis

- Diagnosis is confirmed with a skin biopsy which may also resolve the lesion.

Treatment

Topical Treatment

- Topical 1% propranolol twice daily until resolution
- Imiquimod 5% cream daily until resolution
- Silver nitrate can be used for smaller lesions

Surgical Treatment

- Shave removal or excision followed by electrocautery is sufficient to remove most lesions
- Recurrence is common
- Excision is effective and may provide a lower rate of recurrence
- Desiccation and curettage
- Cryotherapy may be effective for small lesions

Systemic Treatment

- There are no systemic treatments for PG

Management and Patient Education

- PGs are benign, but if not removed, they can persist.
- Refer to a dermatologist, plastic surgeon, or general surgeon for excision and biopsy.
- Reassure the patient and family that these are benign. No follow-up is needed.
- If a PG occurs in a cosmetically sensitive location, use caution when using destructive treatments as scarring can result.

Vascular Malformations

A vascular malformation is an abnormal development of blood vessels that occurs without any endothelial cell growth or proliferation. Vascular malformations are often present at birth, and do not undergo rapid progression, or involution. Thus, vascular malformations are permanent.

Vascular malformations are categorized by the predominant vessel involved, including capillary, venous, and arteriovenous malformations (AVMs).

Pathophysiology

Vascular malformations can be affected by hormonal changes during puberty and pregnancy and can result from fluid or blood accumulating in poorly formed veins or lymphatic channels

Clinical Presentation

Skin Findings

Salmon Patch

* A salmon patch, also known as *nevus simple,* is a common capillary malformation that occurs in 30% to 40% of all newborns.
* *Angel's kiss* refers to salmon patches on the occipital scalp, forehead or eyelids, glabella, nose or nasolabial area while *stork bites* are located on the posterior neck.
* Lesions become more pronounced when infants cry, hold their breath, strain during defecation, or physically exert themselves.

Port Wine Stain

* A port wine stain (PWS) or *nevus flammeus* is the most common type of vascular malformation, highest in Caucasian newborns
* They initially appear as pink patches, then become dark red color over time (Fig. 13.5-3)
* They can occur anywhere on the body but are most common on the face

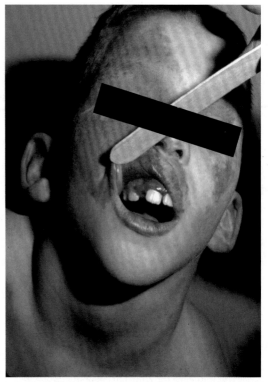

FIG. 13.5-4. Sturge–Weber syndrome. (Photo courtesy of W. Elliot Love.)

* Almost always unilateral
* Can become raised or develop nodules and blebs

Non-Skin Findings

Salmon Patch

* No non-skin findings.

Port Wine Stain

* PWS can affect the growth of underlying tissue.
* They can be associated with Sturge–Weber syndrome (Fig. 13.5-4), Parkes–Weber syndrome, Klippel–Trenaunay syndrome, hyperkeratotic cutaneous capillary-venous malformation, and Proteus syndrome.
* If the PWS is in the trigeminal area, there is a high risk of glaucoma.
* Lesions covering an extremity should be carefully evaluated for risk of venous stasis, varicosities, lymphedema, ulcerations, and Klippel–Trenaunay syndrome.
* Patients with facial PWS may have Sturge–Weber syndrome, glaucoma, or complications of the central nervous system.

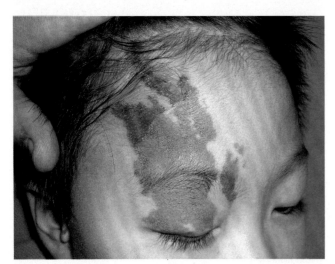

FIG. 13.5-3. Port wine stain.

DIFFERENTIAL DIAGNOSIS	Port Wine Stain
Common	*Uncommon*
• Birth trauma	• Morphea
• Infantile hemangiomas	• Sturge–Weber syndrome
• Salmon patch	• Parkes–Weber syndrome
• Cellulitis	• Klippel–Trenaunay syndrome
• Allergic contact dermatitis	• Hyperkeratotic cutaneous capillary-venous malformation
	• Proteus syndrome

Confirming the Diagnosis

- Capillary malformations can be diagnosed clinically.
- No workup is needed for most lesions.
- Monitor lesions over time for proliferation or involution to help make the diagnosis.
- Ultrasound can be utilized if the diagnosis is uncertain or if there is concern for involvement below the skin.
- If a syndrome is suspected, genetic testing can be performed.
- Skin biopsy would also confirm the diagnosis.

Treatment

- Salmon patches are benign and have no associated developmental risks, and therefore do not require treatment.
- Pulse dye laser can effectively treat PWS.
- The earlier a PWS is treated with laser, the better it responds.
- Laser treatment for PWS requires referral to a cardiovascular or dermatology specialist with experience treating PWS in children.

Management and Patient Education

- The size of the lesion, location, and possible associated syndromes will influence the clinician's plan of care.
- Most PWS are small and benign, require no treatment, and fade slightly over time.
- Reassure and educate parents that lesions become more pronounced during crying, or straining to defecate.
- If there is any suspicion for an associated syndrome, a prompt referral to a dermatologist, neurologist, and ophthalmologist is essential.
- The above-mentioned genetic syndromes are managed by dermatology, ophthalmology, radiology, plastic surgery, and vascular surgery.
- Ninety-five percent of salmon patches on the face fade by age 2 years.
- Some salmon patches on the neck fade over time, while others may remain visible for life.
- Neck lesions are usually covered by hair and are therefore minimally bothersome cosmetically.
- If the PWS is in the trigeminal area, patients must be followed by ophthalmology to monitor for glaucoma.

CLINICAL PEARLS

- Unlike infantile hemangiomas, PWS are static and do not undergo a proliferation phase
- PWS can be indistinguishable from IHs at birth as they can both appear as dark red vascular papules or plaques. Natural evolution differs, so history of the lesion is key to making the correct diagnosis
- Even when not associated with a genetic syndrome, these lesions are almost always of cosmetic importance because of their size and location
- If cosmesis is a concern, the patch can usually be covered with camouflage makeup such as Dermablend

---

VENOUS MALFORMATIONS

Venous malformations (VMs) are the most common of all vascular anomalies. Although they are congenital, they may not be clinically obvious until infancy, childhood, or adulthood.

Pathophysiology

- These are slow-flow vascular malformations resulting from the abnormal development of venules or veins
- The exact etiology is not well understood
- Most appear to be sporadic
- There are familial cases caused by autosomal dominant inheritance (i.e., Klippel–Trenaunay syndrome)
- Some VMs may also present with a lymphatic malformation (LM) and arterionenous malformation (AVM)

Clinical Presentation

Skin Findings

- At birth, a VM may appear as blue or purple nodules, such as in Blue rubber bleb nevus syndrome, which is a genetic condition that causes AVMs in the skin and GI tract (Fig. 13.5-5).
- It may not be detectable for a few years.
- Initially, they are asymptomatic, soft, and compressible.
- Most common on the face, trunk, and extremities.

Non-Skin Findings

- When the limb is in a dependent position, the lesion can become engorged with blood

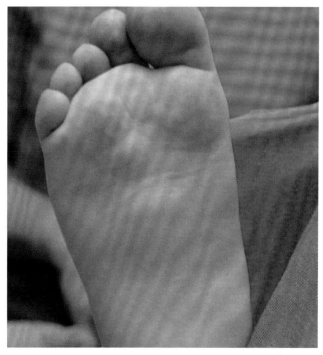

FIG. 13.5-5. Venous malformation. Venous malformation foot. (Used with permission from Gru, A. A., & Wick, M. [2018]. *Pediatric dermatopathology and dermatology.* Wolters Kluwer Health.)

- Localized intravascular coagulopathy
- Blood clots can form following trauma or venous stasis
- Pain may develop as lesions enlarge and apply pressure on surrounding structures.
- Disfigurement and possible psychosocial distress
- Limited mobility
- Infections are quite common
- VM can affect developing bones and cause deformities

DIFFERENTIAL DIAGNOSIS	Venous Malformations
Common	*Uncommon*
• Infantile hemangioma	• Blood clot
• Trauma	• Kasabach–Merritt syndrome
	• Klippel–Trenaunay syndrome

Confirming the Diagnosis

- VMs can be diagnosed with CT scan, MRI, or Doppler ultrasonography.
- VMs lack thrills or bruits on auscultation.
- By comparison, AVMs commonly have a thrill or bruit on auscultation.
- VMs do not pulsate.

Treatment

Topical Treatment

- Compression stockings for VMs of the extremities

Surgical Treatment

- If there are no significant symptoms or risks, surgical treatment is not necessary.
- Sclerotherapy is the gold standard treatment using direct percutaneous puncture with contrast injection performed under fluoroscopy (Behravesh et al., 2016).
- Surgical excision to remove smaller lesions.
- Some authors advocate for early surgical intervention to prevent symptoms and to reduce long-term complications.

Systemic Treatment

- Low-dose aspirin can help prevent thrombotic events

Management and Patient Education

- As lesions enlarge, they can become nodular with swelling and pain
- VMs are difficult to treat and are typically managed by a pediatric vascular anomaly team
- Compression stockings reduce pain, swelling, and risk for blood clots
- Refer patients to a dermatologist and/or surgeon
- Follow-up in a pediatric specialty clinic is advised

Special Considerations

- Orbital VMs can be associated with proptosis, engorged retinal or conjunctival vessels, impaired movement of extraocular muscles, pain, and visual impairment.
- Refer to ophthalmology when diagnosing VMs on the face.
- Klippel–Trenaunay syndrome (VM and LM) often results in abnormal development of the underlying soft tissue and bone growth in the limb.
- Refer to specialists for treatment.
- Inform parents that lesions are difficult to treat.

CLINICAL PEARLS

- There are no thrills or bruits on auscultation
- Lesions on extremities often display more frequent symptoms than those on the trunk
- Extremity lesions are more symptomatic and are more prone to recurrence
- VMs on the extremities are more likely to require treatment
- Chronic localized intravascular coagulopathy can cause coagulopathy or hemorrhage in newborns

Arteriovenous Malformations

AVM is a rare vascular malformation involving both arteries and veins. These are the most serious type of vascular anomaly and can cause functional deformity, cardiovascular compromise, and cosmetic concerns. AVMs may become apparent later in life as blood flow increases through abnormal connections between arteries and veins.

Pathophysiology

- AVMs are high-flow lesions resulting from the shunting between the artery and vein, bypassing the capillaries.
- Lesions are present at birth, but if there is minimal skin involvement, they may not be detected until years later.
- AVMs get larger over time; signs and symptoms of AVMs may not be clinically obvious until the second or third decade of life.

Clinical Presentation

Skin Findings

- AVMs range from small red patches to thin vascular plaques or large pulsating masses (Fig. 13.5-6).
- Overlying skin may be thickened.
- Most start out as a vascular blush that begins to expand and bleed.

Non-Skin Findings

- May have an audible bruit or thrill on auscultation
- Scalp or facial lesions can cause seizures and headaches

DIFFERENTIAL DIAGNOSIS	AVM
Common	*Uncommon*
• Infantile hemangioma	• Venous malformation
• Port wine stain	
• Trauma	

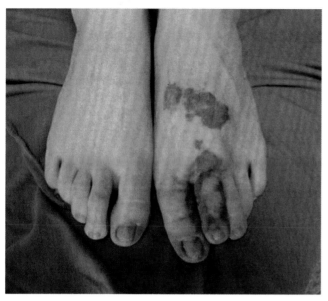

FIG. 13.5-6. AV Malformation. Arteriovenous malformation with associated overgrowth of the left foot. (Used with permission from Gru, A. A., & Wick, M. [2018]. *Pediatric dermatopathology and dermatology.* Wolters Kluwer Health.)

Confirming the Diagnosis

- Ultrasound
- CT
- MRI
- Angiography

Treatment

There are no topical or systemic treatments available for AVMs

Surgical Treatment

- Treatment depends on the age of the patient, comorbidities, and the size, location, and severity of the AVM
- Options include monitoring, excision, amputation, or embolization
- When localized to the skin, excision and embolization can be curative

Management and Patient Education

- Prognosis depends on the location of the AVM.
- Lesions grow faster during puberty or other hormonal changes.
- They can undergo frequent, dramatic, and rapid growth spurts, which are caused by a number of environmental factors.
- They can be life-threatening because of the risk of massive bleeding from cutaneous and internal lesions.
- Refer patients to a multidisciplinary team experienced in managing vascular anomalies.

  Dermatology, cardiology, neurology, and other specialists may be involved.

- Monitor patients regularly for signs and symptoms of AVM reexpansion or cardiovascular compromise.

Special Considerations

Pregnancy

- Although stable in childhood, AVMs may worsen during pregnancy because of increased blood pressure and blood volume.

CLINICAL PEARLS

- Lesions grow faster during puberty or other hormonal changes
- Some AVMs are internal and are only detected when patients become symptomatic

---

READINGS AND REFERENCES

Adegboyega, P. A., & Qui, S. (2005). Hemangioma versus vascular malformation: Presence of nerve bundle is a diagnostic clue for vascular malformation. *Archives of Pathology and Laboratory Medicine, 129*(6), 772–775.

Anderson, L. E., Treat, J. R., Brod, B. A., & Yu, J. (2019). "Slime" contact dermatitis: Case report and review of relevant allergens. *Pediatric Dermatology, 36*(3), 335–337.

Behravesh, S., Yakes, W., Gupta, N., Naidu, S., Chong, B. W., Khademhosseine, A., & Oklu, R. (2016). Venous malformations: Clinical diagnosis and treatment. *Cardiovascular Diagnosis and Therapy, 6*(6), 557–569.

Buckmiller, L. M., Richter, G. T., & Suen, J. Y. (2010). Diagnosis and management of hemangiomas and vascular malformations of the head and neck. *Oral Diseases, 16*(5), 405–418.

Centers for Disease Control and Prevention. (2012). Measles serology. http://www.cdc.gov/measles/lab-tools/serology.html

Cohen, E., & Sundel, R. (2016). Kawasaki disease at 50 years. *JAMA Pediatrics, 170*(11), 1093–1099.

Coughlin, C. C., & Taïeb, A. (2014). Evolving concepts of neonatal skin. *Pediatric Dermatology, 31*(Suppl 1), 5–8.

de Graaf, M., Breur, J. M. P. J., Raphaël, M. F., Vos, M., Breugem, C. C., & Pasmans, S. G. M. A. (2011). Adverse effects of propranolol when used in the treatment of hemangiomas: A case series of 28 infants. *Journal of the American Academy of Dermatology, 65*(2), 320–327.

Eichenfield, L. F., Krakowski, A. C., Piggott, C., Del Rosso, J., Baldwin, H., Friedlander, S. F., Levy, M., Lucky, A., Mancini, A. J., Orlow, S. J., Yan, A. C., Vaux, K. K., Webster, G., Zaenglein, A. L., & Thiboutot, D. M.; American Acne and Rosacea Society. (2013). Evidence-based recommendations for the diagnosis and treatment of pediatric acne. *Pediatrics, 131*(Suppl 3), S163–S186.

Ganguly, S., & Kuruvila, S. (2016). Eczema coxsackium. *Indian Journal of Dermatology, 61*(6), 682–683.

Glitter, J. K., Garzon, M. C., & Lauren, C. T. (2018). "Slime" may not be so benign: A cause of hand dermatitis. *The Journal of Pediatrics, 200*, 288.

Heller, E., Murthy, A. S., & Jen, M. V. (2019). A slime of the times: Two cases of acute irritant contact dermatitis from homemade slime. *Pediatric Dermatology, 36*(1), 139–141.

Hon, K. L., & Leung, A. K. C. (2012). Neonatal lupus erythematosus. *Autoimmune diseases, 2012*, 301274. https://doi.org/10.1155/2012/30127

Kusari, A., Han, A. M., Virgen, C. A., Matiz, C., Rasmussen, M., Friedlander, S. F., & Eichenfield, D. Z. (2019). Evidence-based skin care in preterm infants. *Pediatric Dermatology, 36*(1), 16–23.

Liu, A. S., Mulliken, J. B., Zurakowski, D. Fishman, S. J., & Greene, A. K. (2010). Extracranial arteriovenous malformations: Natural progression and recurrence after treatment. *Plastic and Reconstructive Surgery, 125*(4), 1185–1194.

Martínez-Pérez, M., Imbernón-Moya, A., Lobato-Berezo, A., & Churruca-Grijelmo, M. (2016). Mycoplasma pneumoniae-induced mucocutaneous rash: A new syndrome distinct from erythema multiforme? Report of a new case and review of the literature. *Actas Dermosifiliogr, 107*(7), e47–e51. https://doi.org/10.1016/j.ad.2015.09.02

Melancon, J. M., Dohil, M. A., & Eichenfield, L. F. (2012). Facial port wine stain: When to worry? *Pediatric Dermatology, 29*(1), 131–133.

Miller, P. K., Zain-Ul-Abideen, M., Paul, J., Perry, A. E., Linos, K., Carter, J. B., Kurtzberg, J., & Mann, J. A. (2017). A case of eczema coxsackium with erythema multiforme-like histopathology in a 14-year-old boy with chronic graft-versus-host disease. *JAAD Case Reports, 3*(1), 49–52.

Mishra, A. K., Yadav, P., & Mishra, A. (2016). A systemic review on Staphylococcal scalded skin syndrome (SSSS): A rare and critical disease of neonates. *Open Microbiology Journal, 10*, 150–159.

Northrup, H., & Krueger, D. A.; International Tuberous Sclerosis Complex Consensus Group. (2013). Tuberous sclerosis complex diagnostic criteria update: Recommendations of the 2012 International Tuberous Sclerosis Complex Consensus Conference. *Pediatric Neurology, 49*(4), 243–254.

O'Connor, N. R., McLaughlin, M. R., & Ham, P. (2008). Newborn skin: Part I. Common rashes. *American Family Physician, 77*(1), 47–52.

Paller, A. S., & Mancini, A. J. (2015). A textbook of skin disorders of childhood & adolescence. *Hurwitz clinical pediatric dermatology.* (5th ed.). Elsevier Saunders.

Pride, H. B., Tollefson, M., & Silverman, R. (2013). What's new in pediatric dermatology? Part I. Diagnosis and pathogenesis. *Journal of the American Academy of Dermatology, 68*(6), 885.e1–e12; quiz 897–898.

Pride, H. B., Tollefson, M., & Silverman, R. (2013). What's new in pediatric dermatology? Part II. Treatment. *Journal of the American Academy of Dermatology, 68*(6), 899.e1–e11; quiz 910–912.

Schalock, P. C., & Dinulos, J. G. H. (2009). Mycoplasma pneumoniae-induced cutaneous disease. *International Journal of Dermatology, 48*(7), 673–680; quiz 680–681.

Schwartz, R. A., Janusz, C. A., & Janniger, C. K. (2006). Seborrheic dermatitis: An overview. *American Family Physician, 74*(1), 125–130.

Yang, E. A., & Lee, K. Y. (2017). Additional corticosteroids or alternative antibiotics for the treatment of macrolide-resistant Mycoplasma pneumoniae pneumonia. *Korean Journal of Pediatrics, 60*(8), 245–247.

Zhang, A. J., Boyd, A. H., Asch, S., & Warshaw, E. M. (2019). Allergic contact dermatitis to slime: The epidemic of isothiazolinone allergy encompasses school glue. *Pediatric Dermatology, 36*(1), e37–e38.

Approach to the Wound Patient

Jeremy Honaker

CHAPTER

14

In This Chapter

- Wound Definitions
- How to Approach a Patient with a Wound
- Wounds Differential Diagnosis
- Pressure Injury Staging System
- Phases of Wound Healing

- Impediments to Wound Healing
- Wound Management
- Topical Anti-Microbial/Antiseptics
- Wound Care Dressings
- Common Chronic Wounds

Wound is defined as an injury (e.g., laceration, skin tear) to the body resulting in a break in the skin barrier (open wound) or blunt trauma causing damage to underlying tissue (closed wound). Wounds are often classified by etiology and include traumatic wounds, surgical wounds, thermal injuries (e.g., frostbite, burns), infectious wounds (e.g., abscesses), pressure injuries (PIs), venous ulcers, arterial ulcers, malignancy, and wounds associated with systemic disease. Wounds are further classified as acute (<6 weeks) or chronic (>6 weeks) and can be considered partial (dermal exposure only) or full thickness (subcutaneous, muscle, tendon exposure). An *acute wound* (e.g., surgical, lacerations) is considered to be one that passes through the wound healing process and responds to local treatment within the expected time frame. In contrast, a *chronic wound* is a wound that fails to progress in an orderly fashion through the phases of wound healing. It has been estimated that the prevalence of chronic, non-healing wounds (NHWs) occurs in about 2% of the U.S. population. The overall cost burden of NHWs is estimated conservatively at $35 to $50 billion per year. NHWs can be life-impairing or life-altering for a short period or can continue for many years resulting in significant impact on mental health, financial security, social interactions, and ability to complete activities of daily living. Primary care providers serve as a point of care for patients with wounds.

A working knowledge of the diagnostic approach to the etiology of wounds, wound healing principles, and management is essential. Clinicians must also be mindful of potential complications which may require timely referral.

HOW TO APPROACH A PATIENT WITH A WOUND

Identifying the underlying cause of the wound is the first essential step (Table 14-1). In addition, clinicians must simultaneously identify comorbidities, medications, and other host factors that may delay wound healing (Table 14-2).

Wound History

The initial evaluation for wounds involves a comprehensive history (Box 14-1) and detailed review of systems (see Section 1.3).

TABLE 14-1	Potential Causes/Differential Diagnosis Wound
Trauma	Pressure injury Skin tears Burns
Infections	Bacterial Viral Fungal Atypical mycobacterial
Hypersensitivity	Vasculitis Stevens–Johnson syndrome/toxic epidermal necrolysis
Autoimmune disease	Bullous pemphigoid Pemphigus vulgaris Systemic lupus erythematosus Rheumatoid arthritis

Systemic disease	Diabetes Mellitus
	    Necrobiosis lipoidica
	    Bullosis diabeticorum
	Sarcoidosis
	Pyoderma gangrenosum

Vascular disorders	Venous leg ulcer Arterial ulcer Mixed arteriovenous disease
Malignancy	Lymphoproliferative Basal/squamous cell carcinoma Melanoma Cutaneous metastasis
Psychogenic disorders	Skin picking disease Factitial dermatitis
Vasculopathy	Calciphylaxis Emboli

Adapted from Morton, L. M., & Phillips, T. J. (2016). Wound healing and treating wounds: Differential diagnosis and evaluation of chronic wounds. *Journal of the American Academy of Dermatology, 74*(4), 589–605; quiz 605–606.

521

TABLE 14-2	Host Factors Influencing Wound Healing
Comorbidities	Diabetes Anemia Heart failure Hypertension Peripheral arterial disease Chronic venous insufficiency Deep vein thrombosis Lymphedema Inflammatory bowel disease Peripheral neuropathy Tetraplegia Anxiety Obsessive-compulsive disorder Depression Lower extremity surgery/injury
Medications	Chemotherapeutics Immunosuppressants (prednisone, methotrexate, etc.) Hydroxyurea
Other	Smoking Alcohol Malnutrition

Adapted from Morton, L. M., & Phillips, T. J. (2016). Wound healing and treating wounds: Differential diagnosis and evaluation of chronic wounds. *Journal of the American Academy of Dermatology, 74*(4), 589–605; quiz 605–606.

Physical Examination

While the comprehensive history may elucidate potential wound etiologies or systemic factors that may impair wound healing, a comprehensive wound examination provides additional clues and must be performed and documented at every visit (see Table 14-3).

Documentation for a Comprehensive Wound Examination

See Table 14-3.

- **Location and Distribution**
  - Traumatic wounds can happen anywhere on the body, but favor the face and extremities.
  - Infectious wounds can happen anywhere on the body, but favor face, extremities, and intertriginous areas.
  - Chronic wounds favor a particular location and distribution (see Table 14-4).
  - Psychogenic wounds are absent in areas patients cannot reach.

BOX 14-1	Gathering Wound History

How did the wound(s) occur (spontaneous, trauma, surgical)?
When did the wound(s) occur?
When was the wound noticed?
Does the wound open and close cyclically?
History of previous wounds and locations?
When and what wound dressings, medications, or procedures have been employed?
What, if any, home or alternative remedies have been used?
Has the wound been cultured?
Is there pain, including location, characteristics, occurrence, relievers, triggers?

TABLE 14-3	Documentation of a Comprehensive Wound Examination
Location and distribution	• Single or multiple wounds • Lower extremity • Pressure points • Digits
Wound size and shape	• Measure in centimeters • Length (cm) × width (cm) × depth (cm) Longest length (12–6 o'clock) Head Widest width (3–9 o'clock) Deepest depth Toes • Example 6.2 × 3 × 0.5 cm

Wound bed status	• Color
	  Red—granulation tissue
	  Yellow—slough
	  Black—eschar
	• Anatomy (any visible tendons, muscle, fat, bone)
	• Shape (round, oval, irregular)

Undermining/ sinus tracts	• Document presence and location by using face of clock (e.g., 4–7 o'clock) • Measure deepest depth in centimeters
Wound exudate	• Color • Odor • Volume
Periwound skin	• Maceration • Primary lesions • Secondary lesions • Edema • Heat • Blanchable/nonblanchable erythema
Vascular examination	• Palpate pulses • Lower extremity edema • Capillary refill • Leg elevation • Ankle-brachial index
Neurologic examination	• Light sensation test with 5.07 monofilament • Vibratory sensation with tuning fork • Deep tendon reflexes
Pain examination	• Sharp, ache, burning, tingling • Pain scale

TABLE 14-4	**Comparison of Common Chronic Wounds**			
	PRESSURE INJURY	**VENOUS LEG ULCER**	**ARTERIAL ULCER**	**DIABETIC FOOT ULCER**
Location	Sacrum/coccyx Buttocks Ischial tuberosities Trochanter Heels Lateral malleoli	Medial malleoli Gaiter area	Anterior shin lateral malleoli Pressure points (heels, toes)	Metatarsal heads Heel Mid foot for those with bony deformity Interdigital areas of toes Dorsal and distal aspects of digits
Wound appearance	Round to irregular pattern +/–Eschar/slough	Irregular pattern Red to maroon wound bed Slough > eschar	Irregular to punched out Pale dry wound bed Eschar > slough	Oval to round pattern +Callous +/–Eschar/slough
Skin findings	Blanchable erythema Nonblanchable erythema Nonblanchable purple skin Maceration Denudation	Varicose veins Hemosiderin Telangiectasias Atrophie blanche Pitting edema Lipodermatosclerosis Maceration	Atrophic tissue Hair loss Dependent rubor Pale skin	Diabetic dermopathy Bullous diabeticorum Necrobiosis lipoidica Paronychia Onychomycosis Tinea pedis
Pulses	Normal to diminished	Normal	Diminished to absent	Normal to diminished
Neuropathy	+/–	–	+/–	+
Wound management	• Refer stage III, IV, unstageable, and deep tissue pressure injuries to wound care specialist • Offload pressure by repositioning every 2 h, minimize sitting time to 2 h max, and use of a pressure-reducing mattress/cushion/boot • Avoid foam rings or donuts • Reduce friction/shear by keeping head of bed at minimal height to reduce sliding and/or using soft silicone border/hydrocolloid dressings as a barrier • Reduce moisture-associated skin damage for those with urinary/fecal incontinence by using moisture barrier creams and/or appropriate absorptive products • Nutritional evaluation	• Compression therapy • Leg elevation • Low sodium diet • Avoid prolonged sitting, standing, or crossing of legs • Exercises to promote ankle range of motion and calf muscle strengthening • Pentoxifylline 400 mg 3 times daily • Simvastatin 40 mg daily • Skin substitute dressings (e.g., Apligraf) • Plasma-rich plasma	• Refer to vascular specialist for further evaluation • Avoid cold temperatures • Avoid tight clothing • Should not be debrided until vascular status has been determined • Dry eschar should have Betadine painted on the area left open to air to assist with preventing infection • Hyperbaric oxygen therapy • Patients should be referred urgently if there is the sudden onset of pain, pulselessness, pallor, paralysis, paresthesias, and polar (cold) in the foot (acute limb ischemia)	• Refer to wound care specialist or podiatry • Offload pressure by using total contact cast, cast walkers, therapeutic shoes, or knee walkers • Close monitoring of blood glucose levels to optimize wound healing • Becaplermin 0.01% gel daily • Skin substitutes (e.g., Dermagraft) • Hyperbaric oxygen therapy

- Vasculitis-related wounds typically occur on lower extremities and dependent areas.
- **Size and shape**
  - Wounds should be consistently measured in centimeters with the standard parameters of length, width, and depth.
- **Wound bed status**
  - *Red* wound beds represent the presence of granulation tissue in the wound bed and is a marker of healing. While bright red granulation indicates proliferation; wound beds with dark red to maroon discoloration suggest inflammation (Fig. 14-1).
  - *Yellow* wound beds represents *slough,* which presents as loose or adherent yellow or green necrotic tissue (Fig. 14-2).

- *Black* wound beds represent *eschar, which* presents as black leathery necrotic tissue (Fig. 14-3).
- The identification of exposed anatomy (e.g., tendon, bone) is essential so that appropriate measures can be taken to protect and prevent further desiccation of tissue (Fig. 14-4).
- Probing bone in the base of an open wound may suggest osteomyelitis.
- **Undermining and sinus tracts**
  - *Undermining* represents tissue destruction under the skin around the perimeter of the wound edge (Fig. 14-5).
  - *Sinus tracts* represent tissue destruction extending beyond the wound and underneath intact skin through subcutaneous or muscle tissue (Fig. 14-6).

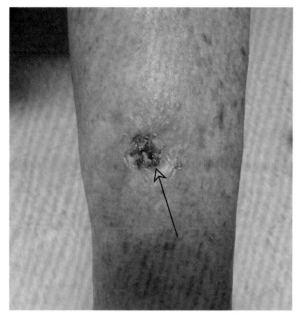

FIG. 14-1. Granulation tissue in a surgical wound (see *arrow*). In photos, granulation tissue can be identified by light reflection.

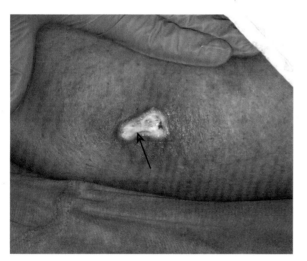

FIG. 14-2. Status post skin infection on the abdomen with adherent slough (see *arrow*).

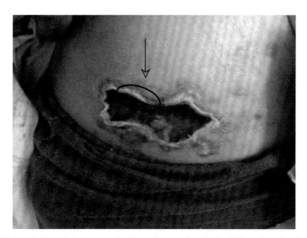

FIG. 14-3. Calciphylaxis wound with mature eschar. Notice lifting of eschar (see *arrow* and *circle*) near wound edge with underlying slough.

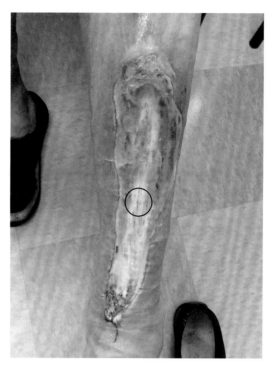

FIG. 14-4. Pyoderma gangrenosum with exposed tendon (see *circle*).

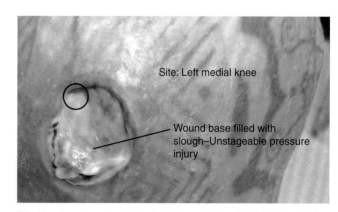

Site: Left medial knee

Wound base filled with slough–Unstageable pressure injury

FIG. 14-5. Unstageable pressure injury tattoo. Note the undermining (see *circle*) on the superior edge of the wound. (Photo courtesy of Dea Kent.)

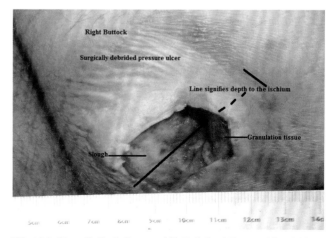

Right Buttock

Surgically debrided pressure ulcer

Line signifies depth to the ischium

Granulation tissue

Slough

FIG. 14-6. Stage IV. (Illustration copyright © National Pressure Ulcer Advisory Panel, 2007.)

- **Wound exudate**
  - *Color* can range from sanguinous (red) to serous (straw colored) to yellow/green. The yellow color occurs as a result of increased death of neutrophils, which can occur in both infection and neutrophilic dermatoses (e.g., pyoderma gangrenosum).
  - *Volume* can range from minimal to copious amounts. The sudden increase in drainage can suggest underlying infection, increased inflammation, or uncontrolled lower extremity edema.
  - *Drainage* is typically odorless, but odor is important to note with each dressing change. While odor can occur with infectious processes, it can also occur as a result of some wound dressings (e.g., hydrocolloid).
- **Primary and secondary lesions in the periwound skin area**
  - The periwound skin can provide insight into wound etiology as there are unique skin findings that manifest with particular chronic wounds (see Table 14-4).
  - *Primary and secondary skin lesions* noted on examination should prompt the use of the morphology algorithm for developing differential diagnosis (see Section 1.3).
  - For venous leg ulcer (VLU) periwound skin findings, see Figs. 14-7 to 14-12.
  - For diabetic ulcer periwound skin findings, see Figs. 14-13 and 14-14 and Sections 6.1 (tinea pedis, onychomycosis), 6.3 (paronychia), and 12.1 (diabetic dermopathy, necrobiosis lipoidica, bullosis diabeticorum).

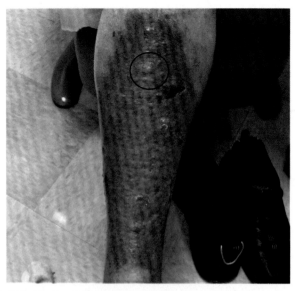

FIG. 14-8. Lipodermatosclerosis. Notice inverted champagne bottle lower extremity with hyperpigmented waxy sclerotic papules (see *circle*) and plaques on the shin.

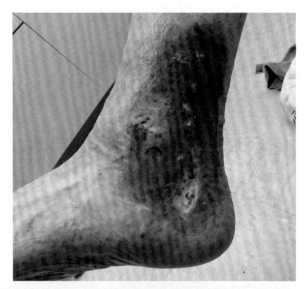

FIG. 14-9. Venous leg ulcer with allergic contact dermatitis due to Neosporin.

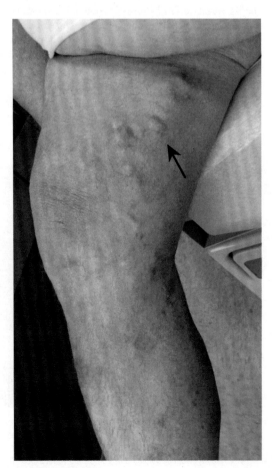

FIG. 14-7. Varicose veins (see *arrow*).

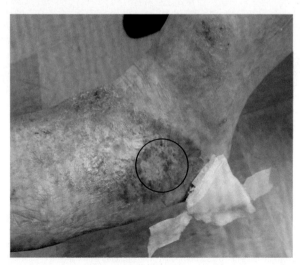

FIG. 14-10. Atrophie blanche (see *circle*) presents as a white atrophic reticulated scar.

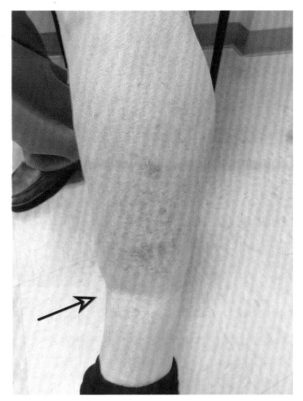

FIG. 14-11. Hemosiderin staining. Tan brown macules coalescing into poorly demarcated patch. Notice indentation (see *arrow*) of skin representing pitting edema from a tight sock.

- *For arterial ulcer periwound skin findings, see Figs. 14-15 and 14-16.*
- **Vascular**
  - A comprehensive vascular examination (e.g., pulses, edema) for extremity wounds is essential to identify any potential underlying vascular disease that could impede wound healing.

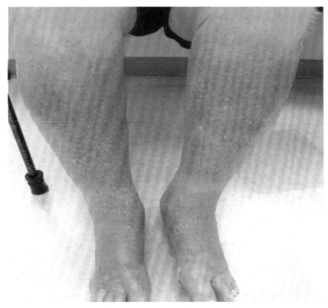

FIG. 14-12. Stasis dermatitis. Notice bilateral erythematous scaly patches. Often mistaken for cellulitis. Stasis dermatitis often presents with bilateral erythematous edematous lower extremities.

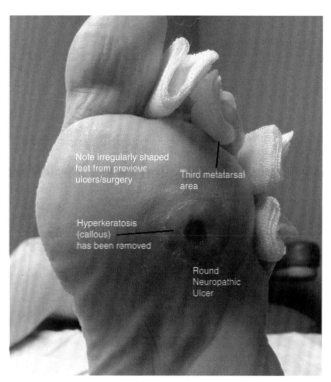

FIG. 14-13. Diabetic foot ulcer, plantar ulcer. Notice hypertrophic callus to periwound skin around the ulcer. (Photo courtesy of Dea Kent.)

- The leg elevation test helps to evaluate for dependent rubor (Fig. 14-16). Dependent rubor is the presence of dark red to red discoloration of the lower extremity when in a dependent position. For patients with arterial disease, elevation of the leg causes the leg to become white or paler.
- **Neurologic**
  - An alteration in light touch sensation (Fig. 14-17), vibratory sensation, or deep tendon reflexes should raise concern for underlying neuropathic etiology (Table 14-4).

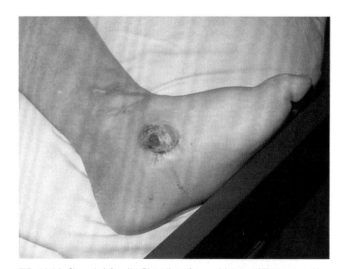

FIG. 14-14. Charcot deformity. Disruption of normal bony architecture resulting in new bony prominences that may ulcerate due to repeated trauma. (Used with permission from Wound, Ostomy and Continence Nurses Society®; Doughty, D. B., & McNichol, L. L. [2015]. *Wound, Ostomy and Continence Nurses Society® core curriculum: Wound management.* Wolters Kluwer.)

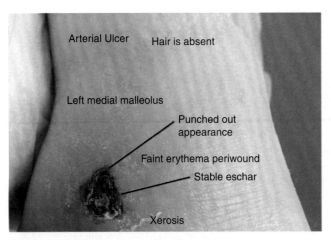

FIG. 14-15. Arterial ulcer.

Arterial Ulcer
Hair is absent
Left medial malleolus
Punched out appearance
Faint erythema periwound
Stable eschar
Xerosis

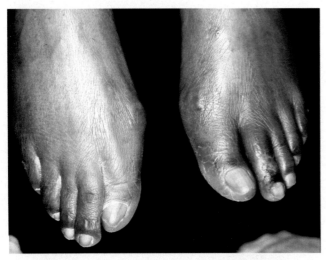

FIG. 14-16. Dependent rubor. Left foot has red or ruddy color when in a dependent position indicating tissue ischemia. When elevated, the ischemic limb will become pale. (Used with permission from Baranoski, S., & Ayello, E. A. [2020]. *Wound care essentials* [5th ed.]. Wolters Kluwer.)

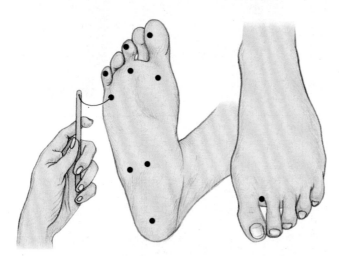

FIG. 14-17. Monofilament testing for peripheral neuropathy. (Used with permission from Baranoski, S., & Ayello, E. A. [2020]. *Wound care essentials* [5th ed.]. Wolters Kluwer.)

- **Pain**
  - Patients with chronic wounds often suffer from wound pain rather at rest or with dressing changes. The severity and character of the pain (e.g., burning) should be determined to identify a possible underlying neuropathic component.
- **Staging**
  - Additional standardized nomenclature can be used for documenting wounds. While several wound staging systems exist, wounds can be generally classified as partial thickness (dermal exposure only) or full thickness (subcutaneous, muscle, tendon exposure). When possible, wound-specific staging systems should be used when documenting the wound. However, staging systems can be nuanced. A review of the diabetic foot ulcer (e.g., Wagner) staging systems is beyond the scope of this textbook; the PI staging system is reviewed below:
    - National Pressure Injury Advisory Panel Pressure Injury Staging system (Table 14-5):
      - For all PIs, a standardized staging system should be used for documentation.
      - When preparing to stage a PI, the wound should be cleansed thoroughly of debris so that a clear examination of the wound anatomy can be performed.
      - The PIs should be staged based on the maximum anatomy identified on examination. For example, an evaluation of a wound reveals subcutaneous tissue, but no ligament, fascia, or muscle would be categorized as a stage III PI.
      - PIs are not reverse staged, meaning, that as a stage IV PI heals, it does not become a stage III or II PI.
      - It is certainly possible to presume the depth of tissue injury, but technically, no classifiable stage can be determined until the wound base is visible.
      - When staging PI in skin of color, inspect the skin for areas of hyperpigmentation in contrast to the *patient's* skin color. Patients with darker skin tones will not exhibit blanching when pressure is applied. Additionally, gently palpate bony prominences to assess areas of increased/decreased temperature, edema, and induration. While gently palpating bony prominences, monitor patient response to determine potential areas of tenderness if patient is not communicative.

WOUND HEALING

Wound healing follows a logical order and cannot progress if there is persistent inflammation. Wounds may be stuck in the inflammatory phase due to underlying etiology, increased bacterial burden, presence of necrotic tissue, impaired cell signaling, imbalance of inflammatory mediators (reactive oxygen species, proteinases, cytokines), or impaired cell division. Furthermore, an inflammatory environment impairs fibroblast and keratinocyte function (Fig. 14-18).

Phases of Wound Healing

Injury/Hemostasis

At the time of wounding, there is a disruption of cells, collagen, and tissues, which causes hemorrhage. Subsequently, there is a series of cellular activities that promote clot formation within minutes of the injury. Within 10 to 15 minutes, this clot is dissolved to allow the next cascade of events to occur, and it is at this point that the inflammatory stage begins.

TABLE 14-5 Pressure Injury Stages (Categories)

Stage I: Nonblanchable Erythema

Stage I pressure injury

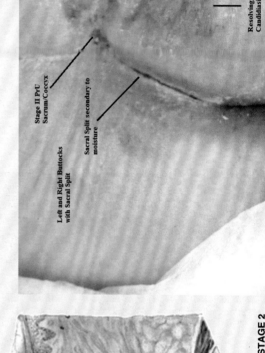

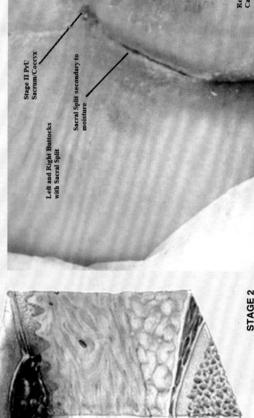

Stage II PrU
Left Lateral Metatarsal
Broken skin =Stage II

Xerosis

Stage I PrU
Left Lateral Foot

Stage I PrU
Left Lateral Malleolus

STAGE 1

NATIONAL
PRESSURE
ULCER
ADVISORY
PANEL

Intact skin with nonblanchable redness of a localized area, usually over a bony prominence.

It can be difficult to identify in darkly pigmented skin as it may not have visible blanching; its color may differ from the surrounding area.

The area may be painful, firm, soft, warmer, or cooler as compared to adjacent tissue. The presence or development may indicate "at-risk" persons.

Stage II: Partial Thickness

Stage II pressure injury

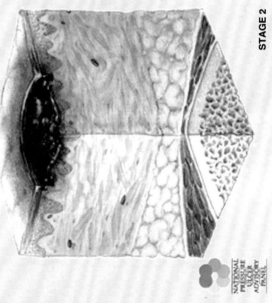

Stage II PrU
Sacrum/Coccyx

Left and Right Buttocks
with Sacral Split

Sacral Split secondary to
moisture

Resolving
Candidiasis

STAGE 2

NATIONAL
PRESSURE
ULCER
ADVISORY
PANEL

Partial-thickness loss of dermis presenting as a shallow open ulcer with a red pink wound bed, without slough.

May also present as an intact or open/ruptured serum-filled or serosanguineous-filled blister.

A shiny or dry, shallow ulcer without slough or bruising indicates deep tissue injury.

This category should not be used to describe skin tears, tape burns, incontinence-associated dermatitis, maceration, or excoriation.

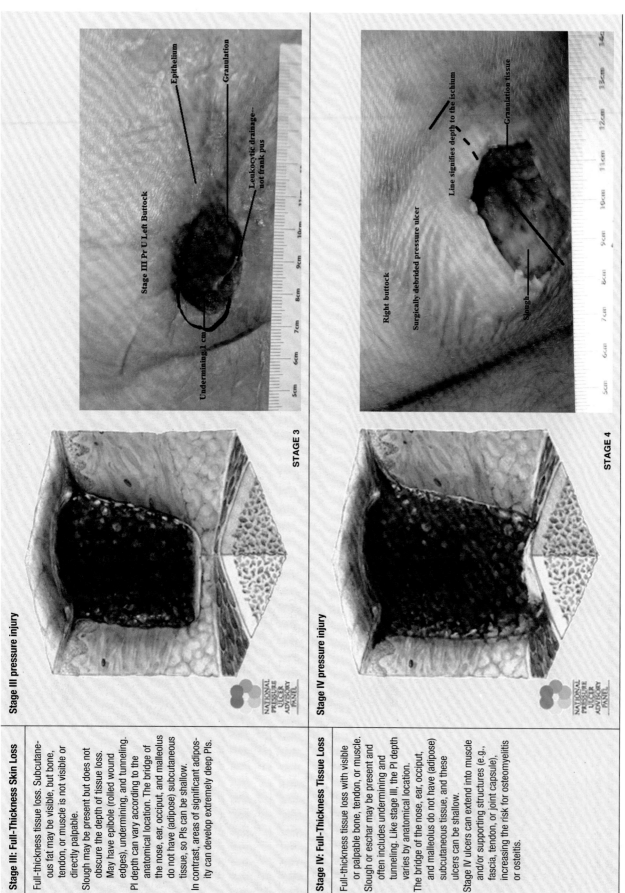

Stage III: Full-Thickness Skin Loss

Stage III pressure injury

Full-thickness tissue loss. Subcutaneous fat may be visible, but bone, tendon, or muscle is not visible or directly palpable.

Slough may be present but does not obscure the depth of tissue loss. May have epibole (rolled wound edges), undermining, and tunneling.

PI depth can vary according to the anatomical location. The bridge of the nose, ear, occiput, and malleolus do not have (adipose) subcutaneous tissue, so PIs can be shallow.

In contrast, areas of significant adiposity can develop extremely deep PIs.

STAGE 3

Stage IV: Full-Thickness Tissue Loss

Stage IV pressure injury

Full-thickness tissue loss with visible or palpable bone, tendon, or muscle. Slough or eschar may be present and often includes undermining and tunneling. Like stage III, the PI depth varies by anatomical location.

The bridge of the nose, ear, occiput, and malleolus do not have (adipose) subcutaneous tissue, and these ulcers can be shallow.

Stage IV ulcers can extend into muscle and/or supporting structures (e.g., fascia, tendon, or joint capsule), increasing the risk for osteomyelitis or osteitis.

STAGE 4

(continued)

529

TABLE 14-5 Pressure Injury Stages (Categories) (*Continued*)

Unstageable: Full-Thickness Skin or Tissue Loss—Depth Unknown

Full-thickness tissue loss in which actual depth of the ulcer is completely obscured by slough (yellow, tan, gray, green, or brown) and/or eschar (tan, brown, or black) in the wound bed.

Until enough slough and eschar are removed to expose the base of the wound, the true depth cannot be determined.

Stable (dry, adherent, intact without erythema, or fluctuance).

Eschar on the heels serves as "the body's natural (biologic) cover" and should not be removed.

Unstageable pressure injury

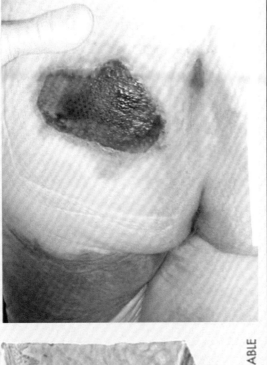

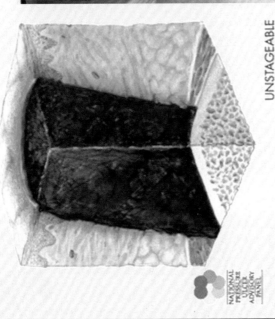

UNSTAGEABLE

Deep Tissue Pressure Injury (DTPI)—Depth Unknown

Intact or nonintact purple, maroon, or deep red localized area of discolored intact skin, nonintact skin, or blood-filled blister due to damage of underlying soft tissue from pressure and/or shear.

The area may be preceded by tissue that is painful, firm, mushy, boggy, warmer, or cooler as compared to adjacent tissue.

DTPI may be difficult to detect in individuals with dark skin tones.

A blister over a dark wound bed may evolve further into thin eschar or resolve without tissue loss.

DTPIs are not be confused with other wounds (e.g., vascular, dermatologic).

Deep Tissue Pressure Injury

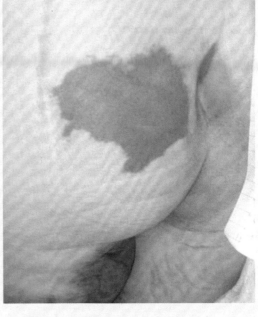

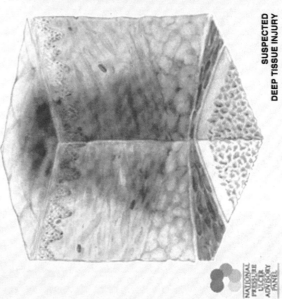

SUSPECTED DEEP TISSUE INJURY

530

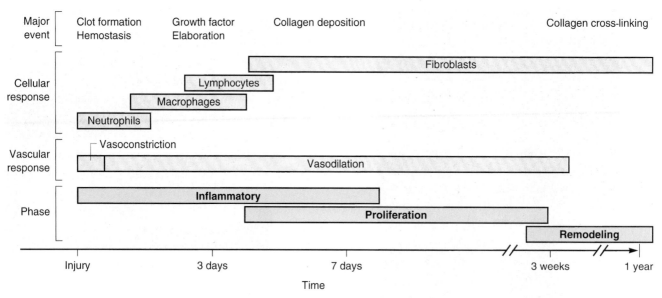

FIG. 14-18. Timeline of phases of wound healing.

Inflammatory Phase

- Initially, the cellular waste products are contained and removed as neutrophils and macrophages arrive.

- There is also a vasodilation process that occurs, which permits plasma and blood cells to pass into the wound bed, bringing growth factors and a host of other cells to the wound.

- Clinical signs of the inflammatory phase may include slough, eschar, friable wound bed, dark red to maroon wound bed (Fig. 14-19), hypergranulation tissue (Fig. 14-20), increased exudate, and periwound erythema, edema, or induration (Fig. 14-21). By days 3 to 5, the inflammatory phase should transition to the proliferative phase.

Proliferative Phase

- During proliferation, collagen and other proteins are deposited in an unorganized fashion in the wound environment by fibroblasts. This produces a scaffolding for cell (fibroblasts, keratinocytes) migration to support development of granulation tissue and reepithelialization of the wound.

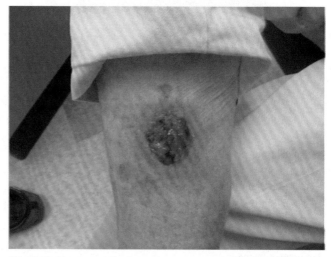

FIG. 14-20. Hypergranulation tissue.

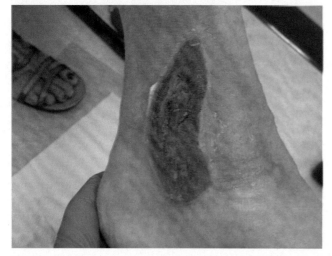

FIG. 14-19. Dark red wound bed with eschar.

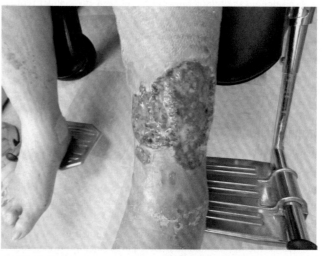

FIG. 14-21. Pyoderma gangrenosum ulcer during inflammatory phase.

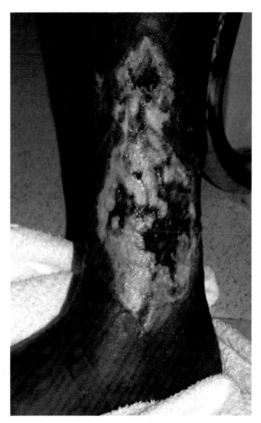

FIG. 14-22. Venous leg ulcer with noted pink tissue representing reepithelialization. (Used with permission from Baranoski, S., Ayello, E. A. [2020]. *Wound care essentials* [5th ed.]. Wolters Kluwer.)

- In addition, myofibroblasts assist in decreasing wound size by causing wound contraction.
- Clinical signs of this phase may include decreased drainage, beefy red granulation tissue (Fig. 14-1), decreased wound size/depth, and pink scar tissue at wound edge representing reepithelialization (Fig. 14-22).

Remodeling Phase

- Remodeling may begin as early as 1 week post injury. At the end of proliferation, the skin has about 20% tensile strength.
- Throughout the remodeling phase, collagen and cellular reorganization continues to occur over the next year.
- Once the remodeling phase has completed, the tensile strength of collagen approaches 80%, therefore scars may reopen more easily with trauma or other injury.
- The clinical sign of remodeling is the presence of a scar (Fig. 14-23).

Impediments to Wound Healing

Tissue/Trauma

- *Necrotic tissue* presents as *slough* or *eschar*.
- *Unrelieved pressure, shear, or friction* results in blanchable or nonblanchable red, purple, or maroon skin, excoriation, or erosions.
- *Expansion of tissue injury* may present as noted by temperature change, induration, nonblanchable purple/maroon discoloration, or blister formation.

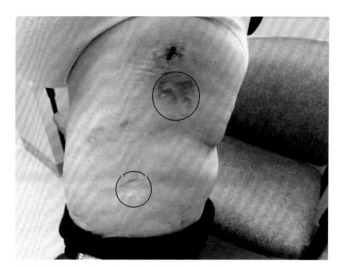

FIG. 14-23. Calcinosis cutis with nonhealing ulcer with scars (see *circles*).

Infection

- Clinical presentation of infection may include increased wound size, wound pain, odor, purulent exudate, necrotic tissue, discolored wound bed (maroon, dark red), friable/bleeding granulation tissue, and periwound erythema, induration, and temperature (Fig. 14-24).
- Subtle signs of infection such as faint halo to periwound skin, delayed wound healing, increased wound size, or wound pain may be the only signs noted in those with malnutrition, immunosuppression, diabetes, anemia, chronic kidney disease, hepatic impairment, malignancy, morbid obesity, and cardiopulmonary disease.
- Systemic signs of infection may include fatigue, malaise, chills, or fever.

Moisture

- *Excessive wound exudate* may present as maceration (Fig. 14-25), irritant contact dermatitis (Fig. 14-9), or hypergranulation tissue.

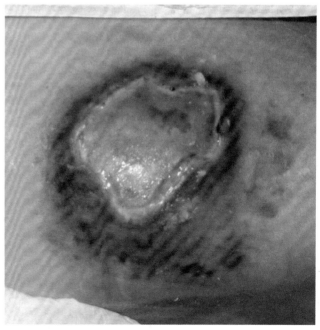

FIG. 14-24. Infected pressure injury.

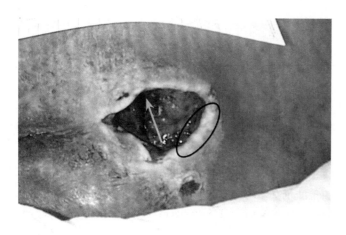

FIG. 14-25. Pressure injury with maceration (*circle*) and undermining (*arrow*).

Wound Edge

- *Hypergranulation* tissue (Fig. 14-20) presents as excessive growth of granulation tissue that above the plane of the wound is friable and often easily bleeds.

- *Malignancy* or fungating tumors may present as excessive growth of granulation tissue, sudden development of red tissue in a focal area of a wound, or as necrotic cauliflower-like growth from a chronic ulcer (Fig. 14-26).

- *Epibole* represents wound edges that have rolled downward and are not connected with the wound bed (see Fig. 14-27).

Nutrition

- A thorough nutritional examination should be performed in those with pressure injuries or multiple ulcerations (see Box 14-2).

Vascular Impairment

- Diminished or absent pulses can be noted in chronic wounds (see Table 14-4).

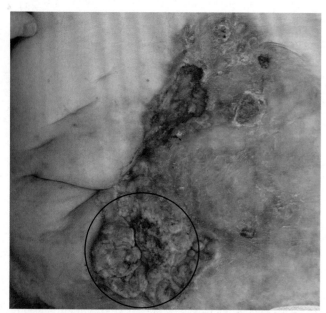

FIG. 14-26. Fungating tumor (see *circle*).

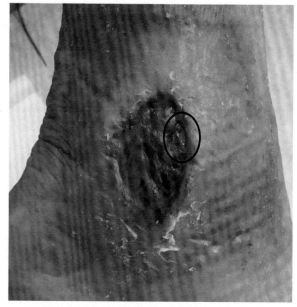

FIG. 14-27. Epibole. Notice rolled wound edge (see *circle*).

While a palpable dorsalis pedis or posterior tibialis suggests a blood pressure of ≥80 mm Hg, there is the possibility that arterial insufficiency exists. ABI, an indirect measure of arterial circulation, should be measured (Box 14-3) if there is a weak or absent pulse and prior to initiating compression therapy.

- Lower extremity edema should raise the suspicion for VLU or mixed arterial-venous ulcer.

BOX 14-2　Guidelines for Nutritional Examination

Visual Assessment—General Appearance
Frail, thin, obese, pale
Poor dentition/no teeth/poor-fitting dentures
Muscle wasting
Flaky skin
Thin, dry, brittle broken hair
Brittle nails
Cracked lips

Body Mass Index
<19 is risk for increased mortality, pressure injury development, undernutrition
>30 is obese, but not necessarily nutritionally healthy

Patient Interview
Recent unplanned weight loss
Recent hospitalization/acute disease
Activity level (e.g., bedbound, walking)
Loss of appetite/decreased food intake
Swallowing/chewing difficulties
Medications (can influence appetite)

Assessment of Weight Loss
Formula: current body weight/usual body weight × 100
Example: current weight: 137 lb; usual body weight: 145 lb
137/145 × 100 = 94.5% or weight loss of 5.5%, which could be significant

Laboratory
Prealbumin level—normal limits, 28–38 mg/dL
Albumin level—3.5–5 g/dL
Serum transferrin—204–360 mg/dL (not widely used)

BOX 14-3   Ankle-Brachial Index (ABI) Testing

Equipment needed	Stethoscope
	Blood pressure cuff
	Doppler (ultrasound) handheld
Procedure	1. The patient should be supine for this procedure.
	2. Obtain brachial pressures in both arms, unless contraindicated.
	3. Place the sphygmomanometer cuff on the leg, just above the ankle.
	4. Locate the dorsalis pedis or posterior tibial pulse—each will be tested.
	5. Apply ultrasound gel to the area of pulse.
	6. Apply a Doppler to pulse area, then inflate cuff until the pulse sound disappears.
	7. Deflate the cuff slowly and listen for the pulse sound to return.
	8. The higher of the two ankle pressures number reading is used in the calculation.
Calculate ABI	Highest ankle pressure/brachial pressure = ABI
	Example: brachial 120, ankle 114, 114/120 = 0.9
ABI interpretation	>1.3 — Get arterial Doppler
	0.9–1.3 — Within normal limits
	≤0.9 — Mild LEAD
	≤0.6–0.8 — Moderate LEAD
	<0.5 — Critical limb ischemia
False-negative results	Untreated hypertension
	Noncompressible vessels
	Diabetes
	Older adults
	Chronic kidney disease

Differential Diagnosis

See Table 14-1 for differential diagnosis for wounds.

Confirming the Diagnosis

Further diagnostic evaluation is warranted when:

- Wounds have an unusual presentation or do not have typical clinical features of VLU, arterial ulcers, PI, or neuropathic ulcers.
- Wounds are associated with primary lesion morphology.
- Wounds fail to respond to appropriate management after 4 to 6 weeks.
- There is a sudden wound change (e.g., increased wound size, abnormal granulation tissue).

Laboratory Studies

Wound Culture

- A wound culture is indicated when there are signs and symptoms of infection (see wound examination section). If the patient is already on an antibiotic, culturing the wound may not be valuable.
- Wound culture can be prepared using tissue, needle aspirate, or swab specimens.
  - *Tissue culture* is considered the gold standard for wound culturing and is collected by harvesting tissue using a sterile scalpel or a punch after cleansing with a nonantiseptic solution (i.e., saline). The tissue should be submitted in a nonantiseptic solution to avoid influence on the culture results.
  - *Needle aspirate* is selected when collected by aspirating exudate directly from an abscess or pustule into a syringe. With this technique, it is permissible to prep the skin with an antimicrobial cleanser, because the aspirate would not be in contact with the antiseptic.
  - *Swab* is the most popular type of culture due to ease of collection and is not invasive. The swab should be rotated over a 1 cm² area in the deepest portion of the wound for 5 seconds with enough pressure to elicit fluid from the wound bed (Levine technique). Once the exudate is collected, the swab is placed in the transport tube carefully as to avoid contamination of the specimen.

Skin Biopsy

- Punch or excisional biopsy should be considered when ruling out malignancy, vasculitis, vasculopathy, or panniculitis.
- Tissue from the wound edge should include ulcer tissue, intact skin, and subcutaneous tissue.
- If considering malignancy, tissue should be collected from suspicious tissue (Fig. 14-26).

Serology

- Complete blood count
  - As hemoglobin is essential for the transportation of oxygen to the tissue, patients with anemia (hemoglobin <12 g/dL) should have their hemoglobin levels optimized.
- Fasting comprehensive metabolic panel
  - Blood glucose levels consistently above 150 mg/dL can delay wound healing.
  - May identify underlying chronic kidney or hepatic disease.
- Hemoglobin A1c may assist with determining glycemic control and potential need for dietary or medication adjustment.
- Albumin (half-life 12 to 23 days) or prealbumin (half-life 2 to 3 days) may be considered for patients with pertinent findings on nutritional examination (Box 14-3).

WOUND MANAGEMENT

Once the underlying etiology of the wound has been addressed and the systemic factors (e.g., vascular status, nutrition) that impact wound healing have been optimized, clinicians need to develop a wound management plan that addresses any impediments to wound healing as noted above.

Tissue/Trauma

- The presence of necrotic tissue in the wound bed prolongs the inflammatory phase of wound healing and provides a medium for excessive bacterial growth. Patients with eschar should be referred to a wound care specialist, general surgeon, or plastic surgeon for debridement management as multiple approaches (e.g., sharp, enzymatic, chemical) for debridement are required if clinically appropriate. Patients with impaired ABI or diminished pulses should be evaluated by a vascular surgeon prior to debridement.
- Unrelieved or repeated episodes of pressure, friction, or shear can cause additional tissue damage and prolong the inflammatory phase. The use of protective dressings such as hydrocolloids, foams, or gauze wrap can provide protection from repeated trauma. Additionally, offloading devices such as foam wedges, chair cushions, or offloading boots can assist with offloading pressure–induced trauma.

Infection

- Most wounds have varying degrees of microorganism colonization (i.e., bacteria, fungi), which can play a role in both healing and tissue damage (infection). An overgrowth of microorganisms or the coordinated development of a biofilm (community of microorganisms encased in a protective extracellular polymeric substance) can promote inflammation, wound expansion, and tissue necrosis as a result of infection.

- If patients are without symptoms of infection and do not have a culture and sensitivity from the wound exudate or tissue, topical and systemic antibiotics should be avoided. The selection of topical and systemic antibiotics should be based on culture and sensitivity. See Sections 1.4 and 6.2 regarding selection of topical and systemic antibiotic agents that cover the most common causes of skin bacteria (e.g., *Staph, Strep* species).

- For topical broad-spectrum antimicrobial dressings and antiseptic solutions, see Table 14-6. Frequency of dressing change could be twice daily to once a week and depends on the dressing type, manufacturer guidelines, and wound exudate volume.

- Wounds that fail to respond to a particular antimicrobial dressing after 10 to 14 days should be switched to an alternate topical antimicrobial dressing.

- As many of the antimicrobial dressings and antiseptic solutions (Table 14-6) may have cytotoxic effects, transitioning to noncytotoxic dressings once the infection is controlled is imperative to support granulation tissue formation.

- General expert consensus is that NHWs are more likely to have biofilms prolonging the inflammatory phase, therefore maintaining sharp debridement is recommended. Referral to a wound care specialist, general surgeon, or plastic surgeon is recommended if sharp debridement is required.

Moisture Management

- Excessive or too little moisture in a wound can impede wound healing and damage periwound skin (e.g., maceration). Chronic wound fluid is composed of proinflammatory cytokines and proteases that prevent wounds from progressing into the proliferative phase. On the other hand, an optimal moist wound environment supports cell signaling and function of growth factors and cytokines, as well as cell migration. Wound dressings have the ability to support an optimal wound healing environment, and some absorptive dressings (e.g., hydrofiber, collagen, oxidized regenerated cellulose) have the capacity to remove proinflammatory mediators from the wound environment. Wound drainage volume can frequently fluctuate which may result in changing wound dressings to accommodate drainage. The correct dressing one week could be the wrong dressing the next week.

- An approach to selecting wound dressings:
  Determine the wound depth.
  Superficial wounds should be covered with a wound dressing. Deep wounds require two dressings, a dressing to fill the cavity and to cover the wound (secondary dressing). Additionally, when filling the wound cavity, clinicians should ensure that undermining and sinus tract spaces should be filled to avoid premature closure and dead space development.
  Determine the wound exudate volume.
  If the wound is dry (minimal to no drainage), use a dressing that will add moisture (Table 14-7). If the wound is wet (moderate to copious drainage), use a dressing that will remove moisture (Table 14-8).

Determine the need for antimicrobial dressings.
Patients with chronic wounds, repeated infections, or higher risk for infection (e.g., immunosuppressed) may benefit from the use of antimicrobial and antibiofilm dressings.
Determine the need for nonadherent dressings.
Wounds and periwound skin that are fragile may be easily traumatized with dressing removal; therefore, the use of nonadherent dressings like petroleum-based gauze or silicone-based contact layers is preferred. Additionally, wounds with exposed tendon or ligaments should be protected with nonadherent dressings. As these dressings do not provide any absorptive capacity, a secondary dressing (e.g., foam, gauze) is necessary. Additionally, nonadherent dressings are well tolerated for patients who experience severe wound pain with dressing changes.
Determine available resources.
Patient capacity to be able to perform dressing changes should be discussed. If the patient is unable to access the wound, identifying available resources (family, neighbors) is essential to support proper wound care in the home setting. When resources are not available, collaborating with Home Health services for assistance with developing a sustainable plan of care or teaching of family or neighbors to perform wound dressings is recommended. Additionally, financial resources should be determined as wound dressings can become costly. Insurance companies often have a list of approved wound products and distributors of wound products.

- Wound specialists should be consulted in the wound dressing selection when wounds deteriorate or fail to show signs of healing (e.g., decreased wound size) by 4 to 6 weeks of appropriate therapy. In some circumstances, wound management systems (i.e., negative pressure wound therapy, skin substitutes) are used, but an overview of specialty wound dressings or wound management systems is beyond the scope of this textbook.

Edge of Wound

- Hypergranulation, also known as "proud flesh," and epibole inhibit keratinocytes from crossing the wound bed. Hypergranulation may occur as a result of overgrowth of bacteria or excessive moisture whereas epibole may occur due to sinus tracts or fistula.

- Patients with epibole or hypergranulation tissue should be referred to a wound care specialist, general surgeon, or plastic surgeon for consideration of chemical cauterization (e.g., silver nitrate) or sharp debridement.

- Patients with malignancy should be referred for surgical excision of the tumor.

Nutrition

- Nutritional impairment can prolong the inflammatory phase of wound healing, and cause cellular transactions to be impaired, delayed, or absent. If the nutritional examination (Box 14-2) or laboratory identifies actual or potential malnutrition, patients should be referred to dietitians for further evaluation, nutritional counseling, and development of patient-centered dietary interventions (e.g., supplements).

Vascular Impairment

- Diminished arterial blood flow can cause impaired healing, tissue ischemia, and necrosis. Due to impaired arterial circulation, tissues are starved of necessary nutrients to support cellular activity and tissue repair. Additionally, the removal of cellular waste products is

TABLE 14-6	Topical Antimicrobial Dressings/Cleansers		
TOPICAL AGENT	**ORGANISMS**	**CYTOTOXIC**	**CLINICAL PEARLS/CAUTION**
Silver: Silver sulfadiazine Silver nitrate 0.5% Silver-releasing dressings (Acticoat, Aquacel Ag)[c]	Gram-positive bacteria Gram-negative bacteria Fungus Candida	Silver sulfadiazine and silver nitrate ≥1% concentrations may be cytotoxic. Silver-releasing dressings may be cytotoxic.	Silver is only released from impregnated dressings in the presence of moisture. If the wound is dry, consider silver hydrogel, silver sulfadiazine, or other antimicrobial. Silver nitrate and silver-releasing dressings (e.g., Acticoat) may cause permanent discoloration (argyria). Silver sulfadiazine may cause pseudoeschar development or reversible neutropenia. Silver nitrate rarely may cause hemoglobinemia or methemoglobinemia.
Bismuth tribromophenate[a] (Xeroform)[c]	Gram-positive bacteria Gram-negative bacteria	No	Dressings are changed daily and require a secondary dressing. Dressings are nonadherent and are excellent in reducing dressing change–associated wound pain. Use of bismuth dressings over large surface areas may cause bismuth toxicity.
Sodium hypochlorite (Dakin solution) Or Hypochlorous acid[b] (Vashe)[c]	Gram-positive bacteria Gram-negative bacteria Fungus Viral	¼ strength (0.125%) to full strength (0.5%) Dakin solution is cytotoxic and can inhibit wound healing when used as a dressing. 0.025% solution retains antimicrobial effects and is not cytotoxic and is applied b.i.d. to wounds with gauze followed by a secondary dressing.	Dakin soaked gauze is applied daily to twice daily based on wound exudate volume. Excellent choice for infected wounds with eschar or slough as Dakin is also considered a chemical-debriding agent.
Iodine: Polyvinylpyrrolidone[b] (Betadine)[c] Or Cadexomer iodine (Iodosorb)[c]	Gram-positive bacteria Gram-negative bacteria Fungus Candida Viruses Protozoa	≥1% iodine solutions or gels are cytotoxic and should be used for nonhealable or maintenance wounds only. Cadexomer iodine dressings are not cytotoxic.	Cadexomer iodine dressing changes every 2–3 days (dressing changes from brown to yellow gray). Must use secondary dressing. May cause transient skin discoloration, burning sensation with dressing application, and irritant/allergic dermatitis. Avoid use in patients with Hashimoto thyroiditis, Graves disease, or nontoxic nodular goiter. Increased risk of thyroid toxicity from ≥1 wk of use, application to large surface area, and in patients with impaired thyroid or renal function. Avoid using during radioiodine diagnostic testing.
Gentian violet 1% solution (Hydrofera Blue)[c]	Gram-positive bacteria Gram-negative bacteria Fungus Candida	No	Dressings are changed daily to every 3 days. Foam dressing may require moistening with sterile water or normal saline before applying.
Honey (Medihoney, Actilite)[c]	Gram-positive bacteria Gram-negative bacteria	No	Do not use over-the-counter honey products due to concerns regarding *Clostridium* bacterial spores. Honey-based dressings can also promote autolytic wound debridement. Patients may experience burning/stinging with initial application.
Chlorhexidine[b,c] Or Polyhexamethylene biguanide (PHMB) (Kendall AMD, Suprasorb X + PHMB)[c]	Gram-positive bacteria Gram-negative bacteria Fungus Candida	No	Dressings do not release PHMB into the wound bed, therefore providing antimicrobial activity above the wound.
Acetic acid 0.5–1% solution	Gram-negative bacteria Gram-positive bacteria	In vitro data suggests cytotoxicity at 0.25%, but no clinical data showing cytotoxicity with 0.5–1% concentrations.	Acetic acid solution–soaked gauze applied daily to 3 times daily based on wound exudate volume. Should not be used with skin grafts. Some patients may experience burning with application, which is more common in higher concentrations.

[a]Bacteriostatic only.
[b]These compounds are only used as cleansers.
[c]Trade names are not all inclusive or exhaustive, and no money was exchanged for inclusion of names in this table. Dressings should always be used per manufacturer's instructions, which may vary by dressing type and function.

TABLE 14-7	Dressings for Wounds with Minimal to No Exudate		
DRESSING TYPE	**GENERAL INFORMATION**	**CAUTION/CONTRAINDICATIONS**	**CLINICAL PEARLS**
Hydrocolloid (Comfeel, DuoDERM)	No secondary dressing required. May be left in place up to 7 days based on manufacturer's instructions.[a] May be used as a secondary dressing. Change if dressing begins to leak or become saturated.	Do not apply to stable eschar on heels. Caution in use on lower extremities and foot in diabetics, or in patients with vascular compromise, as they are more prone to anaerobic proliferation. Do not use in infected wounds.	Promotes autolytic debridement in some patients. When hydrocolloids absorb wound exudate, an odorous yellow drainage forms that can be mistaken for infection.
Hydrogel (Skintegrity, Solosite)	Requires a secondary dressing. Change every 1–3 days depending on the form of dressing, per manufacturer's instructions.[a]	Monitor wound and wound environment for maceration.	Promotes autolytic debridement in some patients.
Film (Tegaderm, Opsite)	Does not require secondary dressing. Can be left in place up to 7 days based on manufacturer's instructions.[a] Can be used as a secondary dressing.	Caution with fragile skin, as removal can promote skin trauma. Remove dressing by stretching it horizontally to break the adhesive; do not pull upward, as this may cause stripping of skin layers. Caution in use on lower extremities and foot in diabetics, or in patients with vascular compromise, as they are more prone to anaerobic proliferation.	Can be used to prevent friction on some bony prominences. Can be used to promote autolytic debridement in selected candidates.

[a]Trade names are not all inclusive or exhaustive, and no money was exchanged for inclusion of names in this table. Dressings should always be used per manufacturer's instructions, which may vary by dressing type and function.

impaired resulting in toxic milieu. Patients with diminished pulses or abnormal ABI should be referred to vascular surgery for further evaluation and management. Additionally, patients who are current smokers should be counseled that a single cigarette can cause up to 90 minutes of vasoconstriction and a 1 pack per day can result in days of impaired circulation. Connecting patients with smoking cessation programs, where available, can provide additional community support for smoking cessation. Furthermore, patients should be counseled to avoid wearing tight garments and limit their exposure to cold temperatures.

TABLE 14-8	Dressings for Wounds with Moderate to Heavy Exudate		
DRESSING TYPE	**GENERAL INFORMATION**	**CAUTION/CONTRAINDICATIONS**	**CLINICAL PEARLS**
Alginate (Kaltostat, Maxorb)	Needs secondary dressing. Can be left in place 1–5 days based on manufacturer's instructions.[a]	Do not pack the rope form into blind cavities. Some alginates turn into a moist substance when saturated, and will not appear in the wound base when changing the dressing. Irrigate the wound to ensure total dressing removal. Do not use for third-degree burns.	Alginate dressings have mild hemostatic effects due to calcium.
Foam (Biatain, Mepilex	May require a secondary dressing if there is not a waterproof backing on the foam. Change every 3–7 days or if dressing becomes saturated per manufacturer's instructions.[a] Can be used with other dressings as a secondary dressing.	None	May also be used as a prevention dressing for high-risk bony prominences.
Gauze	May be used for minimal to heavily exudative wounds with frequency of dressing change occurring 1–3 times daily based on wound exudate volume. May be used alone to absorb or combined with topical antiseptic solutions or hydrogel to add moisture. May be used as a secondary dressing. Change at least daily.	Often promotes pain during dressing changes when used as a primary dressing. Considered "cheap" but actually is more expensive due to frequency and intensity of dressing change.	Good to use for mechanical debridement.

[a]Trade names are not all inclusive or exhaustive, and no money was exchanged for inclusion of names in this table. Dressings should always be used per manufacturer's instructions, which may vary by dressing type and function.

- Tissue edema as a result of trauma, chronic venous insufficiency, or lymphedema can also impair normal cellular activity required to support tissue repair. Patients with noted edema should be managed with compression stockings or compression wraps. Compression wraps support venous return, improve lymphatic circulation, reduce inflammation, and improve microcirculation. Compression therapy should be avoided if ABI of ≤0.5, active thrombus, or uncompensated heart failure with ejection fraction of 20% to 30%. Patients with ≤0.8 ABI should be referred to wound care or vascular specialist for compression therapy management. Single-component compression wraps (Unna boot) are more intended for physically active patients, while multicomponent (Coban 2, Profore) compression wraps are effective in more sedentary patients. Patients who are able to proceed with compression wraps should be followed up in 2 to 3 days for reevaluation, followed by follow-up to the clinic every 5 to 7 days for dressing change and wound evaluation. The application of compression wraps is a skill and can be applied incorrectly resulting in suboptimal or excessive compression. When in doubt, the patient should be referred to a wound clinic or specialist with expertise to avoid unintended injury or worsening of the wound due to incorrect compression wrap application.

Management and Patient Education

- The ability to predict wound healing is complicated and influenced by wound size, wound etiology, and host factors. Small wounds may heal within 2 to 4 weeks, whereas some wounds can take years to heal. In some instances, healing may not be the goal of therapy. When palliative care is the goal, the focus should be on symptom management (e.g., pain), preventing infection, and psychological support.

- Patients with NHW frequently experience severe pain and should be referred to pain management.

- When available, patients should be referred to facility-based or stand-alone wound care clinics where a multidisciplinary team of nurses, physicians, physical therapists, dieticians, vascular specialists, surgeons, podiatrists, and infectious disease specialists aids in the management of NHW.

- Wounds should be referred for further evaluation and management when the following etiologies are suspected: arterial ulcers, VLU, osteomyelitis (bone probed in wound bed), vasculitis, vasculopathy, autoimmune connective tissue disease, or primary dermatologic disease.

Chronic Wounds

While there are numerous wound etiologies that can result in chronic wounds, there are four common chronic wound categories. A comprehensive review of wound etiologies that may result in chronic wounds is beyond the scope of this text. However, an overview of common chronic wound categories is presented in Table 14-4.

ACKNOWLEDGMENT

Jeremy Honaker would like to thank the previous author, Dea Kent. Many of the figures, tables, and photographs have been edited or reused from the previous edition.

READINGS AND REFERENCES

Cambiaso-Daniel, J., Boukovalas, S., Bitz, G. H., Branski, L. K., Herndon, D. N., & Culnan, D. M. (2018). Topical antimicrobials in burn care: Part 1-topical antiseptics. *Annals of Plastic Surgery.* https://doi.org/10.1097/SAP.0000000000001297

Edsberg, L. E., Black, J. M., Goldberg, M., McNichol, L., Moore, L., & Sieggreen, M. (2016). Revised National Pressure Ulcer Advisory Panel Pressure Injury Staging System: Revised pressure injury staging system. *Journal of Wound, Ostomy, and Continence Nursing, 43*(6), 585–597.

Grada, A. A., & Phillips, T. J. (2017). Lymphedema: Pathophysiology and clinical manifestations. *Journal of the American Academy of Dermatology, 77*(6), 1009–1020.

Gupta, S., Andersen, C., Black, J., de Leon, J., Fife, C., Lantis Li, J. C., Neizgoda, J., Snyder, R., Sumpio, B., Tettelbach, W., Treadwell, T., Weir, D., & Silverman, R. P. (2017). Management of chronic wounds: Diagnosis, preparation, treatment, and follow-up. *Wounds : A Compendium of Clinical Research and Practice, 29*(9), S19–S36.

Halstead, F. D., Rauf, M., Moiemen, N. S., Bamford, A., Wearn, C. M., Fraise, A. P., Lund, P. A., Oppenheim, B. A., & Webber, M. A. (2015). The antibacterial activity of acetic acid against biofilm-producing pathogens of relevance to burns patients. *PLoS One, 10*(9), e0136190.

Harries, R. L., Bosanquet, D. C., & Harding, K. G. (2016). Wound bed preparation: TIME for an update. *International Wound Journal, 13*(Suppl 3), 8–14.

Lim, C. S., Baruah, M., & Bahia, S. S. (2018). Diagnosis and management of venous leg ulcers. *BMJ (Clinical Research Ed.), 362*, k3115.

Mervis, J. S., & Phillips, T. J. (2019a). Pressure ulcers: Pathophysiology, epidemiology, risk factors, and presentation. *Journal of the American Academy of Dermatology, 81*(4), 881–890.

Mervis, J. S., & Phillips, T. J. (2019b). Pressure ulcers: Prevention and management. *Journal of the American Academy of Dermatology, 81*(4), 893–902.

Morton, L. M., & Phillips, T. J. (2016). Wound healing and treating wounds: Differential diagnosis and evaluation of chronic wounds. *Journal of the American Academy of Dermatology, 74*(4), 589–605; quiz 605–606.

Panuncialman, J., Hammerman, S., Carson, P., & Falanga, V. (2010). Wound edge biopsy sites in chronic wounds heal rapidly and do not result in delayed overall healing of the wound. *Wound Repair and Regeneration, 18*(1), 21–25.

Percival, S. L., Finnegan, S., Donelli, G., Vuotto, C., Rimmer, S., & Lipsky, B. A. (2016). Antiseptics for treating infected wounds: Efficacy on biofilms and effect of pH. *Critical Reviews in Microbiology, 42*(2), 293–309.

Powers, J. G., Higham, C., Broussard, K., & Phillips, T. J. (2016). Wound healing and treating wounds: Chronic wound care and management. *Journal of the American Academy of Dermatology, 74*(4), 607–625; quiz 625–626.

Sibbald, R. G., Elliott, J. A., Verma, L., Brandon, A., Persaud, R., & Ayello, E. A. (2017). Update: Topical antimicrobial agents for chronic wounds. *Advances in Skin & Wound Care, 30*(10), 438–450.

Sibbald, R. G., Goodman, L., Woo, K. Y., Krasner, D. L., Smart, H., Tariq, G., Ayello, E. A., Burrell, R. E., Keast, D. H., Mayer, D., Norton, L., & Salcido, R. S. (2011). Special considerations in wound bed preparation 2011: An update©. *Advances in Skin & Wound Care, 24*(9), 415–436; quiz 437–438.

Singer, A. J., Tassiopoulos, A., & Kirsner, R. S. (2018). Evaluation and management of lower-extremity ulcers. *The New England Journal of Medicine, 378*(3), 302–303.

Tardáguila-García, A., García-Morales, E., García-Alamino, J. M., Álvaro-Afonso, F. J., Molines-Barroso, R. J., & Lázaro-Martínez, J. L. (2019). Metalloproteinases in chronic and acute wounds: A systematic review and meta-analysis. *Wound Repair and Regeneration, 27*(4), 415–420.

Tripathi, R., Knusel, K. D., Ezaldein, H. H., Honaker, J. S., Bordeaux, J. S., & Scott, J. F. (2019). Incremental health care expenditure of chronic cutaneous ulcers in the United States. *JAMA Dermatology, 155*(6), 694–699.

Wound, Ostomy and Continence Nurses Society (WOCN). (2012). Guideline for management of wounds in patients with lower-extremity neuropathic disease. Mount Laurel: WOCN. NGC:009275.

Wound, Ostomy and Continence Nurses Society (WOCN). (2014). Guideline for management of wounds in patients with lower-extremity arterial disease. Mount Laurel: WOCN. NGC:006521.

Wound, Ostomy and Continence Nurses Society (WOCN). (2019). Guideline for management of wounds in patients with lower-extremity venous disease. Mount Laurel: WOCN. NGC:009276.

Common Dermatologic Procedures

Douglas C. DiRuggiero

In This Chapter

- Postprocedure
- Skin Biopsies Punch, Shave
- Wound Care Instructions
- Skin Tag Removal
- Liquid Nitrogen Cryotherapy
- Cantharidin Application
- Topical Salicylic Acid
- Potassium Hydroxide Preparation
- Fungal Culture
- Wood's Lamp Examination
- Mineral Oil Preparation

The following discussion presents some of the common dermatologic procedures performed in the office setting by primary care and specialty clinicians. Content is provided to serve as a guide to be incorporated into the clinical judgment. Performing these, or any, procedural skills requires the development of competency to optimize patient safety and outcomes. Therefore, it is recommended that clinicians should:

- acquire essential knowledge of the procedure, indications, and complications. However, knowledge alone does not confer competency.
- obtain basic instruction for a skill, including observation.
- demonstrate the skill under the supervision of a trainer or experienced clinician until it can be performed in its entirety without any mistakes or concerns. This should be done in a variety of settings that simulate real patient care.
- perform continuous self-assessment, with patient and peer feedback and educational updates.
- document competency of skills, which is both valuable and required in some health care settings or by regulatory boards.

POSTPROCEDURE

The following postprocedure wound instructions are widely utilized by dermatology providers, but these recommendations should be customized and adapted to your clinic and patient needs.

- Initial bandage may be left in place for 24 hours unless saturated with blood.
- After 24 hours, bathe as normal and wash the biopsy site with gentle soap and water only.
- After drying, apply petrolatum ointment to the suture line and bandage.
- Stay out of oceans, lakes, and swimming pools until after the sutures are removed.

- Return for suture removal as indicated.
  - Face and neck in 3 to 7 days
  - Arms in 7 to 10 days
  - Trunk and legs in 10 to 14 days
- Keep wound moist with petrolatum and cover for 1 to 2 weeks for optimal healing and best cosmetic results.
- The patient should be educated about the signs and symptoms of infection, including redness, warmth, tenderness, and discharge. Contact information should be given in the event that this should occur.
- If bleeding should occur, apply constant pressure for 20 minutes. Contact office if bleeding persists.
- No smoking until wound is completely healed. Smoking constricts blood vessels, causing delayed or improper wound healing.
- Inform patients when and how they will receive the results of their biopsy.
- Arrange for suture removal.

SKIN BIOPSY

Punch Biopsy

Punch biopsy is a *nonsterile* procedure by which sampling of an endophytic skin lesion or full thickness of skin is performed for the purpose of histopathologic examination.

Indications

- "Rashes" in general
- Small pigmented lesions of the skin (nevi or small melanomas)
- Benign skin tumors (i.e., dermatofibroma, neurofibroma)
- Vascular disease of the skin or subcutaneous fat
- Superficial inflammatory or granulomatous diseases
- Papulosquamous disease (i.e., psoriasis)
- Connective tissue disorders (i.e., systemic lupus erythematosus, discoid lupus erythematosus)

Contraindications

- Infection at the biopsy site
- Superficial artery or nerve (i.e., Erb point) at biopsy site
- Pigmented lesion larger than available punches

Equipment

- Alcohol or chlorhexidine prep pads
- Examination gloves and sterile gloves
- Syringe, usually 1 mL or 3 mL
  - 25G to 31G needle depending on site; 31G insulin syringes are helpful for noses and ears
- Lidocaine 1% or 2%, with or without epinephrine, depending on site
- Sterile 4×4 or 2×2 gauze sponges
- Baker-type biopsy punch or equivalent, commercially available in sizes 2 to 12 mm
- Pickup forceps
- Iris scissors or scalpel
- Needle drivers
- Monofilament nonabsorbable suture appropriate for the thickness of skin; 4-0 black nylon on a P-12 needle is useful for most punches
- Absorbable suture for larger punches (8 to 12 mm)
- Formalin in normal saline specimen containers of appropriate size for the specimen prelabeled with the patient's name and medical record number—never label after the fact. A biopsy for direct immunofluorescence should be placed in a container with Michels transport medium
- Hyfrecator for control of bleeding
- Petrolatum-based ointment (like Vaseline or Aquaphor)
- Adhesive dressing of appropriate size (check for allergy)

Preparation

- Procedure details, risks, and alternatives are discussed with the patient. All questions are answered and informed consent is given by the patient and documented in the chart.
- All specimen containers to be used and histology requisitions are labeled and information is verified by patient.
- After gloving, the area to be sampled is cleaned with alcohol or chlorhexidine.

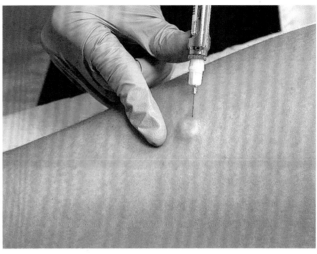

FIG. 15-1. Injection of local anesthetic using a 30G needle that produces a wheal under the lesion for biopsy. Localized blanching will occur when lidocaine with epinephrine is used as anesthetic.

- Lidocaine is injected intradermally below the lesion to be sampled; if done correctly, the lesion will be raised on a wheal (Fig. 15-1).

Procedure

- Sterile gloves are not required for closure with sutures.
- With the nondominant hand, stretch the skin perpendicular to the relaxed skin lines. This will result in an elliptical defect when the tension is released, making for a much more cosmetically acceptable closure.
- With the dominant hand, place the biopsy punch over the lesion and gently apply downward pressure while twisting the punch until you *feel* a slight pop and the punch goes through the dermis (Fig. 15-2A,B).
- Retract the punch from the defect. *Gently* lift the freed skin specimen with the pickups and cut or snip the bottom attachment with the subcutaneous fat (Fig. 15-2C).
- Place the specimen into a container and seal.
- Blot biopsy site with gauze square and apply direct pressure to the site. Electrocautery with a hyfrecator may be used with caution. Proceed when hemostasis is complete.

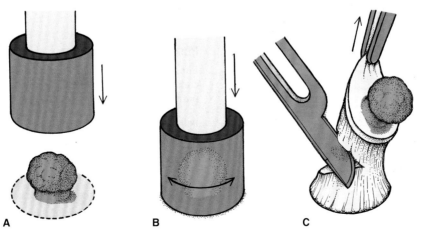

FIG. 15-2. Punch biopsy. **A:** Punch lesion perpendicular to skin. **B:** Use a gentle circular motion to ensure all tissue is released but be mindful of any underlying structures. **C:** Gently grab tissue on the edge of the punch, or at the bottom of the punch, and cut or snip the tissue at the base.

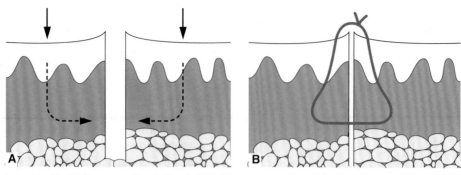

FIG. 15-3. Simple interrupted suture. **A:** Closure for punch biopsy with equal amounts of tissue on both sides of the defect. **B:** Eversion of the wound edges for optimal healing. (Zuber, T. J., & Mayeaux, E. J. Jr. [2004]. *Atlas of primary care procedures.* Wolters Kluwer Health I Lippincott Williams & Wilkins.)

- Suture the defect closed with interrupted sutures; larger defects may also require an absorbable deep cuticular suture to prevent a dead space at the wound base (Fig. 15-3).
- Apply petrolatum ointment to wound after hemostasis is achieved.
- Apply adhesive dressing.

Anticipated Outcomes

- Mild pain at biopsy site
- Possible infection
- Possible bleeding
- Possible separation of the wound edges of punch biopsy
- Scar at the biopsy site. Be sure to emphasize this point when you obtain informed consent.

Aftercare

+ Give patients both verbal and printed aftercare instructions in their preferred language (see wound care instructions below).

Shave Biopsy

Shave biopsy is a *nonsterile* procedure by which sampling of an exophytic or shallow endophytic skin lesion is performed for the purpose of histopathologic examination.

Indications

- Raised lesions
- Dome-shaped nevi and benign tumors
- Nonmelanoma skin cancers

**Suspicious pigmented lesions too large for a single punch biopsy should be excised, but a deeper shave (deep saucerization) which extends into the reticular dermis can be utilized by experienced clinicians to ensure removal of the entire lesion.

Contraindications

- Infection at the biopsy site
- Vascular lesion of unknown extent for depth (cavernous hemangioma)
- Inflammatory rashes are best evaluated by punch biopsy, allowing the pathologist to assess all layers of the skin

Equipment

- Alcohol or chlorhexidine prep pads
- Examination gloves

- Syringe, size as required (usually 1cc or 3cc)
- 25G to 31G needle depending on site. 31G insulin syringes are helpful for noses and ears
- Lidocaine 1% or 2%, with or without epinephrine, depending on site
  - Sterile 4×4 or 2×2 gauze sponges
- Derma Blade, double-sided shave blade, or a no. 15 scalpel blade
- Formalin in normal saline specimen containers of appropriate size for the specimen prelabeled with the patient's name and medical record number—never label after the fact
- Aluminum chloride 20% solution (Drysol), Monsel solution, or hyfrecator
- Cotton-tipped applicators
- Petrolatum-based ointment (Vaseline or Aquaphor)
- Adhesive dressing of appropriate size

Preparation

- Same as for punch biopsy

Procedure

- Using the Derma Blade or scalpel blade, tangentially shave the lesion off the skin with a gentle side-to-side movement (Fig. 15-4). Place the specimen into a container and seal.

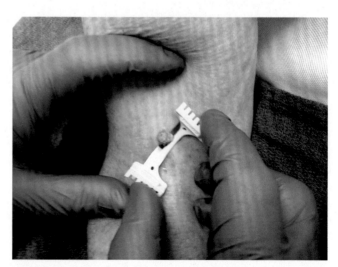

FIG. 15-4. Shave biopsy. Holding the Derma Blade tangentially to the skin surface, the blade can remove a sample of the epidermis and dermis. A deeper saucerization requires a sharper angle to the skin, allowing the blade to scoop deep into the dermis. (Photo courtesy of Theodore Scott.)

- Blot biopsy site with gauze square and use a cotton-tip applicator saturated (not dripping) with the aluminum chloride or Monsel solution to stop mild bleeding. Light electrocautery with a hyfrecator may be needed.
- Apply petrolatum ointment to wound after hemostasis is achieved.
- Apply adhesive dressing.
- Give patients both verbal and printed aftercare instructions in their preferred language.

Anticipated Outcomes

- Same as with punch biopsy

Aftercare

- See wound care instructions below, although shave biopsy has no suture.

Wound Care Instructions

> ### CLINICAL PEARLS
>
> - Avoid epinephrine on fingertips and penile tip.
> - Punch biopsies ≤4 mm can be left open to heal by secondary intention.
> - Alcohol and hydrogen peroxide are no longer used for routine wound care as they are toxic to the keratinocytes.
> - Neomycin, polymyxin, and bacitracin ointments are not recommended as they are potential sensitizers.
> - For all skin diseases other than pigmented lesions, a 4-mm punch will give the pathologist adequate material to make a diagnosis if there is sufficient depth.
> - For pigmented lesions, select a punch that will completely sample the lesion and a slim margin of clear skin.
> - Never perform a shallow shave biopsy of a pigmented skin lesion to avoid the risk of transecting the pigmented lesion. The most predictive factor in the clinical course of melanoma treatment is the depth of invasion on initial biopsy. This information would be lost with a transected specimen.
> - Never take a small punch or several small punches of a large pigmented lesion. A small punch of a large lesion will not provide the most accurate measurement of the depth.
> - If a pigmented lesion is too large to sample comfortably in your clinic, arrange expedient referral to a provider skilled in dermatology or surgery.
> - Avoid Monsel solution and silver nitrate in cosmetically sensitive areas as they can leave a permanent pigmentation.

Skin Tag Removal

Procedure to remove benign skin tags (arcochordon) by various methods

Indications

- Symptomatic (tender, bleeding, or itching)
- Cosmetic concerns

Equipment

Depending on the method used:

- Alcohol swabs
- Gauze 4×4
- Lidocaine, or topical anesthetic

- Small sharp scissors (gradle)
- Forceps (optional)
- Liquid nitrogen
- Hyfrecator

Preparation

- Procedure details, risks, alternatives, and recurrence are discussed with the patient. All questions are answered and informed consent is given by the patient.
- Advise patients that this may be considered a cosmetic procedure and *not* covered by insurance.
- If you have any doubt as to the benign nature of the lesion, *send it for biopsy!*
- Consider anesthesia options: ice for 1 minute prior to removal; a brief spray of liquid nitrogen (LN2); topical anesthetic; lidocaine injection; and no anesthesia, which is very common for clipping, hyfrecation, and cryotherapy.

Procedures

Several techniques, including scissor removal, shave removal, hyfrecation, and cryosurgery.

Scissor Removal

- Grasp the skin tag and slightly extend it upward. Make sure to use sharp tissue scissors to assure a quick and accurate snip at the base of the lesion (Fig. 15-5). Bleeding should be controlled with pressure, as it is the least likely method to result in scarring. Aluminum chloride (Drysol) is irritating but can be used if the pressure is ineffective. If bleeding continues, electrocautery/hyfrecation may be used after assurance of anesthesia. Before using cautery, remove all alcohol and aluminum chloride (flammable) that may be left on the skin.

Shave Removal

- Perform the procedure by gently grasping the acrochordon with forceps, slightly extending the lesion upward. Using a Derma Blade or scalpel, shave the lesion at the base (similar technique as shave biopsy). This is the preferred technique for a larger acrochordon or fibroepithelial polyps. Control bleeding as above.

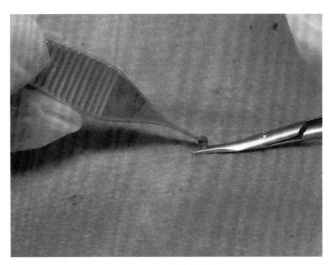

FIG. 15-5. Snip skin tag. (Photo courtesy of M. Bobonich.)

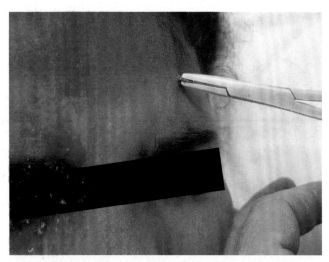

FIG. 15-6. Cryotherapy with needle holder. (Photo courtesy of M. Bobonich.)

Hyfrecation

- Touch the base of the skin tag with the tip of the hyfrecator (high-frequency eradicator) set at lowest frequency. Contact the skin at a few second intervals until the base turns white/gray.
- Limit the contacts to three for each skin tag if possible.

Liquid Nitrogen

- Place the LN2 spray gun nozzle about 1.5 cm from the lesion and aim at the center. Spray until a minimal ice ball encompasses the skin tag. Do up to three freeze and thaw cycles.
- Freeze times that exceed 10 seconds or are performed at very close range may result in significant tissue damage and hyperpigmentation.
- To minimize the risk of spray to the surrounding tissue, cold forceps can be used to apply the therapy. Place the tip of a small needle holder or mosquito forceps into a styrofoam cup of LN2 for 30 seconds, allowing the temperature of the metal instrument to drop. Then grasp the papule, and the cold will transfer to the lesion, creating an ice ball. The effect of cryotherapy can be controlled so that the surrounding skin is not damaged. This method is also used for warts (Fig. 15-6).

Anticipated Outcomes

- Minimal discomfort
- Small blister formation or crust for 5 to 7 days
- Scarring and recurrence

Aftercare

Postprocedure care will depend on the type of technique utilized.

- Advise the patient what to expect post procedure, as the skin tag usually does not fall off immediately with cryotherapy or hyfrecation. It usually takes a week and may darken or turn black before it falls off.
- With snip or shave method, advise wound care with daily cleansing with soap and water, petrolatum, and small bandage as needed.
- Educate patients about the signs of infection and the importance of reporting troublesome changes promptly.
- Patients should understand that skin tags can recur and new ones develop.

Liquid Nitrogen Cryotherapy

LN2 (−198°C) applied directly to warts or other epidermal lesions induces a localized form of frostbite, causing tissue damage to keratinocytes. A blister develops at the dermal–epidermal junction. When the blister dries and erodes, the affected area will slough part or all of the epidermis.

Cryotherapy is not the same as *cryosurgery* which is performed on some nonmelanoma skin cancers by experienced dermatologists.

Indications

- Verruca (warts), molluscum contagiosum, actinic keratoses (AKs), seborrheic keratoses, solar lentigines, keloids, and other benign cutaneous lesions

Contraindications

- Patients with Raynaud's, cold urticaria, cryoglobulinemia
- Be cautious in cosmetic areas, as cryotherapy can result in hypo- or hyperpigmentation and/or scarring

Equipment

- LN2
- Cryogun (Brymill or Cry-Ac spray)
- Insulated storage container (or one-time-use styrofoam cup) with cotton-tipped applicators
- Disposable otoscope tips

Procedure

- Explain the procedure risks, alternatives, and expected course of treatment.
- Using a cryogun or cotton-tipped applicator, LN2 is applied to the lesion (Figs. 15-7 and 15-8).

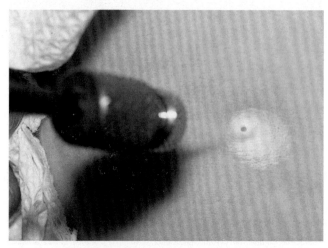

FIG. 15-7. Cryotherapy with spray gun. (Photo courtesy of M. Bobonich.)

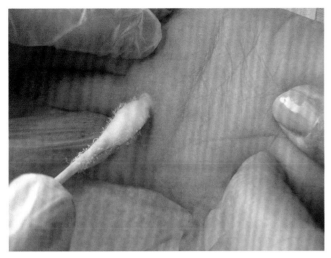

FIG. 15-8. Cryotherapy with cotton applicator.

- The visibly frozen area (ice ball) will turn white and should be maintained for 3 to 5 seconds depending on the type of lesion and location. A 2-mm border surrounding the perimeter of the lesion should be included (Fig. 15-9).
- Placing a disposable otoscope tip directly over the lesion before treating will allow you to confine the freeze to the specific lesion without treating too much surrounding tissue (useful in children).
- The ice ball should thaw in 30 to 60 seconds. The cycle may be repeated up to three cycles, which may lead to a better treatment response in thicker warts.

Actinic Keratosis

- AKs are defined as precancerous lesions in Section 2.2 and therefore special awareness is necessary when treating with LN2.
- AKs are technically confined to the epidermis and should respond nicely to cryotherapy. However, thicker or hypertrophic lesions may represent squamous cell carcinoma in situ, especially on the scalp. Patients should be advised to return for follow-up if the lesion does not completely resolve (Fig. 15-10).
- If a lesion has been treated with LN2 more than once without resolution, it should be biopsied.

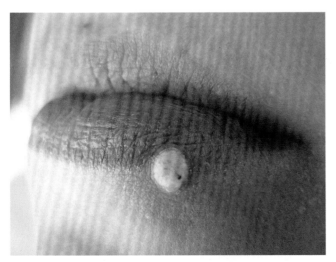

FIG. 15-9. Ice ball from cryotherapy. (Sauer, G. C. [2017]. *Manual of skin diseases* [11th ed.]. Wolters Kluwer.)

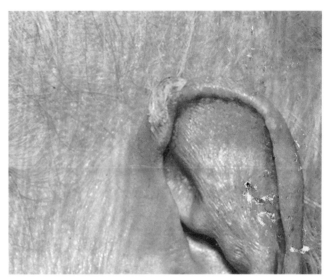

FIG. 15-10. Hypertrophic actinic keratosis, strongly consider biopsy, but if LN2 therapy is utilized, follow carefully to ensure complete resolution. (Photo courtesy of M. Bobonich.)

Anticipated Outcomes

- Patient response can vary from minimal erythema to hemorrhagic blistering.
- Cryotherapy is painful during procedure and in the immediate few minutes post procedure.
- Cryotherapy can result in hypo-, hyper-, or depigmentation, especially in darkly skinned individuals.
- Scarring can occur with intense or extensive cryotherapy treatment.

Aftercare

- Blisters commonly form within days. Plain petrolatum should be applied.
- Warn patients that they may develop blood blisters (especially on the fingers/toes and with repeated freeze–thaw cycles).
- Try to keep blister intact. If necessary, rupture with sterile pin but do not unroof.

CLINICAL PEARLS

- It is better to undertreat a lesion and retreat at a later date than to overtreat and increase risk of dyspigmentation or scarring.
- Use of liquid nitrogen around the nail may cause damage to the nail plate.
- Over-the-counter (OTC) freeze sprays (dimethyl ether) are available but much less effective than liquid nitrogen. If a margin beyond the border of the verruca is not achieved, the patient could develop a "doughnut-shaped" lesion that has central clearing only (Fig. 15-11).
- Cotton-tipped applicator should be used on only one patient, then discarded.
- A pulsing spray or intermittent contact with the applicator maintains the ice ball without causing a spread to healthy tissue.
- Thinner lesions require a shorter treatment time, while thicker lesions should have a longer ice ball and repeated treatment may be needed.
- A fast freeze and slow thaw is the most effective cryotherapy treatment.
- Always biopsy suspicious lesions or those that do not respond to LN2 therapy.

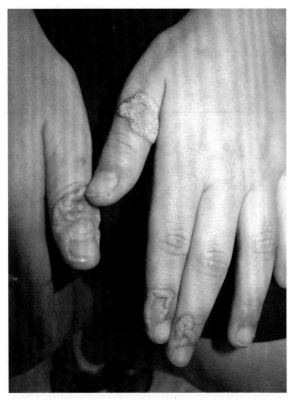

FIG. 15-11. Ring wart. "Doughnut" or ringed warts occurring post cryotherapy. (Used with permission from Gru, A. A., & Wick, M. [2018]. *Pediatric dermatopathology and dermatology.* Wolters Kluwer Health.)

Cantharidin

Cantharidin is a liquid derived from a blistering insect which causes acantholysis (loss of adhesion between keratinocytes). The result is a blister that develops between the epidermal and dermal layers of skin. *Cantharidin is not FDA approved in the United States, but was placed on the FDA's proposed bulk substances list and may only be used in the professional setting. It cannot be prescribed or applied by patients.*

Indications

- Molluscum contagiosum and verruca vulgaris (except mosaic warts)

Contraindications

- Use with caution on the face, digits, skin folds, and genital mucosa.

Equipment

- Cantharidin 0.7%, Cantharone
- Canthacur PS (combination of Cantharone plus podophyllin 5% and salicylic acid [SA] 30%)
- Wooden-tipped applicator or toothpicks (flat end)
- Clear tape

Procedure

- The clinician should carefully apply the liquid directly to the lesion and avoid any contact with the surrounding healthy tissue.
- The wooden end of a cotton-tipped applicator or flat toothpick is helpful in applying minute amounts to 1- to 2-mm lesions. Each applicator is discarded after touching the lesion (Fig. 15-12).

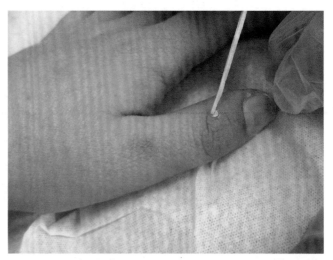

FIG. 15-12. Cantharidin applicator. (Casanova, R., Chuang, A., Goepfert, A. R., Heuppchen, N. A., Weiss, P. M., Beckmann, C. R. B., Ling, F. W., Herbert, W. N. P., Laube, D. W., & Smith, R. P. [2018]. *Obstetrics and gynecology* [8th ed.]. Wolters Kluwer Health | Lippincott Williams & Wilkins.)

- As the liquid dries, it forms a clear film (Canthacur PS produces a white film) over the area. Cover with a nonporous tape.
- There is a large variation in practice regarding the amount of treatment time that cantharidin is left on the skin. Some suggest removing the tape and washing off the film in 2 to 4 hours after application. Others recommend leaving it in place for up to 8 hours.
  - Variation also depends on the location. Thicker skin (plantar surface) may require longer application time.
- Petrolatum should be applied twice daily for comfort and to promote healing.

Anticipated Outcome

- A blister can form within hours after application. At that time, the tape should be removed, and the area washed with soap and water to remove any residual medication.
- Severe blistering can result even with correct application.

Aftercare

- Treat the blister with plain petrolatum twice daily.
- Try to keep blister intact. If necessary, rupture with sterile pin but do not unroof.
- When treating warts, SA or liquid nitrogen may be applied when blisters heal, if wart tissue remains.

CLINICAL PEARLS

- At the first visit, treat only a few lesions and allow only 2 to 3 hours of contact time to assess the patient's response and tolerance.
- A hypersensitivity reaction is rare but possible.
- Severe blistering can occur if cantharidin is applied incorrectly or with long application times.
- Avoid contact with opposing skin (axillae, thighs, gluteal folds, etc.).
- Use a new toothpick for *each application* to prevent contamination of multidose bottles.
- Repeated treatments every 3 to 4 weeks are often required.
- Patient application of topical salicylic acid on warts between visits can accelerate the treatment process.

Topical Salicylic Acid

Salicylic acid (SA) is a keratolytic agent which is intended to soften and thin excess skin which can build up over and around warts, callus, and other benign growths.

Indications (for Use at Home)

- Warts, calluses, and corns

Contraindications

- Pregnancy
- Peripheral neuropathy (diabetes)
- Peripheral artery disease
- Nonintact skin or erosions

Equipment

- SA is available in liquid or plaster forms and with various applicators: Duofilm, Duoplant, Compound W, Wart-off, Occlusal-HP, Trans-Ver-Sal, Virasal, and Mediplast are commonly available.
- Most OTC preparations are 17% SA. OTC plasters with 40% SA are more effective and may shorten treatment.
- Soak the affected area in warm water for 10 to 20 minutes prior to treatment.
- Rub the surface with a nail or foot file to remove loosened skin. There may be some pinpoint bleeding.
- Apply liquid or plaster to the affected area and only a few millimeters border of normal skin.
- Leave in place for 12 to 24 hours, and then remove.
- Repeat daily until lesions resolve.
- If discomfort develops, discontinue for several days until better, then resume for shorter intervals.

Anticipated Outcomes

- *Gradual* destruction and peeling of skin will occur in the treated area.
- It can take weeks or months to eradicate a wart using this method, especially on the plantar surface, but reduction of callus will relieve discomfort.
- Skin may become white and macerated.
- Swelling, tenderness, and secondary infection can occur from overuse.

Aftercare

- Pare down (exfoliate) hyperkeratotic skin with nail file or pumice stone in between treatments to ensure that medication penetrates the affected area.

CLINICAL PEARLS

- Salicylic acid will destroy all skin in which it contacts, so careful application is advised.
- Plain petrolatum can be applied to the normal skin surrounding the wart prior to treatment to prevent damage to normal skin.
- Disposable emery boards may be used for exfoliating the lesion. Discard after use.
- A pumice stone can harbor the virus and recontaminate the skin.
- Occlusion with duct tape is preferred, but a Band-Aid can be used to keep the SA in place.

In-Office Diagnostic Tests

Potassium Hydroxide Preparation

Potassium hydroxide (KOH) prep allows the immediate examination of scale or debris to determine the presence or absence of superficial fungal elements or other organisms. KOH obliterates the cellular components, making fungal elements easier to visualize.

Indications

- Any scaling, vesicular or pustular eruption that could represent a dermatophyte or yeast infection
- Identification of molluscum bodies
- Demodex (mites) infestations

Contraindications

- None

Equipment

- Microscope, glass slides, and coverslip
- No. 10 or 15 blade or curette
- Solution: 10% to 20% KOH; 20% KOH with added dimethyl sulfoxide (DMSO); Swartz-Lamkins stain (SLS) or Chlorazol black E counterstain containing KOH plus dye (makes the fungal elements more visible)
- Alcohol lamp or disposable lighter as heating source (generally not needed for DMSO, SLS, or Chlorazol stains)

Procedure

- *Skin:* scrape the active scaly border of the lesion (area of highest yield) and place scale on a glass slide. For blisters or pustules, the fungus is in the roof of the vesicle. Gently dissect the vesicle and scrape the underside with no. 15 blade and smear on the glass slide.
- *Nails:* collect subungual debris from the distal lateral edge of the nail or the white scale from the underside of the nail surface.
- *Hair:* pull hairs from affected site ensuring that the root or bulb is present. Tape the bulb/proximal shaft portion onto a glass slide, (this is not to be confused with a hair pull test, or trichogram).
- Add a drop or two of KOH or other counterstain preparations to the specimen and place a coverslip over the specimen (Fig. 15-13A,B).
- Heat *gently,* but not to boiling, for 3 to 5 seconds. If using DMSO, SLS, or Chlorazol counterstains, heating is not necessary.
- SLS prep can be examined immediately, but KOH slides of thicker specimens may need to sit for 5 to 10 minutes.
- Place slide on microscope with low-to-medium light. Focus with the low-power objective (4× or 10×) and scan the slide until possible hyphae or spores are identified. Then switch to a higher power (10× or 40×) for a closer examination.
- Dermatophytes will be seen as long, segmented hyphal elements which will be bluish/green if stained with SLS (Fig. 15-14A).
- For tinea versicolor or pityrosporum folliculitis, you will see both hyphae and spores, the classic "spaghetti and meatballs" sign (Fig. 15-14B).
- *Candida* will show mainly budding yeast cells (Fig. 15-14C).

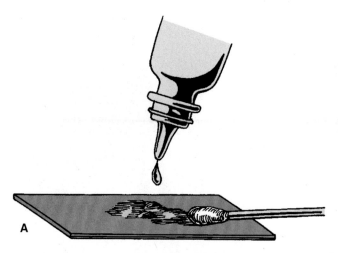

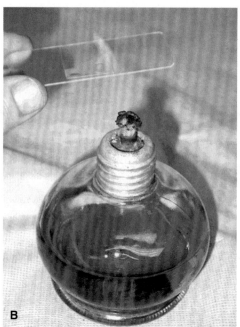

FIG. 15-13. KOH preparations. **A:** The specimen is collected and placed onto a glass slide. A drop of 10% to 20% KOH is also placed on the slide. The preparations are then covered with a cover slide for microscopic viewing. **B:** Gentle heating of a small amount of scale with KOH prep over an alcohol lamp is the key for a useful fungal preparation. (Photos courtesy of Victor Newcomer, MD, Santa Monica, CA.)

- *Hairs* will show clusters of spores either within the hair shaft (endothrix) or clung to the outside of the hair shaft (ectothrix). Visualize under 10–20× magnification.
- Molluscum is seen as spherical bodies within the keratinocytes.

Anticipated Outcome

- This procedure causes minimal discomfort to the patient.
- Confirmation of the presence or absence of spores or hyphae or molluscum bodies helps develop a differential diagnosis.

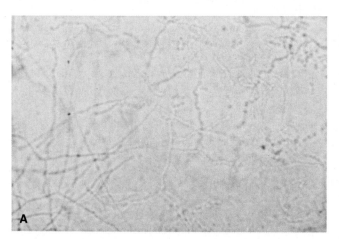

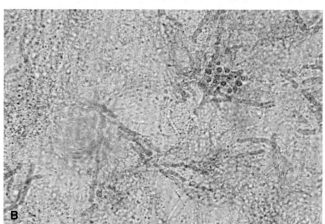

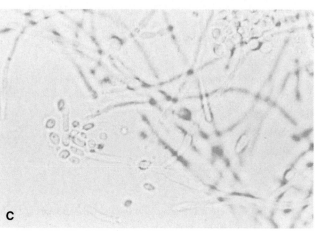

FIG. 15-14. **A:** KOH preparation, with dermatophyte hyphae visualized on microscopic examination. **B:** Tinea versicolor on KOH preparation. Note the short, stubby hyphae ("spaghetti") and the clusters of spores ("meatballs"). The hyphae and spores elements stain blue when using KOH with a Swartz-Lamkins counterstain. **C:** Budding yeast cells of Candida.

- If the KOH prep is negative but there is strong clinical suspicion, repeat the KOH prep and/or perform a fungal culture.

Aftercare

- None

Fungal Culture

Fungal culture of a skin, nail, or hair specimen is performed to detect the presence of superficial fungal elements. This is *not* the appropriate laboratory testing for deep fungal infections.

Indications

- Specimens should be tested for fungus if you are unable to perform a KOH prep; still suspect a fungus even with a negative KOH prep; or need to identify the specific causative fungal organism. Sensitivities may also be ordered and performed.

Contraindications

- None

Equipment

- Sterile transport container or culture media relative to the type of test, such as dermatophyte test medium (DTM), Mycosel agar, or Sabouraud dextrose agar
- Alcohol prep pads
- Instruments to collect sample: nail clippers, curette, no. 10 or 15 scalpel blade, brush (toothbrush)

Procedure

- These are general guidelines for most fungal specimen collection. Fungi can remain viable for days in scale and hair, so no medium is required; and the specimen is sent directly to the laboratory in a sterile culture container.
- If there is a specific test such as DTM or laboratory analysis being used, follow the recommended procedures for collection according to the company (Fig. 15-15).

Skin Specimens

- Collect specimens from areas that are clean and dry. Avoid collecting skin that has topical moisturizers or medications.
- Using a no. 10 or 15 scalpel blade, gently scrape the leading edge of the scaly patch or plaque. Allow the scale to fall into the sterile container or culture medium.

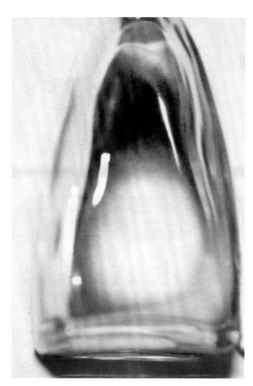

FIG. 15-15. Fungal culture using the DTM. Note the positive result indicated by the color change from yellow to red. (Goodheart, H. P. [2015]. *Goodheart's photoguide of common skin disorders* [4th ed.]. Wolters Kluwer Health | Lippincott Williams & Wilkins.)

Nail Specimens

- Prior to collection, clean the nail and surrounding skin with warm, soapy water. Let dry. Then wipe the area with an alcohol prep pad and air dry.
- Use sterile instruments to trim the free edge of the nail and expose debris.
- Discard the nail.
- Gently wipe with a new alcohol pad and air dry (again).
- Use a sterile curette to remove subungual debris and collect in a sterile specimen container or specific container requested by the laboratory.
- Label appropriately and complete requisition.

Hair Specimens

- Avoid collection of hair with hair care products.
- Identify the area and trim hairs close to the scalp. Pluck hairs with tweezers, forceps, or brush and place in sterile container or on specified culture medium.

Scalp Specimens

- Use a sterile scalpel/blade and/or toothbrush-like tool to scrape over the affected area and transfer scale into collection container. The brush may also be submitted.

Anticipated Outcome

- Minimal discomfort
- Confirmed diagnosis

Aftercare

- None unless there is bleeding, and then small bandages are sufficient.

Wood's Lamp Examination

The Wood's lamp is a safe and inexpensive office tool which is useful to diagnose infections of the skin and disorders of pigmentation. Invented by a Baltimore physician, Robert Wood, in 1903, the Wood's lamp emits black light (long-wave UVR) produced by a high-pressure mercury arc fitted with a compound filter, known as the "Wood's filter." Fluorescence of skin occurs when the Wood's light is absorbed and radiation of a longer wavelength, usually visible light, is emitted.

Indications

- Bacterial skin infections, fungal skin infections, hypopigmentation or depigmentation, hyperpigmentation, melasma, and porphyria

Equipment

- Wood's lamp

Procedure

- Some Wood's lamps need to warm up for about 1 minute.
- The examination room should be completely darkened.
- Topical medications, lint, deodorant, and soap residue should be wiped off from the site being examined, as these can fluoresce under Wood's lamp.
- Hold the Wood's lamp 4 to 5 inches away from the skin. Beginning at the scalp, you can gradually pass the light over the entire surface of the skin in a "windshield wiper" type of motion. Be sure to look at axilla and genital areas, especially if you suspect vitiligo.

Anticipated Outcome

- Fluorescence of normal skin is faint or absent.
- Vitiligo: Lesions are well demarcated and fluorescent under Wood's lamp examination. A blue-white color is noted and varies in intensity depending on decreased or absent melanin (Fig. 15-16).
- Hyperpigmentation: Lesions show an increased border contrast under Wood's lamp.
- Pseudomonas fluoresces green in folliculitis and infected wounds.
- Erythrasma fluoresces coral red because of the *Corynebacterium*.
- Propionibacterium acnes show orange-red in comedones.
- Tinea versicolor: *Malassezia furfur* fluoresces yellowish-white or copper-orange.
- Tinea capitis: blue-green (most *Microsporum* species), sometimes dull yellow (*Microsporum gypseum*) and dull blue (Trichophyton schoenleinii)
- Porphyria: Urine, teeth, and feces may fluoresce pink-red.

Aftercare

- None

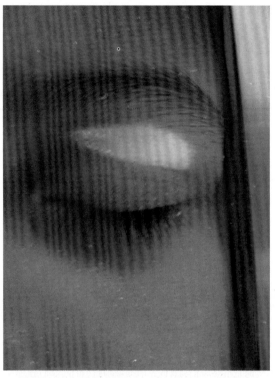

FIG. 15-16. Wood's lamp examination. Note the enhanced coloration of the depigmented area. (Photo courtesy of M. Bobonich.)

Mineral Oil Preparation

Mineral oil mount for microscopic analysis to identify mites, eggs, or scybala (feces)

Indications

- Scabies (Sarcoptes scabiei)

Equipment

- Mineral oil
- Glass microscope slide
- No. 15 surgical blade (nonsterile)
- Slide coverslip
- Microscope

Procedure

- Identify new, nonexcoriated burrow (typically linear) or vesicle. Look for a black dot at one end, which may represent the mite, and scrape at that location + apply a drop of mineral oil onto the center of a glass microscope slide. Dip the edge of a no. 15

surgical blade also in the oil (or apply a drop of oil to the blade). Utilizing the lateral edge of the scalpel blade, at a 45-degree angle, scrape the skin to attain several wide superficial skin scrapings. There may be some pinpoint bleeding.

- After scraping, mix the accumulated debris on the blade into the mineral oil on the slide, and apply a coverslip.

- Scan the slide at low power (4× or 10×) before switching to high power (20×), to look for scabiei mites.

- Eggs may be present as discrete and ovoid-shaped figures, either containing a larval mite or the empty remains of a hatched egg. Scybala, or fecal pellets, will appear as brownish-black, poorly defined globules (Fig. 15-17).

Anticipated Outcome

- Slight discomfort and minimal bleeding are expected with scraping.

Aftercare

- None

CLINICAL PEARLS

- Scabies mites are often few in numbers (except in the case of crusted scabies). The diagnosis can be confirmed with the presence of eggs or scybala alone.

- Scrape from several areas to increase likelihood of positive results.

- If clinical suspicion is high, treat patients and family members for scabies, even if scraping is negative.

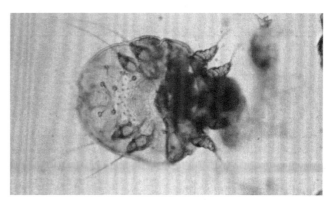

FIG. 15-17. Scabies mite.

ACKNOWLEDGMENT

Special thanks to previous contributors: Theodore D. Scott, Kathleen Haycraft, Kelly Noska, Janice T. Chussil, Katie Brouillard O'Brien, and Melissa E. Cyr.

READINGS

Micromedix. (2020). *Micromedex medication, disease and toxicology management. (Micromedix 2.0).* Truven Health Analytics. www.micromedixsolutions.com

Scott, T. D. (2011). Procedure primer: The potassium hydroxide preparation. *The Journal of the Dermatology Nurses' Association, 3*(5), 304–305.

Sterry, W., Paus, R., & Burgdorf, W. (2006). *Thieme clinical companions: Dermatology* (5th ed.). Thieme.

Usatine, R., Tobinick, E., & Siegel, D. (1998). *Skin surgery: A practical guide.* St. Louis, Mosby.

Index

Note: Page numbers followed by "f", "t", figures, tables, respectively.

ORAL ANTIMICROBIAL AGENTS, MICRO-ORGANISM SUSCEPTIBILITY, AND DOSING FOR SKIN AND SOFT TISSUE INFECTIONS

	PEDIATRIC	ADULT
Penicillins—*Enterococcus faecalis, Staph* spp., *Strep* spp., *Escherichia coli[a], Klebsiella* spp.[a], *Proteus* spp.[a], *Pasteurella* spp., *Erysipelothrix rhusiopathiae, Eikenella corrodens, Cutibacterium acnes*		
Penicillin V	25–50 mg/kg/day divided q.i.d. (Max 2000 mg daily)	250–500 mg q.i.d.
Amoxicillin	25 mg/kg/dose divided b.i.d. (Max 2000 mg per dose)	500 mg t.i.d.
Amoxicillin-Clavulanic acid	25 mg/kg/dose divided b.i.d. (Max 2000 mg per dose)	875/125 mg b.i.d.
Cephalosporins—*Staph* spp., *Strep* spp., *Klebsiella* spp., *Proteus* spp.,[b] *E. coli*,[b] *Vibrio vulnificus*,[b] *Cutibacterium acnes, Aeromonas hydrophila*,[b] *Erysipelothrix rhusiopathiae*		
Cephalexin	25–50 mg/kg/day divided b.i.d.–q.i.d. (Max 2000 mg daily)	250–500 mg q.i.d.
Cefdinir	14 mg/kg/day divided q.d.–b.i.d. (Max 600 mg daily)	300 mg b.i.d.–q.i.d. *or* 600 mg q.d.
Lincosamides—*Staph* spp., *Strep* spp., *Corynebacterium* spp., *Erysipelothrix rhusiopathiae*		
Clindamycin	10 mg/kg/dose divided t.i.d. (Max 450 mg per dose)	300 mg q.i.d. *or* 450 mg t.i.d.
Macrolides—*Strep* spp., *Haemophilus* spp., *Neisseria gonorrhea, Mycobacterium marinum*		
Erythromycin	30–50 mg/kg/day t.i.d.–q.i.d. (Max 2 g daily)	250–500 mg q.i.d.
Azithromycin	10 mg/kg/loading dose (Max 500 mg per dose) then 5 mg/kg dose q.d. (Max 250 mg per dose)	500 mg loading dose followed by 250 mg daily
Fluoroquinolones—*Staph* spp., *Strep* spp., *Enterobacter* spp., *Klebsiella* spp., *E. coli, Serratia* spp., *Vibrio vulnificus, Haemophilus* spp., *Pasteurella* spp., *Eikenella corrodens, Pseudomonas aeruginosa, Aeromonas hydrophila, Erysipelothrix rhusiopathiae*		
Ciprofloxacin	10–20 mg/kg/day divided b.i.d. (Max 500–750 mg per dose)	500–750 mg b.i.d.
Levofloxacin	8–10 mg/kg/dose b.i.d. (Max 750 mg daily)	500–750 mg daily
Folate Pathway Inhibitors—*Staph* spp., *Eikenella corrodens, Pasteurella, Mycobacterium marinum, Enterobacter* spp.		
TMP-SMX	6–12 mg/kg/day divided b.i.d. (Max TMP 160 per dose)	800/160 tablet b.i.d.
Tetracyclines[c]—*Staph* spp., *Enterococcus* spp., *Pasteurella* spp., *Rickettsia* spp., *Vibrio vulnificus, Cutibacterium acnes, Aeromonas hydrophila, Mycobacterium marinum*		
Doxycycline	2 mg/kg/dose divided b.i.d. (Max 100 mg per dose)	100 mg b.i.d.
Minocycline	2 mg/kg/dose divided b.i.d. (Max 100 mg per dose)	100 mg b.i.d.
Aminoglycosides[d]—*Enterococcus* spp., *Enterobacter* spp., *Klebsiella* spp., *Proteus* spp., *Serratia* spp., *Haemophilus* spp., *Pseudomonas aeruginosa, Aeromonas hydrophila*		
Gentamicin	0.1–0.3% cream, ointment t.i.d.–q.i.d.	

Adapted from Gilbertd, D. N., Chambers, H. F., Eliopoulos, G. M., Saag, M. S., Pavia, A. T., Black, D., Freedman, D. O., Kim, K., & Schwartz, B. S. *The Sanford guide to antimicrobial therapy 2019.* Antimicrobial Therapy Inc.; Klein, K. (2020). *Antimicrobial dosing recommendations for pediatric patients (≥2 months of age and post-menstrual age >44 weeks).* C.S. Mott Children's Hospital Michigan Medicine. http://www.med.umich.edu/asp/pdf/pediatric_guidelines/ABX-dosing_PEDS.pdf; Vasagar, B., Jain, V., Germinario, A., Watson, H. J., Ouzts, M., Presutti, R. J., & Alvarez, S. (2018). Approach to aquatic skin infections. *Primary Care, 45*(3), 555–566.
SMP, sulfamethoxazole; TMP, trimethoprim.
Antibiotic medications and their respective micro-organism susceptibilities presented in this table are generally reliable, however local resistance rates and patterns may differ. Bacterial culture provides the more reliable information regarding causative organism and respective sensitivities. For anti-fungal and anti-viral skin and soft tissue infections, please see Sections 6.1 to 6.3, respectively.
[a]Only amoxicillin-clavulanic acid.
[b]Only 3rd- and 4th-generation cephalosporins.
[c]>8 years of age.
[d]Aminoglycosides are only available topically or intravenously.